THE WASHINGTON MANUAL OF SURGICAL PATHOLOGY

2nd Edition

The Lauren V. Ackerman Laboratory of Surgical Pathology
Barnes-Jewish and St. Louis Children's Hospitals
Washington University Medical Center
Department of Pathology and Immunology
Washington University School of Medicine
St. Louis, Missouri

Editors

Peter A. Humphrey, MD, PhD

Louis P. Dehner, MD

John D. Pfeifer, MD, PhD

Wolters Kluwer | Lippincott Williams & Wilkins
Health
Philadelphia · Baltimore · New York · London
Buenos Aires · Hong Kong · Sydney · Tokyo

Senior Executive Editor: Jonathan W. Pine, Jr.
Product Managers: Marian Bellus, Emilie Moyer
Vendor Manager: Bridgett Dougherrty
Senior Manufacturing Manager: Benjamin Rivera
Director of Marketing: Caroline Foote
Design Coordinator: Holly McLaughlin
Production Service: Aptara, Inc.

Library of Congress Cataloging-in-Publication Data

The Washington manual of surgical pathology / editors, Peter A. Humphrey, Louis P. Dehner,
John D. Pfeifer. – 2nd ed.
   p. ; cm.
   Surgical pathology
   Includes bibliographical references and index.
   Summary: "The aim of this book is to provide a practical manual that is helpful to pathologists and
residents in the daily practice of surgical pathology. The text encompasses all anatomic sites in the
human body. Each chapter covers tissue handling, gross examination, gross dissection and diagnosis,
processing, slide preparation, microscopic diagnosis, special studies, and diagnostic reporting. The
format of the book would be modeled after the Washington Manuals for other specialties (such as
Medical Therapeutics, Oncology, and Surgery)"—Provided by publisher.
   ISBN 978-1-4511-1436-2
   I. Humphrey, Peter A. II. Dehner, Louis P., 1940– III. Pfeifer, John D. IV. Title: Surgical pathology.
   [DNLM: 1. Pathology, Surgical—Handbooks. WO 39]
   LC classification not assigned
   617'.07—dc23   2012000549

To purchase additional copies of this book, call our customer service department at (800) 638-3030
or fax orders to (301) 223-2320. International customers should call (301) 223-2300.

Visit Lippincott Williams & Wilkins on the Internet at LWW.com. Lippincott Williams & Wilkins
customer service representatives are available from 8:30 am to 6:00 pm, EST.

CCS0312

10 9 8 7 6 5 4 3 2 1

My wife Kay, and children Tom and Jennifer—P.A.H.

For the continued opportunity, joy, and satisfaction of working with great colleagues and house staff—L.P.D.

P.J., S.M., and L.P.D., for their friendship and support—J.D.P.

Contributors

Ashima Agarwal, MD
Instructor
Department of Pathology and Immunology
Washington University School of Medicine
St. Louis, Missouri

Hussam Al-Kateb, MSc, PhD
Assistant Professor
Associate Director of Cytogenomics and
  Molecular Pathology
Department of Pathology and Immunology
Washington University School of Medicine
St. Louis, Missouri

Craig Allred, MD
Professor
Section Head, Breast Pathology
Department of Pathology and Immunology
Washington University School of Medicine
St. Louis, Missouri

Catalina Amador-Ortiz, MD
Resident
Department of Pathology and Immunology
Washington University School of Medicine
St. Louis, Missouri

Emily A. Bantle, MD
Chief, Dermatopathology
Department of Pathology
David Brant Medical Center
Travis Air Force Base, California

Nils Becker, MD
Resident
Department of Pathology and Immunology
Washington University School of Medicine
St. Louis, Missouri

Elizabeth M. Brunt, MD
Professor
Section Head, Liver/GI Pathology
Department of Pathology and Immunology
Washington University School of Medicine
St. Louis, Missouri

Dengfeng Cao, MD, PhD
Assistant Professor
Department of Pathology and Immunology
Washington University School of Medicine
St. Louis, Missouri

Danielle H. Carpenter, MD
Surgical Pathology Fellow
Department of Pathology and Immunology
Washington University School of Medicine
St. Louis, Missouri

Yumei Chen, MD, PhD
Molecular Genetic Pathology Fellow
Department of Pathology and Immunology
Washington University School of Medicine
St. Louis, Missouri

Rebecca D. Chernock, MD
Assistant Professor
Department of Pathology and Immunology
Washington University School of Medicine
St. Louis, Missouri

Brian Collins, MD
Associate Professor
Section Head, Cytopathology
Department of Pathology and Immunology
Washington University School of Medicine
St. Louis, Missouri

Catherine E. Cottrell, PhD
Assistant Professor
Associate Director of Cytogenomics and
  Molecular Pathology
Department of Pathology and Immunology
Washington University School of Medicine
St. Louis, Missouri

Kimberly G. Crone, MD
Dermatopathologist
Associated Dermatologists of West
  Bloomfield and Commerce
Commerce Township, Michigan

Erika Crouch, MD, PhD
Professor
Department of Pathology and Immunology
Washington University School of Medicine
St. Louis, Missouri

Rosa M. Davila, MD
Medical Director, Clinical Laboratory
Barnes Jewish West County Hospital
St. Louis, Missouri

Louis P. Dehner, MD
Professor of Pathology and Immunology
Professor of Pathology in Pediatrics
Department of Pathology and Immunology
Washington University School of Medicine
St. Louis, Missouri

Samir K. El-Mofty, DMD, PhD
Professor of Oral and Maxillofacial
 Pathology
Associate Professor of Otolaryngology
 and Head and Neck Surgery
Associate Professor of Pathology
Section Head, Head and Neck Pathology
Department of Pathology and Immunology
Washington University School of Medicine
St. Louis, Missouri

John L. Frater, MD
Assistant Professor
Department of Pathology and Immunology
Washington University School of Medicine
St. Louis, Missouri

Joseph P. Gaut, MD, PhD
Instructor
Department of Pathology and Immunology
Washington University School of Medicine
St. Louis, Missouri

Omar Hameed, MD
Associate Professor
Department of Pathology, Microbiology
 and Immunology; Department of Surgery
Vanderbilt University
Medical Director, Surgical Pathology;
 Associate Medical Director, Anatomic
 Pathology
Vanderbilt University Medical Center
Nashville, Tennessee

George J. Harocopos, MD
Assistant Professor of Ophthalmology and
 Visual Sciences
Associate Professor of Pathology and
 Immunology
Department of Ophthalmology and Visual
 Sciences
Washington University School of Medicine
St. Louis, Missouri

Anjum Hassan, MD
Assistant Professor
Department of Pathology and Immunology
Washington University School of Medicine
St. Louis, Missouri

Johann D. Hertel, MD, MA
Resident
Department of Pathology and Immunology
Washington University School of Medicine
St. Louis, Missouri

Jena Beth Hudson, MD
Resident
Department of Pathology and Immunology
Washington University School of Medicine
St. Louis, Missouri

Phyllis C. Huettner, MD
Associate Professor of Pathology and
 Immunology
Associate Professor of Obstetrics and
 Gynecology
Section Head, Gyn Pathology
Department of Pathology and Immunology
Washington University School of Medicine
St. Louis, Missouri

Michael E. Hull, MD
Assistant Professor
Department of Pathology and Immunology
Washington University School of Medicine
St. Louis, Missouri

Peter A. Humphrey, MD, PhD
Ladenson Professor of Pathology and
 Immunology
Chief of Anatomic and Molecular
 Pathology
Department of Pathology and Immunology
Washington University School of Medicine
St. Louis, Missouri

Mohammad O. Hussaini, MD
Resident
Department of Pathology and Immunology
Washington University School of Medicine
St. Louis, Missouri

Michael Isaacs, BS
Director of Information Systems
Department of Pathology and Immunology
Washington University School of Medicine
St. Louis, Missouri

Jason A. Jarzembowski, MD, PhD
Assistant Professor
Department of Pathology
Medical College of Wisconsin
Program Director, Perinatal Pathology
Department of Pathology
Children's Hospital of Wisconsin
Milwaukee, Wisconsin

Jeffery M. Klco, MD, PhD
Research Instructor
Department of Pathology and Immunology
Washington University School of Medicine
St. Louis, Missouri

Michael J. Klein, MD
Professor of Pathology and Laboratory
  Medicine
Department of Pathology and Laboratory
  Medicine
Weill Cornell School of Medicine
Pathologist-in-Chief and Director
Department of Pathology and Laboratory
  Medicine
Hospital for Special Surgery
New York, New York

Friederike Kreisel, MD
Assistant Professor
Department of Pathology and Immunology
Washington University School of Medicine
St. Louis, Missouri

Elise L. Krejci, MD
Staff Pathologist
Sherman Hospital
Elgin, Illinois

Hannah R. Krigman, MD
Associate Professor
Department of Laboratory Medicine and
  Pathology
University of Minnesota
Minneapolis, Minnesota

Shashikant Kulkarni, PhD
Associate Professor
Medical Director, Cytogenomics and
  Molecular Pathology
Department of Pathology and Immunology
Washington University School of Medicine
St. Louis, Missouri

Julie Elizabeth Kunkel, MD
Staff Pathologist
Department of Pathology
San Antonio Military Medical Center
San Antonio, Texas

Kathryn M. Law, MD
Instructor
Department of Pathology and Immunology
Washington University School of Medicine
St. Louis, Missouri

Jochen K. Lennerz, MD, PhD
Pathologist
Institute of Pathology
University Ulm
Ulm, Germany

James S. Lewis, Jr., MD
Assistant Professor
Department of Pathology and Immunology
Washington University School of Medicine
St. Louis, Missouri

Helen Liapis, MD
Professor
Section Head, Renal Pathology
Department of Pathology and Immunology
Washington University School of Medicine
St. Louis, Missouri

Anne C. Lind, MD
Associate Professor
Section Head, Dermatopathology
Department of Pathology and Immunology
Washington University School of Medicine
St. Louis, Missouri

Ta-Chiang Liu, MD, PhD
Resident
Department of Pathology and Immunology
Washington University School of Medicine
St. Louis, Missouri

Dongsi Lu, MD, PhD
Assistant Professor
Department of Pathology and Immunology
Washington University School of Medicine
St. Louis, Missouri

Changqing Ma, MD, PhD
Resident
Department of Pathology and Immunology
Washington University School of Medicine
St. Louis, Missouri

Mitra Mehrad, MD
Resident
Department of Pathology and Immunology
Washington University School of Medicine
St. Louis, Missouri

ILKe Nalbantoglu, MD
Assistant Professor
Department of Pathology and Immunology
Washington University School of Medicine
St. Louis, Missouri

TuDong Nguyen, MD, PhD
Assistant Professor
Department of Pathology and Immunology
Washington University School of Medicine
St. Louis, Missouri

Deborah Novack, MD, PhD
Associate Professor of Internal Medicine
Associate Professor of Pathology and
  Immunology
Washington University School of Medicine
St. Louis, Missouri

Sushama Patil, MD
Department of Pathology and Immunology
Washington University School of Medicine
St. Louis, Missouri

Richard J. Perrin, MD, PhD
Assistant Professor
Department of Pathology and Immunology
Washington University School of Medicine
St. Louis, Missouri

Arie Perry, MD
Professor of Pathology and Neurological
  Surgery
Director of Neuropathology
Department of Pathology, Division of
  Neuropathology
University of California San Francisco
  School of Medicine
San Francisco, California

John D. Pfeifer, MD, PhD
Professor of Pathology and Immunology
Professor of Obstetrics and Gynecology
Vice Chairman for Clinical Affairs
Department of Pathology and Immunology
Washington University School of Medicine
St. Louis, Missouri

Meredith E. Pittman, MD, MSCI
Resident
Department of Pathology and Immunology
Washington University School of Medicine
St. Louis, Missouri

Samuel J. Pruden, II, MD, FACS
Dermatopathology Fellow
Department of Pathology and Immunology
Washington University School of Medicine
St. Louis, Missouri

Jon H. Ritter, MD
Professor
Director of Anatomic and Surgical
  Pathology
Department of Laboratory Medicine and
  Pathology
University of Minnesota
Minneapolis, Minnesota

Souzan Sanati, MD
Assistant Professor
Department of Pathology and Immunology
Washington University School of Medicine
St. Louis, Missouri

Robert E. Schmidt, MD, PhD
Professor
Chief of Neuropathology
Department of Pathology and Immunology
Washington University School of Medicine
St. Louis, Missouri

Kevin Selle, MT, HTL (ASCP)
Lab Supervisor
Department of Surgical Pathology
Barnes-Jewish Hospital
St. Louis, Missouri

Maria F. Serrano, MD
Physician
Department of Pathology
Kaiser Permanente San Rafael Medical
  Center
San Rafael, California

David E. Spence, MD
Pathologist
Department of Pathology
Associated Pathologists at Erlanger
  Hospital
Chattanooga, Tennessee

Kiran R. Vij, MD
Fellow in Clinical Cytogenomics
Department of Pathology and
  Immunology
Washington University School of Medicine
St. Louis, Missouri

Nathan C. Walk, MD
Pathologist/Dermatopathologist
Department of Pathology
Middlesex Hospital
Middletown, Connecticut

Hanlin L. Wang, MD, PhD
Professor
Department of Pathology and Laboratory
  Medicine
David Geffen School of Medicine
  University of California Los Angeles
Los Angeles, California

Joshua I. Warrick, MD
Resident
Department of Pathology and Immunology
Washington University School of Medicine
St. Louis, Missouri

Mark Watson, MD, PhD
Associate Professor
Department of Pathology and Immunology
Washington University School of Medicine
St. Louis, Missouri

Rao Watson, MD
Resident
Department of Pathology and Immunology
Washington University School of Medicine
St. Louis, Missouri

Frances V. White, MD
Associate Professor
Department of Pathology and Immunology
Washington University School of Medicine
Interim Chief of Pathology, St. Louis
  Children's Hospital
St. Louis, Missouri

Heather N. Wright, MD
Surgical Pathology Fellow
Department of Pathology and Immunology
Washington University School of Medicine
St. Louis, Missouri

Lourdes R. Ylagan, MD, FIAC
Associate Professor
Department of Pathology and Laboratory
  Medicine
Roswell Park Cancer Institute
Buffalo, New York

Barbara Zehnbauer, PhD, FACMG
Adjunct Professor of Pathology
Department of Pathology
Emory University School of Medicine
Atlanta, Georgia

Preface

Welcome to the second edition of the *The Washington Manual of Surgical Pathology*. As with the first edition, the book draws on the rich heritage of surgical pathology at Barnes Hospital (now Barnes-Jewish Hospital), which began with Lauren V. Ackerman, MD. When Dr. Ackerman joined the institution in 1948 as director of surgical pathology, he was the first trained and board-certified pathologist to occupy a position previously held by surgeons. Dr. Ackerman initiated the paradigm of diagnostic excellence with a central focus on the patient, and advanced the vital role of the surgical pathologist as a consultant to clinicians. He was keenly aware of the role of surgical pathologists as educators. Dr. Ackerman also emphasized that, as investigators of illness from an observational perspective, surgical pathologists were uniquely qualified to correlate morphologic findings with the clinical behavior of disease. If he were alive today, Dr. Ackerman would likely enthusiastically add that surgical pathologists are also uniquely qualified to correlate morphologic findings with the molecular features of disease.

Although multivolume textbooks as well as subspecialty texts continue to have a central role in education and everyday clinical practice, this book is an attempt to respond to the immediate needs of an ever-accelerating world in which pathology residents and fellows never seem to have enough time to "get it all done." Likewise, pathologists in practice never seem to be able to sign out cases quickly enough to satisfy their clinical colleagues, and clinicians themselves need a ready and available reference in surgical pathology. As with the first edition, it is our goal that this book, continuing in the fast-access *Washington Manual* outline format, will fill a niche in our hectic world.

This edition of the *The Washington Manual of Surgical Pathology* includes several significant revisions and additions. In addition to updates to every chapter, several new sections have been added to the manual, including new subchapters on renal transplant pathology and cystic diseases of the kidney, a new chapter on diseases of the retroperitoneum, and a reorganized chapter on molecular genetic testing. Over 1000 new images have been added, and the text includes the updated AJCC cancer staging schemes released in 2010. As with the first edition, a companion website offers the text and image bank (which now contains over 2850 full-color images) in an electronic and fully searchable format (see the inside front cover for website access information).

As with the first edition, most of the individuals who have contributed to this work had their surgical pathology training in the Lauren V. Ackerman Laboratory of Surgical Pathology at Barnes-Jewish Hospital or are current members of the faculty. As is the tradition of the *Washington Manual* series, residents and fellows have contributed to many of the chapters.

Peter A. Humphrey, MD, PhD
Louis P. Dehner, MD
John D. Pfeifer, MD, PhD

Acknowledgments

The second edition of *The Washington Manual of Surgical Pathology* would not have been possible without the participation of our colleagues, who so willingly and generously provided their time and expertise to the project. All but one of the authors (again, special thanks to Dr. Michael Klein) are, or were, faculty or house staff in the Department of Pathology and Immunology at Washington University School of Medicine, which emphasizes that surgical pathology at Washington University has always been a collaborative venture between the faculty and trainees. The Department's Chairman, Dr. Herbert (Skip) Virgin, has not hesitated to continue to provide the support necessary to maintain the tradition of diagnostic excellence, academic productivity, and education that forms the foundation of academic surgical pathology at our institution.

We extend special thanks to our administrative assistants, Elease Barnes, Jeannie Doerr, and Shari Jackson, who handled most of the logistical and secretarial work required to make the second edition a reality. We also acknowledge the artistic expertise of the staff at MedPIC (the medical illustration service of Washington University School of Medicine), especially Marcy Hartstein and Vicki Friedman, who together revised the figures for the book. Walter Clermont expertly and patiently edited all the electronic figures found at the associated website. We are lucky to continue to have had the opportunity to work with several wonderful people at Lippincott William & Wilkins, including Jonathan W. Pine, Jr. (who enthusiastically suggested at an early stage that we produce a second edition of the manual), Emilie Moyer, Marian Bellus, and Martha Cushman.

And our families. Their love, patience, and support made the book possible, and make it all worthwhile.

Peter A. Humphrey
Louis P. Dehner
John D. Pfeifer

Contents

Head and Neck

Oral Cavity and Oropharynx

Rebecca D. Chernock and James S. Lewis Jr.

I. NORMAL ANATOMY

A. Oral cavity. The anterior aspect of the oral cavity extends from the mucocutaneous junction (vermilion border) of the lips to include the buccal mucosa (inside of cheek), maxillary and mandibular arches (teeth), retromolar trigone, anterior two-thirds of the tongue (oral tongue), floor of mouth, and hard palate. Posteriorly, the oral cavity freely communicates with the oropharynx; the border between the two is marked by the junction of the hard and the soft palate superiorly and the line of circumvallate papillae on the dorsal tongue (border between the anterior two-thirds and posterior one-third of the tongue) inferiorly.

1. The oral tongue is freely mobile and composed mainly of skeletal muscle. It has a dorsal (exposed) surface, ventral surface, and tip. The dorsal surface contains numerous papillae that have specialized taste receptors. The floor of the mouth lies beneath the tongue and is divided into sides by the midline frenulum (mucosal fold) of the tongue. It contains ostia of the submandibular and sublingual salivary glands, whereas the main duct of the parotid gland (Stensen's duct) enters the oral cavity through the buccal mucosa. The hard palate forms the roof of the oral cavity and consists of portions of the maxillary and palatine bones.

2. The oral cavity is lined by stratified squamous mucosa with prominent mucoserous glands in the submucosa. Most of the mucosa is nonkeratinizing with the exception of the hard palate, gingiva, and dorsal tongue, which become keratinized due to the friction of mastication.

B. Oropharynx. The oropharynx is the space posterior to the oral cavity that communicates with the nasopharynx superiorly and the larynx and hypopharynx inferiorly. The soft palate (posterior one-third of the palate) marks the superior aspect of the oropharynx and is suspended from the posterior aspect of the hard palate. In contrast to the hard palate, the soft palate is fibromuscular without a bony skeleton. Whereas the oral aspect is covered with nonkeratinizing stratified squamous epithelium, the nasal surface is covered by pseudostratified ciliated columnar (respiratory-type) epithelium. Numerous mucoserous glands lie in its submucosa. The uvula extends down from the posterior aspect of the soft palate and has an identical histology. The posterior one-third of the tongue is rich in lymphoid tissue (known as the lingual tonsil). The palatine and lingual tonsils, together with the pharyngeal tonsil in the nasopharynx, are collectively known as Waldeyer's ring.

II. GROSS EXAMINATION, TISSUE SAMPLING, AND HISTOLOGIC SLIDE PREPARATION

A. Open and endoscopic biopsies. The majority of specimens from the oral cavity and oropharynx consist of open biopsies of lesions that can be visualized by the naked eye. The small biopsy pieces should be placed immediately into 10% buffered formalin or other appropriate fixative. Processing of the biopsies should include gross description of the tissue fragments with documentation of the number of pieces present; the biopsies should be entirely submitted, with three levels cut from each paraffin block for hematoxylin and eosin (H&E) examination.

B. Resections

1. **Open procedure specimens** are widely variable depending on the location of the tumor. Because many lesions encroach upon or invade the bone of the mandible or maxilla, composite resections with bone and soft tissue are common. As a generalization, all specimens need to be oriented appropriately, the soft tissue margins inked, and mucosal and soft tissue margins evaluated followed by sectioning of the tumor relative to cartilage/bone and tissue margins. Margins should be evaluated by either shave or radial sections, depending on the nature of the specimen. If the tumor is relatively distant from a margin, 1- to 2-mm shave sections are preferred. If the tumor grossly approximates a margin to <1 to 2 mm, radial sections should be taken.

2. **Partial resections** with a CO_2 laser under an operating microscope are becoming more common. Because the inherent approach of this procedure is to excise the tumor piece by piece, the surgeon inks the individual pieces as he/she alone knows what constitutes the true margin. In the gross room all that is therefore required is to measure the pieces provided, describe them, and submit them entirely in sections perpendicular to the ink. If there is an additional orienting marker such as a suture, then one should submit the sections sequentially from that end to the opposite end.

C. Frozen sections are a critical element of surgical therapy for tumors of the head and neck region. Although practices vary, at most institutions shave margins are taken by the surgeon from the periphery of the surgical defect after the tumor has been removed, and separately submitted. In other cases, the surgeon may sample the tumor or suspicious sites to confirm and/or map the lesion, with additional samples from areas where the tumor is felt to be closest to the surgical margin.

For frozen sections, the tissue is submitted in saline to the pathology lab and then frozen in its entirety. The tissue pieces should be evaluated grossly for mucosa (typically the shiny and pink-tan surface of the tissue) and, if mucosa is present, the specimen should be oriented in the frozen section block to demonstrate this surface on edge. It is critical to cut deeply into the block to obtain sections that represent the entire tissue submitted so that small foci of tumor are not missed by inadequate sampling. At our institution, we cut three rather than two H&E frozen section slides to reduce these sampling errors.

The tissue that remains after frozen section is submitted for evaluation by permanent sections, which helps assure adequate sampling. Permanent sections can help resolve a number of issues from frozen section including freezing and cautery artifact, volume of tumor, and orientation (note that the margins of the main resection specimen should also be evaluated throughout their entirety because the separate frozen section specimens almost never cover the entire margins of a resection specimen). The final margin status is then a conglomerate of three sources: frozen section slides, permanent slides of the frozen tissue, and the tissues not submitted for frozen section, and the margins of the main specimen.

III. DIAGNOSTIC FEATURES OF COMMON BENIGN DISEASES

A. Inflammation. Lichen planus, pemphigus vulgaris, and cicatricial pemphigoid are autoimmune disorders that predominantly affect middle-aged adults and occur more frequently in women than men. They are diseases that affect mucosal sites as well as skin, so the oral cavity is sometimes involved as well.

1. **Lichen planus.** This disorder commonly affects the oral mucosa. Whereas skin involvement is usually self-limited, oral lichen planus follows a more protracted waxing and waning course. The oral lesions are typically asymptomatic unless ulceration occurs.

   Any oral mucosal surface may be involved, and several patterns can be seen. The classic pattern is reticular with intersecting white keratotic streaks (Wickham's striae); the lesions are ill-defined, and the background may be erythematous due to mucosal atrophy. Some lesions may be mostly erythematous with minimal keratotic streaks, whereas others may show extensive keratinization and/or ulceration or form bullae. Microscopically, a dense submucosal band of lymphocytes is present, which may be less distinct in ulcerated lesions (e-Fig. 1.1).* The rete ridges may be hyperplastic (saw-toothed) or flattened. There is loosening of the basal layer of the epithelium, with degeneration of individual keratinocytes that may form eosinophilic colloid (dyskeratotic, cytoid, or Civatte) bodies (e-Fig. 1.2). The surface may show hyper- or parakeratosis. Although the histologic findings of lichen planus have been well defined, they are nonetheless not specific; for example, some oral lesions with a similar histologic picture may be due to a contact hypersensitivity reaction. In addition, a lichenoid infiltrate may accompany dysplastic lesions.

   Asymptomatic patients require no treatment, but steroids (particularly topical) are often used for erosive or erythematous lesions. Some data suggest that there is an increased risk of malignant transformation in the erythematous, ulcerative, and bullous forms of oral lichen planus. Although this proposed risk of malignancy is controversial, these lesions at least require closer clinical follow-up.

2. **Pemphigus vulgaris.** This is an uncommon disorder that causes superficial ulceration of the skin and mucous membranes. Involvement of the oral mucosa may precede the development of skin lesions. The disease is caused by autoantibodies to desmogleins 1 and 3, cellular transmembrane proteins involved in the assembly of desmosomes. Cell-to-cell adhesion is impaired in the suprabasal epithelium, leading to clefting and ulceration. Flaccid bullae that easily rupture to form painful erosions can be seen on any oral mucosal surface. The lesions heal without scarring. Microscopically, intraepithelial separation with edema and acantholysis, which imparts a "tombstone" appearance to the remaining attached basal cell layer (e-Fig. 1.3), is seen at the edge of the ulcer. Acute and chronic inflammation are frequently present in the submucosa. Direct immunofluorescence is positive for immunoglobulin G (IgG) along cell membranes throughout the epidermis.

   Paraneoplastic pemphigus, which is associated with an underlying malignancy, may be distinguished from pemphigus vulgaris by the identification of a different pattern of antibody staining by direct immunofluorescence.

3. **Cicatricial or mucous membrane pemphigoid.** This is a rare disease caused by various antibodies that target the basement membrane of mucous membranes and occasionally the skin. The oral mucosa is almost always involved, most commonly the gingiva. In contrast to pemphigus vulgaris, the variably sized bullae are not flaccid, and ruptured bullae heal with scarring. Microscopically, there is clefting between the epithelium and the basement membrane, and the space may be filled with serous fluid containing sparse inflammatory cells. Direct immunofluorescence shows a linear band of IgG and C3 on the

---

*All e-figures are available online via the Solution Site Image Bank.

basement membrane. Treatment is with immunosuppression, but the disease is often progressive despite therapy.

B. Infections. Only a few of the numerous infections that may involve the oral cavity are discussed here.

1. Fungal. *Candida* species cause most of the fungal infections of the oral cavity. Other fungal infections that occur less frequently in the oral cavity include histoplasmosis, blastomycosis, and coccidiomycosis. *Candida* species are a part of the normal oral flora; candidiasis occurs due to overgrowth, usually in the setting of a predisposing factor, and *Candida albicans* is the most frequently isolated species. Local and systemic factors that favor overgrowth include immunosuppression, use of steroids or antibiotics, radiation therapy, xerostomia, use of dentures, and anemia. The extremes of age are more often affected as well, and infection may be acute or chronic. Symptoms include a burning sensation or foul odor, although the infection may be asymptomatic.

Several clinical patterns of oral candidiasis are seen. White plaques that are easily scraped off underlying erythematous mucosa are called pseudomembranous candidiasis (oral thrush). This is the most common type of oral candidiasis. Erythematous candidiasis appears as a red patch due to atrophy of the mucosa. Median rhomboid glossitis is a type of erythematous candidiasis that occurs in a specific location, namely a rhomboid-shaped area on the midline dorsal tongue, which over time may develop a nodular appearance. Angular cheilitis causes red fissuring and scaling at the labial commissures; predisposing factors include drooling and ill-fitting dentures. Chronic hyperplastic candidiasis presents as asymptomatic, white patches (due to the thickened, hyperplastic mucosa) that cannot be removed by scraping. This pattern is more common in immunocompetent individuals and may predispose to the development of carcinoma, although a causal relationship between the two has not been clearly demonstrated.

Microscopically, an intraepithelial infiltrate of neutrophils is seen in all types of candidal infection. The epithelium may be ulcerated, although in chronic hyperplastic candidiasis it is thickened and hyperkeratotic (e-**Fig. 1.4**). Fungal pseudohyphae may be difficult to identify on routine H&E-stained slides. However, methenamine silver or periodic acid-Schiff (PAS) stains will highlight the fungal elements within the keratin and in the superficial squamous epithelium (e-**Fig. 1.4**, inset A).

2. Viral. Oral viral infections are highly prevalent, although frequently asymptomatic.

a. Human papillomavirus (HPV) does not cause specific clinically symptomatic infection but is associated with several benign and malignant neoplasms in the oral cavity and oropharynx including squamous papillomas and squamous cell carcinoma (SCC) (see respective sections to follow).

b. Herpes simplex virus (HSV) causes a common oral viral infection with seroprevalence rates of up to 80% of the population. There are two common serotypes (HSV-1 and HSV-2), and HSV-1 is primarily associated with oral lesions. Gingivostomatitis occurs in 10% of initial infections, predominately in children, and is characterized by fever and a vesicular rash. The virus then latently infects sensory ganglia and may be reactivated periodically throughout life. Recurrent disease is manifested by clusters of vesicles that may cause a burning sensation at the mucocutaneous junction of the lip or the nose. Intraoral lesions can also occur.

Microscopically, the lesional mucosa is often ulcerated and acantholytic, with marked acute and chronic inflammation. There are typically individual necrotic squamous cells. Identification of the classic intranuclear eosinophilic inclusions within squamous epithelial cells is diagnostic of herpes virus infection; the inclusion-harboring cells are often single, detached, and multinucleated with molding of the nuclei to each other (e-**Fig. 1.5**). Immunohistochemical stains may be useful to confirm the diagnosis.

c. **Epstein–Barr virus (EBV).** Acute EBV infection, although frequently asymptomatic, may cause pharyngitis and tonsillitis. The virus enters the host through oral epithelial cells, where it then gains access to and infects B lymphocytes. Acute EBV infection may produce reactive changes in the tonsils and lymph nodes that can mimic a hematopoietic malignancy.

Latent EBV infection is virtually universal in adults and is usually asymptomatic. However, an EBV-driven proliferation of tongue epithelial cells, known as **oral hairy leukoplakia,** occurs in immunosuppressed patients, approximately 80% of whom are HIV positive. The lesions are asymptomatic unless superinfection with *Candida* occurs. Grossly, hairy leukoplakia appears as a flat, white, shaggy plaque on the lateral tongue. Microscopically, the epithelium is acanthotic with hyper- and parakeratosis. Perinuclear clearing forming "balloon cells" is characteristic (e-**Fig. 1.6**), and viral replication may cause "nuclear beading" (e-**Fig. 1.7**). Inflammation is typically sparse. Definitive diagnosis relies on detection of EBV within the lesion by immunohistochemistry or in situ hybridization (e-**Fig. 1.8**). Oral hairy leukoplakia is self-limited with no propensity for malignant transformation.

Latent EBV infection has been implicated in the development of a variety of hematopoietic and nonhematopoietic malignancies as well (see Chaps. 3 and 43).

3. **Bacterial. Cervicofacial actinomycosis ("lumpy jaw").** *Actinomyces* are gram positive, saprophytic anaerobes that are part of the normal oral flora. The organisms are often incidentally found in sections of the tonsillar crypts. Occasionally, they are introduced into the soft tissues through trauma, particularly from dental manipulations, where an acute or chronic infection may ensue. *Actinomyces israeli* is the most common pathogenic species.

Acute infections are suppurative, creating a nontender fluctuant mass. In the chronic phase, infections may form a more extensive firm fibrous mass mimicking a neoplasm. Sinus tracts may exit either the skin or mucosa (e-**Fig. 1.9**) and often discharge yellow clusters of tightly adherent *Actinomyces* bacteria that have the appearance of sulfur granules. Osteomyelitis may develop in adjacent bone. Microscopically, collections of radiating, filamentous organisms are seen in a background of neutrophils with surrounding granulation tissue and/or fibrosis. Cultures are often negative due to overgrowth of other organisms. Treatment with prolonged antibiotics is usually successful, although incision and drainage may be necessary.

C. **Other non-neoplastic lesions**
   1. **Fibrous lesions.** A number of different types of fibrous lesions occur in and around the oral cavity.
      a. **Irritation fibroma.** These are the most common oral mucosal mass lesions. They are painless reactive proliferations of fibrous tissue that develop in response to trauma from teeth or dentures. The lateral tongue and buccal mucosa along the bite line are the most common sites. Multiple fibromas may be seen in inherited syndromes including Cowden' syndrome and tuberous sclerosis. Linear, grooved fibromas occurring in the mucosa opposing the teeth or sulcus of the alveolar ridge are called epulis fissuratum and are denture-related.

      Grossly, irritation fibroma is usually pink to white, dome-shaped, and only a few millimeters in maximal diameter. Microscopically, there is a nodular deposition of dense collagen with associated chronic inflammation and overlying thinned mucosa (e-**Fig. 1.10**). Trauma-related changes such as hyperkeratosis and ulceration may be seen. The fibroblasts are spindled and indistinct. If larger, stellate fibroblasts are present, the lesion is called a **giant cell fibroma**, which, in contrast to irritation fibromas, is not associated with trauma and occurs at a younger age (**e-Fig. 1.11**). Whereas typical irritation fibromas do not recur after simple resection, giant cell fibromas may recur.

b. **Gingival fibromatosis.** This is generalized, but not necessarily symmetrical, enlargement of the gingiva which may be hereditary, drug-induced, related to poor oral hygiene, or idiopathic. When it is drug-induced, it is called **fibrous gingival hyperplasia** and frequently regresses with cessation of the inciting drug.

Grossly, the gums are enlarged, smooth-surfaced, and firm. Microscopically, the submucosa shows dense eosinophilic to slightly basophilic fibrous tissue with associated mild chronic inflammation (**e-Fig. 1.12**). The surface squamous epithelium may have chronic inflammation or extreme elongation of the rete, but is otherwise unremarkable.

2. **Inflammatory papillary hyperplasia** is a denture-associated lesion and is typically located beneath a denture base in the hard palate and alveolar ridges. Occasionally, it is seen in patients without dentures and may be associated with poor oral hygiene.

Clinically, the mucosa looks "pebbly" with numerous, small, papular projections. Microscopically, the mucosa may be atrophic or demonstrate pseudoepitheliomatous hyperplasia. The underlying submucosa may vary from edematous to fibrotic, with mild chronic inflammation. Individual nodules may resemble an irritation fibroma or pyogenic granuloma. The condition is not premalignant, may subside with less denture wear, or may require surgical excision.

3. **Torus palatinus, torus mandibularis, and buccal exostosis** are common developmental anomalies that continue to grow throughout life and typically present in adulthood. They are site-specific. Torus palatinus occurs in the midline of the hard palate, torus mandibularis occurs on the lingual surface of the mandible near the bicuspid teeth, and buccal exostosis is found on the facial surface of the alveolar bone. Any identical appearing bony proliferations at other oral sites are generically termed "bony exostosis" or "osteoma" and are not developmental, but rather trauma-related or true neoplasms that can be associated with Gardner syndrome.

Grossly, these lesions are broad-based, single, or lobulated masses with smooth surfaces (**e-Fig. 1.13**). Microscopically, they are composed of dense lamellar bone with scattered osteocytes and variable amounts of marrow. Ischemic changes with marrow fibrosis and loss of osteocytes from lacunae may be seen. Resection is not necessary except for cosmetic reasons or if the lesions become large. There is little risk of recurrence, and the lesions have no malignant potential.

4. **Fordyce granules.** Sebaceous glands are normally found in the skin associated with hair follicles. When they are ectopically present in the oral mucosa, they are called Fordyce granules. They are common (present in up to 80% of adults) and can occur on any oral mucosal surface, although the buccal mucosa is most common. Most appear as scattered, 1 to 3 mm, white to yellow papules. Microscopically, normal sebaceous glands are present in the submucosa without associated hair follicles; occasionally, Fordyce granules coalesce to form the larger cauliflower-like lesion termed sebaceous hyperplasia. No treatment is necessary unless for cosmetic reasons (biopsies are rarely performed as the diagnosis is usually clinically apparent).

5. **Cysts.** Included here are several of the more common soft tissue true cysts that have an epithelial lining. Odontogenic cysts, bone cysts, and salivary

gland–derived pseudocysts (lacking a true epithelial lining) are discussed in Chapter 4.

a. Epidermoid cyst. Intraoral epidermoid cysts are much less common than their counterparts in the skin and are thought to represent inclusions of surface epithelium or cystic change in odontogenic rests. They often present in teenagers and young adults. The most common site is the gingiva. Clinically, they are small (<1 cm) superficial nodules. When they occur in the midline floor of mouth, however, they can become much larger (>5 cm) and interfere with swallowing. Microscopically, they are lined by thin stratified squamous epithelium, with or without a granular cell layer, and are often filled with keratinous debris. Rupture with spillage of keratinous debris may elicit a granulomatous inflammatory reaction. Treatment is by simple surgical excision.

b. Dermoid cysts. These are similar to epidermoid cysts but contain adnexal structures, such as sebaceous glands or hair follicles, in the cyst wall. If other tissue types are present, the lesion is termed teratoid cyst.

c. Nasolabial cysts. These rare cysts occur at the base of the nostril or at the superior aspect of the upper lip. They are thought to be derived from remnants of the embryonic nasolacrimal duct. Seventy-five percent of cases occur in women. More than 10% are bilateral. They present as slow growing masses, usually <1.5 cm, and they may have irregular contours. Soft tissue swelling with loss of the nasolabial fold or elevation of the nasal ala or floor may occasionally cause nasal obstruction. Pressure erosion of underlying bone is possible.

Microscopically, the cysts may be lined by respiratory type, cuboidal, and/or stratified squamous epithelium with scattered mucus-filled goblet cells, with surrounding chronic inflammation. A fibrous or epithelial connection to the nasal mucosa is almost always present. Simple surgical excision is curative.

d. Lymphoepithelial cysts. These cysts are thought to develop from invaginations of crypt epithelium within accessory tonsillar tissue. Clinically, they are painless submucosal nodules that are almost always <6 mm in diameter and typically occur in teenagers or young adults. Half of cases occur in the floor of the mouth. The lateral and ventral tongue, as well as the soft palate, are also common sites. They do not occur in the alveolar soft tissue.

Microscopically, the cyst lining is an attenuated squamous epithelium with a poorly formed granular layer. The cyst is filled with orthokeratin and surrounded tightly by lymphoid aggregates with variable numbers of germinal centers. The cysts may become dissociated from the epithelium or remain connected, often with keratin plugging. Microscopically, the prominent lymphoid aggregates distinguish this cyst from an epidermoid cyst. Similar appearing cysts can be seen within the tonsils themselves from blockage of the crypt connection with the surface.

6. Pseudoepitheliomatous hyperplasia is a generic term for benign, downward proliferation of the epithelium that is important to distinguish from invasive, well-differentiated SCC. Pseudoepitheliomatous hyperplasia is characteristically seen in association with specific lesions including inflammatory papillary hyperplasia, submucosal granular cell tumors, and fungal infections. It can also be seen adjacent to ulcers or be seen associated with myriad other lesions. Microscopically, irregular and pseudoinfiltrative nests of keratinizing squamous epithelium are sometimes seen beneath a markedly thickened surface epithelium. The papillae of the squamous epithelium may be markedly elongated and extend deeply into the submucosa (e-**Fig. 1.14**). However, in contrast to squamous dysplasia and carcinoma, cytologic atypia is absent.

7. Amalgam tattoo. Amalgam is a material used for dental fillings that is composed of a combination of metals. It can be inadvertently implanted into oral mucosa during a dental procedure, creating a tattoo that may be mistaken clinically for melanoma. The lesions present as painless, blue-gray pigmented macules that are variable in size and location. Microscopically, pigmented particles are seen scattered in the submucosa around vessels and along reticulin fibers (e-**Figs. 1.15** and **1.16**). There is typically no tissue reaction.

IV. NEOPLASTIC LESIONS. The World Health Organization (WHO) classification of tumors of the oral cavity and oropharynx is listed in Table 1.1.

A. Epithelial

1. Benign

a. Squamous papilloma. Squamous papillomas are benign squamous proliferations caused by HPV. They are most common in the larynx but also occur as solitary lesions in the oral cavity and oropharynx.

TABLE 1.1	The WHO Histologic Classification of Tumors of the Oral Cavity and Oropharynx

Malignant epithelial tumors	Myoepithelial carcinoma
Squamous cell carcinoma	Carcinoma ex pleomorphic adenoma
Verrucous carcinoma	**Benign epithelial tumors**
Basaloid squamous cell carcinoma	Pleomorphic adenoma
Papillary squamous cell carcinoma	Myoepithelioma
Spindle cell carcinoma	Basal cell adenoma
Acantholytic squamous cell carcinoma	Canalicular adenoma
Adenosquamous carcinoma	Ductal papilloma
Carcinoma cuniculatum	Cystadenoma
Lymphoepithelial carcinoma	**Soft tissue tumors**
Epithelial precursor lesions	Kaposi's sarcoma
Benign epithelial tumors	Lymphangioma
Papillomas	Ectomesenchymal chondromyxoid tumor
Squamous cell papilloma and verruca	Focal oral mucinosis
vulgaris	Congenital granular cell epulis
Condyloma acuminatum	**Hematolymphoid tumors**
Focal epithelial hyperplasia	Diffuse large B-cell lymphoma (DLBCL)
Granular cell tumor	Mantle cell lymphoma
Keratoacanthoma	Follicular lymphoma
Salivary gland tumors	Extranodal marginal zone B-cell lymphoma
Salivary gland carcinomas	of mucosa-associated lymphoid tissue
Acinic cell carcinoma	(MALT) type
Mucoepidermoid carcinoma	Burkitt lymphoma
Adenoid cystic carcinoma	T-cell lymphoma (including anaplastic
Polymorphous low-grade adenocarcinoma	large cell lymphoma)
Basal cell adenocarcinoma	Extramedullary plasmacytoma
Epithelial–myoepithelial carcinoma	Langerhans cell histiocytosis
Clear cell carcinoma, not otherwise	Extramedullary myeloid sarcoma
specified	Follicular dendritic cell sarcoma/tumor
Cystadenocarcinoma	**Mucosal malignant melanoma**
Mucinous adenocarcinoma	**Secondary tumors**
Oncocytic carcinoma	
Salivary duct carcinoma	

From: Barnes L, Eveson J, Reichart P, Sidransky D, eds. *World Health Organization Classification of Tumours. Pathology and Genetics. Head and Neck Tumours.* Lyon: IARC Press; 2005. Used with permission.

Squamous papillomas are strongly associated with the nononcogenic HPV types 6 and 11, but have a very low infectivity so do not appear contagious. In the oral cavity and oropharynx, they occur in adults between 30 and 50 years of age, most commonly on the hard and soft palate and the uvula.

Squamous papillomas have a characteristic morphology. Grossly, they are soft, exophytic, granular, and pink-red or tan. Microscopically, they consist of arborizing, papillary fronds of thickened but maturing squamous epithelium with nuclei that are slightly enlarged and irregular but not overtly dysplastic. Mitotic activity is usually present but is modest. Sometimes there is slight hyperplasia of the basal layer. Cells in the midlayer often have cytoplasmic clearing, but frank koilocytosis is not regularly observed. Although typically absent, surface keratinization may be seen (e-**Fig. 1.17**).

Squamous papillomas are cured by simple excision. They have limited growth potential, rarely recur, and have essentially no risk of malignant transformation.

b. **Condyloma acuminatum and verruca vulgaris.** Both of these lesions, although much more common on the skin, can also occur in the oral cavity. Condylomas are considered a sexually transmitted disease and usually occur in young adults on the lips and soft palate as clusters of pink nodules that coalesce into more exophytic masses. They have more blunted, papillary fronds and more hyperkeratosis than squamous papillomas.

Verrucae also can occur intraorally, particularly in children, commonly on the lips and anterior tongue. They have a morphology identical to that of verrucae of the skin with a broad base, marked papillomatosis, and hyperkeratosis with parakeratosis.

c. **Verruciform xanthoma.** This is a peculiar lesion of the oral cavity which has no relation to HPV and may be reactive in nature. It occurs in middle-aged to older adults and is most common on the alveolar ridges. Clinically and grossly, it is a well-demarcated, painless, and soft, slightly elevated mass. It may have a yellow or white color with a roughened surface. Microscopically, it consists of broad papillae with intervening cleft-like spaces covered by a slightly thickened, nondysplastic squamous epithelium with hyperkeratosis and parakeratosis. The diagnostic cells, which lie in the superficial submucosa, are foamy macrophages with abundant pale, flocculent cytoplasm and round to oval, bland nuclei (e-**Fig. 1.18**). These cells are filled with lipid and should be distinguished from the eosinophilic granular cells of granular cell tumor (see Section E to follow).

Verruciform xanthoma is treated by conservative excision and has no risk of malignant transformation. Recurrences are rare.

2. **Precursor (premalignant) squamous lesions.** Precursor lesions are defined as altered squamous epithelium with an increased risk of progression to SCC, and are strongly associated with smoking and alcohol use. They may present as leukoplakia (white, thickened epithelium; see e-**Fig. 1.19**), erythroplakia (thin, erythematous, and red epithelium), or speckled erythroplakia (a mixture of both erythroplakia and leukoplakia).

The terms dysplasia or intraepithelial neoplasia should be used for these lesions. The likelihood of malignant change relates to the severity of dysplasia, although carcinoma can develop from any grade of dysplasia (as well as from normal epithelium). Atypia, on the other hand, is not considered synonymous with dysplasia and is used in a more general sense because the term may also describe changes seen in reactive epithelium. There are a number of changes that occur in dysplasia including nuclear abnormalities, architectural/organizational abnormalities, and abnormal keratinization.

TABLE 1.2 Precursor Lesion Classification Schemes

Ljubljana classification squamous intraepithelial lesions (SIL)	Squamous intraepithelial neoplasia (SIN)	2005 WHO classification
Squamous cell (simple) hyperplasia	Not applicable	Squamous cell hyperplasia
Basal/parabasal cell hyperplasia	SIN 1	Mild dysplasia
Atypical hyperplasia	SIN 2	Moderate dysplasia
Atypical hyperplasia	SIN 3	Severe dysplasia
Carcinoma in situ	SIN 3	Carcinoma in situ

Unfortunately, there is poor agreement among pathologists about the minimum histopathologic changes that constitute dysplasia, and about the grading of dysplasia (several grading systems that have been proposed are shown in Table 1.2). The 2005 WHO Classification is most frequently utilized, at least in the United States.

3. **Malignant.** SCC is overwhelmingly the most common malignant tumor of the oral cavity and oropharynx (salivary gland neoplasms are discussed in Chap. 6). SCC has a high male to female ratio (3:1) and a strong relationship to tobacco smoking and alcohol consumption, with a multiplicative rather than additive relative risk. Although not as extreme, the risk of SCC is also increased with the use of snuff and chewing tobacco. Betel quid, commonly used in some parts of the world, is also a major risk factor. Finally, HPV, particularly type 16, has a major causative role in oropharyngeal SCC, leading to carcinomas that usually show a distinct nonkeratinizing morphology and which have less aggressive behavior.

   a. **Conventional or keratinizing-type SCC.** The gross appearance of keratinizing-type SCC is quite variable, ranging from fungating, exophytic tumors to endophytic, ulcerated tumors with raised edges. Most tumors elicit stromal fibrosis, and thus have firm and tan-white cut surfaces. Microscopically, these tumors consist of nests and sheets of cells with squamous differentiation. The cells are typically polygonal in shape and have distinct cell borders, eosinophilic cytoplasm, and round to oval nuclei, often with prominent nucleoli. Well-differentiated tumors retain abundant pink or clear cytoplasm, often show intercellular bridges representing desmosomes, and sometimes show keratin "pearl" formation (e-Fig. 1.20). Moderately differentiated tumors (the majority of cases) have cells with more pleomorphism and a higher nucleus to cytoplasm ratio while still retaining moderate amounts of eosinophilic cytoplasm (e-Fig. 1.21). Poorly differentiated tumors often have single cells or small nests of cells with more mitotic activity and less cytoplasm (e-Fig. 1.22). Grading should be performed but has not been shown to consistently predict clinical behavior. Perineural, lymphatic, and vascular space invasion are commonly seen.

   Treatment for oral cavity SCC typically consists of surgery followed by postoperative radiotherapy, the latter depending somewhat on the stage of disease. Small primary lesions without neck lymph node metastases, or with small lymph node metastases without extracapsular extension, may be effectively treated by surgery alone. Radiotherapy, sometimes with chemotherapy and/or epidermal growth factor receptor (EGFR)-targeted drugs, is sometimes used, particularly for large tumors that are not surgically resectable or for high risk patients after surgical resection. The overall survival for conventional, keratinizing-type SCC of the oral cavity is approximately 50% to 55% at 5 years but varies greatly by tumor stage. For oropharyngeal keratinizing-type SCC, treatment can consist of primary surgery or primary chemoradiotherapy. Approximately 25% are related to high risk HPV, and these have a more favorable prognosis. For the non-HPV related tumors, the prognosis is slightly worse than for such tumors in the oral cavity.

b. **Nonkeratinizing SCC.** This entity is slowly gaining recognition as a specific subtype of head and neck SCC. Tumors with this morphology are almost exclusively seen in the palatine tonsils and base of tongue and are virtually always HPV-associated (high risk HPV in >95% of cases and specifically type HPV16 in >90% of such cases). Patients with nonkeratinizing SCC are, on average, 5 years younger than those with conventional keratinizing-type SCC. A significant minority are non-smokers, and those that do smoke are less likely to be heavy smokers. The most common clinical presentation is as an asymptomatic neck mass. Nonkeratinizing SCC arises in the crypts of the tonsillar tissue, so the tumors tend to be subsurface and thus clinically subtle or totally hidden. This feature, combined with the tumor's strong propensity for early metastasis to cervical lymph nodes, explains why the most common presentation is as a painless neck mass. Better recognition of this tumor type has led to more intensive scrutiny of the tonsils and base of tongue in this clinical setting.

Grossly, nonkeratinizing SCC is endophytic, firm, and tan in most cases. However, because the tumors are often small and do not elicit much desmoplasia in the surrounding stroma, they can be quite difficult to identify grossly. Microscopically, they consist of ribbons of tumor cells lining the crypt epithelium and of nests and sheets of cells with smooth borders in the submucosa. The overlying surface epithelium is typically intact without dysplasia (e-**Fig. 1.23**). The cells are basal in appearance, with round to oval to spindled nuclei, relatively homogeneous chromatin without prominent nucleoli, minimal cytoplasm, and very brisk mitotic activity with abundant apoptosis (e-**Fig. 1.24**). Central (comedo) necrosis is common in the tumor cell nests.

In situ hybridization and/or polymerase chain reaction (PCR) are positive for HPV16 or other high-risk HPV types in almost all cases. More recently, assays specific for high-risk HPV RNA transcripts have been applied which are almost always positive in this tumor type. Immunohistochemistry is positive for cytokeratins and for p16 (a tumor suppressor protein that is aberrantly overexpressed in cells infected by HPV) (e-**Fig. 1.25**). Strong and diffuse p16 immunoreactivity has become increasingly recognized as a clinically useful surrogate marker for HPV-driven SCCs of the oropharynx. Many use this as a single risk stratification test in clinical practice because, when positive, it indicates a tumor with a much more favorable prognosis than for head and neck SCC in general.

Treatment is most often by surgical resection with neck dissection followed by postoperative radiation therapy, although primary chemoradiation therapy is a very effective approach as well. Numerous studies have shown that the prognosis for HPV-related SCC of the oropharynx is better than for keratinizing type SCC, despite the fact that tumors commonly present with lymph node metastases and thus are high stage.

c. **Verrucous carcinoma (VC)** is a specific, well-differentiated and nonmetastasizing variant of SCC. It occurs in the larynx and oral cavity and grossly appears as a well-circumscribed, warty and exophytic, broad-based, white or tan mass (e-**Fig. 1.26**). It can become very large and dramatically invade soft tissues and bone. Microscopically, VC consists of very thick surface squamous epithelium with club-shaped papillae that have a broad pushing base. These blunt and downward-pushing projections have sometimes been likened to elephant's feet. There is usually prominent surface hyperkeratosis, and the sheets of tumor are composed of bland cells with abundant eosinophilic to clear cytoplasm, sometimes described as glassy in appearance. There is no cytologic atypia. The stroma directly beneath the tumor typically demonstrates prominent chronic inflammation, often with abundant plasma cells (e-**Fig. 1.27**).

Pure VC is a tumor type in which the cells have not invaded through the basement membrane, and as such has an excellent prognosis. Although the tumor can be large and locally destructive, complete surgical resection is often curative because the tumor cells cannot spread beyond the local site. Radiation is also an acceptable treatment, particularly in poor surgical candidates. Conventional invasive SCC sometimes arises from VC. When this occurs, the prognosis and behavior are the same as for conventional SCC. Thus, the lesion must be thoroughly sampled histologically before a diagnosis of pure VC is made.

d. **Spindle cell carcinoma (SpCC)** is the head and neck mucosal form of sarcomatoid carcinoma, a variant of SCC consisting of spindled or pleomorphic tumor cells that simulate a true sarcoma. It is clear from ultrastructural, immunohistochemical, and molecular studies that the sarcomatoid cells represent a clone of poorly differentiated, or divergently differentiated, carcinoma cells. SpCC has demographics similar to those of conventional SCC, occurring in the fifth to sixth decade, showing a strong association with smoking and alcohol use, and having a very high male to female ratio. It occurs most commonly in the larynx (particularly the glottis) followed by the oral cavity, hypopharynx, and nasal cavity. Up to 20% of patients have a history of previous radiation to the originating site, which is higher than that for conventional SCC.

Grossly, the vast majority of laryngeal and hypopharyngeal SpCC, and approximately 50% of oral SpCC, have a polypoid growth pattern resulting in an exophytic mass with a smooth and extensively ulcerated surface. Up to 75% of SpCC are biphasic tumors with areas of conventional SCC admixed with areas of spindled and/or pleomorphic tumor cells (e-**Fig. 1.28**). The spindled component usually predominates. The conventional squamous component may take the form of squamous dysplasia, carcinoma in situ, or invasive carcinoma. Because the tumors are usually exophytic with extensive surface ulceration, the noninvasive component may be only a focal finding or may be effaced altogether. SpCC has a wide variety of architectural patterns including fascicular (e-**Fig. 1.29**), storiform, lace-like, or myxoid areas of growth. On occasion, the tumor cells may be widely spaced in an edematous stroma mimicking granulation tissue with cytologic atypia, which is a major diagnostic pitfall. Approximately 5% of tumors will have definable heterologous sarcomatous differentiation, either osteo- or chondrosarcomatous. Immunohistochemistry in the spindle cell component is positive for cytokeratins and/or epithelial membrane antigen in approximately two-thirds of cases, and positive for p63 in a similar percentage. Vimentin is always positive, and a significant minority of tumors will be positive for smooth muscle actin.

Although any malignant spindle cell lesion of the mucosa of the upper aerodigestive tract should be considered an SpCC until proven otherwise, the differential diagnosis includes a true sarcoma, spindle cell melanoma, nodular fasciitis, and ulcers and granulation tissue with reactive atypia (particularly after radiation). When a conventional squamous cell carcinoma component is present intermingled with the spindle cells, the diagnosis of SpCC is confirmed without the need for additional studies.

Because SpCC is inherently a carcinoma, current treatment recommendations are essentially identical to those for conventional SCC, and taking all patients together, the prognosis does not appear different from conventional SCC. However, the prognosis is worse for oral cavity SpCC, and patients with endophytic tumors do worse than those with exophytic tumors.

e. **Papillary SCC** is a rare variant of SCC that is defined as more than 50% of the tumor having an exophytic, papillary growth pattern (e-**Figs. 1.30** and **1.31**). It is more common in the larynx than in the oral cavity and oropharynx, and has a good prognosis.

f. **Adenosquamous carcinoma** is another rare variant consisting of a mixture of SCC and adenocarcinoma with true gland formation, often with mucin production (e-**Fig. 1.32**). The oral cavity and oropharynx are less common sites than the larynx. These tumors are typically more aggressive than conventional SCC.

g. **Basaloid squamous cell carcinoma (BSCC)** is a variant that is rare in the oral cavity but is slightly more common in the oropharynx, larynx, and hypopharynx. It is characterized by molded nests forming a "jigsaw" pattern. The tumor cells are basaloid with hyperchromatic, round to oval nuclei, and scant cytoplasm (e-**Fig. 1.33**). Extracellular mucoid or hyaline material may be present. Abrupt squamous differentiation or overlying squamous dysplasia is seen (e-**Fig. 1.34**). While generally this tumor is an aggressive variant with high rates of distant metastasis, BSCC in the oropharynx is frequently HPV positive and when so, has a better prognosis than BSCC at other sites.

B. Melanocytic. Melanoma is not uncommon in the oral cavity. It occurs in adults with an average age of approximately 60 years, with a very even incidence from age 20 to 80 years. Unlike cutaneous melanoma, in which sun damage underlies the development of most cases, no major etiology has been identified for oral lesions. There is a slight male preponderance and, also unlike cutaneous melanoma, oral lesions occur relatively equally among numerous races. Oral melanomas present as incidental pigmented lesions identified by a dentist or physician, as masses arising in a preexisting pigmented lesion, or most frequently as a new mass growing over a few months. The most common oral site is the hard palate (~40%), followed by the maxillary gingiva (~25%) (e-**Fig. 1.35**), the buccal mucosa, the mandibular gingiva, and the lip. Melanomas of the oropharynx are rare.

Grossly, most tumors are heavily pigmented and heterogeneous, with a brown, gray, or black color. There are sometimes satellite lesions without intervening pigmentation. Microscopically, most melanomas are deeply invasive, but two-thirds retain a surface in situ component as well. Architecturally, the tumors consist of single cells and ill-defined sheets and nests of either epithelioid cells, spindle cells, or both. The large epithelioid cells have abundant cytoplasm (which can be eosinophilic to gray) and round to oval nuclei with a characteristic single, large, cherry red nucleolus (e-**Fig. 1.36**). Melanin pigment is commonly present. Spindle cells are less common and have cigar-shaped nuclei and moderate clear to eosinophilic cytoplasm. Plasmacytoid and rhabdoid cells can also be seen. Intranuclear cytoplasmic inclusions that are typical of melanomas at other sites are uncommon in oral melanomas. By immunohistochemistry, oral melanomas express the same proteins as other melanomas, namely Melan-A, MART-1, HMB-45, S-100, and tyrosinase.

Treatment consists of radical resection with radiation, with or without chemotherapy. Neck dissection is performed only for clinically detected disease. The prognosis is poor. Numerous studies have demonstrated a collective 5-year survival between 15% and 25%. Breslow thickness, unlike cutaneous lesions, is of very limited prognostic utility. Approximately 40% of patients will develop cervical lymph node metastases, and distant metastases are common. Major sites include the lung, the liver, and the brain.

C. Neuroendocrine carcinomas are uncommon tumors in the head and neck region in general, and are very uncommon in the oral cavity and oropharynx. They are essentially all high grade with a small cell morphology, composed of cells with scant cytoplasm, crush artifact, granular chromatin without nucleoli, and extensive necrosis with brisk mitotic activity (i.e., morphologically identical to small cell carcinomas of the lung and other organs) (e-**Fig. 1.37** and e-**Fig. 1.38**). Some are mixed with a component of SCC. In the oropharynx, recent studies have shown that roughly one-half of tumors have been shown to have transcriptionally-active HPV. Carcinoid tumors (low-grade neuroendocrine carcinomas) almost never occur in the oral cavity and oropharynx.

The prognosis for high-grade neuroendocrine carcinoma is very poor, with rapid progression of disease including the development of cervical lymph node metastases and distant metastatic disease. This seems to still hold true for patients with HPV-related oropharyngeal neuroendocrine carcinomas as well.

D. Vascular

1. **Pyogenic granulomas** (or lobular capillary hemangiomas) are benign lesions of the oral cavity that are usually solitary, and are most common on the lips, tongue, and gingival and buccal mucosa. They occur in patients of all ages but have a particular predilection for the gingiva of pregnant women and, thus, are often referred to as a "pregnancy tumor" in this setting. They usually present as small (a few centimeters or less) exophytic masses that bleed easily. They may grow rapidly and cause false clinical concern for a malignant neoplasm.

   Grossly, they are polypoid or pedunculated, pink to red, and have a smooth surface. Microscopically, they consist of lobules of small capillaries with plump endothelial cells that have round to oval nuclei and occasional mitoses (e-**Fig. 1.39**), with larger central "feeder" vessels. Extensive surface ulceration with associated fibrin is usually present. The cells are positive for endothelial immunohistochemical markers such as CD34, CD31, and factor VIII–related antigen.

   Pyogenic granulomas are benign neoplasms that are cured by simple excision. A small percentage may recur. Pregnancy-related lesions often regress postpartum and thus may be hormonally driven.

2. **Hemangioma** and **lymphangioma** are benign tumors composed of abundant blood or lymphatic vessels, respectively. Hemangiomas of the oral cavity usually occur in adults. They occur most commonly on the lip, buccal mucosa, and lateral tongue borders and present as painless, nodular or well-circumscribed, red or blue masses (e-**Fig. 1.40**) measuring <2 cm in maximal dimension. Microscopically, they consist of blood vessels ranging from small capillaries to large cavernous spaces. The endothelial lining cells can be plump and may have mitotic activity, a feature more common in children. There are a number of named histologic variants, most of which have no clinical significance.

   Lymphangiomas (or cystic hygromas) are composed of dilated lymphatic channels. About 75% occur in the head and neck and, when presenting in the oral cavity, they are almost always found in children younger than 3 years. Histologically, they typically consist of very dilated lymphatic channels lined by bland, inconspicuous endothelial cells, with intraluminal eosinophilic material, lymphocytes, and occasional red blood cells. They often are interstitial aggregates of lymphocytes.

   Both hemangioma and lymphangioma are benign lesions cured by conservative excision. Hemangiomas can be treated by sclerotherapy as well. Large lymphangiomas are often debulked, often via serial resections to avoid major morbidity.

3. **Kaposi sarcoma (KS)** is a locally aggressive tumor uniformly associated with human herpesvirus 8 (HHV-8) that predominantly involves the skin but can

also involve mucosal sites. When KS involves the oral cavity, usually as a complication of AIDS, it is most commonly found in the palate, followed by the gingiva and dorsal tongue. Clinically, KS appears as purple, red-blue, or brown macules or plaques. Later in the disease course, the lesions become nodular and may ulcerate.

The three histologic stages of KS (patch, plaque, and nodular; all discussed in more detail in Chap. 39) can all be associated with oral KS (e-Fig. 1.41). There are frequently associated collections of extravasated red blood cells and hemosiderin-laden macrophages. A characteristic feature that is sometimes seen is the pale, eosinophilic hyaline globule, which probably represents degenerating red blood cells. Immunohistochemistry is positive for the common endothelial markers CD34 and CD31.

The behavior of oral KS is variable. It is generally indolent in nonimmunocompromised patients but is more aggressive in patients with AIDS. However, the mortality related to KS is highly dependent on other comorbidities such as opportunistic infections and systemic symptoms.

E. **Neural/neuroectodermal. Granular cell tumors** are benign, slow growing tumors of neural origin that occur at many anatomic sites. Approximately 50% occur in the head and neck region, and half of these occur in the tongue. They also occur in the buccal mucosa, floor of mouth, and palate, are twice as common in women as men, and approximately 10% to 20% are multiple. Grossly, they are smooth, sessile, and firm with a pink or tan-white color. Microscopically, they consist of infiltrative nonencapsulated sheets and cords of bland cells with abundant eosinophilic granular cytoplasm and indistinct cell borders (e-Fig. 1.42). There is usually no significant stromal reaction. The nuclei are small, oval, and hyperchromatic with minimal atypia and no mitotic activity. A common feature is pseudoepitheliomatous hyperplasia of the overlying squamous epithelium, which can closely mimic SCC. Conservative excision is the treatment of choice, with a risk of recurrence of <10%. Malignant granular cell tumors (as covered in the Soft Tissue chapter) are very rare but do occur.

F. **Mesenchymal**

1. **Peripheral ossifying fibroma** is a reactive proliferation of fibrous tissue on the gingiva which shows focal bone formation. It occurs over a broad age range, but young adults are most commonly affected. The lesions range from a few millimeters up to 2 cm in maximal dimension. They are essentially exclusive to the gingiva, particularly along the incisors, and present as sessile pink nodules, usually with surface ulceration. Microscopically, they consist of randomly distributed plump (but not atypical) fibroblasts with foci of mineralization ranging from dystrophic calcification, to cementum-like material, to well-formed bone (e-Fig. 1.43). Rare giant cells can be seen. The lesions should be excised down to the periosteum but will recur in 15% to 20% of cases.

2. **Peripheral giant cell granuloma** is another reactive proliferation of the gingiva, particularly along the incisors, caused by chronic irritation. It presents over a wide age range, particularly in middle-aged to older adults, as a solitary broad-based nodule that is reddish or blue and <2 cm in diameter. Microscopically, it consists of a mixture of multinucleated osteoclast-like giant cells and plump spindled to oval mononuclear cells (e-Fig. 1.44). Hemosiderin, chronic inflammation, and foci of metaplastic bone are frequent. The differential diagnosis includes brown tumor of hyperparathyroidism, cherubism, and central (intraosseous) giant cell granuloma. The lesion is treated by local excision down to the bone. Recurrence occurs in approximately 10% of cases.

3. **Congenital granular cell epulis** is a rare benign mesenchymal tumor that classically arises from the anterior alveolar ridge of a newborn. Girls are more frequently affected than boys by a ratio of 9:1. The tumor presents as a

TABLE 1.3 The 2010 AJCC Staging Guidelines for Tumors of the Oral Cavity and Lip

Primary tumor (T)
Primary tumor cannot be assessed (TX)
No evidence of primary tumor (T0)
Carcinoma in situ (Tis)
Tumor ≤2 cm in greatest dimension (T1)
Tumor >2 cm but not >4 cm in greatest dimension (T2)
Tumor >4 cm in greatest dimension (T3)
Moderately advanced local disease (T4a)
(Oral cavity) Tumor invades adjacent structures only (e.g., through cortical bone[a], into deep [extrinsic] muscle of tongue [genioglossus, hyoglossus, palatoglossus, and styloglossus], maxillary sinus, skin of face)
(Lip) Tumor invades through cortical bone[a], inferior alveolar nerve, floor of mouth, or skin of face (chin or nose)
Very advanced local disease (T4b)
Tumor invades masticator space, pterygoid plates, or skull base and/or encases internal carotid artery

Regional lymph nodes (N)
Regional lymph nodes cannot be assessed (NX)
No regional lymph node metastasis (N0)
Metastasis in a single ipsilateral lymph node, ≤3 cm in greatest dimension (N1)
Metastasis in a single ipsilateral lymph node, >3 cm but not >6 cm in greatest dimension (N2a)
Metastasis in multiple ipsilateral lymph nodes, none >6 cm in greatest dimension (N2b)
Metastasis in bilateral or contralateral lymph nodes, none >6 cm in greatest dimension (N2c)
Metastasis in a lymph node >6 cm in greatest dimension (N3)

Distant metastasis (M)
No distant metastasis (M0)
Distant metastases (M1)

Stage grouping
The overall pathologic AJCC stage is
Tis/N0/M0 (Stage 0)
T1/N0/M0 (Stage I)
T2/N0/M0 (Stage II)
T3/N0/M0 (Stage III)
T1/N1/M0 (Stage III)
T2/N1/M0 (Stage III)
T3/N1/M0 (Stage III)
T4a/N0/M0 (Stage IVA)
T4a/N1/M0 (Stage IVA)
T1/N2/M0 (Stage IVA)
T2/N2/M0 (Stage IVA)
T3/N2/M0 (Stage IVA)
T4a/N2/M0 (Stage IVA)
T4b/Any N/M0 (Stage IVB)
Any T/N3/M0 (Stage IVB)
Any T/Any N/M1 (Stage IVC)

[a]Superficial erosion alone of bone/tooth socket by gingival primary carcinoma is not sufficient to classify a tumor as T4.
From: Edge SB, Byrd DR, Compton CC, et al., eds. *AJCC Cancer Staging Manual.* 7th ed. New York, NY: Springer; 2010. Used with permission.

TABLE 1.4 The 2010 AJCC Staging Guidelines for Tumors of the Oropharynx (Including Base of Tongue, Soft Palate, and Uvula)

Primary tumor (T)

Primary tumor cannot be assessed (TX)

No evidence of primary tumor (T0)

Carcinoma in situ (Tis)

Tumor $\leq$2 cm in greatest dimension (T1)

Tumor >2 cm but not >4 cm in greatest dimension (T2)

Tumor >4 cm in greatest dimension or extension to the lingual surface of the epiglottis (T3)

Moderately advanced local disease (T4a)

Tumor invades the larynx, deep/extrinsic muscle of tongue, medial pterygoid, hard palate, or mandible

Very advanced local disease (T4b)

Tumor invades lateral pterygoid muscle, pterygoid plates, lateral nasopharynx, or skull base, or encases carotid artery

Regional lymph nodes (N)[a]

Regional lymph nodes cannot be assessed (NX)

No regional lymph node metastasis (N0)

Metastasis in a single ipsilateral lymph node, $\leq$3 cm in greatest dimension (N1)

Metastasis in a single ipsilateral lymph node, >3 cm but not >6 cm in greatest dimension (N2a)

Metastasis in multiple ipsilateral lymph nodes, none >6 cm in greatest dimension (N2b)

Metastasis in bilateral or contralateral lymph nodes, none >6 cm in greatest dimension (N2c)

Metastasis in a lymph node >6 cm in greatest dimension (N3)

Distant metastasis (M)

No distant metastasis (M0)

Distant metastases (M1)

Stage grouping

The overall pathologic AJCC stage is

   Tis/N0/M0 (Stage 0)

   T1/N0/M0 (Stage I)

   T2/N0/M0 (Stage II)

   T3/N0/M0 (Stage III)

   T1/N1/M0 (Stage III)

   T2/N1/M0 (Stage III)

   T3/N1/M0 (Stage III)

   T4a/N0/M0 (Stage IVA)

   T4a/N1/M0 (Stage IVA)

   T1/N2/M0 (Stage IVA)

   T2/N2/M0 (Stage IVA)

   T3/N2/M0 (Stage IVA)

   T4a/N2/M0 (Stage IVA)

   T4b/Any N/M0 (Stage IVB)

   Any T/N3/M0 (Stage IVB)

   Any T/Any N/M1(Stage IVC)

[a]Note: Metastases at level VII are considered regional lymph node metastases.
From: Edge SB, Byrd DR, Compton CC, et al., eds. *AJCC Cancer Staging Manual.* 7th ed. New York, NY: Springer; 2010. Used with permission.

smooth, nonulcerated mass about 1 cm in size arising from the gingiva over the lateral incisor/canine area of the maxilla, or less commonly, the mandible. Grossly, it is polypoid and has a homogeneous firm pink or tan cut surface. Microscopically, it consists of sheets of large cells that have abundant, granular, eosinophilic cytoplasm and round to oval, bland nuclei. The surface squamous epithelium is intact and shows no hyperplasia. By immunohistochemistry, the cells are positive only for vimentin, and specifically are negative for S-100.

Congenital granular cell epulis is not the newborn equivalent of a granular cell tumor and shows no neural differentiation. The tumor stops growing at birth and regresses over time, but most cases still require surgical resection. There is no recurrence, even after incomplete removal.

V. PATHOLOGIC REPORTING OF ORAL CAVITY AND OROPHARYNGEAL MALIGNANCIES

A. **Staging.** The American Joint Committee on Cancer (AJCC) staging guidelines for oral cavity and oropharyngeal carcinomas are listed in Tables 1.3 and 1.4. Staging is extremely important for clinical management and establishing prognosis. These staging guidelines are applicable to all forms of carcinoma. Any nonepithelial tumor type is excluded. A specific and very important point in staging involves bone involvement by tumor. To qualify as a T4 lesion, the tumor must erode through the bone cortex. Superficial bone erosion is not sufficient for classification as T4.

It is important to note that mucosal melanomas of the head and neck, including the oral cavity, have their own staging system.

B. **Additional pertinent pathologic features.** As with carcinomas at all upper aerodigestive tract sites, margin status, tumor differentiation, and the presence or absence of perineural or lymphovascular space invasion should be reported. Perineural invasion is particularly common in oral cavity carcinomas and is correlated with a poorer prognosis. The pattern of infiltration as well as the presence or absence of a host inflammatory response should also be reported, because both features have been correlated in many studies with a higher rate of local recurrence, a poorer prognosis, or both. Some recent studies have developed formal grading systems for these features that have promise for clinical implementation, particularly for early stage oral cavity SCC, but these are not ready for active implementation. Depth of invasion, particularly for T1 and T2 tumors, although not reflected in the staging system specifically, is important for clinical management and prognosis, and so should be reported.

SUGGESTED READINGS

Adelstein DJ, Ridge JA, Gillison ML, et al. Head and neck squamous cell cancer and the human papillomavirus: summary of a National Cancer Institute State of the Science Meeting, November 9–10, 2008. *Washington, DC, Head Neck.* 2009;31:1393–1422.

Ang KK, Harris J, Wheeler R, et al. Human papillomavirus and survival of patients with oropharyngeal cancer. *N Engl J Med.* 2010;363:24–35.

Bouquot JE, Muller, S, Nikai H. Lesions of the oral cavity. In: Gnepp DR, ed. *Diagnostic Surgical Pathology of the Head and Neck.* 2nd ed. Philadelphia, PA: W.B. Saunders Publishers; 2009.

Chernock RD, El-Mofty SK, Thorstad WL, et al. HPV-related nonkeratinizing squamous cell carcinoma of the oropharynx: utility of microscopic features in predicting patient outcome. *Head Neck Pathol.* 2009;3:186–194.

Chernock RD, Lewis JS, Jr, Zhang Q, et al. Human papillomavirus-positive basaloid squamous cell carcinomas of the upper aerodigestive tract: A distinct clinicopathologic and molecular subtype of basaloid squamous cell carcinoma. *Hum Pathol.* 2010;41:1016–1023.

Slootweg P, Eveson JW. Tumours of the oral cavity and oropharynx. In: Barnes L, Eveson JW, Reichart P, Sidransky, eds. *Pathology and Genetics Head and Neck Tumours.* Lyon, France: IARC Press; 2005.

Thompson LDR, ed. *Head and Neck Pathology*, 1st ed. New York, NY: Churchill Livingstone; 2006.

2 Larynx

James S. Lewis Jr.

I. NORMAL ANATOMY

A. Macroscopic/gross.
The larynx is a unique organ designed to produce phonation by modulation of the respiratory airstream. It is composed of several cartilaginous structures: the thyroid, cricoid, and arytenoid cartilages and the epiglottis. The hyoid bone sits above and is connected to the larynx by the thyrohyoid membrane (Fig. 2.1). The thyroid (and lesser so, cricoid cartilage) ossifies in adults. In functional terms, the larynx is divided into three subsites. The glottis includes the true vocal folds or cords, below, and the false folds or cords, above. The space between them is called the ventricle, and its deeper recess, the saccule. The true cords, with a hypocellular stroma called Reinke's space, are designed to vibrate for phonation, and the ventricle amplifies this further. The cords are manipulated by muscles that attach to and move the arytenoid cartilages, which sit at the posterior aspect of the vocal folds. The larynx can be divided into three compartments for tumor management and staging purposes: the supraglottis, glottis, and subglottis. The supraglottis includes the epiglottis, aryepiglottic folds, false cords, and ventricle. Glottis refers to the vocal cords from the edge of the ventricle to the free edge of the vocal cord. Subglottis refers to the area from the free edge of the vocal fold to the inferior border of the cricoid cartilage but has a slightly different definition for American Joint Committee on Cancer (AJCC) staging (see later).

B. Microscopic.
The larynx is covered by a mixture of squamous and pseudostratified ciliated columnar (respiratory-type) epithelium. In smokers, however, often the entire endolarynx is covered by squamous epithelium. The true cords themselves are always covered by squamous epithelium. They contain a lamina propria area called Reinke's space, which lies between the epithelium and the vocal ligament and which consists of loose connective tissue with few capillaries, no lymphatics, and sparse seromucinous glands (e-Fig. 2.1).* The false cords and ventricle are typically lined by respiratory-type epithelium.

II. GROSS EXAMINATION, TISSUE SAMPLING, AND HISTOLOGIC SLIDE PREPARATION

A. Endoscopic biopsies.
The majority of specimens from this region consist of endoscopic forcep biopsies. The tissue samples should be placed immediately into 10% buffered formalin or other appropriate fixative. These should undergo gross examination and description documenting the exact number of pieces present and their size, and then be entirely submitted with three levels cut from each paraffin block for hematoxylin and eosin (H&E) examination.

B. Resections

1. Partial. These are widely variable specimens depending on the location of the tumor. Standard procedures include vertical hemilaryngectomy and supraglottic or supracricoid laryngectomy. As a generalization, these specimens need to be oriented, the soft tissue margins inked, and margins demonstrated by shave or radial section followed by sectioning of the tumor relative to cartilage/bone and soft tissue margins. The use of either shave or radial sections depends on the nature of the specimen. If the tumor is relatively distant from a margin, 1- to 2-mm shave sections are preferred. If the tumor approximates a margin to <1 to 2 mm, radial sections are taken.

---

*All e-figures are available online via the Solution Site Image Bank.

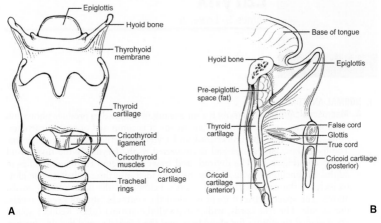

Figure 2.1 Larynx anatomy: **(A)** anterior view; **(B)** sagittal cross section.

Partial resections with a CO_2 laser under an operating microscope are becoming more common because of their low morbidity. Because an inherent part of this procedure is to cut into the tumor or to remove tumor in more than one piece, surgeons ink the individual pieces themselves, as they alone know what constitutes the true margin. In the pathology lab, the pieces are measured, described, and submitted entirely in sections perpendicular to the ink.

2. **Total.** For years, total laryngectomy has been the standard operation for malignancy. However, partial resections with preservation of function are increasingly common. Total laryngectomy is used most often now as salvage therapy for recurrences after partial surgery or after definitive radiation and chemotherapy. Occasionally, patients present with progressive disease that makes total laryngectomy necessary as the initial surgery (**e-Fig. 2.2**).

The usual approach to grossing a total laryngectomy is to initially ink the peripheral nonmucosal soft tissue margins and then open the larynx by a posterior vertical midline cut with scissors, propping it wide open with a small stick or portion of a wooden swab. After overnight formalin fixation, the specimen is ready for prosection. After orientation and measurement in three dimensions, the tumor is measured and described, specifically noting what structures are involved. The specimen typically includes the entire larynx and cartilages, small portions of hypopharyngeal mucosa bilaterally adjacent to the aryepiglottic folds, and the hyoid bone anterosuperiorly. Standard sections (Fig. 2.2) are taken as follows. (i) Margins: shaved inferior tracheal ring; shaved right and left hypopharyngeal mucosa; shaved postcricoid soft tissue; radial sections demonstrating anterior, anterolateral, and base of tongue inked soft tissue margins. (ii) Soft tissue/mucosa: bilateral vertical glottis (including both true and false cords); vertical anterior commissure; vertical midline epiglottis showing pre-epiglottic soft tissue space; bilateral aryepiglottic folds; four sections of tumor if not included in the previous sections. (iii) Cartilage/bone: vertical sections showing tumor and thyroid cartilage (at closest or at sites of gross invasion); sections of right and left wings of the hyoid bone (where closest to or involved by tumor). Typically, all soft tissue and margin sections are taken first, and the entire specimen is

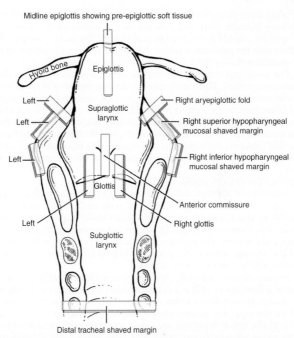

Midline epiglottis showing pre-epiglottic soft tissue

Hyoid bone

Epiglottis

Left

Supraglottic larynx

Left

Right aryepiglottic fold

Right superior hypopharyngeal mucosal shaved margin

Left

Right inferior hypopharyngeal mucosal shaved margin

Glottis

Anterior commissure

Left

Right glottis

Subglottic larynx

Distal tracheal shaved margin

Figure 2.2 Larynx grossing. Standard sections from a total laryngectomy are shown. Additional sections include sections of tumor (4–5 total), right and left postcricoid soft tissue shaved margins, and anterior soft tissue margins (either shaved or radial). Post decalcification, additional sections should include cartilage deep to the tumor showing involvement or nearest approach, any surrounding lymph nodes in neck soft tissue, of the hyoid bone (where closest to tumor or grossly involved by it). If necessary, sections of tracheostomy skin, thyroid lobe(s), and neck skin should also be submitted.

bisected in the midline vertically and decalcified in toto overnight followed by cartilage and/or bone section acquisition.

C. Frozen sections. These are a critical element of surgical therapy for tumors of the head and neck region. Although practices vary, most institutions have margins taken as small pieces by the surgeon from the periphery of the surgical defect after the tumor has been removed. Because laryngeal resections are quite variable, the sites where frozen sections are taken are not standard; with total laryngectomies, sometimes no frozen sections are clinically necessary. The surgeon may sample the tumor or suspicious sites to confirm and/or map the tumor, and then take margins from the area of closest approach after resection of it. The tissue pieces are submitted individually to pathology in saline and frozen in their entirety, with two (and at our institution, three) H&E slides generated at representative levels. It is critical to obtain sections that represent the entire tissue submitted so that small foci of tumor are not missed by "sampling error" (i.e., where tiny foci of tumor are not present on frozen section slides but are seen on permanent sections, due to not "sampling" the tissue well at the time of the frozen). This is best done by making sure that the second and third sections are taken from deep into the tissue. The pieces should be evaluated grossly for mucosa—typically shiny and pink-tan on one surface of the tissue; if present, the specimen should be oriented to demonstrate this surface on one edge of the section with the submucosa below. Additional sections should be cut if needed to assure that two or three quality sections are obtained.

The tissue that remains after frozen section is submitted for evaluation by permanent sections. This process can help resolve a number of issues from frozen section including freezing and cautery artifact, amount of tumor represented, and orientation or embedding issues. The margins of the main resection specimen are also evaluated throughout its entirety because the separate frozen section specimens are small and almost never cover the entire margin of a resection. The final margin status is then a conglomerate of all three sources: frozen section slides, permanent slides of the frozen tissue, and the margins of the specimen itself.

III. DIAGNOSTIC FEATURES OF COMMON DISEASES

A. **Inflammation and infection.** Inflammation of the larynx (laryngitis) is quite common clinically, and can be divided into acute and chronic forms, which are variable by age. Laryngitis rarely necessitates tissue biopsy for pathologic evaluation. Infections can be caused by a myriad of agents including viruses, bacteria, fungi, and parasites. The pathologist must be alert to the possibility of infection, and the immune status of the patient is helpful information, as many of these patients will be immunocompromised.

Inflammation is essentially never present in the normal larynx, so the presence of inflammatory cells is a diagnostic clue. Depending on the organism, the inflammation can take a number of different forms, almost all of which are typical for the type of organism when it presents in other locations. Examples of some of the major infections include cytomegalovirus, herpes simplex virus, tuberculosis, rhinoscleroma (*Klebsiella rhinoscleromatis*), candidiasis, histoplasmosis, blastomycosis, cryptococcosis, coccidiomycosis, or rhinosporidiosis (*Rhinosporidium seeberi*). The resulting inflammation may cause mucosal ulceration, acute and chronic inflammation, necrosis, or granulomas. Special stains (such as Gomori's methenamine silver (GMS), acid-fast bacillus (AFB), or periodic acid–Schiff (PAS)) should be utilized to look for, and characterize, organisms.

B. **Non-neoplastic lesions**

1. **Traumatic**

a. **Vocal cord nodules and polyps.** These are non-neoplastic degenerative stromal lesions of Reinke's space that are usually related to trauma due to misuse or vocal excess. As such, they have been referred to as singer's or screamer's nodules. They are more common in women and are commonly bilateral, characteristically occurring at the junction of the anterior and middle one-third of the vocal cord, as this is the point of maximal vibration during phonation. Macroscopically, they appear as gray or white broad-based nodules or polyps (e-**Fig. 2.3**). Microscopically, they consist of squamous mucosa with or without hyperkeratosis, are only rarely ulcerated, and overlie a sparsely cellular myxoid, edematous, fibrous, fibrinous, or vascular stroma. The myxoid appearance is most common and it may demonstrate small cystic spaces (e-**Figs. 2.4 and 2.5**). So-called vocal cord polyps are histologically identical but clinically present unilaterally, and in men and smokers with more regularity.

b. **Contact ulcer.** Also referred to clinically as *contact granuloma* or just *granuloma*, these occur on the vocal process of the arytenoids classically as a result of forceful vocalization in individuals who must affect a low, deep, forceful voice. However, they also may result after endotracheal intubation or as a result of gastroesophageal reflux disease. They are more common in men, can be unilateral or bilateral, and present as polypoid lesions.

Microscopically, they are essentially granulation tissue polyps with an ulcerated mucosa and a stroma containing abundant small vessels in a haphazard configuration with plump endothelial cells (e-**Fig. 2.6**). The stroma may be rich in lymphocytes, plasma cells, neutrophils, or histiocytes (sometimes including giant cells).

2. **Cysts.** Laryngeal cysts may be divided into three categories: (i) ductal cysts, (ii) laryngoceles, and (iii) saccular cysts. All are cured by simple excision.

   a. **Ductal cysts.** These are the most common and result from obstruction of a minor salivary gland duct. Ductal cysts are typically small "bumps" on endoscopy and have a predilection for the cords, ventricle, aryepiglottic folds, and epiglottis. The cyst lining may be squamous or oncocytic.

   b. **Laryngocele.** A laryngocele is an asymptomatic dilatation of the saccule (the deep aspect of the ventricle). It may remain internal and manifest as a supraglottic mucosal bulge, or may herniate above the thyroid cartilage to project externally into the neck soft tissue and present as a neck mass. Microscopically, it is lined by respiratory-type mucosa (e-**Fig. 2.7**).

   c. **Saccular cyst.** This represents a mucin-filled dilatation of the saccule, either developmental or acquired. It is also typically lined by respiratory-type mucosa, but the lining can be squamous or oncocytic on occasion. It is easily confused with a branchial cleft cyst.

3. **Metabolic**

   a. **Amyloidosis.** The larynx is a well-established, although infrequent, site of localized amyloidosis. It most commonly involves the false cord, followed by the true cord and ventricle. A subset of patients has multifocal disease, with approximately one-third having tracheal disease as well. The majority of patients have only localized disease, but systemic disease also occurs in a subset of patients. All patients should have a workup to rule out systemic amyloidosis with or without an associated plasma cell dyscrasia. The amyloid in localized laryngotracheal amyloidosis is of the AL (or immunoglobulin light chain type) type. It usually macroscopically presents as a polypoid nodule covered by intact mucosa. Microscopically, it consists of sheets and nodular masses of amorphous, hypocellular eosinophilic material in the stroma (e-**Fig. 2.8**), in blood vessel walls, and in the basement membranes of mucoserous glands. The diagnosis is confirmed by Congo red special staining with "apple-green" birefringence on polarized microscopy. Thioflavin T staining with examination under fluorescence microscopy is also sometimes used.

C. **Neoplastic lesions.** The World Health Organization (WHO) classification of tumors of the larynx, hypopharynx, and trachea is listed in Table 2.1.

1. **Benign**

   a. **Squamous papillomas** are squamous proliferations caused by human papilloma virus (HPV) and are the most common benign tumors of the larynx. They are most common in the larynx, but also occur in the trachea and bronchi. They also occur occasionally in the oral cavity and pharynx. There are two separate clinical settings: juvenile or juvenile-onset laryngeal papillomatosis (JOLP) and adult (or adult-onset) laryngeal papillomatosis (AOLP). Juvenile papillomas most often begin before the age of 5 years and are much more likely than adult papillomas to be multifocal and to have an associated clinical impact. In a significant minority of patients, carpeting of the larynx occurs, requiring repeated laser excisions and occasionally tracheostomy or even laryngectomy for control and airway management. Papillomas tend to recur rapidly, but the disease severity usually regresses in early adulthood. In adult papillomas, the peak age is between 20 and 40 years, disease is usually unifocal or limited, and even when multifocal, it is less aggressive. Only occasionally does it present as multifocal disease that recurs after excision.

Malignant epithelial tumors
Squamous cell carcinoma
  Verrucous carcinoma
  Papillary squamous cell carcinoma
  Basaloid squamous cell carcinoma
  Spindle cell carcinoma
  Adenosquamous carcinoma
  Acantholytic squamous cell carcinoma
Lymphoepithelial carcinoma
Giant cell carcinoma
Malignant salivary gland-type carcinomas
  Adenoid cystic carcinoma
  Mucoepidermoid carcinoma

Neuroendocrine tumors
Typical carcinoid
Atypical carcinoid
Small cell carcinoma, neuroendocrine type
Combined small cell carcinoma, neuroendocrine type

Benign epithelial tumors
Papilloma
Papillomatosis
Salivary gland-type adenomas
  Pleomorphic adenoma
  Oncocytic papillary cystadenoma

Soft tissue tumors
Malignant tumors
  Fibrosarcoma
  Malignant fibrous histiocytoma
  Liposarcoma
  Leiomyosarcoma
  Rhabdomyosarcoma
  Angiosarcoma
  Kaposi sarcoma
  Malignant peripheral nerve sheath tumor
  Synovial sarcoma
Borderline tumors/low malignant potential
  Inflammatory myofibroblastic tumor
Benign tumors
  Schwannoma
  Neurofibroma
  Lipoma
  Leiomyoma
  Rhabdomyoma
  Hemangioma
  Lymphangioma
  Granular cell tumor

Hematolymphoid tumors

Tumors of bone and cartilage
Chondrosarcoma
Osteosarcoma
Chondroma
Giant cell tumor

Mucosal malignant melanoma

Secondary tumors

From: Barnes L, Eveson J, Reichart P, Sidransky D, eds. *World Health Organization Classification of Tumours. Pathology and Genetics. Head and Neck Tumours.* Lyon: IARC Press; 2005. Used with permission.

Squamous papillomas are strongly associated with the low risk HPV types 6 and 11, which are thought to be transmitted from the mother to the upper aerodigestive tract (UADT) of the neonate during vaginal delivery, thus explaining the occurrence in childhood. There is minimal risk of transformation to invasive carcinoma.

Regardless of the clinical context, squamous papillomas have a typical morphology. Grossly, they appear as exophytic, granular, and friable pink, red, or tan lesions. Microscopically, they consist of arborizing, papillary fronds of thickened but maturing squamous epithelium with slight hyperplasia of the basal layer (e-Fig. 2.9). Cells in the midlayer often have cytoplasmic clearing, but frank koilocytosis is not regularly observed. The nuclei are slightly enlarged and irregular but do not appear overtly dysplastic, and mitotic activity, while present, is usually limited. Characteristically, there is minimal surface keratinization (e-Fig. 2.10). Frank dysplasia can be seen in some lesions and should be reported and graded as in nonpapillary squamous mucosa (see Section III.C.2). However, there is no consistent correlation of overt dysplasia with the development of subsequent invasive carcinoma.

b. **Granular cell tumors** are benign, slowly growing tumors of neural origin that occur in a multitude of anatomic locations. They are particularly common in the head and neck region with a minority occurring in the larynx. They are slightly more common in African Americans and typically present with hoarseness. Grossly, they are smooth, white polypoid tumors involving the posterior true cords, anterior commissure, false cords, or subglottis. Microscopically, they consist of infiltrative, nonencapsulated sheets and cords of bland cells with abundant eosinophilic granular cytoplasm and indistinct cell borders. There is usually no significant stromal reaction. The nuclei are small, oval, and eccentric with minimal atypia and no mitotic activity. A common feature is pseudoepitheliomatous hyperplasia of the overlying squamous epithelium, which can be quite alarming, can mimic squamous cell carcinoma, and should prompt a search of the submucosa for granular cells (e-Fig. 2.11). Conservative endoscopic excision is the treatment of choice with a less than 10% risk of recurrence.

c. **Paragangliomas** are tumors recapitulating the paraganglia, specialized organs of the autonomic nervous system derived from the neural crest. They occur in numerous locations throughout the body, and their behavior is largely dependent on site. Laryngeal paragangliomas are benign and are divided into two groups: superior and inferior. Superior paragangliomas are much more common and occur in the supraglottic larynx, from the false cord up into the aryepiglottic fold. They are polypoid submucosal lesions. Inferior paragangliomas occur along the cricoid cartilage in the subglottic region and often present as dumbbell-shaped lesions with both intra- and extralaryngeal components.

Microscopically, these tumors are identical to those arising elsewhere. They consist of sheets and nests of polygonal to spindled cells with abundant eosinophilic to slightly basophilic cytoplasm, and round to oval nuclei with a slightly granular chromatin. They are very vascular with stellate large vessels throughout (e-Fig. 2.12). Nuclear pleomorphism may be striking, but there is minimal mitotic activity. They are arranged in nests (classically termed *zellballen*) (e-Fig. 2.13). By immunohistochemistry, they are strongly positive for synaptophysin and chromogranin A, virtually always negative for epithelial markers such as epithelial membrane antigen (EMA) and cytokeratin, and show the typical sustentacular (or supporting) cell staining for S-100 around the periphery of the nests whereas the tumor cells themselves are negative.

TABLE 2.2 Precursor Lesion Classification Schemes

Ljubljana classification squamous intraepithelial lesions (SIL)	Squamous intraepithelial neoplasia (SIN)	2005 World Health Organization classification
Squamous cell (simple) hyperplasia	N/A	Squamous cell hyperplasia
Basal/parabasal cell hyperplasia	SIN 1	Mild dysplasia
Atypical hyperplasia	SIN 2	Moderate dysplasia
Atypical hyperplasia	SIN 3	Severe dysplasia
Carcinoma in situ	SIN 3	Carcinoma in situ

N/A, not applicable.

2. **Precursor (premalignant) squamous lesions** are defined as altered squamous epithelium with an increased risk of progression to squamous cell carcinoma. The term dysplasia or intraepithelial neoplasia should be used for these lesions. Atypia, in contrast, is not considered synonymous with dysplasia or risk of squamous cell carcinoma and is used in a more general sense, and may describe changes seen in reactive epithelium as well.

Unfortunately, there is poor agreement about the histopathologic changes that constitute dysplasia and about its grading. Also, there is poor correlation between the varying grades of dysplasia and subsequent risk of carcinoma. Several grading systems have been proposed (Table 2.2). Precursor lesions are strongly associated with smoking and alcohol use. Most precursor lesions present along the true cords and are often bilateral. This early presentation is likely due to dysfunction of the cords from the dysplasia; at other sites in the larynx, symptoms do not usually develop until there is established invasive malignancy.

There are a number of changes that occur in dysplasia including nuclear abnormalities, architectural/organizational abnormalities, and abnormal keratinization. Hyperplasia manifests as thickening of the epithelium without any cytologic atypia. The changes of dysplasia, particularly mild dysplasia, are difficult to distinguish from hyperplasia or reactive change, and by the same token, the varying degrees of dysplasia are difficult to distinguish from each other. In broad terms, mild dysplasia shows nuclear enlargement, hyperchromasia, and increased nucleus to cytoplasm ratios limited to the lower third of the epithelium (e-Fig. 2.14), moderate dysplasia into the middle third (e-Fig. 2.15), and severe dysplasia into the upper third or full thickness (e-Fig. 2.16). However, severe dysplasia, in particular, may manifest as an expanded basal cell layer with maturation in the upper layers, particularly with bulbous or downstreaming tongues of basal epithelium toward the submucosa (e-Fig. 2.17). The epithelium is usually thickened but sometimes thinned, and hyperkeratosis may or may not be present.

3. **Malignant**

a. **Squamous cell carcinoma** is overwhelmingly the most common malignant tumor of the larynx. It occurs with a peak in the sixth and seventh decades and, just as with other UADT squamous cancers, has a high male-to-female ratio (5:1) and a strong relationship to tobacco use and alcohol consumption, with a multiplicative rather than additive relative risk when both are used. Most cases involve the glottis or supraglottic region. Glottic tumors present earliest and at the smallest size because of functional compromise and symptomology.

The gross appearance of squamous cell carcinoma is quite variable, ranging from fungating, exophytic tumors to endophytic, ulcerated tumors with raised edges. Microscopically, the term "squamous cell carcinoma, keratinizing type" is used to describe the common version of the cancer and to distinguish it clearly from the numerous variant squamous cell carcinoma types that exist. Keratinizing-type squamous cell carcinoma consists of nests and sheets of cells with abundant eosinophilic cytoplasm and round to oval nuclei, often with prominent nucleoli. Well-differentiated tumors retain abundant pink or clear cytoplasm and often show keratin "pearl" formation (e-Fig. 2.9). Moderately differentiated tumors have more pleomorphism and a higher nucleus to cytoplasm ratio in many of the cells while still retaining moderate eosinophilic cytoplasm (e-Fig. 2.10). Poorly differentiated tumors often have single cells or small nests of cells with more mitotic activity and less cytoplasm (e-Fig. 2.11). Grading should be performed, although it has not been shown to consistently predict the clinical behavior of individual tumors. The majority of UADT squamous cell carcinomas are moderately differentiated. Although frank keratin formation is commonly seen in well- and moderately differentiated carcinomas, its presence or absence does not have any clinical significance for laryngeal carcinoma.

i. **Verrucous carcinoma (VC)** is a specific, well-differentiated, and non-metastasizing variant of squamous cell carcinoma. First described by Lauren V. Ackerman in the 1950s, it has thus also been called "Ackerman's tumor." It occurs in the larynx and oral cavity and grossly appears as a well-circumscribed, warty, and exophytic, broad-based white, granular, and friable mass. Microscopically, VC consists of very thick, club-shaped papillae with broad pushing bases. These blunt and downward-pushing projections have sometimes been likened to "elephant's feet." There is usually prominent surface hyperkeratosis, and the sheets of tumor have bland cells with abundant eosinophilic to clear cytoplasm, sometimes described as "glassy" in appearance. There is no cytologic atypia, mitotic activity is very low and basal, and there is a smooth interface with the stroma. This latter feature is because the individual tumor cells have not breached the basement membrane. The stroma directly beneath the tumor typically demonstrates prominent plasma cell rich chronic inflammation (e-Figs. 2.18, 2.19, and 2.20).

The prognosis for pure VC is excellent. Although it can be large and locally destructive, complete surgical resection is often curative. Radiation is also an acceptable treatment, particularly in poor surgical candidates. However, routine invasive squamous cell carcinoma sometimes arises from VC. When this occurs, the prognosis and behavior are the same as for typical squamous cell carcinoma.

ii. **Spindle cell carcinoma (SpCC)** is the term for a poorly differentiated carcinoma that adopts a sarcomatoid, spindled, or mesenchymal-appearing morphology but is, nevertheless, of epithelial origin/differentiation. It is frequently biphasic with a spindled component and intermingled either in situ or invasive squamous cell carcinoma. The tumor has the same demographics as routine squamous cell carcinoma.

Grossly, SpCC is characteristically polypoid with a smooth, ulcerated surface. The glottis is the most common laryngeal site. Microscopically, these tumors can be quite variable, but typically consist of sheets of spindle cells mimicking a fibrosarcoma or malignant fibrous histiocytoma (e-Fig. 2.21). Sometimes they consist of pleomorphic, hyperchromatic cells widely separated in an edematous stroma (e-Fig. 2.22). There is usually brisk mitotic activity and necrosis. Foci of recognizable sarcomatous differentiation such as chondrosarcoma, osteosarcoma, or rhabdomyosarcoma sometimes occur. Most cases are "biphasic," showing some component of in situ or invasive squamous cell carcinoma (e-**Fig. 2.23**), but it may take extensive sectioning to demonstrate the routine squamous component.

If the tumor consists of spindle or pleomorphic cells only, immunohistochemistry for epithelial markers such as pancytokeratin, EMA, and p63 is usually very helpful. These markers are positive in onefourth to one-third of cases. With markedly extended panels utilizing antibodies to more than 10 different individual keratins, approximately three-quarters of tumors will demonstrate staining; however, in everyday practice, utilization of pancytokeratin (AE1/AE3) as well as 34βE12 or 5/6 usually suffices demonstrate keratin expression. SpCC stains for some mesenchymal markers as well, such as vimentin (every case), smooth muscle actin, and muscle-specific actin. Whatever the case, a malignant spindle cell neoplasm involving/arising along the mucosa of the UADT should be considered an SpCC until proven otherwise, because sarcomas are distinctly uncommon at these sites. The differential diagnosis includes a granulation tissue polyp, true sarcoma, or inflammatory myofibroblastic tumor. The positive epithelial marker immunohistochemistry will distinguish SpCC from these other entities.

iii. **Basaloid squamous cell carcinoma (BSCC)** is a variant of squamous cell carcinoma composed almost entirely of basaloid cells giving it a "blue cell" appearance. It has the same demographics as routine squamous cell carcinoma but has a predilection for the supraglottic larynx, the oropharynx, and the hypopharynx, particularly the pyriform sinuses. It typically presents at high stage and is more aggressive than typical squamous cell carcinoma stage for stage, with high rates of distant metastasis.

Grossly, BSCC presents as a centrally ulcerated mass with thickening at the edges, and commonly with extensive submucosal induration and spread at the periphery. Microscopically, there are two components. The first is predominant and consists of rounded nests of basaloid cells with hyperchromatic round nuclei, inconspicuous nucleoli, and scant cytoplasm. Comedo-type central necrosis is common. The second component is typical keratinizing-type squamous cell carcinoma, either in situ or invasive, which is always focal (e-**Fig. 2.24**). The basaloid component of many tumors shows a characteristic hyalinized, eosinophilic basement membrane–like stroma around the tumor cells, and/or as small round nodules within tumor nests akin to that seen in cylindromas of the skin (e-**Fig. 2.25**).

The differential diagnosis includes neuroendocrine carcinoma or the solid variant of adenoid cystic carcinoma. The former expresses neuroendocrine markers in most cases and is negative for highmolecular-weight cytokeratins such as 34βE12 and 5/6. Solid adenoid cystic carcinoma shows some evidence of myoepithelial differentiation upon staining for p63 manifested as scattered staining at the periphery of tumor nests; in contrast, BSCC stains diffusely throughout the tumor (as with squamous epithelium and squamous cell carcinoma, which also show strong staining).

iv. **Papillary squamous cell carcinoma (PSCC)** is an uncommon variant of squamous cell carcinoma which has the same demographics as typical squamous cell carcinoma. The larynx is among the most common sites of involvement, the supraglottis and glottis in particular; only very rarely does the tumor arise in the subglottis. Grossly, it is a soft, polypoid, and friable tumor. Microscopically, it is defined by having a predominantly (>50%) papillary growth pattern with fibrovascular cores lined by full thickness, markedly dysplastic squamous cells, which are most often very immature and basaloid appearing. There is usually minimal keratinization. Stromal invasion may or may not be present, but when it is, it has the appearance of typical squamous cell carcinoma. If frank invasion is not present, the lesion should be termed PSCC in situ.

The differential diagnosis includes squamous papilloma, verrucous carcinoma, and typical squamous cell carcinoma with a partially exophytic growth pattern. The prognosis of PSCC is better than for typical squamous cell carcinoma. PSCC frequent recurs locally, but metastases are infrequent.

v. **Adenosquamous carcinoma.** The larynx is the most common site for adenosquamous carcinoma followed by the oral cavity and sinonasal region. Adenosquamous carcinoma has the same demographics and clinical presentation as typical squamous cell carcinoma. It does not have a unique gross appearance, and is either exophytic or ulcerated with indurated edges. Microscopically, it consists of both true squamous cell carcinoma and adenocarcinoma. The two components are usually close to each other but still have a tendency to segregate. The squamous component, which is usually of the keratinizing type, can be either invasive or in situ and has the same appearance as typical squamous cell carcinoma. It usually predominates in the superficial aspects of the tumor, whereas the adenocarcinoma component, which may either be isolated glands or gland-like structures within larger sheets of tumor, tends to occupy the deeper aspects (e-**Fig. 2.26**). The glands are often "punched out" with round, smooth edges. Mucin production is not required for the diagnosis but is very frequently present (e-**Fig. 2.27**); mucicarmine or other mucin stains can be quite helpful to highlight its presence.

The differential diagnosis includes mucoepidermoid carcinoma, acantholytic or adenoid squamous cell carcinoma, and squamous cell carcinoma invading seromucinous minor salivary gland tissue. Mucoepidermoid carcinoma is the most important consideration (Table 2.3). Adenosquamous carcinomas are more aggressive than typical squamous cell carcinoma, although not markedly so. The literature shows that the prognosis for adenosquamous carcinoma is worse than conventional squamous cell carcinoma.

b. **Neuroendocrine carcinomas.** Neuroendocrine carcinomas of the larynx are relatively uncommon and are divided into three major categories:

TABLE 2.3 Adenosquamous Carcinoma versus Mucoepidermoid Carcinoma: Histologic Features	
Adenosquamous carcinoma	**Mucoepidermoid carcinoma**
Squamous cell carcinoma in situ	No squamous cell carcinoma in situ
Origin from squamous epithelium	Origin from seromucinous glands
Keratin pearls	Limited keratin pearls
Glands at lower invasive parts	Glands widely intermingled
No lobular arrangement	Lobular arrangement
No intermediate cells	Large, clear "intermediate cells"

carcinoid tumor (low-grade neuroendocrine carcinoma), atypical carcinoid tumor (intermediate grade neuroendocrine carcinoma), and small cell carcinoma (high-grade neuroendocrine carcinoma). More recently, large cell neuroendocrine carcinoma similar to that seen in the lung has been defined in the larynx as well. There is a clear spectrum of behavior among the subtypes ranging from very indolent to highly aggressive.

Most neuroendocrine carcinomas of the larynx occur in the sixth to the eighth decade, and there is a strong male predominance. They are almost exclusively supraglottic, and smoking is associated with atypical carcinoid tumors and small and large cell neuroendocrine carcinomas only.

The histology of these tumors directly parallels those within the lung. Carcinoid tumor is characterized by nests, trabeculae, and sheets of round, regular tumor cells with moderate eosinophilic to partially clear cytoplasm. Nuclei are round, regular, and show the typical "salt and pepper" or stippled chromatin. Mitotic activity is less than 2 per 10 high power fields. Atypical carcinoid tumor has a similar appearance but is less organized and shows more cellular pleomorphism, focal necrosis, and more prominent mitotic activity (3–10 per 10 high power fields). Small cell carcinoma is high grade and consists of sheets of blue cells with nuclear molding, crush artifact, and delicate chromatin with indistinct nucleoli (e-**Fig. 2.16**). Large cell neuroendocrine carcinoma is also high grade but has larger cells with generous eosinophilic cytoplasm and frequently a more organized growth pattern with peripheral palisading. There is brisk mitotic activity and prominent necrosis in both forms of high-grade neuroendocrine carcinoma. All of these neoplasms stain with neuroendocrine markers by immunohistochemistry (synaptophysin, chromogranin-A, CD56/N-CAM), but there tends to be less staining with the high-grade tumors. In particular, in small cell carcinoma, the staining can become quite focal and sometimes is only present for one of the several neuroendocrine markers.

Carcinoid tumor has an excellent prognosis despite frequent local recurrence. Metastases are uncommon. Atypical carcinoid tumor is an aggressive tumor with frequent cervical lymph node and distant metastases. Surgery is the treatment of choice for both. The high-grade neuroendocrine carcinomas have a dismal prognosis with frequent neck nodal and distant metastases. Patients are typically treated with radiation and chemotherapy rather than surgery.

c. **Mesenchymal tumors.** A great variety of mesenchymal tumors occasionally occur in the larynx, the most common of which are the cartilaginous tumors chondroma and chondrosarcoma. Chondrosarcomas are the most common sarcoma of the larynx, occur in older adults, and are decidedly more common in men. They originate from the cricoid or thyroid lamina (3:1, cricoid to thyroid) and tend to present differently by site of origin with slowly progressive dyspnea for cricoid tumors, or an anterior neck mass for thyroid tumors. Symptoms are usually present for a long period of time (often several years). Grossly, the neoplasms consist of well-circumscribed, shiny white or gray lobulated masses with gritty areas of calcification and a glistening cut surface (e-**Fig. 2.17**). Microscopically, they consist of lobules of cartilage which, relative to normal, show increased cellularity and nuclear atypia with variability in size, more than one nucleus in individual lacunae, and binucleated cells (e-**Fig. 2.28**). The periphery of the tumor is typically pushing and not infiltrative. The grading system is identical to that for chondrosarcomas elsewhere in the body. With increasing grades, the cellular atypia increases with cells having enlarged nuclei and nucleoli, but mitotic activity is only seen in high-grade

TABLE 2.4	2010 American Joint Committee on Cancer Staging Guidelines for Tumors of the Larynx

Tumor, nodes, and metastases (TNM) categories

PRIMARY TUMOR (T)

TX	Primary tumor cannot be assessed
T0	No evidence of primary tumor
Tis	Carcinoma in situ

Supraglottis

T1	Tumor limited to one subsite of supraglottis with normal vocal cord mobility
T2	Tumor invades mucosa of more than one adjacent subsite of supraglottis or glottis or region outside the supraglottis (e.g., mucosa of base of tongue, vallecula, medial wall of pyriform sinus) without fixation of the larynx
T3	Tumor limited to larynx with vocal cord fixation and/or invades any of the following: postcricoid area, pre-epiglottic space, paraglottic space, and/or inner cortex of the thyroid cartilage
T4a	Moderately advanced local disease. Tumor invades through the thyroid cartilage and/or invades tissues beyond the larynx (e.g., trachea, soft tissues of neck including deep extrinsic muscles of the tongue, strap muscles, thyroid, or esophagus)
T4b	Very advanced local disease. Tumor invades prevertebral space, encases carotid artery, or invades mediastinal structures

Glottis

T1	Tumor limited to the vocal cord(s) (may involve anterior or posterior commissure) with normal mobility
T1a	Tumor limited to one vocal cord
T1b	Tumor involves both vocal cords
T2	Tumor extends to supraglottis and/or subglottis and/or with impaired vocal cord mobility
T3	Tumor limited to larynx with vocal cord fixation and/or invades the paraglottic space and/or inner cortex of the thyroid cartilage
T4a	Moderately advanced local disease. Tumor invades through the outer cortex of the thyroid cartilage and/or invades tissues beyond the larynx (e.g., trachea, soft tissues of neck including deep extrinsic muscles of the tongue, strap muscles, thyroid, or esophagus)
T4b	Very advanced local disease. Tumor invades prevertebral space, encases carotid artery, or invades mediastinal structures

Subglottis

T1	Tumor limited to subglottis
T2	Tumor extends to vocal cord(s) with normal or impaired mobility
T3	Tumor limited to larynx with vocal cord fixation
T4a	Moderately advanced local disease. Tumor invades cricoid or thyroid cartilage and/or invades tissues beyond the larynx (e.g., trachea, soft tissues of neck including deep extrinsic muscles of the tongue, strap muscles, thyroid, or esophagus)
T4b	Very advanced local disease. Tumor invades prevertebral space, encases carotid artery, or invades mediastinal structures

REGIONAL LYMPH NODES (N)

NX	Regional lymph nodes cannot be assessed
N0	No regional lymph node metastasis
N1	Metastasis in a single ipsilateral lymph node, ≤ 3 cm in greatest dimension
N2a	Metastasis in a single ipsilateral lymph node, >3 cm but <6 cm in greatest dimension
N2b	Metastasis in multiple ipsilateral lymph nodes, none >6 cm in greatest dimension
N2c	Metastasis in bilateral or contralateral lymph nodes, none >6 cm in greatest dimension
N3	Metastasis in a lymph node >6 cm in greatest dimension

(continued)

TABLE 2.4	2010 American Joint Committee on Cancer Staging Guidelines for Tumors of the Larynx (*Continued*)

DISTANT METASTASIS (M)

MX	Distant metastasis cannot be assessed
M0	No distant metastasis
M1	Distant metastasis

STAGE GROUPING

The overall pathologic AJCC stage

Stage 0	Tis	N0	M0
Stage I	T1	N0	M0
Stage II	T2	N0	M0
Stage III	T3	N0	M0
Stage III	T1	N1	M0
Stage III	T2	N1	M0
Stage III	T3	N1	M0
Stage IVA	T4a	N0	M0
Stage IVA	T4a	N1	M0
Stage IVA	T1	N2	M0
Stage IVA	T2	N2	M0
Stage IVA	T3	N2	M0
Stage IVA	T4a	N2	M0
Stage IVB	T4b	Any N	M0
Stage IVB	Any T	N3	M0
Stage IVC	Any T	Any N	M1

From: Edge SB, Byrd DR, Compton CC, et al., eds. *AJCC Cancer Staging Manual.* 7th ed. New York, NY: Springer; 2010. Used with permission.

tumors. It can be remarkably challenging to differentiate chondrosarcomas from chondromas, particularly on biopsy specimens. Chondrosarcomas display cytologic atypia with nucleoli in chondrocytes and show at least some areas of more infiltrative growth at the periphery.

The vast majority of laryngeal chondrosarcomas are well differentiated (grade 1). However, grade does not seem to affect prognosis. Surgery is directed at larynx-sparing complete excision, with total laryngectomy reserved for recurrences or uncontrolled local disease. Survival is greater than 95% at 10 years.

IV. PATHOLOGIC REPORTING OF LARYNGEAL CARCINOMA

A. **Staging (AJCC).** Staging of laryngeal carcinomas is extremely important for clinical management and prognosis. For T-staging purposes, the larynx is divided into the supraglottis, glottis, and subglottis (Table 2.4). Although squamous cell carcinoma is the overwhelmingly most common type of malignancy, staging guidelines are applicable to all forms of carcinoma. Any nonepithelial tumor type is excluded. The staging guidelines often require both clinical and pathologic input (e.g., vocal cord fixation or not) for proper classification.

B. **Additional pertinent pathologic features.** As with carcinomas at all UADT sites, margin status, tumor differentiation, and the presence or absence of perineural or lymphvascular space invasion should be reported. In addition, the pattern of infiltration as well as the presence or absence of a host inflammatory response should be reported. All of these features have been correlated in many studies with higher rates of local recurrence, a poorer prognosis, or both.

SUGGESTED READINGS

Brandwein-Gensler MS, Mahadevia P, Gnepp DR. Nonsquamous pathologic diseases of the hypopharynx, larynx, and trachea. In: Gnepp DR, ed. *Diagnostic Surgical Pathology of the Head and Neck*. Philadelphia, PA: W.B. Saunders Publishers; 2009.

Gale N. Benign neoplasms of the larynx, hypopharynx, and trachea. In: Thompson LDR, ed. *Head and Neck Pathology*. New York, NY: Churchill Livingstone; 2006.

Slootweg PJ, Richardson M. Squamous cell carcinoma of the upper aerodigestive system. In: Gnepp DR, ed. *Diagnostic Surgical Pathology of the Head and Neck*. Philadelphia, PA: W.B. Saunders Publishers; 2009.

Thompson LDR. Malignant neoplasms of the larynx, hypopharynx, and trachea. In: Thompson LDR, ed. *Head and Neck Pathology*. New York, NY: Churchill Livingstone; 2006.

Thompson LDR. Non-neoplastic lesions of the larynx, hypopharynx, and trachea. In: Thompson LDR, ed. *Head and Neck Pathology*. New York, NY: Churchill Livingstone; 2006.

Zidar N, Boffetta P. Tumours of the hypopharynx, larynx, and trachea. In: Barnes L, Eveson JW, Reichart P, Sidransky D, eds. *Pathology and Genetics Head and Neck Tumours*. Lyon, France: IARC Press; 2005.

3 Nasal Cavity, Paranasal Sinuses, and Nasopharynx

Heather N. Wright and James S. Lewis Jr.

I. NORMAL ANATOMY

A. Nasal cavity. The normal sinonasal region consists of the central nasal cavity, paired bilateral paranasal sinuses, and the nasopharynx. The nasal cavity consists anteriorly of the nasal vestibule, the small hair-bearing region just inside the nasal ostia, with the remainder representing the nasal antrum; the nasal cavity has four walls, a central dividing septum, and paired upper, middle, and lower turbinates. The nasal vestibule lining is an extension of the surrounding facial skin, and as such has a stratified, keratinizing squamous epithelium with associated dermal appendages and hair. It extends for 1 to 2 cm into the nasal cavity. The nasal antrum is lined by pseudostratified ciliated columnar (respiratory-type) epithelium of ectodermal origin referred to as the Schneiderian membrane (**e-Fig. 3.1**).* The submucosa consists of minor salivary gland mucoserous glands embedded in fibrovascular connective tissue with small ducts that convey their secretions to the surface. The turbinates have a more richly vascular stroma. The roof of the nasal cavity contains the cribriform plate with olfactory mucosa, a modified respiratory-type epithelium with olfactory nerve cells, and supporting cells.

B. Paranasal sinuses. The paranasal sinuses consist of the maxillary (largest), frontal, sphenoid, and ethmoid sinuses. They drain into the nasal cavity and are air filled, intraosseous, and open. The ethmoid sinuses are small and complex (referred to as the ethmoid labyrinth or air cells). All paranasal sinuses are in continuity with the nasal cavity so they have a similar, although thinner, mucosa. The submucosa is also thinner, looser, and less vascular than in the nasal cavity, although it does contain prominent seromucinous glands.

C. Nasopharynx. The nasopharynx is the most cephalad portion of the pharynx and is a cuboidal structure. Its roof is formed by the pharyngeal tonsil. The lateral walls are the most pathologically important because they contain the openings of the Eustachian tubes, and a depression posterior to the torus tubarius called the fossa of Rosenmüller. The fossa of Rosenmüller is the most common site of origin for nasopharyngeal carcinoma (NPC). Since the nasopharynx is surrounded by bone and vital structures, it is poorly accessible for surgery. The epithelial lining consists of a mixture of stratified squamous, intermediate (or transitional), and respiratory-type epithelium.

II. GROSS EXAMINATION, TISSUE SAMPLING, AND HISTOLOGIC SLIDE PREPARATION

A. Endoscopic biopsies. Most of the specimens from this region consist of endoscopic forcep biopsies. The small tissue pieces should be placed immediately into 10% buffered formalin or other appropriate fixative. If there is a suspicion of lymphoma, a minimum of three biopsy passes should be submitted in saline or RPMI medium and send directly for an appropriate hematopathology workup. Standard formalin-fixed specimens should undergo gross examination and description documenting the exact number of pieces present, and then should

---

*All e-figures are available online via the Solution Site Image Bank.

be entirely submitted for histologic examination (three hematoxylin and eosin [H&E] levels cut per block). For very small specimens, or where few pieces are obtained from clinical masses, it is strongly recommended that additional unstained slides be cut from the block on initial submission for potential use for immunohistochemistry or special stains.

B. Functional endoscopic sinus surgery (FESS; "sinus contents"). The tissue consists of fragments of ethmoid and maxillary ostium sinus bone and mucosa, resected inflammatory polyps, and nasal cavity and sinus tissue obtained by suction devices. These samples should be described, measured, and submitted for histologic examination. If firm or dense tissue fragments are identified, they should be submitted as they may represent an unsuspected neoplasm. Otherwise, pieces of intact tissue should be collected from the blood and fluid from the suction device, inspected grossly, and measured in aggregate. Only one cassette of these fragments need be submitted for histologic examination with decalcification in EDTA or formic acid if gross pieces of bone are identified.

C. Resections. Surgical resections for sinonasal tumors are complex and varied, and are guided by tumor location, extent, and type. They always consist of soft tissue, mucosa, and bone. Margins are in large part guided by the separate specimens submitted for frozen section. The main specimen should be oriented, the tumor identified, and mucosal, soft tissue, and bone margins identified. The main specimen should be described and measured; the soft tissue margins are inked and then mucosal and soft tissue margin sections sampled. If the tumor is relatively distant from a margin, 1 to 2 mm thick shave sections are preferred; if the tumor approximates a margin (within 1 to 2 mm), radial sections are taken. After this, the tumor is sectioned and sampled. Four to five sections should be taken from tumors, or if small, tumors should be entirely submitted for histologic examination. Often sectioning requires a saw to cut through bone to demonstrate the relationship of the lesion to the adjacent structures. The bone should be decalcified, and shave sections from the bone margins as well as sections demonstrating tumor involving bone should be taken.

D. Frozen sections are a critical element of surgical therapy for head and neck tumors. Although practices vary, most institutions have margins taken as small pieces by the surgeon from the periphery of the surgical defect after the tumor has been removed. The pieces should be evaluated grossly for mucosa (which is typically shiny and pink-tan on one surface of the tissue); if present, the tissue should be oriented to demonstrate this mucosal surface on one edge of the section. Two (or at our institution, three) high quality sections are obtained with the second and third levels taken deep into the tissue to ensure adequate sampling.

The tissue that remains after a frozen section should be submitted for evaluation on permanent sections. This is done to further assure adequate sampling of the tissue and to help resolve a number of issues from frozen section including freezing and cautery artifact, amount of tumor represented, and orientation/embedding issues. The final margin status is therefore a conglomerate of the frozen section slides, permanent slides of the frozen tissue, and the margins of the resection specimen itself.

III. DIAGNOSTIC FEATURES OF COMMON DISEASES
  A. Inflammation and infection. These processes are extremely common in the United States, necessitating a large amount of medical care and surgery.
   1. Acute rhinosinusitis. Acute sinusitis is rarely seen by the pathologist because it is treated medically. However, typical histologic findings include neutrophils migrating through, and present in, the respiratory-type mucosa with luminal contents showing necrotic material, apoptotic neutrophil nuclear debris, and mucin with abundant neutrophils.
   2. Chronic rhinosinusitis. Chronic inflammation of the nasal cavity can result from allergy, upper respiratory tract infection, or cystic fibrosis. Sinusitis is

thought to occur secondary to obstruction of the outflow of the paranasal sinuses by myriad etiologies such as edema and inflammation, or anatomic abnormalities, particularly in children. Some of the most common obstructing agents are inflammatory polyps, a deviated septum, or concha bullosa (air pocket in the middle turbinate). Finally, rare genetic conditions such as immotile cilia syndrome (Kartagener's syndrome) cause chronic sinusitis. Complications include secondary bacterial infection and, in chronic allergic sinusitis, the development of inflammatory polyps.

Specimens from FESS in chronic sinusitis typically show edema of the submucosa with a mixture of lymphocytes, plasma cells, and eosinophils, the latter sometimes being quite prominent. The abundance and distribution of eosinophils histologically do not have a clinical correlate other than suggesting allergy as an underlying etiology for the sinusitis.

3. **Wegener granulomatosis** is an autoimmune disorder characterized by necrotizing vasculitis that affects the nasal cavity and paranasal sinuses, pulmonary, and/or renal systems. Manifestations of nasal cavity/paranasal sinus involvement include rhinorrhea, sinusitis, headache, nasal obstruction, anosmia, and sometimes middle ear and mastoid symptoms if inflammation obstructs the Eustachian tube.

   Histologically, in biopsies of the sinonasal region, the diagnosis can be quite difficult. Features include mucosal ulceration, acute and chronic inflammation, necrosis, and granulomas. Wegener granulomatosis causes a vasculitis which is often obscured by the inflammation, so elastic stains such as Verhoeff–van Gieson may be helpful to demonstrate the elastic fibers of inflamed vessels. The vasculitis involves arterioles, small arteries, and veins with changes ranging from fibrinoid necrosis with neutrophils and associated extravasated red blood cells and fibrin thrombi, to granulomatous inflammation with multinucleated giant cells and histiocytes (e-**Fig. 3.2**). It is very important to correlate the histologic findings with clinical information and laboratory investigation, which reveals cytoplasmic antineutrophil antibodies (cANCA) in approximately 90% of patients.

4. **Inflammatory polyps.** Sinonasal inflammatory polyps are nonneoplastic mucosal and submucosal projections that arise in longstanding chronic rhinitis, usually associated with allergy or asthma. They are seen most commonly in adults but can be seen in children as well, particularly in those with cystic fibrosis. Symptoms include headache, nasal obstruction, and rhinorrhea. They are multiple, often bilateral, and most commonly arise from the lateral nasal wall. Although nonneoplastic, they are capable of dramatic behavior including deviation of the septum, destruction of bone, and extension into the nasopharynx and rarely the orbit or cranial cavities.

   Grossly, inflammatory polyps can measure up to several centimeters and are boggy, gelatinous, and partially translucent with broad bases. Microscopically, there is a highly edematous or lightly myxoid stroma with a mixed inflammatory infiltrate of lymphocytes, plasma cells, and a variable number of eosinophils. There are few small vessels and minimal, bland, spindled stromal cells. Inflammatory polyps typically are devoid of seromucinous glands, a feature that is particularly helpful in identifying them when they are in fragmented pieces (e-**Fig. 3.3**). The surface mucosa is typically intact and lined by respiratory epithelium with a variably thickened basement membrane, although it occasionally shows squamous metaplasia.

5. **Fungal infections** are relatively frequent and can involve any of the paranasal sinuses. They can be broadly classified as "invasive" and "noninvasive" (Table 3.1).

   a. **Noninvasive.** Immunocompetent patients usually develop noninvasive fungal disease, either allergic fungal sinusitis or mycetoma ("fungus ball").

TABLE 3.1	Fungal Sinusitis		
Entity	**Clinical**	**Histology**	**Organism**
Noninvasive: Allergic fungal sinusitis	Chronic sinusitis; inflammatory polyps; allergic symptoms; pan-sinusitis	Eosinophilic mucus; sheets of degenerating eosinophils; Charcot–Leyden crystals; sometimes fragmented hyphae in mucus	*Aspergillus;* dematiaceous fungi: *Bipolaris, Alternaria, Curvularia, Cladosporium*
Noninvasive: Mycetoma ("fungus ball")	Chronic sinusitis, mass lesion on imaging— usually one sinus cavity; usually nonallergic-type presentation	Large intraluminal collections of fungal hyphae; minimal mucus; minimal inflammation	*Aspergillus;* dematiaceous fungi: *Bipolaris, Alternaria, Curvularia, Cladosporium*
Invasive: Acute invasive fungal sinusitis	Severe acute sinusitis; fever; nasal discharge; ocular or neurologic deficits	Necrosis; thrombosis; hemorrhage; angioinvasive fungal hyphae in viable tissue; minimal inflammation	Common: Mucorales order—*Mucor, Rhizopus, Absidia, Cunninghamella;* Uncommon: *Aspergillus, Curvularia, Alternaria*
Invasive: Chronic invasive fungal sinusitis	Slow, progressive onset; neurologic or orbital deficits; mass on imaging	Necrosis; angioinvasive fungal hyphae; granulomas	*Aspergillus*

Clinically, they have similar presentations with symptoms of chronic sinusitis including headache, nasal discharge, stuffiness, and facial pressure.

Allergic fungal sinusitis patients have asthma (present in >90% of cases), eosinophilia, atopy, and elevated total fungus-specific immunoglobulin E (IgE) concentrations. Endoscopy reveals thick, sticky, greenish or black to brown mucus, often described as the consistency of peanut butter. Microscopically, abundant brightly eosinophilic hypocellular mucin is present, distinct from slightly basophilic normal mucin. The mucin contains sheets of eosinophils that are degenerating and degranulating. These granules may coalesce to form the classic Charcot–Leyden crystals (**e-Fig. 3.4**). The most common causative organisms are dematiaceous fungi such as *Bipolaris* and *Curvularia, Alternaria,* and *Aspergillus.* Fungal hyphae are fragmented and widely scattered in the mucin, so they are rarely visible by H&E. Special stains such as Grocott's Methenamine Silver (GMS) are usually necessary for identification. If the typical histologic picture is present without identifying organisms, the term *allergic mucin* is used. If hyphae are identified, the term *allergic fungal sinusitis* is used.

Patients with mycetoma have chronic sinusitis but usually lack allergic symptoms. On endoscopy, the single affected sinus has mucopurulent, cheesy, or clay-like material that microscopically consists of sheets of fungal hyphae with minimal mucin and inflammatory cells (**e-Fig. 3.5**).

b. **Invasive.** Patients with invasive fungal disease are usually immunocompromised, frequently from diabetes mellitus, bone marrow or solid organ transplantation, and occasionally human immunodeficiency virus (HIV) infection, and are at great risk of morbidity and mortality.

Patients are often severely ill with fever, cough, nasal discharge, headache, and mental status changes. They sometimes have ophthalmologic symptoms or neurologic deficits due to orbital or cranial involvement. On endoscopy, there are dark ulcers on the mucosa and associated black, greasy necrotic tissue. The fungi are angioinvasive, so they cause extensive hemorrhage and necrosis. In the viable tissue, the microscopic findings include minimal inflammation and blood vessels filled with refractile fungal hyphae (e-**Fig. 3.6**). The order *Mucorales* is most common (e.g., *Mucor, Rhizopus, Absidia*), but other fungi including *Aspergillus* species may be causative. The morphology of *Mucor* species includes bizarre, angulated hyphal fragments and elongated hyphae that are wide, irregular, and thick walled. Typically there is 90-degree angle branching without septation. Diabetics may also develop a chronic pattern of invasive fungal disease, often presenting as a slowly progressive orbital mass; microscopically, angioinvasive hyphae or granulomas are often present in these patients.

B. **Nonneoplastic lesions.** Several lesions, developmental or mechanical, can occur in the sinonasal region and can be mass-like and simulate true neoplasms.

1. **Mucous impaction** is an uncommon lesion that occurs mostly in children and young adults with a long history of chronic sinusitis. It represents impaction of a large amount of mucus within the maxillary antrum. Grossly, it consists of translucent gray to pink material. Microscopically, it simply consists of slightly basophilic to eosinophilic extracellular mucin with a mixture of plasma cells, lymphocytes, and neutrophils with desquamated respiratory-type epithelium.

2. **Paranasal sinus mucoceles** are chronic, nonneoplastic cysts that form from the obstruction of the sinus outlet by any of a number of processes. They occur most commonly in the ethmoid and frontal sinuses. Grossly, they consist of a cyst filled with mucoid or gelatinous material. Microscopically, they consist of extracellular mucin with a flattened respiratory-type epithelial lining that may have secondary squamous metaplasia.

3. **Respiratory epithelial adenomatoid hamartoma (REAH)** is a rare, benign, polypoid lesion characterized by an adenomatoid proliferation of respiratory-type epithelium that occurs primarily on the posterior nasal septum. Microscopically, it consists of a polypoid proliferation of variably sized, round to oval glands lined by respiratory-type epithelium with a markedly thickened basement membrane and no cytologic atypia or significant mitotic activity (e-**Fig. 3.7**). The gland-like structures are often in direct continuity with the surface epithelium (e-**Fig. 3.8**). The stroma is edematous and can resemble that of an inflammatory polyp.

C. **Neoplastic lesions.** A wide array of neoplasms occur in the sinonasal region (Table 3.2).

1. **Benign**

a. **Schneiderian papillomas.** The ectodermally derived Schneiderian membrane gives rise to three different types of benign papillomas: exophytic, inverted, and oncocytic (Table 3.3). The distinction of these papillomas is important because of their differences in behavior and risk of carcinoma development. For this reason, it is critical to entirely submit all papilloma tissues for microscopic examination.

i. **Exophytic papilloma (fungiform papilloma).** Most of these occur on the nasal septum, particularly anteriorly, in adults 20 to 50 years old. They

Malignant epithelial tumors
Squamous cell carcinoma
  Verrucous carcinoma
  Papillary squamous cell carcinoma
  Basaloid squamous cell carcinoma
  Spindle cell carcinoma
  Adenosquamous carcinoma
  Acantholytic squamous cell carcinoma
Lymphoepithelial carcinoma
Sinonasal undifferentiated carcinoma
Adenocarcinoma
  Intestinal-type adenocarcinoma
  Nonintestinal-type adenocarcinoma
Salivary gland-type carcinomas
  Adenoid cystic carcinoma
  Acinic cell carcinoma
  Mucoepidermoid carcinoma
  Epithelial–myoepithelial carcinoma
  Clear cell carcinoma not otherwise
    specified
  Myoepithelial carcinoma
  Carcinoma ex pleomorphic adenoma
  Polymorphous low-grade
    adenocarcinoma
Neuroendocrine tumors
  Typical carcinoid
  Atypical carcinoid
  Small cell carcinoma, neuroendocrine
    type

Benign epithelial tumors
Sinonasal papillomas
  Inverted papilloma
  (Schneiderian papilloma, inverted type)
  Oncocytic papilloma
  (Schneiderian papilloma, oncocytic type)
  Exophytic papilloma
  (Schneiderian papilloma, exophytic type)
Salivary gland–type adenomas
  Pleomorphic adenoma
  Myoepithelioma
  Oncocytoma

Soft tissue tumors
Malignant tumors
  Fibrosarcoma
  Malignant fibrous histiocytoma
  Leiomyosarcoma
  Rhabdomyosarcoma
  Angiosarcoma
  Malignant peripheral nerve sheath tumor
Borderline and low malignant potential
  tumors
  Desmoid-type fibromatosis
  Inflammatory myofibroblastic tumor

Glomangiopericytoma
  (Sinonasal-type hemangiopericytoma)
  Extrapleural solitary fibrous tumor
Benign tumors
  Myxoma
  Leiomyoma
  Haemangioma
  Schwannoma
  Neurofibroma
  Meningioma

Tumors of bone and cartilage
Malignant tumors
  Chondrosarcoma
  Mesenchymal chondrosarcoma
  Osteosarcoma
  Chordoma
Benign tumors
  Giant cell lesion
  Giant cell tumor
  Chondroma
  Osteoma
  Chondroblastoma
  Chondromyxoid fibroma
  Osteochondroma (exostosis)
  Osteoid osteoma
  Osteoblastoma
  Ameloblastoma
  Nasal chondromesenchymal hamartoma

Hematolymphoid tumors
  Extranodal natural killer (NK)/T-cell
    lymphoma
  Diffuse large B-cell lymphoma
  Extramedullary plasmacytoma
  Extramedullary myeloid sarcoma
  Histiocytic sarcoma
  Langerhans cell histiocytosis

Neuroectodermal
  Ewing sarcoma
  Primitive neuroectodermal tumor
  Olfactory neuroblastoma
  Melanotic neuroectodermal tumor of
    infancy
  Mucosal malignant melanoma

Germ cell tumors
  Immature teratoma
  Teratoma with malignant transformation
  Sinonasal yolk sac tumor (endodermal
    sinus tumor)
  Sinonasal teratocarcinosarcoma
  Mature teratoma
  Dermoid cyst
Secondary tumors

TABLE 3.3	Schneiderian Papillomas		
Type	**Common location**	**Pathology**	**Behavior**
Exophytic	Nasal septum	Exophytic fronds of bland epithelium—squamous, transitional, or respiratory type; intraepithelial neutrophils and microcysts; thin basement membranes	Local recurrence; essentially no risk of invasive carcinoma
Inverted	Lateral nasal wall; paranasal sinuses	Pushing, endophytic nests of bland epithelium—squamous, transitional, or respiratory type; lesser exophytic component at times; intraepithelial neutrophils and microcysts; thin basement membranes	Local recurrence; ~10% risk of invasive carcinoma
Oncocytic	Lateral nasal wall; paranasal sinuses	Exophytic and endophytic pushing nests of columnar, oncocytic cells with abundant, granular eosinophilic cytoplasm; intraepithelial neutrophils and microcysts	Local recurrence; ~5%–15% risk of invasive carcinoma

are more common in men. Human papillomavirus (HPV; specifically the low risk types HPV 6 and 11) has been detected in a significant number of cases, so the virus may be important for pathogenesis. Exophytic papillomas are usually solitary and discrete, and patients present with epistaxis, unilateral nasal obstruction, or an asymptomatic mass.

Clinically and grossly, they are warty gray-pink, nontranslucent growths with a broad base. Microscopically, they consist of exophytic papillary fronds lined by a variably thickened epithelium that varies from squamous to respiratory type to a transitional form with features of both (e-**Fig. 3.9**). Scattered mucin-containing cells are usually present, and the lining characteristically has abundant intraepithelial neutrophils, some in small collections simulating microabscesses. Surface keratinization is absent except in rare cases in which the lesion has been traumatized. There is minimal mitotic activity and no cytologic atypia.

After complete removal, exophytic papillomas recur locally in <25% of cases. However, there is no significant risk for developing carcinoma.

ii. **Inverted papilloma.** This is the most common type of Schneiderian papilloma and occurs primarily in adults between 40 and 70 years old. These tumors characteristically arise from the lateral nasal wall in the region of the middle turbinate and ethmoid recesses, frequently extending into the sinuses. Only 8% of inverted papillomas arise from the nasal septum. They are only rarely bilateral. HPV, of numerous different serotypes, can be detected in as many as one-half of the cases.

Grossly, the lesion is fleshy, pink-tan, and papillary or polypoid. Microscopically, inverted papillomas are composed of numerous basement membrane–enclosed, rounded ribbons of thickened epithelium identical to that seen in exophytic papillomas, ranging from squamous to transitional to respiratory type (e-**Figs. 3.10** and **3.11**). There is minimal mitotic activity, no significant cytologic atypia, and the epithelium characteristically has abundant intraepithelial neutrophils, singly and in clusters, as well as numerous mucin-filled microcysts. Some inverted papillomas can have a prominent exophytic-appearing component. However, any Schneiderian papilloma with a significant inverted and/or downward pushing component (more than just rare nests) should be diagnosed as an inverted papilloma.

Uncommonly, there is surface keratinization and 5% to 20% of these lesions show varying degrees of dysplasia. Interestingly, dysplasia by itself does not signify malignancy or a different clinical course for the patient, but it does make it important to thoroughly evaluate the lesion for coexisting carcinoma. Approximately 10% to 15% of inverted papillomas are complicated by carcinoma, mostly squamous cell carcinoma. In approximately 60% of cases, the malignancy is synchronous and in 40% of cases, the malignancy is metachronous. A significant number of inverted papillomas will recur, particularly after conservative resection.

iii. **Oncocytic papillomas** are the least common Schneiderian papillomas and have various alternate names including cylindrical cell and columnar cell papilloma. They occur in the same sites as inverted papillomas, namely, the lateral nasal wall and paranasal sinuses. Unlike other Schneiderian papillomas, they have an equal male to female ratio, and studies have not identified HPV in them.

Microscopically, they typically have a mixture of exophytic and endophytic components and are lined by a unique two- to eight-cell layer of tall columnar oncocytic cells that have abundant granular, eosinophilic cytoplasm. The nuclei are slightly more atypical than in other Schneiderian papillomas with a wrinkled, dark to slightly vesicular appearance with small nucleoli. The epithelium contains numerous mucin-filled microcysts and intraepithelial neutrophils (e-**Fig. 3.12**).

Oncocytic papillomas have a risk of local recurrence and carcinoma similar to that of inverted papillomas.

b. **Verruca vulgaris (nasal vestibule).** As the nasal vestibule is essentially an extension of the surrounding nasal skin, verrucae occur here and have the same morphology as elsewhere (see Chap. 38).

2. **Malignant**

a. **Sinonasal undifferentiated carcinoma (SNUC).** This tumor is a clinicopathologically distinct, aggressive form of sinonasal carcinoma. Patients are most commonly in their sixth decade and present with symptoms of short duration, including nasal obstruction and epistaxis, and often have orbital or cranial nerve deficits. The tumor most often arises in the nasal cavity, particularly superiorly, or in the maxillary or ethmoid sinuses. It is usually bulky, often involving contiguous sites.

There are no unique gross features. Tumors are usually larger than 4 cm, poorly defined, and invade bone. Microscopically, different growth patterns can be seen including nested, trabecular, or lobular, although the nests are not usually well defined. The tumor cells are small to moderate in size, have a small to moderate amount of cytoplasm with distinct cell borders, and have nuclei that range from hyperchromatic to vesicular, often with prominent nucleoli. Despite being overtly malignant, the individual tumor cells tend to be remarkably regular in size. There is abundant apoptosis, brisk mitotic activity, and often prominent necrosis (e-**Fig. 3.13**). By definition, there is a lack of definable differentiation.

Immunohistochemistry is positive for pan-cytokeratin and epithelial membrane antigen. More specifically, simple keratins such as 7, 8,

TABLE 3.4	The 2005 WHO Classification of Nasopharyngeal Carcinoma
Histology	**Type**
Keratinizing squamous cell carcinoma	1
Nonkeratinizing carcinoma, differentiated	2a
Nonkeratinizing carcinoma, undifferentiated	2b
Basaloid squamous cell carcinoma	3

and 19 are present, whereas complex keratins such as 5/6 are absent. Neuron-specific enolase (NSE) is positive in up to 50% of cases, but more specific neuroendocrine markers such as chromogranin A and synaptophysin are negative or show very minimal staining.

SNUC is very aggressive with a mean survival of 4 to 18 months despite aggressive surgery and radiation therapy.

b. **Nasopharyngeal carcinoma.** Although still relatively uncommon in the United States, NPC is important because of its relationship to Epstein–Barr virus (EBV) and because of specific geographic predilections (it is particularly common in the so-called "endemic" areas of Asia and North Africa). The World Health Organization (WHO) classification (2005) recognizes four major types: keratinizing, differentiated nonkeratinizing, undifferentiated, and basaloid (Table 3.4). NPC occurs in all age groups, with a peak incidence between 30 and 50 years of age. It is not uncommon in adolescents. Patients present with symptoms of a sinonasal mass, including nasal obstruction and epistaxis but may also have serous otitis media from Eustachian tube obstruction or, not infrequently, an asymptomatic neck mass from metastasis.

The clinical and macroscopic appearance is nondescript. Microscopically, the keratinizing type (WHO Type 1) has a morphology identical to that of keratinizing squamous cell carcinoma elsewhere in the head and neck and is graded similarly, from well to poorly differentiated (e-Fig. 3.14). The differentiated nonkeratinizing type (WHO Type 2a) can have surface disease with stratified cells that have an appearance similar to that of urothelial carcinoma of the urinary bladder. The cells are moderately atypical with well-defined cell borders and a sharp interface of tumor with the surrounding stroma (e-Fig. 3.15). The undifferentiated type (WHO Type 2b) is the most common, most distinctive, and most challenging. It consists of syncytial aggregates/sheets of tumor cells with moderate eosinophilic cytoplasm, large, vesicular nuclei with prominent nucleoli, and a brisk mixed chronic inflammatory infiltrate (e-Fig. 3.16). Occasionally, the cells are dispersed in small clusters or as single cells making the diagnosis of carcinoma difficult. Apoptosis and brisk mitotic activity are invariably present. Finally, basaloid squamous cell carcinoma (WHO Type 3), the least common type, has a morphology identical to that seen in the same tumor in other regions of the head and neck (e-Figs. 3.17 and 3.18).

NPC has a number of interesting clinicopathologic features. First, given the location and anatomy of the nasopharynx, radiation therapy is the first-line treatment modality. Surgery is uncommon and usually reserved for salvage therapy. Second, although EBV is strongly related to the tumorigenesis of nonkeratinizing NPC (Types 2a and 2b), in keratinizing NPC, EBV is usually absent except in endemic areas. Third, nonkeratinizing NPC tends to metastasize to lymph nodes early (60% to 85% overall), often to the posterior triangle (level V), and these tumors have a different staging system that reflects this unique behavior (see AJCC staging below). Finally, despite presenting with advanced disease, nonkeratinizing NPC responds well to systemic therapy (5-year survival of approximately 65% in the United States). Keratinizing NPC, although it more often presents with localized disease, does not respond well to therapy (5-year survival of approximately 20% to 40% in the United States).

c. **Squamous cell carcinoma/nonkeratinizing carcinoma.** Although squamous cell carcinoma is the most common carcinoma in most head and neck anatomic subsites, it constitutes only approximately 65% of carcinomas in the nasal cavity and paranasal sinuses. When it occurs in the nasopharynx, it is designated *keratinizing squamous cell carcinoma* (WHO Type 1; see section III.C.2.b above and Table 3.4). Keratinizing, or typical, squamous cell carcinoma of the nasal cavity and paranasal sinuses has the same morphology as that occurring elsewhere in the upper aerodigestive tract. Squamous cell carcinoma of this subsite, unlike other head and neck subsites, has only a modest association with smoking. However, tumors have been related to other exposures including nickel, chlorophenols, and textile dust.

A distinct variant of nonkeratinizing squamous cell carcinoma occurs in this region, the so-called cylindrical cell (Schneiderian or transitional) carcinoma. The recent WHO classification simply terms it *nonkeratinizing carcinoma*. It has a papillary configuration with ribbons of invaginating tumor composed of pleomorphic cells without keratinization. These ribbons have a smooth border without clear stromal infiltration, which makes identification of frank invasion difficult (e-**Fig. 3.19**). This tumor type has been associated with HPV and is also reported by several authors to have a better prognosis, although the latter contention is still controversial.

d. **Salivary gland–type tumors** constitute a small percentage of sinonasal neoplasms. They arise from submucosal seromucinous glands. The most common are adenoid cystic carcinoma and pleomorphic adenoma, although almost all other types have been described (e-**Figs. 3.20** to **3.22**). They are morphologically identical to their counterparts elsewhere.

e. **Adenocarcinoma.** Primary non-salivary gland–type adenocarcinomas of the sinonasal region are uncommon. The WHO classifies them as intestinal and nonintestinal types, the latter of which are subdivided into high- and low-grade tumors.

i. **Intestinal type.** Primary intestinal-type adenocarcinomas (ITACs) of the sinonasal region typically arise from the ethmoid sinuses or high in the nasal cavity. They have a strong association with long-term occupational exposures, specifically wood dust (in carpenters), leather dust, nickel, or chromium compounds. The latency period is several decades. Microscopically, these tumors recapitulate gastrointestinal adenocarcinomas, including very well–differentiated tumors resembling colonic adenomas, typical "colonic-appearing" tumors with columnar glands with or without mucinous differentiation (e-**Fig. 3.23**), and high-grade tumors with a signet ring cell morphology.

By immunohistochemistry, they are positive for cytokeratin 20, CDX-2, MUC2, and villin, similar to gastrointestinal adenocarcinoma. Cytokeratin 7 is variably positive and carcinoembryogenic antigen (CEA) is usually positive. As such, they stain essentially identical to gastrointestinal adenocarcinomas, so it can be very difficult to separate them from the rare metastasis to this region from a primary gastrointestinal adenocarcinoma.

ITACs should be graded from poorly to well differentiated, and the type (colonic, mucinous, papillary, signet ring cell, or solid) specified, as both have prognostic significance. The mortality rate is approximately 50% overall.

ii. Nonintestinal type. These are uncommon tumors, most of which are low grade and have a predilection for the ethmoid sinuses. Low-grade tumors have a glandular or papillary growth pattern with numerous uniform, small glands arranged back-to-back and lined by a single layer of cuboidal to columnar cells with a moderate amount of eosinophilic to clear cytoplasm and round nuclei. There is only mild nuclear pleomorphism, modest mitotic activity without atypical forms, and no necrosis. Controversy exists as to what defines them as frankly malignant, histologically. Infiltrative growth is usually a critical feature to identify. High-grade tumors typically occur in the maxillary sinus and have similar histologic features, but also have solid areas and show moderate to severe nuclear pleomorphism with brisk mitotic activity and necrosis.

By immunohistochemistry, nonintestinal-type adenocarcinomas are positive for cytokeratin 7 and negative for cytokeratin 20, CDX-2, and MUC2. Smooth muscle actin and p63 are negative. The prognosis for low-grade tumors is excellent, but for high-grade tumors is quite poor.

f. Neuroendocrine carcinomas occasionally arise in the sinonasal region and are morphologically identical to those arising in the lung.

i. Low-grade neuroendocrine carcinoma (i.e., carcinoid tumor) is extremely rare in this region.

ii. Intermediate-grade neuroendocrine carcinoma (i.e., atypical carcinoid tumor) is also extremely rare in this region.

iii. High-grade neuroendocrine carcinoma (small cell carcinoma) is a rapidly proliferating, aggressive neoplasm that presents with epistaxis, nasal obstruction, and exophthalmos. It usually presents at an advanced stage with extensive local disease and lymph node or distant metastases. Microscopically, it consists of nests and sheets of small- to intermediate-sized blue cells with minimal cytoplasm, speckled chromatin, frequent nuclear molding, and crush artifact (e-Fig. 3.24). Apoptosis is abundant, and there is brisk mitotic activity and necrosis. By immunohistochemistry, it is positive for pan-cytokeratin with a "dot-like" paranuclear staining pattern (e-Fig. 3.25A). It is variably positive for the neuroendocrine markers CD56, synaptophysin, and chromogranin A, but in most cases at least one of these markers is positive on careful inspection (e-Fig. 3.25B). The tumor is negative for S-100, CD99 (O13), and cytokeratin 20.

g. Melanoma. Primary malignant melanoma of the sinonasal tract constitutes approximately 1% of all melanomas. It is more common in the nasal cavity than in the paranasal sinuses, and most patients are over 50 years old, with tumors most often occurring on the middle or inferior turbinate, or anterior septum. Although variable, the typical macroscopic appearance is a sessile or polypoid lesion with mucosal ulceration. Most lesions are heavily pigmented with a brown or black color. Microscopically, melanoma has a wide range of appearances, although usually it is composed of high-grade epithelioid cells. Some tumors have a mixture of epithelioid and spindle cells. A junctional component with pagetoid spread of melanocytes in the intact mucosa is also sometimes present.

Immunohistochemistry results are the same as for melanomas at other sites, with virtually all tumors expressing S-100, HMB-45, and melan-A. Cytokeratin reactivity, if present, is only focal.

Metastasis of melanoma to the sinonasal region from another primary site is not particularly uncommon and should always be considered.

Although metastases can recapitulate a primary lesion, a junctional component in the surface mucosa essentially rules out metastasis.

The prognosis for sinonasal melanoma is very poor, with frequent local recurrence and distant metastasis. Sinonasal melanomas have their own AJCC staging system, and, unlike cutaneous melanomas, tumor (Breslow) thickness has not been shown to predict behavior.

h. Olfactory neuroblastoma. This unique tumor arises almost exclusively in the upper nasal cavity from the olfactory mucosa of the cribriform plate, upper lateral nasal wall, and superior turbinate. The presumed cell of origin is the reserve cell that gives rise to neuronal and sustentacular cells of the olfactory mucosa. The tumor occurs at any age but most commonly in the third and fourth decades, with symptoms of nasal obstruction, epistaxis, and anosmia.

The neoplasm is usually a unilateral, polypoid mass, microscopically composed of small, round cells that are slightly larger than lymphocytes. The nuclei are round, with uniform to delicately stippled chromatin without nucleoli. Many tumors have areas with fibrillary eosinophilic material reminiscent of neuropil (e-**Fig. 3.26**). Some tumors have a very lobulated and nested growth pattern, whereas others have a diffuse pattern. Homer-Wright rosettes (that have no central lumen) are relatively common. Mitotic activity is low. Necrosis and dystrophic calcification are uncommon. Some tumors have been reported to show significant nuclear pleomorphism and high mitotic activity. However, this is very uncommon and merits consideration of another neoplasm, particularly high-grade neuroendocrine carcinoma. Rare findings include ganglion cells, melanin-containing cells, and divergent differentiation including glandular, squamous, and teratomatous features.

By immunohistochemistry, olfactory neuroblastoma shows strong cytoplasmic staining for synaptophysin, chromogranin A, and NSE (e-**Fig. 3.27**). S-100 often highlights sustentacular cells at the periphery of tumor nests, but is negative in tumor cells themselves. Although unusual, cytokeratin reactivity has been reported in up to 35% of cases, specifically CAM 5.2 and less often AE1/AE3. The staining is typically weaker and more focal than would be expected in a carcinoma. Recent reports have shown calretinin staining to be positive in olfactory neuroblastoma and negative in many other tumors in the differential diagnosis.

Grading systems, most notably by Hyams, have been proposed, but their correlation with prognosis has not been consistently demonstrated.

i. Mesenchymal tumors

i. Angiofibroma (nasopharyngeal angiofibroma). This unique tumor is thought to arise from a fibrovascular nidus in the posterolateral nasal wall adjacent to the sphenopalatine foramen. It occurs virtually exclusively in boys aged 10 to 20 years. The tumor often presents as a nasopharyngeal mass due to its pushing, well-circumscribed border, which bulges posteriorly into the nasopharynx as it enlarges, causing nasal obstruction and epistaxis.

Grossly, the tumor is gray-white to tan, smooth, and lobulated, with a homogeneous cut surface. Microscopically, it consists of abundant vessels ranging from capillaries to large vessels, the latter often assuming a "staghorn" appearance (e-**Fig. 3.28**). The vessels are lined by a single layer of endothelial cells that can be flat to slightly plump without cytologic atypia. The vessel wall is typically devoid of smooth muscle and blends imperceptively with the stromal component of the tumor, which has regularly distributed, plump, stellate spindle cells embedded in a dense collagenous stroma. The stromal cells have

TABLE 3.5 The 2010 American Joint Committee on Cancer (AJCC) Staging Guidelines for Tumors of the Nasal Cavity and Paranasal Sinuses

Primary tumor (T)

Maxillary sinus

TX	Primary tumor cannot be assessed
T0	No evidence of primary tumor
Tis	Carcinoma in situ
T1	Tumor limited to maxillary sinus mucosa with no erosion or destruction of bone
T2	Tumor causing bone erosion or destruction including extension into the hard palate and/or middle nasal meatus, except extension to posterior wall of maxillary sinus and pterygoid plates
T3	Tumor invades any of the following: Bone of the posterior wall of maxillary sinus, subcutaneous tissues, floor or medial wall of orbit, pterygoid fossa, or ethmoid sinuses
T4a	Moderately advanced local disease. Tumor invades anterior orbital contents, skin of cheek, pterygoid plates, infratemporal fossa, cribriform plate, sphenoid or frontal sinuses
T4b	Very advanced local disease. Tumor invades any of the following: Orbital apex, dura, brain, middle cranial fossa, cranial nerves other than maxillary division of trigeminal nerve V2, nasopharynx, or clivus

Nasal cavity and ethmoid sinus

TX	Primary tumor cannot be assessed
T0	No evidence of primary tumor
Tis	Carcinoma in situ
T1	Tumor restricted to any one subsite, with or without bone invasion
T2	Tumor invading two subsites in a single region or extending to involve an adjacent region within the nasoethmoidal complex, with or without bony invasion
T3	Tumor extends to invade the medial wall or floor of the orbit, maxillary sinus, palate, or cribriform plate
T4a	Moderately advanced local disease. Tumor invades any of the following: Anterior orbital contents, skin of nose or cheek, minimal extension to anterior cranial fossa, pterygoid plates, sphenoid or frontal sinuses
T4b	Very advanced local disease. Tumor invades any of the following: Orbital apex, dura, brain, middle cranial fossa, cranial nerves other than V2, nasopharynx, or clivus

Regional lymph nodes (N)

NX	Regional lymph nodes cannot be assessed
N0	No regional lymph node metastasis
N1	Metastasis in a single ipsilateral lymph node, 3 cm or less in greatest dimension
N2a	Metastasis in a single ipsilateral lymph node, >3 cm but not >6 cm in greatest dimension
N2b	Metastasis in multiple ipsilateral lymph nodes, none >6 cm in greatest dimension
N2c	Metastasis in bilateral or contralateral lymph nodes, none >6 cm in greatest dimension
N3	Metastasis in a lymph node >6 cm in greatest dimension

Distant metastasis (M)

MX	Distant metastasis cannot be assessed
M0	No distant metastasis
M1	Distant metastasis

(continued)

TABLE 3.5	The 2010 American Joint Committee on Cancer (AJCC) Staging Guidelines for Tumors of the Nasal Cavity and Paranasal Sinuses (*Continued*)		
Stage grouping			
The overall pathologic AJCC stage is			
Stage 0	Tis	N0	M0
Stage I	T1	N0	M0
Stage II	T2	N0	M0
Stage III	T3	N0	M0
Stage III	T1	N1	M0
Stage III	T2	N1	M0
Stage III	T3	N1	M0
Stage IVA	T4a	N0	M0
Stage IVA	T4a	N1	M0
Stage IVA	T1	N2	M0
Stage IVA	T2	N2	M0
Stage IVA	T3	N2	M0
Stage IVA	T4a	N2	M0
Stage IVB	T4b	Any N	M0
Stage IVB	Any T	N3	M0
Stage IVC	Any T	Any N	M1

From: Edge SB, Byrd DR, Compton CC, et al., eds. *AJCC Cancer Staging Manual*. 7th ed. New York, NY: Springer; 2010. Used with permission.

vesicular chromatin, sometimes with small nucleoli, but no atypia and minimal mitotic activity. By immunohistochemistry, the stromal cells are positive for vimentin and negative for smooth muscle actin. The endothelial cells are positive for CD34. Otherwise, the tumors are negative for S-100, desmin, and cytokeratin.

Although the tumor is benign, pressure erosion of the adjacent bone is not uncommon. The virtually exclusive occurrence in adolescent boys, with growth around puberty, is consistent with the fact that androgen receptors can be demonstrated in most cases.

ii. **Glomangiopericytoma (sinonasal-type hemangiopericytoma or hemangiopericytoma-like tumor).** This is a somewhat uncommon tumor of perivascular myoid-type cells. All ages can be affected, but patients in their seventh decade predominate. Unilateral nasal cavity involvement is most common, and the tumor is grossly polypoid, beefy-red to gray-pink, and soft. Microscopically, the tumor consists of numerous variably sized vascular channels that classically have a staghorn appearance. The intervascular stroma consists of a proliferation of closely packed cells with round to ovoid nuclei and modest amounts of eosinophilic cytoplasm. The tumor cells grow in short fascicles, sometimes with a storiform pattern. There is minimal nuclear pleomorphism, little mitotic activity, and no necrosis (e-**Fig. 3.29**). By immunohistochemistry, the cells are strongly and diffusely positive for smooth muscle and muscle-specific actins, and for vimentin and factor XIIIa. The tumor cells lack strong, diffuse CD34 staining. The prognosis is excellent, with only a modest recurrence rate and >90% survival at 5 years after surgery.

iii. **Alveolar rhabdomyosarcoma.** Grossly, the lesion has a fleshy to firm tan-gray appearance. Microscopically, the tumor has a "blue cell" apperance, being composed of small- to medium-sized cells with

TABLE 3.6   The 2010 AJCC Staging Guidelines for Tumors of the Nasopharynx

Primary tumor (T)

TX	Primary tumor cannot be assessed
T0	No evidence of primary tumor
Tis	Carcinoma in situ
T1	Tumor confined to the nasopharynx, or tumor extends to oropharynx and/or nasal cavity without parapharyngeal extension[a]
T2	Tumor with parapharyngeal extension[a]
T3	Tumor involves bony structures of skull base and/or paranasal sinuses
T4	Tumor with intracranial extension and/or involvement of cranial nerves, hypopharynx, orbit, or with extension to the infratemporal fossa/masticator space

Regional lymph nodes (N)

NX	Regional lymph nodes cannot be assessed
N0	No regional lymph node metastasis
N1	Unilateral metastasis in cervical lymph node(s), 6 cm or less, above the supraclavicular fossa, and/or unilateral or bilateral, retropharyngeal lymph nodes, 6 cm or less[b]
N2	Bilateral metastasis in cervical lymph node(s), 6 cm or less, above the supraclavicular fossa[b]
N3	Metastasis in a lymph node(s) >6 cm and/or to the supraclavicular fossa[b]
N3a	Greater than 6 cm
N3b	Extension to the supraclavicular fossa[c]

Distant metastasis (M)

MX	Distant metastasis cannot be assessed
M0	No distant metastasis
M1	Distant metastasis

Stage grouping

The overall pathologic AJCC stage is

Stage 0	Tis	N0	M0
Stage I	T1	N0	M0
Stage II	T1	N1	M0
Stage II	T2	N0	M0
Stage II	T2	N1	M0
Stage III	T1	N2	M0
Stage III	T2	N2	M0
Stage III	T3	N0	M0
Stage III	T3	N1	M0
Stage III	T3	N2	M0
Stage IVA	T4	N0	M0
Stage IVA	T4	N1	M0
Stage IVA	T4	N2	M0
Stage IVB	Any T	N3	M0
Stage IVC	Any T	Any N	M1

[a]Parapharyngeal extension denotes posterolateral infiltration by tumor.
[b]Midline lymph nodes are considered ipsilateral.
[c]Supraclavicular zone or fossa is relevant to the staging of NPC and is the triangular region originally described by Ho. It is defined by three points, and this would include caudal portions of levels IV and VB. All cases with lymph nodes (whole or part) in the fossa are considered N3b.
From: Edge SB, Byrd DR, Compton CC, et al., eds. *AJCC Cancer Staging Manual*. 7th ed. New York, NY: Springer; 2010. Used with permission.

TABLE 3.7 The 2010 AJCC Staging Guidelines for Mucosal Melanoma of the Head and Neck

Primary tumor (T)

T3[a]	Mucosal disease
T4a	Moderately advanced disease. Tumor involving deep soft tissue, cartilage, bone, or overlying skin
T4b	Very advanced disease. Tumor involving brain, dura, skull base, lower cranial nerves (IX, X, XI, XII), masticator space, carotid artery, prevertebral space, or mediastinal structures

Regional lymph nodes (N)

NX	Regional lymph nodes cannot be assessed
N0	No regional lymph node metastasis
N1	Regional lymph node metastasis present

Distant metastasis (M)

M0	No distant metastasis
M1	Distant metastasis

Stage grouping

The overall pathologic AJCC stage is

Stage III	T3	N0	M0
Stage IVA	T4a	N0	M0
Stage IVA	T3	N1	M0
Stage IVA	T4a	N1	M0
Stage IVB	T4b	Any N	M0
Stage IVC	Any T	Any N	M1

[a]There is no T1 or T2 classification.
From: Edge SB, Byrd DR, Compton CC, et al., eds. *AJCC Cancer Staging Manual.* 7th ed. New York, NY: Springer; 2010. Used with permission.

hyperchromatic nuclei and scant eosinophilic cytoplasm growing as loosely cohesive sheets separated by fibrous septa (e-**Fig 3.30**). Multinucleated giant cells with peripheral nuclei are patchy but can usually be identified (e-**Fig. 3.31**). Cytodifferentiation may be seen, particularly after treatment, manifesting as cells with more abundant eosinophilic, fibrillary cytoplasm. By immunohistochemistry, the cells are positive for desmin, muscle-specific actin, myoglobin, myoD1, and myogenin (e-**Fig. 3.32**), but negative for cytokeratins. Although the cells may be, confusingly, positive for synaptophysin and chromogranin A, such staining is not indicative of a neuroendocrine neoplasm.

Alveolar rhabdomyosarcoma is nearly always characterized by one of two characteristic translocations, namely t(1;13), resulting in a PAX7-FKHR fusion transcript (approximately 20% of cases) and t(2;13) resulting in a PAX3-FKHR fusion transcript (approximately 80% of cases). The former is thought to be associated with a better prognosis, but only in the setting of metastatic disease.

IV. **PATHOLOGIC REPORTING OF SINONASAL MALIGNANCIES**
  A. **Staging (AJCC).** Clinical staging of sinonasal cancers is important for prognosis and treatment and differs by site. The 2010 Tumor, Node, and Metastasis (TNM) AJCC staging classification is shown in Table 3.5 for the nasal cavity and paranasal sinuses and in Table 3.6 for the nasopharynx. Staging guidelines are applicable to all forms of carcinoma. Any nonepithelial tumor type is excluded. The staging system for mucosal melanoma of the nasal cavity and paranasal sinuses is shown in Table 3.7.

B. Additional pertinent pathologic features. Several pathologic features not reflected in the AJCC staging have been proven important for head and neck squamous cell carcinomas, as well as for numerous other tumor types, including perineural invasion, lymphovascular space invasion, and positive margin status. All of these features have been demonstrated in numerous studies to correlate with a higher risk of local recurrence, a poorer prognosis, or both.

SUGGESTED READINGS

Barnes L, Tse LLY, Hunt JL, et al. Tumours of the nasal cavity and paranasal sinuses. In: Barnes L, Eveson JW, Reichart P, Sidransky D, eds. *Pathology and Genetics Head and Neck Tumours*. Lyon, France: IARC Press; 2005.

Brandwein-Gensler M, Thompson LDR. Non-neoplastic lesions of the nasal cavity, paranasal sinuses, and nasopharynx. In: Thompson LDR, ed. *Head and Neck Pathology*. New York, NY: Churchill Livingstone; 2006.

Chan JKC, Pilch BZ, Kuo TT, et al. Tumours of the nasopharynx. In: Barnes L, Eveson JW, Reichart P, Sidransky D, eds. *Pathology and Genetics Head and Neck Tumours*. Lyon, France: IARC Press; 2005.

Perez-Ordonez B, Thompson LDR. Benign neoplasms of the nasal cavity, paranasal sinuses, and nasopharynx. In: Thompson LDR, ed. *Head and Neck Pathology*. New York, NY: Churchill Livingstone; 2006.

Prasad, ML, Perez-Ordonez B. Nonsquamous lesions of the nasal cavity, paranasal sinuses, and nasopharynx. In: Gnepp DR, ed. *Diagnostic Surgical Pathology of the Head and Neck*. Philadelphia, PA: W.B. Saunders Publishers; 2009.

Thompson LDR. Malignant neoplasms of the nasal cavity, paranasal sinuses, and nasopharynx. In: Thompson LDR, ed. *Head and Neck Pathology*. New York, NY: Churchill Livingstone; 2006.

4

Tumors and Cysts of the Jaws

David E. Spence and Samir K. El-Mofty

I. **NORMAL ANATOMY.** Of all the bones of the skeleton, the jaws are uniquely distinguished by harboring the odontogenic apparatus of the deciduous and permanent dentitions. The teeth germs are composed of three main components: the enamel organ, the dental papilla, and the tooth follicle. The enamel organ is composed of ectodermally derived epithelial cells, the ameloblasts, and is responsible for enamel formation. The dental papilla is of ectomesenchymal origin and produces the dentine. The tooth follicle is also ectomesenchymal; it surrounds the developing tooth and provides the supporting structures of the formed teeth, the periodontium. The odontogenic tissues may also be a source of a bewildering array of odontogenic cysts and tumors. Nonodontogenic cysts and tumors of the jaws will also be discussed in this chapter.

II. **ODONTOGENIC AND NONODONTOGENIC CYSTS.** Odontogenic cysts of the mandible and the maxilla are relatively common and can present over a large age range. Accurate diagnosis is simplified by location, radiographic correlation, and microscopic examination (**e-Fig. 4.1**).* Odontogenic tumors by contrast are uncommon. They may be epithelial, mesenchymal, or mixed; may be noncalcifying; or they may contain hard structures that mimic enamel, dentine, cementum, or bone. Although malignant odontogenic tumors are extremely rare, odontogenic carcinoma, sarcoma, and carcinosarcoma do occur.

A. **Odontogenic cysts.** With the exception of a few cysts that may develop along embryonic lines of fusion (known as "nonodontogenic cysts"), most jaw cysts are lined with epithelium that is derived from the odontogenic epithelium. Odontogenic cysts are classified as either developmental or inflammatory. Various types of odontogenic cysts are listed in Table 4.1.

1. **Developmental odontogenic cysts**

a. **Dentigerous cyst (follicular cyst)** is a unilocular cyst that forms in association with the crown of an impacted tooth and is usually associated with a molar or canine. Patients usually present with an asymptomatic, well-defined, expansive, radiolucent lesion. Microscopic examination shows a thin layer of cuboidal to slightly flattened epithelial cells. Focal keratinization, mucous cells, inflammation, and dystrophic calcification are possible. Enucleation and excision of the associated tooth are the treatment of choice. **Eruption cyst** is a subclass of dentigerous cysts associated with the erupting primary or permanent tooth.

b. **Keratocystic odontogenic tumor (odontogenic keratocyst)** usually presents as an asymptomatic unilocular cyst in the mandible or the maxilla. While more frequent in the second to fourth decades of life, they may be seen at any age. Their incidence is higher in Caucasians, especially in and men, and roughly 5% of patients with odontogenic keratocysts have nevoid basal cell carcinoma (Gorlin) syndrome. Gross examination typically yields a cyst containing keratinous debris. Microscopic examination shows palisading basal cells covered by a few layers of squamous cells under a

---

*All e-figures are available online via the Solution Site Image Bank.

TABLE 4.1	Odontogenic Cysts

Developmental

  Dentigerous cyst and eruption cyst

  Keratocystic odontogenic tumor (odontogenic keratocyst)

  Lateral periodontal cyst

  Gingival cyst of the adult

  Calcifying cystic odontogenic tumor (calcifying odontogenic cyst, Gorlin cyst)

  Glandular odontogenic cyst

Inflammatory

  Periapical (radicular) cyst

  Residual periapical (radicular) cyst

corrugated parakeratotic surface (e-**Fig. 4.2**). A key diagnostic feature is the lack of rete pegs. Satellite cysts and intramural epithelial cell proliferation are more commonly found in the syndrome-associated cases. Exceptionally, dysphasia and carcinoma develop in the cyst. Treatment is surgical excision, and recurrence is common.

c. *Lateral periodontal cyst* generally presents as a well-demarcated radiolucent lesion in asymptomatic patients in their fifth to seventh decades of life. The typical locations are the lateral surface of the roots of the mandibular premolar teeth, although rare presentations in the maxilla may be encountered. Microscopic examination shows a thin layer of nonkeratinized epithelium with focal thickening and possible clear cells (e-**Fig. 4.3**). The adjacent soft tissue is not inflamed. A rare polycystic variant (botryoid odontogenic cyst) is characterized by rapid growth and an elevated probability of recurrence. Simple excision is typically curative.

d. *Gingival cyst of the adult* is an infrequent lesion appearing on the buccal gingiva of the mandible near the premolars and canines. It represents the soft tissue counterpart of the lateral periodontal cyst. The typical age of patients is the fifth to sixth decades of life and they present with a <1-cm gingival cyst that has a normal to bluish overlying mucosal surface. While usually unicystic, rare multicystic gingival cysts (gingival botryoid odontogenic cyst) may be seen. Microscopic examination shows a cyst lined by a thin layer of epithelium with rare focal thickening; the adjacent soft tissue is fibrotic and does not show inflammation. Treatment is simple excision.

e. *Calcifying cystic odontogenic tumor* (calcifying odontogenic cyst, Gorlin cyst) presents as a radiolucent asymptomatic lesion of the maxilla or the mandible. The tumor can be unicystic, multicystic, and occasionally solid. Focal radio-opaque areas may be identified. The incidence peaks in the second and third decades, although cases occur in all age groups. Microscopic examination shows a proliferating layer of columnar palisaded basal cells similar to ameloblasts. The superficial layers frequently have larger ghost cells characterized by eosinophilic cytoplasm without nuclei (e-**Fig. 4.4**). Calcification of the tumor and adjacent soft tissue can be identified in some cases. Treatment is surgical excision and recurrence is uncommon.

f. *Glandular odontogenic cyst* is a recently defined lesion that has also been referred to as sialo-odontogenic cyst. The majority occur as a radiolucent cyst in the anterior mandible or the anterior maxilla. Patients typically present with pain and swelling, but some cases are asymptomatic. Microscopic examination demonstrates a unilocular/multilocular cyst with nonkeratinized epithelium, mucous producing cells, and focal solid areas (e-**Fig. 4.5A** and **B**). Hyaline bodies, ghost cells, and ciliated cuboidal eosinophilic cells may be present. Care should be taken to differentiate between a glandular odontogenic cyst and a central mucoepidermoid carcinoma. Surgical excision is the treatment of choice.

2. **Inflammatory odontogenic cysts.** *Radicular (periapical) cysts* are associated with a nonviable carious teeth. The usual location is the apical third of the tooth root, with occasional cases involving the lateral root surface. The cyst is more common in the mandible. The typical age of patients is the third to sixth decades of life. The most common presentation is pain and swelling, but presentation as an incidental finding on routine radiographic examination is not unusual. Microscopic examination reveals an inflamed, nonkeratinizing, stratified epithelium. Cholesterol crystals, foamy macrophages, dystrophic calcifications, and intraepithelial hyaline bodies (Rushton bodies) may be identified (e-**Fig. 4.6A and B**). The *residual cyst* is a variant of radicular cyst that is seen at the site of an extracted tooth.

B. **Nonodontogenic cysts.** This class of lesions includes a group of epithelium-lined cysts as well as non–epithelium-lined bone cysts. The epithelial-lined cysts are believed to arise from epithelial remnants entrapped along embryonic lines of fusion and are referred to as fissural cysts (e-**Fig. 4.7**).

1. **Epithelial-lined nonodontogenic cysts (fissural cysts)**

   a. *Nasopalatine duct cyst (incisive canal cyst)* is the most common of the fissural cysts. It is believed to arise from remnants of the nasopalatine duct. The cyst can develop almost at any age, but it is most common in the fourth to sixth decades of life. Most studies show a slight male predilection. The most common presenting symptoms include swelling of the anterior palate, drainage, and pain.

   Radiographs usually demonstrate a well-circumscribed radiolucency, in or near the midline of the anterior maxilla, between and apical to the central incisor teeth. The lesion most often is round oval or pear-shaped. Microscopically, the epithelial lining of the cyst may be stratified squamous, pseudostratified columnar, simple columnar, or cuboidal. Commonly, more than one epithelial type is present. Because the cyst arises within the incisive canal, moderate-sized nerves and small muscular arteries and veins are usually found in the cyst wall (e-**Fig. 4.8**). Surgical enucleation is the treatment of choice.

   b. *Globulomaxillary cyst* is believed to develop from epithelium entrapped during fusion of the globular portion of the medial nasal process with the maxillary process, although its origin continues to be a subject of debate.

   The cyst classically develops between the lateral incisor and cuspid teeth, although occasionally it has been reported between the central and lateral incisors. Radiographically, the cyst presents as well-circumscribed unilocular radiolucency between and apical to the teeth. The radiolucency is often pear-shaped. As the cyst expands, tilting of the adjacent teeth may occur. Microscopically, many of the cysts are lined with stratified squamous epithelium. Occasionally, however, the lining epithelium is of pseudostratified columnar ciliated type. Enucleation is the treatment of choice.

   c. *Median palatal cysts (median palatine cysts)* are rare fissural cysts. They are believed to develop from epithelium entrapped along the embryonic line of fusion of the lateral palatal shelves of the maxilla. The cyst may be difficult to distinguish from the nasopalatine duct cysts, and some cases may actually represent a posteriorly placed nasopalatine duct cyst.

   Clinically, the cyst presents as a firm or fluctuant swelling in the midline of the hard palate, posterior to the incisive papilla. It is more frequent in young adults and is often asymptomatic. The average size is 2 × 2 cm, but these cysts may become quite large. Radiographs demonstrate a well-circumscribed lucency in the midline of the hard palate. Microscopically, the cyst is commonly lined by stratified squamous epithelium, but areas of pseudostratified columnar epithelium may be seen. Surgical removal is the treatment of choice.

2. Non–epithelial-lined nonodontogenic bone cysts of the jaws

   a. *Simple bone cysts* are known by multiple names including unicameral bone cyst, solitary bone cyst, progressive bony cavity, hemorrhagic cyst, and traumatic bone cyst. The typical patient is younger than 20 years of age and has a well-demarcated osteolytic solitary lesion in the posterior mandible. Unusual cases have been seen in the maxilla. The cyst cavity is lined by fibrovascular tissue with hemosiderin-laden macrophages. Reactive bone and osteoclasts may be identified.

   b. *Aneurysmal bone cyst* is a rapidly enlarging blood-filled cystic lesion usually identified in the first three decades of life. The majority are well-demarcated, unilateral pseudocysts located in the mandible (60%) and the maxilla (40%). Aneurysmal bone cyst may be identified alone or in conjunction with another lesion (e.g., chondroblastoma, osteoblastoma.) CT and MRI studies show characteristic layering of blood cells and serum. Microscopic examination shows a fibrotic stroma with giant cells, macrophages, and hemosiderin granules (e-**Fig. 4.9A** and **B**). Areas of ossification may be present. Treatment is curettage and enucleation, and about 25% of the lesions recur.

III. ODONTOGENIC TUMORS. Odontogenic tumors are classified according to their composition into epithelial, mesenchymal, or mixed. Epithelial odontogenic tumors are composed of only odontogenic epithelium, whereas mesenchymal odontogenic tumors are composed principally of ectomesenchymal elements. Mixed odontogenic tumors contain epithelial and ectomesenchymal tissues. Inductive interactive action between the epithelial and ectomesenchymal elements may mimic normal odontogenesis and thus dental hard tissues may, on occasions, be found in these tumors. As stated above, malignant odontogenic tumors are rare, but carcinomas, sarcomas, and carcinosarcomas do occur.

Odontogenic tumors are listed in Table 4.2.

A. Epithelial odontogenic tumors

   1. *Ameloblastoma* is the most common clinically significant odontogenic tumor. Its relative frequency equals the combined frequency of all other odontogenic tumors, excluding odontoma. Ameloblastoma is slow-growing, locally invasive neoplasm. The tumor is encountered over a wide age range; it is rare in children and is most prevalent in the third to seventh decades of life. There is no gender predilection. Some studies show an increased frequency in blacks.

   About 85% of ameloblastomas occur in the mandible, most often in the molar-ascending ramus area. About 15% of ameloblastomas occur in the maxilla, usually in the posterior region. Painless swelling or expansion of the jaw is the usual clinical presentation. If untreated, the lesion may grow slowly to massive or grotesque proportions. Pain and paresthesia are uncommon, even in large tumors. Radiographically, the most typical feature is that of a multilocular radiolucent lesion. Cortical expansion is frequently present. Microscopically, the lesion may present several patterns; these microscopic patterns have no bearing on the behavior of the tumor, and large tumors often show a combination of patterns.

   The follicular pattern is the most common and recognizable. It is composed of nests of epithelium that resemble the enamel organ of the developing teeth, dispersed in a mature fibrous connective tissue stroma. The core of the nests is composed of loosely arranged angular cells that resemble the stellate

TABLE 4.2 WHO Histological Classification of Odontogenic Tumors[a]

BENIGN TUMORS
Odontogenic epithelium with mature fibrous stoma without odontogenic ectomesenchyme
Ameloblastoma, solid/multicystic type
Ameloblastoma, extraosseous/peripheral type
Ameloblastoma, desmoplastic type
Ameloblastoma, unicystic type
Squamous odontogenic tumor
Calcifying epithelial odontogenic tumor
Adenomatoid odontogenic tumor
Keratocystic odontogenic tumor

Odontogenic epithelium with odontogenic ectomesenchyme, with or without hard tissue formation
Ameloblastic fibroma
Ameloblastic fibrodentinoma
Ameloblastic fibro-odontoma
Odontoma
  Odontoma, complex type
  Odontoma, compound type
Odontoameloblastoma
Calcifying cystic odontogenic tumor
Dentinogenic ghost cell tumor
Mesenchyme and/or odontogenic ectomesenchyme with or without odontogenic epithelium
Odontogenic fibroma
Odontogenic myxoma/myxofibroma
Cementoblastoma

MALIGNANT TUMORS
Odontogenic carcinomas
Metastasizing (malignant) ameloblastoma
Ameloblastic carcinoma—primary type
Ameloblastic carcinoma—secondary type (dedifferentiated), intraosseous
Ameloblastic carcinoma—secondary type (dedifferentiated), peripheral
Primary intraosseous squamous cell carcinoma—solid type
Primary intraosseous squamous cell carcinoma derived from keratocystic odontogenic tumor
Primary intraosseous squamous cell carcinoma derived from odontogenic cysts
Clear cell odontogenic carcinoma
Ghost cell odontogenic carcinoma

Odontogenic sarcomas
Ameloblastic fibrosarcoma
Ameloblastic fibrodentino- and fibro-odontosarcoma

[a]Modified from Barnes L, Eveson J, Reichart P, et al., eds. *World Heath Organization Classification of Tumours. Pathology and Genetics. Head and Neck Tumours.* Lyon: IARC Press; 2005. Used with permission.

reticulum of the enamel organ. A single layer of tall columnar ameloblast-like cells surrounds the central core. The nuclei of these cells are placed away from the basement membrane (so-called reversed polarity) (e-**Fig. 4.10**). Cyst formation is common and may vary from microcysts forming within the follicles to large macroscopic cysts that may be several centimeters in diameter.

The plexiform type of ameloblastoma consists of long anastomosing cords or large sheets of odontogenic epithelium bound by ameloblastic cells as seen in the follicular pattern, with similar stellate reticulum-like cores. Cyst formation is rare (e-**Fig. 4.11**).

Unless removed in its entirety, ameloblastoma has a high recurrence rate. The tumor cells tend to infiltrate the surrounding marrow spaces, and the actual margin of the tumor often extends beyond its apparent radiographic or clinical margin. Marginal resection is therefore the most widely used treatment, but it is still associated with recurrence rates of up to 15%, and thus many surgeons advocate that the margin of resection should be at least 1.0 cm past the radiographic limit of the tumor.

2. *Calcifying epithelial odontogenic tumor (Pindborg tumor)* is a rare tumor that presents as a slowly growing painless expansive lesion that favors the posterior mandible. The peak age of incidence is the third to seventh decades of life, and the male/female ratio is equal. The radiographic appearance of the tumor changes over time. Early on, the tumor appears as a radiolucent lesion that can be mistaken for a cyst. As the lesion ages, it develops a poorly demarcated border and multiple radio-opaque foci. The lesion may be multilocular.

On microscopic examination, the tumor is characterized by clusters of pleomorphic polyhedral epithelial cells with a well-defined cell border and dense nuclear staining. The cells show mild to moderate nuclear pleomorphism, rare mitotic figures, and may contain multiple nuclei. Layered calcifications and amyloid-like globules are usually present (e-Fig. 4.12). Calcifying epithelial odontogenic tumors are generally treated surgically. Because they tend to be infiltrating tumors, treatment should include removal with a border of clinically and radiographically normal bone.

3. *Adenomatoid odontogenic tumor (adenoameloblastoma)* typically presents as a slowly growing asymptomatic mass in the anterior portion of the maxilla or the mandible in patients younger than 30 years. Women are affected twice as often as men. Radiographic examination demonstrates a radiolucent, well-defined lesion involving the crown of an unerupted/impacted tooth. Adjacent teeth may show root divergence without root resorption. Gross examination reveals a well-defined encapsulated mass of soft tissue with focal cystic and granular areas. Microscopic examination shows a well-defined fibrotic capsule surrounding a multinodular mass of eosinophilic spindle and polyhedral cells. Scattered among these cells are amphophilic globules with variable levels of calcification and lamination; these globules are periodic acid-Schiff (PAS) positive and diastase resistant. In addition to the globules, small cystic spaces lined by a single layer of cuboidal to columnar cells with foamy cytoplasm and basally orient nuclei are present (e-Fig. 4.13). Treatment is enucleation, and recurrence is extremely rare.

4. *Squamous odontogenic tumors* are benign lesions that occur in patients over a wide age distribution. Patients generally present with tooth loosening in the absence of periodontal disease. Radiology demonstrates a radiolucent mass in the anterior maxilla or the posterior mandible with tooth root involvement. Microscopic examination shows that the lesion is characterized by nodules of bland squamous cells with peripheral flattening of the basal cells, separated by a fibrous stroma (e-Fig. 4.14). Treatment is surgical excision with associated tooth removal.

5. *Malignant ameloblastoma and ameloblastic carcinoma.* Very rarely, ameloblastoma exhibits frank malignant behavior with development of metastasis. The frequency of such an event is difficult to determine but probably occurs in far less than 1% of all ameloblastomas.

By definition, malignant ameloblastoma is a tumor that shows histomorphologic features of a benign ameloblastoma, yet metastasizes. Metastasis is most often to the lungs, which has been regarded as aspiration or implant metastasis. In such cases, the first evidence of metastasis is often discovered 1 to 30 years after surgical treatment of the primary lesion.

The term "ameloblastic carcinoma" should be reserved for an ameloblastoma that has the cytologic features of malignancy in the primary tumor, in a recurrence, or in any metastatic deposit (e-**Fig. 4.15**). These lesions typically follow a markedly aggressive local course but metastasis does not always occur.

B. Mesenchymal odontogenic tumors

1. ***Odontogenic myxoma*** is a benign tumor that has the potential for local infiltration with extensive bone destruction and a relatively high recurrence rate. It is thought to be derived from the ectomesenchyme. Microscopically, it resembles the dental papilla of a developing tooth. Myxomas are most common in the second and third decades of life; although they occur in patients aged 5 to 72 years, they are uncommon in patients younger than 10 years or older than 50 years. Some studies show a female predilection. The lesion may be found at any location in the jaws, although some studies show a predominance of maxillary tumors.

   Myxomas vary in their radiographic appearance, from small and unilocular to large and multilocular, with a "soap bubble" appearance. Tooth displacement and cortical expansion are common in larger lesions. Maxillary tumors often extend into the maxillary sinus. Microscopic examination reveals a bland, monotonous, hypocellular proliferation of loose mesenchymal fibrous tissue. The cells are spindled or stellate, with long cytoplasmic processes. The nuclei are small and may be hyperchromatic. Mitoses are scarce. Small nests of odontogenic epithelium may be present but are not necessary for the diagnosis (e-**Fig. 4.16A** and **B**).

   Because of their lack of encapsulation and infiltrative growth, myxomas tend to extend beyond their clinically anticipated boundaries. Recurrence rates are as high as 25%, and thus close follow-up is recommended (recurrences are usually due to incomplete excision). Some recurrences occur years after excision.

2. ***Benign cementoblastoma (true cementoma)*** is a distinctive mesenchymal odontogenic tumor which is intimately associated with the roots of teeth. It is characterized by the formation of calcified cementum-like tissue deposited on the tooth root, most commonly mandibular molars. Although the tumor is detected in patients over a wide age range, it most commonly affects teenagers and young adults. Pain is a frequent symptom. The radiographic appearance of cementoblastoma is characteristic and is almost pathognomonic, namely, a radio-opaque mass that obliterates the radiographic details of the root of the affected tooth.

   On microscopic examination, the peripheral part of the tumor resembles osteoblastoma. Centrally, thick trabeculae of cementum, which are strongly basophilic, are deposited on the intact or partially resorbed tooth root. Peripherally, bone-like trabeculae are rimmed with plump cementoblasts. The intervening fibrovascular tissue shows dilated vessels and occasional clusters of multinucleated osteoclast-like giant cells (e-**Fig. 4.17**).

   Cementoblastoma is a slowly growing benign neoplasm, but it may attain a large size if not treated. The recommended treatment is surgical excision with extraction of the affected tooth. Recurrence is usually a result of incomplete removal.

3. ***Cemento-ossifying fibroma* (COF)** of the jaws is synonymous with ossifying fibroma and cementifying fibroma. It is a benign odontogenic neoplasm that is limited to the tooth-bearing areas of the jaws. COF is more often seen in the mandible (90%) and in women (83%). Most patients are in their third to fourth decades of life, and they present with a small asymptomatic expanding bone mass that does not erode the adjacent cortical bone. Larger lesions may present with facial deformation and pain. Radiographic

examination demonstrates a well-circumscribed radiolucent lesion with patchy focal radio-opaque areas that does not encase the teeth roots. Tooth displacement, resorption, and root divergence may be seen.

Microscopic examination shows a lesion characterized by a fibrous stroma with bone trabecula and associated variable mineralized material that resembles dental cementum; either component may dominate in an individual lesion. The stroma is usually hypercellular; the bone trabeculae are usually woven but lamellar bone may also be seen. Osteoblastic rimming may vary in extent (e-Fig. 4.18).

Most COFs are small tumors that can be shelled out or curetted out of the jawbone with relative ease. Recurrence after adequate removal is seldom. Incompletely excised tumors continue to grow slowly but may attain a large size.

C. Mixed odontogenic tumors

1. *Odontomas* represent the most highly differentiated of the mixed odontogenic tumors. They are considered by some pathologists to be hamartomas. Two types of odontomas are recognized, *compound* and *complex*. Compound odontoma is composed of many, sometimes even dozens, of small miniature teeth that are surrounded by a dental follicle, the same tissue that surrounds a normal developing tooth. This form of odontoma shows the highest degree of histodifferentiation and morphodifferentiation (e-Fig. 4.19). In contrast, the complex odontoma is composed of a mass of intermixed enamel and dentine with no resemblance to normal or miniaturized teeth (e-Fig. 4.20).

Compound odontoma occurs most often in the anterior segment of the jaws, particularly the canine area in association with an impacted canine tooth. It is the most common odontogenic tumor. It is found most often in the second decade of life and is more common in males than in females by a 3:2 ratio.

Complex odontomas occur most often in the posterior segment of the jaws, primarily in association with an impacted third molar tooth. They are the second most common odontogenic tumors and are usually discovered in the early third decade of life. Like compound odontomas, there is a male gender predilection of 2:1.

Odontomas are typically discovered when radiographic examination is performed because of a delay in eruption of a tooth. They may be mostly radiolucent with areas of opacity and may be associated with an odontogenic cyst (particularly dentigerous cyst) or with calcifying odontogenic cyst. They are treated by surgical excision.

2. *Ameloblastic fibroma* is a true neoplasm composed of both epithelial and mesenchymal types of tissues but without calcified structures. The tumor is typically seen in adolescent patients. The average age is 14 years and there is an equal male/female distribution. About 80% of patients present with a well-defined unilocular or multilocular lesion in the mandible. Association with an unerupted tooth is common. Gross examination demonstrates a smooth well-defined lesion with a tan white cut surface. Microscopic examination demonstrates a lesion characterized by a background of immature connective tissue that resembles dental papilla with cords, strands, and nests of cuboidal to columnar epithelial cells. The epithelial nests are indistinguishable from those seen in follicular ameloblastoma, with a central stellate reticulum-like component and peripheral palisaded columnar cells showing reversed nuclear polarity. A prominent basement membrane separates the epithelial cells from the stroma (e-Fig. 4.21). Treatment is by enucleation and thorough curettage and, if necessary, extraction of the involved tooth. Recurrence is uncommon. Malignant transformation is extremely rare but has been documented.

3. **Ameloblastic fibrosarcoma and odontogenic carcinosarcoma.** Sarcomatous transformation of the mesenchymal component of ameloblastic fibroma, in association with benign epithelial elements, is designated **ameloblastic fibrosarcoma.**

Tumors with both sarcomatous and carcinomatous components are termed "**odontogenic carcinosarcoma.**"

Ameloblastic fibrosarcoma typically presents as an expansive mandibular mass measuring 4 to 6 cm in maximum dimension in an adolescent or young adult. The tumor has high propensity for recurrence if conservatively treated and can occasionally metastasize. Death more frequently results from aggressive local growth.

Microscopically, the architecture of ameloblastic fibrosarcoma resembles ameloblastic fibroma, albeit with a malignant connective tissue component. The epithelial cords and nests are widely separated by a hypercellular stroma. The fibroblast cells are round or fusiform and pleomorphic, with hyperchromatic nuclei and a high mitotic rate (**e-Fig. 4.22**). Ameloblastic fibrosarcoma can arise in an existing or recurrent ameloblastic fibroma. Multiple recurrences are usually associated with increasingly malignant cytologic features.

Odontogenic carcinosarcoma is extremely rare. One case developed in a preexisting ameloblastic fibroma in a 19-year-old pregnant woman, exhibited sudden growth, and was painful to palpation. The lesion was radiolucent and extended from the left body of the mandible into the ramus, reaching the condyle. Microscopically, areas of benign ameloblastic fibroma were associated with malignant epithelial and mesenchymal components. Interestingly, Ki67 labeling scores differed significantly between the two components of the tumor; the carcinosarcoma's score was much higher than that of the ameloblastic fibroma. The tumor was resected en bloc with no evidence of recurrence after 2 years of follow-up.

IV. **NONODONTOGENIC TUMORS.** The jaws, like other bones in the skeleton, can be a site of a wide variety of benign and malignant bone tumors. These entities are discussed in other parts of this manual. This chapter will mainly address tumors and tumorlike lesions that occur predominantly or exclusively in the jaws (Table 4.3).

A. **Benign fibro-osseous lesions** are a group of lesions that share similar histomorphologic features although they have differing clinical and radiographic presentations and behavior. Microscopically, fibro-osseous lesions are composed of fibrous connective tissue stroma containing mineralized structures which may

---

TABLE 4.3	Nonodontogenic Tumors

Benign fibro-osseous lesions
Fibrous dysplasia
Juvenile ossifying fibroma
   Trabecular
   Psammomatoid
Cemento-osseous dysplasia
   Periapical
   Florid

Giant cell lesions
Central (intro-osseous) giant cell granuloma
Brown tumor of hyperparathyroidism
Cherubism
Aneurysmal bone cyst

be bone or cementum. Proper diagnosis requires correlation of historical, clinical, and radiographic findings. The more important types of fibro-osseous lesions of the jaws are discussed here.

1. **Fibrous dysplasia** is a skeletal anomaly in which normal bone is replaced by poorly organized and inadequately mineralized immature woven bone and fibrous connective tissue. Fibrous dysplasia is separated into two forms: the polyostotic form involves multiple bones, whereas the monostotic form is limited to a single site. Polyostotic fibrous dysplasia is less common, and a few of these cases may be associated with skin pigmentation and endocrine anomalies, a condition known as the "McCune-Albright syndrome." The craniofacial skeleton is involved in 20% to 25% of cases of monostotic fibrous dysplasia, particularly the mandible and the maxilla.

   Craniofacial fibrous dysplasia is not strictly monostotic but may extend by continuity to adjoining bones across suture lines. The maxilla is involved more often than the mandible. Most patients present in their second to third decades of life with a painless expanding bone mass. The mass does not involve the overlying bone cortex and growth halts when the patient reaches skeletal maturity. The radiographic appearance can be variable, but the majority of patients present with a poorly defined lesion that is radiolucent when small but becomes radio-opaque as it enlarges, often described as having a ground glass appearance. The lesion blends imperceptibly with the surrounding bone.

   Microscopic examination demonstrates a bland fibrovascular stroma with numerous irregular trabeculae of woven bone merging to form complex shapes described as resembling Chinese letters. The bone trabeculae are not rimmed with osteoblasts and lamellar bone is rarely identified (e-**Fig. 4.23**). Repair of the deformity is usually attempted after the cessation of growth with skeletal maturity. Radiation is contraindicated because of the elevated risk of radiation-induced sarcomas.

2. **Juvenile ossifying fibroma** (JOF), also known as "juvenile active and juvenile aggressive ossifying fibroma," is used in the literature to describe two distinct clinicopathologic entities: *trabecular JOF (TrJOF)* and *psammomatoid (PsJOF)*.

   a. **Trabecular juvenile ossifying fibroma (TrJOF).** The great majority of the patients are children and adolescents, with an equal gender distribution. Clinically, the lesions are characterized by progressive and sometimes rapid expansion. The maxilla is more commonly affected than the mandible. Radiographically, the tumor is expansive and may be fairly well demarcated, with cortical thinning and perforation. Depending on the amount of calcification, the lesion may show varying degrees of radiodensity.

   Microscopically, TrJOF is composed of a cell-rich fibrous stroma containing bundles of cellular osteoid and bone trabeculae, without osteoblastic rimming. Aggregates of multinucleated giant cells are invariably present in the stroma (e-**Fig. 4.24**). Cystic degeneration and aneurysmal bone cyst formation may occur. The clinical course of TrJOF following conservative treatment is characterized by recurrence; eventual complete cure can be achieved by reexcision without resorting to radical surgery. Malignant transformation has not been reported.

   b. **Psammomatoid juvenile ossifying fibroma (PsJOF).** Unlike TrJOF, PsJOF is a lesion that affects predominantly the extragnathic skull bones, particularly the periorbital bones. Occasional cases are encountered in the jaws, particularly the mandible. Affected patients tend to be older than those who have TrJOF. There is no sex predilection.

On radiographic examination, the tumor appears expansive with well-defined borders that may be corticated. Sclerotic changes within the lesion may impart a ground glass appearance. The tumors vary in size from 2 to 8 cm. Cystic changes are not uncommon and present as areas of low density in the CT scans.

Microscopically, the tumor is noteworthy for multiple, round, uniform, small ossicles that are basophilic and resemble psammoma bodies. The psammomatoid structures are embedded in relatively cellular stroma composed of stellate and spindle-shaped cells (e-Fig. 4.25). Aneurysmal bone cyst formation is not uncommon. Surgical excision is the treatment of choice; multiple recurrences are not unusual. No malignant changes are observed.

3. *Cemento-osseous dysplasia* of the jaws is a nonneoplastic, presumably dysplastic, fibro-osseous lesion of the tooth-bearing areas of the jaws. Two types are recognized: *periapical cemento-osseous dysplasia* and *florid cemento-osseous dysplasia*.

a. *Periapical cemento-osseous dysplasia (PCOD),* also known as "periapical cementoma," is a relatively common condition, particularly in middle-aged black female patients. The anterior mandibular teeth are typically the site of this lesion. The condition is nonexpansive, asymptomatic, and is typically identified in routine dental radiographs as "periapical radiolucencies," which becomes progressively mineralized in older lesions. Microscopic examination shows a poorly demarcated lesion consisting of fibrovascular stroma with trabeculae of bone and smooth globular masses of cementum-like material (e-Fig. 4.26). The bone and cementum may merge with adjacent bone but will not involve adjacent teeth. No treatment is required. It is of importance to distinguish PCOD from periapical inflammatory disease.

b. *Florid cemento-osseous dysplasia (FCOD)* is uncommon. It usually presents in middle-aged or older black women, is usually asymptomatic, and may be incidentally discovered on routine radiographic examination. Pain is rarely manifested. Radiographically, FCOD is characterized by extensive sclerotic areas often involving the posterior quadrants of the mandible and the maxilla bilaterally in the tooth-bearing areas, usually symmetrically (e-Fig. 4.27). Microscopically, FCOD and PCOD are analogous. However, large sclerotic masses are hypocellular, extremely dense, and have small marrow spaces and are more likely to form in FCOD. It is of importance to recognize the clinical radiographic features of FCOD so that the patient is not subject to surgical intervention. In fact, surgery is contraindicated because it may result in local infection, pain, and a complicated clinical course.

B. **Giant cell lesions of the jaws.** Giant cell lesions of the jaws are heterogeneous clinical entities that share similar microscopic features.

1. *Central giant cell granuloma (CGCG),* or intraosseous granuloma of the jaws, is also known as "giant cell reparative granuloma." It is a localized osteolytic lesion of the mandible (66% of cases) and the maxilla (33% of cases). The majority of patients are younger than 30 years, and women outnumber men by a ratio of 2:1.

Giant cell granulomas are typically nonaggressive and present on routine dental radiographs as a small radiolucent expansive masses that do not erode into the cortex. The majority of CGCGs occur in the anterior mandible, commonly crossing the midline. Microscopically, the lesions are unencapsulated and are composed of focal or evenly dispersed aggregates of multinucleated osteoclast-like giant cells in a richly vascular stroma, with little collagen deposition (e-**Fig. 4.28**). Two types of mononuclear stromal cells are identified: spindle-shaped fibroblastic cells and polygonal macrophage-like cells. Areas of ossification and hemosiderin granules may be present.

A rare aggressive variant characterized by pain, rapid growth, and cortical perforation with a marked tendency for recurrence may be an example of "true" giant cell tumor of bone. The lesion may show increased mitotic activity and evenly distributed larger giant cells that have an increased number of nuclei.

CGCG of the jaws is usually treated by curettage. Recurrent lesions often respond to further conservative surgery. A number of alternative nonsurgical approaches have been used in recent years, including intralesional corticosteroids injections, subcutaneous calcitonin injections, and interferon alpha therapy.

2. ***Brown tumor of hyperparathyroidism*** is an osseous lesion that develops in bones affected by primary or secondary hyperparathyroidism. It is currently less frequently encountered since the diagnosis of hyperparathyroidism is now often made on the basis of elevated serum calcium levels in asymptomatic adults.

The lesions may be solitary or multifocal, and the mandible is a common site of involvement. Radiographically, brown tumors are well-defined lytic lesions that are microscopically identical to CGCG. Treatment is aimed at correction of the hyperparathyroid state; complete resolution usually occurs within 6 months after removal of a parathyroid adenoma.

3. ***Cherubism*** is a rare dominant genetic disease with complete male penetrance and 50% to 70% penetrance in women. It typically presents as painless bilateral symmetric jaw expansion in children aged 1 to 5 years, which slowly increases in size until puberty; at puberty, the lesion undergoes variable regression. The lesions may be unilocular or multilocular, with a "soap bubble" appearance on radiographic examination.

Microscopically, the lesions are essentially similar to CGCG. However, the giant cells in cherubism tend to be less numerous and placed in a less cellular stroma. The pathologic process in cherubism is self-limited and treatment is dictated by cosmetic and functional needs. Curettage and contouring of bone are the treatments of choice.

SUGGESTED READINGS

Delair D, Bejarano P, Peleg M, et al. Ameloblastic carcinosarcoma of the mandible arising in ameloblastic fibroma: a case report and review of literature. *Oral Surg Oral Med Oral Pathol Oral Radiol Endod.* 2007;103:516–520.

El-Mofty SK. Bone lesions. In: Gnepp DR, ed. *Diagnostic Surgical Pathology of the Head and Neck.* 2nd ed. Philadelphia: WB Saunders Co; 2009:729–784.

El-Mofty SK. Cemento-ossifying fibroma and benign cementoblastoma. In El-Mofty SK Guest editor. *Semin Diag Pathol.* 1999;16:302–307.

El-Mofty SK. Psammomatoid and trabecular juvenile ossifying fibroma of the craniofacial skeleton: two distinct clinicopathologic entities. *Oral Surg Oral Med Oral Pathol Oral Radiol Endod.* 2002;93:269–304.

El-Mofty SK, Kyriakos M. Soft tissue and bone lesions. In: Gnepp DR, ed. *Diagnostic Surgical Pathology of the Head and Neck.* Philadelphia: WB Saunders Co; 2001:505–604.

Nevill BW, Damm DD, Allen CM, et al, eds. Odontogenic cysts and tumors. *Oral and Maxillofacial Pathology.* 3rd ed. Philadelphia: WB Saunders Co; 2009:589–642.

Philipsen HP, Reichart PA, Slootweg PJ, et al. Odontogenic tumors. In: Barnes L, Eveson JW, Reichart P, et al, eds. *Pathology and Genetics Head and Neck Tumors.* Lyon: IARC Press; 2005.

Slootweg PJ, El-Mofty SK. Ossifying fibroma. In: Barnes L, Eveson JW, Reichart P, et al, eds. *Pathology and Genetics Head and Neck Tumors.* Lyon: IARC Press; 2005.

The Eye

George J. Harocopos

I. DISEASES OF THE CONJUNCTIVA

A. Degenerative. Two benign degenerative lesions on the conjunctiva are the **pinguecula** and the **pterygium,** which are manifestations of chronic actinic damage to the interpalpebral bulbar conjunctiva. The pinguecula is confined to the conjunctiva, appearing clinically as a yellowish nodule, whereas the pterygium extends onto the peripheral cornea, appearing clinically as a vascular, wing-shaped lesion. Histologically, a pinguecula shows elastotic (actinic) degeneration and may show variable degrees of chronic inflammation (**e-Fig. 5.1**).* The pterygium may show these same findings, but the most prominent feature is congested vessels (**e-Fig. 5.2**).

B. Inflammatory. A variety of infectious and noninfectious conditions may cause conjunctivitis.

1. **Sarcoidosis** often affects the conjunctiva, manifesting clinically as small, tan nodules in the inferior forniceal conjunctiva, often in non-injected, asymptomatic eyes. Sarcoidosis may also cause symptomatic inflammation in all parts of the eye, including conjunctivitis, uveitis, retinal phlebitis, optic neuritis, and so on. Conjunctival biopsy may provide the most expedient way of diagnosing this systemic disease, even in cases where there are no visible nodules clinically, though the diagnostic yield is highest when an obvious nodule is present.

   Histology shows noncaseating granulomatous tubercles in the stroma, with a variable (but usually minimal) cuff of lymphocytes and plasma cells (**e-Fig. 5.3**).

2. **Ocular cicatricial pemphigoid (OCP)** is a form of cicatrizing conjunctivitis that typically also involves other mucous membranes and sometimes involves the skin. When conjunctival biopsy is performed to establish the diagnosis, half the specimen should be submitted in formalin for routine histology, and half in Michel's medium or saline for immunofluorescence studies. Histology shows epithelial bullae (or blebs) and a subepithelial band of chronic inflammation composed predominantly of plasma cells (**e-Fig. 5.4**). Immunofluorescence demonstrates IgG, IgA, and/or IgM immunoglobulins, and complement (C3) positivity in the epithelial basement membrane zone. The sensitivity of immunofluorescence may be as low as 50%, and accordingly, a negative result does not rule out OCP.

C. Neoplasms of the conjunctiva fall mostly into one of the three categories: squamous (surface epithelium), melanocytic, or lymphoid.

1. Neoplasms arising from the surface epithelium range from benign **papillomas** (**e-Fig. 5.5**) to **ocular surface squamous neoplasia (OSSN)** which is further subdivided into **conjunctival intraepithelial neoplasia (CIN)** (**e-Fig. 5.6**) versus invasive **squamous cell carcinoma** (**e-Fig. 5.7**). Histologic sections of a papilloma show finger-like projections of hyperplastic epithelium draped over fibrovascular cores. The epithelium may exhibit loss of goblet cells and surface keratinization if the lesion was exposed (i.e., not covered adequately by the tear film due to its size).

---

*All e-figures are available online via the Solution Site Image Bank.

TABLE 5.1	Carcinoma of the Conjunctiva

Definition of TNM. These definitions apply to both clinical and pathologic staging.

Primary tumor (T)

TX	Primary tumor cannot be assessed
T0	No evidence of primary tumor
Tis	Carcinoma in situ
T1	Tumor ≤5 mm in greatest dimension
T2	Tumor >5 mm in greatest dimension, without invasion of adjacent structures
T3	Tumor invades adjacent structures, excluding the orbit
T4	Tumor invades orbit with or without further extension
T4a	Tumor invades orbital soft tissues, without bone invasion
T4b	Tumor invades bone
T4c	Tumor invades adjacent paranasal sinuses
T4d	Tumor invades brain

Regional lymph nodes (N)

NX	Regional lymph nodes cannot be assessed
N0	No regional lymph node metastasis
N1	Regional lymph node metastasis

Distant metastasis (M)

M0	No distant metastasis
M1	Distant metastasis

Anatomic stage/prognostic groups
No stage grouping is presently recommended.

From: Edge SB, Byrd DR, Compton CC, et al., eds. *AJCC Cancer Staging Manual.* 7th ed. New York, NY: Springer; 2010. Used with permission.

OSSN histologically exhibits epithelial hyperplasia with loss of goblet cells, nuclear hyperchromasia, and cellular pleomorphism, and often shows surface keratinization, dyskeratosis, and increased mitotic figures. In the most severe cases, squamous eddies or keratin whorls/pearls may be seen. There is frequently a subepithelial chronic inflammatory response. The most important distinction histologically in terms of prognosis is whether the lesion is confined by the epithelial basement membrane, (i.e., CIN) versus whether the lesion has broken through the basement membrane and invaded the stroma, (i.e., invasive squamous carcinoma). The staging scheme for conjunctival squamous carcinoma is given in Table 5.1. Treatment options for OSSN include excision with 3 to 4 mm margins and cryotherapy to the edges of excision versus topical chemotherapy with agents such as interferon (IFN) alpha-2b, 5-fluorouracil (5-FU), or mitomycin C (MMC). Topical chemotherapy may also be used as pre- or post-operative adjuvant treatment.

2. Melanocytic lesions of the conjunctiva range from benign to malignant.
   a. Conjunctival **melanocytic nevi** (e-Fig. 5.8) are benign lesions that bear similarities to cutaneous melanocytic nevi. Clinically, they may be pigmented or amelanotic. On histology, as with melanocytic nevi of the skin, the melanocytes are typically arranged in nests which may be junctional, intrastromal, or compound. Another important feature generally seen in conjunctival nevi is epithelial inclusion cysts in association with the melanocytes.
   b. Intraepithelial melanocytic lesions of the conjunctiva include **benign acquired melanosis** (BAM) (also known as racial melanosis) (e-Fig. 5.9),

which appears clinically as bilateral, flat, patchy brown pigmentation in darkly skinned individuals, and **primary acquired melanosis (PAM)** which has a similar clinical appearance except that it is generally unilateral in Caucasians. Histologically, BAM appears as a lentiginous proliferation of normal-appearing melanocytes confined to the basal layer of the epithelium, similar to lentigo simplex of the skin.

PAM is subdivided into PAM without atypia, which appears histologically identical to BAM (and accordingly has no to minimal risk of future malignant transformation) versus PAM with atypia (e-**Fig. 5.10**). In PAM with atypia (similar to melanoma in situ of the skin), the melanocytic proliferation extends into the more superficial epithelial layers to varying degrees, and the melanocytes exhibit discohesiveness and may have epithelioid morphology; however, the lesion is still confined by the epithelial basement membrane. There is frequently a subepithelial chronic inflammatory response. In the ophthalmic nomenclature on conjunctival neoplasms, the term *melanoma* in situ is generally reserved for PAM with severe atypia involving at least 75% of the epithelial thickness. PAM with atypia carries a significant risk of future malignant transformation, with the risk being proportional to the degree of atypia. It is therefore generally treated via complete excision with 4 mm wide margins and cryotherapy to the edges of excision, similar to squamous neoplasms. Topical chemotherapy may also be a treatment option for very extensive lesions deemed too large for excision, though the success rate with this treatment is not as high as with squamous lesions.

c. **Melanoma** of the conjunctiva (e-**Fig. 5.10**) generally arises from PAM with atypia, may arise de novo, or, less commonly, may arise from a nevus. When melanoma arises from PAM with atypia, histology demonstrates an area where the melanocytic proliferation violates the epithelial basement membrane and invades the stroma. Particularly when the focus of invasion is relatively small, immunostains such as melanA-red may be helpful in distinguishing the focus of invasion from the surrounding chronic inflammatory response, and in delineating the deep margin of invasion. The staging scheme for melanomas of the conjunctiva is given in Table 5.2. Conjunctival melanoma is generally treated via complete excision with at least 4 mm margins and cryotherapy to the edges of excision.

TABLE 5.2	Malignant Melanoma of the Conjunctiva

Definition of TNM

Clinical classification (cTNM)

Primary tumor (T)

TX	Primary tumor cannot be assessed
T0	No evidence of primary tumor
T(is)	Melanoma confined to the conjunctival epithelium
T1	Malignant melanoma of the bulbar conjunctiva:
T1a	Less than or equal to 1 quadrant
T1b	More than 1 but ≤2 quadrants
T1c	More than 2 but ≤3 quadrants
T1d	Greater than 3 quadrants
T2	Malignant melanoma of the nonbulbar (palpebral, forniceal, caruncular) conjunctiva:

(continued)

TABLE 5.2	Malignant Melanoma of the Conjunctiva (*Continued*)
T2a	No caruncular, ≤ 1 quadrant
T2b	No caruncular, >1 quadrant
T2c	Any caruncular, with ≤ 1 quadrant
T2d	Any caruncular, with >1 quadrant
T3	Any malignant conjunctival melanoma with local invasion:
T3a	Globe
T3b	Eyelid
T3c	Orbit
T3d	Sinus
T4	Tumor invades the central nervous system

Regional lymph nodes (N)

NX	Regional lymph nodes cannot be assessed
N0a (biopsied)	No regional lymph node metastasis, biopsy performed
N0b (not biopsied)	No regional lymph node metastasis, biopsy not performed
N1	Regional lymph node metastasis

Distant metastasis (M)

M0	No distant metastasis
M1	Distant metastasis

Pathologic classification (pTNM)

Primary tumor (pT)

pTX	Primary tumor cannot be assessed
pT0	No evidence of primary tumor
pT(is)	Melanoma of the conjunctiva confined to the epithelium
pT1a	Melanoma of the bulbar conjunctiva not more than 0.5 mm in thickness with invasion of the substantia propria
pT1b	Melanoma of the bulbar conjunctiva more than 0.5 mm but not more than 1.5 mm in thickness with invasion of the substantia propria
pT1c	Melanoma of the bulbar conjunctiva >1.5 mm in thickness with invasion of the substantia propria
pT2a	Melanoma of the palpebral, forniceal, or caruncular conjunctiva not more than 0.5 mm in thickness with invasion of the substantia propria
pT2b	Melanoma of the palpebral, forniceal, or caruncular conjunctiva more than 0.5 mm but not >1.5 mm in thickness with invasion of the substantia propria
pT2c	Melanoma of the palpebral, forniceal, or caruncular conjunctiva >1.5 mm in thickness with invasion of the substantia propria
pT3	Melanoma invading the eye, eyelid, nasolacrimal system, sinuses, or orbit
pT4	Melanoma invading the central nervous system

Regional lymph nodes (pN)

pNX	Regional lymph nodes cannot be assessed
pN0	No regional lymph node metastasis
pN1	Regional lymph node metastasis present

Distant metastasis (pM)

cM0	No distant metastasis
pM1	Distant metastasis

Anatomic stage/prognostic groups

No stage grouping is presently recommended.

3. Lymphocytic lesions of the conjunctiva include **lymphoid hyperplasia** and **lymphoma,** either of which may be unilateral or bilateral. Lymphomas can range from primary localized lesions (even if bilateral), to lesions associated with systemic disease. Most conjunctival/orbital lymphomas are low-grade B-cell lymphomas, with the single most common type being extranodal marginal zone lymphoma (e-**Fig. 5.11**), which is generally localized to the conjunctiva. Histologically, marginal zone lymphoma shows a sheet of lymphocytes infiltrating the subepithelial region of the substantia propria (stroma) without well-defined follicles; scattered lymphocytes may extend into the epithelium. Immunohistochemistry for B- and T-cell markers (e-**Fig. 5.12**) as well as in situ hybridization (ISH) for kappa and lambda light chains (e-**Fig. 5.13**) are very helpful diagnostically. Other techniques for establishing clonality such as IgH gene rearrangement testing by PCR and flow cytometry are also useful, particularly in cases where ISH proves insufficient. Fluorescence in situ hybridization (FISH) may also be used if needed to test for specific genetic translocations.

Follicular and mantle cell lymphomas are also seen in the conjunctiva. More rarely, diffuse large B-cell, Burkitt, Hodgkin, plasmacytoma, or T-cell lymphoma may also occur. Lower-grade lymphomas are more often localized to the conjunctiva, whereas higher-grade lymphomas are more likely to be associated with systemic disease. If the lymphoma is localized to the conjunctiva, the treatment is generally orbital radiation. Another treatment option is subconjunctival injections of IFN or intravenous rituximab. In contrast, if systemic lymphoma is present, then it is treated accordingly with chemotherapy; if systemic remission is achieved, the conjunctival lesion(s) will likewise resolve. The staging scheme for conjunctival/orbital lymphoma is given in Table 5.3.

4. Other neoplasms. **Oncocytoma,** also known as **apocrine cystadenoma** or **oxophilic cystadenoma** (e-**Fig. 5.14**), is a benign lesion that arises most commonly in the caruncle of elderly females. Histologically, it is an adenoma composed of apocrine or accessory lacrimal gland epithelial cells which exhibit distinctive eosinophilic cytoplasm and surround gland-like spaces.

Any neoplasm seen in the orbit may also occasionally arise in the conjunctiva, including neural, vascular, fibrous, and muscular tumors. Additionally, metastatic lesions to the conjunctiva rarely occur.

II. **DISEASES OF THE CORNEA.** The host tissue from a corneal transplant procedure is traditionally referred to as a corneal "button"; the surgical procedure itself is a keratoplasty (KP). Most often, full-thickness cornea is removed, (i.e., penetrating keratoplasty or PKP). More recently, however, surgical techniques have been developed such that, for certain disorders, only the diseased layer(s) of the cornea need be transplanted, for example, deep anterior lamellar keratoplasty (DALK), in which only the epithelium and stroma are removed, versus Descemet's stripping endothelial keratoplasty (DSEK), in which only Descemet's membrane and endothelium are removed. In the gross room, corneal buttons are bisected, and each half is embedded with the cut side down. The most common reasons for keratoplasty to be performed are Fuchs endothelial dystrophy, pseudophakic/aphakic bullous keratopathy, keratoconus, infectious keratitis (especially herpetic), and graft failure.

A. **Fuchs endothelial dystrophy** (e-**Fig. 5.15**) exhibits an autosomal dominant inheritance pattern or may be sporadic, generally becoming symptomatic in middle-aged to older individuals. The corneal endothelial cells diminish in number significantly faster than is normal for aging, ultimately leading to chronic edema of the cornea. If conservative therapy is unsuccessful, then keratoplasty (either PKP or DSEK) is necessary. Histologically, Fuchs dystrophy demonstrates loss of the endothelial cells and the presence of anvil-shaped excrescences, known

TABLE 5.3   Ocular Adnexal Lymphoma

Definition of TNM. These definitions apply to both clinical and pathologic staging.

Primary tumor (T)

TX	Lymphoma extent not specified
T0	No evidence of lymphoma
T1	Lymphoma involving the conjunctiva alone without orbital involvement:
T1a	Bulbar conjunctiva only
T1b	Palpebral conjunctiva +/– fornix +/– caruncle
T1c	Extensive conjunctival involvement
T2	Lymphoma with orbital involvement +/– any conjunctival involvement:
T2a	Anterior orbital involvement (+/– conjunctival involvement)
T2b	Anterior orbital involvement + lacrimal involvement (+/– conjunctival involvement)
T2c	Posterior orbital involvement (+/– conjunctival involvement +/– anterior involvement +/– any extraocular muscle involvement)
T2d	Nasolacrimal drainage system involvement (+/– conjunctival involvement but not including nasopharynx)
T3	Lymphoma with preseptal eyelid involvement +/– orbital involvement +/– any conjunctival involvement
T4	Orbital adnexal lymphoma extending beyond orbit to adjacent structures such as bone and brain:
T4a	Involvement of nasopharynx
T4b	Osseous involvement (including periosteum)
T4c	Involvement of maxillofacial, ethmoidal, and/or frontal sinuses
T4d	Intracranial spread

Regional lymph nodes (N)

NX	Involvement of lymph nodes not assessed
N0	No evidence of lymph node involvement
N1	Involvement of ipsilateral regional lymph nodes (preauricular, submandibular, or cervical)
N2	Involvement of contralateral or bilateral regional lymph nodes
N3	Involvement of peripheral lymph nodes not draining ocular adnexal region
N4	Involvement of central lymph nodes

Distant metastasis (M)

M0	No evidence of involvement of other extranodal sites
M1a	Noncontiguous involvement of tissues or organs external to the ocular adnexa (e.g., parotid glands, submandibular gland, lung, liver, spleen, kidney, breast, etc.)
M1b	Lymphomatous involvement of the bone marrow
M1c	Both M1a and M1b involvement

Anatomic stage/prognostic groups
No stage grouping is presently recommended.

From: Edge SB, Byrd DR, Compton CC, et al., eds. *AJCC Cancer Staging Manual.* 7th ed. New York, NY: Springer; 2010. Used with permission.

as guttae, along a thickened Descemet's membrane. Often secondary epithelial bullae are seen (i.e., bullous keratopathy).

B. **Pseudophakic bullous keratopathy** (e-Fig. 5.16) is the term used when endothelial cell decompensation follows (usually months or years later) cataract extraction with intraocular lens implantation. Endothelial decompensation following cataract surgery without lens implantation is referred to as **aphakic bullous keratopathy.** Generally, around 5% of endothelial cells are lost during an anterior segment procedure, but occasionally 50% or more of the endothelial cells may be lost if the surgery is highly complex/traumatic. The endothelium may then decompensate, either immediately if the residual endothelial cells are too few, or sometime later, after the endothelial cell population declines further with age. Keratoplasty (either PKP or DSEK) may ultimately be required. Although cataract surgery is the most common intraocular procedure performed, bullous keratopathy may similarly occur following other intraocular procedures, for example, multiple glaucoma surgeries or retinal surgeries. Histologically, endothelial cell loss is seen, but without guttae of Descemet's membrane; epithelial bullae are present.

C. **Keratoconus** is a condition generally presenting in teenagers and young adults in which the cornea is more ectatic (i.e., cone shaped) than normal, causing myopia and astigmatism. Both genetic and environmental/acquired factors may be involved, since keratoconus is associated with both hereditary connective tissue disorders such as Marfan syndrome, as well as with excessive eye rubbing such as in chronic atopic conjunctivitis or chronic blepharitis associated with Down syndrome. In the early phases of the disease, the patient may be managed with spectacle or contact lens correction, but if the condition progresses to the extent that a corneal stromal scar forms at the apex of the cone (by which time the patient is often middle aged), then keratoplasty (either PKP or DALK) is required for visual rehabilitation. The corneal button shows central thinning; breaks in Bowman's layer; and often loss of Bowman's layer with anterior stromal fibrosis at the apex of the cone correlating with the apical scar seen clinically (e-**Fig. 5.17**).

D. Corneal buttons with **ulcerative keratitis** may or may not reveal the offending microorganism when special stains are performed (e.g., Gram for bacteria; Gomori's Methenamine Silver [GMS] and periodic acid-Schiff [PAS] for fungi; GMS and PAS for *Acanthamoeba*). Lack of microorganisms on histology despite a history of positive cultures is generally attributable to antecedent anti-microbial therapy, as an attempt is generally made to sterilize the ulcer prior to keratoplasty. This scenario is frequently encountered with bacterial corneal ulcers, whereas fungi (e-**Fig. 5.18**) and amoebal cysts (e-**Fig. 5.19**) are often more difficult to eradicate with medical treatment and are therefore generally still present on histology. Herpes simplex keratitis has a characteristic histopathologic appearance including patchy loss of Bowman's layer, stromal fibrosis and vascularization, interstitial keratitis (consisting of plasma cells and lymphocytes in the corneal stroma), and often granulomatous inflammation near Descemet's membrane (e-**Fig. 5.20**).

E. When a PKP fails (e.g., due to immunologic rejection, infectious ulcerative keratitis, or most commonly, simply gradual loss of endothelial cells over time), a regraft may be necessary. On histology, the button may be identified as a regraft by peripheral discontinuities in Bowman's layer and peripheral stromal scars (e-**Fig. 5.21**) that represent the entry sites of sutures and sometimes the graft–host interface (i.e., if the surgeon chose to make the regraft of a slightly larger diameter than the prior graft). Residual suture material may be present, or may be absent if all the sutures were removed at some point after the initial procedure. Chronic inflammatory cells are often present along the suture tracks. The most essential histologic feature of graft failure is generally endothelial cell loss. In many cases there is also a fibrous retrocorneal membrane.

F. Other rare entities for which a PKP is performed include hereditary stromal dystrophic diseases, for example, macular dystrophy (due to acid mucopolysaccharide accumulation), granular dystrophy (due to hyaline deposition), lattice dystrophy (due to amyloid), and combined granular–lattice (Avellino) dystrophy, in which both hyaline and amyloid deposits are seen (e-**Fig. 5.22**).

III. VASCULAR, INFLAMMATORY, AND INFECTIOUS DISEASES AND TRAUMA. Eyes are often removed when they become "blind and painful." The reasons for an eye becoming blind and painful are numerous, but often the final common pathway involves the development of secondary angle-closure glaucoma and/or chronic retinal detachment, and optic nerve atrophy. The antecedent event can range from previous accidental trauma or previous surgical trauma to specific disease entities such as retinal vascular disease (including diabetes, or central retinal artery or vein occlusion), intraocular infection (endophthalmitis), chronic inflammatory disease, or primary retinal detachment. Surgical methods of removing an eye include enucleation, in which the entire eye is removed intact, or evisceration, in which only the intraocular contents (lens, retina, uvea) and possibly cornea are removed with retention of the sclera in the eye socket to house the orbital implant. Exenteration, in which the eye along with surrounding orbital soft tissues are removed, is sometimes required to achieve complete excision of an eyelid/orbital tumor (see later).

A. Secondary glaucoma. The key histopathologic finding in most cases of secondary glaucoma is an anterior chamber angle closed by peripheral anterior synechiae. The term "closed angle" means that the anatomical angle normally formed by the cornea and iris, and occupied by the trabecular meshwork (the main outflow channel for aqueous humor), is occluded by the peripheral iris. If this occlusion is chronic, then permanent adhesions form between the peripheral iris and the trabecular meshwork, that is, peripheral anterior synechiae (e-**Fig. 5.23**). These adhesions may be induced by chronic inflammation, such as in various forms of chronic uveitis, or by the abnormal proliferation of capillaries (neovascular glaucoma), as seen in proliferative diabetic retinopathy or retinal vascular occlusion (see later). Occasionally, in contrast to the closed-angle appearance, post-contusion angle recession may be seen in cases of blunt trauma. The retina in glaucoma exhibits atrophy of the nerve fiber layer and loss of ganglion cells; the optic nerve shows cupping (e-**Fig. 5.24**) and atrophy.

B. Chronic retinal detachment. Retinal detachment may be idiopathic, trauma induced, related to inflammation or infection, or secondary to proliferative retinopathy of various etiologies (diabetic, post-vascular occlusion, and so on). Often an attempt is made to repair the detachment surgically, but severe cases in which surgery fails or the detachment repeatedly recurs may ultimately be treated by enucleation (e-**Fig. 5.25**).

C. Retinal vascular diseases. Eyes with severe retinal vascular disease (most commonly diabetic retinopathy, or central retinal arterial or venous occlusion) often exhibit both secondary angle closure due to neovascularization of the iris (e-**Fig. 5.26**) and angle (neovascular glaucoma), as well as chronic tractional retinal detachment due to proliferative retinopathy. In cases of diabetic retinopathy, microscopic examination of the retina reveals the key features of diabetes: lipoproteinaceous exudates, intraretinal hemorrhages, and neovascularization of the inner surface of the retina (proliferative diabetic retinopathy) (e-**Fig. 5.27**), often with tractional retinal detachment and hemorrhage into the vitreous. In cases of old central retinal vein or artery occlusion, the retina exhibits atrophy and cystoid degeneration of the inner two-thirds of the retina, lipoproteinaceous exudates, and in the case of venous occlusion, often a persistence of hemorrhage. There may also be a neovascular epiretinal membrane with tractional retinal detachment and vitreous hemorrhage. As with neovascular glaucoma of any etiology, eyes with severe diabetic retinopathy or central retinal vascular occlusion also exhibit atrophy and possibly cupping of the optic nerve.

D. Intraocular inflammation and infection. Endophthalmitis most commonly occurs via an exogenous source (e.g., following a surgical procedure, trauma, or perforated corneal ulcer), or may arise from an endogenous source (e.g., secondary to bacteremia or fungemia). Endophthalmitis is generally treated with intravitreal antibiotics and/or antifungals, and possibly vitrectomy surgery to clear the abscess. However, in severe cases treatment may not be successful, and evisceration or enucleation may ultimately be performed. On histology (e-Fig. 5.28), such cases demonstrate intraocular abscess formation and retinal detachment/destruction; depending on the degree of chronicity, optic nerve atrophy may also be seen.

Other severe inflammatory or infectious diseases that can lead to a blind and painful eye include diffuse uveitis of unknown etiology; juvenile rheumatoid arthritis-associated uveitis or uveitis associated with other collagen vascular/autoimmune diseases; diffuse granulomatous uveitis secondary to sympathetic ophthalmia (e-Fig. 5.29), sarcoidosis, or toxoplasmosis; and necrotizing retinitis (as seen in cytomegalovirus [CMV] retinitis or herpetic retinitis).

E. **Trauma.** Many eyes are enucleated because of severe trauma. If there is no attempt at repair by the ophthalmologist because the rupture is too extensive, the pathology specimen usually consists of a ruptured globe with massive intraocular hemorrhage and total retinal detachment (e-Fig. 5.30). Often there is loss of intraocular contents such as the lens and a portion of the uvea, and possibly also the retina. If an attempt has been made by the surgeon to salvage the ruptured globe, but the eye later has to be enucleated because it has become blind and painful, the histopathologic findings vary depending on the degree of chronicity; in cases of recent rupture, the findings may be the same as described above (i.e., massive intraocular hemorrhage, total retinal detachment, and loss of intraocular contents) or may also include additional findings such as endophthalmitis. In cases with a more distant history of rupture, there may be total retinal detachment with gliosis and loss of intraocular contents, intraocular granulation tissue or fibroconnective tissue emanating from the rupture site, and often osseous metaplasia of the retinal pigment epithelium (see later). Angle closure or post-contusion angle recession may also be present depending on the location of the rupture and the nature of the traumatic forces. Optic nerve atrophy is generally also seen.

F. **Phthisis bulbi.** When an eye has undergone a previous insult such as severe trauma, complications of surgery, proliferative retinopathy, or chronic inflammation, and has a chronic total retinal detachment, a gradual degenerative process eventually ensues in which the eye undergoes shrinkage, that is, phthisis (from the Greek verb "to wither"). Clinically, the eye has hypotony (very low intraocular pressure) and is visibly shrunken. Histologically, the retina is totally detached, with marked diffuse atrophy and architectural distortion of all layers of the eye including such severe retinal gliosis as to render the retina barely recognizable. Often the retinal pigment epithelium undergoes osseous metaplasia, and bone may occupy a significant portion of the intraocular cavity (e-Fig. 5.31). Choroidal effusion may be seen. The optic nerve is atrophic.

IV. **INTRAOCULAR NEOPLASMS**

A. Gross room processing of enucleated globes follows a standard protocol to generate the pupil–optic nerve (p.o.) section, as shown in Figure 5.1. Larger cassettes are required for processing. The figure shows the standard transverse plane that is often used for cutting the section, but the globe may be opened along any plane that best captures the particular area of interest. For eyes enucleated due to intraocular tumors, especially primary uveal melanoma, the tumor may be localized by transillumination prior to cutting the eye. Transillumination is achieved by shining onto the cornea a very bright light source that is about 1 cm or less in diameter. The normal uvea will not block the transmission of light, and hence the sclera will glow. However, a uveal tumor will block light transmission, thereby casting a shadow over the corresponding portion of sclera.

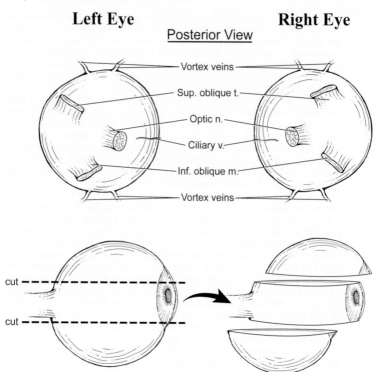

Figure 5.1 The globe is identified as to right eye or left eye using anatomic landmarks (*upper panel*). Two cuts (traditionally referred to as the p.o. sections) are then made in a transverse plane, passing in relation to the pupil and optic nerve as shown (*lower panel*). The superior cap (also known as the superior calotte) and inferior cap are usually not processed unless abnormalities are seen or the eye has an intraocular tumor.

B. The most common primary intraocular neoplasm is **melanoma of the uvea** (choroid, ciliary body, or less commonly, iris). Melanomas usually occur in adults of light complexion. Melanomas of the iris have a better prognosis than do melanomas of the ciliary body and/or choroid. Although some intraocular melanomas can be treated by excision or brachytherapy, some patients do not seek medical attention until the melanoma has become so large that the only course of management is enucleation of the globe. If the diagnosis is in doubt, fine-needle aspiration biopsy (FNAB) may be performed to confirm the diagnosis (e-**Fig. 5.32**). In cases of medium-sized melanomas treated with radioactive plaque brachytherapy, some ocular oncologists routinely perform FNAB at the time of plaque placement so as to obtain a sample for gene expression profiling, as this provides useful prognostic information.

Large uveal melanomas are generally treated with enucleation. Primary uveal melanoma usually arises from the ciliary body or choroid as an ellipse or almond-shaped mass (e-**Figs. 5.33 and 5.34**) which eventually breaks through Bruch's membrane and becomes mushroom shaped (e-**Fig. 5.35**). Microscopically, intraocular melanomas are composed of cells ranging from spindle to

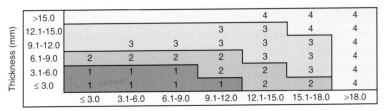

Figure 5.2 Size categories for ciliary body and choroidal melanoma based on thickness and diameter.

epithelioid, with the latter having a worse prognosis (e-**Figs. 5.36** and **5.37**). Other histopathologic features that predict prognosis are size (e-**Fig. 5.38**), extrascleral extension (e-**Fig. 5.38**), and location (those arising from the iris have a better prognosis, whereas those involving the ciliary body [e-**Fig. 5.39**] or peripapillary region have a poorer prognosis). Other factors associated with a worse prognosis include necrosis and mitotic figures. The staging scheme for melanoma of the uvea is described in Table 5.4 and Figure 5.2.

C. **Retinoblastoma** is the most common ocular neoplasm in children. The usual age for clinical presentation in nonfamilial cases is 1 year, whereas familial cases are generally screened within the first few weeks of life and therefore present earlier. The usual clinical appearance is leukocoria (white pupil). In nonfamilial cases, the tumor is generally large and unilateral and accordingly treated with enucleation. In familial cases, tumors are generally seen bilaterally. The tumor may be much larger in one eye than the other, in which case the eye with the large tumor is enucleated, whereas the eye with smaller tumor(s) may be salvaged via laser or cryotherapy applied to the tumor foci, possibly with antecedent adjuvant systemic chemotherapy. A few centers utilize intra-arterial chemotherapy (delivered to the ophthalmic artery) to treat unilateral or bilateral tumors, thereby potentially salvaging eyes that would otherwise need to be enucleated. Some centers utilize periocular injection of chemotherapy.

Histopathologically, retinoblastoma arises from the retina (e-**Fig. 5.40**) and is composed of small blue cells intermingled with anastomosing pools of pink necrosis giving rise to the traditional description of "islands of blue tumor in a sea of pink necrosis" (e-**Fig. 5.41**). Scattered flecks of purple calcium are often seen. Cytologically, the tumor is composed of cells with hyperchromatic, oval-shaped nuclei with scant cytoplasm; the nuclei are densely packed together and thus show nuclear molding. There are many apoptotic bodies and numerous mitotic figures. More differentiated retinoblastomas often exhibit Flexner–Wintersteiner rosettes (e-**Fig. 5.42**). Extension into the optic nerve, and especially presence of tumor at the surgical margin of the nerve, predicts a poor prognosis (e-**Fig. 5.43**). The other factor predictive of poor prognosis is massive invasion of the choroid. If optic nerve invasion past the lamina cribrosa or massive choroidal invasion is seen on histology, then the patient is treated with adjuvant systemic chemotherapy. (Some practitioners have a lower threshold for adjuvant chemotherapy than others; the optimal algorithm for post-enucleation chemotherapy has not been established). The staging scheme for retinoblastoma is given in Table 5.5.

V. **DISEASES OF THE LACRIMAL GLAND AND LACRIMAL SAC**
   A. Lacrimal gland lesions are similar to lesions of the parotid gland (see Chap. 6). Infiltrative lesions include dacryoadenitis, sarcoidosis, lymphoid hyperplasia, and lymphoma. Intrinsic lesions of the lacrimal gland include pleomorphic

TABLE 5.4 Malignant Melanoma of the Uvea

Definition of TNM. These definitions apply to both clinical and pathologic staging.

Primary tumor (T)

All uveal melanomas

TX	Primary tumor cannot be assessed
T0	No evidence of primary tumor

Iris

T1	Tumor limited to the iris:
T1a	Tumor limited to the iris not >3 clock hours in size
T1b	Tumor limited to the iris >3 clock hours in size
T1c	Tumor limited to the iris with secondary glaucoma
T2	Tumor confluent with or extending into the ciliary body and/or choroid
T2a	Tumor confluent with or extending into the ciliary body and/or choroid with secondary glaucoma
T3	Tumor confluent with or extending into the ciliary body and/or choroid with scleral extension
T3a	Tumor confluent with or extending into the ciliary body with scleral extension and secondary glaucoma
T4	Tumor with extrascleral extension
T4a	Tumor with extrascleral extension ≤5 mm in diameter
T4b	Tumor with extrascleral extension >5 mm in diameter

Ciliary body and choroid

T1	Tumor size category 1[a]:
T1a	Tumor size category 1 without ciliary body involvement or extraocular extension
T1b	Tumor size category 1 with ciliary body involvement
T1c	Tumor size category 1 without ciliary body involvement but with extraocular extension ≤5 mm in diameter
T1d	Tumor size category 1 with ciliary body involvement and extraocular extension ≤5 mm in diameter
T2	Tumor size category 2[a]:
T2a	Tumor size category 2 without ciliary body involvement or extraocular extension
T2b	Tumor size category 2 with ciliary body involvement
T2c	Tumor size category 2 without ciliary body involvement but with extraocular extension ≤5 mm in diameter
T2d	Tumor size category 2 with ciliary body involvement and extraocular extension ≤5 mm in diameter
T3	Tumor size category 3[a]:
T3a	Tumor size category 3 without ciliary body involvement or extraocular extension
T3b	Tumor size category 3 with ciliary body involvement
T3c	Tumor size category 3 without ciliary body involvement but with extraocular extension ≤5 mm in diameter
T3d	Tumor size category 3 with ciliary body involvement and extraocular extension ≤5 mm in diameter
T4	Tumor size category 4[a]:
T4a	Tumor size category 4 without ciliary body involvement or extraocular extension
T4b	Tumor size category 4 with ciliary body involvement

(continued)

TABLE 5.4   Malignant Melanoma of the Uvea (*Continued*)

T4c	Tumor size category 4 without ciliary body involvement but with extraocular extension ≤5 mm in diameter
T4d	Tumor size category 4 with ciliary body involvement and extraocular extension ≤5 mm in diameter
T4e	Any tumor size category with extraocular extension >5 mm in diameter

Regional lymph nodes (N)

NX	Regional lymph nodes cannot be assessed
N0	No regional lymph node metastasis
N1	Regional lymph node metastasis

Distant metastasis (M)

M0	No distant metastasis
M1	Distant metastasis
M1a	Largest diameter of the largest metastasis ≤3 cm
M1b	Largest diameter of the largest metastasis 3.1–7.9 cm
M1c	Largest diameter of the largest metastasis ≥8 cm

Histopathologic type. The histopathologic types are as follows:
Spindle cell melanoma (>90% spindle cells)
Mixed cell melanoma (>10% epithelioid cells and >10% spindle cells)
Epithelioid cell melanoma (>90% epithelioid cells)

Histopathologic grade (G)

GX	Grade cannot be assessed
G1	Spindle cell melanoma
G2	Mixed cell melanoma
G3	Epithelioid cell melanoma

Anatomic stage/prognostic groups

Stage I	T1a	N0	M0
Stage IIA	T1b–d	N0	M0
	T2a	N0	M0
Stage IIB	T2b	N0	M0
	T3a	N0	M0
Stage IIIA	T2c–d	N0	M0
	T3b–c	N0	M0
	T4a	N0	M0
Stage IIIB	T3d	N0	M0
	T4b–c	N0	M0
Stage IIIC	T4d–e	N0	M0
Stage IV	Any T	N1	M0
	Any T	Any N	M1a–c

[a]See Figure 5.2.
From: Edge SB, Byrd DR, Compton CC, et al., eds. *AJCC Cancer Staging Manual.* 7th ed. New York, NY: Springer; 2010. Used with permission.

adenoma, adenoid cystic carcinoma, and mucoepidermoid carcinoma. The staging scheme for lacrimal gland carcinoma is given in Table 5.6.

B. Generally occurring in middle-aged to elderly individuals, a stone (dacryolith) may form in the lacrimal sac, causing obstruction of the nasolacrimal drainage system which generally presents as chronic severe watering of the eye (epiphora). Lacrimal sac dacryolithiasis often contains *Actinomyces* organisms. (e-**Fig.** 5.44). Alternatively, *Streptococcal* or fungal organisms may be

TABLE 5.5   Retinoblastoma

Definition of TNM

Clinical classification (cTNM)

Primary tumor (T)

TX	Primary tumor cannot be assessed
T0	No evidence of primary tumor
T1	Tumors no more than 2/3 of the volume of the eye with no vitreous or subretinal seeding
T1a	No tumor in either eye is >3 mm in largest dimension or is located closer than 1.5 mm to the optic nerve or fovea
T1b	At least one tumor is >3 mm in largest dimension or located closer than 1.5 mm to the optic nerve or fovea. No retinal detachment or subretinal fluid beyond 5 mm from the base of the tumor
T1c	At least one tumor is >3 mm in largest dimension or located closer than 1.5 mm to the optic nerve or fovea, with retinal detachment or subretinal fluid beyond 5 mm from the base of the tumor
T2	Tumors no more than 2/3 the volume of the eye with vitreous or subretinal seeding. Can have retinal detachment:
T2a	Focal vitreous and/or subretinal seeding of fine aggregates of tumor cells is present, but no large clumps or "snowballs" of tumor cells
T2b	Massive vitreous seeding and/or subretinal seeding is present, defined as diffuse clumps or "snowballs" of tumor cells
T3	Severe intraocular disease:
T3a	Tumor fills more than 2/3 of the eye
T3b	One or more complications are present, which may include tumor-associated neovascular or angle-closure glaucoma, tumor extension into the anterior segment, hyphema, vitreous hemorrhage, or orbital cellulitis
T4	Extraocular disease detected by imaging studies:
T4a	Invasion of optic nerve
T4b	Invasion into the orbit
T4c	Intracranial extension not past chiasm
T4d	Intracranial extension past chiasm

Regional lymph nodes (N)

NX	Regional lymph nodes cannot be assessed
N0	No regional lymph node involvement
N1	Regional lymph node involvement (preauricular, cervical, submandibular)
N2	Distant lymph node involvement

Metastasis (M)

M0	No metastasis
M1	Systemic metastasis:
M1a	Single lesion to site other than CNS
M1b	Multiple lesions to sites other than CNS
M1c	Prechiasmatic CNS lesion(s)
M1d	Postchiasmatic CNS lesion(s)
M1e	Leptomeningeal and/or CSF involvement

Pathologic classification (pTNM)

Primary tumor (pT)

pTX	Primary tumor cannot be assessed
pT0	No evidence of primary tumor
pT1	Tumor confined to eye with no optic nerve or choroidal invasion
PT2	Tumor with minimal optic nerve and/or choroidal invasion:

(continued)

TABLE 5.5	Retinoblastoma (*Continued*)
pT2a	Tumor superficially invades optic nerve head but does not extend past lamina cribrosa *or* tumor exhibits focal choroidal invasion
pT2b	Tumor superficially invades optic nerve head but does not extend past lamina cribrosa *and* tumor exhibits focal choroidal invasion
pT3	Tumor with significant optic nerve and/or choroidal invasion:
pT3a	Tumor invades optic nerve past lamina cribrosa but not to surgical resection line *or* tumor exhibits massive choroidal invasion
pT3b	Tumor invades optic nerve past lamina cribrosa but not to surgical resection line *and* tumor exhibits massive choroidal invasion
pT4	Tumor invades optic nerve to resection line or exhibits extraocular extension elsewhere:
pT4a	Tumor invades optic nerve to resection line but no extraocular extension identified elsewhere
pT4b	Tumor invades optic nerve to resection line and extraocular extension identified elsewhere

Regional lymph nodes (pN)

pNX	Regional lymph nodes cannot be assessed
pN0	No regional lymph node involvement
pN1	Regional lymph node involvement (preauricular, cervical)
pN2	Distant lymph node involvement

Metastasis (pM)

cM0	No metastasis
pM1	Metastasis to sites other than CNS
pM1a	Single lesion
pM1b	Multiple lesions
pM1c	CNS metastasis
pM1d	Discrete mass(es) without leptomeningeal and/or CSF involvement
pM1e	Leptomeningeal and/or CSF involvement

Anatomic stage/prognostic groups
No stage grouping is presently recommended.

From: Edge SB, Byrd DR, Compton CC, et al., eds. *AJCC Cancer Staging Manual.* 7th ed. New York, NY: Springer; 2010. Used with permission.

seen. Tumors of the lacrimal sac include papillomas, nonkeratinizing squamous cell carcinoma, and other rare entities such as plasmacytoma or lymphoma.

VI. **DISEASES OF THE ORBIT.** Lesions of the orbit include all the aforementioned lesions of the lacrimal gland; lesions elsewhere in the orbit include lymphoma, cavernous hemangioma in young to middle-aged adults, capillary hemangioma in children, idiopathic orbital inflammation (also known as inflammatory pseudotumor), schwannoma, neurofibroma, infectious abscess, dermoid cyst, and lymphangioma. Less common lesions include rhabdomyosarcoma, granular cell tumor, Rosai–Dorfman disease, optic nerve glioma, meningioma of the optic nerve sheath or of the sphenoid wing, alveolar soft part sarcoma, fibrous histiocytoma, melanoma, plasmacytoma, and metastatic carcinoma.

The morphologic features of all these lesions are the same as when they occur in other soft tissue sites. The staging scheme for sarcomas of the orbit is given in Table 5.7.

VII. **DISEASES OF THE EYELID.** The common benign and malignant lesions of the eyelid are identical to those that occur at other cutaneous sites. The staging scheme for carcinoma of the eyelid is given in Table 5.8. Sometimes basal cell, squamous cell, or sebaceous gland carcinomas of the eyelid become so extensive as to invade the

TABLE 5.6 Carcinoma of the Lacrimal Gland

Definition of TNM. These definitions apply to both clinical and pathologic staging.

Primary tumor (T)

TX	Primary tumor cannot be assessed
T0	No evidence of primary tumor
T1	Tumor 2 cm or less in greatest dimension, with or without extraglandular extension into the orbital soft tissue
T2	Tumor more than 2 cm but not more than 4 cm in greatest dimension[a]
T3	Tumor more than 4 cm in greatest dimension[a]
T4	Tumor invades the periosteum or orbital bone or adjacent structures:
T4a	Tumor invades periosteum
T4b	Tumor invades orbital bone
T4c	Tumor invades adjacent structures (brain, sinus, pterygoid fossa, temporal fossa)

Regional lymph nodes (N)

NX	Regional lymph nodes cannot be assessed
N0	No regional lymph node metastasis
N1	Regional lymph node metastasis

Distant metastasis (M)

M0	No distant metastasis
M1	Distant metastasis

Anatomic stage/prognostic groups
No stage grouping is presently recommended.

[a]Note: As the maximum size of the lacrimal gland is 2 cm, T2 and greater tumors will usually extend into the orbital soft tissue.
From: Edge SB, Byrd DR, Compton CC, et al., eds. *AJCC Cancer Staging Manual*. 7th ed. New York, NY: Springer; 2010. Used with permission.

TABLE 5.7 Sarcoma of the Orbit

Definition of TNM. These definitions apply to both clinical and pathologic staging.

Primary tumor (T)

TX	Primary tumor cannot be assessed
T0	No evidence of primary tumor
T1	Tumor 15 mm or less in greatest dimension
T2	Tumor more than 15 mm in greatest dimension without invasion of globe or bony wall
T3	Tumor of any size with invasion of orbital tissues and/or bony walls
T4	Tumor invasion of globe or periorbital structure, such as eyelids, temporal fossa, nasal cavity and paranasal sinuses, and/or central nervous system

Regional lymph nodes (N)

NX	Regional lymph nodes cannot be assessed
N0	No regional lymph node metastasis
N1	Regional lymph node metastasis

Distant metastasis (M)

M0	No distant metastasis
M1	Distant metastasis

Anatomic stage/prognostic groups
No stage grouping is presently recommended.

From: Edge SB, Byrd DR, Compton CC, et al., eds. *AJCC Cancer Staging Manual*. 7th ed. New York, NY: *Springer*; 2010. Used with permission.

TABLE 5.8 Carcinoma of the Eyelid

Definition of TNM. These definitions apply to both clinical and pathologic staging.

Primary tumor (T)

TX	Primary tumor cannot be assessed
T0	No evidence of primary tumor
Tis	Carcinoma in situ
T1	Tumor 5 mm or less in greatest dimension
	Not invading the tarsal plate or eyelid margin
T2a	Tumor more than 5 mm, but not more than 10 mm, in greatest dimension
	Or, any tumor that invades the tarsal plate or eyelid margin
T2b	Tumor more than 10 mm, but not more than 20 mm, in greatest dimension
	Or, involves full-thickness eyelid
T3a	Tumor more than 20 mm in greatest dimension
	Or, any tumor that invades adjacent ocular or orbital structures
	Any T with perineural tumor invasion
T3b	Complete tumor resection requires enucleation, exenteration, or bone resection
T4	Tumor is not resectable due to extensive invasion of ocular, orbital, craniofacial structures, or brain

Regional lymph nodes (N)

NX	Regional lymph nodes cannot be assessed
cN0	No regional lymph node metastasis, based upon clinical evaluation or imaging
pN0	No regional lymph node metastasis, based upon lymph node biopsy
N1	Regional lymph node metastasis

Distant metastasis (M)

M0	No distant metastasis
M1	Distant metastasis

Anatomic stage/prognostic groups

Stage 0	Tis	N0	M0
Stage IA	T1	N0	M0
Stage IB	T2a	N0	M0
Stage IC	T2b	N0	M0
Stage II	T3a	N0	M0
Stage IIIA	T3b	N0	M0
Stage IIIB	Any T	N1	M0
Stage IIIC	T4	Any N	M0
Stage IV	Any T	Any N	M1

From: Edge SB, Byrd DR, Compton CC, et al., eds. *AJCC Cancer Staging Manual.* 7th ed. New York, NY: Springer; 2010. Used with permission.

orbit and ocular surface, in which case exenteration may be required to achieve complete excision. Exenteration is sometimes also required for tumors arising in the orbit/sinuses. In processing an exenteration specimen, the eye should be dissected out of the surrounding soft tissue; the soft tissue should then be processed in the usual fashion for soft tissue tumors, and the eye should be placed separately in fixative for at least 24 hours. The eye may then be processed as described previously under gross room processing of enucleated globes. In such cases, there may be varying degrees of optic atrophy due to optic nerve compression by the tumor, but the intraocular contents are often normal on histology.

SUGGESTED READINGS

Eagle RC. *Eye Pathology, an Atlas and Text*. 2nd ed. Philadelphia, PA: Lippincott Williams & Wilkins; 2011.

Font RL, Croxatto JO, Rao NA. In: *AFIP Atlas of Tumor Pathology, Series 4*. Vol 5. Washington, DC: ARP Press; 2006.

Smith ME, Kincaid MC, West CE. In: Krachmer JH, ed. *The Requisites in Ophthalmology*. St. Louis, MO: Mosby; 2002; chapters 3–9, 23.

Yanoff M, Sassani JW. *Ocular Pathology*. 6th ed. Philadelphia, PA: Elsevier/Mosby; 2009.

6

Salivary Glands

Joshua I. Warrick, Elise L. Krejci,
and James S. Lewis Jr.

I. NORMAL ANATOMY

A. Macroscopic/gross. The salivary glands are exocrine organs that secrete components of saliva to both break down carbohydrates and lubricate the passage of food. There are three major paired salivary glands: the parotid, the submandibular, and the sublingual. There are also numerous minor salivary glands located in the submucosa of the entire upper aerodigestive tract (UADT), from the lips and nasal cavity to the major bronchi.

The parotid glands are the largest major salivary glands and are located between the ramus of the mandible and the mastoid process. Each gland is composed of a superficial lobe and a smaller deep lobe, and the facial nerve is intimately associated with both lobes. Each gland normally contains approximately 20 intraglandular lymph nodes. The secretions of the parotid gland empty via Stensen's duct into the buccal mucosa of the oral cavity near the second maxillary molar.

The submandibular glands (also referred to as the submaxillary glands) are located just medial to the body of the mandible, and are smaller than the parotid glands. Their secretions drain through Wharton's duct into the floor of the mouth.

The sublingual glands are the smallest of the major salivary glands and are located in the floor of the mouth between the genioglossus muscle and the mandible. Their secretions drain into the floor of the mouth directly via small ducts or through the larger (Bartholin's) duct which drains into Wharton's duct.

B. Microscopic. The major salivary glands are enclosed by a connective tissue capsule and divided into lobules composed of ducts and acini, whereas the minor salivary glands are unencapsulated. The acini are composed of mucinous and/or serous epithelial cells surrounded by a layer of myoepithelial cells which contract to aid in the movement of glandular secretions. Myoepithelial cells are inconspicuous in normal salivary gland sections.

A single acinus may be composed of a mixture of serous and mucous cells. Serous cells are pyramidal in shape and contain basophilic periodic acid-Schiff (PAS)-positive granules within their cytoplasm. Mucous cells are more rounded, have basally oriented nuclei, and contain abundant clear mucin. The parotid gland is almost exclusively serous, the sublingual gland almost exclusively mucinous, and the submandibular gland is mixed serous and mucinous (e-Figs. 6.1 to 6.3).* The acini secrete fluid into the intercalated ducts, which are lined by a low simple cuboidal epithelium. Intercalated ducts are also the source of reserve cells that can repopulate the acinar system. The intercalated ducts join to form striated ducts, which merge to form interlobular ducts, which ultimately empty into the large named ducts.

II. GROSS EXAMINATION, TISSUE SAMPLING, AND HISTOLOGIC SLIDE PREPARATION

A. Biopsies of many salivary gland lesions are taken prior to surgery to characterize the lesion and direct management.

1. Fine needle aspiration (FNA) is the procedure of choice for initial characterization of salivary gland lesions for many reasons (see cytology section that follows).

---

*All e-figures are available online via the Solution Site Image Bank.

2. Core needle and incisional biopsies of the parotid gland can damage the facial nerve branches so are rarely performed.

B. **Resections.** Some salivary gland masses are removed in their entirety without a previous tissue diagnosis. Superficial parotidectomy remains the initial procedure of choice for benign parotid gland tumors. Submandibular gland resections are usually performed without taking any significant periglandular soft tissue, although more tissue may be included with the specimen for submandibular or parotid tumors that are known or suspected to be malignant. The rare sublingual gland tumors necessitate a resection of the floor of mouth that is qualitatively similar to those performed for mucosal-based squamous carcinomas of the same area.

In general, salivary gland specimens are small enough to prosect the day of receipt. The gland should be described, and its dimensions recorded. The deep (covered by muscle and fascia) and superficial (covered by subcutaneous fat) surfaces of the parotid gland can sometimes be discerned, and should be differentially inked. The specimen should be serially sectioned, and any mass or focal lesion described including dimensions, color, texture, and distance to the margins. Four to five sections of the tumor, including representative areas of the closest inked margins, should be taken. At least one section of the normal surrounding gland should also be taken. For the parotid gland, the surrounding gland and any periglandular soft tissue should be thoroughly searched for lymph nodes, which should be separately submitted.

III. **DIAGNOSTIC FEATURES OF COMMON DISEASES**

A. **Inflammation and infection.** Sialadenitis, or inflammation of the salivary glands, can be divided into bacterial causes, viral causes, and autoimmune disease.

1. **Bacterial sialadenitis** is rare and is generally a result of obstruction by stones (sialolithiasis). The causative organism is usually *Staphylococcus aureus,* followed by *Streptococcus viridans* and gram-negative rods. Surgical specimens from bacterial sialadenitis are almost never seen. However, sialadenitis may lead to an abscess that requires surgical drainage. Gross specimens may show a purulent exudate or a relatively intact gland. Microscopic sections can show abscesses, cystic degeneration, and/or bacterial colonies.

2. **Viral sialadenitis** is most commonly caused by mumps (paramyxovirus), but can also be associated with Epstein–Barr, coxsackie, influenza A, and parainfluenza viruses. Surgical specimens are rarely encountered. Grossly infected glands are boggy and edematous, and chronic inflammation may be seen microscopically.

3. **Autoimmune sialadenitis** is relatively common, and usually presents as Sjögren's syndrome, characterized by facial swelling, dry mouth, and dry eyes (termed Sicca syndrome) with inflammatory arthritis and elevated autoantibodies. On physical examination, bilateral, symmetric enlargement of the salivary and lacrimal glands is seen. Diagnosis may be facilitated by a minor salivary gland biopsy, typically taken from the inner lip.

Grossly, the major glands usually have a discrete, tan nodularity. Microscopically, in early disease, there is a lymphoplasmacytic septal inflammatory infiltrate with little to no abnormality of the parenchyma. The so-called "focus score," a nodular collection of >50 lymphocytes, is considered diagnostic of autoimmune sialadenitis in the appropriate clinical context. In larger glands or in more severe disease, there is typically an extensive lymphoid infiltrate with germinal centers (e-Fig. 6.4). The acini are often atrophic, and interstitial fibrosis may be present. In late disease, acini may be completely absent leaving only isolated residual ducts, termed "epimyoepithelial islands," with an associated dense intraepithelial lymphocytosis. In Sjögren's syndrome, the lymphocytic infiltrate is polyclonal, in contrast to the monoclonal lymphoid proliferation seen in mucosa-associated lymphoid tissue (MALT) lymphoma.

4. **Chronic sialadenitis** (or chronic sclerosing sialadenitis) is usually unilateral and clinically can mimic a true salivary gland neoplasm. When it occurs in the submandibular gland, it is known as a Kuttner tumor. Chronic sialadenitis most commonly results from sialolithiasis with obstruction, although some cases may be due to radiation therapy or duct strictures. It can have no structural or obvious etiology and recently most of these cases have been shown to be an autoimmune-related IgG4-related sclerosing disease similar to that occurring in the pancreas. Grossly, it is characterized by a very hard, fibrotic gland with lobulation and septation (e-**Fig. 6.5**). Histologic examination of the gland early in the disease process shows dilated ducts filled with secretions with an associated lymphocyte and plasma cell–rich infiltrate, occasionally with germinal center formation. As the disease progresses, fibrosis surrounds the ducts and results in lobulation of the gland (e-**Fig. 6.6**) with acinar atrophy and broad fibrous bands. Surgical excision may be required, either to definitively rule out a neoplasm or just for symptom relief.

5. **Necrotizing sialometaplasia** is a rare inflammatory/destructive lesion that simulates malignancy and is thought to occur because of ischemic injury. Although it can occur anywhere along the UADT, the vast majority of cases occur in the hard palate. Men are slightly more commonly affected, and the average patient age is 46 years. Clinically, the lesion consists of a sharply defined and deep ulcer that develops rapidly (over a few days) and can persist for months. Grossly, the lesion consists of loose tissue with a surface ulcer and no distinguishing mass lesion. Microscopically, the most typical feature is coagulative necrosis of the minor salivary gland lobules with a prominent associated inflammatory response. There is extensive squamous metaplasia of the ducts (an alarming feature), but the lesion retains its overall lobular architecture (e-**Fig. 6.7**). The surface squamous mucosa may show pseudoepitheliomatous hyperplasia. The lack of peripheral infiltration and the retained lobular architecture are keys to recognizing the lesion as benign. No specific therapy is indicated because the lesion is self-healing.

B. **Cystic lesions**

1. **Acquired immune deficiency syndrome (AIDS)-related parotid cysts (ARPCs)** are benign lymphoepithelial cysts. Patients present with unilateral or bilateral, painless, slowly enlarging parotid masses. They sometimes have associated cervical lymphadenopathy and/or nasopharyngeal swelling. Grossly, these lesions have multiple cystic spaces usually containing serous fluid. Microscopically, ARPCs consist of cysts that most often have a thin, mature squamous epithelial lining, although the lining is sometimes cuboidal or columnar with goblet cells. Below the epithelium, the cyst wall has dense lymphoid tissue with germinal centers. Occasionally, lesions within the gland can lack cystic change and appear similar to epimyoepithelial islands.

Unlike autoimmune sialadenitis, the vast majority of human immunodeficiency virus (HIV) patients with ARPC have no autoimmune symptoms, no Sicca syndrome from glandular dysfunction, and no serum autoantibodies. The etiology of ARPC is thus unclear. Patients usually have bilateral disease by radiologic examination, even if there are no symptoms and no clinical mass in the contralateral gland. If the diagnosis is established by radiologic imaging and cytology, surgery is not necessary for other than cosmetic reasons.

2. **Benign lymphoepithelial cysts** are unifocal lesions that occur in patients in their fifth and sixth decades. They most commonly involve the parotid gland, but are occasionally seen in the oral cavity. There is no association with systemic disease. Grossly, they consist of well-circumscribed unilocular cysts with contents ranging from serous to mucoid to caseous; keratinous debris may be present. Microscopically, they consist of a cyst lined by thin, mature squamous epithelium without papillary projections. In rare cases, the lining is cuboidal or columnar with goblet cells. Below the epithelium, the cyst

wall has dense lymphoid tissue with germinal centers (e-Fig. 6.8). Excision is curative, and the lesion does not recur.

3. **Mucoceles** are the most common non-neoplastic lesion of salivary gland tissue and are defined as pooling of mucin in a cystic cavity. Two types are recognized. In the retention type, the mucin is within a dilated duct. In the extravasation type, the mucin accumulates in the soft tissue. The lower lip is the most common site for mucoceles, followed by the tongue, the floor of the mouth (where the lesion is termed a "ranula"), and the buccal mucosa. The peak incidence of mucoceles is in the third decade. Grossly, a mucocele presents as a cystic cavity in the connective tissue that is filled with glistening fluid. Microscopically, the cyst wall may or may not have an epithelial lining, depending on the type. Those of the retention type have a lining and usually no surrounding inflammation, whereas those of the extravasation type consist of mucin with surrounding inflammatory cells and no lining. Some late lesions consist only of a collection of foamy histiocytes containing mucin (e-Fig. 6.9), which can be confirmed by PAS or mucicarmine stains. Surgical excision is usually curative.

IV. **NEOPLASMS.** Neoplasms of the salivary gland can be roughly classified based on the cell type(s) of the normal salivary gland toward which they differentiate: acinar, myoepithelial, or ductal. However, most neoplasms have dual differentiation because almost all show of those with ductal differentiation also have some myoepithelial differentiation. Most benign neoplasms have a malignant counterpart. The World Health Organization (WHO) classification of tumors of the salivary gland is listed in Table 6.1.

A. **Benign neoplasms**

1. **Pleomorphic adenoma (PA)** is the most common neoplasm of the salivary glands. Ninety percent of PAs occur in the parotid gland and PAs represent 60% of parotid gland neoplasms; the majority of the remaining cases occur in the hard palate or submandibular gland. The tumor occurs over a wide age range, but the peak incidence is in the fourth and fifth decades. The tumor presents as a slow-growing, painless mass that usually is between 2 and 5 cm in diameter. On gross examination, these tumors appear well-circumscribed but are not usually encapsulated. They are never encapsulated when occurring in minor salivary glands. Sectioning reveals a rubbery, myxoid, tan-white mass (e-Fig. 6.10). The microscopic appearance, as the name suggests, is highly variable, but always shows an intimate admixture of epithelial and mesenchymal elements. The epithelial component consists of ductal structures with an associated myoepithelial layer but also may contain collections of myoepithelial cells that can range from spindled to clear, plasmacytoid, or basaloid. The mesenchymal, or stromal, component is typically myxoid, hyaline, or chondroid (e-Fig. 6.11). Although defined subcategories have no clinical significance, pleomorphic adenomas have been divided into a myxoid type (>80% mesenchymal-type tissue), cellular type (>80% epithelial-type tissue), and mixed or classic type (generally an equal mix of components).

Treatment requires complete excision because PAs are likely to recur if tumor is left behind or transected. Multinodular growth is uncommon in primary tumors but is frequent in recurrent disease, yielding a so-called "buckshot" pattern (e-Fig. 6.12). Therapy for recurrence is consequently more difficult.

2. **Warthin tumor** (papillary cystadenoma lymphomatosum) is the second most common benign salivary gland tumor and is found exclusively in the parotid gland. It is the most common bilateral or multifocal salivary gland tumor, usually presents in the sixth or seventh decade, and is associated with smoking. Grossly, it presents as a soft, brown or yellow mass that is composed of cysts that are classically filled with viscous brown fluid. Microscopically, the

TABLE 6.1   WHO Histologic Classification of Tumors of the Salivary Glands

Malignant epithelial tumors
Acinic cell carcinoma
Mucoepidermoid carcinoma
Adenoid cystic carcinoma
Polymorphous low-grade adenocarcinoma
Epithelial–myoepithelial carcinoma
Clear cell carcinoma, not otherwise specified
Basal cell adenocarcinoma
Sebaceous carcinoma
Sebaceous lymphadenocarcinoma
Cystadenocarcinoma
Low-grade cribriform cystadenocarcinoma
Mucinous adenocarcinoma
Oncocytic carcinoma
Salivary duct carcinoma
Adenocarcinoma, not otherwise specified
Myoepithelial carcinoma
Carcinoma ex pleomorphic adenoma
Carcinosarcoma
Metastasizing pleomorphic adenoma
Squamous cell carcinoma
Small cell carcinoma
Large cell carcinoma
Lymphoepithelial carcinoma
Sialoblastoma

Benign epithelial tumors
Pleomorphic adenoma
Myoepithelioma
Basal cell adenoma
Warthin's tumor
Oncocytoma
Canalicular adenoma
Sebaceous adenoma
Lymphadenoma
  Sebaceous
  Non-sebaceous
Ductal papillomas
  Inverted ductal papilloma
  Intraductal papilloma
  Sialadenoma papilliferum
Cystadenoma

Soft tissue tumors
Hemangioma

Hematolymphoid tumors
Hodgkin's lymphoma
Diffuse large B-cell lymphoma
Extranodal marginal zone B-cell lymphoma

Secondary tumors

From: Barnes L, Eveson J, Reichart P, Sidransky D, eds. *World Health Organization Classification of Tumours. Pathology and Genetics. Head and Neck Tumours.* Lyon: IARC Press: 2005. Used with permission.

TABLE 6.2 Major Architectural Patterns of Basal Cell Adenoma

Tubular
Solid
Trabecular
Membranous ("dermal anlage tumor")

lesion has a characteristic and highly reproducible morphology with papillary projections into cystic spaces which have an epithelial lining composed of two layers of cells with oncocytic features (e-Fig. 6.13). The epithelium overlies a dense, polyclonal, lymphoid component with germinal centers. Warthin tumors may show a giant cell reaction, fibrosis, or squamous metaplasia from trauma and/or cyst rupture. Surgical excision is almost always curative as recurrence is rare. Associated malignancy is also very rare and is usually either squamous cell carcinoma or lymphoma.

3. **Basal cell adenomas** are benign tumors that are composed of small basaloid cells. They generally occur in adults, and 75% occur in the parotid gland. They usually present as an asymptomatic, slowly growing mass. The membranous subtype ("dermal anlage tumor") may be multicentric. The occurrence of numerous basal cell adenomas, dermal cylindromas, and trichoepitheliomas is called Brooke–Spiegler Syndrome.

On gross examination, these tumors are usually solid, well-circumscribed, and pink to brown. Some may be cystic. Microscopically, four patterns are recognized: tubular, solid, trabecular, and membranous (Table 6.2). In all patterns, the tumor is composed of two cell types. Small cells with little cytoplasm typically lie at the neoplasm's edge, frequently show peripheral palisading, and give the tumor its basaloid appearance. Polygonal basaloid cells with slightly more cytoplasm and round to oval nuclei with more open chromatin usually lie in the center of the nests. The trabecular and membranous patterns have a "jigsaw puzzle" appearance with rounded nests of tumor cells shaped like puzzle pieces (e-Fig. 6.14). The membranous pattern additionally shows hyalinized, eosinophilic, linear, or nodular basement membrane–like material around the nests (e-Fig. 6.15). The tubular pattern consists of tubular, gland-like structures (eFig. 6.16). The solid pattern consists of solid nests of cells. The tumor cells express ductal and myoepithelial markers including pan-cytokeratin, S-100, smooth muscle actin, and p63.

The differential diagnosis for basal cell adenoma includes basal cell adenocarcinoma and adenoid cystic carcinoma, both of which, unlike basal cell adenoma, show infiltrative growth and/or perineural invasion. Simple excision of basal cell adenoma is usually curative and recurrence is rare, except in the membranous type, where the recurrence rate approaches 25%.

4. **Canalicular adenomas** are benign salivary tumors thought to arise from the excretory ducts of the minor salivary glands, particularly of the upper lip. They are frequently multifocal (e-Fig. 6.17). Women and African Americans are more commonly affected, and the peak incidence is in the seventh decade. Canalicular adenomas present clinically as an asymptomatic, fluctuant or firm 1- to 2-cm submucosal nodule that grows slowly.

On gross examination, they are well-circumscribed but unencapsulated, and have a tan to pink, cystic or solid cut surface. Histologically, canalicular adenomas are composed of long strands or tubules of columnar epithelial cells in a loose, collagenous stroma (e-Fig. 6.18). There are typically two rows of columnar cells situated opposite each other; the rows may take on a "beaded appearance" with tubules coming together and then separating. The epithelial cells lining the tubules usually have eosinophilic cytoplasm and range from cuboidal to columnar. There is no significant pleomorphism, and mitotic activity is low. The epithelial cells express cytokeratin and S-100, but are negative for calponin.

The differential diagnosis for canalicular adenoma includes pleomorphic adenoma and basal cell adenoma. However, the pattern of growth of canalicular adenoma is virtually always distinctive enough to make the diagnosis. Simple local excision is performed with an attempt to obtain clear margins. Recurrence is rare.

5. **Myoepitheliomas** are benign tumors composed of myoepithelial cells. These tumors occur with approximately equal frequency in the parotid gland and minor salivary glands, particularly the hard and the soft palate, and present as slowly growing, painless masses in adults. Men and women are affected equally.

Grossly, these neoplasms are well-circumscribed and encapsulated with a tan to white cut surface. Histologically, they are composed almost exclusively of sheets and cords of myoepithelial cells, though ductal cells may comprise a small percentage (<10%) of individual tumors. In this regard, myoepitheliomas are sometimes considered to lie at one end of a biologic spectrum, with pleomorphic adenoma in the middle, and basal cell adenoma at the opposite end. The tumors can be classified into four major subtypes, based on myoepithelial cell morphology: spindle cell, hyaline, plasmacytoid, and clear cell. All subtypes commonly have a collagenous or myxoid stroma. The spindle cell type shows an interlacing, fascicular pattern of growth (e-Fig. 6.19). Loosely cohesive myoepithelial cells with eosinophilic cytoplasm and eccentric round nuclei are present in the plasmacytoid variant (e-Fig. 6.20). The clear cell type is composed of sheets and aggregates of clear cells (e-Fig. 6.21). The tumor cells express typical myoepithelial markers such as S-100, pan-cytokeratin, smooth muscle actin, and p63.

Simple excision is generally the treatment of choice unless malignant features, such as infiltrative growth or perineural invasion, are encountered, in which the diagnosis is myoepithelial carcinoma. Myoepitheliomas have a slightly lower recurrence rate than pleomorphic adenomas.

B. Malignant neoplasms

1. **Mucoepidermoid carcinoma** is the most common salivary gland malignancy. The major salivary glands account for more than half of all cases, with most arising in the parotid gland. These tumors also arise from minor salivary glands in the oral cavity, particularly in the hard palate, buccal mucosa, lip, and retromolar trigone. They may also develop intraosseously in the mandible and maxilla, but such tumors are considered odontogenic in origin and have a different clinical behavior. Mucoepidermoid carcinomas are slightly more common in women, and the mean age of affected patients is approximately 45 years. The tumor also occurs in children and is the most common pediatric salivary gland carcinoma. Patients usually present with a painless, slowly growing mass, but may also present with a blue-red superficial nodule along the oral mucosa mimicking a mucocele or vascular lesion.

Grossly, both solid and cystic components may be present, often with mucinous material within the cysts. Microscopically, the hallmark of these tumors is the presence of the three different cell types: mucous, squamoid (epidermoid), and intermediate, although frequently squamoid cell are inconspicuous. These three cell types are present in variable proportions in individual tumors and form sheets, nests, duct-like structures, or cysts. Intermediate cells frequently predominate, and range from small basal cells with minimal basophilic cytoplasm to larger oval cells with pale eosinophilic cytoplasm. The mucous cells occur singly or in clusters and have pale, foamy cytoplasm, distinct cell membranes, and eccentric small nuclei (e-Fig. 6.22). They frequently line cystic spaces and are positive with mucicarmine and PAS stains. Squamoid cells have abundant eosinophilic cytoplasm and vesicular nuclei with open chromatin. They are not truly squamous as they lack intercellular bridges, and only very rarely is there true keratinization. A population of glycogen-rich clear cells is often scattered throughout the tumor.

The differential diagnosis includes necrotizing sialometaplasia, which is discerned by its residual normal lobules of minor salivary gland tissue, presence of necrosis, associated dense inflammatory infiltrate, and lack of cytologic atypia. Adenosquamous carcinoma and squamous cell carcinoma are also in the differential, but both have true squamous differentiation with intercellular bridges or keratinization, and are frequently associated with surface squamous dysplasia or carcinoma in situ. Many mucoepidermoid carcinomas possess a t(11;19)(q21;p13) translocation which appears to be quite specific for this tumor type. Tumors that carry the rearrangement have better clinical outcomes, but they are also usually smaller and of lower grade, although recent studies have increasingly found the translocation in many high-grade tumors as well. The clinical utility of testing for this translocation has yet to be established.

Prognosis is highly dependent on the grade of the tumor, and the grade is in turn dependent on the relative amounts of the various cell types. Low-grade lesions are markedly cystic and have abundant well-differentiated mucous cells. High-grade lesions are more solid with squamoid and intermediate cells predominating. Different grading systems have been proposed with inconsistent results, although the Brandwein-Gensler grading system (Table 6.3) has gained acceptance for its reproducibility and ability to stratify for outcomes.

Wide local excision is recommended. Radiation therapy has not been shown to be beneficial except for palliation of unresectable or recurrent disease. The prognosis for low-grade tumors is excellent (>90% survival at 5 years) but drops greatly for high-grade tumors (about 50% survival at 5 years).

2. **Polymorphous low-grade adenocarcinoma (PLGA)** arises exclusively from the minor salivary glands and accounts for 25% of all minor salivary gland tumors. The tumor's most common site is the palate, particularly at the junction of the hard and soft palate. Less common sites include the upper lip, buccal mucosa, and base of the tongue. PLGA arises more commonly in women and tends to present in the fourth to sixth decades, often as a very slowly growing mass that may be present for years before coming to clinical attention.

On gross examination, PLGA is a circumscribed, nonencapsulated, and pale yellow or tan mass that generally ranges from 1 to 3 cm. Microscopically, the architectural features are quite variable, as the name suggests, showing

TABLE 6.3	Brandwein-Gensler Grading System for Mucoepidermoid Carcinoma	
Parameter		**Point value**
Cystic component <25%		+2
Tumor front invades in small nests and islands		+2
Pronounced nuclear atypia		+2
Lymphatic and/or vascular invasion		+3
Neural invasion		+3
Necrosis		+3
4 or more mitoses/10 high power fields		+3
Bony invasion		+3
Grade		**Point score**
Low		0
Intermediate		2–3
High		4 or more

Adapted from *Am J Surg Pathol.* 2001;25:835.

solid nests, lobules, cribriform gland-like structures, duct-like arrangements, or a characteristic concentric whorling of the cellular nests in a single file arrangement that has been termed "the eye of the storm." Stromal hyalinization with a grayish-blue hue is characteristic. The periphery of the tumor shows markedly infiltrative growth, and perineural invasion is common (e-Fig. 6.23). Cytologically, in contrast to the architecture, the tumor cells are very uniform with moderate eosinophilic cytoplasm and characteristic round to oval nuclei with open chromatin (e-Fig. 6.24). There is minimal mitotic activity and no necrosis. The differential diagnosis includes pleomorphic adenoma, which usually exhibits myxochondroid areas that are not seen in PLGA, and adenoid cystic carcinoma, which consists of basaloid cells with more hyperchromatic nuclei than those of PLGA and which has a much "tighter" cribriform pattern with a much more obvious myoepithelial component.

Conservative resection is the treatment of choice. Recurrence occurs in 10 to 15% of patients. Neck dissection is only recommended for clinical adenopathy or proven metastasis because lymph node metastases are uncommon. Distant metastases are even less common. Patients have an excellent long-term prognosis even in the presence of recurrent/metastatic disease, and deaths due to PLGA are quite rare.

3. **Acinic cell carcinoma** accounts for only 1% to 3% of salivary gland tumors. It occurs evenly through the second to seventh decades and can be seen in childhood (in fact, it is the second most common childhood salivary gland malignancy). About 80% of cases arise in the parotid gland, usually presenting as a slowly growing mass which is occasionally painful.

Grossly, acinic cell carcinoma presents as a single, usually circumscribed, solid mass that can undergo cystic degeneration. Histologically, the architecture can be solid/lobular, microcystic, papillary-cystic, or follicular. Mixed architectural patterns are common as is a background inflammatory infiltrate with germinal center formation (e-Fig. 6.25A). Small tumors can be easily missed because the acinar cells may be very well differentiated. The acinic cell is characteristic (and requisite for the diagnosis) and has the appearance of a salivary acinar cell with abundant granular, basophilic cytoplasm and a small, round, somewhat eccentrically placed nucleus (e-Fig. 6.25B). PAS stains will highlight the cytoplasmic zymogen granules, which are resistant to diastase digestion. A number of other cell types can also be present including eosinophilic, clear, and vacuolated cells. The periphery of the tumor may not be infiltrative, but this should not be interpreted as a finding of benignancy. There is no acinic cell adenoma. The differential diagnosis differs depending on the architecture and predominant cell type, and includes normal parotid gland, oncocytoma/oncocytic carcinoma, and clear cell carcinoma. The papillary variant of acinic cell carcinoma must be differentiated from cystadenoma/adenocarcinoma. In addition, a new entity, the mammary analogue secretory carcinoma, has similar features but has no true serous granules and has intraluminal secretory material.

Recurrence after excision occurs in approximately one-third of cases. Although classically regarded as a low-grade malignancy, 10% to 15% of these tumors will metastasize to regional lymph nodes or distantly, particularly to the lungs and bones. This has been more clarified by recent literature which shows that approximately 15–20% of cases with have high grade areas with mitotic activity higher than 2 per 10 high power fields and/or with necrosis (e-Fig. 6.26). The higher grade areas usually lose their acinic cell (serous granules) features. The older term for this was "de-differentiation" although more recently, authors have favored the terms "high grade" or "with high grade transformation." Tumors with these features consistently have progressive disease with poor outcomes and are the ones responsible for the 10–15% of metastatic cancers noted above. For this reason, grading is actually

TABLE 6.4	Grading of Adenoid Cystic Carcinoma
Predominant pattern	**Grade**
Tubular	I
Cribriform	II
Solid	III

very important. The tumors lacking these histologic features may recur locally, but rarely spread and rarely result in death.

4. **Adenoid cystic carcinoma** is one of the most recognizable salivary gland tumors. It comprises 10% of all salivary gland malignancies, and is the most common malignancy of the minor salivary glands. Although the tumor occurs in patients over a wide age range, the peak incidence is between 40 and 60 years of age. The tumor is slow growing, but nonetheless relentlessly progressive. Perineural invasion is extremely common, so cranial nerve involvement, including facial nerve palsy, may be the presenting symptom, with or without associated pain.

Grossly, the tumor is solid, light tan, firm, and well-circumscribed. Histologically, several architectural patterns are found including cribriform, tubular, and solid. Most are a mixture of patterns, however. Tumors are graded based on the predominant pattern (Table 6.4). The tubular pattern consists of double cell-lined ducts with inner epithelial and outer myoepithelial layers (e-**Fig. 6.27**). The most common and recognizable pattern is cribriform (e-**Fig. 6.28**) which consists of nests of cells arranged around gland-like spaces filled with reduplicated basement membrane material, which appears either as pink and hyaline, or as glycosaminoglycans, which appear basophilic and mucoid. The solid pattern consists of rounded nests of basaloid tumor cells with no, or virtually no, tubule formation (e-**Fig. 6.29**). The cells in adenoid cystic carcinoma are basaloid, with little cytoplasm, and have round to oval nuclei that are dark and hyperchromatic usually without prominent nucleoli. The cells are usually regular with little mitotic activity, except in the solid type, in which mitotic activity may be prominent. Perineural invasion is seen in the majority of cases, particularly at the tumor's periphery. The tumors are composed of epithelial cells, which express pan-cytokeratin and EMA, and much less prominent myoepithelial cells, which express S-100, SMA, calponin, and p63, particularly as scattered cells at the periphery of the nests (e-**Fig. 6.30**). The myxoid stromal material in and around the nests will stain for collagen type IV and laminin.

The differential diagnosis for low-grade (tubular) tumors most importantly includes polymorphous low-grade adenocarcinoma, epithelial–myoepithelial carcinoma, and basal cell adenocarcinoma. None of these tumors will show the basaloid and hyperchromatic nuclei characteristic of adenoid cystic carcinoma. High-grade neuroendocrine carcinomas and basaloid squamous cell carcinoma enter the differential diagnosis for solid-type adenoid cystic carcinoma. Adenoid cystic carcinoma lacks neuroendocrine staining and lacks squamous differentiation. Solid adenoid cystic carcinoma will have a patchy p63 staining pattern with positive cells at the periphery of the nests, while in basaloid squamous cell carcinoma the staining is diffuse.

Despite its somewhat bland-appearing morphology, adenoid cystic carcinoma is overtly malignant and usually causes progressive disease. Five- and ten-year survival rates are only 62% and 40%. Local recurrence is extremely common, particularly in the first 5 years after surgery, although late recurrences also occur. Involvement of bone, submandibular gland origin, and solid histologic type (grade III) all adversely affect prognosis. Identification of perineural invasion may adversely affect prognosis as well.

5. **"Malignant mixed tumor"** is a broad term that is used to encompass true malignant mixed tumors, carcinoma ex pleomorphic adenoma, and metastasizing mixed tumor.

   a. **True malignant mixed tumor** (or carcinosarcoma) is a malignant neoplasm that is composed of both carcinomatous and sarcomatous components, and is exceedingly rare. The mean age is 58 years, and one-third of patients have evidence of a preexisting pleomorphic adenoma. Approximately two-thirds of cases arise in the parotid gland, 15% in the submandibular gland, and 15% in the minor salivary glands of the palate.

   Grossly, there is typically a firm, tan-white mass with hemorrhage, necrosis, and, on occasion, grittiness or calcification. Microscopically, there is an intimate admixture of the two components. The carcinomatous component typically takes the form of high-grade salivary duct carcinoma or undifferentiated carcinoma (e-**Fig. 6.31**). The sarcomatous component is usually chondrosarcoma or osteosarcoma, but fibrosarcoma, leiomyosarcoma, and even liposarcoma occur rarely. Treatment consists of wide local excision combined with radiotherapy. The tumors are very aggressive, with up to two-thirds of patients dying of disease, usually within 30 months.

   b. **Carcinoma ex pleomorphic adenoma** is defined as a mixed tumor in which carcinoma is present. This tumor accounts for >95% of malignant mixed tumors, and is most common in the parotid gland, followed by the minor salivary glands, submandibular gland, and sublingual gland. Most patients are in their sixth or seventh decade, which is approximately 1 decade older than the age of most patients who have pleomorphic adenomas. The classic history is a patient with a longstanding mass that undergoes rapid growth over a period of several months.

   Grossly, these can reach up to 25 cm in diameter, and the average size is more than twice that of pleomorphic adenomas. The carcinomatous component is usually an infiltrative, hard, white to tan-gray mass with hemorrhage and necrosis. Microscopically, the proportions of the carcinoma and pleomorphic adenoma are quite variable, and the pleomorphic adenoma component may be replaced by scarring or may be overgrown by the malignant component. The malignant component most often is a poorly differentiated adenocarcinoma not otherwise specified (e-**Figs 6.32** and **6.33**), salivary duct carcinoma, or undifferentiated carcinoma. Low-grade carcinomas such as myoepithelial carcinoma occasionally occur.

   Prognosis and management are highly dependent on the type of carcinoma and extent of invasion. The malignant component should be classified as noninvasive (intracapsular), minimally invasive (≤ 1.5 mm in greatest extent), or widely invasive (>1.5 mm). Wide resection is the treatment of choice, with lymph node dissection and radiation therapy reserved for widely invasive tumors or tumors with obvious cervical lymph node metastases.

   c. **Metastasizing mixed tumor** is the least common form of malignant mixed tumor. These tumors have the same bland morphology of a pleomorphic adenoma, but metastasize either to local lymph nodes or distantly, usually to bone and lung. Often, there is a protracted clinical course with many recurrences at the primary site before nodal or distant metastases develop. Overall mortality due to the tumor is 40%.

6. **Salivary duct carcinoma** is one of the most aggressive primary salivary gland tumors and accounts for <10% of salivary gland tumors. Men are more commonly affected in a ratio of 4:1. Patients generally present in the sixth decade with a rapidly growing parotid mass with facial nerve involvement.

   Grossly, the tumors are solid and white with hemorrhage, necrosis, and cystic areas. Infiltration of the surrounding tissue is usually apparent.

Microscopically, it resembles high grade ductal carcinoma of the breast. Ductal carcinoma in situ is often present, and frequently shows a cribriform pattern often with comedo-type necrosis (e-**Fig. 6.34**). The tumor's invasive component consists of large cells with abundant eosinophilic cytoplasm and large, round nuclei with vesicular chromatin and prominent nucleoli (e-**Fig. 6.35**). The neoplasm shows marked tissue infiltration with stromal desmoplasia and brisk mitotic activity, and vascular and perineural invasion are common. Salivary duct carcinomas express low- and high-molecular-weight cytokeratins, carcinoembryogenic antigen (CEA), androgen receptors, and human epidermal growth factor receptor 2 (HER2/neu), for which the gene is amplified in up to 1/3rd of cases. The differential diagnosis includes metastatic breast carcinoma, poorly differentiated squamous cell carcinoma, and mucoepidermoid carcinoma. The presence of intraductal carcinoma is an important finding that argues strongly for a diagnosis of a primary salivary duct carcinoma rather than metastasis.

Salivary duct carcinoma is the most aggressive salivary gland tumor. Approximately one-third of patients develop local recurrence, half develop distant metastases, and 65% of patients die of their disease, most within 4 years of diagnosis. Wide local excision with neck dissection and postoperative radiotherapy is the treatment of choice.

7. **Epithelial–myoepithelial carcinoma** is a low-grade carcinoma that accounts for 0.5% to 1% of salivary gland neoplasms. It arises in the parotid gland, and occasionally from the minor salivary glands of the larynx or paranasal sinuses.

   Grossly, the tumor is firm and well-demarcated, averaging 2 to 3 cm in diameter. Microscopically, the tumor is usually partially encapsulated, with invasion by tumor into the adjacent parenchyma. The classic morphology is of ductal structures lined by an inner layer of eosinophilic epithelial cells and an outer layer of clear myoepithelial cells (e-**Fig. 6.36**), which lie in an eosinophilic, hyaline stroma. In rare cases, the myoepithelial cell component may be present as large sheets or nests of cells with only focal ductal differentiation. The individual tumor cells are bland with minimal mitotic activity. The epithelial cells express low-molecular-weight cytokeratins, and the myoepithelial cells express calponin, smooth muscle actin, and p63. The differential diagnosis includes pleomorphic adenoma, myoepithelioma/myoepithelial carcinoma, and the tubular variant of adenoid cystic carcinoma.

   Epithelial–myoepithelial carcinoma is a moderately aggressive tumor with a recurrence rate of 40%. Metastases to lymph nodes, lung, or liver occur in 15% of patients, and overall survival at 5 years is about 80%. Treatment is wide local excision with or without radiotherapy.

8. **Squamous cell carcinomas** only rarely as primary tumors of the salivary gland. Metastases to the intraparotid lymph nodes from primary skin cancers of the head and neck, particularly of the scalp, ear, and face, are much more common. Most patients are in their sixth to eighth decades. About 80% of tumors arise in the parotid gland and 20% in the submandibular gland. The tumors typically are high stage at the time of diagnosis. By definition, the diagnosis of primary squamous cell carcinoma is restricted to the large salivary glands, because tumors arising in the minor salivary glands cannot be reliably distinguished from primary squamous carcinoma of the surrounding mucosa.

   Grossly, the neoplasm is a firm, white, infiltrative, and nonencapsulated mass. Microscopically, it is identical to typical squamous cell carcinomas of the UADT, although cases arising in a salivary gland tend to be well-differentiated. Prominent desmoplasia is common, and perineural invasion and extension of the tumor into periglandular soft tissue are frequently present.

The differential diagnosis most importantly includes metastatic squamous cell carcinoma. High-grade mucoepidermoid carcinoma can have a largely squamoid appearance but lacks keratinization, has a more heterogeneous cell population, and almost always demonstrates mucous cells.

Primary squamous carcinomas are aggressive tumors, and the 5-year survival of patients is approximately 25%. Treatment involves radical surgery, neck dissection, and radiotherapy.

9. **Malignant counterparts** to benign salivary gland tumors are relatively uncommon and microscopically resemble benign salivary gland tumors in differentiation and cellular components but show aggressive features such as an invasive growth, perineural invasion, lymphvascular invasion, cellular anaplasia, necrosis, and/or metastasis. The more common types are basal cell adenocarcinoma (e-**Fig. 6.37**) and myoepithelial carcinoma (e-**Fig. 6.38**), although the majority of benign salivary gland tumors have a reported malignant counterpart.

10. **Metastasis** to the salivary glands or, more commonly, to intra- or periglandular lymph nodes, is a frequent occurrence.

    The parotid contains an average of 20 lymph nodes which drain the scalp, face, ear skin, external auditory canal, and tympanic membrane. Skin tumors such as squamous cell carcinoma and melanoma, therefore, account for approximately 80% of metastases to the gland. The remaining metastases are from non–head and neck primary tumors, most commonly lung, kidney, and breast carcinomas.

    The opposite distribution of metastases is seen for the submandibular gland, which does not contain intraglandular lymph nodes. More than 85% of metastases arise from infraclavicular primary tumors, most commonly breast, kidney, and lung carcinomas, particularly pulmonary small cell carcinoma.

11. **Pediatric tumors** are uncommon. Hemangioma is the most frequent, but most salivary gland neoplasms that occur in adults can also occur in children. There are two congenital tumors that are worth mentioning here.

    a. **Sialoblastoma** is an extremely rare, potentially aggressive neoplasm that recapitulates the embryonic stage of salivary gland development and is thought to develop from retained blastomatous cells. Clinically, it is seen in the perinatal to the neonatal period, usually involving the parotid gland. This tumor may grow quickly and cause skin ulceration or airway compromise.

       Grossly, the mass is lobulated and partially circumscribed. Microscopically, it is composed of nests or nodules of basaloid cells with scanty cytoplasm, round to oval nuclei, and fine chromatin with small nucleoli. The mitotic rate is highly variable and can be quite high. Complete surgical excision with a rim of normal tissue is the treatment of choice. Although local recurrence is relatively common, occurring in up to 30% of cases, metastasis is extremely uncommon.

    b. **Salivary anlage tumor,** also referred to as a congenital pleomorphic adenoma, occurs in male neonates in the first 2 weeks of life and is associated with respiratory obstruction or difficulty feeding. Sometimes the mass is spontaneously passed or inadvertently removed by airway suctioning. On examination, a mass attached by a thin stalk to the posterior nasal mucosa or nasopharynx is sometimes present.

       Grossly, salivary anlage tumors are firm and tan-yellow with a smooth surface. Microscopically, the tumor's surface shows nonkeratinizing squamous epithelium, with a deeper stroma composed of bland spindled cells and intervening squamous islands. The overall histology suggests a hamartoma rather than a true neoplasm. The treatment is simple excision of the mass, and the lesion does not recur or spread.

TABLE 6.5 Tumor, Node, Metastasis (TNM) Staging Scheme for Tumors of the Major Salivary Glands

Primary tumor (T)

TX	Primary tumor cannot be assessed
T0	No evidence of primary tumor
T1	Tumor ≤2 cm in greatest dimension without extraparenchymal extension[a]
T2	Tumor >2 cm but not >4 cm in greatest dimension without extraparenchymal extension[a]
T3	Tumor >4 cm and/or tumor having extraparenchymal extension[a]
T4a	Moderately advanced disease####
	Tumor invades skin, mandible, ear canal, and/or facial nerve
T4b	Very advanced disease
	Tumor invades skull base and/or pterygoid plates and/or encases carotid artery

Regional lymph nodes (N)

NX	Regional lymph nodes cannot be assessed
N0	No regional lymph node metastasis
N1	Metastasis in a single ipsilateral lymph node, ≤3 cm in greatest dimension
N2a	Metastasis in a single ipsilateral lymph node, >3 cm but not >6 cm in greatest dimension
N2b	Metastasis in multiple ipsilateral lymph nodes, none more than 6 cm in greatest dimension
N2c	Metastasis in bilateral or contralateral lymph nodes, none >6 cm in greatest dimension
N3	Metastasis in a lymph node, >6 cm in greatest dimension

Distant metastasis (M)

MX	Distant metastasis cannot be assessed
M0	No distant metastasis
M1	Distant metastasis

Stage grouping

The overall pathologic AJCC stage is

Stage I	T1	N0	M0
Stage II	T2	N0	M0
Stage III	T3	N0	M0
Stage III	T1	N1	M0
Stage III	T2	N1	M0
Stage III	T3	N1	M0
Stage IVA	T4a	N0	M0
Stage IVA	T4a	N1	M0
Stage IVA	T1	N2	M0
Stage IVA	T2	N2	M0
Stage IVA	T3	N2	M0
Stage IVA	T4a	N2	M0
Stage IVB	T4b	Any N	M0
Stage IVB	Any T	N3	M0
Stage IVC	Any T	Any N	M1

[a] Note: Extraparenchymal extension is clinical or macroscopic evidence of invasion of soft tissues. Microscopic evidence alone does not constitute extraparenchymal extension for classification purposes. From: Edge SB, Byrd DR, Compton CC, et al., eds. *AJCC Cancer Staging Manual.* 7th ed. New York, NY: Springer; 2010. Used with permission.

V. PATHOLOGIC REPORTING OF MALIGNANT SALIVARY GLAND TUMORS

A. **Staging: American Joint Committee on Cancer (AJCC).** Clinical staging of salivary gland cancers is important for prognosis and treatment decisions. The 2010 Tumor, Node, Metastasis (TNM) AJCC staging classification is provided in Table 6.5. Minor salivary gland carcinomas are staged according to the anatomic site of origin (e.g., oral cavity, sinus, larynx). Staging guidelines are applicable to all forms of carcinoma. Any nonepithelial tumor type is excluded.

B. **Additional pertinent pathologic features.** Pathologic features such as tumor grade, positive resection margins, and skin or bone invasion have been demonstrated in numerous studies to correlate with a higher risk of local recurrence, a poorer prognosis, or both, and so should always be reported. Perineural and lymphovascular space invasion should also always be reported when observed, because they have been correlated with distant metastases in some studies, even though they are not necessarily correlated with recurrence or poorer prognosis.

Cytopathology of the Salivary Glands

Brian Collins

The parotid and minor salivary glands are superficially located and palpable, and so salivary gland lesions are readily amenable to percutaneous FNA. A pattern approach is typically utilized for the evaluation of FNA specimens for diagnosis, classification, and clinical management of patients.

I. NON-NEOPLASTIC CONDITIONS

A. **Chronic sialadenitis.** Chronic inflammation can cause diffuse or focal enlargement which by palpation can be indistinguishable from a neoplasm. However, chronic sialadenitis is very tender on FNA, which can be a helpful clue to diagnosis. Aspiration smears are hypocellular with benign ductal epithelial groups which have a minimal degree of nuclear atypia. Acinar elements can be scant or absent due to the underlying destructive nature of the process. A variable mixture of large and small lymphocytes is present. Acinic cell carcinoma is an important differential diagnostic consideration when presented with bland acinar–type cells and lymphocytes on aspirate smears.

B. **Lymph nodes.** The parotid is a common site of intra-parenchymal lymph nodes which can be clinically difficult to distinguish from a neoplasm. Aspirate smears will show a mixture of lymphocytes in the pattern typically seen with reactive lymphoid hyperplasia.

II. BENIGN NEOPLASMS

A. **Warthin tumor.** This tumor commonly arises in the parotid gland and by aspiration shows a mixture of lymphocytes and cohesive groups of oncocytic-type epithelial fragments (e-Figs. 6.39 and 6.40). The lymphoid elements are intimately admixed with the oncocytic cells, and the background usually shows cystic change and with macrophages and granular debris.

B. **Pleomorphic adenoma.** Aspiration smears can show a wide variety of patterns and cellular elements. Commonly, there is a mixture of bland epithelial, spindled, and myoepithelial-like cells which occur as single cells and are intimately admixed with a variable amount of fibromyxoid stroma (e-Figs. 6.41 and 6.42). The relative proportions of these elements can vary significantly between cases. Diff-Quik staining of smears helps to highlight the metachromatic fibromyxoid stroma. When present in the customary pattern, a definitive diagnosis can be rendered.

C. Basal cell adenoma. Aspiration smears are cellular and contain small uniform basaloid cells with scant cytoplasm and round to oval nuclei with indistinct nucleoli. The dense extracellular material present, usually less than that seen in pleomorphic adenoma, tends to be arranged in globules and trabecular–tubular configurations (e-**Fig. 6.43**). This pattern typically is classified as a basaloid neoplasm and the differential diagnosis includes adenoid cystic carcinoma, since the cytomorphologic pattern on aspiration does not permit definitive classification.

III. MALIGNANT NEOPLASMS

A. Adenoid cystic carcinoma. Aspiration shows small basaloid cells with globules of dense matrix material. The cells are monomorphic with round to oval nuclei, even chromatin, indistinct nucleoli, and scant cytoplasm. Aspirates are usually cellular with cell groups arranged in syncytial and three-dimensional fragments. The extracellular matrix consists of dense amorphous material with tubular and/or globular shapes (e-**Figs. 6.44** to **6.46**). Classically, the cells appear to surround the round globules. Because of the cytomorphologic overlap with other basaloid tumors, definitive classification is not possible.

B. Mucoepidermoid carcinoma. These neoplasms vary in their cellular composition, and this difference is reflected in the patterns and cellular elements encountered by FNA. For low-grade neoplasms, aspiration smears are hypocellular and contain thick mucoid-like material with granular debris. The three cell types that characterize the tumor (squamoid or epidermoid), mucous, and intermediate are all present, and they can be arranged separately or be admixed. The nuclear features of all three cell types are bland (e-**Figs. 6.47** and **6.48**). For high-grade neoplasms, aspirate smears are cellular with groups and sheets of cells with a squamoid appearance. Nuclei are large with coarse chromatin and prominent nucleoli; the cytoplasm is dense, and moderate in amount with well-defined cell borders. Mucin cells with intracytoplasmic vacuoles are usually few and can be difficult to identify (e-**Figs. 6.49** and **6.50**).

C. Acinic cell carcinoma. Aspirate smears are cellular with a mixture of single cells, small groups of cells, and three-dimensional clusters. The cells are intermediate in size with monomorphic round bland nuclei with nucleoli. The cytoplasm is critical in the diagnosis and will demonstrate features of acinar differentiation with delicate vacuoles and granules (e-**Figs. 6.51** and **6.52**). While usually clean, the background can show the features characteristic of cystic lesions and show significant lymphoid elements.

SUGGESTED READINGS

Eveson JW. Malignant neoplasms of the salivary glands. In: Thompson LDR, ed. *Head and Neck Pathology*. New York, NY: Churchill Livingstone; 2006.

Eveson JW, Auclair P, Gnepp DR, et al. Tumors of the salivary glands. In: Barnes L, Eveson JW, Reichart P, Sidransky D, eds. *Pathology and Genetics Head and Neck Tumors*. Lyon, France: IARC Press; 2005.

Faquin WC, Powers CN. *Salivary Gland Cytopathology: Essentials in Cytopathology*. New York, NY: Springer; 2008.

Gnepp DR, Henley JD, Simpson RHW, et al. Salivary and lacrimal glands. In: Gnepp DR, ed. *Diagnostic Surgical Pathology of the Head and Neck*. Philadelphia, PA: W.B. Saunders Publishers; 2009.

Layfield L. *Cytopathology of the Head and Neck*. Chicago: ASCP Press; 1997.

Powers CN, Frable WJ. *Fine Needle Aspiration Biopsy of the Head and Neck*. Boston: Butterworth Heinemann; 1996.

Richardson MS. Non-neoplastic lesions of the salivary glands. In: Thompson LDR, ed. *Head and Neck Pathology*. New York, NY: Churchill Livingstone; 2006.

Torske K. Benign neoplasms of the salivary glands. In: Thompson LDR, ed. *Head and Neck Pathology*. New York, NY: Churchill Livingstone; 2006.

Wenig BM. Major and minor salivary glands. In: Wenig BM, ed. *Atlas of Head and Neck Pathology*. Philadelphia, PA: Saunders Elsevier; 2008.

7 The Ear

Peter A. Humphrey and Rebecca D. Chernock

I. **NORMAL ANATOMY.** The ear is composed of the external ear, the middle ear, and the inner ear. The external ear is made up of the auricle, which leads to the external auditory canal. The auricle has a supporting plate of elastic cartilage, which also helps form the outer two-thirds of the external auditory canal. Skin covers both the auricle and the canal; the main distinctive histologic features of this skin are that the squamous lining of the inner half of the canal is thinned, and that modified apocrine glands called ceruminal glands are present in the outer third of the canal. The clustered ceruminal glands are lined by cuboidal epithelial cells that have an eosinophilic cytoplasm that often harbors a granular golden-yellow pigment (e-**Fig. 7.1**).*

The middle ear, or tympanic cavity, lies within the temporal bone. It is separated from the external auditory canal by the tympanic membrane, a thin fibrous sheet that has an external keratinizing squamous epithelial lining and an inner cuboidal cell lining. The middle ear contains the three auditory ossicles (malleus, incus, and stapes), ossicle ligaments, tendons of the ossicular muscles, the auditory tube, the tympanic cavity itself, and the epitympanic recess, the mastoid cavity, and the chorda tympani of the facial nerve (cranial nerve VII). The auditory or eustachian tube connects the tympanic cavity with the nasopharynx. The tympanic cavity is lined by a single layer of flattened to cuboidal respiratory epithelium, whereas most of the auditory tube is lined by low ciliated epithelium.

The inner ear is located within the petrous portion of the temporal bone and is composed of a membranous labyrinth surrounded by an osseous labyrinth. The membranous labyrinth houses the cochlea and the vestibular apparatus, both of which are supplied by cranial nerve VIII. There are several parts to the cochlea: the cochlear duct with the organ of Corti (the end organ of hearing), and the scala vestibuli and scala tympani, which hold the perilymph. The organ of Corti has thousands of neurotransmitting hair cells. The vestibular apparatus, which functions in motion and position sensing, consists of three semicircular canals and the utricle and the saccule. The ampullae of the canals have a sensory end organ, the crista ampullaris, with neurosensory hair cells. The utricle and the saccule also possess a sensory end organ, the macula, which has neurosensory hair cells and otoliths. There is also a blind sac in the membranous labyrinth known as the endolymphatic sac, which is lined by tall columnar epithelium arranged on papillae.

II. **GROSS EXAMINATION AND TISSUE SAMPLING**

A. **External ear.** Biopsy and excision specimens should be handled as skin specimens from other anatomic sites (see Chaps. 38–40).

B. **Middle and inner ear.** Samples from the middle ear are often obtained in cases of suspected cholesteatoma. For these cases, it should be noted whether bone fragments are present. Standard hematoxylin and eosin (H&E) slide preparation is sufficient. Ossicles from the middle ear can be processed by gross examination only unless microscopic examination is requested by the surgeon. For middle ear and inner ear neoplasms, which are uncommon, use of ink to mark the peripheral margins is not usually necessary because these specimens are typically received as small fragments. In those rare cases in which the patient has a history of

---

*All e-figures are available online via the Solution Site Image Bank.

lymphoma or lymphoma is suspected clinically, fresh tissue should be processed according to the standard lymphoma work-up protocol. For all other middle ear samples, all tissue should be submitted for histologic examination, with H&E slide generation.

III. COMMON DISEASES OF THE EXTERNAL EAR

A. **Nonneoplastic diseases.** The common diseases of skin that involve the pinna and the external ear canal are covered in the chapters on skin (Chaps. 38–40). Some diseases have a particular predilection for the skin of the ear, including gout, keloids (often secondary to ear piercing), relapsing polychondritis, angiolymphoid hyperplasia with eosinophilia (epithelioid or histiocytoid hemangioma), and chondrodermatitis nodularis (the latter is discussed below).

1. **Congenital anomalies of the ear** that may be seen by the surgical pathologist include accessory tragi, branchial cleft abnormalities, congenital aural sinuses, and salivary gland ectopia.

   a. **Accessory tragi** are found at birth and clinically and macroscopically are most often solitary, sessile, or pedunculated polyps in the preauricular area. Microscopically, skin, hair follicles, and a central fibrofatty core with or without cartilage are observed (e-**Fig. 7.2**). They should not be misdiagnosed as a papilloma, fibroma, or chondroma.

   b. **Anomalies of the first branchial cleft** present near the ear as cysts, sinuses, and fistulas. The epithelial lining can be squamous or respiratory; type I or pure squamous cell–lined cysts can be confused with keratinous cysts histologically. Lymphoid tissue in the wall (e-**Fig. 7.3**) is less frequently found in the first branchial cleft cysts than in the much more common second branchial cleft cysts, which arise in the lateral neck. Type II defects can harbor skin including adnexal structures or cartilage (e-**Fig. 7.4**); associated salivary gland tissue may also be present when the process extends into or near the parotid gland.

   c. **Congenital aural sinuses** are distinguished from branchial cleft anomalies by location: Branchial cleft abnormalities are found in infra- or postauricular sites, whereas congenital aural sinuses are present in a preauricular location.

2. **Chondrodermatitis nodularis helicis** is a condition of uncertain etiology that occurs on the skin of the external ear, usually on the upper part of the helix. Clinically, middle-aged or older, typically male, patients present with a small (<1 cm) painful nodule that can be ulcerated and can exhibit a crust. This appearance can clinically simulate actinic keratosis or squamous cell carcinoma. Microscopically, there is a somewhat funnel-shaped ulcer with associated dermal collagen edema and degeneration. There may be surrounding pseudoepitheliomatous squamous cell hyperplasia (e-**Fig. 7.5**), granulation tissue and fibrosis, and a predominantly lymphocytic inflammatory cell infiltrate, although the infiltrate can be mixed. A perichondritis with destruction of cartilage can be seen but is uncommon. Superficial or shave biopsies may show only a few of the above findings. Curettage and cautery are used for treatment, with recurrence in a minority of patients.

3. **Otitis externa** is inflammation of the external auditory canal and/or pinna and is very common in clinical practice. Biopsy is generally not indicated.

4. **Necrotizing (malignant) otitis externa** is usually caused by *Pseudomonas aeruginosa* infecting diabetic patients, but fungi can also be the causative agent. Microscopically, the response is one of necrotizing inflammation.

B. **Neoplasms of the external ear.** The 2005 World Health Organization (WHO) histologic classification of tumors of the ear is given in Table 7.1. The most common neoplasms of the external ear are **basal cell carcinoma** and **squamous cell carcinoma** of the skin of the ear. Of the tumors of the external ear, only

TABLE 7.1   The 2005 WHO Histologic Classification of Tumors of the Ear

Tumors of the external ear
Benign tumors of ceruminous glands
   Adenoma
   Chondroid syringoma
   Syringocystadenoma papilliferum
Cylindroma
Malignant tumors of ceruminous glands
   Adenocarcinoma
   Adenoid cystic carcinoma
   Mucoepidermoid carcinoma
Squamous cell carcinoma
Embryonal rhabdomyosarcoma
Osteoma and exostosis
Angiolymphoid hyperplasia with eosinophilia

Tumors of the middle ear
Adenoma of the middle ear
Papillary tumors
   Aggressive papillary tumor
   Schneiderian papilloma
   Inverted papilloma
Squamous cell carcinoma
Meningioma

Tumors of the inner ear
Vestibular schwannoma
Lipoma of the internal auditory canal
Hemangioma
Endolymphatic sac tumor
Hematolymphoid tumors
B-cell chronic lymphocytic leukemia/small lymphocytic lymphoma
Langerhans cell histiocytosis

Secondary tumors

From: Barnes L, Eveson J, Reichart P, Sidransky D, eds. *World Health Organization Classification of Tumours. Pathology and Genetics. Head and Neck Tumours.* Lyon: IARC Press: 2005. Used with permission.

the rare ceruminous gland tumors are specific for this site and are discussed below.

1. **Benign ceruminous gland tumors** include ceruminous adenoma, chondroid syringoma, and syringocystadenoma papilliferum. The latter two entities have the same histopathologic features as when they occur at other sites. Ceruminous adenomas are rare, and are seen in adult patients who present with a painless mass of the outer half of the external auditory canal (*Am J Surg Pathol.* 2004;28:308). Grossly, they are 0.4- to 4-cm polypoid growths. Microscopically, there are regular oxyphilic glands and small cysts lined by an inner ceruminous cell layer and an outer spindled to cuboidal myoepithelial cell layer (**e-Fig. 7.6**). Cerumen pigment, cytokeratin (CK)7 expression in ceruminal cells, and p63 and CK5/6 expression in the myoepithelial cells can be helpful in the distinction from adenocarcinoma and middle ear adenoma. There is about a 10% recurrence rate, which is associated with incomplete excision.

2. **Malignant tumors of ceruminous glands** include adenocarcinoma, adenoid cystic carcinoma, and mucoepidermoid carcinoma. The latter two are histologically identical to those arising in salivary glands. Ceruminous adenocarcinomas show infiltrative growth and range from cytologically bland to markedly atypical with an increase in mitotic activity. Perineural invasion is uncommon, but can be a useful diagnostic clue favoring adenocarcinoma when detected, especially in small biopsy samples. Ceruminous adenocarcinomas are locally aggressive.

3. **Other unusual neoplasms and tumorlike conditions of the external ear** include malignant melanoma, benign fibro-osseous lesion, osteoma and exostosis, and idiopathic pseudocystic chondromalacia (which is a nonneoplastic swelling of the pinna due to fluid accumulation within the cartilage of the ear).

IV. COMMON DISEASES OF THE MIDDLE EAR

A. **Nonneoplastic middle ear diseases.** The common disorders include choristoma, inflammation, infection, cholesterol granuloma, cholesteatoma, and otosclerosis.

1. **Choristomas** (heterotopic tissues) in the middle ear are composed of benign salivary gland, glial, or sebaceous gland tissue. Glial heterotopia is histologically identical to the more commonly occurring encephalocele; the two must be distinguished clinically (e-**Fig. 7.7A** and **B**).

2. **Otitis media** is one of the most common diseases of childhood. Most acute purulent cases are due to bacterial infection by *Streptococcus pneumoniae* or *Haemophilus influenzae*. Tissue samples are not usually procured, but in chronic cases tissue may be removed. Microscopically, granulation tissue, scar tissue, chronic inflammation, calcific debris, and sclerotic or reactive bone can be seen. Occasionally, neutrophils and foreign body–type giant cells are present. There may be associated polypoid granulation tissue, cholesterol granulomas, cholesteatoma, or tympanosclerosis. Entrapped metaplastic glands should not be mistaken for neoplastic glands.

3. **Cholesterol granulomas** are found in a number of chronic ear diseases. Cholesterol clefts, a foreign body–type giant cell reaction, and hemosiderin deposition are characteristic (e-**Fig. 7.8**).

4. **Cholesteatoma** may be congenital or acquired (*Eur Arch Otorhinolaryngol.* 2004;261:6). The congenital form is found in infants and young children, is defined as occurring in the presence of an intact tympanic membrane, and may result from an epidermoid cell rest (epidermoid formation). In the more common acquired form, seen mainly in older children and adults, there is an association with severe otitis media and a perforated tympanic membrane. Histologically, there are three major elements: keratin (e-**Figs. 7.9** and **7.10**), stratified squamous epithelium, and fibrous and/or granulation tissue. Since squamous epithelium is not normally found in the middle ear, the diagnosis is usually straightforward. Downgrowth of the epithelium into underlying subepidermal connective tissue may be appreciated. Marked vascular congestion and abscess formation may also be found. Cholesteatoma is not a neoplasm, but can be locally destructive; ossicle(s) and the bony wall of the middle ear can be eroded. There is an increased cell proliferation index in the squamous epithelium of cholesteatoma (*Acta Otolaryngol.* 2003;123:377) and overexpression of cathepsin enzymes (*Laryngoscope.* 2003;113:808), abnormalities that may be related to the local growth but are not required for diagnosis.

5. **Otosclerosis** is a disease of unknown etiology that leads to progressive fixation of the stapes footplate and, as a result, conductive hearing loss. The onset is typically in adulthood and women are more often affected than men.

The initial histologic changes include resorption of bone and replacement by cellular fibrovascular tissue. Over time, this is replaced by dense sclerotic bone (e-Fig. 7.11). Patients are treated with stapedectomy.

B. **Neoplasms of the middle ear** include paraganglioma, adenoma of the middle ear, papillary tumors, meningioma, and squamous cell carcinoma (Table 7.1).

1. **Paraganglioma** (also known as glomus tumor, glomus tympanicum, or chemodectoma) is the most common tumor of the middle ear (but is nonetheless still rare). It usually presents clinically with hearing loss or tinnitus in patients in the fifth and sixth decades of life. The neoplasm can be solitary or part of a familial paraganglioma–pheochromocytoma syndrome caused by germline mutations in *SDHB, SDHC,* or *SDHD* genes; the head and neck paragangliomas in this syndrome are bilateral/multicentric. Clinically, paraganglioma is bulging, red, pink, or bluish (and not white like a cholesteatoma). Biopsy may result in brisk bleeding.

   Microscopically, sections usually demonstrate the classical "zellballen" appearance with nests of small uniform epithelioid cells that have a peripheral layer of flattened cells (e-Figs. 7.12 and 7.13). Sclerosis and vascularity can be pronounced in some tumors; in the former circumstance, the nested pattern may not be apparent (e-Fig. 7.14). Immunohistochemical stains can be confirmatory and particularly contributory in small biopsy samples, which may display significant crush artifact. Chromogranin A and synaptophysin immunostains are positive, whereas carcinoembryogenic antigen and keratin immunostains are negative. Only a few S-100–positive peripheral sustentacular cells may be present. These tumors grow slowly and can recur after surgery and/or radiation treatment. Intracranial extension develops in a small minority of patients, and about 1% to 2% of patients suffer from metastatic spread. It is not possible to predict aggressive behavior based on histopathologic features.

2. **Adenoma of the middle ear** is a benign glandular neoplasm with variable neuroendocrine and mucin-secreting differentiation (*Arch Pathol Lab Med.* 2006;130:1067). The typical clinical presentation is in an adult (mean age in the 40s) with muffled hearing, tinnitus, and/or a sensation of pressure and/or fullness. The neoplasms are variably colored and only uncommonly penetrate through the tympanic membrane. Microscopic architectural patterns include closely packed small glands with solid and/or trabecular arrangements (e-Fig. 7.15). The glands lack a myoepithelial layer. Cytologically, the cuboidal to columnar glandular cells are bland, with uniform small nuclei and rare nucleoli (e-Fig. 7.16). Mitoses should not be present. The immunoprofile includes positivity for cytokeratin and neuroendocrine markers such as chromogranin and synaptophysin. In the past, this immunophenotype was viewed as being indicative of a carcinoid tumor of the middle ear, but it is now recognized that expression of neuroendocrine markers is a characteristic feature of most middle ear adenomas. Recurrence has been reported in a small minority of cases, usually after incomplete surgical excision.

3. **Papillary tumors of the middle ear** include aggressive papillary tumor, Schneiderian papilloma, and inverted papilloma, although only a few cases of the latter two neoplasms have been described. Aggressive papillary tumors are more common (*Adv Anat Pathol.* 2006;13:131), and are also known as low-grade papillary adenocarcinomas and endolymphatic sac tumors (Heffner tumor). Typically, patients in their fourth decade present with hearing difficulty and vertigo; 15% of patients have a family history of von Hippel–Lindau syndrome. Microscopically, there are complex interdigitating papillae with fibrous cores covered by cuboidal to columnar cells that have bland nuclear cytology and eosinophilic cytoplasm. Mitoses are absent. The papillae may

overlie the granulation tissue causing diagnostic confusion with reactive processes. Cystic spaces with a colloid-like material simulating thyroid follicles can also be present. Immunostains show positivity for keratin, with variable S-100, glial fibrillary acid protein (GFAP), and synaptophysin immunoreactivity; thyroglobulin immunostaining is negative. Despite the bland histologic appearance, the tumor is a slowly growing, locally aggressive, but nonmetastasizing neoplasm. Temporal bone invasion is common, and the tumor may extend into the cerebellum. Outcome is related to size of the tumor and adequacy of excision; radical surgical excision affords the best chance for cure. Recurrence is seen in about 20% of cases, with tumor-specific death in about 13% of patients.

4. **Meningioma** in the middle ear is a rare neoplasm that is more likely to represent secondary extension from an intracranial meningioma than from a primary middle ear meningioma. Patients with primary middle ear meningiomas present at a mean age of 50 years with hearing changes and sometimes otitis and pain (*Mod Pathol.* 2003;16:236). The histopathologic features are similar to intracranial meningiomas, with meningothelial meningioma predominating (**e-Fig. 7.17**). Vimentin, progesterone receptor, and epithelial membrane antigen immunostains are positive, and cytokeratin immunostains are negative. Meningiomas are slowly growing neoplasms and can recur following incomplete surgical excision. The 5-year survival is 83%.

5. **Squamous cell carcinoma** in the middle ear is uncommon and is typically advanced at presentation. Its development is not clearly related to chronic otitis media and is not related to cholesteatoma. Microscopically, the carcinoma is keratinizing and displays a variable degree of differentiation. Outcome is related to tumor extent and margin status at surgery, but not histologic grade. The 5-year survival is roughly 50% (*Int J Radiat Oncol Biol Phys.* 2007;68:1326).

6. **Other rare neoplasms of the middle ear** include embryonal rhabdomyosarcoma (**e-Fig. 7.18**), lipoma, hemangioma, osteoma, ossifying fibroma, and teratoma.

7. **Metastasis** to the ear is uncommon, accounting for only 2% to 6% of all neoplasms of the ear. Most patients have known, widely disseminated cancer. The middle ear is the most common site for metastatic spread. Breast, lung, and prostate are, in order, the common primary sites of origin for the metastatic deposits.

V. **NEOPLASMS OF THE INNER EAR.** Vestibular schwannoma, lipoma, and hemangioma are the most common neoplasms of the inner ear. Endolymphatic sac tumors also arise in the inner ear (the aforementioned aggressive papillary tumor of the middle ear is thought to represent an endolymphatic sac tumor with extension into the middle ear).

A. **Vestibular schwannoma (acoustic neuroma)** is relatively common. Unilateral vestibular schwannoma accounts for 5% to 10% of all intracranial tumors, and has been found in about 1% of autopsies. Bilateral vestibular schwannoma, found in 5% of all vestibular schwannoma cases, is characteristic of neurofibromatosis type 2 (an autosomal dominant disease due to mutations in the *NF2* gene on 22q12). Patients, usually in their 40s or 50s, present with progressive hearing loss and tinnitus. Grossly, the size range of the tumor is a few millimeters up to 6 cm in maximal dimension. The smaller tumors are round to oval, whereas large tumors can assume a mushroom shape. The cut surfaces are yellow, and can exhibit hemorrhage and cystic change. Microscopically, the attributes are the same as in soft tissue schwannomas (**e-Fig. 7.19**), with Antoni A regions with Verocay bodies, and Antoni B areas. Mitotic figures should be rare. Degenerative nuclear atypia should not be taken as a sign of malignancy. S-100 immunoreactivity is strong.

B. Lipomas of the internal auditory canal resemble lipomas at other anatomic sites, except that cranial nerve VII or VIII or their branches may be present in the lipoma.

SUGGESTED READINGS

Barnes L. The ear. In: Silverberg SG, ed in chief, *Silverberg's Principles and Practices of Surgical Pathology and Cytopathology*. Philadelphia, PA: Churchill Livingstone Elsevier; 2006:2268–2287.

Barnes L, Eveson JW, Reichart P, Sidransky D, eds. Tumors of the Ear, Chapter 7. In: *Pathology and Genetics Head and Neck Tumours*. Lyon, France: IARC Press; 2005.

Wenig BM. Diseases of the External Ear, Middle Ear and Temporal Bone. Chapter 9. In: Barnes L, ed. *Surgical Pathology of the Head and Neck*. New York, NY: Informa Healthcare; 2009:423–474.

Thorax

Lung
Jon H. Ritter and Hannah R. Krigman

I. **NORMAL ANATOMY.** The lung is defined by airway branching, first into right and left lobes, then segments, and finally, the functional unit of the lung, the lobule. Arteries follow the airways, while veins and lymphatics flow toward lobular septa and finally to the hilum and main pulmonary veins. Bronchi are lined by a pseudostratified respiratory epithelium that includes goblet cells, which is separated by basement membrane from a delicate submucosa. Larger airways have a smooth muscle wall that contains minor salivary glands and a cartilaginous skeleton; bronchioles have lost the latter components. Each lobule has a central bronchovascular bundle; the interstitial space between the pulmonary artery branches and the bronchioles is eventually continuous with the alveolar interstitium. Lymph nodes occur within the lung, and also are discontinuous along the bronchi.

   Progressive branching of the airways leads to the alveolar ducts, from which alveoli spring. Normal alveolar walls are very delicate and have a fine elastic tissue matrix. The barrier between the blood in capillaries and air in the alveolar space consists of the endothelial cell, the basement membrane, the wispy alveolar interstitium, epithelial cell basement membrane, and the flattened type 1 pneumocyte. Type 2 pneumocytes can proliferate to replace injured type 1 cells.

   The visceral pleura consists of an inner vascular layer that abuts the alveolar tissue, a connective tissue layer, and an outer layer of mesothelium. The visceral pleura is reflected back at the hilum and becomes continuous with the parietal pleural layer that lines the chest cavity.

II. **SPECIMEN HANDLING AND REPORTING**

   A. **Samples.** Biopsies of lung tissue for diagnosis are obtained endoscopically (transbronchial or endobronchial biopsy), via radiologically guided procedures (usually needle core biopsies), or for peripheral disease, via wedge biopsies. Resections can involve a single lobe (lobectomy), two lobes (bilobectomy), or an entire lung (pneumonectomy.)

   B. **Gross examination and sampling**

   1. **Endoscopic biopsies** are usually submitted in a single cassette. The fragments are small; use of a nylon mesh bag or a filter paper wrap is preferable to submission on biopsy sponges since tissue can be compressed or lost in the pores of sponges. The number of fragments, range of size, and color should be recorded. Three hematoxylin and eosin stained levels should be examined. For smaller biopsies, additional unstained levels may be cut at the time of initial sectioning in case special stains are needed.

Core biopsies of nodules presumed to represent neoplasms are obtained under CT guidance. They should be processed as for endoscopic biopsies.

2. **Wedge resections** are performed for either non-neoplastic or neoplastic processes. The specimen should be measured in three dimensions and weighed. Assessment of alveolar architecture may be improved by gently inflating the specimen by injection of formalin at multiple sites. If the specimen is inflated, the gross description should include this fact. Wedge biopsies generally have multiple staple lines, which should be cut off as close to the staples as possible; ideally, sections are taken perpendicular to the staple line. The entire specimen should be submitted in non-neoplastic cases; levels are usually not necessary. If the specimen is obtained for diagnosis of a neoplasm, the presence and dimensions of any masses should be described, as well as the distance to the staple line(s).

3. **Lung resections** should be described as lobectomy, bilobectomy, or right or left pneumonectomy. The specimen should be measured in three dimensions and weighed. Any additional designation by the surgeon (e.g., sutures) should be described. If a portion of chest wall is attached to the specimen, its size in three dimensions and the number of ribs or other attached structures should be noted. For lobectomy and pneumonectomy specimens, insufflation by injection of formalin into the bronchial orifices improves fixation and visualization of changes. Occasionally, obstruction of bronchi by tumor makes this technique ineffective, in which case the lung can be expanded by injection of formalin at multiple sites. The pleural surface should be described; areas of puckering, dullness, or adhesions should be noted, as should adhesions of lobes together in multilobe resections. Areas of pleural distortion over a mass should be marked with ink. The hilar area should be examined and the number and size of bronchial stumps noted. The lung can be sectioned in either parasagittal or in coronal planes; it is important to choose planes to highlight the extent of tumor, pleural invasion, invasion of adjacent structures, proximity to the hilum, and relationship to major airways and vessels. At least four sections of tumor should be taken, including one or two with the closest pleural surface (which may be at the hilum). If tumor is invading structures such as a rib, chest wall, or mediastinal soft tissue, a section that shows tumor in the lung in continuity with the involved structure should be taken. Other sections should include normal appearing lung, areas distal to the tumor that show obstructive pneumonia, and any additional nodules or lesions. Vascular and bronchial margins, hilar lymph nodes, and peribronchial lymph nodes should be submitted as well.

C. **Adjunct Information.** For both non-neoplastic and neoplastic samples, the radiographic findings are an important adjunct to diagnosis. Either review the radiograph directly, or review its interpretation; old films may provide information on the pace of disease. The distribution of abnormalities, the presence of lymphadenopathy, and the extent of disease all contribute to the final diagnosis. For non-neoplastic cases, a review of the clinical history, including the presence of systemic illnesses, medications, exposures; laboratory data including cultures and serologic studies; and pulmonary function tests all assists in interpretation of the findings.

D. **Microscopic description**

1. A description of small biopsies includes the number of pieces and their constituent elements: alveolar tissue, bronchial wall, alveolar tissue, and superficial detached fragments of epithelium. The number of fragments is not insignificant; six fragments are considered to be representative of lung. The low power impression of normal or abnormal alveolar architecture should be included. Expansion of the alveolar septa may be by inflammatory tissue, cellular tissue, or acellular fibrosis. Alveolar spaces may be

empty, or filled with blood, histocytes, or exudates. The vasculature may be unremarkable, thickened, show inflammation or vasculitis, or contain tumor or thromboemboli. The bronchial epithelium can be columnar, squamous, or dysplastic. The absence or presence and type of granulomas should be described. Inflammatory cells should be noted and characterized as to type and distribution, whether alveolar, septal, peribronchial, perivascular, or diffuse. The results of special stains for organisms or fibrosis should be reported.

Biopsies for a neoplasm should include the same quantitation of the biopsy fragments as for non-neoplastic samples, as well as a description of the neoplasm. An in situ or dysplastic component should be described, if present. Detectable vascular space invasion should be noted.

2. The pathology report of wedge resections for non-neoplastic processes should contain the same information as for smaller biopsies, but should also include additional assessment of larger airways and vessels, and distribution of any non-neoplastic processes. Fibrosis, for example, can be diffuse, peripheral, or sparing the periphery. Similarly, inflammation or granulomas can be perivascular, peribronchial, or distributed along septa.

3. Definitive resections of neoplasms, from wedge resections to pneumonectomies, should provide as much information as possible. Prior sampling (endoscopic biopsy, mediastinoscopies, or previous wedge resections) and prior treatment (chemotherapy or irradiation) should be included in the pathology report. Margins should be evaluated, and the non-neoplastic lung should be described.

III. NON-NEOPLASTIC DISEASE

A. **Acute lung injury patterns.** When evaluating lung biopsies taken for medical diseases, identification of patterns of acute lung injury should be a major point of emphasis. These patterns represent the response of the lung to an acute injury, and immediately switch the diagnostic considerations away from the chronic fibrosing interstitial lung diseases. The commonly recognized patterns of acute lung injury include diffuse alveolar damage (DAD), bronchiolitis obliterans/organizing pneumonia, and acute interstitial pneumonia (AIP). All three processes share key findings: they all feature fibrosis characterized by loose, fibroblast-rich, new fibrous tissue; they are temporally uniform; and they may be potentially reversible, at least before significant collagen fibrosis develops.

1. **DAD** is the prototypical pattern of acute lung injury (**e-Fig. 8.1**).* It is the pattern of histologic changes underlying the clinical syndrome of acute respiratory distress syndrome (ARDS), the clinical triad of diffuse lung infiltrates, hypoxemia, and decreased pulmonary compliance. DAD has myriad causes, as detailed in Table 8.1. DAD is caused by cellular injury to pulmonary epithelial and endothelial cells. The initial insult causes edema from leaky capillaries, and the sloughed cellular material and fibrinous exudate form hyaline membranes; there is often surprisingly little inflammation in this early phase, known as the exudative stage. By six to seven days after the initializing injury, the edema and hyaline membranes begin to disappear, and hyperplastic and regenerative type 2 pneumocytes are prominent. By seven days, the process of organization is well underway, with interstitial and airspace fibroblastic proliferations; this stage is known as the proliferative or organizing phase. During organization, the alveolar exudates may be incorporated into the alveolar wall if proliferating type 2 pneumocytes grow on top of the exudate rather than along original alveolar basement membrane. Likewise, alveolar collapse may lead to further remodeling of prior

---

*Alle-figures are available online via the Solution Site Image Bank.

TABLE 8.1	Etiology of Diffuse Alveolar Damage
Category	**Selected agents**
Infectious	Viruses
	Mycoplasma
	Other infections in immunocompromised patients
Inhaled toxins	Oxygen
	Smoke
Drugs	Chemotherapeutic agents
	Amiodarone
	Nitrofurantoin
Shock	Traumatic
	Cardiogenic
	Other
Sepsis	Any organism
Miscellaneous	Radiation
	Burns
	Cardiopulmonary bypass
	Pancreatitis
	Lupus

airspaces. This process of organization and fibrosis may resolve at some point, or can continue along the path of fibrosis leading to the appearance of honeycomb lung within 3–4 weeks.

The hallmark of biopsies with DAD is spatial and temporal uniformity; that is, the process is similar across all areas of the tissue because the inciting injury is diffuse. By the time most patients are sick enough to come to biopsy, this process has been present for at least several days, and hence is in the organizing phase. A search for such etiologic clues as viral inclusions or fungus by silver stains is important, but the identification of the etiology for DAD is generally a clinicopathologic correlation exercise. When patients recover, they may be essentially normal, or may be left with some degree of lung impairment. Trichrome or similar stains may be helpful when reviewing these biopsies. Cases that show cellular fibrosis but in which trichrome stains do not show significant collagen deposition are thought to be reversible; however, once significant collagen is present in the areas of fibrosis, the process is not likely to resolve.

2. **AIP** is histologically similar to DAD, but has no definable cause and could thus also be considered as idiopathic DAD. The patients, often young adults, present with rapid onset of respiratory failure. There is often a history of a flu-like illness, and some studies have suggested that a Herpes-like virus may be present in some cases. By the time patients come to biopsy, the lung almost always shows a picture identical to that of organizing phase DAD. Most patients die of disease within 2 months. This rapid form of interstitial lung disease was classically described as Hamman–Rich syndrome.

3. **Bronchiolitis obliterans-organizing pneumonia (BOOP)** is another manifestation of acute lung injury (e-Fig. 8.2). Some authors now advocate the substitution of the term cryptogenic organizing pneumonia (COP). Causes are detailed in Table 8.2. Idiopathic cases tend to present in older adults with fever, cough, and some dyspnea; there may be an antecedent respiratory infection. Radiographs show patchy, peripheral air-space filling opacities that may appear in different areas of the lung over time. Histologic sections show a very distinctive pattern of immature fibroblastic tissue within

TABLE 8.2	Process Associated with Bronchiolitis Obliterans-Organizing Pneumonia (BOOP) Response

- Idiopathic BOOP
- Collagen Vascular diseases
- Toxins
- Organizing infection
- Proximity to a variety of space-occupying lesions including neoplasms, granulomas, infarcts, and abscesses
- Distal to bronchiectasis
- Acute infection
- Immune mediated pneumonidites

terminal bronchioles and alveolar ducts, which often has an elongated or hook-like configuration; these are often referred to as Masson bodies and can also be seen in peribronchiolar alveolar spaces. Because of the luminal filling of terminal bronchioles, there is often an associated localized obstructive pneumonia in the form of accumulation of lipid-filled macrophages. Since BOOP is centered on terminal airways, low-power views of wedge biopsies show a somewhat nodular configuration in contrast to the diffuse nature of injury in DAD. Thus, BOOP shares the temporal uniformity of DA, but not the homogeneous spatial appearance; nonetheless, the basic lesion of epithelial and endothelial cell injury is identical to that seen in DAD. It is important to emphasize that many, if not most, cases of BOOP are secondary to some other process. Consequently, the finding of a pattern of BOOP on a biopsy should lead to a careful search of the tissue for lesions that can be associated with BOOP, such as granulomas, vasculitis, or viral inclusions indicative of viral infection.

While the distinction between nodular versus diffuse involvement (and consequently, distinction between BOOP and DAD/AIP) may be obvious in wedge biopsies, transbronchial biopsies may show features such as organizing airspace fibrosis and type 2 pneumocyte hyperplasia without a clear indication of the spatial distribution of the process. In such cases, a more generic diagnosis of "organizing acute lung injury" may be used. This conveys the essential information for patient care—that is, the diagnosis defines the patient as having an acute injury with attendant lung response, as opposed to a chronic idiopathic interstitial lung disease.

B. Idiopathic Interstitial Pneumonitis

1. **Usual interstitial pneumonitis (UIP)** is the prototypical chronic interstitial pneumonitis. It is so named because it represents the underlying pathology in at least 80% of cases that fall under the clinical term of idiopathic pulmonary fibrosis. UIP is most often a disease of older adults, but has been reported in all age groups, including children. By the time of diagnosis, patients have often had several years of slowly developing shortness of breath. Pulmonary function tests show restrictive disease corresponding to the small lungs seen by chest X-ray examination. CT scans demonstrate honeycombing, most commonly at the lung bases and lung periphery, as well as traction bronchiectasis (e-**Fig. 8.3**). Gross examination shows coarse sponge-like lung corresponding to the honeycombing seen on radiograph. Microscopically, the disease is characterized by spatial and temporal heterogeneity. Temporal heterogeneity refers to the coexistence of old honeycomb scars (defined as cystic spaces lined by bronchiolar type epithelium) with areas of ongoing fibrosis (fibroblastic foci). The fibroblastic foci represent small areas of developing fibrosis, consistent with the insidious progression

of this disease. Acute inflammation is often restricted to the honeycomb areas, which may contain mucoid debris. Spatial heterogeneity refers to the finding that the most severe fibrosis is in the subpleural areas and along lobular septa; more central parts of the pulmonary lobule typically show less severe disease. Chronic inflammation is mild and patchy within areas of fibrosis; autoimmune or connective tissue disorders (CTDs) should be considered in cases with more extensive chronic inflammation. Related changes in the lung include secondary pulmonary hypertension and type II pneumocyte hyperplasia. The clinical course both before and after diagnosis is variable; most patients die within five years of diagnosis, although some patients have a more protracted course. In the process known as acute exacerbation of UIP, histologic sections show DAD superimposed on a background of UIP; the precise etiology for acute exacerbation of UIP is not known (which parallels the fact that the etiology of UIP itself is generally unknown).

2. **Non-specific interstitial pneumonitis (NSIP)** is the second most common form of idiopathic interstitial pneumonitis. As with UIP, patients tend to be middle aged or older adults. Many patients have underlying CTDs such as rheumatoid arthritis or lupus. Pulmonary function tests show a restrictive pattern. CT scans disclose significant differences from those in UIP; honeycombing is rarely a prominent feature in NSIP, but ground glass opacities, linear opacities, and small nodular infiltrates are frequently present (e-**Fig. 8.4**).

   Microscopically, the process has a more homogeneous appearance than UIP. Biopsies usually lack subpleural accentuation, but instead show more uniform involvement of both central and peripheral parts of the lobule. The process is generally more cellular than UIP with a mixed interstitial acute and chronic inflammatory infiltrate. Cases may show features of organizing pneumonia or BOOP, and small non-descript granulomas may be seen in some cases. Honeycombing, if seen on microscopic sections, is usually more focal and should not be a dominant pattern. The forgoing findings are characteristic of the cellular or mixed patterns of NSIP; since they bear significant resemblance to processes such as chronic hypersensitivity pneumonia or unresolved or slowly resolving organizing pneumonia, it is not clear that cases labeled as NSIP do not represent some unusual variants of the latter groups. A third pattern of NSIP, namely the sclerotic variant, consists of hyaline-like interstitial fibrosis. Although the full characterization of NSIP is still evolving, the one unifying feature of NSIP is that the patients survive longer, and with less disability than those patients whose biopsies show UIP.

3. **Desquamative interstitial pneumonia and related lesions (DIP)** is a rare form of interstitial pneumonia characterized by abundant macrophage exudates that fill the alveolar spaces. In most patients, this process is related to cigarette smoking, although rare examples have been reported in non-smokers; most patients are middle aged to older adults. Radiographic studies are dominated by ground glass opacities reflective of the filling of alveolar spaces, and microscopic sections feature dramatic filling of the alveolar spaces by macrophages, which tend to be light brown due to smoking-related pigment (e-**Fig. 8.5**). DIP is spatially homogeneous in that virtually any microscopic field from involved lung will show identical features. The alveolar walls may be thin and delicate, or may show some mild inactive hyaline fibrosis. Honeycomb changes are rare. DIP has an excellent prognosis; in cases related to cigarette use, the primary therapy is smoking cessation.

   Less dramatic findings along the same spectrum of smoking-related changes include respiratory bronchiolitis (RB) and respiratory bronchiolitis associated interstitial lung disease (RB-ILD). RB shows similar macrophages as in DIP, but limited to the lumen of terminal airways; it is often most prominent in the upper lobes and is thought to be the precursor of centriacinar emphysema (e-**Fig. 8.6**). RB-ILD is similar with the addition of mild interstitial fibrosis surrounding the terminal bronchioles.

4. **Lymphoid interstitial pneumonitis (LIP)** is another rare idiopathic form of interstitial pneumonitis. LIP can occur in patients of any age. When LIP occurs in children, it is often a harbinger of HIV infection; similarly, LIP has been described in immunocompromised patients as a manifestation of EBV infection. Some cases of LIP are related to Sjögren syndrome. Chest radiographs demonstrate infiltrates of a variety of patterns. Microscopically, there is diffuse expansion of the pulmonary interstitium by a mixed inflammatory cell infiltrate that includes small lymphocytes, plasma cells, germinal centers, and histiocytes. There may be some associated interstitial fibrosis. Many cases previously described as LIP likely represent examples of pulmonary MALToma or related neoplasms. Immunostains should show a mixed pattern of CD3-positive T-cells and CD20-positive B-cells. In cases of suspected LIP, flow cytometry or molecular studies to assess clonality are very useful to exclude lymphoma.

5. **Giant cell interstitial pneumonitis** is very rare. Most cases are now known to represent a reaction to various heavy metals. Consequently, optimum diagnosis is made by the combination of accurate history and spectrophotometric analysis of lung tissue.

6. **Smoking-related interstitial fibrosis (SRIF)** is a recent addition to list of smoking-related lung diseases (*Hum Pathol.* 2010;41:316–325). SRIF is often found in lobectomy specimens of resected lung carcinomas, in patients with no pre-operative clinical symptoms or imaging diagnosis of interstitial lung disease. The fibrosis typically has a hyaline or sclerotic appearance that somewhat resembles the sclerotic form of NSIP. Also, the fibrosis is usually superimposed on significant emphysema.

C. **Other non-infectious, non-neoplastic pulmonary processes**

1. **Connective tissue disorders.** Lung involvement in CTDs is extremely common and variable. Prominent patterns of involvement for selected disorders are summarized in Table 8.3. There is significant overlap among these entities and assignment to a specific entity should not be made on the basis of pulmonary findings. Also, many of the lung findings in CTDs overlap with the idiopathic interstitial lung diseases.

2. **Drug-induced pulmonary changes.** Prominent pathologic findings associated with drug reactions are listed in Table 8.4. It is clear from this list that drug reactions can mimic virtually any non-neoplastic condition, which emphasizes the need for accurate history and correlation with the clinical setting.

   a. **Amiodarone.** Perhaps 5%–10% of patients treated with amiodarone experience a pulmonary complication. The drug inhibits phospholipase, so the hallmark of exposure is accumulation of phospholipids, which in the lung manifests as accumulations of foamy macrophages (e-**Fig. 8.7**); note that accumulation of foamy macrophages is seen in almost all patients on the drug to varying degrees, and does not by itself indicate toxicity. Toxicity occurs as early as 1 month after initiation of therapy, with an average of 10–12 months, and is associated with higher doses. Patients present with a variety of symptoms, such as cough, dyspnea, chest pain, fever, and myalgias. Radiographs can show a mixture of airspace infiltrates, interstitial disease, or even isolated collections. Microscopically, toxicity has several manifestations, including a cellular chronic interstitial pneumonitis characterized by chronic inflammation in the interstitium, pneumocyte hyperplasia, and fibrosis; foamy alveolar

TABLE 8.3 Pulmonary Manifestations of Connective Tissue Disorders

Disease	Pleural changes	Pulmonary changes
Rheumatoid Arthritis	Non-specific pleuritis	Interstitial pneumonia and fibrosis
	Necrobiotic nodules	Bronchiolitis
		Necrobiotic nodules
		Vasculitis
		Pulmonary hypertension
		Systemic amyloidosis
Systemic Lupus	Fibrinous pleuritis	Chronic interstitial pneumonia
Erythematosus	Effusions	Diffuse alveolar damage
	Pleural fibrosis	Intra-alveolar hemorrhage
		Vasculitis, both large vessel and capillaritis
		Pulmonary hypertension
Scleroderma		Interstitial fibrosis with UIP-like pattern
		Interstitial fibrosis with NSIP-like pattern
		Pulmonary hypertension
Polymyositis and		Interstitial fibrosis
dermatomyositis		Bronchiolitis obliterans-organizing pneumonia
Sjogren Syndrome		Lymphocytic inflammation of tracheobronchial glands, atrophy of glands
		Peribronchiolar lymphocytic inflammation
		Lymphoid hyperplasia/Lymphoid interstitial pneumonitis
		Lymphomas including MALToma

macrophages are also present, as is lipid within pneumocytes and within cells in the interstitium. Rarer cases show a dose-independent reaction that resembles hypersensitivity pneumonitis. Still other cases show a pattern of DAD and/or BOOP-like injury.

b. **Methotrexate therapy** is also commonly complicated by pulmonary toxicity in perhaps 5%–10% of patients, and does not seem to be related to total dose. Radiographically, patients have diffuse infiltrates. Microscopically, there are multiple patterns of injury including (1) cellular interstitial pneumonia with nodular collections of lymphocytes, plasma cells, histiocytes, eosinophils, and poorly formed granulomas; (2) hypersensitivity pneumonitis (many of these patients are on low-dose therapy); and (3) BOOP (with poorly formed granulomas), DAD, and severe pulmonary edema.

3. **Hypersensitivity pneumonitis (HP)**, also known as extrinsic allergic alveolitis (EAA), is a disease caused by exposure to organic antigens. Classically the

TABLE 8.4 Pulmonary Manifestations of Drug Reactions

- Chronic interstitial pneumonia
- Diffuse alveolar damage
- Bronchiolitis obliterans-organizing pneumonia
- Obliterative bronchiolitis
- Eosinophilic pneumonia
- Pulmonary hemorrhage
- Pulmonary edema
- Pulmonary veno-occlusive disease
- Large and small vessel vasculitis

| TABLE 8.5 | Agents Implicated in Hypersensitivity Pneumonitis |

- Thermophillic Actinomyces
- Molds
- Animal proteins
- Rarely, exposure to drugs (i.e. methotrexate, amiodarone)

exposure is to thermophilic *Actinomyces*, but a variety of organic agents have been implicated (Table 8.5). Acute HP occurs with exposure to large amount of antigen; within 4–6 hours dyspnea, cough, fever, and diffuse infiltrates develop. Pulmonary function tests show moderate to severe restriction and decreased DLCO; severe hypoxemia is also present. Radiology studies show airspace disease, ground glass opacities, and some small nodular opacities. Symptoms improve in 12–18 hours, and within 2–3 days the radiographic findings resolve. Microscopically, acute inflammation, edema, and exudates may be seen, but because of the rapid course of the disease, it is rarely biopsied.

Chronic HP is due to repeated or prolonged exposure to small amounts of antigen; it is typically due to episodic exposure to some organic antigen, but the offending antigen is eventually identified in only 1/3 to 1/2 of cases. Chronic HP has several histopathologic characteristic (e-Fig. 8.8) including chronic interstitial inflammation with many CD8+ T-cells, vague granulomas or giant cells in the interstitium, and chronic bronchiolitis, sometimes with BOOP. Eosinophils are not part of the disease, despite the hypersensitivity label. Most patients respond to therapy or have stable disease, with a minority progressing to fibrosis and end-stage lung disease. There is overlap between chronic HP and some cases labeled as NSIP, and the two diseases may actually be the same process.

4. **Sarcoidosis** is a systemic disease of uncertain etiology. While some molecular genetic studies suggest that sarcoid represents a hypersensitivity-like reaction to mycobacterial infection, standard stains and cultures do not show organisms. There is frequent lung involvement, although it is usually mild and as many as 2/3 of patients are asymptomatic. Most cases involve the hilar and mediastinal nodes as well as the lung, but isolated involvement of either site can occur. In symptomatic patients, pulmonary function tests show mixed restriction and obstruction and decreased DLCO; lung volumes tend to be preserved.

The basic histologic lesion of sarcoid is a non-caseating granuloma with enveloping fibrosis (e-Fig. 8.9). The individual granulomas can coalesce to form larger nodules. The granulomas follow the lymphatic routes and so are present along airways; for this reason, transbronchial lung biopsies produce a diagnosis in up to 80% of cases. The giant cells in the granulomas may contain various structures, including Schaumann bodies, asteroid bodies, and oxalate crystals (the latter are produced endogenously by the giant cells, and thus polarizable material in the giant cells should not be taken as evidence of foreign body exposure). Sarcoid also includes varying degrees of interstitial lymphoid infiltrates. Stains for fungi and mycobacteria should be performed in all cases. Some cases otherwise typical for sarcoid show minimal central fibrinoid material in the granulomas; however, true caseation should raise concern about that the diagnosis is not sarcoidosis.

Unusual clinicopathologic features of sarcoid include massive pleural effusions associated with chest pain suggesting mesothelioma or pleural tumors, or one large nodule or multiple nodules with cavitation mimicking primary or metastatic tumor within the lung. Rare cases of sarcoidosis produce peripheral infiltrates that simulate eosinophilic pneumonia, or granulomatous vascular impingement that can simulate veno-occlusive disease. End-stage cases often are dominated by the presence of apical bullous disease; the granulomas at this stage may be largely "burnt-out" and replaced by hyalinized fibrous tissue that tracks along the lymphatic routes.

The differential diagnosis of sarcoid is always granulomatous infection, and it is important to note that up to 10%–15% of biopsies with granulomas and negative special stains are culture-positive. Infection should always be suspected if the granulomas are necrotizing. The differential diagnosis also includes a drug reaction, berylliosis, and aluminum exposure.

5. **Pulmonary eosinophilic granuloma** (also called Langerhans cell histiocytosis, or histiocytosis X) is a disease of adults, with most cases presenting in the third and fourth decades of life. There is a history of cigarette smoking in almost 90% of cases, indicating that this disease should be considered as another facet of smoking-induced lung disease. Patients with pulmonary eosinophilic granuloma (EG) have disease limited to lung; although some are asymptomatic, most complain of cough, dyspnea, fever, or weight loss. Pneumothorax is another documented presentation of EG. Radiologic studies show an upper lobe predominance; cysts and small stellate nodules can be seen by high-resolution CT scans. Because of the smoking history, there is often co-existent emphysema, desquamative interstitial pneumonitis, RB, or RB-ILD.

The characteristic histologic picture of EG (e-Fig. 8.10) is a stellate interstitial collection, often near small airways, of eosinophils and Langerhans cells. Langerhans cells feature a unique convoluted nucleus and a moderate amount of cytoplasm; some bi-nucleated forms may also be present. An admixture of pigmented alveolar macrophages ("smoker's macrophages") is also often present. Langerhans cells can be easily demonstrated by immunostains for S-100 and CD1a; alveolar macrophages stain for CD68 but not S-100 or CD1a. In contrast to the cellular lesions just described, resolved or "burnt out" lesions in chronic disease may consist only of hyalinized stellate scars in the upper lung zones; immunostains may highlight a few Langerhans cells in these scars, or may be completely negative. About 10%–20% of cases progress to fibrosis, but most patients improve with cessation of smoking; rare patients develop severe pulmonary hypertension. Eosinophilic pneumonia is one important differential consideration in small biopsies, but can be easily dismissed by correlation with radiographic and clinical features; in addition, the macrophages in eosinophilic pneumonia will be negative for S-100 and CD1a. Eosinophilic pleuritis may develop after pneumothorax, and may raise concern for EG in the lung, but reactive mesothelial cells are negative for S-100 and CD1a.

6. **Lymphangioleiomyomatosis (LAM)** is a disease that essentially occurs only in woman of reproductive age. Although classified as an interstitial disease, it features preserved lung volumes, unlike most fibrosing diseases. CT scans show diffuse involvement of the lung by cysts of rather uniform size that feature some mural thickening around the cystic spaces, a finding that serves to distinguish LAM from processes such as emphysema. In fact, high resolution CT images are so characteristic that the first pathologic specimen seen in many patients is explanted lungs. Patients present with obstructive lung symptoms or spontaneous pneumothorax, and also may demonstrate large chylous pleural effusions. Microscopic sections of LAM (e-Fig. 8.11) show a proliferation of abnormal smooth muscle-like cells in the lung. In many cases these cells seem to swirl away from the native smooth muscle of airways and vessels. Vascular compromise is linked to microhemorrhages, and so many cases show abundant hemosiderin within the lung. While

LAM is centered in the lung, it also involves lymph nodes in the pulmonary hilum, mediastinum, and abdomen in most cases. The smooth muscle-like cells stain with vimentin, desmin, and smooth muscle actin, and also may express estrogen and progesterone receptor. LAM also shows cross-lineage staining with melanoma markers including HMB-45 and melan-A. In this regard, the cells of LAM share the staining attributes of the members of the PEComa family (including the sugar tumor of lung), renal angiomyolipomas, and some soft tissue tumors (see Chap. 46). LAM also shows overlap with tuberous sclerosis (TS) in that some TS patients develop an identical cystic lung disease, and both LAM and TS share an association with angiomyolipomas in the kidney and elsewhere. The course of the disease is unpredictable; transplantation has been the only long term option for those with severe disease.

7. **Alveolar proteinosis** refers to a peculiar accumulation of intra-alveolar eosinophilic, granular PAS-positive protein and phospholipid. It was initially reported as an idiopathic process, but a relation to immune deficiency, hematologic malignancies, infections, and various exposures is now recognized. Classic exposure-related cases are associated with massive acute silica exposure, which is believed to poison the alveolar macrophages and thus inhibit their ability to clear alveolar debris.

Clinically, patients present with slowly progressive alveolar infiltrates and complain of dyspnea, cough, or sputum production with fever; CT scans show "crazy-paving" with alveolar infiltrates and septal line thickening. The diagnosis is often apparent from the milky appearance of lavage fluid; biopsies show complete filling of the alveolar spaces by granular eosinophilic debris that is PAS-positive and diastase-resistant (e-Fig. 8.12). Findings often include cholesterol clefts (acicular clefts), globular eosinophilic debris, and macrophages. In most cases the underlying alveolar structure appears normal, although some chronic cases may eventually show fibrosis. Secondary infection of the fluid by *Nocardia,* mycobacteria, and fungi has been reported. *Pneumocystis* infection can microscopically mimic alveolar proteinosis, although the material in alveolar proteinosis lacks the frothy appearance characteristic of *Pneumocystis* infection.

D. "Allergic" diseases

1. **Eosinophilic pneumonia** can be divided into acute and chronic forms. The acute forms include the "simple form" also known as Loeffler syndrome; this is an acute, self-limited process with fleeting infiltrates and peripheral blood eosinophilia and is rarely biopsied. The tropical form is usually linked to filaria infection, and also presents as an acute illness. The chronic form is more likely to require biopsy for diagnosis.

Chronic eosinophilic pneumonia (CEP) has a variable presentation from acute illness with fever, dyspnea, and weight loss, to vague respiratory complaints. Many patients have a history of asthma, and laboratory tests reveal elevated blood IgE and peripheral blood eosinophilia. Chest radiographs show patchy non-segmental infiltrates, often peripheral, that may cross fissures, a pattern that is sometimes described as the "photographic negative of pulmonary edema." There are myriad underlying causes; major categories include drugs (antibiotics such as nitrofurantoin, sulfonamides, penicillins, anti-inflammatory agents, and chemotherapeutics), fungus (*Aspergillus* and *Candida*), parasites, nickel vapor, and idiopathic cases. Histologic sections of CEP (e-Fig. 8.13) show an alveolar-filling process consisting of a mixture of eosinophils and macrophages. Necrosis of eosinophils may be present, forming an eosinophilic abscess. Charcot–Leyden crystals will also be present, as well as interstitial and perivascular eosinophils, lymphocytes, plasma cells, and areas of BOOP.

2. **Mucoid impaction of bronchi (MIB)** is the filling of bronchi by viscous mucus, usually caused by another underlying disease such as asthma, cystic fibrosis, or chronic bronchitis. Patients present with evidence of lobar collapse or an irregular branching mass-like density. Histologic sections of the impacted material in most cases show "allergic mucin" that consists of laminated collections of eosinophils, eosinophil debris, and mucinous exudates. Fungal hyphae, most often *Aspergillus* (e-**Fig. 8.14**), may also be present in a pattern that overlaps with allergic bronchopulmonary aspergillosis (ABPA). A related process is plastic bronchitis which is impaction of airways by neutrophilic debris.

3. **ABPA** is a related form of hypersensitivity to fungal organisms, most often *Aspergillus*. The disease almost always occurs in asthmatic patients, and is usually diagnosed by a combination of clinical features that include pulmonary infiltrates and proximal bronchiectasis, skin testing that shows reaction to fungal antigens, precipitating antibodies to fungal antigen, elevated IgE levels, and peripheral blood eosinophilia. Tissue sections show a combination of eosinophilic pneumonia, MIB, and bronchocentric granulomatosis (granulomatous destruction of bronchioles).

4. **Pulmonary amyloidosis occurs in several forms**
   a. **Tracheobronchial amyloidosis** is rare, and features focal or diffuse amyloid deposition in the airway submucosa and around bronchial glands. The amyloid may show calcification or ossification. The patients may have symptoms of wheezing, lobar collapse, or recurrent infections, and the airways are prone to bleeding. This form does not feature systemic involvement.
   b. **Nodular pulmonary amyloid** is also typically confined to lung, with no systemic disease. Patients are usually asymptomatic but have a well circumscribed peripheral nodule or nodules evident on radiographic studies. Grossly, the mass is often described as waxy or lardaceous. Microscopic sections show nodules of amyloid with an associated foreign body reaction, lymphoplasmacytic infiltrate, and foci of calcification and metaplastic bone formation (e-**Fig. 8.15**).
   c. In contrast to the previous types of pulmonary amyloid, the **diffuse septal form** is most often seen with disseminated primary amyloidosis. Patients present with dyspnea, hypoxemia, and an increased A/a gradient. Chest radiographs show diffuse fine reticulonodular infiltrates. Microscopic sections show deposits in the alveolar interstitium, around vessels, and sometime in the airways and pleura (e-**Fig. 8.16**).

E. **Vasculitis and related disease.** Vasculitis and related diseases constitute an important collection of lung diseases, many of which have been historically included together in the category of "angiitis and granulomatosis." Patients with vasculitis and related lesions often present alveolar hemorrhage, the causes of which can be categorized (Table 8.6) based on the histologic finding of

TABLE 8.6	Pulmonary Hemorrhage Syndromes	
Syndrome	**Capillaritis**	**Immunofluorescence**
Goodpasture's	+/−	+, Linear staining
Idiopathic hemosiderosis	−	−
Wegener's	+	−
Microscopic polyarteritis	+	−
Collagen vascular disease (SLE)	+	−
Idiopathic rapidly progressive GN	+	+, Granular staining
Toxins	−	−

TABLE 8.7	Differential Diagnosis of Pulmonary Large Vessel Vasculitis
Involvement by systemic vasculitidies	Polyarteritis nodosa, Behcets, Takayasu's, giant cell arteritis
Classic causes	Wegener's, Necrotizing sarcoid granulomatosis, Churg-Strauss syndrome
Other primary entities with large vessel vasculitis	Collagen vascular disease, malignancy, toxins and drugs
Secondary	Infection, pulmonary hypertension, others

capillaritis (see below) and the immunofluorescent findings. Large pulmonary vessels may also be involved by vasculitis (e-Fig. 8.17); common etiologies of large vessel pulmonary artery vasculitis are presented in Table 8.7.

1. **Wegener granulomatosis** is the prototypical lung vasculitis. It most often presents in middle age with pulmonary symptoms including cough, hemoptysis, and fever. Other patients present with upper respiratory complaints or renal failure, depending on the dominant sites of disease. Chest radiographs may show alveolar filling due to hemorrhage, multiple nodules with cavitation, or even a single massive nodule. Microscopic features in the lung reflect a classic triad of findings (e-Fig. 8.17): (1) Vasculitis which involves arteries, veins, and capillaries (capillaritis). Acute vascular lesions show fibrinoid necrosis; chronic lesions may show only vascular scarring or perivascular chronic inflammation. Capillaritis consists of neutrophils, nuclear dust, and fibrin microthrombi in lung capillaries, analogous to leukocytoclastic vasculitis in the skin. (2) Necrosis that is often described as geographic necrosis, and classically has an abscess-like appearance with a hematoxyphilic hue, surrounded by palisaded histiocytes. (3) Granulomatous inflammation comprised of palisades of histiocytes, scattered giant cells, and poorly formed granulomas.

   Other microscopic features can include acute or chronic alveolar hemorrhage; airway bronchocentric granulomatosis-like lesions, BOOP, chronic bronchitis, and bronchiolitis; interstitial lesions including fibrosis and nonspecific chronic inflammation; DAD; and pleural lesions such as fibrinous pleuritis, granulomas, or chronic inflammation. Serology studies in most cases reveal c-ANCA positivity; the anti-neutrophil antibodies will show a cytoplasmic pattern of staining, and PR3 is usually the antigen. Rarely, p-ANCA will be positive.

2. **Microscopic polyarteritis** is the lung equivalent of leukocytoclastic vasculitis. It is often associated with p-ANCA and has many other associations including drug-related cases, infection (e.g., hepatitis B, bacteria), Henoch-Schönlein purpura, collagen vascular disease, cryoglobulinemia, and idiopathic. The basic lesion is capillaritis, which has two main features: neutrophils in the alveolar septae and capillary walls with neutrophilic nuclear dust, and microscopic fibrin thrombi in capillaries (e-Fig. 8.18). Arteriolitis or venulitis is also often present. Since the differential diagnosis includes acute lung injury or acute pneumonia, microscopic polyarteritis is a diagnosis of exclusion.

3. **Churg–Strauss syndrome** (allergic angiitis and granulomatosis) is another ANCA-related vasculitis. Nearly all patients have a history of asthma. Many patients also have skin lesions, neuropathy, CNS disease, or heart failure; most cases are diagnosed by biopsy of sites other than lung. The histopathologic findings are a combination of two features: (1) Vasculitis that can affect both arteries and veins, with giant cell infiltration of vessel walls. There may also be transmural eosinophilia with fibrinoid necrosis and small palisaded

TABLE 8.8	Causes of Obliterative Bronchiolitis
• Idiopathic	• Rheumatoid arthritis
• Chronic lung allograft rejection	• Post-infection (viruses)
• Graft versus host disease	• "Pop-corn lung"
• Immunodeficiency states	• Inhaled toxins
• Drugs (penicillamine)	

granulomas. (2) Eosinophilic infiltrates that resemble eosinophilic pneumonia consisting of a combination of histiocytes and eosinophils that fill alveoli.

F. **Bronchiolitis**

1. **Obliterative bronchiolitis** (constrictive bronchiolitis, bronchiolitis obliterans), though it has a name that is similar to BOOP, is a completely different disease that is characterized by the progressive narrowing and luminal compromise of small airways by sub-epithelial fibrosis. Conditions associated with this process are listed in Table 8.8, many of which have some immunologic basis. Patients present with insidious onset of shortness of breath and obstructive pulmonary functions with air-trapping. Wedge biopsies are often required for diagnosis, and it is common to see a spectrum of small airway changes in such biopsies ranging from virtually normal, to partial scarring, to total luminal obliteration by fibrous tissue (e-**Fig. 8.19**). Inflammation is variable, and there will be mucus trapped distal to areas of severe luminal compromise. Although the disease may stabilize for some time, the changes are generally irreversible.

2. **Cellular bronchiolitis** is a descriptive name given to forms of bronchiolitis that feature marked acute and chronic bronchiolar inflammation. Conditions associated with this lesion are listed in Table 8.9.

IV. **INFECTIOUS PROCESSES**

A. **Viral infections.** Typically, viral infections of the lung are self limited and do not require biopsy for diagnosis. However, in the setting of immunocompromise or severe pulmonary dysfunction from infection, an attempt to identify the etiology of pneumonia by tissue biopsy is often made. Viral cultures may require 1–4 weeks for growth, and so in some instances a biopsy can provide a specific diagnosis in far less time. In addition to the findings in H&E stained slides, immunostains, electron microscopy, and serology can be used to increase diagnostic sensitivity.

1. **Cytomegalovirus** typically affects immunocompromised patients; since most people are exposed to cytomegalovirus (CMV) in childhood, many cases represent activation of latent infection. Patients may develop fever, cough, or shortness of breath. Chest X-rays show diffuse infiltrates, and biopsies show interstitial pneumonitis as well as DAD or nodular inflammation. Enlarged cells with nuclear and/or cytoplasmic inclusions are pathognomic for CMV infection. In H&E stained sections, nuclear inclusions have an eosinophilic core (6 μm) with a surrounding cleared zone, while the cytoplasmic deposit

TABLE 8.9	Conditions Associated with Cellular Bronchiolitis
• Infections: bacteria, viral, mycoplasma	• Collagen vascular diseases (i.e., Sjogren's)
• Toxin/fume exposures	• Wegener's granulomatosis
• Asthma	• Transplant rejection/graft versus host disease
• Bronchiectasis	• Diffuse pan-bronchiolitis (Homa's disease)
• Central obstruction	

is basophilic (e-**Fig. 8.20**). Epithelial cells, vascular cells, and even stromal cells can exhibit inclusions. Immunohistochemistry for CMV will decorate the enlarged cells; electron microscopy demonstrates virions in the inclusions, while a PAS stain with diastase highlights the cytoplasmic deposits.

2. **Herpesvirus (HSV).** Both HSV types I and II can induce pneumonitis, and immunocompromised hosts are more prone to Herpes viral pneumonia. Clinically, HSV pneumonia may result from extension of upperway disease with primarily bronchiolar inflammation, or from systemic infection which presents as multiple small perivascular inflammatory nodules. Three findings are characteristic of HSV: necrosis, individual cells with inclusions (e-**Fig. 8.21**) (featuring eosinophilic nuclear inclusions with perinuclear clearing; amphophilic nucleoplasm in single cells may represent early inclusions or giant cell formation), and herpes viral giant cells (which contain two or more nuclei with ground glass central nuclear clearing and coarsely granular, sharply defined nuclear borders; the nuclei are often molded against one another). Immunohistochemistry using antibodies to HSV decorates the giant cells and the individual cells with inclusions.

3. **Varicella zoster (VZV)** is the causative agent for chicken pox and shingles. Primary infection in healthy adults and immunocompromised children can result in pneumonia. The underlying lung injury pattern can be either DAD with hyaline membranes and proteinaceous exudates, or nodular inflammation with central necrosis that calcifies and persists on chest radiographs. Biopsies of VZV infections show giant cells similar to those of HSV.

4. **Adenovirus** infection generally presents with symptoms typical of an upper respiratory infection; pneumonia develops in a small percentage of healthy and immunocompromised children and adults. Two patterns of infection evolve. Some patients develop necrotizing bronchiolitis and pneumonia, while others respond with DAD with hyaline membranes and exudates. In adenoviral infections both alveolar lining cells and bronchial epithelial cells may exhibit blurred and hyperchromatic nuclear chromatin (so-called smudge cells) (e-**Fig. 8.22**). The bronchial damage of adenovirus may result in fibrosis or constricting bronchiolitis.

5. **Respiratory syncytial virus (RSV)** affects primarily small children and infants; premature infants and immunocompromised children are particularly prone to infection. RSV infection exhibits some seasonality, and is more common in fall and winter. RSV can induce bronchiolitis with symptoms of cough, wheezing, and respiratory distress. Biopsies show necrotizing bronchiolitis and/or interstitial pneumonia.

6. **Measles virus.** With the advent of vaccination, infection by measles virus is rare, and evolution to pneumonia rarer. Most patients are immunocompromised, and the characteristic skin rash is present. The underlying pathology is DAD, with associated individual and giant cells with viral inclusions; the alveolar spaces may contain exudates, and necrosis may be present. Both eosinophilic intranuclear and cytoplasmic inclusions develop in both alveolar and vascular lining cells. Measles pneumonia features a distinctive multinucleate giant cell thought to derive from coalescence of type II pneumocytes, the Warthin-Finkeldey giant cell, which contains up to 60 nuclei.

7. **Parainfluenza and influenza** generate non-specific patterns, consisting of varying degrees of DAD, bronchial necrosis, and peribronchial inflammation.

B. **Bacterial infections**

1. **Mycoplasma** induces acute and chronic bronchiolitis, with necrosis and denudment of bronchial epithelium. The bronchial lumina may contain acute inflammatory cells admixed with denuded epithelium. Acute and

chronic inflammatory cells often traverse the bronchial wall. Alveolar spaces may exhibit bronchopneumonia, with BOOP or DAD.

2. **Mycobacterial infections** are typically grouped into tuberculosis and other (atypical) mycobacterial infections. The most common stain used to demonstrate organisms in tissue sections is the Ziehl–Neelsen stain; immunofluorescent (auramine-rhodamine) and immunohistochemical stains can also be used to identify mycobacteria. PCR based genetic methods can also be used to detect (and speciate) the organism in tissue sections.

   a. **Tuberculosis (TB).** Multidrug resistance has emerged in this organism and consequently the pathologic spectrum of tubercular infection is expanding. The causative organism is *Mycobacterium tuberculosis*, which is transmitted via inhalation of organisms. Histologically, the tubercular granuloma is a classic palisaded necrotizing granuloma. Granulomas may caseate and coalesce, creating nodules with central necrosis, or even cavitary masses. Organisms may be found in multinucleate giant cells or at the periphery of necrosis (e-**Fig. 8.23**). Lymph nodal involvement may be present. Miliary tuberculosis is unlikely to be sampled in biopsy or resection specimens.

   b. **Atypical mycobacterial infection.** *Mycobacterium avium intracellulare* (MAI) is the most common of the atypical mycobacterial infections, and is more common among immunocompromised patients where it presents with non-specific fever and malaise. Radiographs show diffuse or patchy infiltrates. Histologic findings vary from more typical non-necrotizing punctuate granulomas, to necrotizing granulomatous pneumonia, to diffuse pneumonitis (in which abundant pneumocytes or interstitial cells contain abundant organisms by acid fast stains).

C. **Fungal Infections**

1. ***Candida*** infection arises in several contexts. Mucocutaneous candidiasis can arise in immunocompetent adults, but arises more frequently in immuno-compromised patients; the trachea or bronchial tree can have plaques of fungus admixed with desquamated cells and neutrophils. Impaired host defenses potentiate invasive disease; in the lungs, vascular invasion results in hemorrhagic necrosis. Direct inoculation into the bloodstream from iatrogenic sources (catheters, surgery) or other inoculation (drug abuse) results in disseminated disease. Transplant patients can develop infection at the sites of anastomosis. *C. albicans* is the most prevalent species; other species more often infect compromised hosts. All species exhibit the same basic morphology: non-branching, aseptate pseudohyphae forming "box-car" like chains of cells; yeast forms bud from pseudohyphae (e-**Fig. 8.24**). Yeast forms are visible on H&E, PAS, or silver stains.

2. **Mucormycosis.** Several members of the Phycomycetes result in clinically and morphologically identical disease, including *Mucor, Absidia,* and *Rhizopus,* among others. Almost all cases occur in the setting of diabetic ketoacidosis (sinonasal or rhinocerebral disease) or immunosuppression from hematologic malignancies. Lung involvement may be the primary focus, or develop secondary to head and neck disease. Lung lesions are typified by hemorrhagic pneumonia; fungal thrombi with distal infarction are often present. The dual circulation of the lung (bronchial and pulmonary arterial systems) results in perfusion of infarcted areas with resulting hemorrhagic necrosis, associated with varying amounts of inflammation. A key to recognition of the infection is identification of wide, ribbon-like non-septate hyphae with irregular wide angle branching. The pseudohyphae are often described as "empty" and stain poorly with most special stains.

3. ***Aspergillus*** species cause a wide spectrum of disease, dependent on both host immune status and site of growth. Colonization with *Aspergillus* can

induce an allergic response, including ABPA, sinusitis, and hypersensitivity pneumonitis; *Aspergillus* can also colonize mucus or grow in a pre-existing cavity, and sinus or cavitary lung lesions both can harbor fungus balls. Transplant anastomoses are also prone to colonization by *Aspergillus* species (e-**Fig. 8.25**). The characteristic lung lesion is the target lesion with a sharply delineated hemorrhagic border, which reflects the fact that the fungus is frequently vasoinvasive and produces hemorrhagic infarcts. In well-preserved areas, organisms have relatively uniform septa, which are thinner than those of *Mucor*. The hyphae branch at ~45 degrees; the reproductive form (fruiting body) is only rarely seen in tissues. Degenerate hyphae can be mistaken for *Mucor*, with empty or dilated forms; acute angle branching, occasional septa, and more intact forms indicate the correct diagnosis.

4. ***Cryptococcus.*** The most common pathogen of this genus is *C. neoformans*, which is usually an opportunistic infection but rarely also infects normal hosts after massive exposure. The common portal of entry is the lungs; patients remain virtually asymptomatic while the fungus spreads to other sites. The organism is present in the lung as "naked masses of organisms," to intracellular forms resembling those of histoplasmosis, to granulomas with surrounding fibrosis (so-called cryptococcomas) (e-**Fig. 8.26**). The organisms are much larger than *Candida* or *Histoplasma* with an average diameter of 4–10 μ; only yeast forms are found in tissue. The diameter of cryptococcal forms varies in large part with capsule thickness, a function of host immune status, and mucicarmine stains the capsule strongly (generally considered a diagnostic feature). Capsule-deficient forms are common in cancer or AIDS patients, and may be much more difficult to diagnose definitively.

5. **Blastomycosis** is generally seen in the middle of the United States. Infection usually involves lungs and skin; spore inhalation is the mode of transmission for virtually all cases. Pulmonary blastomycosis takes several forms; the most common is a solitary focus of infection with variable associated lymph nodal disease, which heals and leaves a fibrous scar. Progressive disease is less common, in which infection spreads throughout the lung as miliary foci which range from neutrophil-rich abscesses to tubercle-like granulomas. The causative agent maintains a variably sized yeast form in tissue ranging from 5 to 25 μ, and has a thick, refractile, double-contoured wall; unlike *Cryptococcus*, this wall is negative or very weakly mucin-positive (e-**Fig. 8.27**).

6. **Histoplasmosis.** In the United States, infection is usually caused by *H. capsulatum* from bird or bat droppings. In tissue, the fungus reverts to a primitive yeast, 2–5 μ in diameter with occasional unequal budding. Primary histoplasmosis produces a mild, self-limited febrile illness in most cases, with hyalinized granulomas the result (e-**Fig. 8.28**) but can result in a progressive, disseminated, fatal disease. Cases with active disease can also produce a granulation-tissue like pattern, with vague granulomas. The organism can also induce secondary scarring forms of inflammation, such as sclerosing mediastinitis with calcified granulomas in which organisms are often not identified.

7. **Coccidiomycosis** is caused by *Coccidioides immitis*, a soil borne saprophyte typically found in the southwestern United States. Patients typically have travel histories to that region, and present with an acute febrile illness (some infections are asymptomatic). Infection develops in both immunocompetent and immunocompromised individuals. The inhaled organisms transform into spherules, thick walled sacs 60–80 μ in diameter containing multiple endospores (e-**Fig. 8.29**); reproduction in tissue results from rupture of the spherule with release of endospores. Microscopically, the organisms create a

nodule, typically with non-caseating granuloma formation; cavitation may occur. Lymph nodal involvement may be present and disseminated infection may result. The organisms can be demonstrated with GMS or PAS stains.

8. **_Pneumocystis carinii_ pneumonia (PCP).** _Pneumocystic carinii_ was formerly considered a protozoan, but genetic analysis suggests that it is best classified as a fungus. Infection is generally seen among immunocompromised patients. The chest radiograph classically shows diffuse infiltrates, which correspond to the diffuse alveolar infiltrates that are almost diagnostic microscopically (e-**Fig. 8.30**). Cytologically, the infiltrate exfoliates in lavage specimens as alveolar casts. PCP can induce interstitial pneumonitis or granulomatous inflammation; these variant forms are often seen in chronic disease or with partially treated disease, may progress to cavitating or cystic disease in the upper lobes, and are associated with extra-pulmonary disseminated disease. The cysts stain well with GMS in most cases; in degenerate cases, immunostains may be of some help. The organism has a helmet or cup shape, often referred to as a "dented ping-pong ball."

D. Parasite Infections

1. **Dirofilariasis.** _Dirofilaria_ are nematodes, the most common pathogen of which is _D. immitis_, the common dog heartworm. While this parasite does not have a life cycle in the human host, occasional infection can develop with adult nematodes via transmission by a mosquito bite. Infection can result in non-caseating granulomas presenting as a nodule in the lung (or other organ). Cross sections of the organism's refractile cuticle (10–14 μ in greatest diameter) may be seen in histologic sections. Endovascular thrombi with organisms have been reported as well.

V. SELECTED PNEUMOCONIOSES

A. Asbestosis.
Asbestosis is an interstitial lung disease caused by asbestos. It usually occurs in workers heavily exposed, for a prolonged period of time. There is often a long latency period, usually at least 15 years, between exposure and the disease. Mild disease shows no symptoms; with increasing severity, patients complain of dyspnea, dry cough, weight loss, and chest pain. Radiographic findings are characterized by small irregular opacities, most prominent in the bases of the lung. The American Thoracic Society has defined six clinical criteria a clinical diagnosis of asbestosis, including exposure, a latency period, rales, decreased lung volumes and DLCO by PFTs, and chest radiograph infiltrates. Thankfully, pathologic criteria include just two required findings: the presence of peribronchiolar fibrosis (*fibroelastosis*), and associated asbestos bodies (e-**Fig. 8.31**). Grading of asbestosis can be performed: grade 1: fibrosis confined to respiratory bronchioles; grade 2: fibrosis involves alveolar ducts, or two tiers of alveoli; grade 3: fibrosis involves all alveoli between two bronchioles; grade 4: honeycombing. The lungs show a high fiber burden: 98%–99% of cases have at least 2000 asbestos bodies per gram of wet lung tissue; most have 10,000 to 100,000 or more asbestos bodies per gram of wet lung tissue which correlates with at least several asbestos bodies per tissue slide in the majority of cases (iron stains often help to demonstrate asbestos bodies). If pathologic examination of biopsy or lung resections suggests asbestosis, or if there is clinical suspicion for asbestosis, it is prudent to set tissue aside for fiber analysis (fiber studies on either fresh lung tissue or formalin fixed and embedded tissue), although it is not required for diagnosis in most cases. Classically, asbestosis is required to attribute pulmonary carcinomas to asbestos exposure; asbestosis plus smoking increases the risk for lung carcinomas by a multiplicative factor, to perhaps 50X non-smoking, non-asbestotic controls. Pleural plaques and mesothelioma, which are also asbestos-related pleuropulmonary lesions, are discussed in the chapter on serosal membranes (Chap. 11).

B. **Silicosis.** Silicosis is produced by silica deposition in the lung. Occupations at risk include sand-blasting, grinding, mining, plastering, and masonry, among many others. Silicosis typically produces infiltrates in the mid-lung zones, in contrast to other types of pulmonary fibrosis. Lymph nodes in the chest will also show characteristic "egg-shell" calcifications on X-ray. The characteristic lung lesion is the silica nodule; nodules have a lymphangitic distribution, so are seen along the bronchovascular tree and in the pleura (e-**Fig. 8.32**). Early nodules are cellular and composed of a swirling collection of fibrohistiocytic cells; birefringent particles can be seen in these nodules with polarized microscopy. Older lesions become progressively hyalinized; they may coalesce to form irregular masses that can mimic pulmonary neoplasms. The relationship of silicosis to the development of pulmonary neoplasms is debated, but appears to be a small risk, if present at all. Nodules may also include other material such as iron or carbon, in which case a diagnosis of mixed dust fibrosis is appropriate.

VI. PULMONARY TRANSPLANTATION

A. **Gross processing of transplant specimens.** Pulmonary transplantation is now a well established therapy for various end-stage lung diseases including emphysema/chronic obstructive pulmonary disease, cystic fibrosis, LAM, pulmonary hypertension, and pulmonary fibrosis of various causes. Examination of the explanted, native lungs should include thorough documentation of the underlying disease process. A minimum of one section per lobe should be submitted for diffuse processes, as well as sections of the hilar lymph nodes; cases of pulmonary hypertension may require additional sections to document plexiform lesions, and any mass or focal abnormality should be sampled thoroughly. Examination should be comprehensive enough to exclude foci of malignancy, or infections which may recur due to the immunocompromise of transplant recipients.

The allograft is surveyed by transbronchial biopsy, and occasional wedge biopsies, both at scheduled protocol intervals, as well as in response to changes in clinical condition. A minimum of five pieces of alveolar tissue is considered adequate for assessment in this setting. In general, three levels of H&E stained sections are obtained; some institutions employ protocols with adjunct special stains for infectious organisms on all biopsies.

B. **Microscopic features of transplant biopsies**

1. **Preservation injury** is the first change seen in post-transplant biopsies. This change reflects ischemic damage that develops in the lung in the interval between removal from the donor and re-implantation. Preservation injury produces a picture of classic lung injury that may exhibit features of DAD or BOOP (e-**Fig. 8.33**). The appearance sometimes suggests viral infection, but for biopsies taken in the first 1–2 weeks after transplant, it is generally too early for opportunistic infections to become manifest. One important differential diagnosis for early acute graft injury is humoral or hyperacute rejection (discussed below).

2. **Opportunistic infections.** Biopsies after the first week or two must be surveyed for opportunistic infections, the most frequent of which is CMV, the features which are detailed above (e-**Fig. 8-20**). Important clues of CMV infection include interstitial neutrophils and alveolar fibrin exudates, findings which warrant immunostains for CMV since transplant patients may not always develop classic inclusions. CMV may produce perivascular inflammation, a finding that mimics acute rejection (see below). Other viral infections often seen include Herpes virus (e-**Fig. 8.21**) and Adenovirus (e-**Fig. 8.22**), and a variety of non-specific pneumonitis patterns may actually represent responses to other viral pathogens. The results of culture, serologic, and molecular tests for infectious organisms must be integrated with biopsy data by the transplant clinician.

TABLE 8.10	Revised Scheme for Lung Allograft Rejection[a]

A: Acute rejection

AO: None
A1: Minimal
A2: Mild
A3: Moderate
A4: Severe

B. Small airway inflammation/lymphocytic bronchiolitis

BO: None
B1R: low grade (previous B1, B2)
B2R: high grade (previous B3, B4)
BX: ungradable

C: Chronic airway rejection—Bronchiolitis obliterans

CO: absent
C1: present

D: Chronic vascular rejection

[a]Stewart S, Fishbein MC, Snell GI, et al. Revision of the 1996 Working Formulation for the Standardization of nomenclature in the diagnosis of lung rejection. *J Heart Lung Trans.* 2007;26:122.

Since most transplant patients currently receive prophylactic therapy against *Pneumocystis* infection, PCP is a rare complication. Fungal infections seen more commonly are due to *Aspergillus* or *Candida* colonization of the bronchial tissue in the region of the airway anastomosis, likely related to tissue ischemia (e-**Fig. 8.25**); invasive growth within the lung is much less common. The presence of foamy macrophages in a transbronchial biopsy may be an indicator of fungal infection and should be followed with silver stains to exclude intra-histiocytic organisms such as *Histoplasma*.

3. **Acute rejection** is a primary concern in all follow-up biopsies. The 2007 revised lung allograft rejection scheme is provided in Table 8.10. The basic lesion of acute rejection is lymphocytic infiltration surrounding blood vessels and airways. The perivascular inflammation is reflected in the "A" scores (e-**Fig. 8.34**). T-cells are the main cell type present in acute rejection; more severe rejections feature larger, more activated cells, and will also show eosinophils and neutrophils. Table 8.11 presents more details of the histologic patterns of rejection.

   Airways are the other target of rejection and are reflected in the "B" scores (e-**Fig. 8.35**, Table 8.11). Airway inflammation is less specific for rejection, and can be seen with chronic airway infections, obstruction, and preservation injury among other causes. In general, A and B grades tend to follow each other, although they can be discordant, particularly if small biopsies are obtained.

4. **Humoral rejection** is a form of acute rejection that has been recognized more recently. It often occurs in cases that show donor-recipient cross match positivity in which the recipient has anti-donor antibodies. The most dramatic example of antibody-mediated rejection is **hyperacute rejection,** where there may be immediate graft dysfunction, noted even in the operating room, as a result of extensive vascular thrombosis and acute inflammation; histologic features of hyperacute rejection include neutrophil infiltrates in the interstitium and fibrinoid vasculitis that leads to necrosis and hemorrhage. In contrast, cases of humoral rejection seen outside of the immediate postoperative period are characterized by more subtle disease; although lesions may include features similar to hyperacute rejection with capillaritis and necrosis, in many cases the only lesion detected in biopsies will be acute interstitial inflammation or a lung injury pattern such as DAD or BOOP. In analogy to renal or cardiac transplantation, it has been suggested that immunostains for C4d may be helpful to identify cases of humoral rejection.

TABLE 8.11 Key Characteristics/Features in the Grading of Allograft Cellular Rejection

"A" lesions

Grade	Circumferential perivascular infiltrates	Cytologic features of infiltrate	Endothelialitis	Airway infiltrate
A0	None	N/A	N/A	Usually absent
A1	Rare, hard to see at scanning power, 1–2 cell thick cuffs	Small, "resting" lymphocytes	Usually absent	Often modest
A2	More vessels with infiltrate, easily seen at scanning power, 2–5 cell thick cuffs	More "activated" lymphocytes, also eosinophils	Sometimes	Common
A3	Often many vessels, infiltrates into adjacent septa, "stellate"	More activated, many eosinophils, can be neutrophils	Almost always	Usually present
A4	May be confluent, associated lung injury	Similar to A3	Almost always, vasculitis-like	Usually present, severe

"B" lesions

Grade	Severity	Epithelial damage
B0	None	N/A
B1R	Mild	No
B2R	Moderate to severe	Yes, individual cell apotosis, to ulcers, total denudation of epithelium

The postulated pattern of positivity is diffuse capillary staining; however, the role of C4d immunostaining in the lung remains to be clarified.

5. **Chronic airway rejection** is a major problem in lung transplantation. Bronchiolitis obliterans syndrome (BOS) is the clinical feature of chronic airway rejection, defined by a drop of FEV below 80% of the post-transplant maximum value. Chronic airway rejection is reflected in the "C" score. The pathologic lesion is subepithelial fibrosis of airways that leads to a picture of obliterative bronchiolitis (e-Fig. 8.36). This subepithelial fibrosis pushes the mucosa toward the center of the lumen, with progressive luminal compromise; the findings in individual airways range from partial eccentric thickening, to complete obliteration of the airway resulting in a small fibrous scar next to an accompanying artery. Features of localized obstructive pneumonitis may also be seen due to bronchiolar dysfunction. The development of chronic rejection is correlated with increasing episodes of acute rejection, and also with the severity of the lymphocytic infiltrate around airways, although the mechanisms of chronic rejection are still poorly understood.

6. **Post-transplant lymphoproliferative disorder (PTLD)** is another serious post-transplant process. Changes in immunosuppressive regimens have resulted in a decreased incidence of the disease. In lung transplant patients there is a propensity for PTLD to develop in the transplanted lung, although lymph nodes, the gastrointestinal tract, and tonsils appear to be other preferred sites. The vast majority of cases, in particular those that occur early in the transplant course, are EBV-positive with a B-cell phenotype. There should be a high index of suspicion for PTLD in any lung allograft biopsy that shows an intense infiltrate with cytologic atypia or necrosis, or where the clinical

history suggests nodules or a mass. Cases usually fall into three general categories: plasma cell hyperplasia, consisting of cases that show low-grade findings; polymorphous PTLD, which is comprised of a mixed population of atypical lymphoid cells; and monomorphous PTLD, consisting of cases that consist of a monotonous population of high grade, malignant-appearing cells (e-Fig. 8.37). Monomorphous cases are much less likely to regress following diminution of immunosuppression as compared with the lower grade lesions; thus, higher grade cases are likely to require cytotoxic therapy. In allograft biopsies, if there is a question of PTLD versus a rejection-related infiltrate, a simple panel of CD3, CD20/CD79a, and EBV immunostains will provide dichotomous results: the infiltrate in severe rejection or infections is almost always a CD3 predominant infiltrate, while the infiltrate in PTLD is positive for CD20 and CD79a, as well as EBV, in the great majority of cases. Adjunctive studies to indicate clonality may also be of value in terms of diagnosis, classification, and prognosis. It is important to note that rare examples of PTLD may have the morphology of Hodgkin disease, and that late cases of EBV negative lymphoid neoplasms (4 or 5 years after transplant) which resemble non-Hodgkins lymphomas can also develop.

7. **Recurrent disease.** With the exception of a few cases of sarcoid, recurrence of the native lung disease in allografts is not a significant problem. There are reports of occasional cases of carcinoma arising in transplanted lungs, as well as in the native lung in the setting of unilateral transplant; these patients fare poorly.

VII. **NEOPLASMS.** The WHO classification of lung neoplasms is presented in Table 8.12. Malignancies of the lung are the most common cause of cancer-related mortality in the United States. Despite decades of warnings, cigarette smoking remains the predominant risk factor for the development of pulmonary carcinoma. There has been speculation that a shift in location and cell type for pulmonary carcinomas is related to changes in cigarette usage. Some data suggest that filtered cigarettes, which remove larger tar particles, have allowed carcinogens to penetrate to more distal parts of the lung and produce peripheral adenocarcinomas instead of central squamous carcinomas or small cell carcinomas caused by larger particles. Changes in tobacco formulation over the years may also have played some role in these changes. Other risk factors for lung carcinoma, either proven or speculative, include asbestos exposure, radiation, various chemicals, heavy metals, viral infection, fibrosing lung diseases, immunosuppression, and genetic syndromes. Outside of these causes, there remain some cases of lung carcinomas for which there is no clear etiologic factor.

Up to 10% of patients with head and neck carcinomas may harbor a concurrent lung primary carcinoma; therefore, the finding of a lung nodule in a head and neck cancer patient should not automatically be assumed to represent metastatic disease. Similarly, 2%–5% of lung carcinoma patients present with apparent synchronous lung primary tumors (which may be due to the greatly improved resolution of CT techniques which can now detect additional small nodules in patients with a dominant lung masses); histologic sampling of these lesions often shows alveolar proliferations with varying degrees of atypia, which may represent precursor lesions in the peripheral lung similar to squamous dysplasia in the more central airways.

A. **Pathologic reporting.** The important data to be included in a diagnostic report of a primary pulmonary neoplasm are summarized in Table 8.13. Generally, tumor size is assessed by gross examination, and this measurement suffices unless there is confounding fibrosis or peritumoral pneumonia. The extension of tumor through the pleura covering the lung (visceral pleura) or into the pleura lining the chest wall (parietal pleura) should be noted; an elastin stain can delineate these layers in some cases. Lymphatic and venous invasion should

TABLE 8.12 WHO Histological Classification of Tumors of the Lung

Malignant epithelial tumors
Squamous cell carcinoma
    Papillary
    Clear cell
    Small cell
    Basaloid
Small cell carcinoma
    Combined small cell carcinoma
Adenocarcinoma
    Adenocarcimoma, mixed subtype
    Acinar adencocarcinoma
    Papillary adenocarcinoma
    Bronchioloalveolar carcinoma
        Non-mucinous
        Mucinous
        Mixed non-mucinous and mucinous or indeterminate
    Solid adenocarcinoma with mucin production
    Fetal adenocarcinoma
    Mucinous ("colloid") carcinoma
    Mucinous cystadenocarcinoma
    Signet ring adenocarcinoma
    Clear cell adenocarcinoma
Large cell carcinoma
    Large cell neuroendocrine carcinoma
        Combined large cell neuroendocrine carcinoma
    Basaloid carcinoma
    Lymphoepithelioma-like carcinoma
    Clear cell carcinoma
    Large cell carcinoma with rhabdoid phenotype
Adenosquamous carcinoma
Sarcomatoid carcinoma
    Pleomorphic carcinoma
    Spindle cell carcinoma
    Giant cell carcinoma
    Carcinosarcoma
    Pulmonary blastoma
Carcinoid tumor
    Typical carcinoid
    Atypical carcinoid
Salivary gland tumors
    Mucoepidermoid caricinoma
    Adenoid cystic carcinoma
    Epithelial–myoepithelial carcinoma
Preinvasive lesions
    Squamous carcinoma in situ
    Atypical adenomatous hyperplasia
    Diffuse idiopathic pulmonary neuroendocrine cell hyperplasia
Messenchymal tumors
    Epithelioid haemangioendothelioma
    Angiosarcoma
    Pleuropulmonary blastoma

(continued)

TABLE 8.12   WHO Histological Classification of Tumors of the Lung (*Continued*)

Chondroma
Congenial peribronchial myofibroblastic tumour
Diffuse pulmonary lymphangiomatosis
Inflammatory myofibroblastic tumour
Lymphangioleiomyomatosis
Synovial sarcoma
   Monophasic
   Biphasic
Pulmonary artery sarcoma
Pulmonary vein sarcoma

Benign epithelial tumors
Papillomas
Squamous cell papilloma
   Exophytic
   Inverted
Glandular papilloma
Mixed squamous cell and glandular papilloma
Adenomas
Alveolar adenoma
Papillary adenoma
Adenomas of the salivary gland type
   Mucous gland adenoma
   Pleomorphic adenoma
   Others
Mucinous cystadenoma

Lymphoproliferative tumors
Marginal zone B-cell lymphoma of the MALT type
Diffuse large B-cell lymphoma
Lymphomatoid granulomatosis
Langerhans cell histiocytosis

Miscellaneous tumors
Harmatoma
Sclerosing hemangioma
Clear cell tumor
Germ cell tumors
   Teratoma, mature
   Immature
   Other germ cell tumors
Intrapulmonary thymoma
Melanoma

Metastatic tumors

From: Travis WD, Brambilla E, Müller-Hermelink HK, Harris CC, eds. *World Health Organization Classification of Tumours. Pathology and Genetics. Tumours of the Lung, Pleura, Thymus and Heart.* Lyon: IARC Press; 2004. Used with permission.

be noted separately. The status of the margins of resection should be listed, and any abnormalities in the adjacent lung should be described. The AJCC pathologic staging of lung carcinomas is provided in Table 8.14.

In the past, therapy of non-small cell lung carcinomas (SCLCs) was largely independent of histology. However, recent developments in the therapy make histologic classification important. Therapy with pemetrexed has been demonstrated to be efficacious in pulmonary adenocarcinomas, and bevucizamid

TABLE 8.13	Diagnostic Features To Be Reported with Lung Carcinoma Resections
• Tumor type	• Margins
• Grade	• Associated Conditions in Non-Neoplastic Lung
• Tumor Size	• T stage
• Pleural Involvement	• N stage
• Lymphatic Invasion	• M data
• Venous Invasion	• Overall stage (AJCC)

is contraindicated in squamous carcinomas due to bleeding complications. Furthermore, mutation testing is indicated in high-stage adenocarcinomas. Thus, it is now vital that cases with such features as glandular formation, mucin production, or keratinization should be classified as adenocarcinoma or squamous carcinoma. Cases which have less defined features may be classified by immunostaining; napsin and TTF-1 are largely restricted to adenocarcinoma, while p63 or cytokeratin 5/6 are largely seen in squamous tumors; however, immunohistochemical classification is still an evolving area, as different experts have recommended various panels in this context (*Am J Surg Pathol.* 2011;35:15, *Mod Pathol.* 2011; May 27 [epub ahead of print], *Pathol.* 2011;43:103). Also, it remains to be seen whether cases classified only by immunostaining produces the same therapeutic implications as for cases that can be classified on histology alone, which was the method of classification in the chemotherapy trials discussed above.

B. Non-small cell carcinomas

1. Adenocarcinoma is now the most common subtype of lung carcinoma, accounting for 40% or more of all primary lung carcinomas. This subtype is relatively more common in women. More than two-thirds of cases arise in the periphery of the lung, often in a sub-pleural location, often with an associated scar (e-Fig. 8.38). Pulmonary acinar adenocarcinoma, sometimes designated as adenocarcinoma of no special type, represents the most common form of pulmonary adenocarcinoma. This variant of adenocarcinoma features a glandular, tubular, or solid growth pattern. The cytologic features range from very bland and well differentiated to highly anaplastic. Subtypes of adenocarcinoma include papillary, invasive micropapillary, mucinous, enteric-like, clear cell, glassy cell, and bronchioloalveolar carcinoma (BAC) (see below). Because of the peripheral location of the most adenocarcinomas, they have a higher rate of resectability than many other non-small cell carcinomas, and also tend to involve the visceral pleura. Finally, since lymphatic and vascular invasion, with consequent lymph node metastases, are quite common, relatively small peripheral adenocarcinomas may have mediastinal lymph node involvement.

Electron microscopic and immunostaining studies show that pulmonary adenocarcinomas can resemble the many different respiratory cell types, including bronchial cells, goblet cells, Clara cells, and alveolar pneumocytes. Immunostains show consistent positivity for epithelial membrane antigen (EMA), various cytokeratins including cytokeratin 7, various surfactants and related proteins, and the nuclear marker thyroid transcription factor-1 (TTF-1) (e-Fig. 8.39). TTF-1 has been shown to be quite useful in differentiating primary pulmonary adenocarcinomas from lung metastases of adenocarcinomas from a variety of other origins, and can also identify metastatic pulmonary adenocarcinomas in distant sites. Since very poorly differentiated adenocarcinomas, as well as some mucinous pulmonary carcinomas, do not express TTF-1, TTF-1 negativity does not provide definitive evidence that a tumor is not of pulmonary origin; such a determination must

TABLE 8.14 TNM Classification of the Lung

Primary Tumor (T)

TX	Primary tumor cannot be assessed, or tumor proven by the presence of malignant cells in sputum or bronchial washings but not visualized by imaging or bronchoscopy
T0	No evidence of primary tumor
Tis	Carcinoma in situ
T1	Tumor 3 cm or less in greatest dimension, surrounded by lung or visceral pleura, without bronchoscopic evidence of invasion more proximal than the lobar bronchus (i.e., not in the main bronchus)[a]
T1a	Tumor 2 cm or less in greatest dimension
T1b	Tumor more than 2 cm but 3 cm or less in greatest dimension
T2	Tumor more than 3 cm but 7 cm or less or tumor with any of the following features (T2 tumors with these features are classified T2a if 5 cm or less); Involves main bronchus, 2 cm or more distal to the carina; Invades visceral pleura; Associated with atelectasis or obstructive pneumonitis that extends to the hilar region but does involve the entire lung
T2a	Tumor more than 3 cm but 5 cm or less in greatest dimension
T2b	Tumor more than 5 cm but 7 cm or less in greatest dimension
T3	Tumor more than 7 cm or one that directly invades any of the following: parietal pleural (PL3) chest wall (including superior sulcus tumors), diaphragm, phrenic nerve, mediastinal pleura, parietal pericardium; or tumor in the main bronchus <2 cm distal to the carina[a] but without involvement of the carina; or associated atelectasis or obstructive pneumonitis of the entire lung or separate tumor nodule(s) in the same lobe
T4	Tumor of any size that invades any of the following: mediastinum, heart, great vessels, trachea, recurrent laryngeal nerve, esophagus, vertebral body, carina; separate tumor nodule(s) in a different ipsilateral lobe

Regional Lymph Nodes (N)

NX	Regional lymph nodes cannot be assessed
N0	No regional lymph node metastasis
N1	Metastasis in ipsilateral peribronchial and/or ipsilateral hilar lymph nodes and intrapulmonary nodes, including involvement by direct extension
N2	Metastasis in ipsilateral mediastinal and/or subcarinal lymph node(s)
N3	Metastasis in contralateral mediastinal, contralateral hilar, ipsilateral or contralateral scalene, or supraclavicular lymph node(s)

Distant Metastasis (M)

M0	No distant metastasis
M1	Distant metastasis
M1a	Separate tumor nodule(s) in a contralateral lobe tumor with pleural nodules or malignant pleural (or pericardial) effusion
M1b	Distant metastasis

(continued)

be based on all available clinical, radiographic, and pathologic information. In addition, TTF-1 is not specific for pulmonary adenocarcinoma and may be expressed by thyroid carcinomas and neuroendocrine carcinomas arising at a variety of other anatomic sites. As mentioned below, napsin is a marker typically present in lung adenocarcinomas. As expected in many adenocarcinomas, pulmonary adenocarcinoma also expresses many generic

TABLE 8.14 TNM Classification of the Lung (*Continued*)

ANATOMIC STAGE/PROGNOSTIC GROUPS

Occult carcinoma	Tx	N0	M0
Stage 0	Tis	N0	M0
Stage 1A	T1a	N0	M0
	T1b	N0	M0
Stage 1B	T2a	N0	M0
Stage IIA	T2b	N0	M0
	T1a	N1	M0
	T1b	N1	M0
	T2a	N1	M0
Stage IIIB	T2b	N1	M0
	T3	N0	M0
Stage IIIA	T1a	N2	M0
	T1b	N2	M0
	T2a	N2	M0
	T2b	N2	M0
	T3	N1	M0
	T3	N2	M0
	T4	N0	M0
	T4	N1	M0
Stage IIIB	T1a	N3	M0
	T1b	N3	M0
	T2a	N3	M0
	T2b	N3	M0
	T3	N3	M0
	T4	N2	M0
	T4	N3	M0
Stage IV	Any T	Any N	M1a
	Any T	Any N	M1b

[a]The uncommon superficial spreading tumor of any size with its invasive component limited to the bronchial wall, which may extend proximally to the main bronchus, is also classified as T1a.
From: Edge SB, Byrd DR, Compton CC, et al., eds. *AJCC Cancer Staging Manual.* 7th ed. New York, NY: Springer; 2010, Used with permission.

carcinoma markers including carcinoma embryonic antigen (CEA), the B72.3-related antigen, CD15, and MOC31.

a. **Molecular diagnostics** play increasingly import role in the evaluation of lung adenocarcinoma (*Cancer Treat Rev.* 2010;36(suppl 3):S21). It has now been convincingly shown that adenocarcinomas with EGFR-activating mutations will respond, sometimes very impressively, to EGFR-inhibitors such as erlotinib. In multiple trials, such therapy is superior to cytotoxic chemotherapy with markedly decreased side effects, and thus EGFR inhibitor therapy is now the recommended first-line therapy for stage III and IV adenocarcinomas with *EGFR* mutations. While studies suggest that *EGFR*-mutated adenocarcinomas tend to occur more often in Asian populations, never- or light-smokers, and women, the emergence of *EGFR* inhibitor therapy and the presence of mutated cases outside of the Asian/female/non-smoking population has made testing of all high stage adenocarcinomas for *EGFR* mutations essentially standard of care. The validity of this approach is emphasized by the fact that approximately 15% of lung adenocarcinomas harbor *EGFR* mutations. A single activating mutation in exon 19 accounts for most clinically important *EGFR* mutations; the clinical value of rigorous testing for more uncommon mutations is currently less clear.

Crizotinib is another tyrosine kinase inhibitor that targets lung adenocarcinomas harboring the *EML4-ALK* translocation. This translocation tends to occur in tumors with mucinous or signet ring histology, but can occur more rarely in other histotypes. Overall, 4%–5% of lung adenocarcinomas harbor this translocation, and detection by FISH analysis is the current methodology of choice.

K-ras mutations are also found in a subset of adenocarcinomas. It has been shown that *K-ras*, *EGFR*, and *ALK* mutations are essentially mutually exclusive, and thus some experts advocate the following approach: Initial genetic analysis should consist of testing for *K-ras* mutations, which can be easily and rapidly accomplished. If a *K-ras* mutation is found, testing is essentially complete; if *K*-ras is wild type, *EGFR* testing should be performed, since *EGFR* mutations are more prevalent than *ALK* mutations. *ALK* testing can be performed in the *K-ras* negative, *EGFR* negative cases. A number of other targets for directed therapy are currently under investigation (such as COX-2, BRAF, met, IGF), but at this time as there is no accepted therapy currently tied to these targets and such testing is, therefore, not part of routine clinical analysis of lung adenocarcinomas. Similarly, multi-gene expression assays and whole genome sequencing are under investigation and may in the near future provide additional prognostic and therapeutic information, but are not currently part of routine clinical analysis.

b. **BAC** is a specialized form of pulmonary adenocarcinoma. With the relative and absolute increase of peripheral lung carcinomas, as discussed above, an increasing number of primary lung cancers present as ground glass opacities on chest imaging. Clinicians and radiologists often characterize these as BAC, but the morphologic diagnosis of BAC is somewhat rare because the restrictive WHO guidelines demand that BAC maintain an alveolar architecture. WHO criteria specify that BAC grow primarily in a lepidic pattern; cases with any significant component of destructive invasion, as indicated by desmoplasia, should be classified as invasive adenocarcinomas. Pure BAC, therefore, is rare; it develops relatively more often in women and in non-smokers. It is much more common as a peripheral component of an invasive adenocarcinoma, in which case it is best reported as adenocarcinoma with bronchioloalveolar features. Emerging thought suggests that the degree of invasion in peripheral adenocarcinomas is an important feature. Tumors with no invasive component are "pure BACs," and are analogous to in situ carcinoma. Cases with a large BAC component and 5 mm or less of invasion also have an excellent prognosis, while cases with >5 mm of invasive tumor behave closer to classical invasive adenocarcinomas. Thus, reporting of the total tumor size, and the constituent size of BAC and invasive components is suggested.

BAC may present as a solitary peripheral nodule, multiple nodules, with lobar consolidation that mimics pneumonia, or rarely with diffuse involvement of the entire lung. BACs are well-differentiated neoplasms. The tumor cell nuclei are often only modestly atypical, but are abnormal by their monotonous nature, and may be differentiated from reactive alveolar processes in part by this cellular uniformity. So-called sclerosing BAC may have some expansion of the alveolar interstitium by fibrosis without invasion, but many postulated examples of this tumor are actually invasive adenocarcinoma. Because BAC grows very slowly, there may be a central elastotic scar that is degenerative or involutional and

TABLE 8.15	Atypical Alveolar Hyperplasia Versus Bronchioloalveolar Carcinoma	
	Atypical Alveolar hyperplasia	**Bronchioloalveolar carcinoma**
Size	Small, usually <5 mm	5 mm
Clinical presentation	Often unsuspected, may be found in sections of grossly "normal" lung or in sections of margins	Radiographic and gross lesion is present
Cytologic features	Mildy atypical, but polymorphous	Mildly atypical, monomorphous

so should not be labeled as invasive growth; these scars may feature calcification or even metaplastic bone. Some example of BAC can have extensive lymphocytic infiltrates, often with a nodular pattern. BAC has been classically divided into type I and Type II.

  i. **Type I BACs** are mucinous and may resemble pulmonary goblet cells, gastric mucous cells, or intestinal epithelium, both morphologically and in terms of mucin types (e-**Fig. 8.40**). Mucinous BAC is often multifocal and may present with bronchorrhea. The cells grow along alveoli, often with a discontinuous appearance, and mucin and muciphages may fill the involved alveolar spaces. Invasive mucinous carcinomas, including signet ring lesions, are often found in continuity with mucinous BAC. Another type of adenocarcinoma closely related to mucinous BAC is so-called enteric type adenocarcinoma, which closely resembles colonic or other gut carcinomas. Finally, the so-called mucinous cystadenoma may be associated with mucinous BAC; this rare low grade mucinous lung lesion resembles mucinous cystadenomas in other sites, and so is best considered as a lesion of low malignant potential. Metastatic adenocarcinoma of gastric, pancreatic, or intestinal origin is the most important differential consideration for mucinous BAC.

  Mucinous BAC and related invasive adenocarcinomas of the lung often show immunohistochemical co-expression of cytokeratins 7 and 20 (e-**Fig. 8.41**), but may be negative for TTF-1. CDX2 staining may be of some utility, as most pulmonary mucinous neoplasms do not react with this immunostain. Adequate clinical history and correlation with the appearance and stage of the primary tumor is of great importance in this differential diagnosis.

  ii. **Type II BAC** cells can resemble several bronchial and alveolar type cell types including type II pneumocytes and Clara cells (e-**Fig. 8.42**). Type II tumors, as compared with Type I tumors, are more likely to present as solitary mass although multiple type II tumors do occur. Tumors with type II pneumocyte differentiation commonly have intranuclear pseudoinclusions, while Clara cell lesions may show PAS-positive apical granules.

  c. **Atypical alveolar hyperplasia (AAH)** is a lesion closely related to BAC. In fact, molecular genetic studies show virtually identical abnormalities in cases of AAH and BAC. Key features in the separation of these lesions are presented in Table 8.15. AAH and BAC are best considered as the peripheral lung equivalents of dysplasia and carcinoma in situ, with a postulated role as precursors of invasive peripheral adenocarcinomas.

2. **Squamous cell carcinoma (SCC)** is most frequently a central lesion arising in larger airways although peripheral lesions do occur; primarily endobronchial tumors are unusual. Post obstructive pneumonia has been reported in up to one-half of SCC. SCC is prone to central necrosis,

and cavitation is a common radiologic finding. Squamous dysplasia and carcinoma in situ not infrequently accompany SCC and may be the only material retrieved by endoscopic biopsy. The histology of SCC does not differ significantly from SCC that occurs at other body sites; both keratinizing and non-keratinizing variants occur, as well as basaloid and clear cell forms (e-**Fig. 8.43**).

Poorly differentiated SCC should not be confused with small cell carcinoma; SCC lacks the individual cell necrosis, crush artifact, and nuclear molding seen in small cell carcinoma. The distinction between small cell carcinoma and SCC can be facilitated by immunostains for p63; SCC generally reacts with antibodies to p63 while small cell carcinoma does not. SCC also seems to be somewhat less prone to nodal metastasis.

3. **Large cell carcinoma** is an undifferentiated epithelial neoplasm. Neither squamous differentiation (keratin, cytoplasmic bridges) nor glandular features (mucin, acinar formation) are seen by light microscopy, although ultrastructural studies show both squamous and glandular elements. Exhaustive and expensive attempts to subclassify undifferentiated large cell carcinoma into a specific diagnostic category offers no clinical utility; the finding of a tumor so poorly differentiated that standard sampling and diagnostic techniques cannot demonstrate clear cut squamous or glandular differentiation provides prognostic information in itself. These tumors are generally aggressive. Large randomized clinical trials have shown that demonstration of neuroendocrine markers in non-small neoplasms in general, and large cell neoplasms in particular (outside of the defined neuroendocrine tumor types delineated below), does not denote responsiveness to small-cell carcinoma specific chemotherapeutic regimens.

4. **Giant cell carcinoma** is a unique variant of large cell carcinoma. The tumor grows as a large bulky peripheral mass, and often invades the pleura and chest wall. Giant cell carcinoma is composed of large epithelioid cells, many of which are multi-nucleated (e-**Fig. 8.44**). The cells grow in large sheets and are loosely cohesive. An intense acute and chronic inflammatory cell infiltrate almost always permeates giant cell carcinoma. A spindle cell component often mixes with the giant cell pattern, producing what has sometimes been designated as pleomorphic carcinoma. Unique aspects of giant cell carcinoma include a propensity to metastasize to abdominal sites including the small bowel, and an association with leukemoid reaction. Immunoreactivity for epithelial markers including cytokeratin and EMA are generally maintained; documentation of these markers in a giant cell carcinoma distinguishes this tumor from such possible mimics as malignant fibrous histiocytoma, anaplastic large cell lymphoma, or choriocarcinoma.

5. **Clear cell carcinoma** does not represent a distinct primary form of pulmonary carcinoma; rather, lung carcinomas with cytoplasmic clearing represent variants of other forms of non-small cell carcinoma. Clearing has been reported in 25% or more of all pulmonary adenocarcinomas, squamous carcinomas, and even large cell carcinomas (e-**Fig. 8.45**). Of course, a pulmonary clear cell neoplasm should raise concern for a metastatic clear cell carcinoma, typically of renal origin, as well as the rare pulmonary clear cell tumor (see below).

6. **Adenosquamous carcinoma** is an uncommon variant of pulmonary carcinoma. These tumors are generally associated with a smoking history. The diagnosis should be reserved for tumors in which there is clearly recognizable differentiation into squamous (intercellular bridges, and possibly keratinization) and glandular elements (acini). Solid adenocarcinomas with minimal squamoid differentiation or foci of cytoplasmic eosinophilia should not be interpreted as adenosquamous carcinoma; similarly, SCC s that

TABLE 8.16	Features of Pulmonary Neuroendocrine Neoplasms					
WHO Terminology	**Alternative Terminology**	**Cell Size**	**Nuclear Atypia**	**Mitoses**	**Necrosis**	**Malignant Potential**
Carcinoid	Grade 1 NEC	Medium to large	None	<2/hpf	None	Low
Atypical Carcinoid	Grade 2 NEC	Medium to large	Mild	2-10/hpf	Focal	Intermediate
Large Cell Neuroendocrine Carcinoma	Grade 3 NEC, Large Cell type	Large	Marked	>10/hpf	Extensive	High
Small Cell Neuroendocrine Carcinoma	Grade 3 NEC, Small Cell type	Small	Marked	High	Extensive	High

contain rare droplets of intracytoplasmic mucin are better classified as SCC s. High grade mucoepidermoid carcinomas in the lung are probably best classified as adenosquamous carcinomas

7. **Other rare types** of lung carcinoma include lymphoepithelial-like carcinoma (e-Fig. 8.46), non-small cell carcinoma with rhabdoid features, and invasive micropapillary carcinoma.

C. **Neuroendocrine neoplasms.** Neuroendocrine neoplasms (see Table 8.16) constitute a spectrum of neoplasms, from lesions of little clinical significance to highly malignant tumors. The exact origin of these neoplasms remains speculative. Although the airways contain neuroendocrine cells known as Kulchitsky cells, the idea that all neuroendocrine tumors arise from pre-existing neuroendocrine cells is probably not true; neuroendocrine differentiation may simply be a reflection of the totipotential nature of malignant neoplasms. In general, better differentiated tumors show greater variety in secretory products and have greater number of neuroendocrine granules on ultrastructural examination.

1. **Neuroendocrine cell hyperplasia** is the simplest neuroendocrine lesion seen in the lungs. As its name implies, this process consists of an increased number of neuroendocrine cells in the bronchial and bronchiolar epithelium. This lesion is often not apparent by standard histology and only visualized through the use of immunostains for neuroendocrine markers. The lesion likely represents a reactive process and may be associated with conditions that cause airway inflammation or injury, and is of little or no clinical significance. It is the one lung neuroendocrine lesion that can be safely thought of as benign in essentially all cases.

2. **Carcinoid tumors** should be considered grade 1 neuroendocrine carcinomas. Carcinoids can be divided into central lesions which have an association with cartilaginous airways (often designated as typical carcinoids), and peripheral types which lack such an association. Carcinoid tumors tend to occur on average as much as one to two decades earlier than other type of lung carcinomas. In addition, they do not show any convincing relationship to cigarette smoking (in contrast to higher grade neuroendocrine tumors). The clinical presentation of patients with carcinoid tumors varies based on the tumor's location. Central tumors, which are slowly growing, often present with airway-related symptoms such as wheezing, recurrent pneumonias, and cough (e-Fig. 8.47). In contrast, peripheral carcinoids are often asymptomatic and are discovered incidentally as a pulmonary "coin lesion." Unlike small bowel carcinoids, they essentially will never be

associated with the carcinoid syndrome, although cases of Cushing syndrome have been reported due to ACTH release.

Grossly, central carcinoid tumors usually present as yellow-tan polypoid intraluminal masses covered by normal respiratory tract mucosa; they almost always measure <5 cm. Microscopic sections show a variety of architectural patterns including trabecula, rosettes, papillary formations, and areas of solid growth (e-Fig. 8.48). The tumors have vascular stroma, which can also feature elements including amyloid and bone. The individual cells tend to have moderate to abundant cytoplasm, which is often granular and eosinophilic. The tumor cells have nuclei that are regular, and round to oval; the chromatin is granular, and often referred to as having a "salt and pepper" character. Mitotic activity should be essentially absent; the most recent WHO standard is ≤2 mitosis per 10 high power fields. Necrosis should be absent. Peripheral carcinoid tumors are morphologically identical to central tumors, although peripheral carcinoid tumors often exhibit a spindled morphology. Tumors with a peripheral location and spindled pattern should not be designated automatically as atypical carcinoid tumors (see below).

Carcinoid tumors (which can also be referred to as well differentiated neuroendocrine carcinomas) contain abundant neurosecretory granules, and show strong expression of chromogranin and synaptophysin; they are also immunopositive for epithelial markers such as cytokeratin. Carcinoid tumors have a low malignant potential. Only about 5% of patients present with lymph node metastases; <5% of cases develop distant metastases disease with spread to the liver, brain, bones, and skin. Long-term survival is in excess of 95%.

a. **Carcinoid tumorlets** are microscopic proliferations (4 mm or less in size) that are otherwise histologically and immunophenotypically identical to carcinoid tumors (e-Fig. 8.49); distinction is based solely on size. Tumorlets tend to occur in distal airways, and may be single lesions incidentally discovered in resection specimens. Rare patients may have hundreds of these lesions in their distal airways. Multiple carcinoid tumorlets have some association with chronic airway diseases. Tumorlets have little or no clinical significance.

b. **Paraganglioma** features nested cells, a fine fibrovascular stroma, cells with eosinophilic to granular cytoplasm and some spindling, and regular nuclei, and so it can be difficult to distinguish paraganglioma from carcinoid tumor. Although paraganglioma shows immunopositivity for chromogranin and synaptophysin, it is not reactive with antibodies to cytokeratin; in addition, the tumor contains S-100 positive sustentacular cells that are not present in carcinoid tumors.

c. **Chemodectomas.** Multiple pulmonary chemodectomas were once considered a variant of paraganglioma, but now are known to have no relationship to paraganglioma. Chemodectomas consist of 1–2 mm stellate proliferations that fill the pulmonary interstitium and feature bland epithelioid cells in a whirling pattern. These tumors share immunoreactivity for EMA and vimentin, and have been labeled as "minute meningothelial-like nodules." They are of no clinical significance.

3. **Atypical carcinoid tumor,** better designated as grade 2 neuroendocrine carcinoma, is more rare than carcinoid tumor, and more evenly divided between central and peripheral locations (e-Fig. 8.50). Because more tumors are peripheral, airway-related symptoms are less common. In addition, there is a closer relationship to cigarette smoking. These tumors tend to be slightly larger than grade 1 lesions at the time of diagnosis, but it is microscopic features that distinguish grade 2 neuroendocrine carcinoma (atypical

carcinoid) from grade 1 neuroendocrine carcinoma (carcinoid). The tumor cells tend to be slightly smaller than those of classic carcinoid tumors, and some modest nuclear pleomorphism is also usually present. Spindling of the cells is also more common than with grade 1 cases, and mitotic activity is more frequent; up to 10 mitoses in 10 high power fields is an accepted criterion. Necrosis may be present, but is usually limited. Because the cells are moderately differentiated, neuroendocrine immunostains tend to be positive.

Atypical carcinoids show significantly greater malignant potential than classic carcinoids. About 25% of patients with atypical carcinoid tumor have lymph nodal metastases at presentation, and approximately 25% of patients are dead of disease at 5 years after diagnosis.

4. **Large cell neuroendocrine carcinoma** (large cell NEC) can also be designated grade 3 neuroendocrine carcinoma. It is an extremely lethal form of lung carcinoma, and is the most recent variant of neuroendocrine carcinoma to be described. The demographics of LCNEC are similar to those of other lung carcinomas; almost all cases have been reported in cigarette smokers. The vast majority of the tumors are found in the periphery of the lung, and thus they tend to present with the same sort of non-specific symptoms as do other lung carcinomas. The gross of appearance of the tumor is similar to that of other lung carcinomas, and may include necrosis or cavitation (e-Fig. 8.51).

The microscopic features of LCNEC are quite distinctive. The tumor has an organoid appearance in which large solid nests of tumor are separated by scant fibrovascular stroma. In some cases, the tumor seems to fill up the preexisting alveolar spaces. Tumors may show palisading of tumor cells at the periphery of the nests, and spindling or rosettes may also be present. The dominant feature in most cases is extensive necrosis, which may make up the bulk of the tumor mass. The tumor cells themselves are generally polygonal and have a significant amount of cytoplasm. LCNEC can be distinguished from small cell neuroendocrine carcinoma based on several factors: at lower power microscopy, the nuclei of the tumor do not touch (as do the nuclei in small cell carcinomas, see below); the nuclear–cytoplasmic ratio is significantly lower than that of small cell carcinoma; the nuclear chromatin may be vesicular and nucleoli are often prominent; and finally, crush artifact and nuclear molding are not usually seen.

Mitotic activity is one of the key features of this tumor; the tumor should feature at least 10 mitoses per 10 high power fields, although the actual rate is generally far higher. Combined with the extensive necrosis described above, it is generally relatively straightforward to separate large cell NEC from lower grade tumors such as atypical carcinoid. In fact, large cell NEC probably has greatest overlap with non-small cell carcinomas such as poorly differentiated squamous carcinomas. Thus, immunostains can be quite helpful in diagnosis. Large cell NEC shows reliable staining with pancytokeratin antibodies (because of the increased amount of cytoplasm in the tumor, cytokeratin stains do not show the dot-like pattern that is typical of small cell carcinoma, but rather show strong circumferential cytoplasmic staining). The majority of cases of large cell NEC also show positive staining for chromogranin, synaptophysin, CD56, and CD57, although the more poorly differentiated nature of LCNEC is reflected in more focal reactivity for these neuroendocrine markers. Large cell NEC often also shows positive staining for p53.

The prognosis for large cell NEC is quite poor. Although the great majority of patients present with node negative lesions at diagnosis, most patients rapidly develop recurrent or metastatic disease. The overall survival at five and 10 years is poor, approximately 20% and 10%, respectively.

5. **SCLC** is classically described as high grade neuroendocrine carcinoma. The incidence of SCLC is decreasing, but SCLC still accounts for at least 10% of all primary lung carcinomas. This tumor type has a very strong association with cigarette smoking. At least 95% of patients present with a central mass comprised of hilar and/or mediastinal adenopathy; the adenopathy often is larger than any radiographically definable intra-pulmonary mass (e-**Fig. 8.52**). The bulky tumor in the mediastinum leads to a variety of clinical presentations, including cough, hemoptysis, lobar collapse, shortness of breath from pleural effusions, chest pain, hoarseness from recurrent laryngeal nerve invasion, or superior vena cava syndrome. A significant number of patients also present with signs or symptoms referable to distant spread, such as neurologic symptoms (brain metastases), bone lesions, or symptoms due to abdominal organ involvement. Paraneoplastic syndromes are common, including the syndrome of inappropriate secretion of anti-diuretic hormone (Eaton–Lambert syndrome) and Cushing syndrome (related to ACTH production).

Since small cell carcinomas are rarely resected, the gross features of the tumor are seldom seen in the surgical pathology laboratory. These features include a large central mass that tends to spread along the bronchial tree, with involvement of hilar lymph nodes often in a contiguous fashion with the primary tumor. Some cases show an endobronchial lesion; <5% of cases present as a peripheral pulmonary nodule.

The microscopic appearance of small cell carcinoma varies with the method of sampling (e-**Fig. 8.53**). Endobronchial biopsies commonly have the so-called "oat cell" appearance characterized by small cells (about twice the diameter of a resting lymphocyte) with dark hyperchromatic nuclei. There is scant to barely visible cytoplasm, and crush artifact and nuclear molding are prominent; nucleoli are not usually prominent. Individual apoptotic cells are often seen, and more extensive confluent necrosis may be present. Mitotic figures are frequent. The cells tend to stream through the tissue in irregular sheets, although some cases may show rosettes, palisades, or trabecular growth patterns. Small cell carcinoma often has a slightly different appearance in larger tissue samples, such as resected primary tumors or lymph node biopsies. The cells are oftentimes slightly larger (up to four times the diameter of a resting lymphocyte), but still feature dark hyperchromatic nuclei, often with nucleoli. Crush artifact and nuclear molding may be less prominent. Necrosis is often widespread; one well-known feature of small cell carcinoma with excessive necrosis is the so-called Azzopardi effect, which is the coating of blood vessel walls by nucleic acid to produce dark blue ring-like structures in the midst of otherwise eosinophilic necrotic areas.

Immunostains can be helpful in the diagnosis of small cell carcinoma. Cytokeratin immunostains often produce a dot-like perinuclear pattern of positivity due to the small amount of cytoplasm and the condensation of cytoskeletal elements in the tumor cells. Stains for CD45 can exclude lymphoma. In cases with classic morphology, this simple panel (cytokeratin and CD45) is sufficient for the diagnosis of small cell carcinoma. If additional immunostains are requested to confirm neuroendocrine differentiation, it should be noted that small cell carcinomas have very few neurosecretory granules, and hence chromogranin stains are relatively insensitive. Similarly, synaptophysin and CD57 stains are positive in only approximately 50%–60% of cases. Stains for NCAM (CD56) are more sensitive, and stains TTF-1 are also positive in the majority of cases of pulmonary small cell carcinoma. The cells of small cell carcinoma may also express CD99, bcl2, p53, and CEA, although these stains generally are not obtained in a diagnostic context.

Since small cell carcinoma has spread extensively at the time of diagnosis in most cases, treatment is generally non-surgical. Survival remains poor. Modern chemotherapy and radiation regimens produce significant disease remissions in the majority of patients, but relapse within a few months is common. Overall 5 year survival is in the range of 5% to 10%.

Neuroendocrine carcinoma may also be mixed with non-small cell carcinoma. This combination is rarely if ever seen with low grade lesions, but is seen in a small minority of cases of large cell NEC and small cell carcinoma. Admixed non-small cell components are rarely seen in bronchial biopsy specimens, but are detected in up to 10% of resected small cell cancer cases; this discrepancy is probably related to sampling volume. When recurrences occur after treatment of small cell carcinoma, a dominant non-small cell component may be present; it is likely that this shift in phenotype represents selective survival of a previously minor admixed non-small cell component not targeted by treatment directed against small cell carcinoma.

D. **Sarcomatoid carcinoma and related neoplasms.** A subset of primary pulmonary carcinomas have sarcoma-like features. These tumors have been given a variety of names, including carcinosarcoma and spindle cell carcinoma; sarcomatoid carcinoma is the currently preferred designation for all carcinomas with sarcoma-like features. Patients with sarcomatoid carcinoma have a similar age and smoking history as those with other forms of pulmonary carcinoma. Sarcomatoid carcinoma, however, presents in two distinct patterns. Some cases present as a polypoid intraluminal mass within a large central airway; these tumors tend to be small, most likely because patients present with airway-related symptoms early in the course of the tumor's growth. In contrast, other patients present with a bulky peripheral mass, often with pleural and chest wall invasion. Microscopic sections show malignant spindled tumor cells (e-**Fig. 8.54**) which may transition from areas of non-small cell carcinoma. Various heterologous elements such as malignant cartilage or osteoid may also be seen.

The major differential is with true pulmonary sarcomas and sarcomatoid mesotheliomas. In order to diagnose sarcomatoid carcinoma, the sarcoma-like tumor must be proven to show some evidence of an epithelial lineage. This can be accomplished by immunostaining; reactivity for cytokeratins, EMA, p63, or other generic carcinoma markers such as carcinoembryonic antigen will be present in the majority of (although not all) examples of sarcomatoid carcinoma. Electron microscopy, with identification of epithelial features such as cell junctions, may be quite useful in this context. In many cases, extensive sampling is enough to demonstrate an epithelial component by showing transition from sarcoma-like areas to classic areas of squamous carcinoma or adenocarcinoma; the finding of such a transition provides definitive evidence as to the nature of the neoplasm. Differentiation from mesothelioma may be difficult in that immunophentoypes may overlap; WT1 and calretinin expression would favor mesothelioma. Clinical presentation as a single intrapulmonary mass may be a critical feature that favors sarcomatoid carcinoma, since mesothelioma tends to present as a diffuse pleural neoplasm.

The behavior of sarcomatoid carcinomas varies with the clinical presentation. Cases presenting as a small intraluminal polypoid airway lesion have a fair prognosis. In contrast, those cases occurring as large bulky peripheral tumors have a poor outcome since high stage disease at presentation is common.

TABLE 8.17	Blastoma-like Lung Neoplasms					
Tumor type	Age at diagnosis	Smoking history	Size	Malignant glands	Malignant stroma	Prognosis
Monophasic pulmonary blastoma	third–fourth decade	yes	small	yes	no	excellent
Biphasic pulmonary blastoma	3rd–4th decade	yes	Large, fleshy	yes	yes	poor
Pleuropulmonary blastoma	Children (rare adults)	no	Large, solid and/or cystic	no	yes	Variable, dependent on type

E. **Fetal adenocarcinoma** is also known as monophasic pulmonary blastoma. It is a tumor of adults, although it occurs on average several decades earlier than other non-small cell carcinomas. Most patients are smokers. The tumors generally are found in the periphery of the lung, average 4 to 5 cm, and are usually well-circumscribed. Microscopically, the tumor is composed of closely packed glands and tubules with scant intervening stroma (e-Fig. 8.55). Cribriform and vaguely papillary patterns can also be seen. The tumor is composed of cytologically bland columnar cells with cytoplasmic clearing that resemble secretory endometrium. The glandular lumina are often filled with solid morules; the cells of these morules have nuclear clearing. Ultrastructural and immunohistochemical studies of fetal adenocarcinomas show pneumocyte-like differentiation, including expression of surfactants and Clara cell antigens. In addition, the glandular and morular cells contain neurosecretory granules with immunoexpression of neuroendocrine markers. The prognosis for this tumor is excellent; more than 80% of patients are cured by surgical resection, an outcome that contrasts markedly with the poor prognosis of biphasic pulmonary blastoma.

F. **Biphasic pulmonary blastoma.** Like sarcomatoid carcinoma, biphasic pulmonary blastoma features both a malignant glandular and malignant stromal component. Biphasic pulmonary blastoma must be distinguished from pleuropulmonary blastoma (PPB) (see Table 8.17 and below). Despite the designation as a blastoma, biphasic pulmonary blastoma occurs almost exclusively in adults, albeit at a younger age (third or fourth decade of life) than most non-SCLCs. Most patients are cigarette smokers and present with a large peripheral mass often accompanied by a pleural effusion and/or adenopathy. On gross examination the tumors are fleshy, and may show necrosis, cystic change, or hemorrhage. Microscopic examination shows a characteristic biphasic pattern with endometrioid-type glands similar to those of monophasic blastoma, although the epithelial component may also be more poorly differentiated and consist of ill-defined cords and sheets of cells without obvious differentiation (e-Fig. 8.56). The malignant stromal component may resemble the blastemal component of Wilms tumor, or can include ill-defined spindle cells as well as malignant elements such as chondrosarcoma, osteosarcoma, or a myogenic sarcoma. In contrast to monophasic blastoma, the outcome is poor, with most patients dying within 2 years of presentation.

G. **PPB** arises almost exclusively in children, although very rare cases have been described in young adults. There is a familial component to many cases of PPB, and many patients have relatives with a variety of other childhood and adult neoplasms. The tumors present in the lung, most often in the sub-pleural area.

PPB is subclassified on the basis of gross features: predominately cystic (type 1), solid and cystic (type 2), or solid (type 3) (e-**Fig. 8.57**). When cystic, the legion is often confused with a variety of benign cystic conditions including cystic adenomatoid malformation; the misdiagnosis is often discovered when the lesion recurs. Microscopic sections of the cystic cases show that the cysts are lined by benign epithelium with an underlying stroma that can have a variety of appearances, ranging from mature fibroblastic cells to overtly malignant cells with a sarcomatous appearance. The more solid cases similarly show sarcomatous-like malignant cells; rhabdomyoblasts and malignant cartilage may be included. Unlike monophasic and biphasic pulmonary blastoma, PPB does not include a malignant epithelial component. The majority of patients with completely excised cystic lesions that are confined to the lung demonstrate long-term survival; the prognosis is much more guarded for predominantly solid lesions.

H. **Salivary gland tumors.** Minor salivary glands are present all along the tracheobronchial tree. Consequently, the airway can be the site of any of the neoplasms that can occur in the salivary glands. Although rare examples of pleomorphic adenoma (e-**Fig. 8.58**), acinic cell tumor (Fechner tumor), and oncocytoma have been reported, two salivary gland type neoplasms occur with a high enough frequency to warrant further discussion.

1. **Mucoepidermoid carcinoma.** Low grade forms of this tumor tend to present as a polypoid intraluminal mass, and cases have been described in both adults and children. Histologic sections show a mixture of mucus producing cells, clear cells, and squamous cells (e-**Fig. 8.58**). There is minimal mitotic activity and necrosis is lacking. Many cases have abundant mucus-filled cystic areas. The tumor is generally indolent; local invasion and local recurrence are the primary concerns, and local resection is often curative. The major differential diagnostic considerations include mucus gland adenoma (which lacks the locally invasive character of mucoepidermoid carcinoma) and squamous carcinoma (which tends to show more extensive keratinization and less mucus production). High grade forms of mucoepidermoid carcinoma similar to those described in the salivary glands also occur in the lung; since such high grade tumors have a prognosis similar to other forms of non-small cell carcinoma, by convention they are generally considered to represent adenosquamous carcinomas.

2. **Adenoid cystic carcinoma (ACC)** also occurs in the tracheobronchial tree. It is more common in the trachea, but also arises in the larger bronchi. Most tumors are found in middle aged to older adults, and many patients present with a long history of airway symptoms such as wheezing; the long history reflects the indolent nature of these tumors. ACC is usually 2 to 5 cm at the time of diagnosis. The tumor may grossly appear well circumscribed, but microscopically most cases extend beyond the area of gross disease. The histology of the tumor in the lung is identical to the analogous tumor of the salivary glands, with uniform, modestly atypical polygonal cells arranged in nests, cribriform patterns, and solid sheets (e-**Fig. 8.59**). Many of the tumor nests contain characteristic eosinophilic matrix material. As in the salivary glands, perineural invasion is common. Immunostains are consistent with the proposed myoepithelial origin of this tumor, demonstrating immunopositivity for cytokeratin, vimentin, actin, and S100. Many cases are CD117 positive (it is not clear whether this finding has any therapeutic implications). Positive resection margins are common because of the infiltrative growth pattern; postoperative radiation therapy may help control incompletely resected tumors for extended periods of time. Intra-pulmonary metastasis eventually occurs in many cases as a late complication; even

these metastases tend to be slow growing and many patients survive with metastatic disease for an extended period of time.

I. **Sarcomas.** Primary sarcomas of the lung are distinctly uncommon. Before concluding that a tumor is a primary pulmonary sarcoma, primary pulmonary sarcomatoid carcinoma and a sarcoma metastatic to the lung must be excluded. It is, therefore, important to know details of the clinical history and radiographic findings before labeling a lung tumor as a primary lung sarcoma. Fibrohistiocytic, fibroblastic, smooth muscle, and vascular sarcomas have been reported as primary lung sarcomas, as have primary neurogenic, osteogenic, and cartilaginous sarcomas. Small blue cell tumors of the lung include members of the Ewing sarcoma/primitive neuroectodermal tumor (EWS/PNET) family and rhabdomyosarcoma. Lung sarcomas are essentially identical in appearance to their soft tissue counterparts.

1. **Synovial sarcoma i**s a tumor that has recently been recognized to occur in both the lung and pleural spaces. It occurs in relatively younger adults than do primary lung carcinomas. The tumor may show calcifications on radiographs, but otherwise has few defining clinical or radiographic features (e-**Fig. 8.60**). Histologic sections show features identical to synovial sarcomas of the soft tissue (see Chap. 46). Immunostains are tremendously helpful for averting a misdiagnosis; synovial sarcomas of the lung demonstrate expression of cytokeratin and EMA staining in both the glandular and spindle cell areas, and the tumor cells may also be positive for CD34 and CD99. The differential diagnosis includes other biphasic pulmonary tumors such as sarcomatoid carcinoma and biphasic mesothelioma. Molecular demonstration of a t(X;18) translocation can be a helpful aid in diagnosis. As with synovial sarcoma arising in other locations, recurrence or metastasis may take many years to develop, but the ultimate prognosis is poor, with the majority of patients eventually dying of the disease.

2. **Epithelioid hemangioendothelioma (EH)** was originally termed intravascular bronchioloalveolar tumor. EH presents most commonly in women of young to middle age. Patients may be asymptomatic, or present with cough or shortness of breath. Radiology typically shows multiple small pulmonary nodules. Histologic sections show nodules containing pale-staining, hyaline to myxoid stroma in which the preexisting alveolar structure is often still apparent. The neoplastic cells are present within this stoma; they are small and epithelioid and often contain an intracytoplasmic lumen which represents a primitive attempt at vessel formation (e-**Fig. 8.61**). Ultrastructural studies show endothelial cell features such as Weibel-Palade bodies; the cells also react with antibodies for vascular markers, including CD31 and CD34. Although the tumor grows slowly, most patients eventually develop progressive disease with respiratory failure.

3. **Kaposi sarcoma (KS)** is another vascular tumor that may involve the lung. Pulmonary involvement occurs almost exclusively in the setting of immunocompromise, predominantly HIV/AIDS, and rarely in solid organ transplant recipients. Pulmonary KS most often co-exists with cutaneous disease. Radiographic studies show nodular infiltrates and a pleural effusion may be present; symptoms include cough, fever, and hemoptysis. KS spreads via lymphovascular routes and thus is seen along the bronchial tree, along pulmonary vessels, and along the pleural and lobular septa. Histology shows typical lesions of KS, with spindled cells arranged to form slit-like vascular spaces, extravasated erythrocytes, and hemosiderin (e-**Fig. 8.62**). Patients who have pulmonary KS have a poor prognosis, determined not only by the response of KS to chemotherapy but also by the course of the underlying HIV infection.

4. **Pulmonary artery sarcoma** is another rare but deadly lung sarcoma. Patients tend to be middle aged or older, and typically present with shortness of breath or signs of right-sided heart failure. Imaging studies often show intravascular filling of the pulmonary artery trunk which may be interpreted as thromboembolic disease. The tumor may be situated in the main pulmonary artery trunk or in one or both of the main right and left artery branches; the sarcoma may extend distally into progressively smaller branches within the lung. The histologic features of pulmonary artery sarcoma are variable, including smooth muscle, fibrohistiocytic, endothelial, and even chondroid or osteoid differentiation. The prognosis of pulmonary artery sarcoma is poor; even in cases with complete resection, distal recurrences within the ipsilateral lung are the rule. To date, radiation and chemotherapy have not been particularly effective in treating this sarcoma.

5. **Thoracopulmonary small cell tumor,** also known as Askin tumor, is now known to be a member of the EWS/PNET family of neoplasms. This highly malignant tumor most often occurs in children and young adults and is typically very large at presentation; it may literally fill an entire hemithorax (e-**Fig. 8.63**). The exact site of origin is often unclear, although most tumors probably originate from the chest wall with secondary invasion into the lung. The tumor consists of a classic small blue cell proliferation, growing in sheets or rosettes. Necrosis may be prominent. The tumor shows membrane staining for CD99 as well as various neuroendocrine markers. Most cases demonstrate a characteristic t(11;22) translocation (see Chap. 46).

J. MISCELLANEOUS NEOPLASMS

1. **Pulmonary hamartoma** (chondroid hamartoma) is a benign proliferation usually seen in adults. The tumor usually occurs as a solitary peripheral mass with a radiographic appearance of a so-called "coin lesion." A minority of cases involve the more central airways, or even the trachea. Chondroid hamartomas may be part of a heritable syndrome in some cases; Carney triad consists of pulmonary hamartomas, gastric stromal tumors, and extraadrenal pheochromocytomas. Grossly, the tumor is a well circumscribed, nodular lesion (e-**Fig. 8.64**). Histologic sections disclose a mixture of benign mesenchymal components, including cartilage, mature adipose tissue, and smooth muscle. Bronchial type epithelium is usually present within the lesion, although this is thought to represent entrapped tissue rather than a true component of the proliferation. Radiographic diagnosis of this lesion can be confidently made based on the presence of adipose tissue and calcifications within the cartilaginous component; for this reason, hamartomas are often not resected.

2. **Pulmonary clear cell tumor,** or sugar tumor, is a unique pulmonary tumor composed of cells with clear cytoplasm. The tumor generally arises in adults and presents as a well circumscribed, nodular mass; most are found incidentally in asymptomatic patients. The tumor usually measures <5 mm in greatest dimension. Histologic sections show epithelioid cells with bland nuclei and abundant clear cytoplasm (e-**Fig. 8.65**). The cells grow either in nests separated by fine fibrovascular stroma or in a more sheet-like pattern. PAS stains are positive due to abundant intracellular glycogen, as confirmed by ultrastructural studies which may also show pre-melanosomes within the tumor cells. Immunostains show a unique pattern of vimentin positivity, as well as positivity with melanocyte markers such as HMB-45 and melan-A, with expression of actin and CD117 as well.

   The histogenesis of this tumor has long been debated. Most recently it has been suggested that the tumor is a member of the family of tumors known as perivascular epithelioid cell tumors, or PEComas. The most important neoplasm in the differential diagnosis is metastatic renal cell carcinoma; in this regard, it is important to emphasize that pulmonary clear cell tumors uniformly lack expression of epithelial markers such as cytokeratin and EMA. The behavior of pulmonary clear cell tumor has generally been considered to be benign, although rare tumors show malignant behavior.

3. **Inflammatory myofibroblastic tumor (IMT)** has traditionally been given a variety of names, including inflammatory pseudotumor and plasma cell granuloma. IMT is the most common benign lung tumor in children, but occurs in adults as well. The most common presentation is as a relatively small solitary peripheral nodule; IMT also occurs as an endobronchial lesion. Patients may be asymptomatic, or may present with a variety of systemic signs and symptoms, including fever, anemia, and polyclonal hypergammaglobulinemia; systemic manifestations usually resolve with removal of the tumor. In most cases, the tumor is confined to the lung, although occasional cases may exhibit more aggressive local behavior, including invasion of mediastinal structures.

Microscopic sections show a proliferation of spindled myofibroblastic cells with a haphazard pattern of vague fascicles (see Chap. 46) (e-**Fig. 8.66**). The spindle cells are characteristically bland and mitotic figures are rare, without abnormal mitotic figures; necrosis is unusual. There is often a marked inflammatory cell infiltrate in the lesion that may include plasma cells, lymphocytes with lymphoid follicles, neutrophils, and eosinophils. The stroma varies from myxoid to densely collagenized and keloid-like. Immunohistochemical stains show that the spindle cells are positive for vimentin and smooth muscle actin, and are negative for cytokeratin, CD34, and desmin. ALK-1 is variably expressed in IMTs of the lung, corresponding to those cases that harbor a rearranged *ALK* gene (see Chap. 46). The plasma cells are polyclonal by light chain studies. The immunophenotype of IMT can be used to rule out several tumors in the differential diagnosis such as spindle cell carcinoma, solitary fibrous tumor, and fibrohistiocytic neoplasms.

IMT of the lung is usually cured by surgery. Recurrence is rare, but more common if the lesion has invaded adjacent structures at the time of resection. Extremely unusual cases of malignant transformation to a high grade fibroblastic or round cell neoplasm have been reported.

It must be emphasized that non-neoplastic inflammatory processes occur in the lung, which are also capable of producing a mass-like lesion, such as organizing pneumonia, infarcts, scars, and confluent granulomas. These processes must always be included in the differential diagnosis of IMT.

K. **HEMATOLYMPHOID LESIONS.** Hematolymphoid neoplasms and pseudoneoplasms can involve the lung, both primarily and as part of systemic disease. Fresh tissue should be set aside for flow cytometry whenever possible. In cases for which only fixed tissue is available, a variety of molecular studies including gene rearrangement analysis can also be used to evaluate clonality. By definition, primary pulmonary lymphomas should not have evidence of disease outside of the lung or hilar lymph nodes.

1. **MALToma.** Lymphomas of mucosal associated lymphoid tissue, so called MALTomas, commonly arise in the lung and constitute the most common form of primary pulmonary lymphoma. MALTomas for the most part correspond to marginal zone lymphoma, and many harbor a t(8;11) translocation which may be relatively specific for lung MALTomas. Most cases occur in adults; there is no specific relationship to infection or autoimmune disorders. Pulmonary MALToma may have a nodular or diffuse appearance, with an infiltrate comprised of small lymphocytes, monocytoid cells,

and plasmacytoid cells (e-**Fig. 8.67**) that may replace or disrupt the appearance of pre-existing germinal centers. The cells also infiltrate the bronchial mucosa with production of lymphoepithelial lesions as are seen with MAL-Toma in other sites. The infiltrating cells are positive for CD19, CD20, and bcl-2, but negative for CD5, CD10, CD23, and cyclin D1.

2. **Large Cell Lymphoma.** Pulmonary large cell lymphoma generally presents as a solitary mass lesion involving a single lobe of the lung. These masses may develop central necrosis. Pulmonary large cell lymphomas are usually either of diffuse large cell type or immunoblastic, and are of B-cell lineage (e-**Fig. 8.68**).

3. **Lymphomatoid granulomatosis (LYG)** is the name for a lung lesion now recognized to be a malignant lymphoma, now also known as angiocentric immunoproliferative lesion (AIL). It is an Epstein-Barr virus (EBV)-related B-cell proliferation analogous to post-transplant lymphoproliferative disorder or AIDS related lymphoma. In fact, patients with LYG often have some underlying immunodeficiency. LYG usually is seen in middle aged and older adults, and shows multiple nodules that may suggest metastatic disease; concomitant skin and CNS involvement is quite common. Patients have respiratory symptoms such as cough or dyspnea, or may have constitutional symptoms. Microscopically, vasculocentric and angio-destructive lymphoid infiltrates that involve all layers of the vessel are the hallmark of LYG (e-**Fig. 8.69**); this vascular infiltration is hypothesized to result in infarct-like necrosis of the lung seen in the higher grade cases. Grade 1 lesions have infiltrates composed mainly of small T-cells, plasma cells, and histiocytes; CD20 and EBV stains show only rare atypical B-cells (<5 per hpf). Grade 2 cases show a greater number of atypical B-cells (5-20 per hpf). Grade 3 cases have abundant large, atypical B-cells.

4. **Leukemic infiltrates.** The lung may be the site of acute leukemic infiltrates in cases of acute myelogenous leukemia (AML), representing a granulocytic sarcoma or extra-medullary myeloid tumor. Infiltration of airways, interstitial infiltrates, or nodular parenchymal masses are possible manifestations. Histologic clues to a diagnosis of AML include blast-like cells and the presence of immature eosinophilic precursors. Many cases are initially thought to represent a large cell lymphoma; one of the first clues to the correct diagnosis is the absence of expression of both B- or T-cell markers in the presumed lymphomatous cells.

The lung may also show extensive involvement by chronic lymphocytic leukemia/small lymphocytic lymphoma. In this setting, the infiltrate presents as nodular expansions along lymphatic routes in the lung.

5. **Other hematolymphoid diseases.** The lung has been the reported primary site of a variety of hematolymphoid lesions, including Hodgkin disease, intravascular lymphomatosis, plasmacytomas (e-**Fig. 8.70**), and Castleman disease. However, it should be reiterated that secondary involvement of the lung in patients with advanced hematolymphoid disease is very common, can occur with essentially all entities, and so must always be excluded.

6. **Pseudolymphoma.** Small nodular lymphoid deposits in the lung have traditionally been called pseudolymphoma. However, with the advent of more specific diagnostic techniques, many of these lesions have been shown to be lymphomas, such as MALTomas. For lesions that can be demonstrated to be polyclonal, the term lymphoid hyperplasia is more appropriate.

L. **Metastatic tumors.** It is prudent to include metastatic disease in the differential diagnosis of every lung tumor. Metastases should be suspected when a tumor type is encountered that would be unusual as a lung primary tumor. Also, presentation as multiple nodules, the finding of a tumor that is predominantly within lymphatics or vessels, and a tumor that appears very well circumscribed without a host stromal and inflammatory reaction should also raise suspicion for a secondary lung tumor. Clinical history, liberal use of special stains, and radiologic consultation can all be used to evaluate the possibility of metastatic disease.

Cytopathology of the Lung

Hannah R. Krigman

I. **SAMPLE TYPE.** Cytology is an appropriate diagnostic modality for both neoplastic and non-neoplastic conditions of the lung. Exfoliative techniques include preparations of sputum, fluid from bronchial washing or lavage, and bronchial brushing. Fine needle aspiration of pulmonary processes can be via a transthoracic, transbronchial, or transesophageal approach. The sensitivity of cytopathologic evaluation depends on the type of procurement technique used. Sputum specimens yield the lowest quantity of exfoliated cells, FNA specimens yield the highest; endobronchial and transthoracic FNA for central and peripheral lung masses, respectively, both yield similarly cellular specimens.

II. **SPECIMEN ADEQUACY AND PREPARATION**

A. **Exfoliate endoluminal samples (sputum, bronchial washing, bronchioalveolar lavage, and bronchial brushing).** Bronchial washing, brushing, and lavage specimens are adequate if sufficient alveolar macrophages are present, or if diagnostic findings are present. Sputum must contain macrophages to be adequate; if sputum does not contain macrophages, then the cells are likely of oropharyngeal origin. For bronchial brushing specimens, bronchial epithelial cells are also required (e-**Fig. 8.71**). Samples can be submitted fresh or in liquid fixative for the monolayer technique. Mucus in sputum can be dispersed by mechanical disruption or by lytic agents. Airdried cytospins can be stained by a Romanowsky technique; alcohol fixed samples can be Pap stained. Brushing samples can be smeared directly on a slide, but care must be taken to fix smears immediately or air-dry artifact will render the slides uninterpretable. Brushes may be fixed in fluid, and cell block or Pap stained specimens can be made from material dislodged from the brush into the fluid.

B. **Fine needle aspirates** of lung masses, whether obtained via endoscopic or transthoracic approaches, are DiffQuik and Papanicolaou stained.

C. **Pleural effusions** are generally submitted fresh, in toto, from which a well-mixed portion (generally 2–300 ml) is used to prepare both a cytospin DiffQuik and ThinPrep Papanicolaou stained slide preparation. Benign mesothelial cells are generally found in these specimens (e-**Fig. 8.72**), with or without inflammation.

III. **DIAGNOSTIC CATEGORIES**

A. **Negative for malignancy.** This diagnosis is rendered when the specimen shows only alveolar macrophages, benign bronchial epithelial cells, and mixed inflammatory cells. This diagnosis is also used when fungal elements are identified, or when viral cytopathic changes are seen.

B. **Atypical cytology.** This diagnosis is rendered when the specimen shows bronchial epithelial cells which can be interpreted as reactive, but in which there is the absence of evidence of an underlying lesion. A repeat aspirate or tissue biopsy is usually suggested. An aspirate which shows markedly reactive bronchial epithelial cells which may be interpreted as positive for carcinoma should be repeated if the cells are adjacent to ciliated bronchial epithelium (e-**Fig. 8.73**).

C. **Suspicious for malignancy.** This diagnosis is rendered when rare malignant cells are present, but the quantity is insufficient for a definitive diagnosis of malignancy. This diagnosis usually prompts a repeat diagnostic procedure before definitive surgical treatment.

D. **Positive for malignancy.** This diagnosis is rendered when both the quality and quantity of malignant cells are sufficient for an unequivocal diagnosis of malignancy. Diagnoses of malignancy are best considered a function of both quality and quantity of atypical cells; either rare markedly atypical cells or an abundance of only minimally atypical cells can suggest malignancy.

IV. **NON-NEOPLASTIC CONDITIONS**
   A. **Infections**
      1. **Viral.** The radiologic correlates to viral infection typically include diffuse pulmonary infiltrates. Cytopathologically, viral changes are best appreciated on bronchial washing and bronchioloalveolar lavage specimens. The viral cytopathic changes seen in Herpes virus infections include multinucleate and single infected cells that have large nuclei with clear to faintly basophilic centers and peripheralized chromatin; the nuclei are molded with one another. CMV infected cells have both nuclear and cytoplasmic inclusions that are PAS positive. Adenovirus, which yields a typical "smudged" appearance on histologic section, shows a polygonal nuclear inclusion and multinucleate cells. Measles shows a characteristic multinucleate giant cell.

      2. **Fungal.** The chest X-ray of patients with fungal infection can exhibit either a mass effect, multiple nodules, or, on occasion, diffuse infiltrates.
         a. The cytologic features of *Pneumocystis jiroveci* are well described. Alveolar casts containing fibrin and the organisms have a bubbly or foamy look on Papanicolaou-stained materials. Romanowsky stained preparations show a central organism and a clear coat. Methenamine silver stains can highlight the organism, and the stain can be applied to formalin-fixed paraffin embedded cell blocks, or to cytospins. Patients taking prophylactic antibiotics for *Pneumocystis* may not have alveolar casts, and their samples may have rare, cup shaped organisms located within macrophages.
         b. Fragments of *Rhizopus* or *Aspergillus* species can be seen in washings, either from cavitary masses or in ABPA. In the latter, concretions of allergic type mucin or Charcot Leyden crystals may be noted.
         c. *Histoplasma* infection rarely shows detectable organisms; however, a granulomatous reaction may be present in aspirations of pulmonary masses or of involved lymph nodes.
         d. *Cryptococcus, Coccidiomycosis,* and *Blastomycosis* can all induce solitary masses, which can be sampled by aspiration. The yeast forms are best appreciated on Romanowsky stains; often the organisms are clear. Again, cell blocks, direct smears, or cytospins can be stained with traditional techniques to better highlight the organisms.

      3. **Bacterial**
         a. The prototypical bacterial infection for which cytologic sampling is pursued is tuberculosis. Infection with *M. tuberculosis* can yield both diffuse infiltrates, as in military tuberculosis, or mass-like lesions, occasionally with cavitation.
            Washings or lavage may be pursued primarily for obtaining material for culture, molecular laboratory test to detect the organism, or antibody-mediated studies. Cytopathologically, washings or lavage fluid can show no significant changes or may exhibit necrosis and acute inflammation. Cavitary lesions can have secondary squamous metaplasia, which may be atypical; for this reason, the possibility of a false positive cytology should always be considered in the setting of a cavitary lung mass. Patients with *M. tuberculum* infection can also have extensive hilar adenopathy,

which may sway the less confident reviewer to a spurious diagnosis of malignancy. Finally, because tuberculosis can present as a mass lesion, FNA may be obtained; frequently, multinucleate giant cells are present, again in a setting of acellular necrotic debris and acute inflammation.

   b. **Community acquired bacterial pneumonias** are less often sampled, but again, fluids from such cases exhibit acute inflammation, macrophages, and respiratory epithelial cells.

B. **Sarcoidosis.** Sarcoidosis is a diagnosis of exclusion, and fine needle aspiration from patients with infiltrates and adenopathy may be used as a minimally invasive technique for evaluation. Washings and lavage do not have a high yield for diagnosis. Aspiration of lymph nodes form patients with hilar adenopathy yields fragments of granulomas, rare multinucleate giant cells, and a background of mixed chronic inflammatory cells.

C. **Pulmonary alveolar proteinosis (PAP).** Bronchioloalveolar lavage is both diagnostic and therapeutic in patients with PAP. The gross features of PAP cytology specimens are fairly typical in that lavage fluid is white to milky and may have a surface lipid layer. Cytologically, washing samples contain granules and fragments of PAS positive, diastase resistant material that is pale on Pap stain and basophilic on Romanowsky stain. The background contains mixed acute and chronic inflammatory cells, with variable numbers of eosinophils.

D. **Hemosiderosis.** Alveolar hemorrhage from any cause can result in the presence of hemosiderin laden macrophages, highlighted by iron stain. Detection of hemosiderin pigment in 20% of macrophages on bronchoalveolar lavage reportedly correlates with alveolar hemorrhage. Hemosiderosis requires a combination of radiographic and clinical features and is best diagnosed on open biopsy, after exclusion of other causes of alveolar hemorrhage.

V. NEOPLASMS

A. **Squamous cell carcinoma (SCC),** a type of non-small cell carcinoma, consists of cells with varying degrees of keratinization, inconsistent size and shape, polygonal to amphophilic cytoplasm, and dark pyknotic nuclei. The background usually shows so-called dirty necrosis with abundant keratinized cellular debris (e-**Fig. 8.74**).

B. **Adenocarcinoma,** another type of non-small cell carcinoma, shows cells with fine foamy to vacuolated cytoplasm, and vesicular nuclei with prominent nucleoli. There is typically no background necrosis unless the tumor is large (e-**Fig. 8.75**).

   Immunohistochemistry has been proposed as an effective adjunct to cytologic examination in separating SCC from adenocarcinoma. Performed on formalin fixed, paraffin embedded cell blocks, immunohistochemical stains generally show expression of thyroid transcription factor 1 (TTF-1) in adenocarcinomas but not in SCC s. Care must be to distinguish between tumor groups and incidentally obtained normal pulmonary epithelial elements which retain TTF-1 expression. In general, SCC s express cytokeratin 5/6 and p63, while adenocarcinomas do not express these antigens.

C. **Neuroendocrine carcinoma.** Small cell carcinomas and large cell neuroendocrine tumors must be distinguished from non-small cell carcinomas since they respond differently to chemotherapy.

   1. **Carcinoid tumor** has both polygonal cells with rounded nuclei and spindle cells with elongate nuclei. Nucleoli are not prominent. Aspirate smears can have some nuclear molding and crush artifact, but aspirates should contain some areas where the cells show the morphology of typical carcinoid.

   2. **Large cell neuroendocrine tumor** has flattened cohesive groups of cells with large round to polygonal nuclei that have prominent nucleoli and vesicular nuclear chromatin. Cytoplasm is sparse.

   3. **Small cell carcinoma** is composed of cells with only a small amount of cytoplasm. Nuclei show a molding pattern, fine granular chromatin, and streaming. Apoptotic debris and cellular necrosis are prominent (e-**Fig. 8.76**).

D. Hematopoietic malignancies. Both high and low grade non-Hodgkin lymphomas occur in the lung, either as solitary pulmonary nodules or associated with adenopathy. The cytologic features are similar to those of lymphomas aspirated at other sites. High grade lymphomas contain a discohesive single cell population with fragmented lymphocytes in the background; individual cells have sparse cytoplasm. Prominent chromocenters are present. Low grade lymphomas are composed of a monotonous mature lymphoid population. For most lymphomas, some of the FNA passes should be reserved for flow cytometry to characterize the malignant cell population. If the background inflammation is mixed and contains eosinophils, material should be reserved for a cell block to identify the Reed Sternberg cells of Hodgkin disease or for gene rearrangement studies for T-cell lymphoma.

E. Mesothelioma is usually seen in association with a pleural effusion. Cytologically, the cells show variability in size, with those in clusters having scalloped edges. A cell-in-cell arrangement is often present. Enlarged and convoluted nuclei, with or without nucleoli, are typical (**e-Fig. 8.77**). Appropriate immunohistochemical stains to rule out adenocarcinoma should be performed. Asbestos fibers (**e-Fig. 8.78**) may be seen in bronchioalveolar lavage specimens from these patients.

F. Metastases to the lung are common and should be evaluated on the basis of the patient's clinical history. The diagnostic approach to tumors of unknown origin presenting as lung metastases is the same as for tumors of unknown origin presenting at other sites (*Semin Oncol.* 1993;20:206).

SUGGESTED READINGS

Churg A, Green FYH, eds. *Pathology of Occupational Diseases.* New York, NY: Igaku-Shoin; 1988.

Churg AM, Myers JL, Tazelaar HD, et al. *Thurlbecks Pathology of the Lung.* 3rd ed. New York, NY: Thieme; 2005.

Colby TV, Koss MN, Travis WD. AFIP Atlas of Tumor Pathology. Series III. In: *Tumors of the Lower Respiratory Tract.* Armed Forces Institute of Pathology; 1996

Katzenstein AA. *Katzenstein and Askin's Surgical Pathology of Non-Neoplastic Lung Disease*, 4th ed. Philadelphia, PA: WB Saunders Company; 2006.

Papanicolaou Society of Cytopathology Task Force on Standards of Practice. Guidelines of the Papanicolaou Society of Cytopathology for the Examination of Cytologic Specimens Obtained from the Respiratory Tract. *Diagnostic Cytopathology.* 1999;21:61–69.

Tomashefski TF, Cagle PT, Farver CF, et al. *Dail and Hammar's Pulmonary Pathology. Vol. 1 Non-neoplastic Lung Disease*, 3rd ed. Springer Verlag; 2008.

Travis WD, Brambilla E, Müller-Hermelink HK, et al. *Pathology & Genetics of Tumours of the Lung, Thymus And Heart (World Health Organization Classification of Tumours).* WHO Press; 2004.

Travis WD, Colby TV, Koss MN, et al. AFIP Atlas of Non-Tumor Pathology. Series I: *Non-Neoplastic Disorders of the Lower Respiratory Tract.* Washington, DC: American Registry of Pathology and the Armed Forces Institute of Pathology; 2002.

Wick MR, Leslie KG. *Practical Pulmonary Pathology: A Diagnostic Approach.* 2nd ed. Churchill Livingstone; 2010.

Cardiovascular System

Jochen K. Lennerz and John D. Pfeifer

HEART

I. **NORMAL ANATOMY.** The normal weight of the **adult heart** is 300 to 350 g (male) and 250 to 300 g (female). Cardiomegaly above a critical weight of 500 g is associated with ischemic changes (see later) and is termed *cor bovinum*. The normal ventricular thickness is 0.3 to 0.5 cm on the right and 1.2 to 1.5 cm on the left (**e-Fig. 9.1**),* measured at the base of the papillary muscles (Fig. 9.1). The heart is composed of three layers: the epicardium (including the serous or visceral pericardium, and the main branches of the coronary arteries), the muscular myocardium, and the endocardium (with an ill-defined subendocardial layer that contains many Purkinje fibers).

Microscopically, the normal myocardium is a functional syncytium of myocardial fibers (cardiac myocytes) that have centrally located nuclei (**e-Fig. 9.1**). Cardiac myocytes are a specialized form of striated muscle; faint dark eosinophilic intercalated discs between the myocytes form the mechanical and electrical couplings. Numerous capillaries with sparse interstitial tissue are found between the myocardial fibers (**e-Fig. 9.1**).

The atrioventricular valves (mitral and tricuspid) are composed of an annulus, leaflets, chordae tendineae, and papillary muscles. The semilunar valves (aortic and pulmonic) are composed of three cusps (each with a sinus), which meet at the three commissures (corpora arantii, **e-Fig. 9.2**). Valves are relatively avascular, and are lined by endothelial cells on a thin layer of collagen and elastic tissue on the atrial/arterial side, a thicker layer of dense collagen on the ventricular side, and loose myxoid connective tissue (zona spongiosa) in between. The fibrous and spongiotic regions are normally of equal thickness (**e-Fig. 9.2**).

The **conduction system** is composed of specialized myocytes, with fewer intercalated discs and higher glycogen content. Masson trichrome, Verhoeff–van Gieson, and Alcian Blue stains can be used to demonstrate the conduction system (**e-Fig. 9.3**). Exact knowledge of the topographic anatomy and correct sampling techniques are paramount (**e-Fig. 9.4**).

II. **GROSS EXAMINATION AND TISSUE HANDLING**

A. **Endomyocardial biopsies** are usually taken via a right-sided cardiac catheter; the most common indications are monitoring of heart transplant rejection, and grading of Adriamycin toxicity. To avoid sampling errors, a minimum of three, preferably four, samples of myocardium are recommended (**e-Fig. 9.5**). The tissue fragments should be counted and measured during gross examination; their color and consistency should be noted. The tissue should be placed between foam pads or wrapped in filter paper for routine processing. Examination of at least three levels is recommended; some laboratories keep the intervening sections for additional stains if required to assess myocyte damage and fibrosis. Histologically, an adequate biopsy contains at least 50% myocardium, excluding previous biopsy sites (**e-Fig. 9.5**). Occasional cases require fresh frozen tissue or glutaraldehyde fixation for special techniques such as molecular diagnostics

---

*Alle-figures are available online via the Solution Site Image Bank.

Coronary Arteries - Bypasses - Sectioning

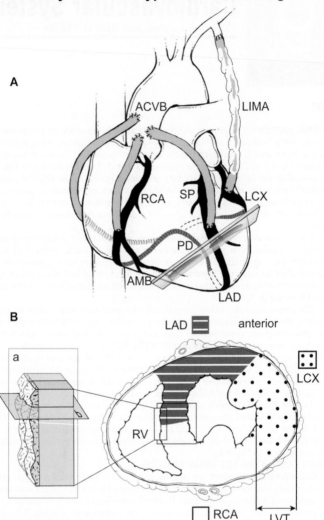

Figure 9.1 Coronary arteries, bypasses, sectioning of the ventricles. (**A**) The left coronary artery branches into LCX (left circumflex) and LAD (left anterior descending), the latter supplies the anterior septum via SP (septal perforators). The RCA (right coronary artery) supplies the AV node (not shown), branches into the AMB (acute marginal branch) and the PD (posterior descending artery). The origin of the PD determines the distribution type (right vs. left). Examples of ACVB (aorto-coronary venous bypass) and LIMA (left internal mammary artery) grafts are displayed in gray. (**B**) Slice from section illustrated in A. The myocardium displays the supplying arteries for mapping of myocardial infarctions. The left ventricular thickness (LVT) is measured on the level of the anterior papillary muscle. The large septal square illustrates a section to determine myocyte disarray. The small rectangle close to the right ventricle (RV) illustrates a myomectomy specimen, which are sectioned perpendicular to the endocardial surface; preferred is horizontal (a) or vertical (b).

or electron microscopy (see later), respectively. Adipose tissue between myocardiocytes is a normal finding and does not indicate ventricular perforation (e-**Fig. 9.5**).

B. **Cardiac valves** are often removed because of calcific degeneration or perforation as a sequela of bacterial endocarditis (e-**Fig. 9.2**). Most valves are received in fragments; if possible, the description should include the distribution of vegetations (e-**Fig. 9.6**) and presence or absence of non–surgery-related leaflet destruction. In cases of calcific degeneration, slow acid decalcification after fixation may be necessary. Sections are taken from the free edge to the annulus.

Prosthetic valves are typically removed because of thrombosis, anastomotic or valvular leakage, mechanical failure, or infection. Evaluation of the prosthetic valve ring attachment is, therefore, critical as infective endocarditis typically affects this region. For most mechanical heart valves, it is not possible to submit any tissue for histology, unless vegetations are present. For bioprosthetic valves, however, the valve cusp is submitted.

Valves from patients treated with the appetite-suppressant drug Fen-Phen (a combination of fenfluramine and phentermine) show patterns of changes that resemble carcinoid valve disease with superficial layers of myofibroblastic proliferation on otherwise normal valve architecture.

C. **Myomectomy specimens,** from ventricular aneurysm repair or septal myomectomy procedures should be measured, weighed, and sectioned at 3-mm intervals, perpendicular to the endocardial surface (Fig. 9.1). All layers of the heart should be described. For cardiac tumors, appropriate sections should assess the inked specimen resection margins (see later).

D. **Heart explant specimens** should be weighed, described, and dissected as outlined (Fig. 9.2). In addition, the valves (circumference or diameter) and walls (Fig. 9.1) should be measured. The septal and ventricular configuration (concentric vs. dilatative ventricular hypertrophy) should be described. Usually the inflow tract of the donor heart is dissected to match the recipient's anatomy; thus, fragments of donor tissue are frequently submitted in the same container.

III. **DIAGNOSTIC FEATURES OF COMMON DISEASES OF THE HEART**

A. **Disorders of the Endocardium**

1. **Infective endocarditis** is characterized by bacterial colonization of the valve forming vegetations that are red, irregular (e-**Fig. 9.6**), and composed of granulation tissue and thrombus; their friability explains the propensity for associated septic embolization (e-**Fig. 9.2**). The myocardium is typically not involved. *Staphylococcus aureus* typically produces acute endocarditis, whereas *Streptococcus viridans* produces subacute endocarditis. Several organisms normally found in the oral cavity are also causative, and have been referred to as the gram-negative HACEK organisms (*Hemophilus aphrophilus*, *Actinobacilus actinomycetemcomitans*, *Cardiobacterium hominis*, *Eikenella corrodens*, and *Kingella kingii*). *Staphylococcus epidermidis* also causes infective endocarditis, more common in the setting of prosthetic valves. Healed infective endocarditis leaves residual valve damage, often fenestrations, usually with a hemodynamic jet lesion and adjacent endocardial fibrosis.

2. **Nonbacterial thrombotic endocarditis** (*marantic endocarditis*) produces small (rarely >0.5 cm), pink, bland, and sterile vegetations attached to the valve surface at the lines of closure (e-**Fig. 9.6**). It is typically seen in cachectic patients with a hypercoagulable state (e.g., Trousseau syndrome).

3. **Libman–Sacks endocarditis** is seen in 4% of cases of systemic lupus erythematosus and is characterized by flat, pale tan, spreading bands of vegetations located on both surfaces of the valves or chordae tendineae (e-**Fig. 9.6**). Affected, in order of frequency, are the tricuspid, mitral, pulmonic, and aortic valves.

Dissection Techniques of the Heart

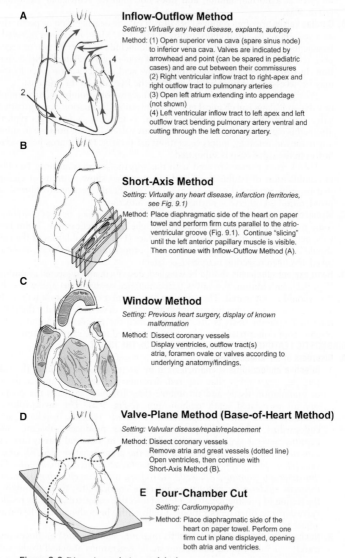

A

Inflow-Outflow Method

Setting: Virtually any heart disease, explants, autopsy

Method: (1) Open superior vena cava (spare sinus node) to inferior vena cava. Valves are indicated by arrowhead and point (can be spared in pediatric cases) and are cut between their commissures
(2) Right ventricular inflow tract to right-apex and right outflow tract to pulmonary arteries
(3) Open left atrium extending into appendage (not shown)
(4) Left ventricular inflow tract to left apex and left outflow tract bending pulmonary artery ventral and cutting through the left coronary artery.

B

Short-Axis Method

Setting: Virtually any heart disease, infarction (territories, see Fig. 9.1)

Method: Place diaphragmatic side of the heart on paper towel and perform firm cuts parallel to the atrio-ventricular groove (Fig. 9.1). Continue "slicing" until the left anterior papillary muscle is visible. Then continue with Inflow-Outflow Method (A).

C

Window Method

Setting: Previous heart surgery, display of known malformation

Method: Dissect coronary vessels
Display ventricles, outflow tract(s)
atria, foramen ovale or valves according to underlying anatomy/findings.

D

Valve-Plane Method (Base-of-Heart Method)

Setting: Valvular disease/repair/replacement

Method: Dissect coronary vessels
Remove atria and great vessels (dotted line)
Open ventricles, then continue with Short-Axis Method (B).

E Four-Chamber Cut

Setting: Cardiomyopathy

Method: Place diaphragmatic side of the heart on paper towel. Perform one firm cut in plane displayed, opening both atria and ventricles.

Figure 9.2 Dissection techniques of the heart.

4. **Rheumatic heart disease (RHD)** is a sequela of rheumatic fever (RF) caused by *Streptococcus pyogenes* (group A or β-hemolytic streptococcus). Aschoff nodules (ANs) are a characteristic feature and appear as interstitial collections of plump mononuclear cells with occasional neutrophils arranged in a granuloma-like formation, although the presence or the number of ANs does not correlate with clinical course or activity of the rheumatic process. The most characteristic cellular component of ANs is the Aschoff giant cell, which has two or more nuclei with prominent nucleoli; another characteristic feature is the presence of Anitschkow cells, which are mononuclear histiocytes that are often arranged in a palisade around the center of the granuloma. The macroscopic pattern is variable (e-**Fig. 9.6**).

   The valvular disease characteristic of chronic RHD is usually the result of multiple recurrent episodes of acute RF, and typically develops many decades after the initial insult. RHD is the most common cause of mitral stenosis, and in up to 75% of cases, the mitral valve is the only valve affected. In 25% of cases, the mitral and aortic valves are affected. Progressive fibrosis leads to thickening of the valve and chordae that eventually leads to fusion of the mitral leaflets at the commissures, producing the classic "fish mouth" appearance.

5. **Endocardial fibroelastosis** is an uncommon condition that can result in restrictive cardiomyopathy. Pearly-white fibroelastic thickening, caused by accumulation of collagen and elastic fibers typically in the left ventricular endocardium (e-**Fig. 9.3**), is often associated with aortic valve obstruction. The disease occurs either focally or diffusely in children from birth to 2 years of age.

6. **Loeffler endocarditis** is also known as fibroelastic parietal endocarditis with blood eosinophilia. Classically, three stages (acute necrotic myocarditis, organizing thrombus, and endomyocardial fibrosis) are distinguished. The cardiac lesions are associated with dense eosinophilic infiltration of other organs, and the disease is usually rapidly fatal.

B. **Disorders of the Valves**

1. **Myxoid change** is stromal accumulation of glycosaminoglycans as a sign of degeneration (e-**Fig. 9.2**). The layered architecture is preserved; if the architecture is absent or distorted, the differential diagnosis should include RHD. The chordae tendineae are thinned and elongated in myxomatous degeneration, whereas in RHD they are shortened and thickened.

2. **Mitral valves** are removed for acquired post-inflammatory stenosis (e.g., RHD) and may show commissural fusion, cusp scarring, and dystrophic calcification (e-**Fig. 9.2**). RHD vegetations are composed mainly of fibrin and are usually no more than 2 mm in size. Cases of mitral insufficiency or myxomatous degeneration show a floppy valve with redundant and ballooned leaflets with abundant myxoid change.

3. **Tricuspid valves** are most commonly removed for insufficiency or infective endocarditis.

4. **Aortic valves** are removed for stenosis and are typically heavily calcified, sometimes with commissural fusion (senile calcific aortic stenosis), post-inflammatory scarring, or calcification due to a congenitally bicuspid valve (present in 1% of the population).

5. **Pulmonary valves** are usually excised because of stenosis due to congenital heart disease (most commonly as a component of tetralogy of Fallot).

C. **Disorders of the Myocardium**

1. **Myocarditis** is the underlying etiology in about 10% of patients with new-onset cardiac dysfunction. If not fatal, myocarditis often proceeds to dilated cardiomyopathy. Findings in subsequent biopsies, using the first specimen as a reference point, include ongoing/persistent myocarditis, resolving/healing

myocarditis (damage substantially reduced), and resolved/healed myocarditis (damage no longer present). The so-called Dallas criteria (*Hum Pathol.* 1987;18:619) are often used to categorize myocarditis mainly on histopathologic findings, although it has been suggested that the criteria are no longer adequate. The WHO defines myocarditis as a minimum of 14 infiltrating leukocytes per square millimeter, preferably T-cells, with as many as four macrophages (also known as the Marburg criteria; see *Circulation.* 1996;93:841). The diagnosis of *active myocarditis* classically requires the presence of an inflammatory infiltrate (usually lymphocytic) and myocyte necrosis/degeneration or damage not characteristic of an ischemic event; *borderline myocarditis* indicates the absence of necrosis or damage and can be applied to any form of inflammatory infiltrate.

a. **Primary viral myocarditis** accounts for most cases of myocarditis in developed countries. Cardiac involvement typically follows the primary viral infection by several days. The most commonly associated agents are enteroviruses (Coxsackie A and B), adenovirus, echovirus, and poliovirus, influenza viruses A and B, and HIV. The infiltrate is composed mainly of lymphocytes with associated myocyte damage (e-**Fig. 9.7**). Eosinophils are typically not seen. Primary viral myocarditis includes four clinical pathological manifestations: fulminate, chronic active, eosinophilic, and giant cell myocarditis.

b. **Fulminant myocarditis** has a distinct onset within 2 weeks of presentation of profound left ventricular dysfunction without dilatation. Biopsy shows multiple foci of active inflammation and necrosis. Patients usually show complete histologic and functional recovery, or die within 2 weeks.

c. **Chronic active myocarditis** has an indistinct onset with moderate ventricular dysfunction and active or borderline myocarditis. Ongoing inflammation and fibrosis may result in the development of restrictive cardiomyopathy with 2 to 4 years after presentation.

d. **Eosinophilic myocarditis** can be attributed to eosinophilic syndromes or allergic reactions that result in left ventricular compromise. Eosinophils and myocyte damage are present in the biopsy (e-**Fig. 9.7**). This entity sometimes referred to as *hypersensitivity myocarditis* is linked to treatment with methyldopa, antibiotics (penicillin, sulfonamides, and streptomycin), anticonvulsants, and antidepressants, and also shows eosinophils and occasional giant cells. The myocardium has little myocyte necrosis, and the inflammatory infiltrate is lymphohistiocytic and predominantly perivascular (e-**Fig. 9.7**). In some cases, the infiltrate is subendocardial or appears as poorly formed granulomas.

   The differential diagnosis of eosinophilia in the myocardium includes parasitic infection, allergy, a hypereosinophilic syndrome, and hematologic malignancies. Cytomegalovirus infection should enter the differential diagnosis in an immunosuppressed patient.

e. **Idiopathic giant cell myocarditis,** also known as Fiedler's myocarditis, is associated with autoimmune diseases (e.g., inflammatory bowel disease, hypothyroidism) and is rapidly fatal if untreated. It typically occurs in young, healthy, white adults and presents as congestive heart failure. Diffuse, geographic myocardial necrosis with a mixed inflammatory infiltrate including eosinophils and multinucleated giant cells in the absence of granulomas is typical (e-**Fig. 9.8**). The giant cells have the immunohistochemical profile of histiocytes.

f. **Other** organisms associated with myocarditis include bacteria, fungi, spirochetes (especially *Borrelia burgdorferi*), Rickettsiae, *Chlamydia*, parasites (including *Toxoplasma gondii* in immunocompromised patients), and helminths (trichinosis).

g. **Chagas disease,** the most common form of protozoal myocarditis, is caused by the hemoflagellate *Trypanosoma cruzi* and is uncommon in the USA. However, in endemic regions of South and Central America, it accounts for 25% of all deaths of 25- to 40-year-olds; up to 80% of patients with Chagas disease develop myocarditis. Histologically, myofibers contain parasites with an associated mild chronic inflammatory infiltrate. In the acute phase, dense inflammation with myocyte necrosis and trypanosome amastigotes in myocytes is characteristic, whereas the chronic phase shows interstitial and perivascular lymphoplasmacytic infiltrate without fibrosis.

h. **Secondary myocarditis** can occur in the setting of collagen vascular diseases, RF, drugs, heat stroke, and radiation.

i. **Granulomatous myocarditis** (e-Fig. 9.9) can be seen in tuberculosis or sarcoidosis.

j. **Cardiac sarcoidosis** shows non-necrotizing granulomas (e-Fig 9.9) in a background of fibrosis and necrosis. Cardiac involvement, though present in 25% of systemic cases of sarcoidosis, is usually patchy and, therefore, a single negative endomyocardial biopsy does not exclude the disease. The differential diagnosis in cases of suspected cardiac sarcoidosis includes idiopathic giant cell myocarditis, amyloid, Chagas disease, and Fabry disease.

2. **Cardiomyopathy**

a. **Ischemic cardiomyopathy** is usually secondary to severe coronary artery disease (e-Fig. 9.10).

b. **Hypertrophic cardiomyopathy** is typically seen in healthy individuals less than 30 years old, but can be seen at almost any age. Affected individuals suffer from angina, exertional dyspnea, or sudden cardiac death as a result of diastolic dysfunction due to ventricular thickening. In hypertrophic obstructive cardiomyopathy, there is classically asymmetric ventricular septal hypertrophy (with a wall thickness of 15 to 30 mm), with associated fibrous endocardial plaques and mitral valve thickening. Microscopically, disarray of myofibers (e-Fig. 9.11), myofiber hypertrophy, basophilic degeneration, and interstitial fibrosis are characteristic, although nonspecific.

Currently, over 450 disease-causing mutations in 16 genes encoding myocardial contractile proteins have been implicated in hypertrophic cardiomyopathy, a spectrum of genetic changes that suggests that so-called next generation sequencing (see Chap. 60) is a viable diagnostic approach. However, as isolated findings, many causal mutations have limited implications in risk stratification and prognostication, and so the role of DNA sequencing for genetic screening remains unsettled (*Eur J Clin Invest.* 2010;40:360).

c. **Dilated cardiomyopathy,** also known as congestive cardiomyopathy, presents as cardiac failure due to progressive cardiac dilatation with systolic dysfunction. Hypertrophy (increased weight with normal or reduced wall thickness) and marked dilatation of all chambers is typical (e-Fig. 9.12). Histologic examination shows nonspecific abnormalities; in about 50% of the cases, leukocytic infiltrates are present in endomyocardial biopsies. A significant number of cases are thought to be post-viral, or associated with alcohol use or chemotherapeutic agents. Pheochromocytoma is also associated with dilated cardiomyopathy. Dilated cardiomyopathy occurring in the peripartum period (up to 6 months after delivery) is known as peripartum cardiomyopathy. About 90% of familial cases show autosomal dominant inheritance, and 5% to 10% are X-linked; in addition to the genes affected by hypertrophic cardiomyopathy, additional mutations in cytoskeletal, nuclear envelope, and mitochondrial proteins have been found (*Circulation.* 2002;66:219).

d. Restrictive (obliterative) cardiomyopathy is uncommon in developed countries. The ventricles are normal or slightly enlarged and are not dilated; in contrast, the atria exhibit relative bilateral dilatation. Patchy or interstitial fibrosis is found histologically (e-**Fig. 9.13**). The eosinophilic form shows an eosinophil-rich myocardial infiltrate, whereas the noneosinophilic form (more common in USA) shows nonspecific findings. Restrictive cardiomyopathy is typically caused by endomyocardial fibrosis or hemochromatosis, but is often idiopathic.

e. Infiltrative cardiomyopathy is descriptive for a broad panel of metabolic diseases, and can be assigned to any disorder that restricts ventricular filling.

   i. Cardiac amyloidosis histologically shows amorphous, eosinophilic, extracellular material (e-**Fig. 9.14**). Cardiac amyloidosis is associated with restrictive features due to associated decreased ventricular compliance and so presents with diastolic dysfunction. Grossly, the myocardium appears stiff, and rubbery or waxy. The diagnosis of amyloid is confirmed by demonstrating apple-green birefringence with polarized light using a Congo red stain and/or electron microscopy (e-**Fig. 9.14**), or by immunohistochemistry (e-**Fig. 9.15**).

   ii. Hereditary hemochromatosis is a homozygous autosomal recessive disorder resulting from *HFE* gene mutations. The mutation results in unregulated uptake of iron in the small intestine, leading to iron deposition in the liver (hepatomegaly), pancreas (diabetes mellitus), skin (hyperpigmentation), or heart (dilated or restrictive cardiomyopathy). In the heart, myocytes and interstitial macrophages contain abundant brown pigment (e-**Fig. 9.16**), which can be demonstrated to be iron by the Prussian blue stain, but there is little correlation between the amount of cardiac iron and systolic dysfunction. Increased cardiac iron must be distinguished from lipofuscin; the latter is more finely granular, derived from normal intracellular lipid peroxidation, and is not stained by Prussian blue (e-**Fig. 9.16**). Iron overload is not specific for hereditary hemochromatosis but can also be seen in the setting of thalassemia, multiple transfusions, hemosiderosis, or hemolytic anemia.

   iii. Other infiltrative cardiomyopathies include Loeffler endocarditis, endocardial fibroelastosis, and mitochondrial myopathies.

f. Arrhythmogenic right ventricular cardiomyopathy is also known as right ventricular dysplasia, parchment right ventricle, and Uhl's anomaly. This uncommon variant of familial cardiomyopathy shows replacement of the myocardium by adipose and fibrous tissue, predominantly in the inferior and infundibular wall, without associated coronary artery sclerosis. The genetics of the disease have recently begun to be characterized (*J Cardiovasc Electrophysiol.* 2005;16:927).

g. Drug-/radiation-induced cardiomyopathy (*Cancer Treatm Rev.* 2004;30:181) is caused by drugs such as Adriamycin and cyclophosphamide and shows primarily subcellular changes that are best seen by electron microscopy.

   i. Adriamycin (doxorubicin) toxicity is characterized by dose-dependent changes, predominately in the subendocardial region. It frequently occurs after lifetime doses above 500 mg/m^2. Vacuolization of myocytes (mainly due to marked dilatation of the sarcoplasmic reticulum) is initially present (e-**Fig. 9.17**), followed by the appearance of typical "adria cells" that show loss of cross striations, myofilamentous bundles, and accompanying homogeneous basophilic staining (corresponding to ultrastructural fragmentation of sarcomeres). There is no accompanying inflammation. Since the microscopic features are not specific for Adriamycin toxicity, clinical correlation is required (*Environ Health Perspect.* 1978;26:181 and *Int J Cardiol.* 2007;117:6).

    ii. Cyclophosphamide toxicity may produce hemorrhagic necrosis, interstitial hemorrhage, extensive capillary thrombosis, fibrin deposition, and necrosis of myocardial fibers.

    iii. Radiation enhances the changes seen with chemotherapy. Constrictive pericarditis, myocardial fibrosis, and coronary artery lesions are also associated with radiation therapy.

3. Myocardial ischemia—ischemic heart disease

    a. The appearance of a myocardial infarct is dependent on the age of the infarct (e-**Fig. 9.18**). Following acute ischemia, the histologic changes include waviness of fibers (after 1 to 3 hours), progressing to contraction band necrosis (after 4 to 12 hours) (e-**Fig. 9.19**) and infiltration by neutrophils (after 2 to 24 hours). In cases of reperfusion, contraction band necrosis can be seen after 18 to 24 hours as the cells begin to lose cross striations and nuclear detail. Total coagulative necrosis can be seen by 24 to 72 hours.

    b. Chronic ischemic heart disease culminates in diffuse myocardial atrophy (brown atrophy) with patchy perivascular and interstitial fibrosis, with progressive ischemic necrosis. The heart is small with chocolate-colored myocardium that shows excessive lipofuscin deposition within the fibers.

    c. Microscopic arteriopathy is a term used to designate the changes in peripheral coronary arteries that undergo sclerotic changes (e-**Fig. 9.20**) resulting in a small lumen (>75% reduction in cross-sectional area). The disease is typically seen in chronic hypertension or with cocaine-induced cardiomyopathy, but will to some degree occur in chronic heart transplant rejection where it becomes the rate-limiting step to long-term survival.

D. Disorders of the Pericardium

  1. Acute pericarditis (e-**Fig. 9.21**) is idiopathic in 90% of cases, but can be caused by viruses (Coxsackie B, echoviruses, influenza, mumps, Epstein–Barr virus) or bacteria (*Staphylococcus aureus, Streptococci,* or *Haemophilus influenza*). Acute serous pericarditis can be secondary to acute RF, connective tissue disorders (e.g., systemic lupus erythematosus), uremia, metastatic malignancy, and renal transplantation. In contrast, acute fibrinous or serofibrinous pericarditis can be secondary to myocardial infarction (typically after 1 to 3 days), uremia, chest radiotherapy, RF, systemic lupus erythematosus, cardiac surgery, pneumonia, pleural infection, and cardiac trauma. Caseous pericarditis is usually due to *Mycobacterium tuberculosis* infection. Healed acute pericarditis usually results in a focal pearly thickened epicardial plaque, also known as a "soldier's plaque."

  2. Chronic pericarditis can lead to constrictive pericarditis where the heart is encased by a thick layer of fibrous tissue. Constrictive pericarditis can follow caseous pericarditis or radiotherapy, but is usually idiopathic.

  3. Neoplasms. Although primary neoplasms of the pericardium are very rare (including mesothelioma, germ cell tumors, and angiosarcoma), pericardial involvement is present in up to about 10% of patients with disseminated malignancy.

  4. Pericardial effusions. Effusions can be as large as 500 mL in some settings, such as congestive heart failure and hypoproteinemia. However, in acute cardiac tamponade, rapid accumulation of as little as 200 to 300 mL can cause cardiac compression and death.

IV. NEOPLASMS OF THE HEART. The four most common cardiac primary tumors (and tumor-like conditions) are all benign and account for 70% of cardiac neoplasms.

Primary malignancies of the heart are very rare; involvement of the heart by a malignancy is far more likely to represent metastasis by lung carcinoma, breast carcinoma, melanoma, lymphoma, leukemia, renal cell carcinoma, and choriocarcinoma. In cases of metastatic spread to the heart, the pericardium is often involved.

A. **Cardiac myxoma** is the most common primary tumor of the heart. In the sporadic form, the tumor typically occurs in middle-aged women, and is grossly a spherical, soft gray-white, gelatinous, lobulated tumor 1 to 10 cm in maximal dimension, typically attached by a stalk to the left atrium near the fossa ovalis (e-Fig. 9.22). In familial cases (e.g., Carney complex, NAME syndrome [Nevi, Atrial myxoma, Myxoid neurofibroma, and Ephelides], or LAMB syndrome [Lentigines, Atrial myxomas, Mucocutaneous myxomas, and Blue nevi]), the mean age of patients is mid-20s, and the tumor is more often attached to the right atrium or is multicentric. Microscopically, myxomas consist of plump spindled or stellate cells in abundant loose myxoid stroma (e-Fig. 9.22). Heterologous elements including cartilage, foci of ossification (petrified myxoma), or gland formation (glandular myxoma) can be seen, but have no prognostic significance (e-Fig. 9.22).

B. **Papillary fibroelastoma** occurs typically on the ventricular surface of the semilunar valves or the atrial surface of the AV valves. The tumor accounts for 75% of all valvular tumors, and can be up to 7 cm in greatest dimension. In children, the right side is predominantly affected. The branching avascular papillae are composed of fibroelastic myxoid stroma and are lined by hyperplastic endothelium (e-Fig 9.22).

C. **Lipomas** typically have a subendocardial location in the left ventricle.

D. **Rhabdomyoma** presents as a single (10% of cases) or multiple (90% of cases) well-circumscribed gray-white firm myocardial nodule up to 6 cm in size that often protrudes into the ventricle. The tumor is often discovered in the first year of life, and is the most common cardiac tumor in the pediatric age group. Patients usually present with heart failure or arrhythmias. Microscopically, the tumor is composed of mixtures of round and polygonal cells with glycogen-rich vacuoles (e-Fig. 9.22) that are separated by strands of cytoplasm radiating from the center of the cell (the so-called "spider-cells"). Rhabdomyoma is mitotically inactive, noninvasive, and nonmetastasizing; some tumors even regress spontaneously after the first year of life. The tumor is thought to be hamartomatous and is associated with tuberous sclerosis. Rhabdomyoma cells are immunopositive for vimentin, desmin, actin, and myoglobin; focal HMB45 positive cells can be present.

E. **Intramural cardiac fibroma** usually occurs as a single, white, rubbery lesion (e-Fig. 9.22). The tumor cells are typically immunopositive for vimentin and smooth muscle actin, indicating myofibroblastic origin; immunoreactivity for the muscle-specific markers desmin and myoD1 is absent.

F. **Other benign tumors** include mesothelial/monocytic incidental cardiac excrescences (also known as cardiac MICE; e-Fig. 9.21), calcified amorphous tumor of the heart (also known as cardiac CAT), lipomatous hypertrophy of the atrial septum, mesothelioma of the atrioventricular node, adenomatoid tumor, epithelioid or histiocytoid hemangioma, paraganglioma (extra-adrenal pheochromocytoma), schwannoma, and granular cell tumor.

G. **Angiosarcoma** is the most common primary malignant tumor of the heart. It typically involves the right atrium as a large mass with intracavitary extension, and may also infiltrate the myocardium. Primary angiosarcoma of the heart is typically more poorly differentiated than elsewhere (e-Fig. 9.22). Other rare primary cardiac sarcomas include Kaposi sarcoma, leiomyosarcoma, liposarcoma, and rhabdomyosarcoma.

H. **Carcinoid heart disease,** seen in ~50% of patients with carcinoid syndrome, typically affects the heart's right side, particularly the ventricular outflow tract and pulmonic valve. Gross findings include prominent hypertrophy and plaque-like thickening of the endocardium. Microscopically, the valvular cusps show proliferation of smooth muscle and collagen deposition, without valve destruction. There are no carcinoid tumor cells in the lesion.

V. CARDIAC TRANSPLANTS

A. The most sensitive method for the evaluation of **cellular rejection** is microscopic examination of an adequate myocardial biopsy. Often the sample will be taken from a previous biopsy site and show healing foci of ischemic injury with varying degrees of inflammatory infiltrates, changes which should not be confused with acute rejection. The revised and original grading scheme for acute cellular rejection (Fig. 9.3) refers to the histologic findings (e-**Fig. 9.23**); however, the presence or absence of myocyte necrosis should always be documented (*J Heart Lung Transplant*. 2005;24:1710).

B. **Antibody mediated rejection** (AMR, also known as humoral or vascular rejection) occurs in 10% to 20% of cardiac transplants, and is associated with hemodynamic compromise, development of cardiac allograft vasculopathy (see later), poor overall graft survival, and death in 20% to 50% of patients. Specific vascular and cardiomyocyte changes associated with AMR in endomyocardial biopsies have been described, but alone may not be a reliable method for diagnosis. In contrast, strong staining of the endothelium of small vessels and the myocardial capillary network (e-**Fig. 9.24**) by immunohistochemistry for the complement component C4d has been shown to correlate with abnormal cardiac hemodynamics due to AMR (*J Heart Lung Transplant*. 2008;27:372). The diagnosis of AMR, therefore, rests on a combination of histopathologic findings (light microscopic features and identification of diffuse capillary C4d immunostaining) and clinical findings (clinical evidence of anti-donor (HLA) antibodies and graft-dysfunction).

C. **Quilty effect** (e-**Fig. 9.25**) refers to the presence of a dense subendocardial lymphocyte infiltrate (*Am J Cardiovasc Pathol*. 1988;1:139), composed of predominately B-cells. Quilty A lesions are limited to the endo/subendocardium, while Quilty B lesions extend into underlying myocardium where there is often associated myocyte damage (*Curr Opin Cardiol*. 1997;12:146). There is no consensus as to the pathogenesis or clinical significance of Quilty B lesions since up to 20% of post-transplant biopsies show this finding (also known as cyclosporine effect). Quilty lesions have no known adverse prognostic effect, and are not associated with EBV infection responsible for post-transplant lymphoproliferative disorders. Quilty effect is, therefore, classified as one of four nonrejection findings.

Given the location of Quilty B lesions within the myocardium, and the potential for associated myocyte damage, it is often difficult to distinguish the lesions from conventional cellular rejection. However, since Quilty effect is characterized by a collar of T-cells surrounding a central aggregate of B-cells, immunostains for CD3 and CD20 can be used to help classify problematic cases (e-**Fig. 9.26**). It has recently been demonstrated that a compact network of follicular dendritic cells is also present in the center of Quilty lesions (*Am J Surg Pathol*. 2006;30:1008) which can be highlighted by an immunostain for CD21 (e-**Fig. 9.27**).

D. **Ischemic injury** is the second nonrejection finding. It presents either early (up to 6 weeks post-transplant) or late, and is related to allograft coronary disease. Ischemic injury must be differentiated from preservation injury, which develops as a result of the lack of organ perfusion between harvest and implantation. Preservation injury is a common incidental finding in endocardial biopsies during the week or two following transplantation and is characterized by necrosis of the most superficial regions of the endocardium with associated overlying organizing fibrin (e-**Fig. 9.28**). Similarly, artifacts of endomyocardial biopsy

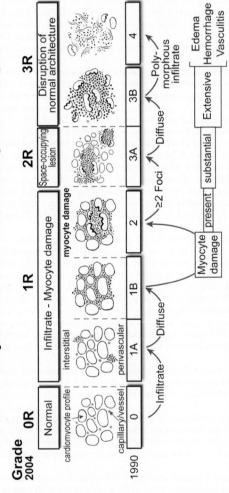

Figure 9.3 Grading of cellular rejection in heart transplant biopsies. The grading is illustrated from left to right. Comparison of original (1990) and revised grading (2004) schemes is schematically illustrated (see also e-Fig. 9.23). Open circles represent cardiomyocyte profiles, small dots represent vessels or inflammatory infiltrate. The main diagnostic feature of each grade is provided. The diagnostic features required for the 1990 grading are provided below the scheme. (Note: diagnosis is based on the highest grade findings present; see *J Heart Transplant.* 1990;9:587; *J Heart Lung Transplant.* 2005;24:1710; *Heart Transplant Pathol.* 2007;131:1169.)

processing that simulate contraction band necrosis (e-Fig. 9.19) must not be confused with true ischemic injury.

E. **Infection and lymphoproliferative disorders** are the two other nonrejection findings in biopsies, characterized by diffuse infiltration by small to medium-sized lymphocytes in a pattern resembling rejection (*J Heart Lung Transplant.* 2005;24:1710).

F. The so-called **transplant arteriopathy** or **cardiac allograft vasculopathy** is characteristic of chronic rejection. It features concentric luminal narrowing of small vessels by intimal thickening and medial proliferation with relative preservation of the internal elastic lamina, a pattern thought to represent an accelerated form of atherosclerosis. In cases with complete vascular obstruction ischemic damage can be found, although ischemic events are clinically silent due to the lack of cardiac reinnervation after transplantation.

VESSELS

I. **NORMAL ANATOMY.** The luminal endothelial cell layer defines vessels and **arteries** have three layers (e-Fig. 9.20): the intima (composed of the endothelium, internal elastic lamella, and subendothelial connective tissue), media (smooth muscle), and adventitia (connective tissue). Venous vessels have the same three layers, but a thinner media and a thicker adventitia.

Endothelial cells are characterized by immunoreactivity for CD34, CD31, vimentin, endothelin, and von Willebrand factor. Endothelium also stains for Factor VIII–related antigen and *Ulex europaeus* I lectin, both stronger in blood vessels in comparison to lymphatic vessels. The smooth muscle cells of the media express desmin. Depending on the anatomic site, pericytes and smooth muscle or glomus cells are located along the outside of the vessel; these cells show immunoreactivity for actin, vimentin, and myosin.

The size of arterial vessels is typically defined in relation to vessels in the kidney. The aorta is categorized as a large artery, the renal and lobar arteries as medium-sized arteries, and the arcuate and interlobular arteries as small arteries (Fig. 9.4). The next smallest arterial vessels, arterioles, are defined by a media that has two to five layers of smooth muscle cells, or as having a luminal radius that equals the wall thickness.

II. **GROSS EXAMINATION AND TISSUE HANDLING.** **Temporal artery biopsies** are typically about 2 to 3 cm long. Because arteritis can have a patchy distribution with the so-called skip areas (see later), proper tissue handling is essential to ensure a maximum diagnostic yield from the biopsy. The external aspect of the vessel should be inked (which is used to ensure that the microscopic sections include the entire wall); the vessel should then be serially sectioned at 3-mm intervals. After processing, embedding of the vessel segments should result in tissue sections with complete ring-like profiles that have an inked external surface. At least three levels should be examined. Orienting the vessel segments in agar before processing (*Ann Diagn Pathol.* 2001;5:107) is a simple way to ensure that proper orientation is achieved during embedding.

Although **embolectomy** specimens are easy to gross, the submission of all tissues can have tremendous clinical impact, because the pathologist may ascertain the exact source of an embolus (e.g., endocarditis, atrial myxoma) in a minute piece of tissue.

III. **DIAGNOSTIC FEATURES OF COMMON DISEASES.** Vascular diseases affect all organs and contribute to the histopathologic presentation of a variety of diseases.

A. **Vasculitides.** Vasculitis is a noninfectious inflammatory disease of the vessel wall and surrounding tissue. The Chapel Hill classification system for vasculitis based on the size of the vessels (Fig. 9.4) is widely used (*Arthritis Rheum.* 1994;37:187).

Vascular Tree and Distribution of Typical Vasculitides

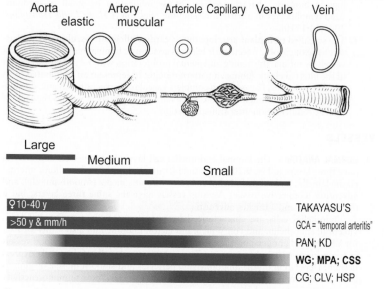

Figure 9.4 Overview of the vascular tree and typical vasculitides. TA = Takayasu's arteritis; GCA = giant cell arteritis = temporal arteritis; PAN = Panarteritis nodose; KD = Kawasaki disease; WG = Wegener's granulomatosis; MPA = microscopic polyangiitis; CSS = Churg–Strauss syndrome; CG = cryoglobulemia; CLV = cutaneous leucocytoclastic vasculitis; HSP = Henoch–Schönlein Purpura. Boldface type indicates ANCA-positive. See also e-**Fig.** 9.20 and e-**Fig.** 9.29.

1. **Large vessel vasculitides**
   a. **Giant cell arteritis (also known as temporal arteritis).** Three of the following five diagnostic criteria by the American College of Rheumatology (ACR) are required for a diagnosis of giant cell arteritis: over 50 years of age, recent localized headache, temporal artery tenderness, ESR 50 mm/h, and a temporal artery biopsy demonstrating vasculitis (e-**Fig.** 9.29). It is worth noting that up to 60% of patients with clinical features of giant cell arteritis show no evidence of vasculitis by arterial biopsy (*Baillieres Clin Rheumatol.* 1991;5:387).

   There are four key diagnostic features of the vasculitis associated with giant cell arteritis: transmural inflammation, giant cells in close relation to disrupted elastic lamellae, intimal thickening, and marked intimal edema. Giant cells are not required for the diagnosis, but typically are present if a substantial or granulomatous inflammatory infiltrate is present. Non-contiguous foci of inflammation, the so-called skip areas, are occasionally present; patches of arteritis can be less than 0.3 mm long, which emphasizes the importance of microscopic examination of multiple tissue levels (*Arch Ophthalmol.* 1976;94:2072).

   The diagnosis of **healed** (e-**Fig.** 9.29) or **subacute cranial arteritis** is an indication for prolonged steroid therapy, and so is an important differential diagnosis. Focal aggregates of lymphocytes and/or macrophages in the media, irregular fibrosis and scarring of the media, breaks of the internal elastic lamella (involving up to 25% of the circumference), and irregular intimal fibrosis are the histologic hallmarks. Since the media does not contain blood vessels in normal arterial vessels, medial neovascularization is a useful indicator of previous inflammation.

Normal changes in the arteries of the elderly can complicate diagnosis. However, arteriosclerosis typically does not include inflammation, and the associated intimal and medial fibrosis is concentric and not irregular. While the internal elastic lamella may show fragmentation, long breaks are uncommon.

b. Takayasu's arteritis. Clinical findings and vascular distribution are necessary to distinguish Takayasu's arteritis from giant cell arteritis because both diseases show identical morphologic features. In more than 80% of cases, Takayasu's arteritis affects women in the age range of 10 to 40 years. The aorta and typically the left mid to proximal subclavian artery are affected, although in 50% of patients the pulmonary arteries and abdominal aorta are involved. In contrast, giant cell arteritis occurs in patients over 50 years of age and typically involves the external carotid artery branches.

2. Medium vessel vasculitides

a. Polyarteritis nodosa is a rare systemic, necrotizing vasculitis that is not associated with glomerulonephritis. The lesions are segmental, and may be only partially circumferential. The inflammation may cause weakening of the arterial wall, with subsequent aneurysmal dilatation and localized rupture.

b. Kawasaki disease is febrile illness of childhood of unknown etiology that is characterized by a self-limited acute vasculitic syndrome. Microscopically, the vasculitis consists of an acute necrotizing arteritis similar to polyarteritis nodosa. Differentiation from polyarteritis nodosa is based on the distinctive clinical picture and age at presentation.

3. Small vessel vasculitides.

This group of diseases is subclassified on the basis of the presence or absence of anti-neutrophil cytoplasmic antibodies (ANCA). Since cytoplasmic ANCA (c-ANCA) mainly recognize proteinase 3 and perinuclear ANCA (p-ANCA) mainly recognize myeloperoxidase, the terms PR3-ANCA and MPO-ANCA, respectively, are now in common use (*Arch Intern Med.* 1996;156:440). ANCA-associated small vessel vasculitides are the most common vasculitides in adults.

a. ANCA-positive. There are four ANCA-positive small vessel vasculitides, Wegener granulomatosis, microscopic polyangiitis, Churg–Strauss syndrome, and drug-induced small vessel vasculitis.

The absence of granulomas defines microscopic polyangiitis. When granulomas are present, the distinction between Churg–Strauss syndrome and Wegener granulomatosis is made on the basis of the presence or absence of asthma and eosinophilia, respectively.

b. ANCA-negative. There are three main ANCA-negative small vessel vasculitides, Henoch–Schönlein purpura, cryoglobulinemia, and the so-called non-ANCA small vessel diseases.

The presence of IgA-dominant immune deposits in small vessels (*N Engl J Med.* 1997;337:1512) is indicative of Henoch–Schönlein purpura, the most common vasculitis in children (**e-Fig. 9.29**). The absence of IgA deposits, together with the presence of serum cryoglobulins is diagnostic of cryoglobulinemia. In the absence of both IgA and cryoglobulins, the differential diagnosis includes various non-ANCA small vessel vasculitides including paraneoplastic small vessel vasculitis, inflammatory bowel disease vasculitis, and immune complex small vessel vasculitis (a category which itself includes lupus vasculitis, rheumatoid arthritis,

Goodpasture's syndrome, Sjögren disease, drug-induced immune complex vasculitis, Behçet disease, and infection-induced immune complex vasculitis). The diagnostic criteria for this group of vasculitides have been well described (*Am Fam Physian. 2002;65*:1615 and *N Engl J Med.* 1997;337:1512).

B. Amyloid angiopathy. The deposition of waxy, extracellular, amorphous, weakly eosinophilic material in the absence of an inflammatory reaction, without intimal myofibroblasts or collagen deposits, is the hallmark of amyloid angiopathy.

IV. NEOPLASMS OF THE VESSELS

A. Benign

1. Leiomyoma is the most common benign tumor of veins, and usually arises in the peripheral veins. Leiomyomas that arise in the inferior vena cava have a prominent luminal component, and often represent extension of a uterine leiomyoma in the setting of intravascular leiomyomatosis.

2. Rare benign neoplasms of the large arteries include inflammatory pseudotumor and benign fibrous histiocytoma. Paragangliomas occur within the aortic adventitia.

3. Benign lesions of the endothelium are covered in the chapter on soft tissue tumors (see Chap. 46).

B. Malignant

1. **Leiomyosarcoma** is the most common malignant neoplasm of veins, and is thought to arise from the smooth muscle cells of the media (e-**Fig. 9.30**). The tumor usually shows extension into the adjacent soft tissues; only rarely is the tumor confined to the vascular lumen. Most cases arise in the inferior vena cava, in women (the female to male ratio is over 4:1) in their sixth decade. Microscopically, the tumor has the same morphologic features as leiomyosarcomas that occur at other sites.

2. **Aortic intimal sarcoma** is the most common malignant neoplasm of large arteries, and is thought to arise from the pluripotent mesenchymal cells of the intima. By definition the tumor is luminal (e-**Fig. 9.30**), although some cases show focal extension into or through the media. Most cases arise within the abdominal aorta in patients in their seventh decade. Microscopically, the tumor is poorly differentiated and shows myofibroblastic or fibroblastic differentiation, although rare cases show specific histologic differentiation such as angiosarcoma or osteosarcoma. Cytologically, the tumor cells are usually spindle-shaped with marked atypia and pleomorphism.

An analogous rare tumor, intimal pulmonary sarcoma, involves the pulmonary arteries, usually in patients in their fifth decade who present with symptoms suggestive of recurrent pulmonary emboli. As with aortic intimal sarcoma, a subset of cases has the morphology of a specific sarcoma type.

SUGGESTED READINGS

Anderson RH, Becker AE. *Cardiac Anatomy: An Integrated Text and Color Atlas.* London: Gower Medical Publishing; 1980.

Bharati S, Lev M. *The Pathology of Congenital Heart Disease.* New York, NY: Futura Publishing Company; 1996.

Bloom S, ed. *Diagnostic Criteria for Cardiovascular Pathology: Acquired Diseases.* Philadelphia, PA: Lippincott-Raven Publishers; 1997.

Bowker TJ, Wood DA, Davies MJ, et al. Sudden, unexpected cardiac or unexplained death in England: a national survey. *Q J Med.* 2003;96:269.

Cooper, LT. Myocarditis. *N Engl J Med.* 2009;360:1526.

Silver MD, Gotlieb AI, Schoen FJ. *Cardiovascular Pathology.* 3rd ed. Philadelphia, PA: Churchill Livingstone; 2001.

10 Mediastinum

Louis P. Dehner

I. **GROSS ANATOMY.** The mediastinum is located in the thoracic cavity and is generally divided into superior, anterior, middle, and posterior compartments and is bounded by the pleura laterally. Generally, the first rib defines its superior limit and the diaphragm its inferior border. The sternum, ribs, and thoracic vertebrae (T1 through T11–12) constitute the skeletal confines of the mediastinum. The thymus, heart and great vessels, lungs, and esophagus are among the most obvious organs which occupy the anterior (thymus), middle (heart), and posterior (esophagus and aorta) mediastinum. The aortic arch and the proximal segment of the aorta (ascending and proximal aorta) are located in the superior mediastinum, which is bounded by the manubrium sterni anteriorly and thoracic vertebrae 1 through 4. The embryological aspects of the mediastinum are basically those of the organs and structures which occupy this compartment.

The definition of the mediastinum relates to the structures and organs with observable pathology on imaging studies and the associated differential diagnosis. For instance, the anterior mediastinum is the site of the thymus with its varied associated pathology from Hodgkin and non-Hodgkin lymphoma (NHL), to thymoma, to germ cell neoplasms. The pathology of the posterior mediastinum is dominated by a variety of neurogenic neoplasms and bronchoenteric developmental cysts.

II. **GROSS EXAMINATION, TISSUE SAMPLING, AND HISTOLOGIC SLIDE PREPARATION**

A. **Fine needle aspiration (FNA) biopsy.** FNA is generally performed as an image-guided or endoscopically directed procedure on suspected pathology in the anterior or middle mediastinum. These specimens are processed in the same manner as other FNA specimens, and are commonly examined for adequacy so that the results can be transmitted contemporaneously with the procedure. Given the broad range of pathologic processes in the anterior and middle mediastinum, an advanced level of experience is recommended for FNA interpretation of specimens from these sites.

One of the more common specimens is a lymph node with the differential diagnosis of an infectious and/or granulomatous process, metastasis, or lymphoma. Metastasis, usually a carcinoma of the lung or elsewhere (most often squamous cell carcinoma of the head and neck, papillary thyroid carcinoma, or renal cell carcinoma), accounts for over 50% of the diagnoses. NHL (lymphoblastic lymphoma and mediastinal large B-cell lymphoma) and Hodgkin lymphoma (HL) are the most common primary malignant neoplasms of the mediastinum; however, while strong suspicion about an NHL can be voiced in the case of a lymphoblastic lymphoma, both the large B-cell lymphoma and HL of the nodular sclerosis subtype have a considerable fibrous component, which may complicate the ability to obtain a sufficiently cellular FNA specimen for diagnosis.

Biopsy. Tissue samplings from the anterior mediastinum are generally small (<1 cm) and often consist of multiple fragments which have been obtained via mediastinoscopy. These specimens, commonly intrathoracic lymph nodes, are submitted for intraoperative frozen section consultation to ascertain their metastatic status for purposes of operability of a nonsmall cell carcinoma of the lung. Often biopsies that show no evidence of malignancy contain granulomas in varying stages of activity and type (including the so-called naked granulomas of sarcoidosis), or simply a carpet of pigmented macrophages.

165

Mediastinal biopsies in those cases with a clinical suspicion of a disease process other than the metastatic carcinoma present the intraoperative dilemma of performing a frozen section or not when the biopsy consists of only a small amount of tissue; however, a discussion with the surgeon is helpful in these cases. When lymphoma is suspected, tissue should be set aside for flow cytometry, but necrosis and fibrosis often limit the evaluation. When the lymphoma is a suspected HL, every fragment of the tissue is critical in the search for Reed–Sternberg cells and their subsequent confirmation by immunohistochemistry (in this case, prospective sectioning through the entire formalin-fixed paraffin tissue block is recommended, with mounting of the unstained sections for additional studies; however, the alternative approach of returning to the block later results in a high risk of loss of potentially diagnostic tissue during refacing of the block).

Both benign and malignant processes in the mediastinum may be accompanied by a substantial fibroinflammatory reaction, which encases the underlying pathology. It is therefore necessary in these cases to recommend a re-biopsy when the only findings are those of chronic inflammation and fibrosis.

B. Resection. Surgical resections of mediastinal contents are restricted in most cases to mass lesions in the anterior mediastinum with thymic-related neoplasms, the thymus gland in cases of myasthenia gravis or a germ cell neoplasm (which may or may not be associated with the thymus). An enlarged substernal adenomatous thyroid or parathyroid adenoma may also present in the anterior superior mediastinum; however, the examination of these latter two specimen types should follow the recommendation in Chapters 24 and 25, respectively. The other compartments with resectable specimens include cysts of the middle mediastinum (most commonly a bronchogenic cyst) and enteric duplication cysts of the posterior mediastinum, as well as the entire morphologic spectrum of neurogenic neoplasms from neuroblastoma to schwannoma and paraganglioma (as discussed below).

A resected thymus may be represented by nondescript fibroadipose or adipose tissue which upon sectioning fails to demonstrate any mass lesion (*Thorac Surg Clin*. 2011;21:191). On the other hand, a mass lesion may be clearly evident by its size, shape, and weight; these three characteristics should be noted upon the initial gross examination before any sectioning takes place. The external surface should be described as to whether it is smooth and/or glistening, or irregular by virtue of apparent fibrosis; the latter may reflect the presence of adhesions between the mass and contiguous structures such as the pericardium, lung, or pleura which may be included as part of the resection specimen. Because surgical margins are important in pathologic staging, especially in the case of a thymoma, the surface of the tumor should be marked in such a manner that the resection margins can be identified microscopically. If the superior and inferior poles of the specimen can be identified, then the specimen can be bisected along that plane and the surface exposed to describe the salient features including any apparent capsule or pseudocapsule; circumscription or lack thereof; diffuse or lobulated appearance; uniform or heterogeneous character; solid, solid and cystic, or cystic appearance; hemorrhage or necrosis; and any identifiable portion or remnant of uninvolved organs. The selection of blocks for microscopic section should include a thorough sampling of the margins; sections of the apparent tumor should include any regional variations in the appearance of the mass.

If the mass is predominantly cystic, the differential diagnosis is teratoma, thymic cyst, or cystic thymoma. A solid, or solid and cystic, mass may represent a thymoma, thymic carcinoma, seminoma, or mixed germ cell neoplasm, HL, Castleman disease (CD), mediastinal large B-cell lymphoma, Langerhan cell histiocytosis, granulocytic sarcoma (acute myeloid or monocytic leukemia), or localized sclerosing-fibrosing mediastinitis.

III. MEDIASTINAL SOFT TISSUES

A. Inflammation (mediastinitis)

1. **Acute and chronic inflammation.** Acute mediastinitis with a purely neutrophilic reaction is a consequence of a contiguous infection, rupture-perforation of the esophagus, penetrating trauma, congenital duplication, or foregut cyst (*Thorac Surg Clin.* 2009;19:37). A peritonsillar abscess, suppurative thyroiditis, periodontal abscess, and post-sternotomy infection, notably by methicillin-resistant *Staphylococcus aureus,* are other causes. In addition to the acute inflammatory reaction, the tissues may have a necrotizing appearance especially in those cases with the spread of an infection from the head and neck region into the mediastinum by the so-called acute descending necrotizing mediastinitis (*Heart Lung Circ.* 2008;17:124). With the passage of time, acute inflammation is accompanied by a mixed inflammatory response with macrophages, a fibroblastic reaction, and microvascular proliferation.

2. **Chronic fibroinflammatory process (fibrosing-sclerosing mediastinitis).** This uncommon but well-documented clinicopathologic entity comes to attention with a persistent cough and fever in young to middle-aged adults (*Semin Respir Infect.* 2001;16:119). A mass lesion is usually present in the right paratracheal or subcarinal region, often associated with punctuate calcifications. Less frequently, the presentation is as more diffuse infiltrative mass, which is no longer confined to the middle mediastinum. An abnormal host response to the antigens of *Histoplasma capsulatum* is thought to account for cases in regions endemic for the infection. A needle or wedge biopsy is the usual type of specimen for pathologic evaluation. Infrequently, fibrosclerotic lesions may be present elsewhere in the mesentery or retroperitoneum as manifestations of the IgG4-related diseases (*Am J Surg Pathol.* 2010;34:211).

There are several microscopic stages through which this fibroinflammatory process evolves from a reactive fibroblastic stage with an edematous background resembling nodular fasciitis, to a dense hyalinized collagen stage of the interstitium and thickened blood vessels showing similar hyalinized features (e-Fig. 10.1).* A dispersed population of lymphocytes and plasma cells is present throughout the biopsy. Granulomas are not a feature in most cases despite the association with *Histoplasma.* Dystrophic calcifications may or may not be present. A similar pathologic process occurs in the lung as pulmonary hyalinizing granulomas.

The differential diagnosis includes HL and NHL, inflammatory myofibroblastic tumor, calcifying fibrous pseudotumor, and fibromatosis (desmoid tumor). Appropriate immunohistochemical studies are helpful in the differential diagnosis if diagnostic or suspected cells are found in the biopsy (Table 10.1).

3. **Granulomatous mediastinitis.** A number of infectious etiologies are responsible for granulomatous inflammatory reactions in the mediastinum. It is generally the case that other sites in the thoracic cavity including the lungs and regional lymph nodes also harbor the particular infection, which is usually either tuberculous or fungal in nature. The active, infectious granulomas show the presence of caseous necrosis. The granulomas are hyalinized with or without dystrophic calcifications when the infection is inactive. The most common organism in addition to *Mycobacterium tuberculosis* is *H. capsulatum;* other rare causative fungal organisms include *Cryptococcus, Blastomyces, Coccidioides,* and the *Rhizopus* group. Sarcoidosis typically involves hilar lymph nodes without direct involvement of the mediastinal soft tissues,

---

*All e-figures are available online via the Solution Site Image Bank.

TABLE 10.1	Immunohistochemical Phenotypes of Fibroinflammatory Lesions of the Mediastinum				
	CD15	CD30	ALK1	Smooth muscle actin	Factor XIIIa
Fibrosing mediastinitis	−	−	−	±	−
Hodgkin lymphoma	+	+	−	±	−
Inflammatory myofibroblastic tumor	−	−	+	+	−
Calcifying fibrous pseudotumor	−	−	−	±	+
Mediastinal large B-cell lymphoma	−	+	−	−	−
Fibromatosis (desmoid)	−	−	−	+	−

except in rare cases (*Respiration.* 2010;79:341). HL of the nodular sclerosis type may have a prominent granulomatous reaction which can overshadow the isolated Reed–Sternberg cells.

IV. **MEDIASTINAL NEOPLASMS.** Intrathoracic, extrapulmonary, and nonmetastatic neoplasms arising in one of the mediastinal compartments qualify as uncommon to rare in the general experience of most institutions. No more than 5% to 10% of the intrathoracic neoplasms originate in the mediastinum independent of the lung, heart, and great vessels. However, the different tumor types are a microcosm of neoplasms, which are seen not only in intrathoracic sites, but also in extrathoracic organs and locations (*Lancet Oncol.* 2004;5:107). The distribution and frequency of the different types of mediastinal tumors relate to the definition of particular lesions as neoplastic or nonneoplastic, especially in the case of some of the cysts, and whether the series includes both benign and malignant tumors or only the latter. Approximately 30% to 35% of the mediastinal tumors are derived from thymic epithelium, followed by HL and NHL (25% to 30%), germ cell neoplasms (10% to 15%), neurogenic tumors (10% to 15%), and a miscellaneous category (15%) consisting of soft tissue neoplasms of virtually all types. If discussion is limited to those mediastinal tumors presenting in the first two decades of life, the general experience is that HL and NHL account for 40% to 80% of the cases, with neurogenic (20% to 25%) and germ cell (15% to 20%) neoplasms accounting for the remainder (*Semin Thorac Cardiovasc Surg.* 2004;16:201; *Thorac Surg Clin.* 2009;19:47). Nongerm cell thymic neoplasms are rare in children, but a variety of soft tissue neoplasms exclusive of schwannoma are, however, observed in this age group. The WHO classification of mediastinal tumor is shown in Table 10.2.

A. **Thymic neoplasms.** This category of neoplasms includes thymoma, thymic carcinoma, and neuroendocrine carcinoma including thymic carcinoid. These tumors arise from the thymic epithelium. Within the category of thymic neoplasms, approximately 80% to 85% are thymomas, 10% are thymic carcinomas, and 5% are pure neuroendocrine carcinomas.

1. **Thymoma.** Many approaches to the pathologic classification of thymoma have been taken, surprising in that thymomas are an uncommon category of neoplasm whose estimated incidence is <0.15 per 100,000 person-years. In thymomas, the neoplastic thymic epithelium usually appears deceptively bland even though the tumor may have invaded surrounding anatomic structures and even metastasized; tumors that have histologic features of a carcinoma in the traditional sense of cellular enlargement with hyperchromatic and mitotically active nuclei are classified as thymic carcinoma (see below). Considerable data are available on the molecular genetics of thymic neoplasms which broadly correlate with the histologic type of thymoma or thymic carcinoma (*J Thorac Oncol.* 2010;5:S313; *J Thorac Oncol.* 2010;5:S286).

Thymomas are neoplasms which tend to maintain to a greater or lesser degree the overall architectural and mixture of cell types, which are present

TABLE 10.2	WHO Histologic Classification of Tumors of the Mediastinum

Epithelial tumors

Thymoma
  Type A (spindle cell; medullary)
  Type AB (mixed)
  Type B1 (lymphocyte-rich; lymphocytic;
    predominantly cortical; organoid)
  Type B2 (cortical)
  Type B3 (epithelial; atypical; squamoid;
    well-differentiated thymic carcinoma)
  Micronodular thymoma
  Metaplastic thymoma
  Microscopic thymoma
  Sclerosing thymoma
  Lipofibroadenoma
Thymic carcinoma (including neuroendocrine
  epithelial tumors of the thymus)
  Squamous cell carcinoma
  Basaloid carcinoma
  Mucoepidermoid carcinoma
  Lymphoepithelioma-like carcinoma
  Sarcomatoid carcinoma (carcinosarcoma)
  Clear cell carcinoma
  Adenocarcinoma
  Papillary adenocarcinoma
  Carcinoma with t(15;19) translocation
  Well-differentiated neuroendocrine
    carcinomas (carcinoid tumors)
    Typical carcinoid
    Atypical carcinoid
  Poorly differentiated neuroendocrine
    carcinoma
    Large cell neuroendocrine carcinoma
    Small cell carcinoma, neuroendocrine type
  Undifferentiated carcinoma
  Combined thymic epithelial tumors,
    including neuroendocrine carcinomas

Germ cell tumors (GCTs) of the mediastinum

GCTs of one histological type (pure GCTs)
  Seminoma
  Embryonal carcinoma

  Yolk sac tumor
  Choriocarcinoma
  Teratoma, mature
  Teratoma, immature
GCTs of more than one histological type
  (mixed GCT)
GCTs with somatic-type malignancy
GCTs with associated hematologic
  malignancy

**Mediastinal lymphomas and
  hematopoietic neoplasms**

B-cell lymphoma
T-cell lymphoma
Hodgkin lymphomas of the mediastinum
"Gray zone" between Hodgkin and
  non-Hodgkin lymphomas
Histiocytic and dendritic cell tumors
Myeloid sarcoma and extramedullary
  acute myeloid leukemia

**Mesenchymal tumors of the thymus and
  mediastinum**

Thymolipoma
Lipoma of the mediastinum
Liposarcoma of the mediastinum
Solitary fibrous tumor
Synovial sarcoma
Vascular neoplasms
Rhabdomyosarcoma
Leiomyomatous tumors
Tumors of the peripheral nerves

Rare tumors of the mediastinum

Ectopic tumors of the thymus
  Ectopic thyroid tumors
  Ectopic parathyroid tumors

**Metastasis to thymus and anterior
  mediastinum**

Modified from: Travis WD, Brambilla E, Müller-Hermelink HK, Harris CC, eds. *World Health Organization Classification of Tumours. Pathology and Genetics. Tumours of the Lung, Pleura, Thymus and Heart.* Lyon: IARC Press; 2004. Used with permission.

in the normal thymus (e-**Figs. 10.2** and **10.3**). Most thymomas have a multilobular growth pattern which is accentuated by the presence of fibrous bands that enclose the epithelial islands (e-**Fig. 10.4**). In the past, thymomas were differentiated on the basis of the prominence of the lymphocytic and/or epithelial elements. This descriptive classification was systematized in the World Health Organization (WHO) classification into a series of letter designations which denote the morphology (i.e., type) and in turn

TABLE 10.3 WHO Classification of Thymomas (A, B1, B2, B3, AB and C system)

Type	% Total	% Invasive	Microscopic features
A	8	10	Spindle to ovoid epithelial cells with diffuse or hemangiopericytoma-like pattern, no lymphocytes
B1	16	45	Resembles normal thymus with cortex-like features of immature thymocytes and scattered epithelial cells, with or without Hassall's corpuscles
B2	28	70	Lobules of large polygonal epithelial cells separated by immature T-lymphocytes
B3	11	85	Lobules of large polygonal epithelial cells in sheets with a minimal lymphocytic component; presence of mild epithelial atypia may raise the possibility of thymic carcinoma
AB	31	40	Lobules with mixed patterns of type A (lymphocyte poor) and type B (lymphocyte rich) patterns with small spindled to ovoid shaped epithelial cells; overall, lymphocytes more numerous than in type A; type A and B equally represented or one pattern may dominate over the other.
C	5	5	Any pattern of carcinoma with squamous, lymphoepithelial, clear cell, mucoepidermoid, basaloid, sarcomatoid, papillary, and mucinous features

Modified from: Travis WD, Brambilla E, Müller-Hermelink HK, Harris CC, eds. *World Health Organization Classification of Tumours. Pathology and Genetics. Tumours of the Lung, Pleura, Thymus and Heart.* Lyon: IARC Press; 2004. Used with permission.

correlate with the prognosis (Table 10.3), although pathologic staging in some studies is the more significant determinant of outcome. There is also some correlation between the WHO type and the locally aggressive behavior with invasion into or through the capsule. Types A, AB (e-**Fig. 10.5**), and B1 demonstrate invasive features in approximately 10%, 40%, and 45%, respectively whereas types B2 and B3 (e-**Fig. 10.6**) are invasive in 70% and 85% of the cases, respectively. Although uncommon, type A (e-**Fig. 10.7**) or spindle cell thymoma may demonstrate invasive behavior (*Am J Clin Pathol.* 2010;134:793). Thymic carcinoma or type C is regarded as separate and distinct from thymoma, and for this reason not all clinical series of thymic neoplasms include type C; similarly, neuroendocrine carcinoma (or thymic carcinoid as it was initially designated) is classified as an entity separate from thymic carcinoma.

Regardless of the pathologic type, thymic neoplasms tend to have macroscopic features of a solid circumscribed mass with an apparent well-encapsulated appearance. Gross or microscopic evidence that the capsule has been invaded, or that the tumor has extended through the capsule into surrounding tissues of the mediastinum, is an important feature. If the thymoma has invaded the lung, pleura, pericardium, or great vessels, this finding is usually documented at the time of surgery with or without biopsy confirmation.

Some additional challenges in the pathologic diagnosis of a thymoma include the distinction of a type A or spindle cell thymoma from a soft tissue neoplasm like a hemangiopericytoma or monophasic synovial sarcoma (*Appl Immunohistochem Mol Morphol.* 2011;19:329); the spindle cell thymoma may have a papillary or pseudopapillary and adenomatoid patterns (*Am J Surg Pathol.* 2011;35:372l; *Am J Surg Pathol.*

TABLE 10.4	Clinicopathologic Staging of Thymoma According to Masaoka	
Stage	**Qualifying features**	**5-year survival (%)**
I	Completely encapsulated without invasion of capsule	95–100
II	Gross invasion into surrounding soft tissues or mediastinal pleural and/or microscopic invasion into capsule	80–85
III	Gross invasion of pericardium, lung, and great vessels (established by biopsy or excision or intraoperative confirmation)	60–70
IVa	Dissemination to pericardium and/or pleura without contiguous spread as in stage III	40–50
IVb	Distant site metastasis (lung, skin, bone, liver)	25–30

2010;34:1544). Type B3 thymoma and type C or thymic carcinomas are not always readily differentiated from each other in a biopsy, but MUC1 expression in thymic carcinoma has been reported as a useful distinguishing marker (*Virchow Arch.* 2011;458:615).

As discussed above, the clinical and/or pathologic staging of thymoma is complicated by the lack of standardization, but the National Cancer Institute website (www.cancer.gov) has included the Masaoka staging system (Table 10.4) which was first proposed over 25 years ago, and is widely utilized in published clinical series despite its perceived shortcomings (*Chest.* 2005;127:755). Masaoka has recently re-evaluated his staging system, compared it with several other systems, and concluded that it maintains its prognostic importance without the need for revision (*J Thorac Oncol.* 2010;5:S304). Nonetheless, there are complications of the Masaoka staging scheme, including the uncertainty that may arise between stages II and III regarding the gross invasion of surrounding soft tissues since invasion observed by the surgeon may not be documented by a biopsy.

The approximate 5-year survival without consideration of the specific histologic type is summarized in Table 10.4. Local control of tumor is a major impediment to long-term survival, although only a small proportion of patients presents with stage IVb disease. Multivariate analysis has shown that tumor size, complete resection, histologic subtype, and stage are the significant variables (*J Thorac Cardiovasc Surg.* 2003;126:1134).

2. **Thymic carcinoma.** Only 5% or less of all primary thymic neoplasms are carcinomas. These neoplasms arise de novo in the thymus, but there are rare examples which may have evolved from a preexisting thymoma. These tumors may present as a multilocular cyst (*Am J Surg Pathol.* 2011;35:1074). Unless the tumor has been biopsied before resection, the carcinomatous nature may not be appreciated until microscopic examination. A solid, poorly differentiated carcinoma with or without squamous differentiation is the most common histologic appearance, but there is considerable diversity in the particular carcinomatous pattern (e-Figs. 10.8 and 10.9) including basaloid, adenoid cystic, papillary, clear cell, lymphoepithelial-like (EBER-positive), and adenocarcinoma. In some cases, the distinction from an atypical appearing thymoma or carcinoma of the lung may be problematic. Immunohistochemistry may provide assistance in the differential diagnosis (Table 10.5), as well as review of imaging studies. The immunophenotype of thymoma and thymic carcinoma show the following patterns: CK7 (strongly expressed in Type A), CD15 (strongly expressed in Type A), bcl2 (strongly expressed in Type A and C), CK 5/6 and CK7 (no discrimination between thymoma and thymic carcinoma), and CK18, CD5, CD117, MUC1, and GLUT-1 (all uniformly

TABLE 10.5	Differential Diagnosis of Atypical Thymoma, Thymic Carcinoma, and Pulmonary Carcinoma						
	CK7	CD5	CD117	CD1a	TTF-1	CD205	FOXN1
Thymoma	+	−	−	+[a]	−	+	+[b]
Thymic carcinoma	+	+	+	−	−	+	±
Lung carcinoma	±	−	−	−	+	±	−

[a]CD1a positivity in immature thymic T-lymphocytes.
[b]FOXN1 nuclear staining is diffuse in thymoma and focal in thymic carcinoma.

expressed in thymic carcinomas) (*Mod Pathol.* 2009;22:1341). All thymic epithelial neoplasms have genetic alterations in 6q25 and 6p21.3; thymomas except Type A may have alterations in 5q21, 7p15 and 8p11; and numerical alterations are present in thymic carcinomas (1q+, 17q+, 18p+, 3p−, 6−, 16q− and 17p−) (*J Thoracic Oncol.* 2010;5:S286).

Following is a list of some important points to remember about thymic epithelial neoplasms, their diagnosis, and potential pitfalls:

a. Because the lymphocytes in a thymoma are immature T-lymphocytes, they can be mistaken for lymphoblasts as in lymphoblastic lymphoma. These cells are immunopositive for CD1a and CD99.

b. While putative thymomas can measure only 1 to 2 mm in greatest dimension (micro-thymoma), caution is warranted in thymic resections in cases of myasthenia gravis; residual involuted thymus must be excluded.

c. Sharply angulated predominantly lymphoid lobules surrounded by fibrous stroma and widened perivascular spaces containing individual and small aggregates of lymphocytes are characteristic features of thymoma.

d. Ectopic thymomas can present in the neck or on the pleura and are primary tumors in both sites.

e. When a lymphocyte-rich thymoma metastasizes, the lymphocytes may be present in the metastatic focus.

f. Primary thymic hyperplasia can resemble type B1 thymoma. However, the presence of lymphoid follicles with germinal centers in the medulla is a useful differentiating feature in thymic hyperplasia (although not present in all cases).

g. Pathologic staging of thymic carcinoma does not reliably predict the behavior of the tumor in the same sense as thymoma because the carcinoma has a great potential to metastasize that is not necessarily correlated with pathologic stage.

h. A thymoma may be a purely cystic mass. Thymomas with liquefied, degenerated, and necrotic material within cystic spaces present the problem of demonstration of viable tumor to confirm the diagnosis.

i. A multicystic or multilobular thymic lesion may represent a multilocular thymic cyst, cystic thymoma, HL, mature cystic teratoma, or seminoma–germinoma.

j. A small biopsy of an anterior mediastinal mass especially in an adolescent or young adult may consist of thymic tissue which is normal thymus and not a thymoma.

k. Thymomas can be present on the pleura and in the lung as apparent primary tumors, but these are also favored sites for recurrent and metastatic disease (*Cases J.* 2009;2:9149; *Arch Pathol Lab Med.* 1997;121:79; *Am J Surg Pathol.* 1995;19:304).

I. A thymoma can be rarely present in an ectopic site, most commonly in the neck, where the ectopic thymoma may or may not be associated with a cyst, with or without accompanying parathyroid.

3. **Neuroendocrine carcinoma.** This primary neoplasm of the thymus constitutes ≤5% of all thymic epithelial neoplasms (*Semin Diagn Pathol.* 2005;22:223). Cushing syndrome is one of the known clinical presentations, as is a manifestation of multiple endocrine neoplasia type I. These tumors are typically large and have usually invaded into the surrounding mediastinal tissues. The histologic features (e-Fig. 10.10) are those of neuroendocrine carcinomas elsewhere including organoid profiles and/or rosette-like formations of uniform cells with finely distributed nuclear chromatin and central coagulative necrosis to a small cell carcinoma resembling its pulmonary counterpart (in the latter case, imaging studies are a reliable method to localize the mass to the hilum or thymus). It is worth noting that rosette-like profiles are seen in thymoma and mediastinal large B-cell lymphoma. The combination of thymoma and neuroendocrine carcinoma patterns in the same tumor argues to the point that the latter neoplasm is fundamentally derived from thymic epithelium.

B. **Germ cell tumors (GCTs).** The mediastinum, typically the anterior compartment, is one of the more common extragonadal primary sites for this group of neoplasms accounting for 10% to 15% of all the GCTs (*Adv Anat Pathol.* 2007;14:69). GCTs represent approximately 15% to 20% of all primary mediastinal neoplasms, as a category of malignancies that includes seminoma, endodermal sinus tumor, embryonal carcinoma, choriocarcinoma, or a mixture of these patterns with or without teratomatous elements. Individuals with Klinefelter syndrome are at an increased risk for mediastinal GCTs of various histologic types from teratomas to mixed GCTs, which may be heralded by the development of precocious puberty. Primary malignant GCTs of the mediastinum have a marked male predilection (80% or more of the cases), whereas mature and immature teratomas do not have a similar male preference. Metastatic GCTs from the testis more often than the ovary can present as an apparent primary mediastinal neoplasm.

1. **Teratomas,** usually of the mature cystic type, and **seminoma (germinoma)** are the two most common single pattern GCTs arising in the mediastinum, and together represent 50% to 60% of all the mediastinal GCTs. **Endodermal sinus tumor (yolk sac tumor)** is next in frequency as a pure pattern GCT. Pure **choriocarcinomas** occur almost exclusively in males. The remaining tumors have a mixture of teratomatous, seminomatous, and nonseminomatous features in a fashion similar to malignant mixed GCTs of the testis, and thus it is important to widely sample any GCT of the mediastinum. The mediastinum is one site in which a GCT may engender a sarcomatous component including embryonal rhabdomyosarcoma (ERMS), angiosarcoma, and other sarcomatous patterns. Finally, granulocytic sarcoma and other hematologic malignancies (true malignant histiocytosis) are also known to occur in this pathologic setting.

Mature cystic teratoma presents over a broad age range from the neonatal period into early adulthood. The pathologic findings are as with the ovarian counterpart (e-Figs. 10.11 and 10.12). As with teratomas elsewhere, especially in young children, the somatic components may have immature or fetal-like features, most commonly found in the neuroepithelium with embryo-like neural tubes and neuroblastic foci; however, this finding should not be viewed with any more concern than as in a sacrococcygeal teratoma in an infant. In an older child, adolescent, or young adult, a more cautious approach to the same finding is appropriate.

Seminoma, unlike teratoma, can present a diagnostic dilemma from other somewhat similar appearing neoplasms in the anterior mediastinum. Sheets of uniform polygonal tumor cells with a central round nucleus and clear cytoplasm accompanied by lymphocytes and granulomas is the classic microscopic appearance of a seminoma in the mediastinum, as in the testis. However, the lymphocytic infiltrate or granulomas can obscure the tumor cells (e-Fig. 10.13). The differential diagnosis can include mediastinal large B-cell lymphoma, HL, sarcoidosis, and primary or metastatic clear cell carcinoma.

Immunohistochemistry can be extremely helpful in most cases since mediastinal seminoma has a distinctive phenotype including CAM5.2 and vimentin (dot-like pattern, 70% to 80%), SALL4 (100%), placental-like alkaline phosphatase (80% to 90%), CD117 (>70%), CD30 (variable), and OCT4 (90% to 100%) positivity. Cytokeratins AE1/AE3 and 7 are expressed in only approximately 5% of the seminomas. If the seminoma is immunopositive for one or another cytokeratins; if the seminoma has arisen in the thymus; or if a thymoma, thymic carcinoma, or non-small cell carcinoma of the lung are other possibilities, then the diagnostic evaluation is more problematic (as discussed above).

C. **Lymphoid neoplasms (lymphomas).** Lymphomas of all categories account for only approximately 15% of all the mediastinal neoplasms overall, but for 50% to 60% of malignancies in the mediastinum (*Histopathology.* 2009;54:69).

1. **HL** of the nodular sclerosis type is the most common, with a particular predilection for adolescent and young adult females (e-Figs. 10.14 and 10.15). When there is extensive sclerosis–fibrosis, a definitive diagnosis can be difficult to establish as previously discussed above in the section on sclerosing–fibrosing mediastinitis.

2. **Lymphoblastic lymphoma** in children presents most commonly as a mediastinal mass (50% of the cases) (*Semin Pediatr Surg.* 1999;8:69). With the exception of infrequent precursor B-cell lymphoblastic lymphomas, nearly all the cases are examples of T-lymphoblastic lymphoma. If the bone marrow is involved, there is generally no need to biopsy the mediastinal mass.

3. **Mediastinal large B-cell lymphoma (MLBCL)** is specific to the mediastinum and is thought to be derived from thymic medullary B-cells (*Arch Pathol Lab Med.* 2011;135:394). It is a neoplasm which, like HL, has a preference for young females. In fact, the differential diagnosis from HL may not be entirely clear as is indicated by the small subset of cases referred to as "mediastinal gray zone lymphoma" that have hybrid features of nodular sclerosing HL and MLBCL. CD23 positivity discriminates HLBCL from HL (*Int J Surg Pathol.* 2010;18:121).

4. The unicentric form of **castleman disease (CD)** (70% to 75% of all the cases) has two microscopic patterns: hyaline vascular and plasma cell types (*Curr Opin Hematol.* 2007;14:354). Approximately 6% to 10% of all the unicentric cases present in the anterior mediastinum as a well circumscribed mass consisting of one or more matted lymph nodes resembling nodular sclerosis HL (e-Fig. 10.16). Microscopically, a penetrating small blood vessel extends into a germinal center composed of follicular dendritic cells surrounded by a mantle zone of concentrically arranged small lymphocytes in the hyaline vascular type of CD. In contrast, the follicles have hyperplastic germinal centers and mature plasma cells occupying the interfollicular zone in the plasma cell variant. The histologic features of multicentric CD resemble the plasma cell variant. The mantle zone lymphocytes are known to harbor HHV-8.

D. **Neurogenic and neuroblastic neoplasms.** These neoplasms in aggregate account for 20% to 25% of all the mediastinal neoplasms, and virtually all types present in the posterior mediastinum. In children, these tumors are neuroblastic and

TABLE 10.6	Pathologic Types of Neuroblastic Tumors
Type	**Histologic features**
Undifferentiated NB (UF)	High grade malignant round cell neoplasm with high MKI and need for immunohist-ochemistry to differentiate from other malignant round cell tumors
Poorly differentiated NB (UF or FH on basis of age and MKI)	Malignant cells smaller than undifferentiated NB, with neurofibrillary processes, variable rosettes, low or high MKI, and absence of neuromatous or Schwannian stroma
Diffuse or intermixed ganglioneuroblastoma (FH)	Individual nests or lobular foci of neuroblasts with prominent neurofibrillary processes, ganglion cell differentiation, and neuromatous stroma.
Nodular GN (UH)	Distinct nodules of poorly differentiated neuroblasts with high or low MKI in a ganglioneuroma.
Maturing ganglioneuroma (FH)	Microscopic foci of neuroblasts in an otherwise mature ganglioneuroma
Mature ganglioneuroma (FH)	Absence of neuroblasts

NB, neuroblastoma; MKI, mitotic karyorrhectic index; UF, unfavorable histology; FH, favorable histology.

range from neuroblastoma to ganglioneuroma, whereas in adults schwannoma, neurofibroma, and ganglioneuroma are the most common tumors (*Semin Thorac Cardiovasc Surg.* 2004;16:201; *Pediatr Blood Cancer.* 2010;54:895).

1. **Neuroblastoma** presenting in the posterior mediastinum represents 15% to 20% of all the neuroblastic tumors in children of all anatomic sites. These tumors tend to have favorable stages (stages 1, 2A, and 2B), histology (poorly differentiated neuroblastomas, low mitotic karyorrhectic index (MKI), diffuse pattern ganglioneuroblastoma; e-Fig. 10.17), and biologic markers (non-amplified MYCN and no aberrations in chromosomes 1p and 11q) (Table 10.6).

2. **Ganglioneuroma** is often detected incidentally as a paraspinal, posterior mediastinal mass in later childhood and into adulthood. The presence of microscopic nests of neuroblasts in an otherwise ganglioneuromatous background is an example of the favorable histology maturing ganglioneuroma or intermixed ganglioneuroblastoma. Neuroblasts are not found in the mature ganglioneuroma.

V. **CYSTIC LESIONS.** Cysts of the mediastinum are a histogenetically diverse category, ranging from cystic teratoma and thymoma (as discussed above), to developmental cysts including bronchogenic and duplication cysts as manifestations of the so-called bronchopulmonary foregut or bronchoenteric malformation complex (Table 10.7). Another example of a foregut malformation is the extralobar sequestration presenting in either the anterior or posterior mediastinum (*Ann Thorac Surg.* 2009;88:291). Myxopapillary ependymoma may rarely present in the posterior mediastinum (*Ann Diagn Pathol.* 2006;10:283).

A **bronchogenic cyst** is typically unilocular and arises in any one of the three mediastinal compartments (as well as in the heart, neck, or retroperitoneum). The cyst is characterized by a ciliated respiratory type epithelium on the surface and smooth muscle, accessory glands, and cartilage in the wall, although it is important to note that the latter is not identified in all the cases, and that the mucosal lining may have an enteric-like or an indeterminant simplified epithelial appearance.

TABLE 10.7	Cysts and Cystic Lesions of the Mediastinum	
Bronchogenic cyst (50–60% of cases)	Parathyroid cyst
Enteric duplication (foregut) cyst	Thyroglossal duct cyst
Pericardial (coelomic) cyst	Aneurysmal bone cyst (chest wall)
Echinococcal cyst	Multilocular thymic cyst
Thoracic duct cyst	Cystic thymoma
Pancreatic pseudocyst	Cystic adenomatoid tumor
Mullerian (Hattori) cyst	Pleuropulmonary blastoma (type I or II)
Neuroenteric cyst	Cystic teratoma

An **enteric duplication cyst of the esophagus** is an intramural unilocular cyst lined by a squamous or enteric type mucosa. About 20% of all the enteric duplications are found in the esophagus. As a type of foregut malformation, the cyst may be associated with anomalies of the upper airway including a bronchogenic cyst, tracheoesophageal fistula, or a communication of one type or another with the stomach.

VI. **SOFT TISSUE NEOPLASMS.** Soft tissue neoplasms unrelated to the heart or lungs but presenting within the thoracic cavity in one of the mediastinal compartments are exceedingly uncommon. That having been noted, virtually every soft tissue neoplasm of benign, indeterminant, or malignant type has been reported in the mediastinum as a single case or small series.

Lipoma and schwannoma are the most common benign tumors arising, respectively, in the anterior and posterior mediastinum. Lipomatous involvement of the thymus results in the so-called thymolipoma whose pathogenesis as a hamartoma or neoplasm remains uncertain. Myoid cells have been observed in this lesion, which like lipoma, can attain impressive dimensions. Both lymphangioma and hemangioma of various subtypes are also found in the mediastinum. Malignant peripheral nerve sheath tumor, angiosarcoma, leiomyosarcoma, liposarcoma, Ewing sarcoma-primitive neuroectodermal tumor (*Hematol Oncol Stem Cell Ther.* 2009;2:411), malignant rhabdoid tumor (*Pediatr Radiol.* 2009;39:819), desmoplastic small round cell tumor, and ERMS are just some of the soft tissue sarcomas that have been reported in the mediastinum (*Radiographics.* 2002;22:621). In the case of ERMS, the differential diagnosis includes pleuropulmonary blastoma (PPB) in a child under 10 years of age, or a nongerminal malignancy emerging from mediastinal teratoma in an older child, adolescent, or young adult. Synovial sarcoma is well documented as a primary neoplasm arising in the chest as a seeming mediastinal mass, although it actually originates from the pleura and/or lung (*Radiographics.* 2006;26:923). Solitary fibrous tumor has also been reported in the mediastinal soft tissues and thymus (*Internact Cardiovasc Thorac Surg.* 2010;11:382). In a child 6 years old or less, the solid or solid and cystic PPB with its complex multi-patterned sarcoma may extend into one or more mediastinal compartments.

SUGGESTED READINGS

Shimosato Y, Mukai K. *Tumors of the Mediastinum.* Washington DC: Armed Forces Institute of Pathology; 1997.

Travis WD, Brambilla E, Müller-Herkelink H, et al. *Pathology and Genetics of Tumors of the Lung, Pleura, Thymus and Heart.* Lyon: IARC Press; 2004.

11

Serosal Membranes
Jon H. Ritter and John D. Pfeifer

I. **INTRODUCTION.** The serosal membranes are derived from the mesoderm, and form the visceral and parietal surfaces of the pleural cavity, peritoneal cavity, pericardium, and tunica vaginalis testis. Histologically, the serosal membranes consist of a single layer of flat mesothelial cells that rest on a basement membrane, below which is a poorly delimited connective tissue layer. The parietal surfaces of the serosal membranes are perforated by numerous narrow stomas, the so-called lymphatic lacuna, that connect with the extensive lymphatic plexus which drains the enclosed cavities. Under an electron microscope, mesothelial cells show characteristic long, slender surface microvilli; their demonstration can be used to support a mesothelial origin for a neoplasm that is indeterminate by other histopathologic methods.

II. **SPECIMEN PROCESSING**

A. **Biopsy** samples, from procedures performed for diagnosis or in the context of staging procedures, are usually small tissue fragments in the range of 1 to 5 mm in maximal dimension. Detailed gross descriptions are unnecessary, although documentation of the number and size of the fragments is important to ensure that they are adequately represented on the slides. The tissue should be submitted in its entirety, and three hematoxylin and eosin (H&E) stained levels should be examined microscopically.

B. **Excision** specimens, from procedures performed for benign or malignant diseases, include tissue from pleural decortication procedures (stripping procedures to remove thick visceral pleural peels that encase the lung and decrease ventilatory function), debulking procedures, and resections. The aggregate size of the tissue should be described, as well as its color and texture. The presence of gross lesions should also be documented. Gross abnormalities should be thoroughly sampled. When no gross lesions are identified, as a general rule, at least one section per centimeter of aggregate tissue should be submitted for microscopic examination.

III. **NONNEOPLASTIC LESIONS OF THE SEROSAL MEMBRANES**

A. **Acute serositis**

1. **Acute pleuritis** is usually infectious in origin and is most commonly associated with pneumonia. Gram-positive bacteria are most commonly isolated, although a wide variety of pathogens can be responsible. Spontaneous bacterial pleuritis occurs occasionally in patients who have cirrhosis. Autoimmune pleuritis, although sterile, can produce clinical and pathologic findings that resemble infectious pleuritis.

2. **Acute peritonitis** is usually associated with a perforated viscus. If it is due to gastric, biliary, or pancreatic rupture, it has a chemical etiology; on the other hand, if it is due to intestinal rupture, it has a bacterial etiology. Spontaneous bacterial peritonitis also occurs, usually in children, immunocompromised patients, or patients with cirrhosis. Localized acute peritonitis is a feature of pelvic inflammatory disease.

3. **Acute pericarditis** can have an infectious etiology or can be a manifestation of autoimmune disease.

B. **Granulomatous serositis** can present in a number of different patterns; studding of the serosa by innumerable small nodules can be especially worrisome clinically for disseminated tumor.

177

1. **Infectious.** Although special stains can often demonstrate the offending pathogen, microbiologic cultures are a more sensitive and specific method for identification of the causative organism. Common causes include mycobacteria, fungi (including *Histoplasma, Cryptococcus,* and *Coccidioides*), and parasites (including *Schistosoma, Echinococcus,* and *Ascaris*).

2. **Noninfectious** etiologies include a reaction to foreign material from a prior surgical procedure (such as starch granules and sutures) or from a perforated organ. In women, additional causes include retrograde introduction of foreign material through the fallopian tube (e.g., douche fluid, lubricants, radiographic contrast agents), and spillage of amniotic fluid following a Cesarean section.

   Peritoneal granulomas can form as a response to implants of keratin produced by a neoplasm of the female reproductive tract, including mature cystic teratoma, endometrioid adenocarcinoma with squamous differentiation (of either endometrial or ovarian origin), squamous cell carcinoma of the cervix, or even atypical polypoid adenomyoma of the uterus. Microscopically, laminated deposits of keratin (sometimes including the so-called ghost squamous cells) are present in the granulomas, but in the absence of viable tumor, these granulomas have no prognostic significance.

3. **Autoimmune** causes include Crohn disease and sarcoidosis.

4. **Meconium peritonitis** in a neonate can lead to a serosal granulomatous reaction.

C. **Mesothelial Hyperplasia** is commonly seen in response to chronic serosal injury. Microscopically, hyperplasia has a number of different patterns, including solid, tubular, trabecular, papillary, or tubulopapillary, and often shows limited extension into the underlying connective tissue (e-**Fig. 11.1**).* The hyperplastic cells are often disbursed in linear, parallel, or thin layers in associated organizing fibrinous tissue. Cytologically, mild-to-moderate nuclear pleomorphism is present, and mitotic figures and even occasional multinucleated cells can be identified.

   Given these architectural and cytologic features, mesothelial hyperplasia can be difficult to distinguish from well-differentiated diffuse malignant mesothelioma (DMM), especially epithelioid mesothelioma. The distinction is based on the degree of cellular proliferation and atypia. Mesothelioma should be suspected when deep infiltration of the underlying soft tissue is present, or when areas of necrosis are present. Knowledge of the clinical setting can be used to guide the diagnosis, although it is well established that slowly growing mesothelioma can initially present as a lesion that cannot be distinguished from mesothelial hyperplasia.

D. **Metaplasias** are predominantly a feature of the peritoneal serosal surfaces in women. Most originate from the so-called secondary Müllerian system, which by convention includes the pelvic and lower abdominal mesothelium and underlying mesenchyme. The close embryologic relationship of the mesothelium in these areas and the Müllerian ducts (which arise from invaginations of coelomic epithelium) provides an explanation for the fact that many of the metaplasias produce tissues that are a normal component of the female reproductive tract.

1. **Endometriosis** is thought to arise via a metaplastic process, through retrograde implantation of menstrual endometrium (the so-called metastatic theory), or as a developmental anomaly. Rare cases of pleural endometriosis have been reported, as have cases of endometriosis in men who have been

---

*All e-figures are available online via the Solution Site Image Bank.

treated with long-term estrogen therapy (usually in the setting of adenocarcinoma of the prostate).

When endometriosis develops in association with the viscera, such as the wall of the intestine, adjacent to the ureter, the wall of the bladder, and so on, it can clinically present with signs and symptoms that resemble malignancy. Microscopically, the findings include endometrial glands and stroma, often associated with chronic inflammation, hemosiderin laden macrophages, dense fibrosis, and adhesions (e-Fig. 11.2). Since a number of different malignancies, most commonly endometrioid adenocarcinoma and clear cell adenocarcinoma, can develop in endometriosis, areas of endometriosis in biopsy and excision specimens must be carefully examined.

2. **Endosalpingiosis** typically occurs in women during their reproductive years. Microscopically, multiple dilated cysts lined by a single layer of fallopian tube-type epithelium are present. The lack of endometrial-type stroma distinguishes endosalpingiosis from endometriosis.

3. **Endocervicosis,** consisting of benign glands with an endocervical type epithelium, and **squamous metaplasia,** are both rare. Both occur in women, and are primarily metaplasias of the peritoneal mesothelium.

4. **Ectopic decidual reaction** is an incidental finding in women who are pregnant or on high-dose progestogen therapy. Most lesions are not evident grossly, but when they are, they consist of small gray-white nodules which may be hemorrhagic, and often stud the peritoneal surfaces. Microscopically, the metaplasia involves the submesothelial stroma, and consists of large epithelioid cells with prominent cell borders and abundant amphophilic cytoplasm (e-Fig. 11.3) morphologically identical to the cells comprising the decidual reaction characteristic of the fallopian tube, cervix, and upper vagina in pregnant women. Diagnostic difficulty can arise on the rare occasions when the decidual cells assume a signet-ring appearance.

5. **Walthard nests,** usually found on the serosal surfaces of the fallopian tubes or in the mesovarium as yellow-white nodules, are usually only several millimeters in the greatest dimension. They may show cystic change, and are usually lined by mesothelial cells that have undergone transitional (urothelial) metaplasia.

6. **Disseminated peritoneal leiomyomatosis** (leiomyomatosis peritonealis disseminata) is an uncommon multifocal proliferation of smooth muscle-like cells that is thought to represent a hormone-induced metaplasia of the multipotential submesothelial mesenchymal cells of the peritoneum. Grossly, it appears as widely scattered nodules that often suggest metastatic malignancy. Microscopically, the lesion is characterized by cytologically bland, benign spindle cells centered in the submesothelial connective tissue (e-Fig. 11.4). A conservative approach to treatment is indicated, since the condition tends to spontaneously regress.

E. **Fibrosis**

1. **Pleura**

a. **Reactive pleural fibrosis** is usually a consequence of prior inflammation or surgery. Often, the fibrosis is associated with formation of dense adhesions. Because reactive mesothelial cells are entrapped within the fibrous tissue, careful microscopic examination with knowledge of the clinical history is required to avoid over-interpretation as mesothelioma.

b. **Pleural plaques,** which primarily occur on the parietal pleura of the thoracic cavity, are raised, discrete, white to gray-white lesions that range from several millimeters to over 6 cm in diameter. When pleural plaques are bilateral, they are almost always related to prior asbestos exposure, even very low fiber levels. Causes of unilateral plaques include asbestos, as well as any process that features pleural chronic effusions. Microscopically, they consist of pauci-cellular dense collagenous connective tissue with a basket-weave pattern, sometimes associated with overlying organizing fibrinous deposits. Asbestos bodies are essentially never seen within the plaques. Mesothelial cells are not a prominent component of the lesion; any significant cellularity in a putative pleural plaque should raise concern for desmoplastic mesothelioma. Finally, since mesothelioma and plaques may occur in the same individual, it is not uncommon for blind biopsies to sample plaques; in this setting, additional biopsies are indicated if there is strong clinical suspicion for a pleural malignancy.

    c. **Diffuse visceral pleural fibrosis** has a number of etiologies. It is a feature of several occupational exposures (e.g., silicosis), and occurs as an advanced hypersensitivity reaction, as a component of connective tissue diseases, and as a sequela of bacterial pneumonia (especially as a result of empyema). Grossly, diffuse visceral pleural fibrosis may be difficult to distinguish from desmoplastic mesothelioma. Microscopically, the fibrosis does not infiltrate the subjacent soft tissue and has a zonated appearance, with more cellular areas near the surface while the deeper tissues tend to be more paucicellular; mesothelioma has the reverse pattern. Nonetheless, careful microscopic examination, often accompanied by immunohistochemical studies, can be required to exclude mesothelioma.

2. Peritoneum

    a. **Reactive peritoneal fibrosis** is usually a consequence of recurrent bouts of peritonitis (often associated with long-term peritoneal dialysis), decompensated cirrhosis, or surgery, and is often associated with formation of dense adhesions. As is true with reactive pleural fibrosis, reactive mesothelial cells entrapped within the fibrous tissue must not be over-interpreted as mesothelioma.

    b. **Localized plaques,** composed of dense hyalinized fibrous tissue, are frequent incidental findings on the splenic capsule.

    c. **Sclerosing peritonitis** is due to hyperplasia of submesothelial mesenchymal cells, and manifests as diffuse sheets of white, thickened visceral peritoneum that encase the small bowel and also involve the diaphragmatic, hepatic, and splenic peritoneum. Known etiologies include peritoneal dialysis, infections, autoimmune disorders, therapy with the beta adrenergic blocker practolol, and the carcinoid syndrome. Many cases are idiopathic.

F. Cysts

    1. Emphysematous bulla are the most frequent cystic lesion that involves the pleural cavity.

    2. Peritoneal inclusion cysts characteristically occur in the peritoneal cavity in women of reproductive age (although they also rarely occur in males, and also rarely occur in the pleural cavity). They are usually incidental findings at the time of surgery, and consist of single or multiple, thin-walled, translucent, unilocular cysts lined by a single layer of bland, flattened mesothelial cells.

    3. The so-called **pericardial cyst** is the most common cyst associated with the pericardium. It can achieve dimensions of 15 cm or more. Microscopically, it is lined by bland mesothelial cells.

G. Splenosis is an incidental finding, and usually represents implantation of splenic tissue as a result of traumatic splenic rupture. Grossly, innumerable red–blue nodules ranging from several millimeters to over 5 cm in diameter are scattered widely through the abdomen.

H. Eosinophilic peritonitis arises in the context of a variety of medical diseases including childhood atopy, autoimmune disorders (especially collagen vascular diseases), and the hypereosinophilic syndrome. It also occurs in association with lymphoma and metastatic carcinoma. Other causes include a ruptured hydatid cyst, and in association with peritoneal dialysis.

IV. BENIGN SEROSAL NEOPLASMS

A. **Adenomatoid tumor** is of mesothelial origin, and usually arises in the peritoneum, also rarely from the pleura. It most commonly involves the serosal surfaces of the uterus or fallopian tubes, or paratesticular regions. Grossly, the tumor usually forms a tan 1 to 2 cm well-circumscribed nodule. Microscopically, the tumor is composed of tubular and slit-like spaces lined by a single layer of flattened cuboidal cells with bland cytology (e-**Fig. 11.5**). The cells are immunopositive for cytokeratin, calretinin, WT1, and vimentin expression, but immunonegative for factor VIII-related antigen and CD31 expression, a profile that can be used to distinguish the tumor from metastatic carcinoma and vascular tumors. Adenomatoid tumor is clinically asymptomatic and complete excision is the appropriate management.

B. **Multicystic peritoneal inclusion cyst** usually arises in the pelvis in women and is typically associated with lower abdominal pain. It forms a palpable mass adherent to the pelvic organs that can grossly be indistinguishable from a cystic ovarian tumor, although a subset of cases arises in the upper abdominal cavity, in a hernia sac, or even in the retroperitoneum. Most cases are associated with a history of previous abdominal operation, endometriosis, or pelvic inflammatory disease (*Obstet Gynecol Surg.* 2009;64:321).

Microscopically, the neoplasm consists of numerous thin-walled cysts lined by a single layer of bland, flat-to-cuboidal mesothelial cells. The septa and walls between the cysts are composed of loose fibrovascular connective tissue. The constitutive cells are immunophenotypically identical to other mesothelial cell lesions.

Some confusion exists regarding the proper classification of multicystic peritoneal inclusion cyst, as demonstrated by the fact that the lesion is also known as multicystic mesothelioma. Tumors in which the mesothelium has bland cytologic features with no significant atypia have an indolent course (*Cancer.* 1989;64:1336), although very rare cases may progress to conventional malignant mesothelioma (*Am J Surg Pathol.* 1988;12:737; *J Surg Oncol.* 2002;79:243). However, cases in which the cysts are lined, even focally, by markedly atypical mesothelial cells and/or that harbor areas of conventional malignant mesothelioma are best considered low-grade mesotheliomas from the outset (see below).

V. MALIGNANT PLEURAL NEOPLASMS. The World Health Organization (WHO) classification of tumors of the pleura is shown in Table 11.1.

A. **Mesothelial**

1. **Diffuse malignant mesothelioma** (DMM). The WHO recommends the terminology DMM when referring to malignant neoplasms arising from mesothelial cells. The association of the tumor with asbestos exposure is well established (*Ann Occup Hyg.* 2000;44:565). There is usually a long latency period between asbestos exposure and the onset of mesothelioma, usually 30 to 40 years. While sequences from the highly oncogenic SV40 virus have been reported in some cases (*Clin Lung Cancer.* 2003;5:177), an association with latent viral infection has yet to be established. Rare cases may be related to therapeutic radiation exposure or chronic pleural infections.

Patients with mesothelioma usually present with dyspnea, chest wall pain, and a significant pleural effusion. Constitutional symptoms include weight loss, malaise, chills, sweats, weakness, and fatigue. While the tumor may begin as multiple small nodules on the parietal and visceral pleura, it eventually encases the lung, invades the soft tissue of the chest wall, and often extends into the mediastinum with encasement of the pericardial sac

| TABLE 11.1 | WHO Histologic Classification of Tumors of the Pleura |

Mesothelial tumors
Diffuse malignant mesothelioma
  Epithelioid mesothelioma
  Sarcomatoid mesothelioma
  Desmoplastic mesothelioma
  Biphasic mesothelioma
Localized malignant mesothelioma
Other tumors of mesothelial origin
  Well-differentiated papillary mesothelioma
  Adenomatoid tumor

Lymphoproliferative disorders
Primary effusion lymphoma
Pyothorax-associated lymphoma

Mesenchymal tumors
Epithelioid hemangioendothelioma
  Angiosarcoma
Synovial sarcoma
  Monophasic
  Biphasic
Solitary fibrous tumor
Calcifying tumor of the pleura
Desmoplastic small round cell tumor

From: Travis WD, Brambilla E, Müller-Hermelink HK, Harris CC, eds. *World Health Organization Classification of Tumours. Pathology and Genetics. Tumours of the Lung, Pleura, Thymus and Heart.* Lyon: IARC Press; 2004. Used with permission.

and other midline structures. DMM of the pleura remains a lethal disease, with essentially 100% mortality. Selected early stage cases may benefit from extrapleural pneumonectomy and aggressive adjuvant therapy, although the role for therapy other than supportive care is controversial. The staging scheme for pleural DMM is shown in Table 11.2.

Several histopathologic types of mesothelioma have been described. While recognition of the various patterns is important for diagnosis, they carry no clear prognostic significance. Immunohistochemically, DMM expresses calretinin, WT1, and cytokeratin 5/6, but does not express CEA (monoclonal), Ber72.3, and MOC-31. This panel of markers makes it possible to distinguish mesothelioma from adenocarcinoma of pulmonary or extrapulmonary origin in most cases (*Hum Pathol.* 2002;33:953; *Am J Surg Pathol.* 2003;27:1031).

Nonetheless, despite exhaustive study, no markers are available to reliably distinguish reactive from malignant mesothelial proliferations (*Histopathology.* 2009;54:55). It is this latter observation that suggests that a diagnosis of DMM based strictly on effusion cytology samples is difficult, since definitive stromal invasion cannot be definitively identified in such specimens. Given the gravity of the diagnosis of DMM, it is prudent to demand a tissue specimen in which invasion can be identified.

Recently, there has been interest in the identification of novel biomarkers that may aid risk stratification, or that can be used to direct therapy (*Pathology.* 2011;43;201). Some DMM have been shown to respond to histone deacetylase inhibitors (*J Thorac Oncol.* 2010;5:275) but no reliable markers yet exist to identify this subgroup of tumors.

a. Epithelioid mesothelioma, as its name implies, has an epithelioid morphology, usually consisting of rather bland cells with abundant eosinophilic

| **TABLE 11.2** | **TNM Staging Classification for Pleural Mesothelioma** |

Primary tumor (T)

TX	Primary tumor cannot be assessed
T0	No evidence of primary tumor
T1	Tumor involves ipsilateral parietal pleura with or without mediastinal pleura and with or without diaphragmatic pleural involvement
T1a	No involvement of the visceral pleura
T1b	Tumor also involving the visceral pleura
T2	Tumor involving each of the ipsilateral pleural surfaces (parietal, mediastinal, diaphragmatic, and visceral pleural) with at least one of the following: –Involvement of diaphragmatic muscle –Extension of tumor from visceral pleura into the underlying pulmonary parenchyma
T3	Locally advanced but potentially resectable tumor. Tumor involving all of the ipsilateral pleural surfaces (parietal, mediastinal, diaphragmatic, and visceral pleura) with at least one of the following: –Involvement of the endothoracic fascia –Extension into the mediastinal fat –Solitary, completely resectable focus of tumor extending into the soft tissues of the chest wall –Nontransmural involvement of the pericardium
T4	Locally advanced technically unresectable tumor. Tumor involving all of the ipsilateral pleural surfaces (parietal, mediastinal, diaphragmatic, and visceral pleura) with at least one of the following: –Diffuse extension or multifocal masses of tumor in the chest wall, with or without associated rib destruction –Direct transdiaphragmatic extension of tumor to the peritoneum –Direct extension of tumor to the contralateral pleura –Direct extension of tumor to mediastinal organs –Direct extension of tumor into the spine –Tumor extending through to the internal surface of the pericardium with or without a pericardial effusion or tumor involving the myocardium

Regional lymph nodes (N)

NX	Regional lymph nodes cannot be assessed
N0	No regional lymph node metastasis
N1	Metastasis in the ipsilateral bronchopulmonary or hilar lymph nodes
N2	Metastases in the subcarinal or the mediastinal lymph nodes including the ipsilateral internal mammary and peridiaphragmatic nodes
N3	Metastases in the contralateral mediastinal, contralateral internal mammary, ipsilateral or contralateral supraclavicular lymph nodes

Distant metastasis (M)

MX	Distant metastasis cannot be assessed
M0	No distant metastasis
M1	Distant metastasis present

Stage grouping

Stage 1	T1	N0	M0
Stage IA	T1a	N0	M0
Stage IB	T1b	N0	M0
Stage II	T2	N0	M0
Stage III	T1, T2	N1	M0
	T1, T2	N2	M0
	T3	N0, N1, N2	M0
Stage IV	T4	Any N	M0
	Any T	N3	M0
	Any T	Any N	M1

cytoplasm, although in some cases the cells have more anaplastic features. Architecturally, sheet-like, microglandular (adenomatoid), and tubulopapillary patterns are common (e-**Figs. 11.6 and 11.7**). Psammoma bodies are occasionally encountered.

b. **Sarcomatoid mesothelioma** is composed of spindle cells that have a haphazard distribution (e-**Fig. 11.8**). Some cases resemble fibrosarcoma, others have a pattern that resembles undifferentiated pleomorphic sarcoma. Immunohistochemically, sarcomatoid mesothelioma is less likely to express cytokeratin 5/6; areas of chondrosarcomatous or osteosarcomatous differentiation may show positive staining for actin, desmin, vimentin, and/or S100. Many cases retain expression of calretinin. The potential overlap of histologic and immunohistologic features of sarcomatoid mesothelioma with sarcomatoid carcinoma and various soft tissue sarcomas highlights the necessity for correlation with clinical and radiographic findings; a solitary mass should raise concern for another nonmesothelial sarcomatoid process. Sarcomatoid mesothelioma is generally thought to have a more aggressive course than the epithelioid varieties, and so patients with this subtype are generally excluded from consideration for surgical therapy.

c. **Desmoplastic mesothelioma.** By definition, this type of sarcomatoid mesothelioma consists of scattered atypical cells in a storiform or nonspecific pattern in >50% of the tumor, set in a dense collagenous background. This subtype is the most likely to be misdiagnosed as organizing pleuritis in small biopsy specimens.

d. **Biphasic mesothelioma.** This subtype contains a combination of the other patterns, in most cases a combination of the epithelioid and sarcomatous patterns (e-**Fig. 11.9**). By definition, each component should comprise at least 10% of the tumor.

2. **Well-differentiated papillary mesothelioma** is a rare type of mesothelioma that occurs in a wide range of patients, although most patients are elderly. An association with asbestos exposure has not been established. Patients usually present with dyspnea or a recurrent pleural effusion, but rarely with chest pain. At presentation, the tumor may be either solitary and localized, multifocal, or widespread.

Microscopically, the tumor features fibrovascular cores (that often have a myxoid stroma) covered by a single layer of bland, cuboidal-to-flattened mesothelial cells. Focal areas of limited stromal invasion may be present. In cases with widespread invasion, DMM with papillary architecture must be excluded. The distinction is important, since when strictly defined, well-differentiated papillary mesothelioma has an indolent course with prolonged patient survival.

3. **Localized malignant mesothelioma** is a circumscribed nodular lesion attached to the parietal or visceral pleura that is usually <10 cm in the greatest dimension. It is usually discovered incidentally on imaging studies. Microscopically, the tumor has architectural patterns that are identical to DMM. Some cases are cured by surgical excision. It is interesting to note that recurrent tumors often metastasize in a pattern more typical of sarcomas, without spread along the pleura surfaces.

B. **Mesenchymal**

1. **Epithelioid hemangioendothelioma** (termed intravascular bronchioloalveolar tumor when it arises in the lung) is a low-grade malignant neoplasm of endothelial cells that can develop at virtually any anatomic site. Primary cases arising from the serosal surfaces occur, albeit rarely (*Int J Surg Pathol.* 2006;14:257).

Microscopically, the lesion is characterized by cords, short strands, and solid nests of bland, round-to-slightly spindled endothelial cells that have an epithelioid or histiocytoid morphology and a low mitotic rate (e-**Fig. 11.10**). Endothelial differentiation is evident by the formation of intracytoplasmic lumina (said to "blister" the cells), but distinct vascular channels are rarely formed. The neoplastic cells are classically embedded within a chondroid-like to hyalinized stroma. Immunohistochemically, epithelioid hemangioendothelioma typically expresses a variety of vascular antigens including CD31, CD34, and *Ulex Europaeus* antigen; expression of von Willebrand factor is more variable. Of note, 25% to 30% of the cases show focal cytokeratin expression, which can lead to an incorrect diagnosis of metastatic signet-ring cell carcinoma. In problematic cases, electron microscopy can be used to confirm the tumor's vascular origin by the demonstration of Weibel–Palade bodies.

2. **Solitary fibrous tumor** is classically considered a pleural tumor, although it is now recognized to occur at virtually any anatomic location. Most cases, in fact, occur in extrapleural sites. The tumor is most common in patients between 20- and 70 years old. It is classified as a tumor of intermediate (rarely metastasizing) biologic potential (see Chap. 46).

Grossly, pleural solitary fibrous tumors can be >20 cm in the greatest dimension, although most tumors are <8 cm. The tumor is usually well circumscribed although not encapsulated, and has a firm white cut surface which may show hemorrhage and areas of myxoid degeneration. Microscopically, the tumor is composed of bland plump spindled cells with a so-called patternless architecture that surround branching blood vessels of the type typically associated with hemangiopericytoma (e-**Fig. 11.11**). The cellularity often varies within individual tumors, and the background stroma can show areas of myxoid change or fibrosis. Immunohistochemically, the tumor cells express CD34 and CD99; in a subset of tumors, the cells also show immunoreactivity for smooth muscle actin, BCL2, and epithelial membrane antigen; focal immunoreactivity for desmin, cytokeratin, and/or S100 may even be present. Significant cytokeratin expression should raise concern for sarcomatoid mesothelioma or carcinoma.

Malignant solitary fibrous tumors show an increased mitotic rate (≥ 4 mitoses per 10 high power fields), areas of necrosis, increased cellularity, and focal marked cytologic atypia, usually with infiltrative margins (*Am J Surg Pathol*. 1998;22:1501). However, the clinical behavior of an individual tumor is not absolutely correlated with its histologic features.

C. **Lymphoid**

1. **Primary effusion lymphoma** is a subtype lymphoma that has a distinct clinical pathologic setting, presenting as an effusion without an associated tumor mass. It is defined by the presence of human herpesvirus 8 (*Adv Cancer Res*. 2001;80:115) and most cases arise in immunodeficient individuals in the setting of HIV AIDS. Immunohistochemically, primary effusion lymphoma is usually of null phenotype, although occasional cases express B-cell or T-cell markers (*Cancer*. 2007;111:224).

2. **Pyothorax-associated lymphoma** is a diffuse large B-cell lymphoma that usually presents as a pleura mass in elderly individuals. As the name implies, it occurs in patients who have a longstanding history of pyothorax, usually in the setting of pulmonary tuberculosis or tuberculous pleuritis, and is strongly associated with Epstein–Barr virus infection. Immunohistochemically, representative B-cell markers other than CD20 are frequently negative, while aberrant expression of T-cell markers such as CD2 is present (*Adv Anat Pathol*. 2005;12:324).

TABLE 11.3 WHO Histologic Classification of Tumors of the Peritoneum

Mesothelial tumors
   Diffuse malignant mesothelioma
   Well-differentiated papillary mesothelioma
   Multilocular peritoneal inclusion cyst
   Adenomatoid tumor

Smooth Muscle tumor
   Leiomyomatosis peritonealis disseminata

Tumor of uncertain origin
   Desmoplastic small round cell tumor

Epithelial tumors
   Primary peritoneal adenocarcinoma (specify type)
   Primary peritoneal borderline tumor (specify type)
   Others

From: Travis WD, Brambilla E, Müller-Hermelink HK, Harris CC, eds. *World Health Organization Classification of Tumours. Pathology and Genetics. Tumours of the Lung, Pleura, Thymus and Heart.* Lyon: IARC Press; 2004. Used with permission.

  D. Uncertain origin
    1. Desmoplastic small round cell tumor was originally described as a peritoneal tumor (see the section on malignant peritoneal tumors below). However, it is now recognized that the tumor arises at a wide variety of sites outside the peritoneum, including the pleura.
    2. Synovial sarcoma. Both monophasic and biphasic primary pleural synovial sarcomas occur (despite the tumor's name, no biologic or pathologic relationship between synovial sarcoma and synovium has been demonstrated). Patients with biphasic tumors tend to be younger (third decade of life) than patients with monophasic tumors (fifth decade of life). The tumor is usually localized at presentation. Tumors that arise in the pleura have the same pathologic features as those that arise in the soft tissue (see Chap. 46).
  E. Secondary neoplasms. Although virtually any type of carcinoma can metastasize to the pleural serosal surfaces, secondary involvement is usually due to a peripheral adenocarcinoma of the lung. In western countries, the ovary, large intestine, pancreas, breast, thyroid, and stomach are as a group the second most common site of origin for metastatic tumors. Leukemias and lymphomas form the third most common group of tumors that secondarily involve the pleura. Since metastases to the thoracic cavity vastly outnumber mesotheliomas, metastatic malignancy must always enter into the differential diagnosis of a pleural tumor.
VI. MALIGNANT PERITONEAL NEOPLASMS. The WHO classification of tumors of the peritoneum is shown in Table 11.3.
  A. Mesothelial. The low-grade tumors such as well-differentiated papillary mesothelioma and multicystic mesothelioma are far more common than DMM. DMM and well-differentiated papillary mesothelioma appear to have an association with asbestos exposure.
    1. Well-differentiated papillary mesothelioma is often discovered incidentally; about 80% of the cases occur in women, usually of reproductive age. Grossly, the tumor is typically a solitary to multifocal, gray to white, nodular to papillary mass <2 cm in greatest dimension. Microscopically, papillary fronds with a fibrous core are covered by a single layer of bland cuboidal-to-flattened mesothelial cells.
       When the diagnosis is restricted to lesions with bland cytologic features and no invasion, well-differentiated papillary mesothelioma has an

indolent course (*Cancer.* 1990;65:292). However, those cases that show evidence of invasion of organ walls or fat (emphasizing the need for thorough microscopic sampling) are associated with progressive disease and a worse prognosis, and so should be classified as DMM.

2. **Multicystic mesothelioma** is also known as **multicystic peritoneal inclusion cyst.** As suggested by the two very different names, there is confusion regarding the biologic potential of the neoplasm. Tumors in which the cysts are lined by mesothelium with bland cytologic features with at most only reactive atypia have an indolent course, consistent with a designation as multicystic peritoneal inclusion cysts (as discussed above). However, cases in which the cysts are lined, even focally, by markedly atypical mesothelial cells and/or that harbor areas of conventional malignant mesothelioma are best considered low-grade mesotheliomas (*Hum Pathol.* 1991;22:856).

3. **DMM** arising in the peritoneum is rare; the ratio of pleural to peritoneal mesothelioma is approximately 10:1 in the United States.

   a. The epithelioid subtype is most common (**e-Fig. 11.12**). Rare cases, designated the deciduoid type, have a morphology that resembles an exuberant ectopic decidual reaction (*Am J Surg Pathol.* 2000;24:285). Immunohistochemically, peritoneal epithelioid mesothelioma expresses calretinin, thrombomodulin, WT1, and cytokeratin 5/6, but does not express MOC-31, Ber72.3, Ber-EP4, CA19–9, and CD15 (Leu-M1); this panel of markers is the most useful for distinguishing peritoneal epithelioid mesothelioma from peritoneal and ovarian serous carcinomas (*Am J Surg Pathol.* 1998;22:1203; *Mod Pathol.* 2006;19:34; *Cytopathology.* 2011;22:5).

   b. The sarcomatoid and desmoplastic subtypes are very uncommon in the peritoneum.

B. **Epithelial tumors of Müllerian type.** The architectural and cytologic features of these tumors are identical to those of their counterparts that arise within the ovary, fallopian tube, endometrium, and cervix. Their morphology is thought to represent another manifestation of the close embryologic relationship between the mesothelium and the secondary Müllerian system.

   The criteria for diagnosis of a tumor as of primary peritoneal origin include the following. First, the ovaries must be of normal in size, or enlarged only as a result of a benign process. Second, the extraovarian involvement must be greater than the surface involvement of either ovary. Third, ovarian involvement must be absent, confined to the ovarian surface epithelium without stromal invasion, or involve the cortical stroma with a maximal tumor dimension of less than 5×5 mm^2 (*Cancer Res.* 2000;60:1361).

   Primary peritoneal epithelial tumors are currently staged according to the scheme used for ovarian tumors (Table 31.3).

1. **Primary peritoneal carcinoma** occurs virtually only in women; the mean age of the affected patients is the seventh decade. The most common type is serous adenocarcinoma (**e-Fig. 11.13**), but clear cell adenocarcinoma (**e-Fig. 11.14**), endometrioid adenocarcinoma, transitional cell carcinoma, and even squamous cell carcinomas occur. Primary peritoneal carcinoma should possibly be included as a phenotype in familial breast and ovarian cancer syndromes, although the pattern of genetic abnormalities in primary peritoneal carcinomas seems to be distinct from the pattern that is characteristic of ovarian tumors.

2. **Primary peritoneal borderline tumors** (tumors of low malignant potential) are diagnosed by the same criteria as for their borderline counterparts arising in the ovary (see Chap. 31). Serous borderline tumors are by far the most common histologic type.

C. **Uncertain origin. Desmoplastic small round cell tumor** was originally described as a peritoneal tumor that arises in young men in their second or third decade.

However, the spectrum of disease is now known to include primary tumors arising at a wide variety of sites outside the peritoneum, including the pleura, extremities, viscera, bone, and brain, in patients of all ages.

Microscopically, the tumor is a primitive sarcoma with a growth pattern that includes variably sized sheets and nests of cells separated by a strikingly desmoplastic stroma (e-**Fig. 11.15**). Cytologically, the individual cells are small, round, and have minimal cytoplasm. Immunohistochemically, the cells show unique multilineage differentiation, including immunoreactivity for cytokeratins, EMA, vimentin, desmin, and neuron specific enolase.

The t(11;22) translocation that produces an *EWS-WT1* gene fusion is characteristic of the tumor. Demonstration of the translocation by molecular genetic techniques, or the encoded fusion protein by immunohistochemistry, can be used to aid diagnosis.

D. Secondary Neoplasms

1. **Carcinomas** and **adenocarcinomas** from virtually any primary site can metastasize to the peritoneal serosal surface. By far, the most common group of metastatic tumors in women is epithelial tumors of the reproductive tract, including the ovary, fallopian tube, endometrium, and cervix. Other tumors that commonly secondarily involve the peritoneum are carcinomas of the breast, pancreas, and biliary tract; upper and lower gastrointestinal tract; lung; and sarcomas arising in the female reproductive tract.

2. **Pseudomyxoma peritonei** is the clinical term used to designate masses of jelly like mucus in the pelvis and abdomen. The tumor producing the mucus originates from a low-grade mucinous neoplasm of the appendix in the vast majority of cases; less commonly, the stomach, pancreas, or hepatobiliary tract is the site of origin (*Anat Pathol.* 1997;2:198). It has been shown that classification of pseudomyxoma peritonei based on the cytologic features of the neoplastic epithelium (e-**Fig. 11.16**) provides important prognostic information (*Am J Surg Pathol.* 1995;19:1390). Cases in which the epithelium is benign or shows only mild atypia, classified as peritoneal adenomucinosis, have the best prognosis. Cases in which the epithelium is frankly malignant, classified as peritoneal mucinous carcinomatosis, are more often associated with metastatic spread to lymph nodes and liver, and have a much poorer prognosis.

   In all cases of presumed pseudomyxoma peritonei, the surgeon should be instructed to excise the appendix, regardless of its appearance. Even if grossly normal, the appendix should be entirely submitted for microscopic examination. The surgeon should also be instructed to evaluate the pancreas, hepatobiliary tract, stomach, and intestines for any evidence of a primary neoplasm.

VII. MALIGNANT PERICARDIAL NEOPLASMS.
The WHO classification of tumors of the pericardium is shown in Table 11.4.

A. Mesothelial.
By definition, the diagnosis of primary DMM of the pericardium is reserved for those cases in which there is no tumor outside the pericardium except for lymph node metastases. Histologically, DMM of the pericardium has

---

TABLE 11.4   WHO Histologic Classification of Tumors of the Pericardium

Solitary fibrous tumor
Malignant mesothelioma
Germ cell tumors
Metastatic pericardial tumors

From: Travis WD, Brambilla E, Müller-Hermelink HK, Harris CC, eds. *World Health Organization Classification of Tumours. Pathology and Genetics. Tumours of the Lung, Pleura, Thymus and Heart.* Lyon: IARC Press; 2004. Used with permission.

the same histologic types as tumors arising from the pleura. The development of pericardial mesothelioma is also associated with asbestos exposure.

B. Germ cell tumors. Intrapericardial germ cell tumors are rare, but occur over a wide age range, from neonates to the elderly. Intrauterine presentations are increasingly being recognized in second and third trimester gestations due to the widespread use of prenatal ultrasound examination. Germ cell tumors of the pericardium, as with extragonadal germ cell tumors at other sites, are thought to arise from germ cells that lodge in midline structures early in embryogenesis along the normal route of migration from the yolk sack to the gonad.

Teratomas account for the vast majority of pericardial germ cell tumors. Over 75% of the cases occur in children under the age of 15 years. Teratomas can achieve remarkable sizes, up to 15 cm in the greatest dimension. Grossly, they usually have a lobulated, smooth surface. Histologically, the vast majority are mature teratomas that resemble their counterparts arising in the gonads or mediastinum, in which case the differential diagnosis includes a bronchogenic cyst. While teratomas are benign, tumors that contain other germ cell elements (e.g., embryonal carcinoma, choriocarcinoma, endodermal sinus tumor) are malignant. They are exceedingly rare, and most cases arise in adults.

C. Secondary neoplasms. Metastases are the most common tumor of the pericardium. In a significant percentage of cases, a biopsy (often performed to establish the cause of pericarditis or life-threatening tamponade), provides the first evidence that the patient has a malignancy. The most common primary tumors that metastasize to the pericardium, in decreasing order of frequency, are carcinoma and adenocarcinoma of the lung, breast, and thyroid; lymphoma; and sarcoma. Although lymphatic or hematogenous spread is the most common route of involvement, direct extension (e.g., by pleural mesothelioma or malignant thymoma) also occurs.

VIII. MALIGNANT TUNICA VAGINALIS TESTIS NEOPLASMS

A. DMM occasionally arises from the tunica, and rarely, even from hernia sacs. Grossly, the tumor forms nodules or papillary excrescences. Microscopically, the most common pattern consists of a prominent papillary architecture with associated tubular and solid areas.

B. Epithelial tumors of Müllerian type have been reported.

C. Secondary neoplasms. The tunica, as well as the lining of hernia sacs, can be involved by metastatic carcinoma. In some cases, the involvement of the tunica or hernia sac is the first manifestation of metastatic disease.

SUGGESTED READINGS

Battifora H, McCaughey WTE. *Tumors of the Serosal Membranes. Atlas of Tumor Pathology, 3rd Series, Fascicle 15.* Washington, DC: Armed Forces Institute of Pathology; 1995.

Clement PB. Diseases of the peritoneum. In: Kurman RJ, ed. *Blaustein's Pathology of the Female Genital Tract,* 5th ed. New York: Springer; 2002.

Tavassoli FA, Devilee P, eds. *Pathology and Genetics of Tumors of the Breast and Female Genital Organs. World Health Organization Classification of Tumors.* Lyon: IARC Press; 2003.

Travis WD, Brambilla E, Müller-Hermelink HK, et al. eds. *Pathology and Genetics of Tumors of the Lung, Pleura, Thymus and Heart. World Health Organization Classification of Tumors.* Lyon: IARC Press; 2004.

SECTION III

GI Tract

12 The Esophagus
Danielle H. Carpenter and Elizabeth M. Brunt

I. **NORMAL ANATOMY.** The esophagus, a tubular structure that connects the pharynx to the stomach, is composed of cervical, thoracic, and abdominal segments. It begins at the level of the cricoid cartilage and ends at the gastroesophageal junction (GEJ). The GEJ is the junction of the tubular esophagus and the saccular stomach, and is distinct from the squamocolumnar junction.

By endoscopy, the esophagus is measured beginning 16 cm distal to the incisors and extends 35 to 40 cm to the GEJ. Precise anatomic location within the esophagus is a significant parameter in the differential diagnoses of various pathologic processes, as well as for staging squamous carcinoma.

The esophageal mucosa is composed of stratified squamous epithelium that extends distally to the squamocolumnar junction; this overlies paucicellular lamina propria and is delimited by thin muscularis mucosae that have a rich network of lymphatics (the latter allows for early metastases of relatively superficial malignancies). The deeper submucosa also has a rich lymphovascular network as well as submucosal glands connected to the lumen by ducts. The deep muscularis propria is composed of an inner circular layer and outer longitudinal layer; the proximal third of the muscularis is striated, the distal third is smooth muscle, and the middle third is a mixture. There is no serosal surface on the esophagus, but rather an adventitia.

II. **GROSS EXAMINATION AND TISSUE HANDLING**
   A. **Endoscopic biopsy.** The standard endoscopic biopsy consists of several small (1 to 5 mm) unoriented pieces of mucosa with varying amounts of attached muscularis mucosae. In some cases, the endoscopist may use "jumbo forceps" to obtain larger fragments (4 to 8 mm); submucosa may be present in these biopsies. All fragments are submitted and three hematoxylin and eosin (H&E)-stained slides are examined.
   B. **Endoscopic mucosal resection (EMR).** EMR is a more conservative approach than esophagectomy for resection of superficial malignant and premalignant lesions. These en bloc resections of 1 to 2 cm lesions are obtained by elevation of the mucosa with submucosal saline injection, followed by removal of the mucosa with variable amounts of attached submucosa. The specimens range from 1 to 4 cm in the longest dimension and up to 1 cm in thickness.

   EMR specimens are carefully pinned flat for fixation, all deep and radial margins inked, and the specimen serially sectioned and submitted entirely to assess not only the mucosal lesion, but also the deep and radial margins (Fig. 12.1). Initially, at least three H&E levels are evaluated.

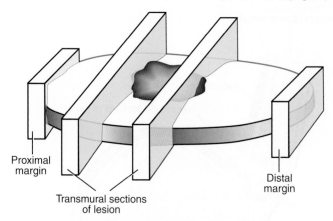

Figure 12.1 Sectioning of endoscopic mucosal resection specimens.

C. Esophagectomy. Esophagectomy specimens consist of esophagus, proximal stomach, and attached soft tissue with lymph nodes. The radial soft tissue margins are inked and the specimen opened longitudinally, avoiding transection of the lesion if possible; the specimen is pinned flat for fixation. The pertinent gross measurements include the overall length, diameter, and thickness of the esophagus and stomach; length, width, and thickness of the lesion and other mucosal abnormalities; and location of the lesion in relation to the proximal, distal, and radial margins, as well as in relation to the GEJ. The general appearance of the lesion (polypoid, ulcerated, and indurated) is important, as is that of the surrounding mucosa.

The standard sections (Fig. 12.2) should include a shave or *en face* section of the proximal esophageal margin (often submitted for frozen section and assessed intraoperatively) and distal stomach margin. A full thickness section of the lesion at its deepest point of invasion including the inked adventitial (radial) margin should also be taken; sections of tumor with closest adjacent proximal and distal margins should also be submitted as appropriate. When the tumor closely approximates the distal margin, the distal margin is entirely submitted radially to best assess distance from tumor to margin. In instances of preoperative radiation and/or chemotherapy, the lesion may be difficult to visualize grossly, and only a shallow ulcer or induration may be present; in such cases, the entire area should be serially sectioned and submitted for histologic examination. All lymph nodes visualized or palpated in the attached soft tissue are dissected and submitted.

III. NONNEOPLASTIC PROCESSES

A. Benign histologic changes

1. **Glycogenic acanthosis.** This asymptomatic, incidental finding is grossly characterized by white nodules or plaques and can be found throughout the length of the esophagus. Microscopically, glycogenic acanthosis is seen as a squamous epithelial layer thickened by clear epithelial cells in which the cytoplasm is distended by glycogen accumulation. The H&E appearance is characteristic, although the presence of glycogen can be confirmed with a Periodic acid–Schiff (PAS) stain.

2. **Gastric heterotopias.** Also known as the "inlet patch," this lesion is a well-circumscribed, small (<2 cm) patch of gastric mucosa in the cervical

Proximal shave margin

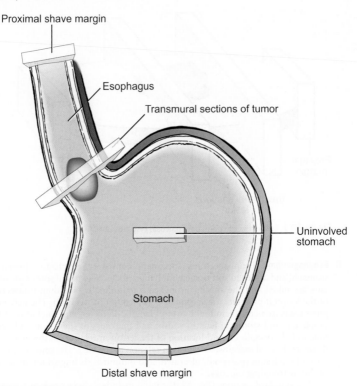

Esophagus

Transmural sections of tumor

Uninvolved stomach

Stomach

Distal shave margin

Figure 12.2 Sectioning of esophagectomy specimens excised for malignancy.

esophagus. Histologically, it can be antral, fundic, or cardiac type mucosa and is often inflamed (e-Fig. 12.1).*

3. **Ectopic tissue.** Other ectopic tissues have been described in the cervical esophagus including thyroid and parathyroid. Sebaceous glands have been described at all levels of the esophagus; they may be a type of metaplasia rather than ectopia.

B. Mucosal injury

1. **Reflux esophagitis.** In patients with gastroesophageal reflux disease (GERD), the distal esophagus may have a range of appearances from minimal erythema, to hemorrhage with ulceration. Histologically, the damage from the GERD is seen as intraepithelial inflammation with reactive changes (e-Figs. 12.2 to 12.4) characterized by an increased basal layer, elongation of the papillae, and intra- and intercellular edema; in severe cases, however, erosion can be observed as well.

Chronic gastroesophageal reflux with mucosal injury can also lead to the development of intestinal metaplasia (Barrett esophagus); this is discussed under section on "Epithelial Neoplasms and Preneoplasms."

2. **Chemical injury.** Secondary to exposure to damaging or caustic agents, chemical injury is seen as mucosal damage ranging from mucosal erythema and

---

*All e-figures are available online via the Solution Site Image Bank.

TABLE 12.1 Clinicopathologic Features of Eosinophilic and Reflux Esophagitis

	Eosinophilic esophagitis	Reflux esophagitis
Age	More common in children	More common in adults
Sex	More common in male	Equally in both sexes
Main symptom	Dysphagia	Heartburn
Endoscopic findings	Stricture, ring	Variable
Involvement	Entire esophagus	Distal esophagus
Microscopic finding	>20 eosinophils/hpf; eosinophilic microabscesses	<5 eosinophils/hpf
Therapy	Topical steroids	Anti-reflux
Complications	Stricture	Barrett esophagus; stricture

friability, to frank necrosis with perforation. Histologically, there is epithelial necrosis with or without inflammation, although usually to a lesser extent than would be expected for the degree of epithelial damage present.

3. **Pill esophagitis** is usually a focal irregular erosion in areas of the esophagus where there is a natural external compression. Certain patients (elderly) with certain habits (taking pills without liquid) and certain medications (e.g., tetracycline, NSAIDs, large pills) are most commonly associated and the diagnosis can usually be made from a careful history. Histologically, the findings include inflammation, reactive changes, and erosion, and may include foreign pill material (e-**Figs. 12.5** and **12.6**).

4. **Radiation injury.** Acute radiation injury can share many features of other esophagitides and is usually clinically diagnosed due to its temporal relation to radiation therapy. Chronic radiation injury can be subtle clinically and show pale mucosa, a stricture, or chronic ulceration. Histologically, the findings include vascular changes consisting of ectasia and intimal fibrosis with resultant ischemic damage and erosion, as well as radiation fibroblasts and atypically enlarged (nucleus and cytoplasm) stromal cells (e-**Figs. 12.7** to **12.9**).

5. **Eosinophilic esophagitis (EE).** Clinically, EE shows a ridged or furrowed esophagus, and commonly involves the midesophagus. The histologic findings in EE may overlap with reflux esophagitis, although the intraepithelial inflammation is predominantly eosinophils (>20/hpf) and eosinophilic microabscesses are often seen (e-**Figs. 12.10** to **12.12**). Since reflux predominantly affects the distal esophagus, biopsies of both mid and distal esophagus are standard in suspected cases of EE. Table 12.1 presents differentiating clinicopathologic features of EE and reflux. The differential diagnosis of EE also includes hypereosinophilic syndrome and eosinophilic gastroenteritis, an allergic reaction to specific food antigens or drugs, or parasitic infection.

6. **Graft versus host disease (GVHD)** is uncommon in the esophagus, but is similar to GVHD in the skin. The squamous mucosa may desquamate, and submucosal fibrosis and stricture formation may develop. Histologically, basal vacuolation and apoptosis, with or without lymphocytic infiltration, are noted.

7. **Infectious esophagitis**
   a. ***Candida.*** Candidiasis is classically seen as white exudative patches over the length of the esophagus with relatively normal appearing intervening mucosa. Histologically, there is a necroinflammatory background with yeast and pseudohyphae present in the superficial epithelial layers (e-**Figs. 12.13** and **12.14**). PAS and Grocott's methenamine silver (GMS) stains highlight infiltrative fungal organisms (e-**Fig. 12.15**).

b. **Herpes simplex virus (HSV).** The classic lesion of HSV esophagitis is shallow ulceration, ranging from millimeters to centimeters in diameter. Viral cytopathic change, characterized by multinucleation, molding of nuclei, and margination of chromatin, are seen most frequently at the edges of the ulcer (e-**Figs. 12.16** to **12.18**). Immunohistochemistry (IHC) is confirmatory in this regard.

c. **Cytomegalovirus (CMV).** Focal, discrete ulceration in the distal esophagus occurs in CMV esophagitis. Granulation tissue from the ulcer *base* (as opposed to the *edge* in HSV) is optimal for identifying viral cytopathic change in endothelial and stromal cells. Large eosinophilic nuclear and/or cytoplasmic inclusions can be seen on routine H&E stained sections, although immunostains for CMV can highlight or confirm the virus.

IV. **BENIGN POLYPS**

A. **Fibrovascular polyps** are elongate, often large ("giant fibrovascular polyp"), pedunculated intraluminal growths that can fill the esophagus and present as an intraoral mass if regurgitated. Histologically, these polyps are composed of an edematous, loose stroma with a rich vascular network covered by benign squamous mucosa.

B. **Inflammatory polyps.** Often related to GERD, inflammatory polyps are present near the squamocolumnar junction and may endoscopically resemble adenocarcinoma. However, histologically they are benign and composed of inflamed squamous and/or foveolar mucosa.

C. **Squamous papilloma.** Also often related to GERD, squamous papillomas can have a filiform appearance microscopically, if not grossly. Delicate fibrovascular cores are covered by benign reactive squamous epithelium with varying degrees of inflammation (e-**Fig. 12.19**). Although rare cases of virus-related papillomas of the esophagus have been reported in immunocompromised patients, squamous papillomas are most often seen in patients with GERD.

V. **EPITHELIAL NEOPLASMS AND PRENEOPLASMS.** The current World Health Organization (WHO) histologic classification of esophageal tumors is given in Table 12.2. The AJCC Staging guidelines for esophagus and esophagogastric junction are applied to primary esophageal and esophagogastric junction mucosal tumors, including the proximal 5 cm of stomach (Table 12.3).

A. **Squamous dysplasia.** Endoscopic evidence of squamous dysplasia may be subtle and most likely identified in association with plaque-like, mass-forming lesions. Dysplastic squamous mucosa has cells with enlarged, hyperchromatic nuclei and increased nuclear to cytoplasmic ratios, as well as overall dysmaturity of the epithelium. Unlike squamous carcinoma, dysplasia is limited by the basement membrane; however, unlike benign reactive changes, dysplasia lacks cytologic uniformity and orderly epithelial maturation.

B. **Squamous cell carcinoma (SCC)** has a range of gross appearances, from erythematous eroded mucosa, to plaque-like growths, to mass-forming exophytic lesions. It is most commonly found in the middle third of the esophagus, followed by the lower then upper thirds. By definition, neoplastic cells extend through the basement membrane into the lamina propria ("carcinoma in situ" is a term no longer used; it has been replaced by "high grade dysplasia") (e-**Figs. 12.20** and **12.21**). Depending on tumor grade, there are varying degrees of keratin formation in SCC of the esophagus (e-**Fig. 12.22**), although the various subtypes of SCC (basaloid, spindle cell, and verrucous) often seen in other body sites can also occur in the esophagus. In addition to tumor, lymph node, metastasis, and grading characterizations, tumor location also factors into tumor staging (Table 12.3).

C. **Barrett esophagus.** A diagnosis of Barrett esophagus entails endoscopic findings of salmon-colored mucosa of any length above the GEJ with correlating histologic findings of a specialized columnar epithelium with goblet cells.

TABLE 12.2 WHO Classification of Tumors of the Esophagus

Epithelial tumors
Premalignant lesions
Squamous
   Intraepithelial neoplasia, low grade
   Intraepithelial neoplasia, high grade
Glandular
   Dysplasia, low grade
   Dysplasia, high grade
Carcinoma
Squamous cell carcinoma
Adenocarcinoma
Adenoid cystic carcinoma
Adenosquamous carcinoma
Basaloid squamous cell carcinoma
Mucoepidermoid carcinoma
Spindle cell (squamous) carcinoma
Verrucous (squamous) carcinoma
Undifferentiated carcinoma
Neuroendocrine neoplasms
Neuroendocrine tumor (NET)
   NET G1 (carcinoid)
   NET G2
Neuroendocrine carcinoma (NEC)
   Large-cell NEC
   Small-cell NEC
Mixed adenoneuroendocrine carcinoma

Mesenchymal tumors
Granular cell tumor
Hemangioma
Leiomyoma
Lipoma
Gastrointestinal stromal tumor
Kaposi sarcoma
Leiomyosarcoma
Melanoma
Rhabdomyosarcoma
Synovial sarcoma

Lymphoma

Secondary tumors

From: Bosman FT, Carneiro F, Hruban RH, Theise ND, eds. *World Health Organization Classification of Tumours of the Digestive System.* Lyon: IARC Press; 2010. Used with permission.

Cytoplasmic distension with mucin alone is not diagnostic for goblet cells; true goblet cells also exhibit a basally oriented nucleus and have mucin that is blue-tinged and acidic (blue stain by PAS/AB at pH 2.5). Occasionally, gastric foveolar cells may show expanded cytoplasm with a goblet contour, although they contain neutral mucin (e-**Fig. 12.23**); additionally, some gastric epithelial cells (aptly named "tall blue cells") without a goblet shape may also contain blue mucin (e-**Fig. 12.24**). In Barrett esophagus, goblet cells are often dispersed among gastric foveolar cells (incomplete intestinal metaplasia; (e-**Figs. 12.25** and **12.26**) or flanked by epithelial cells with brush borders identical to absorptive cells of the small intestine (complete intestinal metaplasia; e-**Fig. 12.27**). It

TABLE 12.3 TNM Staging Scheme for Esophagus and Esophagogastric Junction

Primary tumor (T)

TX	Primary tumor cannot be assessed
T0	No evidence of primary tumor
Tis	High-grade dysplasia
T1	Tumor invades lamina propria, muscularis mucosae, or submucosa
T1a	Tumor invades lamina propria or muscularis mucosae
T1b	Tumor invades submucosa
T2	Tumor invades muscularis propria
T3	Tumor invades adventitia
T4	Tumor invades adjacent structures
T4a	Resectable tumor invading pleura, pericardium, or diaphragm
T4b	Unresectable tumor invading other adjacent structures, such as aorta, vertebral body, trachea, etc.

Regional lymph nodes (N)

NX	Regional lymph nodes cannot be assessed
N0	No regional lymph node metastasis
N1	Metastases in 1–2 regional lymph nodes
N2	Metastases in 3–6 regional lymph nodes
N3	Metastases in seven or more regional lymph nodes

Distant metastasis (M)

M0	No distant metastasis
M1	Distant metastasis

Histologic grade (G)

GX	Grade cannot be assessed – stage grouping as G1
G1	Well differentiated
G2	Moderately differentiated
G3	Poorly differentiated
G4	Undifferentiated – stage grouping as G3 squamous

Stage grouping for esophageal carcinomas

Squamous cell carcinoma

Stage	T	N	M	Grade	Location
Stage 0	Tis/HGD	N0	M0	1, X	Any
Stage IA	T1	N0	M0	1, X	Any
Stage IB	T1	N0	M0	2–3	Any
	T2–3	N0	M0	1, X	Lower, X
Stage IIA	T2–3	N0	M0	1, X	Upper, mid
	T2–3	N0	M0	2–3	Lower, X
Stage IIB	T2–3	N0	M0	2–3	Upper, mid
	T1–2	N1	M0	Any	Any
Stage IIIA	T1–2	N2	M0	Any	Any
	T3	N1	M0	Any	Any
	T4a	N0	M0	Any	Any
Stage IIIB	T3	N2	M0	Any	Any
Stage IIIC	T4a	N1–2	M0	Any	Any
	T4b	Any	M0	Any	Any
	Any	N3	M0	Any	Any
Stage IV	Any	Any	M1	Any	Any

Adenocarcinoma

Stage	T	N	M	Grade
Stage 0	Tis/HGD	N0	M0	1, X
Stage IA	T1	N0	M0	1–2, X
Stage IB	T1	N0	M0	3
	T2	N0	M0	1–2,X
Stage IIA	T2	N0	M0	3
Stage IIB	T3	N0	M0	Any
	T1–2	N1	M0	Any
Stage IIIA	T1–2	N2	M0	Any
	T3	N1	M0	Any
	T4a	N0	M0	Any
Stage IIIB	T3	N2	M0	Any
Stage IIIC	T4a	N1–2	M0	Any
	T4b	Any	M0	Any
	Any	N3	M0	Any
Stage IV	Any	Any	M1	Any

TABLE 12.4	Histologic Findings: Barrett Esophagus

Category	Features
Negative for dysplasia (**e-Figs. 12.28** and **12.29**)	• Cytologically bland with intact nuclear polarity; abundant goblet cells • Normal glandular architecture overall • Any minimal cytologic or architectural atypical features are limited to the deeper portion of the glands, maturation at the surface
Indefinite for dysplasia (**e-Fig. 12.30**)	• Cytologic and architectural alterations present but insufficient for unequivocal diagnosis of dysplasia • For example, in some cases distinction between inflammation-related regenerative change and dysplasia may be difficult • In some cases, the relationship of the surface and deeper glands cannot be assessed due to tangential sectioning
Low-grade dysplasia (**e-Figs. 12.31** and **12.32**)	• Cytologic atypia: stratified, pencil-shaped, and hyperchromatic nuclei with irregular nuclear membranes, but intact polarity and lack of nucleoli; loss of mucin • Mild architectural alterations: minimal glandular crowding may be present • Cytologic atypia, loss of mucin, and minimal glandular crowding focally extend to the surface such that the deeper glands and surface appear similar at low power. Reminiscent of tubular adenomas of the colon
High-grade dysplasia[a] (**e-Figs. 12.33** and **12.34**)	• Cytologic atypia: markedly enlarged, round-to-ovoid hyperchromatic nuclei with extensive stratification and loss of polarity; abnormal mitotic figures may be present • Architectural alterations: glandular crowding with minimal intervening lamina propria; irregularly shaped, budding, branching, cribriforming, or cystically dilated glands; villiform surface common • Only cytologic or architectural features extending to the surface are necessary to diagnose HGD, though both are often present
Intramucosal carcinoma[a] (**e-Figs. 12.35–12.37**)	• Cytologic atypia: as above in high-grade dysplasia • Architectural alterations: invasion through the gland basement membrane into the lamina propria or muscularis mucosae; often seen with extensive cribriform, back-to-back, or complex syncytial growth pattern, and individual dysplastic cells or small clusters of dysplastic cells in the lamina propria; desmoplasia not present

[a]Documented consensus diagnosis by at least two pathologists with special interest/training in GI pathology strongly recommended.

has been suggested that Barrett esophagus with incomplete intestinal metaplasia is more prone to develop dysplasia.

The categories of dysplasia in Barrett esophagus are described in Table 12.4.

D. **Adenocarcinoma** occurs predominantly in the setting of Barrett esophagus and endoscopically can be indistinguishable from surrounding dysplasia, often presenting as a small polypoid, elevated, flat, occult, or even depressed lesion. These tumors are usually located close to the GEJ. Previous ambiguity over classification as esophageal or gastric in origin has been diminished in the current AJCC

TABLE 12.5 Neuroendocrine Neoplasms in the Esophagus

Tumor/frequency	Proliferative indices	Histologic findings
NET G1 (carcinoid)/rare	<2 mit/10 hpfs, ≤2% Ki67 index[a]	Uniform bland tumor cells; insular growth pattern
NET G2/more common	2–20 mit/10 hpfs, 3%–20% Ki67 index[a]	Solid, acinar, or trabecular growth pattern; necrosis
NEC	>20 mit/10 hpfs, >20% Ki67 index[a]	Large-cell (more common) or small-cell features
MANEC/very rare	>20 mit/10 hpfs, >20% Ki67 index[a]	Neuroendocrine and adenocarcinoma or SCC combined

[a]Mitotic count is averaged over 50 hpfs; Ki67 index (using MIB antibody) is calculated as from number of positive nuclear staining tumor cells out of 500 to 2000 tumor cells in areas of strongest labeling. From: Bosman FT, Carneiro F, Hruban RH, Theise ND, eds. *World Health Organization Classification of Tumours of the Digestive System.* Lyon: IARC Press; 2010. Used with permission.

Staging scheme that includes tumors in the proximal 5 cm of the stomach with esophageal and esophagogastric tumors; the current AJCC staging information is given in Table 12.3.

Histologically, esophageal adenocarcinoma consists of infiltrative tubular or papillary structures (e-**Figs. 12.38** to **12.44**). Signet-ring cells and mucin production may be seen (e-**Figs. 12.45** and **12.46**), but signet-ring cell carcinoma (>50% of the tumor composed of signet-ring cells) is more typical of primary gastric tumors. Adenocarcinoma of the gastrointestinal (GI) tract is graded into well-differentiated (>95% of the tumor composed of glands), moderately differentiated (50% to 95%), and poorly differentiated (<50%). Well-differentiated adenocarcinoma may pose a diagnostic challenge in biopsy specimens. More than 90% of the esophageal adenocarcinomas express K7, but 40% also express K20.

E. **Neuroendocrine neoplasms** of the esophagus are classified according to the common criteria for all GI and pancreatic neuroendocrine neoplasms (Table 12.5). These neoplasms more frequently occur in the distal esophagus. Neuroendocrine tumors (NETs) are typically small and polypoid, while neuroendocrine carcinomas (NECs; including mixed adenoneuroendocrine carcinoma, MANEC) can be large, fungating, ulcerated, and deeply invasive masses (e-**Figs. 12.47** and **12.48**).

F. **Salivary gland-type neoplasms.** Thought to arise from the submucosal glands lining the esophagus, mucoepidermoid carcinoma, pleomorphic adenoma, and adenoid cystic carcinoma can be seen in the esophagus.

VI. **MESENCHYMAL NEOPLASMS**

A. **Leiomyoma** is the most common mesenchymal neoplasm of the esophagus. It is seen as an intramural, well-circumscribed nodule in the middle-to-distal esophagus. The firm white-gray cut surface microscopically shows whorls of benign smooth muscle cells.

B. **Granular cell tumor (GCT)** typically presents as an incidental submucosal lesion. Microscopically, GCT is composed of nested sheets of bland cells with granular, S100 and PAS-positive cytoplasm. The overlying epithelium can show pseudoepitheliomatous hyperplasia that should not be mistaken for epithelial dysplasia (e-**Figs. 12.49** to **12.51**).

C. **Vascular tumors.** Hemangiomas present as polypoid intraluminal masses and are of capillary or cavernous types. Lymphangiomas are small, sessile-to-pedunculated growths in the middle-to-lower esophagus with a cavernous histologic pattern.

D. **Gastrointestinal stromal tumor (GIST).** In contrast to the stomach, where leiomyoma is rare and GIST is common, in the esophagus leiomyoma is common and GIST is rare. Esophageal GISTs typically present as intraluminal masses in the distal esophagus. GISTs are KIT(CD117)-positive spindle-cell neoplasms, with *KIT* mutations similar to those in the stomach (e-**Figs. 12.52** to **12.54**).

E. **Other benign and malignant mesenchymal tumors.** Rare benign mesenchymal tumors in the esophagus include glomus tumor, lipoma, and Schwannoma. Rare malignant mesenchymal tumors include rhabdomyosarcoma, synovial sarcoma, and Kaposi sarcoma. All such tumors have features identical to corresponding primary tumors of soft tissue (see Chap. 46).

VII. **OTHER NEOPLASMS**

A. **Melanoma.** Primary melanoma of the esophagus occurs as a pigmented, polypoid lesion in the middle-to-distal esophagus.

B. **Lymphoma.** Primary lymphoma of the esophagus is rare. The most common type is diffuse large B-cell lymphoma, although Mucosa-associated lymphoid tissue, lymphoma and T-cell lymphomas have been described.

C. **Metastasis.** Although uncommonly a site for metastatic disease, breast, lung, and melanoma are the most common malignancies to metastasize to the esophagus.

Cytopathology of the Esophagus

Julie Elizabeth Kunkel

I. **INTRODUCTION.** Indications for esophageal cytologic examination include a suspected neoplasm, an infection, or for surveillance of Barrett esophagus. Mucosal abnormalities are best sampled with endoscopic brushing for circumferential sampling; endoscopic ultrasound-guided fine needle aspiration (EUS–FNA) may be employed to sample targeted mucosal lesions, intramural masses, and for staging of esophageal carcinoma via transmural sampling of paraesophageal lymph nodes. EUS–FNA is the accepted nodal staging modality for esophageal cancer and has an 81% to 97% sensitivity, 83% to 100% specificity, and 83% to 97% accuracy for malignancy (*Ann Thorac Cardiovasc Surg.* 2003;9:2).

II. **INFECTION/REACTIVE ATYPIA.** Brushings are employed in the setting of infection, usually in a patient with esophagitis, erosions, or ulcers. As in other squamous epithelial sites, reactive and reparative atypia are characterized by cohesive two-dimensional (2D) sheets of cells that have slightly enlarged nuclei, smooth nuclear contours, and conspicuous nucleoli. Features worrisome for dysplasia such as marked nuclear crowding or a single-cell distribution pattern are lacking. A background of acute inflammation and some debris are typically present. GERD is generally not an indication for brushings, but some reactive atypia related to epithelial repair may be noted.

Reactive atypia is also present in radiation esophagitis. However, radiation esophagitis will also show the features characteristically present after radiation therapy, such as large, bizarre cells, multinucleation, and biphasic cytoplasm.

A. **Candidal esophagitis** displays pseudohyphae and yeast form (e-**Fig. 12.55**). Oral contamination should be excluded, especially in the absence of inflammation.

B. **Herpetic esophagitis** (almost always HSV-1) and shows herpes viral cytopathic effect, characterized by ground glass chromatin, thick nuclear membranes, multinucleation, and nuclear molding (e-**Fig. 12.56**). Cowdry type A viral inclusions (distinct eosinophilic nuclear inclusions surrounded by a clear halo and a thick nuclear membrane are present (e-**Fig. 12.57**).

C. **CMV esophagitis** demonstrates significantly enlarged mononuclear cells with a large intranuclear inclusion separated from a thickened nuclear membrane by a clear halo. Occasional cytoplasmic granular inclusions are also present.

III. **BARRETT ESOPHAGUS.** Cytological diagnosis relies on the identification of goblet cells within sheets of benign glandular cells. The goblet cells exhibit a single large cytoplasmic vacuole that displaces the nucleus, creating a crescent-shaped nucleus. The diameter of the vacuole is at least three times the width of a normal columnar cell (*Am J Clin Pathol.* 1988;89:493; *Hum Pathol.* 1997;28:465).

For dysplasia in Barrett esophagus, brushing cytology as a screening tool offers the advantage of sampling a wider area of abnormal mucosa as compared with biopsy. The presence of dysplasia and malignancy is evaluated based on architectural irregularities, cell cohesion, and cytological atypia. As interobserver discrepancy is high, any dysplasia identified in cytology specimens should be confirmed by biopsy (*Hum Pathol.* 1997;28:465). Dysplastic changes are categorized as low grade and high grade; high-grade lesions contain more severe cytologic atypia including an increased nuclear:cytoplasmic ratio, nuclear enlargement, hyperchromasia, and nuclear contour irregularity.

IV. **NEOPLASMS**

A. **Intramural neoplasms** include GIST, Schwannoma, and leiomyoma. The cellularity of the specimen is usually low. Findings include microfragments composed of spindle-shaped cells with oval-to-spindled nuclei, fine chromatin, and delicate cytoplasm. The distinction among these low-grade spindle cell neoplasms rests on IHC (*Am J Clin Pathol.* 2003;119:703).

Granular cell tumor may present as a circumscribed or infiltrative process, is characterized by squamous hypertrophy of the overlying mucosa. The tumor cells themselves are polygonal with granular, eosinophilic cytoplasm. Immunoreactivity for S-100 may be helpful in establishing the diagnosis (*J Gastrointest Cancer.* 2008;39:107).

B. **Adenocarcinoma.** The specimen is highly cellular, consisting of haphazardly arranged 3D clusters and abundant isolated atypical cells (**e-Fig. 12.58**). The nuclear atypia and pleomorphism are marked. Necrosis may be present. The distinction from high-grade dysplasia is difficult by cytomorphology alone, and is quantitative rather than qualitative (*Cancer.* 1992;69:8; *Hum Pathol.* 1997;28:465).

C. **Squamous cell carcinoma (SCC).** Well-differentiated SCC displays abundant isolated cells with hyperchromatic and pyknotic nuclei, keratinized cytoplasm with sharp cytoplasmic borders, spindle- and tadpole-shaped malignant cells, and necrosis (**e-Fig. 12.59**). Poorly differentiated SCC shows crowded groups and isolated cells with enlarged nuclei and coarsely clumpy chromatin; distinction from poorly differentiated adenocarcinoma may be difficult due to lack of keratinization.

D. **Secondary tumors and metastases.** The most common form of secondary tumor spread to the esophagus is by direct extension of a thyroidal, pulmonary, or laryngeal carcinoma. Rarely, hematogenous metastases to the esophagus have been reported, usually arising from the stomach, breast, larynx, or pancreas. The diagnostic work-up rests on recognition of cytomorphology not native to the esophagus coupled with immunohistochemical studies.

13 The Stomach

Kathryn M. Law and Elizabeth M. Brunt

I. **NORMAL ANATOMY.** The stomach, a distensible, J-shaped organ, is traditionally divided into five regions: cardia, fundus, body, antrum, and pylorus. The cardia is a poorly defined region extending up to 3 cm distal to the gastroesophageal junction. The fundus is the region that curves lateral and superior to the level of the gastroesophageal junction. Below the gastroesophageal junction in continuation with the cardia and fundus is the body, which extends to the incisura. The antrum encompasses the distal third of the stomach, begins at the incisura, and extends to the pylorus. This region grossly and endoscopically has more flattened and firmly anchored mucosa than the fundus or the body. The pylorus is a muscular zone of the stomach controlling passage of food into the duodenum.

The mucosal lining is of two types: antral (antrum, pylorus, cardia) and oxyntic (fundus, body). Antral-type foveolar mucosa demonstrates a 1:1 relationship of surface to deeper mucus secretory glands separated by lamina propria (e-Fig. 13.1).* Oxyntic foveolar mucosa has a 1:4 pit to gland relationship (e-Fig. 13.2). The mucus neck cells midway along the foveolar fold harbor the regenerative cells of the stomach. The underlying glands are composed of gastric parietal cells, which produce acid and intrinsic factor, and chief cells, which produce pepsinogen. In the antrum, endocrine cells are located just below the surface foveola and include gastrin-producing G-cells, serotonin-producing enterochromaffin (EC) cells, and somatostatin-producing D-cells. In the fundus, endocrine cells are located at the base of the crypts and consist of histamine-producing enterochromaffin-like (ECL) cells and a small number of EC cells. The lamina propria of the stomach normally contains a few inflammatory cells including lymphocytes, plasma cells, eosinophils, and mast cells. The muscularis mucosae, submucosa, muscularis propria, and serosa of the stomach are histologically similar to that of the intestines.

II. **GROSS EXAMINATION AND TISSUE HANDLING**

A. **Endoscopic biopsies.** Endoscopic findings and pertinent history assist in histopathologic interpretation. The gross description should include the number of fragments and overall specimen dimensions to ensure all material has been analyzed microscopically; three levels stained by hematoxylin and eosin (H&E) should be prepared for routine microscopic analysis. Some laboratories order *Helicobacter pylori* stains at the time of processing; others prefer to evaluate the specimens for specific features of infection (see below) before ordering special stains.

B. **Gastrectomy.** Gastrectomies may be partial (often including a portion of the duodenum or esophagus) or total. When the specimen is received, the serosal surface should be examined for evidence of tumor penetration and the area overlying the tumor inked (e-Fig. 13.3). After opening longitudinally along the greater curvature without transecting the tumor (e-Fig. 13.4), the specimen should then be pinned on Styrofoam (with the mucosal surface facing out) and fixed in formalin overnight to ensure well-fixed and oriented sections. Standard measurements include the length of the greater and lesser curvatures, circumferences at the resection margins, and wall thickness. If a tumor is grossly identified, its location, shape, maximal dimension, and distance from the margins

---

*All e-figures are available online via the Solution Site Image Bank.

should be recorded. The tumor should be cross-sectioned and an estimate of the depth of invasion recorded (e-Fig. 13.5). The presence of any other mucosal abnormalities should also be recorded. Three to four sections of the tumor should be submitted to include the deepest invasion and relationship of tumor to uninvolved mucosa. Sections from other mucosal lesions, and uninvolved antrum and body, should also be submitted.

If a previously diagnosed adenocarcinoma cannot be confirmed by a grossly visible lesion, careful examination of the gastric mucosa should be performed to identify subtle mucosal alterations including erosions and effacement of folds. Multiple sections should be taken of any of the abnormalities noted, and a diagram of the sections constructed for later reference.

If the tumor is distant from the margins, a single shave section from the proximal and distal margins is adequate. However, if the tumor approaches the margins, multiple radial sections demonstrating the relationship of tumor to margin should be taken. A careful lymph node dissection should be performed; all perigastric lymph nodes are considered regional lymph nodes.

III. DIAGNOSTIC FEATURES OF NONNEOPLASTIC CONDITIONS OF THE STOMACH

A. **Gastritis.** The classification of gastritis lacks universal standardization. The most recent attempt at standardization is the updated Sydney System, which combines topographical, morphologic, and etiologic information to arrive at a theoretically reproducible and clinically usable diagnosis (*Am J Surg Pathol.* 1996;20:1161). However, in most settings, there is not enough information or sampling to fulfill the requirements of this classification system. Nonetheless, the system describes several parameters that should be evaluated in a gastric biopsy including the presence and degree of neutrophilic (active) inflammation, chronic inflammation, and atrophy (intestinal metaplasia). Additional features to be noted are surface epithelial damage, lymphoid follicles, foveolar hyperplasia, pseudopyloric metaplasia, pancreatic metaplasia, and endocrine cell hyperplasia.

1. **Chronic gastritis** is the most common pathologic diagnosis in gastric biopsies. The diagnosis is associated with a lymphoplasmacytic infiltrate in the lamina propria, and in many cases is attributable to *H. pylori.* However, the number of lymphocytes and plasma cells normally present within gastric biopsies varies with different patient populations, and it is therefore difficult to determine how much inflammation constitutes clinically significant chronic gastritis. Certain histologic features suggest a diagnosis of *H. pylori* associated gastritis, including lymphoid follicles with germinal centers and the presence of neutrophils within the lamina propria, epithelium, or gland lumens (which is termed "active" rather than "acute" gastritis) (e-Fig. 13.6). Patchy or focal activity may be seen with *H. pylori* but can also be seen in inflammatory bowel disease, especially in children with Crohn's disease (e-Fig. 13.7).

   H. pylori can best be identified on routine H&E stain in pits near foci of exocytosis or surface mucin (e-Fig. 13.8). However, if needed, histochemical (Giemsa) and/or immunohistochemical (IHC) stains can be used to enhance detection of the organisms (e-Figs. 13.9 and 13.10). The chance of finding organisms diminishes in the absence of active inflammation or in regions of intestinal metaplasia, as the organisms do not colonize this type of epithelium. Additionally, in patients on proton pump inhibitors (PPIs), antral inflammation is milder and *H. pylori* may relocate deeper in the oxyntic glands. Finally, treatment with other antibiotics, while not eradicating the organism, may nonetheless hinder the ability to detect *H. pylori.*

   After treatment for *H. pylori,* neutrophils disappear within 6 to 8 weeks. However, the lymphoplasmacytic infiltrates can persist for longer (up to a

TABLE 13.1	Clinicopathologic Features of Autoimmune and Nonautoimmune Atrophic Gastritis	
	Autoimmune	**Nonautoimmune**
Patient population	Mainly older white women	Universal
Etiology and pathogenesis	Autoantibodies to parietal cells and intrinsic factor	*Helicobacter pylori*, other environmental factors
Clinical manifestations	Hypochlorhydria, achlorhydria, pernicious anemia	Abdominal pain, dyspepsia, upper GI bleeding
Gastric involvement	Body and fundus only	Mainly antrum, or multifocal
Microscopic findings	Chronic gastritis, progressive destruction of fundic glands, intestinal metaplasia, pyloric metaplasia, ECL cell hyperplasia	Chronic gastritis, intestinal metaplasia, pyloric metaplasia if body is involved
Serum gastrin level	Elevated	Normal or low
Tumor development	Carcinoid, adenocarcinoma	MALT lymphoma

GI, gastrointestinal; ECL, enterochromaffin-like; MALT, mucosa-associated lymphoid tissue.

year in the body and 2 to 4 years in the antrum). Lymphoid follicles and intestinal metaplasia may remain indefinitely.

Atrophic gastritis is a form of chronic gastritis that can be a consequence of *H. pylori* gastritis, or occur as an autoimmune process (e-**Fig. 13.11**). Associated findings include intestinal metaplasia and ECL cell hyperplasia (e-**Figs. 13.12** and **13.13**). Dysplasia, adenocarcinoma, and carcinoid tumor may develop in this background. Table 13.1 summarizes the clinicopathologic features distinguishing autoimmune from nonautoimmune atrophic gastritis. It is worth noting that atrophy may be more difficult to recognize in the antrum than in the body or fundus since atrophic fundic/body mucosa may resemble antral mucosa on H&E stain; hence, knowledge of the location of the biopsy site is important. If necessary, a positive gastrin stain can confirm the antral origin of a biopsy.

2. **Lymphocytic gastritis** is defined as prominent lymphocytic infiltration of the surface and foveolar epithelium (>25 lymphocytes per 100 epithelial cells) with infiltration of the lamina propria (e-**Fig. 13.14**), features that should be present away from lymphoid follicles. Conditions that are associated with increased intraepithelial lymphocytes in the stomach include *H. pylori* gastritis, celiac disease, syphilis, Ménétrier's disease, and Crohn's disease, all of which should be considered secondary gastric epithelial lymphocytosis.

3. **Collagenous gastritis** is an exceedingly rare diagnosis that has been associated with celiac disease and collagenous colitis in some patient populations. Histologically, it is similar to the large intestinal counterpart with a subepithelial collagen layer exceeding 10 μm in thickness, which may be patchy (e-**Fig. 13.15**).

4. **Eosinophilic gastritis** is usually associated with eosinophilic gastroenteritis. Peripheral eosinophilia may be present. Presenting symptoms vary depending on which layers of the bowel wall are involved; while mucosal involvement is most common, the process can involve any layer of the bowel wall, and the diagnosis may therefore be missed on endoscopic mucosal biopsy. Mucosal involvement is characterized by a prominent eosinophilic infiltrate with cryptitis and crypt abscesses (e-**Fig. 13.16**). However, it is important to exclude certain medications as well as inflammatory and infectious conditions such as Crohn's disease and parasitic infection, which can also result in eosinophilic infiltrates.

5. **Granulomatous gastritis.** Granulomas in gastric mucosal biopsies are not specific findings. Although they may be associated with gastric involvement in Crohn's disease (e-Fig. 13.17), they can also be found in a number of other conditions including sarcoidosis, infections, foreign/endogenous material, and less commonly with vasculitis or xanthogranulomatosis.

6. **Infectious gastritis.** A number of bacterial (e.g., mycobacteria, *Treponema pallidum*), viral (e.g., cytomegalovirus, Epstein–Barr virus), fungal (e.g., *Candida, Histoplasma, Mucoraceae*), and rarely parasitic (e.g., *Cryptosporidium, Giardia, Strongyloides, Anisakis*) organisms can infect the stomach (e-Figs. 13.18 and 13.19). Some of these infections can be associated with eosinophilic infiltrates and granulomas.

7. **Ischemic gastritis.** As the stomach has a rich vascular supply from five arteries, ischemic gastritis is very rare. It can be seen in the setting of hypoperfusion with findings of erosion, hemorrhage, necrosis, or ulceration (e-Fig. 13.20).

8. **Graft versus host disease (GVHD)** in the stomach, as in other parts of the gastrointestinal (GI) tract, shows gland apoptosis and destruction (e-Fig. 13.21).

B. Miscellaneous conditions

1. **Foveolar hyperplasia** is not a specific finding. It may be seen in antral biopsies of chronic gastritis and is characterized by edematous, elongated, villiform foveolar lining of the mucosa (e-Fig. 13.22).

2. **Reactive or chemical gastropathy** is characterized by foveolar hyperplasia with tortuous gland outlines and smooth muscle fibers within the lamina propria (e-Fig. 13.23). Although focal activity may be present, inflammation is typically mild to absent. However, these histologic features are nonspecific and can also be associated with bile reflux or with medications, particularly nonsteroidal anti-inflammatory drugs (NSAIDs), which can also cause erosions.

3. **Ménétrier's disease** is endoscopically characterized by giant gastric folds mainly involving the body and fundus. The histologic findings include marked foveolar hyperplasia and glandular atrophy (loss of oxyntic mucosa in the body and fundus), and may be reminiscent of hyperplastic polyps (HPs). Clinically, patients present with protein-losing gastropathy and low acid production.

4. **Parietal cell hyperplasia** due to PPI use or Zollinger–Ellison (ZE) syndrome presents secondary to hypergastrinemia, with an increase in size and number of parietal cells resulting in enlarged mucosal folds in the body and fundus (e-Fig. 13.24). Parietal cells can be found as high as the junction with the foveolar epithelium. Some of the glands may be cystically dilated reminiscent of fundic gland polyps. Foveolar hyperplasia is absent. Hypergastrinemia also causes endocrine cell hyperplasia and can result in neuroendocrine tumors (NETs). The final distinction of PPI use or ZE syndrome is based on the clinical setting.

5. **Gastric antral vascular ectasia,** also known as watermelon stomach because of its endoscopic appearance, is characterized by dilatation of mucosal capillaries in the gastric antrum with or without fibrin thrombi (e-Fig. 13.25), with associated mucosal smooth muscle fibers. Similar changes can be seen in portal hypertension. However, portal hypertensive gastropathy involves the body and fundus and does not classically show fibrin thrombi.

6. **Mucosal calcinosis.** Calcifications are usually found incidentally in mucosal biopsies from patients with renal failure or in organ transplant recipients (e-Fig. 13.26).

7. **Pseudomelanosis** results from iron deposition in mucosa in patients taking ferrous sulfate (surface mucosa) or in patients with hemochromatosis (full

thickness or deep) (e-**Figs. 13.27** and **13.28**). In iron pill gastritis, there may be mild inflammation or erosions (e-**Fig. 13.29**).

8. **Xanthelasma or xanthoma** is characterized by collections of lipid-laden foamy macrophages in the lamina propria and is significant for its potential confusion with poorly differentiated signet ring cell adenocarcinoma on biopsy (e-**Fig. 13.30**). In problematic cases, the diagnosis can be clarified with IHC stains; positivity for pan-cytokeratins and CDX2 is seen in most adenocarcinomas, whereas positivity for CD68 and CD163 would favor xanthoma.

IV. DIAGNOSTIC FEATURES OF COMMON GASTRIC POLYPS

A. **Hyperplastic Polyps (HPs)** are composed of elongated, dilated, branching foveola in association with inflamed, edematous lamina propria. These polyps can show surface erosions, regenerative changes, and intestinal metaplasia (e-**Fig. 13.31**). In addition, foci of dysplasia or invasive carcinoma are present in ~2% of HPs. The likelihood of these findings increases with polyp size, especially in those >2 cm. HPs may occur in a subset of patients with Osler–Weber–Rendu syndrome.

B. **Fundic gland polyps** are composed of cystically dilated spaces partially lined by parietal cells which may be hyperplastic or attenuated (e-**Fig. 13.32**). They can be syndromic, where they represent the most common gastric lesion of familial adenomatous polyposis (FAP), or sporadic. A significant proportion of syndromic fundic gland polyps are associated with low grade or indefinite dysplasia. However, high-grade dysplasia and invasive carcinoma are exceedingly rare. Sporadic fundic gland polyps are sometimes associated with PPI treatment for gastroesophageal reflux.

C. **Inflammatory fibroid polyp (IFP)** is most commonly found in the gastric antrum and consists of a submucosal collection of bland spindle cells, which are characteristically CD34 positive and c-kit negative, in a background of dilated vascular channels and mixed inflammation, which often contains abundant eosinophils (e-**Figs. 13.33** to **13.35**).

D. **Hamartomatous polyps** can be seen in patients with Peutz–Jeghers syndrome, juvenile polyposis, and Cowden's disease. The histologic features of many of these polyps may be reminiscent of hyperplastic gastric polyps.

V. DIAGNOSTIC FEATURES OF COMMON NEOPLASMS OF THE STOMACH. The World Health Organization (WHO) histologic classification of gastric tumors is given in Table 13.2. The American Joint Committee on Cancer (AJCC) staging schema is given in Table 13.3. Molecular tests used in the work-up of stomach specimens are listed in Table 13.4.

A. **Adenoma and dysplasia.** Unlike colonic adenomas, most gastric adenomas are not sporadic but rather arise in the setting of chronic gastric injury. Adenoma and dysplasia are distinguished by architecture: polypoid = adenoma, flat = dysplasia. Both can contain either low-grade (e-**Fig. 13.36**) or high-grade dysplasia (e-**Fig. 13.37**) defined by cytologic features and architectural complexity.

There are three types of stomach adenomas: intestinal type (e-**Fig. 13.38**), resembling those in the colon and containing goblet cells and/or Paneth cells, and two gastric types, foveolar- and pyloric-type adenomas. Foveolar-type adenomas are composed of foveolar epithelial cells containing neutral mucin with apical mucin caps, stain positively for MUC5AC, and are sometimes associated with FAP. Pyloric gland adenomas are composed of tightly packed pyloric gland-type tubules with a single layer of cuboidal to low columnar epithelium that shows round nuclei and pale to eosinophilic ground glass cytoplasm, and that stains for MUC5AC and MUC6 (e-**Fig. 13.39**). Pyloric gland adenomas have been shown to occur more commonly in women and are more frequently associated with autoimmune atrophic gastritis (*Am J Surg Pathol.* 2009;33:186; *Virchows Arch.* 2003;442:317). Pyloric gland adenomas, as is the case with intestinal-type adenomas, are also associated with a higher rate of dysplasia and malignant transformation than gastric foveolar-type adenomas (*Am J Surg Pathol.* 2002;26:1276).

| TABLE 13.2 | WHO Histologic Classification of Gastric Tumors |

Epithelial tumors

Premalignant lesions

Adenoma

Intraepithelial neoplasia (dysplasia), low grade

Intraepithelial neoplasia (dysplasia), high grade

Carcinoma

Adenocarcinoma

   Papillary adenocarcinoma

   Tubular adenocarcinoma

   Mucinous adenocarcinoma

   Poorly cohesive carcinoma (including signet ring cell carcinoma and other variants)

   Mixed adenocarcinoma

Adenosquamous carcinoma

Carcinoma with lymphoid stroma (medullary carcinoma)

Hepatoid carcinoma

Squamous cell carcinoma

Undifferentiated carcinoma

Neuroendocrine neoplasms

Neuroendocrine tumor (NET)

   NET G1 (carcinoid)

   NET G2

Neuroendocrine carcinoma (NEC)

   Large cell NEC

   Small cell NEC

Mixed adenoneuroendocrine carcinoma

EC cell, serotonin-producing NET

Gastrin-producing NET (gastrinoma)

Mesenchymal tumors

Glomus tumor

Granular cell tumor

Leiomyoma

Plexiform fibromyxoma

Gastrointestinal stromal tumor

Kaposi sarcoma

Leiomyosarcoma

Synovial sarcoma

Lymphomas

Secondary tumors

From: Bosman FT, Carneiro F, Hruban RH, Theise ND, eds. *World Health Organization Classification of Tumours of the Digestive System.* Lyon: IARC Press; 2010. Used with permission.

B. **Adenocarcinoma of the stomach.** Gastric adenocarcinomas have classically been divided according to the Lauren classification into intestinal and diffuse types. Intestinal-type adenocarcinomas resemble colorectal carcinoma in their glandular pattern and may be exophytic or ulcerated. Diffuse-type adenocarcinomas are characterized by relatively diffuse growth of loosely cohesive tumor cells without clear gland formation, as is seen in linitis plastica. In many cases, the cells of diffuse-type gastric adenocarcinoma are of the signet ring morphology (e-**Figs 13.40** and **13.41**). Adenocarcinomas arising in the gastric cardia have

TABLE 13.3	Tumor, Node, Metastasis (TNM) Staging Scheme for Gastric Carcinoma

Primary tumor (T)

TX	Primary tumor cannot be assessed
T0	No evidence of primary tumor
Tis	Carcinoma in situ: intraepithelial tumor without invasion of the lamina propria
T1	Tumor invades lamina propria, muscularis mucosae or submucosa
T1a	Tumor invades lamina propria or muscularis mucosae
T1b	Tumor invades submucosa
T2	Tumor invades muscularis propria[a]
T3	Tumor penetrates subserosal connective tissue without invasion of visceral peritoneum or adjacent structures[b,c]
T4	Tumor invades serosa (visceral peritoneum) or adjacent structures[b,c]
T4a	Tumor invades serosa (visceral peritoneum)
T4b	Tumor invades adjacent structures

Regional lymph nodes (N)

NX	Regional lymph nodes cannot be assessed
N0	No regional lymph node metastasis[d]
N1	Metastasis in 1–2 regional lymph nodes
N2	Metastasis in 3–6 regional lymph nodes
N3	Metastasis in seven or more regional lymph nodes
N3a	Metastasis in 7–15 lymph nodes
N3b	Metastasis in 16 or more regional lymph nodes

Distant metastasis (M)

MX	Distant metastasis cannot be assessed
M0	No distant metastasis
M1	Distant metastasis

STAGE GROUPING

Stage 0	Tis	N0	M0	Stage IIIA	T4a	N1	M0
Stage IA	T1	N0	M0		T3	N2	M0
Stage IB	T2	N0	M0		T2	N3	M0
	T1	N1	M0	Stage IIIB	T4b	N0	M0
Stage IIA	T3	N0	M0		T4b	N1	M0
	T2	N1	M0		T4a	N2	M0
	T1	N2	M0		T3	N3	M0
Stage IIB	T4a	N0	M0	Stage IIIC	T4b	N2	M0
	T3	N1	M0		T4b	N3	M0
	T2	N2	M0		T4a	N3	M0
	T1	N3	M0	Stage IV	Any T	Any N	M1

[a]A tumor may penetrate the muscularis propria with extension into the gastrocolic or gastrohepatic ligaments, or into the greater or lesser omentum, without perforation of the visceral peritoneum covering these structures. In this case, the tumor is classified as T3. If there is perforation of the visceral peritoneum covering the gastric ligaments or the omentum, the tumor should be classified T4.
[b]The adjacent structures of the stomach include the spleen, transverse colon, liver, diaphragm, pancreas, abdominal wall, adrenal gland, kidney, small intestine, and retroperitoneum.
[c]Intramural extension to the duodenum or esophagus is classified by the depth of the greatest invasion in any of these sites, including the stomach.
[d]A designation of pN0 should be used if all examined lymph nodes are negative, regardless of the total number removed and examined.
From: Edge SB, Byrd DR, Compton CC, et al., eds. *AJCC Cancer Staging Manual.* 7th ed. New York, NY: Springer; 2010. Used with permission.

TABLE 13.4	Molecular Testing Performed in Evaluation of Stomach Specimens
Test	**Purpose**
GIST *c-kit/PDGFRA* mutation analysis	Confirm diagnosis in problematic cases. Certain mutations provide prognostic information regarding expected response to treatment and prognosis.
Microsatellite instability testing	Identify patients with HNPCC and associated cancer risks.
HER-2 testing by IHC or FISH	In gastric adenocarcinoma to predict response to trastuzumab in addition to standard chemotherapy
Kras mutation analysis	Treatment planning in patients with metastatic disease
E-cadherin mutation analysis	Evaluate for HDGC in patient's meeting criteria who may be candidates for prophylactic gastrectomy.

GIST, gastrointestinal stroma tumor; PDGFRA, platelet-derived growth factor alpha; IHC, immunohistochemistry; FISH, fluorescent in situ hybridization; HNPCC, hereditary nonpolyposis colon cancer; HDGC, hereditary Diffuse Gastric Cancer.

been shown to behave more like esophageal adenocarcinomas arising in the gastroesophageal junction, as reflected in the AJCC staging system.

The molecular/genetic events that lead to intestinal-type gastric carcinogenesis involve a complex interplay between host factors and environmental factors, including *H. pylori* infection and other inflammatory conditions. A number of genetic alterations have been described, many with unclear significance. In general, adenocarcinomas occur in older patients associated with atrophic gastritis, intestinal metaplasia, and dysplasia. HER2 is upregulated in up to 34% of gastric tumors, which has led to clinical trials showing that trastuzumab (Herceptin) in addition to standard chemotherapy improves overall survival in HER2-positive tumors (*Lancet.* 2010;376:687).

In contrast, diffuse-type gastric cancers tend to occur in younger patients and involve mutations affecting E-cadherin (kindreds with familial diffuse-type gastric adenocarcinomas harbor E-cadherin mutations).

C. **NETs.** Gastric NETs have been divided into groups based on etiology. Type I gastric NETs occur in the setting of chronic atrophic gastritis (e-**Fig. 13.42**), in which hypergastrinemia induces ECL cell hyperplasia. The cutoff between nodular ECL hyperplasia and gastric NET is 0.5 mm, although tumors associated with metastasis to lymph nodes or liver are generally >1 cm in size. However, in the setting of Type I gastric NET, the prognosis is excellent even in the presence of metastasis. Type II gastric NETs occur in association with ZE syndrome and almost always in patients with multiple endocrine neoplasia (MEN) Type I. Finally, Type III gastric NETs are sporadic and the most aggressive gastric NETs (e-**Fig. 13.43**).

Histologically, gastric NETs are similar to NETs arising at other GI sites with microglandular, ribbonlike, trabecular, or insular growth patterns and finely granular chromatin, and are graded using the same criteria (e-**Fig. 13.44**). The diagnosis is confirmed with IHC stains for neuroendocrine markers. Table 13.5 contains the AJCC staging system for gastric NETs.

D. **Gastrointestinal stromal tumors (GIST).** The stomach is the most common site for GISTs (60% of cases are gastric), and tumors occurring in the stomach overall tend to behave more indolently than those in the remainder of the GI tract. The tumors are typically relatively well-circumscribed and centered in the submucosa. On cut surface, they are typically tan-white to pink and may show foci of hemorrhage, central cystic degeneration, or necrosis. Morphologically, GISTs are divided into spindle cell (70%) (e-**Fig. 13.45**), epithelioid (20%) (e-**Fig. 13.46**), and mixed types (10%). With treatment, the tumors may

TABLE 13.5	Tumor, Node, Metastasis (TNM) Staging Scheme for Gastric Neuroendocrine Tumors

Primary tumor (T)

TX	Primary tumor cannot be assessed
T0	No evidence of primary tumor
Tis	Carcinoma in situ/dysplasia (tumor size <0.5 mm), confined to mucosa
T1	Tumor invades lamina propria or submucosa and ≤1 cm in size
T2	Tumor invades muscularis propria or >1 cm in size
T3	Tumor penetrates subserosa
T4	Tumor invades visceral peritoneum (serosal) or other organs or adjacent structures
	For any T, add (m) for multiple tumors

Regional lymph nodes (N)

NX	Regional lymph nodes cannot be assessed
N0	No regional lymph node metastasis
N1	Regional lymph node metastasis

Distant metastasis (M)

M0	No distant metastasis
M1	Distant metastasis

Stage grouping

Stage 0	Tis	N0	M0
Stage I	T1	N0	M0
Stage IIA	T2	N0	M0
Stage IIB	T3	N0	M0
Stage IIIA	T4	N0	M0
Stage IIIB	Any T	N1	M0
Stage IV	Any T	Any N	M1

From: Edge SB, Byrd DR, Compton CC, et al., eds. *AJCC Cancer Staging Manual.* 7th ed. New York, NY: Springer; 2010. Used with permission.

develop decreased cellularity, sclerosis, and myxoid changes (e-**Fig. 13.47**). The differential diagnosis of GIST varies depending on the predominant pattern but includes neural tumors, sarcomatoid carcinoma, tumors of fibrohistiocytic origin, smooth muscle tumors, and other soft tissue tumors (e-**Figs. 13.48** and **13.49**). Immunohistochemically, 95% of GISTs express c-kit (CD117); however, the pattern of staining may be membranous (e-**Fig. 13.50**), cytoplasmic (e-**Fig. 13.51**), or cytoplasmic dot-like (e-**Fig. 13.52**). Approximately 5% of GISTs are c-kit negative by IHC, the majority of which are gastric GISTs with an epithelioid morphology. Other markers which may be positive in GIST include CD34 (80% of gastric GIST), smooth muscle actin (30%), and desmin (5%). Expression of cytokeratin or S-100 is rare in GIST. DOG1 is a promising sensitive and specific marker for GIST, and has been shown to stain up to a third of c-kit negative GISTs. In the end, however, a small percentage of tumors morphologically compatible with GIST remain difficult to characterize by IHC. It is important to note that tumors that are c-kit negative by IHC may still respond to tyrosine kinase inhibitor (TKI) therapy.

The role of molecular testing in GIST remains undefined. The most commonly mutated gene is *c-kit*; mutations of *platelet-derived growth factor alpha (PDGFRA)* are less common. Together, mutations in *c-kit* or *PDGFRA* are present in 85% of GISTs. The mutations are tyrosine kinase activating

TABLE 13.6	Proposed Guidelines for Assessing the Malignant Potential of Gastric GISTs

Tumor	Predicted biologic behavior
≤2 cm, ≤5 mitoses/50 HPFs	Benign, metastasis rate or tumor-related mortality: 0
>2 ≤10 cm, ≤5 mitoses/50 HPFs	Very low malignant potential, metastasis rate or tumor-related mortality: <3%
>10 cm, ≤5 mitoses/50 HPFs, or ≤5 cm, >5 mitoses/50 HPFs	Low to moderate malignant potential, metastasis rate or tumor-related mortality: 12–15%
>5 cm, >5 mitoses/50 HPFs	High malignant potential, metastasis rate or tumor-related mortality: 49–86%

GISTs, gastrointestinal stromal tumors; HPFs, high-power fields.

mutations, which stimulate downstream events that regulate cell proliferation, adhesion, motility, and survival. Studies have shown varying responses to the TKI imatinib based on mutation status; *c-kit* exon 11 mutations predict better response rates, *PDGFRA* exon 18 mutants show primary resistance, and other *c-kit* and *PDGFRA* mutants fall in between.

Individuals with familial *c-kit* mutations develop GISTs at a slightly younger age and may have multifocal disease. GIST can also be seen in patients with Carney triad/dyad and neurofibromatosis Type I, and these tumors tend to be

TABLE 13.7	Tumor, Node, Metastasis (TNM) Staging Scheme for Gastric GIST

Primary tumor (T)

TX	Primary tumor cannot be assessed
T0	No evidence of primary tumor
T1	Tumor 2 cm or less
T2	Tumor >2 cm but not >5 cm
T3	Tumor >5 cm but not >10 cm
T4	Tumor >10 cm in greatest dimension

Regional lymph nodes (N)

NX	Regional lymph nodes cannot be assessed
N0	No regional lymph node metastasis
N1	Regional lymph node metastasis

Distant metastasis (M)

M0	No distant metastasis
M1	Distant metastasis

Stage grouping				Mitotic rate
Stage IA	T1 or T2	N0	M0	Low
Stage IB	T3	N0	M0	Low
Stage II	T1	N0	M0	High
	T2	N0	M0	High
	T4	N0	M0	Low
Stage IIIA	T3	N0	M0	High
Stage IIIB	T4	N0	M0	High
Stage IV	Any T	N1	M0	Any rate
	Any T	N0	M1	Any rate

Low mitotic rate: 5 or fewer per 50 HPFs; High mitotic rate: over 5 per 50 HPFs.
From: Edge SB, Byrd DR, Compton CC, et al., eds. *AJCC Cancer Staging Manual.* 7th ed. New York, NY: Springer; 2010. Used with permission.

c-kit mutation negative. Pediatric GISTs, though often show positive for c-kit expression by IHC, also tend to be *c-kit* mutation negative.

Many gastric GISTs behave in an overall indolent manner, and those <2 cm are almost universally benign. However, GISTs do have a propensity to metastasize, which can occur even 10 to 20 years after initial surgery. A number of nomograms have been developed to risk stratify GIST, and proposed guidelines based on a study of >1500 gastric GISTs with long-term follow-up are listed in Table 13.6 (*Am J Surg Pathol.* 2005;29:52). The AJCC staging for gastric GISTs is in Table 13.7.

E. **Marginal zone B-cell lymphoma of mucosa-associated lymphoid tissue (MALT) type** is an extranodal lymphoma composed of morphologically heterogeneous small B-cells (e-**Fig. 13.53**). Up to one-third of gastric MALTs may show plasmacytoid differentiation. The GI tract is the most common site for MALT lymphoma (50% of cases) and the stomach is the most common GI site (85% of cases).

Table 13.8 describes characteristics useful in distinguishing MALT lymphoma from chronic gastritis (e-**Fig. 13.54**). Gastric MALT lymphomas are typically positive for CD20 (e-**Fig. 13.55**), CD79a, CD21, and CD35, but negative for CD5, CD10, and CD23. Some gastric MALT lymphomas are CD43 positive (e-**Fig. 13.56**). Demonstration of light chain restriction is helpful in discriminating MALT lymphoma from reactive lesions. Gastric MALT lymphomas have been associated with *H. pylori* infection; however, the chance of detecting *H. pylori* decreases with progression to lymphoma, and some seropositive individuals will be negative for *H. pylori* in histopathologic studies. The

TABLE 13.8	Comparison of Histologic Features Between MALT Lymphoma and Chronic Gastritis	
Histologic feature	**MALT lymphoma**	**Chronic gastritis**
Lymphoid follicle	Frequent	May be present
Follicular colonization	May be present	Absent
Interfollicular lymphocytes	Small to intermediate in size, irregular nuclear contour, monocytoid	Small and round, mature
B lymphocytes (positive for CD20)	Predominant, present in lymphoid follicles and interfollicular spaces, may coexpress CD43	Sparse, usually limited to lymphoid follicles, do not coexpress CD43
T lymphocytes (positive for CD3)	Variable in number, scattered	Predominant, diffusely involve the lamina propria and interfollicular spaces
Plasma cells	Variable in number, usually seen beneath the surface lining epithelium, show light chain restriction	Usually prominent, diffusely present in the lamina propria, lack light chain restriction
Lymphoepithelial lesion	Usually prominent, the infiltrative lymphoid cells are B cells and form clusters, glandular destruction evident	Rare and inconspicuous, the infiltrative lymphoid cells are T cells and individually distributed, glandular destruction not evident
Helicobacter pylori microorganisms	May be present	May be present
Infiltration of muscularis mucosae by lymphoid cells	May be present	Absent

MALT, mucosa-associated lymphoid tissue.

most common recurrent cytogenetic abnormality in gastric MALT is t(11;18), which has also been associated with resistance to *H. pylori* eradication therapy. MALT lymphomas tend to be indolent, slow to disseminate, and responsive to radiation therapy. Even involvement of multiple sites and the bone marrow do not portend a worse prognosis. However, if solid areas or sheets of large cells are present, the tumor is more appropriately diagnosed as diffuse large B-cell lymphoma.

Cytopathology of the Stomach

Julie Elizabeth Kunkel

I. **INTRODUCTION.** The indications for cytologic sampling of the stomach include the presence of an inflammatory process or a neoplasm. Mucosal lesions can be sampled by endoscopic brushing cytology, and intramural lesions by endoscopic ultrasound-guided fine needle aspiration (EUS-FNA). Brushing cytology for malignancy has a sensitivity of 85% to 93% and a specificity of 99%, both comparable to the sensitivity and specificity of endoscopic biopsy. However, brushing cytology and biopsy are best considered complementary for detection of malignancy (*Acta Cytol.* 1988;32:461; *Acta Cytol.* 1990;34:217). EUS-FNA for malignancy has a lower sensitivity and specificity (*Gastroenterology.* 1997;112:1087), which most likely reflects limitations of the technique due to inadequate sampling.

II. **INFLAMMATORY PROCESSES.** Antral mucosa brushing cytology with Papanicolaou stain is a sensitive, accurate, and simple procedure for investigating the presence of *H. pylori* infection in cases of gastritis. The bacteria presents as curved and S-shaped rods with basophilic staining properties (*World J Gastroenterol.* 2005;11: 2784).

III. **NEOPLASMS**

   A. **Adenocarcinoma.**

   1. The smear of **intestinal-type adenocarcinoma** is hypercellular, consisting of haphazardly arranged three-dimensional cell groups and atypical single cells. The malignant cells show nuclear enlargement, hyperchromasia, and irregular nuclear membrane contours (**e-Fig. 13.57**). A necrotic, dirty background is often present.

   2. The cytologic diagnosis of **diffuse-type adenocarcinoma** is difficult due to scarcity of the malignant cells; when present, the characteristic signet ring cells demonstrate an intracytoplasmic vacuole that indents the nucleus into a concave shape (**e-Fig. 13.58**), with associated nuclear hyperchromasia. The differential diagnosis of the atypical cells in diffuse-type adenocarcinoma includes histiocytes and goblet cells (*Diagn Cytopathol.* 2006;34:177).

   B. **Gastrointestinal stromal tumor (GIST).** The smear shows microfragments and sheets of spindle cells with moderate to high cellularity (**e-Fig. 13.59**), intact single spindle cells, and abundant stripped nuclei. The spindle cells have spindle to oval nuclei, fine chromatin, and abundant delicate cytoplasm with indistinct borders (**e-Fig. 13.60**). Nuclear atypia, mitosis, and necrosis may be identified occasionally. The epithelioid variant demonstrates large epithelioid cells with round nuclei and distinct cell borders. GIST cannot be graded based on cytologic specimens. Immunostains are required for a definitive diagnosis to exclude other submucosal spindle cell neoplasms that possess similar cytomorphology (*Cancer.* 2001;93:269; *Am J Clin Pathol.* 2003;119:703).

   C. **Neuroendocrine Tumor G1 (Carcinoid).** The cytomorphology of carcinoid tumor (low-grade neuroendocrine carcinoma) is identical to that of the tumor at other sites. The smears are cellular and composed of loosely cohesive clusters and isolated cells with characteristic salt-and-pepper chromatin. Focal and variable endocrine atypia are easily identified.

D. Malignant lymphoma. The cytomorphology varies among the subtypes of gastric lymphoma. In general, the smears show isolated lymphoid cells exhibiting different degrees of atypia and monotony (the detailed cytomorphology of different lymphomas is discussed in the cytology section of Chap. 43). Precise diagnosis and classification require ancillary studies, which can be applied to EUS-FNA material (*Acta Cytol.* 1994;38:169).

14

The Intestines, Appendix, and Anus

ILKe Nalbantoglu and Elizabeth M. Brunt

I. NORMAL ANATOMY

A. The small intestine is 6 to 7 m long and divided into the duodenum, jejunum, and ileum. It begins at the distal gastric pylorus and ends at the ileocecal valve and is lined throughout its length by villous mucosa. The individual villus is a slender, fingerlike projection with a variable length-to-crypt ratio ranging from 3:1 to 5:1 (**e-Fig. 14.1**).* The epithelium consists predominantly of tall, columnar absorptive cells that have basally situated nuclei, eosinophilic cytoplasm, and an apical brush border. The absorptive cells rest on a visible, refractile terminal bar. Other cell types of the intestine include goblet cells, crypt cells, basal cells, Paneth cells, and endocrine cells; the granules of Paneth cells are refractile, eosinophilic, and supranuclear, whereas those of endocrine cells are smaller, eosinophilic but nonrefractile, and infranuclear. The lamina propria contains mixed inflammatory cells including plasma cells, although neutrophils are restricted to vascular channels. Peyer's patches, which are lymphoid aggregates, are distributed throughout the small intestine mucosa. Intraepithelial lymphocytes (IELs) are normally rare (no more than one per five enterocytes at the tips of the villi), although an increased IEL density may be seen in epithelium overlying lymphoid aggregates or Peyer's patches in the distal ileum where the associated villi may be shortened or even flattened. Shortened and broadened villi may also be seen in duodenal mucosa overlying Brunner's glands.

B. The large intestine, or colon, is 1 to 1.5 m long and consists of the right and left colon. The right colon is further subdivided into the cecum, ascending, and proximal transverse colon; the left colon consists of the distal transverse, descending, and sigmoid colon, and the rectum. The mucosa contains evenly spaced, nonbranching crypts arranged perpendicularly to the lumen and extending from the surface to the muscularis mucosae (**e-Fig. 14.2**). Occasional branching crypts or slight crypt architectural distortion may be seen in the rectum and sigmoid colon, and in areas adjacent to lymphoid aggregates. Paneth cells may be seen until the mid-transverse colon and, as noted earlier, IELs can be prominent in epithelium overlying lymphoid aggregates. However, there are no villi, the lining epithelium has no microvilli and does not rest on a terminal bar, and goblet cells are more numerous (particularly in the left colon). The lamina propria components are similar to those of the small intestine, although the lamina propria is denser in the right colon, and muciphages (mucin-containing macrophages) are more common in the lamina propria of the left colon.

The entire small and large bowel mucosa rest on muscularis mucosae. This smooth muscle layer delineates the lamina propria from the submucosa which comprises loose fatty tissue with a rich angiolymphatic supply. The inner and outer layers of the muscularis propria lie below the submucosa and are separated by the ganglio-neuronal Auerbach plexus. The entire surface of the

---

*All e-figures are available online via the Solution Site Image Bank.

intestines is covered by visceral peritoneum (serosa) up to the distal portion of the rectum.

C. **The appendix** is a tubular organ that extends from the cecum. It has an average length of 7 to 10 cm and has a mucosa that is similar to the large intestine, except for the presence of more prominent lymphoid aggregates which often have well-formed germinal centers. The appendix also has a poorly developed muscularis mucosae that may be interrupted by lymphoid aggregates.

D. **The anal canal,** the terminal 3 to 4 cm of the gastrointestinal (GI) tract, is an anatomically complex area (**e-Fig. 14.3**). This chapter employs the surgical anal canal terminology as defined by the most current WHO classification of tumors (discussed later). The mucosa lining the upper portion of the anal canal is a direct extension of the rectal mucosa (colorectal mucosa). The mucosa lining the middle portion of the anal canal (the so-called anal transitional zone (ATZ), a 0.5- to 1-cm segment above the dentate line) has the features of both metaplastic squamous mucosa and urothelium. Submucosal and intramuscular anal glands open into the ATZ via anal ducts that are also lined by ATZ epithelium. The mucosa of the distal anal canal, which extends from the dentate line to the anal verge, consists of specialized nonkeratinizing squamous mucosa with melanocytes. It is distinguished from the perianal skin by the lack of skin appendages.

II. GROSS EXAMINATION AND SPECIMEN HANDLING

A. **Endoscopic biopsy.** When processing the specimen, it is important to record pertinent clinical history and endoscopic findings. Biopsies are typically small fragments of mucosal tissue in the range of 1 to 5 mm in greatest dimension that do not need to be inked or subdivided. Important gross descriptors are the number, size, and the size range of the biopsy fragments. In cases where numerous fragments are present, an estimate for the number and the dimensions in aggregate should be given (documentation of the number and size is important to ensure that the biopsies are adequately represented on the slides). Routine microscopic examination of endoscopic biopsies usually entails examination of three hematoxylin and eosin (H&E)-stained levels.

B. **Suction biopsy** of the rectum, which makes possible sampling of the submucosa, is used for evaluation of Hirschsprung's disease. After processing, the tissue is serially sectioned in its entirety, but initially only every third level is H&E-stained; if no ganglion cells are identified in these slides, the remaining sections are stained and examined. In some labs, frozen sections are performed for histochemical staining by the acetylcholinesterase reaction to identify proliferating nerve fibers in the lamina propria and muscularis mucosae.

C. **Polypectomy specimens** should be described and measured. The need for inking of the resection margin is a controversial topic; in practice, it is often difficult to do since the stalk retracts and thus may be hard to identify grossly (although the cauterized base can be easily identified microscopically). The specimen is bisected or serially sectioned depending on its size, and entirely submitted. Sectioning should follow the vertical plane of the stalk to maximize the evaluation of the polypectomy margin. At least three H&E levels are examined.

D. **Endoscopic mucosal resections** can be single or multiple fragments. All dimensions are recorded and the mucosal surface described. Inking of the margins is a matter of choice since cautery artifact will be noted at the time of microscopic evaluation for deep and mucosal margins, and since ink may actually artifactually extend along non-marginal mucosa. The entire specimen is serially sectioned, and the fragments are oriented and entirely submitted.

E. **Bowel resection.**

1. **Neoplastic.** Tumor resections include segmental resection of a portion of small or large bowel, ileocolectomy, low anterior resection (LAR), abdominoperineal resection (APR), total colectomy, and total mesorectal

excision (TME). The portion of resected bowel is oriented, and the length, diameter (or circumference), and wall thickness are measured. The length and diameter of the appendix and the dimensions of mesentery are also measured, if present. The external surface (serosa in most cases) of the bowel is inspected for tumor involvement, perforation, adhesion, and fat wrapping. For TME specimens, the grossly observable completeness of the mesorectum is evaluated as "complete," "near complete," or "incomplete" before opening the bowel (see College of American Pathologists Cancer Protocols for Colon and Rectum at www.cap.org). The bowel is opened longitudinally along the antimesenteric border, unless this would mean cutting through the tumor.

The maximal size of the tumor and the distance to the proximal and distal resection margins, or to the closest margin in unoriented specimens, are documented. After fresh tissue is collected for biobanking (as needed), the specimen is pinned out on a wax board (mucosal side up) and fixed by submerging in 10% formalin overnight. The tumor is then sectioned to assess the depth of invasion; blocks for microscopic examination are taken to include the area of deepest penetration and the relationship to adjacent, grossly nonneoplastic mucosa. Additional sections include proximal and distal resection margins; if tumor approximates the margin, such as in APR or LAR specimens, the margin should be inked and multiple sections perpendicular to the margin submitted; if the inked radial margin is not included in the tumor sections, one separate radial margin section should be submitted. One random section from normal-appearing bowel, and sections from any additional gross lesions (such as separate polyps), should also be submitted. If the appendix is present, it is handled as an appendectomy specimen as described later.

The mesentery and soft tissue are also dissected for lymph nodes (many nodes are located along large vessels), and the number and size range of identified nodes are recorded. Small lymph nodes can be submitted in toto without sectioning. Larger nodes are serially sectioned and the cut surfaces examined; if metastatic carcinoma is grossly appreciated, as evidenced by a white and hard cut surface, the size of the metastatic deposit should be recorded, and one representative section from each grossly positive node should be submitted. If the cut surfaces of the nodes are tan, soft, homogeneous, and lack gross evidence of metastasis, the entire node should be submitted for microscopic evaluation. Although a minimum of 12 nodes is required by established staging criteria, all nodes that can be found should be submitted. Fewer nodes may be acceptable for small specimens, for cases that have received preoperative chemoradiation, and for APR or LAR specimens (because lymph nodes are less numerous below the peritoneal reflection). However, when fewer than 12 nodes are identified, a second attempt to dissect lymph nodes is strongly recommended (and should be documented in the pathology report).

2. **Nontumor bowel resections**
   a. For **polyposis** specimens, pinning and gross examination are similar as for tumor specimens. Sampling focuses on the largest lesions, lesions with a distinct or worrisome gross appearance (including firmness, ulceration, and adherence to the wall), and flat and depressed areas of mucosa.
   b. Resections for **inflammatory bowel disease** (IBD), particularly for ulcerative colitis (UC), require sequential sections spaced every 10 cm. The sections include transition regions between normal-appearing and diseased segments, distal and proximal margins, and representative inflammatory polyps. Any focal lesions (such as areas with raised mucosa), fistula tracts, and strictures are sampled. The appendix, if present, is handled

as an appendectomy specimen, as described later. Representative lymph nodes are submitted, but there is no need for extensive sampling unless a carcinoma is suspected or identified.

c. **Miscellaneous resections.** In the case of ischemic necrosis, the mesenteric vessels should be carefully examined and sampled to evaluate the possibility of thrombosis, embolization, or vasculitis. For penetrating traumatic injuries, inspection for possible entry and exit wound sites is important. It is also important to grossly and microscopically examine the proximal and distal resection margins for tissue viability.

When proctectomy or rectosigmoid resection is performed for Hirschsprung's disease, the distal margin is usually indicated by the surgeon. Sequential sections every 1 to 2 cm from distal to proximal should be submitted to achieve an accurate estimation of the aganglionic region.

F. For **appendectomy** specimens, the length, diameter, surface appearance, and dimensions of the specimen, including the mesoappendix, are recorded. For a nonneoplastic appendix, one half of the longitudinally bisected tip, the proximal margin, and two cross-sections are submitted in a single cassette, to include the mid-portion and any possible perforation. For a neoplastic appendix, after photography and gross description, the specimen is bread loafed and submitted in its entirety. In cases of pseudomyxoma peritonei, any associated mucin is also submitted in toto.

G. **Anal biopsy** is treated similarly to other GI biopsies.

H. **Endomucosal resection (EMR)** specimens are processed as are esophageal EMR specimens (as discussed earlier).

I. **Hemorrhoidal excision** requires one section.

III. **DIAGNOSTIC FEATURES OF NONNEOPLASTIC CONDITIONS OF THE SMALL INTESTINE**

A. **Congenital anomalies**

1. **Heterotopic gastric mucosa** typically presents as a small nodule or sessile polyp in the duodenal bulb and consists of full-thickness fundic-type oxyntic mucosa. It differs from foveolar surface metaplasia in which the surface epithelium of the duodenal mucosa is replaced by gastric foveolar cells (e-**Fig. 14.4**), and which is often associated with duodenitis secondary to *Helicobacter pylori* infection.

2. **Heterotopic pancreas** presents as a mass lesion in the duodenum and is composed of ducts and acini, with or without islets.

3. **Meckel's diverticulum** results from persistence of the proximal portion of the vitelline duct and is always located on the antimesenteric border of the ileum. Associated heterotopic pancreatic tissue or gastric mucosa is common. Congenital diverticulum is a rare occurrence in the duodenum and jejunum (e-**Figs. 14.5** and **14.6**).

4. **Malrotation, stenosis, atresia, duplication, and defects of the musculature** are rare. Duplications can be cystic or tubular; about 75% are not contiguous with the lumen of the associated bowel segment. Duplications contain all the layers of the segment from which they have arisen, although mucosal heterotopias may occur. Any segment of the GI tract may be involved, and duplications are not associated with other anomalies. Neuroenteric remnants most commonly occur in the cervicothoracic or lumbosacral regions and also contain all the layers of the originating segment; however neuroenteric remnants originate from the dorsal midline and are associated with other congenital anomalies. Neural elements may be observed, primarily in lesions approximating the spinal cord.

B. **Malabsorptive disorders**

1. **Celiac disease,** also known as gluten-sensitive enteropathy, celiac sprue, or nontropical sprue, is an immune-mediated disorder secondary to hypersensitivity to α-gliadin. Classic histologic features include villous atrophy, crypt

TABLE 14.1	Conditions That Can Mimic Gluten-Sensitive Enteropathy

Celiac disease/gluten-sensitive enteropathy
Tropical sprue
Autoimmune enteropathy
HIV enteropathy
Common variable immunodeficiency
Viral enteritis
Giardiasis
Bacterial overgrowth
Infectious enteritis
Food allergies
Crohn's disease
Zollinger–Ellison syndrome
Systemic autoimmune diseases
Dermatitis herpetiformis
Nonsteroidal anti-inflammatory drugs
Helicobacter pylori infection

hyperplasia, intraepithelial lymphocytosis, a dense lamina propria lympho-plasmacytic infiltrate, and enterocyte damage. Villous atrophy ranges from partial blunting or broadening to complete flattening, but the overall thickness of the mucosa may not be reduced significantly due to crypt hyperplasia (e-**Figs. 14.7** and **14.8**). Eosinophils and neutrophils may be present in the infiltrate but are usually not prominent. Enterocyte damage is evidenced by flattening and/or cytoplasmic vacuolization. The Marsh–Oberhuber classification scheme describes five histologic lesions of gluten-sensitive enteropathy but is not widely used in routine practice.

An increased number of IELs in villous tips is an important diagnostic feature that has also been described as "loss of the decrescendo pattern." Although the increase is defined as >40 lymphocytes per 100 enterocytes, a formal count or immunostaining for T lymphocytes is usually unnecessary since lymphocytosis is typically diffuse and evenly distributed along the entire length of the villi (if the mucosa is not completely flattened).

Increased IELs may be the only histologic finding in early, latent, or partially treated celiac disease; serologic tests should be suggested in these cases. However, since many other conditions in addition to celiac disease can result in IEL, the pathologic diagnosis should remain descriptive (Table 14.1). The vast majority of patients with celiac disease have HLA-DQ2 or HLA-DQ8 and their absence almost excludes the diagnosis (*Arch Pathol Lab Med.* 2010;134:826).

2. **Refractory sprue** refers to unresponsiveness to a gluten-free diet or relapse of symptoms despite gluten restriction. It is histologically indistinguishable from classic celiac disease; some gastroenterologists regard it as a type of T-cell lymphoma. Neutrophils may be more numerous.

3. **Collagenous sprue** is characterized by villous flattening and subepithelial collagen deposition.

4. **Autoimmune enteropathy** shares many clinical and histopathologic features with celiac disease but often involves both the small and the large intestines. A biopsy typically exhibits villous flattening and dense lamina propria lymphoplasmacytic infiltrates (e-**Figs. 14.9** and **14.10**). In contrast to celiac disease, intraepithelial lymphocytosis and crypt hyperplasia may not be evident, and neutrophils may be more numerous. Apoptotic bodies may be

apparent. A complete lack of goblet cells and/or Paneth cells may be seen in some cases. Although some patients have anti-enterocyte and/or anti-goblet cell antibodies, serologic tests are not routinely employed. A clinical response to steroids may help establish the diagnosis.

5. **Eosinophilic gastroenteritis** involving the small intestine exhibits histologic features similar to those described for eosinophilic gastritis (e-**Fig. 14.11**). There may or may not be villous blunting, but IELs are usually not increased. Parasitic infestations, food allergy including cow's milk protein intolerance, a drug reaction, connective tissue disorders, and a neoplasm should be excluded.

6. **Common variable immunodeficiency** is characterized by the absence of lamina propria plasma cells (e-**Fig. 14.12**). Other features may include a variable degree of villous blunting, intraepithelial lymphocytosis, and lymphoid aggregates. Infectious agents, particularly *Giardia,* should be searched for in these biopsies.

7. **Microvillus inclusion disease** is a rare autosomal recessive disease causing intractable diarrhea in infancy. The hallmark of the disease is the loss of a normal brush border on the luminal surface of the enterocytes. Instead, the brush border is incorporated into the cytoplasm as apical microvillus inclusions. The microscopic features can be best demonstrated by periodic acid–Schiff (PAS) stain, electron microscopy, and immunostains for carcinoembryogenic antigen, CD10, or villin. Diffuse villous atrophy is also present, but an inflammatory response and intraepithelial lymphocytosis are not evident.

8. **Lymphangiectasia,** either primary (congenital) or secondary (due to obstruction), may present as a localized mass lesion or diffusely involve the bowel (e-**Fig. 14.13**). The presence of secondary lymphangiectasia is concerning for an unsampled underlying mass lesion as the source of obstruction, which should be mentioned in the report.

9. **Abetalipoproteinemia** features lipid accumulation in enterocytes giving rise to a clear or foamy appearance. The normal villous architecture is well preserved.

C. Infectious diseases

1. **Tropical sprue and bacterial overgrowth** simulate celiac disease but may involve the entire small intestine with more severe disease distally. Clinical history, including any travel history, is important in establishing the diagnosis.

2. **Giardiasis** does not induce significant villous architectural change or an inflammatory response. The diagnosis is based on the identification of pear-shaped trophozoites at the luminal surface of normal-appearing mucosa (e-**Fig. 14.14**), which can be mistaken as cytoplasmic debris. The organisms can be highlighted by trichrome and Giemsa stains.

Whipple disease exhibits distended villi due to lamina propria accumulation of foamy macrophages stuffed with the diastase-resistant, PAS-positive (e-**Fig. 14.15**), rod-shaped bacterium *Tropheryma whippelii.* The microorganisms can also be detected by polymerase chain reaction (PCR) analysis and electron microscopy. Gomori's methenamine silver (GMS), acid-fast bacilli (AFB), or Fite stains should be performed on these biopsies to rule out fungal (histoplasmosis) or mycobacterial (due to *Mycobacterium avium intracellulare*) infections because the morphology of these infections are quite similar to Whipple disease on H&E stain.

3. **Cryptosporidiosis** is characterized by uniform, spherical, 2- to 4-μm bodies attached to the brush border that appear bluish on H&E stain (e-**Fig. 14.16**). The organisms may be confused with mucin droplets.

4. **Strongyloidiasis** is diagnosed by identification of larvae, eggs, and adult worms embedded in the crypts (e-Fig. 14.17). Eosinophils, sometimes with Charcot–Leyden crystals, may be prominent. The nematodes most commonly infect the small intestine, but also rarely infect the stomach and colon. Gastric strongyloidiasis may sometimes be associated with infection by human T-lymphotropic virus type 1, a virus that causes adult T-cell lymphoma/leukemia.

IV. **DIAGNOSTIC FEATURES OF POLYPS AND NEOPLASMS OF THE SMALL INTESTINE.** The WHO classification scheme of tumors of the small intestine is given in (Table 14.2)

A. **Brunner's gland hyperplasia, hamartoma, and adenoma** may actually be variants of the same process and consist of expanded lobules of benign Brunner's glands separated by delicate fibrous septa. They are typically located in the submucosa, but penetration into the mucosa is common. Cystic degeneration may occur, which has been termed Brunner's gland cyst.

B. **Peutz–Jeghers polyp,** while most common in the small intestine, also occurs in the colon and stomach. It is a hamartomatous polyp characterized by an arborizing network of smooth muscle supporting benign-appearing mucosa that may be hyperplastic (e-Fig. 14.18). Most polyps occur as part of an inherited cancer syndrome, but sporadic cases may be encountered. Because syndromic polyps carry an increased risk of cancer, they should always be assessed for dysplasia.

C. **Adenomyoma of the ampulla of Vater** exhibits an orderly arranged lobular pattern of benign pancreaticobiliary ducts in a background of proliferating smooth muscle. It may coexist with heterotopic pancreas.

D. **Adenomas** are rare in the small intestine and usually occur in the duodenum. Multiple adenomas are almost always associated with familial adenomatous polyposis (FAP). Histologically identical to their colorectal counterparts, they are classified into tubular, tubulovillous, and villous types. The differential diagnosis includes gastric surface metaplasia and reparative change.

E. **Adenocarcinoma** of the small intestine is rare, accounting for only 2% of all primary GI tumors despite the fact that the small intestine constitutes about 75% of the length and about 90% of the mucosal surface of the GI tract (Table 14.3). Adenocarcinoma of the small intestine is morphologically indistinguishable from colorectal adenocarcinoma, but most cases are cytokeratin 7 (CK7)-positive which may help resolve the differential diagnosis.

F. **Ampullary carcinoma** is actually a heterogeneous group of tumors. It arises in the vicinity of the ampulla of Vater and includes the most common intestinal-type adenocarcinoma as well as the pancreaticobiliary type. The former has a more favorable outcome than the latter, although the overall survival of ampullary carcinoma is better than that of pancreatic ductal carcinoma (which probably reflects differences in respectability). However, distinguishing the site of origin is sometimes a challenge (Table 14.4).

G. **Neuroendocrine tumor (NET)** accounts for one-third of small intestinal tumors. Duodenal NETs are derived from endocrine cells of the foregut and tend to be <2 cm in greatest dimension and asymptomatic. Gastrin-producing NETs are associated with ZES (Zollinger–Ellison syndrome) in 40% to 50% of cases. Distal jejunum and ileal NETs are derived from cells of the midgut; 25% to 30% are multifocal, and clinically they are more aggressive than proximal NET.

Microscopically, small intestinal NET are similar to NET arising elsewhere (e-Fig. 14.19) and have a very bland cytomorphology; invasion into or beyond the muscularis propria and/or distant metastasis are the main criteria for determining malignant behavior. In contrast, poorly differentiated NET exhibit overt histologic features of malignancy. Tables 14.5 and 14.6 summarize the current WHO classification and AJCC staging schemes, respectively.

TABLE 14.2	WHO Histologic Classification of Tumors of the Small Intestine

Epithelial tumors
Adenoma
   Tubular
   Villous
   Tubulovillous
Dysplasia (intraepithelial neoplasia), low grade
Dysplasia (intraepithelial neoplasia), high grade
Hamartomas
   Peutz–Jeghers polyp
   Juvenile polyp
Carcinoma
Adenocarcinoma
   Mucinous adenocarcinoma
   Signet-ring cell carcinoma
Squamous cell carcinoma
Adenosquamous carcinoma
Medullary carcinoma
Undifferentiated carcinoma

Neuroendocrine neoplasms
Neuroendocrine tumor (NET)
   NET, G1 (carcinoid)
   NET, G2
Neuroendocrine carcinoma (NEC)
   Large cell NEC
   Small cell NEC
Mixed adenoneuroendocrine carcinoma (MANEC)
EC cell, serotonin-producing NET
Gangliocytic paraganglioma
Gastrinoma
L-cell, glucagon-like peptide and PP/PYY-producing NETs
Somatostatin-producing NET

Mesenchymal tumors
Lipoma
Leiomyoma
Gastrointestinal stromal tumor
Leiomyosarcoma
Angiosarcoma
Kaposi sarcoma
Others

Lymphomas
Burkitt lymphoma
B-cell lymphoma, unclassifiable, with features intermediate between diffuse large B-cell
   lymphoma and Burkitt lymphoma
Diffuse large B-cell lymphoma
Immunoproliferative small intestinal disease (includes α-heavy chain disease)
Follicular lymphoma
Marginal zone lymphoma of mucosa-associated lymphoid tissue (MALT lymphoma)
Mantle cell lymphoma
T-cell lymphoma
Enteropathy associated T-cell lymphoma (EATL)

Secondary tumors

WHO, World Health Organization; EC, enterochromaffin; PP, pancreatic polypeptide; PYY, polypeptide YY.
From: Bosman FT, Carneiro F, Hruban RH, Theise ND, eds. *World Health Organization Classification of Tumours of the Digestive System.* Lyon: IARC Press; 2010. Used with permission.

TABLE 14.3	Tumor, Node, Metastasis (TNM) Staging Scheme for Small Intestinal Carcinomas

Primary tumor (T)

TX	Primary tumor cannot be assessed
T0	No evidence of primary tumor
Tis	Carcinoma in situ
T1a	Tumor invades lamina propria
T1b	Tumor invades submucosa[a]
T2	Tumor invades muscularis propria
T3	Tumor invades through the muscularis propria into the subserosa, or into nonperitonealized perimuscular tissue (mesentery or retroperitoneum) with extension 2 cm or less[a]
T4	Tumor perforates the visceral peritoneum or directly invades other organs or structures (includes other loops of small intestine, mesentery, or retroperitoneum >2 cm, and abdominal wall by way of serosa; for duodenum only, invasion of pancreas or bile duct)

Regional lymph nodes (N)

NX	Regional lymph nodes cannot be assessed
N0	No regional lymph node metastasis
N1	Metastasis in 1–3 regional lymph nodes
N2	Metastasis in 4 or more regional lymph nodes

Distant metastasis (M)

M0	No distant metastasis
M1	Distant metastasis

Stage grouping

Stage 0	Tis	N0	M0
Stage I	T1	N0	M0
	T2	N0	M0
Stage IIA	T3	N0	M0
Stage IIB	T4	N0	M0
Stage IIIA	Any T	N1	M0
Stage IIIB	Any T	N2	M0
Stage IV	Any T	Any N	M1

[a]The nonperitonealized perimuscular tissue is, for jejunum and ileum, part of the mesentery and, for duodenum in areas where serosa is lacking, part of the retroperitoneum.
From: Edge SB, Byrd DR, Compton CC, et al., eds. *AJCC Cancer Staging Manual.* 7th ed. New York, NY: Springer; 2010. Used with permission.

H. **Gangliocytic paraganglioma** occurs almost exclusively in the periampullary region and is benign in the majority of cases. As in other locations, the tumor consists of a mixture of ganglion-like cells, Schwannian cells, and epithelioid endocrine-like cells (**e-Fig. 14.20**). S-100 positivity is a useful marker to differentiate the neoplasm from a gastrointestinal stromal tumor (GIST).

I. **GIST** of the small intestine accounts for 30% to 40% of all GISTs of the GI tract and tends to be more aggressive than its gastric counterpart (Table 14.7) (*Am J Surg Pathol.* 2006;30:477–89). Table 14.8 summarizes the current AJCC staging scheme of GIST arising outside of the stomach.

J. **Immunoproliferative small intestinal disease (IPSID)** is a distinct type of extranodal marginal zone B-cell lymphoma (mucosa-associated lymphoid tissue [MALT] lymphoma), typically seen in young adults in Middle Eastern and Mediterranean countries. About half of patients exhibit characteristic α-heavy

TABLE 14.4	Tumor, Node, Metastasis (TNM) Staging Scheme for Ampullary Carcinoma

Primary tumor (T)

TX	Primary tumor cannot be assessed
T0	No evidence of primary tumor
Tis	Carcinoma in situ
T1	Tumor limited to ampulla of Vater or sphincter of Oddi
T2	Tumor invades duodenal wall
T3	Tumor invades pancreas
T4	Tumor invades peripancreatic soft tissues or other adjacent organs or structures

Regional lymph nodes (N)

NX	Regional lymph nodes cannot be assessed
N0	No regional lymph node metastasis
N1	Regional lymph node metastasis

Distant metastasis (M)

M0	No distant metastasis
M1	Distant metastasis

Stage grouping

Stage 0	Tis	N0	M0
Stage IA	T1	N0	M0
Stage IB	T2	N0	M0
Stage IIA	T3	N0	M0
Stage IIB	T1	N1	M0
	T2	N1	M0
	T3	N1	M0
Stage III	T4	Any N	M0
Stage IV	Any T	Any N	M1

From: Edge SB, Byrd DR, Compton CC, et al., eds. *AJCC Cancer Staging Manual.* 7th ed. New York, NY: Springer; 2010. Used with permission.

TABLE 14.5	Classification and Grading of Neuroendocrine Neoplasms of the GI Tract

Classification	Grade	Definition
Neuroendocrine tumor (carcinoid)	I	Cytologically bland, mitotic count <2 per 10 high power fields (HPFs) and/or 2% ≤Ki 67 index[a]
	II	Cytologically bland, mitotic count 2–20 per 10 HPFs and/or 3–20% Ki 67 index
Neuroendocrine carcinoma (NEC)	III	Mitotic count >20 per 10 HPF and/or >20% Ki 67 index
MANEC		
Hyperplastic and preneoplastic lesions		Tumor displaying at least 30% of adenocarcinoma or NEC

GI, gastrointestinal.
[a]Grading requires mitotic count in at least 50 HPFs and Ki67 percentage in at least 500–2000 cells within the areas of strongest nuclear labeling.
From: Bosman FT, Carneiro F, Hruban RH, Theise ND, eds. *World Health Organization Classification of Tumours of the Digestive System.* Lyon: IARC Press; 2010. Used with permission.

TABLE 14.6	Tumor, Node, Metastasis (TNM) Staging Scheme for Neuroendocrine Tumors of Duodenum/Ampulla/Jejunum/Ileum

Primary tumor (T)

TX	Primary tumor cannot be assessed
T0	No evidence of primary tumor
T1	Tumor invades lamina propria or submucosa and ≤ 1 cm[a] in size (small intestinal tumors); tumor ≤ 1 cm (ampullary tumors)
T2	Tumor invades muscularis propria or >1 cm in size (small intestinal tumors); tumor >1 cm (ampullary tumors)
T3	Tumor invades through the muscularis propria into subserosal tissue without penetration of overlying serosa (jejunal or ileal tumors) or invades pancreas or retroperitoneum (ampullary or duodenal tumors) or into nonperitonealized tissues
T4	Tumor invades visceral peritoneum (serosa) or invades other organs
	For any T, add (m) for multiple tumors
	[a]Tumor limited to ampulla of Vater for ampullary gangliocytic paraganglioma

Regional lymph nodes (N)

NX	Regional lymph nodes cannot be assessed
N0	No regional lymph node metastasis
N1	Regional lymph node metastasis

Distant metastasis (M)

M0	No distant metastasis
M1	Distant metastasis

Stage grouping

Stage 0	Tis[a]	N0	M0
Stage I	T1	N0	M0
Stage IIA	T2	N0	M0
Stage IIB	T3	N0	M0
Stage IIIA	T4	N0	M0
Stage IIIB	Any T	N1	M0
Stage IV	Any T	Any N	M1

[a]Tis applies only to stomach.
From: Edge SB, Byrd DR, Compton CC, et al., eds. *AJCC Cancer Staging Manual.* 7th ed. New York, NY: Springer; 2010. Used with permission.

TABLE 14.7	Proposed Guidelines for Assessing the Malignant Potential of Small Intestinal GISTs

Tumor	Predicted biologic behavior
≤ 2 cm, ≤ 5 mitoses/50 HPFs	Benign, metastasis rate or tumor-related mortality: 0
$>2 \leq 5$ cm, <5 mitoses/50 HPFs	Low malignant potential, metastasis rate or tumor-related mortality: 4%
$>5 \leq 10$ cm, ≤ 5 mitoses/50 HPFs	Moderate malignant potential, metastasis rate or tumor-related mortality: 25%
>10 cm, or >5 mitoses/50 HPFs	High malignant potential, metastasis rate or tumor-related mortality: 50–90%

GIST, gastrointestinal stromal tumor; HPFs, high-power fields.
Modified from *Am J Surg Pathol.* 2006;30:477–89.

TABLE 14.8 Tumor, Node, Metastasis (TNM) Staging Scheme Gastrointestinal Stromal Tumors (Excluding Stomach)

Primary tumor (T)

TX	Primary tumor cannot be assessed
T0	No evidence of primary tumor
T1	Tumor 2 cm or less
T2	Tumor >2 cm but not >5 cm
T3	Tumor >5 cm but not >10 cm
T4	Tumor >10 cm in greatest dimension

Regional lymph nodes (N)

NX	Regional lymph nodes cannot be assessed
N0	No regional lymph node metastasis
N1	Regional lymph node metastasis

Distant metastasis (M)

M0	No distant metastasis
M1	Distant metastasis
M1a	Lung
M1b	Other distant sites

Stage Grouping

				Mitotic rate
Stage IA	T1 or T2	N0	M0	Low
Stage II	T3	N0	M0	Low
Stage IIIA	T1	N0	M0	High
	T4	N0	M0	Low
Stage IIIB	T2	N0	M0	High
	T3	N0	M0	High
	T4	N0	M0	High
Stage IV	Any T	N1	M0	Any rate
	Any T	Any N	M1	Any rate

Low mitotic rate: 5 or fewer per 50 HPFs; high mitotic rate: over 5 per 50 HPFs.
From: Edge SB, Byrd DR, Compton CC, et al., eds. *AJCC Cancer Staging Manual.* 7th ed. New York, NY: Springer; 2010. Used with permission.

chain paraproteinemia without associated light chains (α-heavy chain disease). Patients present with malabsorption and diarrhea. Some patients progress to diffuse large B-cell lymphoma.

K. **Enteropathy-type T-cell lymphoma** typically develops in the setting of refractory sprue and ulcerative jejunitis or jejunoileitis, and most commonly affects the jejunum. It is characterized by dense infiltration of atypical T lymphocytes in association with epithelial destruction.

V. **DIAGNOSTIC FEATURES OF NONNEOPLASTIC CONDITIONS OF THE LARGE INTESTINE**

A. **Neuromuscular disorders**

1. **Hirschsprung's disease** affects approximately 1 in 5000 live births, mainly males. Even though mutations of *RET* (located on 10q11.2) are the most common genetic abnormality associated with this condition, mutations of other genes including but not limited to *EDRNB* (13q22), *SOX10* (22q13), *SIP1* (2q22), and *PHOX2B* (4p12) are also associated with this disease (*J Med Genet.* 2008;45:1). All these genes play a central role in pathogenesis, which is due to failure of neural crest cells to appropriately migrate to the rectum or rectosigmoid colon; rarely the entire colon is affected. The aganglionic segment is narrowed, whereas the upstream segment is dilated due to the functional obstruction. The diagnosis is established by microscopic

demonstration of an absence of ganglion cells in the submucosa on a rectal suction biopsy. Since hypertrophic nerve fibers are also present (e-Fig. 14.21), demonstration of acetylcholinesterase-positive nerve twigs in the muscularis mucosae and lamina propria in frozen sections aids in confirmation of the diagnosis.

The biopsy should be taken at least 2 cm above the pectinate line as the distal 1.5- to 2-cm zone of the rectum is physiologically hypoganglionotic and may have prominent nerve fibers. Thus, biopsies containing squamous or anal canal transitional mucosa are considered inappropriate. The biopsy must contain an adequate thickness of submucosa, generally considered to be a thickness equal to that of the mucosa.

A potential diagnostic pitfall is due to the fact that neonates may have immature ganglion cells with small nuclei, scanty cytoplasm, and inconspicuous nucleoli, which makes their recognition difficult. Immunohistochemical staining for neuron-specific enolase (NSE) or other neuronal markers may aid in their identification.

2. **Pseudo-obstruction syndrome** encompasses a heterogeneous group of neuromuscular disorders characterized by colonic inertia and constipation. The diagnosis is challenging. There may be histologic clues in nerves or muscle fibers of the muscularis propria that require careful evaluation with special stains and clinical correlation.

B. **Ischemic bowel disease.** Although the blood supply to the small bowel is generally protective of ischemia, the large bowel may undergo ischemic injury, particularly in watershed areas such as the splenic flexure. The distal large bowel is more susceptible than the proximal, but the rectum is rarely involved. Ultimately, however, any portion of the colon may be affected, and ischemic injury can occur in young individuals. The etiologic processes that ultimately lead to decreased blood flow in cases of ischemic injury are numerous and presented in Table 14.9. Table 14.10 gives histopathologic differential diagnosis.

TABLE 14.9	Causes of Intestinal Ischemia

Acute vascular occlusion
  Thrombosis
  Embolism
Nonocclusive mesenteric ischemia
  Pig bel
  Necrotizing enterocolitis
Vasculitides and vasculopathies
Hypercoagulable states
Drug effects
Vascular compression
  Volvulus
  Intussusception
  Celiac axis compression
Infection[a]
Amyloidosis
Radiation damage
Diabetes mellitus

[a]Clostridium difficile, Escherichia coli 0157:H7, Staphylococcal enterocolitis, Cytomegalovirus, Aspergillus and Candida species.
Modified from Noffsinger A, Fenoglio Preiser C, Maru D, et al. Gastrointestinal Diseases. Washington, DC: Armed Forces Institute of Pathology, American Registry of Pathology, p. 256, tables 7.1, and 7.3; 2007. Used with permission.

TABLE 14.10	Differential Diagnosis of Histologic Findings of Mucosal Ischemic Colitis

Clostridium difficile colitis
Enterohemorrhagic *Escherichia coli*
NSAID damage
Crohn's colitis
Radiation colitis
Collagenous colitis

Modified from Iacobuzio Donohue CA, Montgomery EA. *Gastrointestinal and Liver Pathology*, p. 332; 2005. Used with permission.

Histologic findings vary, but the mucosa is always involved. In some cases, the key histologic finding is pauci-inflammatory hyalinization of the lamina propria. In other cases, the deepest portion of the crypts may be architecturally intact, but superficial crypts and surface epithelium are either "ghosts" or totally absent; it is important to recognize the enlarged nuclei in these crypts as regenerative and not dysplastic. In some cases, a pseudomembrane is present, erupting from the dying crypts and covering the luminal surface. If the specimen includes full thickness bowel, there may be full thickness infarction with clotted vessels in the adjacent submucosa and/or mesentery, or there may only be subtle findings of early ischemic necrosis with cell shrinkage and pyknotic nuclei within the muscularis propria layers (e-**Fig. 14.22**). Submucosal edema is common.

Chronic ischemia results in similar but less dramatic findings. The mucosal changes are hyalinization of the lamina propria with "withering" of the crypts and shrunken muscle fibers in the muscularis propria. Strictures are common (e-**Figs. 14.23** and **14.24**).

Neonatal necrotizing enterocolitis (NEC) is a special form of ischemic bowel disease that has a high mortality rate and typically occurs in the first week of life in premature infants. It classically affects the terminal ileum and the right colon with gangrenous necrosis. Pneumatosis intestinalis and segmental absence of the muscularis propria may be seen.

C. **IBD**, an idiopathic chronic inflammatory process with a genetic predisposition, refers to Crohn's disease and UC. The diseases are characterized by chronicity and architectural alterations of the crypts, as well as basal plasmacytosis, basal lymphoid aggregates, mucosal atrophy, Paneth cell metaplasia (defined as the presence of Paneth cells beyond the mid-transverse colon), and pyloric metaplasia. Crypt architectural distortion is more pronounced in UC than Crohn's disease and may manifest as branching, shortening, irregular shape, irregular spacing, size variation, and disarray (e-**Figs. 14.25** and **4.26**). Pyloric metaplasia is more common in the small bowel in Crohn's disease but also occurs in the colon in UC (e-**Fig. 14.27**).

The lamina propria in IBD is usually densely infiltrated by mixed inflammatory cells, predominantly lymphocytes and plasma cells, but eosinophils can be abundant. Because of crypt shortening, a bandlike inflammatory infiltrate is often seen in the space above the muscularis mucosae, a finding referred to as basal plasmacytosis; lymphoid aggregates may also be present in this space in some cases. Active disease is defined by exocytosis of neutrophils into the crypts (cryptitis) and crypt lumens (crypt abscesses) (e-**Fig. 14.28**). An increased number of neutrophils in the lamina propria raise a concern of infectious colitis. In some institutions, the inflammatory activity is graded as minimal, mild, moderate, or severe. In the absence of neutrophilic infiltration, the disease is characterized by crypt architectural distortion and is referred to as quiescent or inactive. Treated IBD may be normal. Cytomegalovirus (CMV) inclusions have been described in refractory UC, which otherwise mimics active disease (e-**Fig. 14.29**).

1. **Crohn's disease** may involve any portion of the GI tract. Roughly, about 40% of patients have small bowel disease only, about 40% have small and large bowel involvement, and about 20% have colonic disease only. On the basis of the clinical behavior and pattern of disease, Crohn's disease is divided into three categories: inflammatory, fistulizing, and fibrostenotic. Grossly, the involved bowel segment typically has a rigid, strictured, or thickened wall with creeping fat. Upon opening, the segment usually grossly maintains its cylindrical shape (e-**Fig. 14.30**). The mucosa may show cobble stoning due to linear and transverse ulcers with intervening edematous mucosa. Deep fissuring ulcers and fistula tracts are common. The muscle layer is thickened.

   The microscopic hallmark of Crohn's disease is transmural inflammation with a lack of homogeneous involvement, that is, skip lesions (areas of active disease separated by normal bowel) are present. In resection specimens, lymphoid aggregates may be present in all layers of the bowel wall but are characteristically located in the subserosal fat along the vasculature in a "necklace" pattern (e-**Fig. 14.31**). Granulomas, seen in up to 40% of cases, may be found in the mucosa, submucosa, and subserosa. In the mucosa, Crohn's granulomas are typically small, well-formed, nonnecrotizing, and lack multinucleated giant cells (e-**Fig. 14.32**). A diagnostic pitfall is the so-called crypt granuloma, which represents a pericryptal histiocytic response to mucin from ruptured crypts (e-**Fig. 14.33**), that occasionally includes foreign body-type giant cells. Granulomas within the muscularis mucosae can be overlooked because of similarity to smooth muscle bundles. In the subserosa, granulomas can be larger, can contain giant cells, and are frequently associated with lymphoid aggregates (e-**Fig. 14.34**).

   It should be emphasized that Crohn's disease is a clinical diagnosis. Although supportive histopathologic findings in mucosal biopsies include a lack of uniformity of involvement of all fragments, or a lack of uniformity within of a given fragment, focal colitis is not specific for Crohn's disease. Focal colitis is also commonly seen in other conditions, including infectious colitis, drug toxicity (particularly with nonsteroidal anti-inflammatory drug [NSAID] treatment), and partially treated UC. Consequently, it is prudent to avoid labeling a patient with Crohn's disease at the first biopsy, but rather to give a descriptive diagnosis (such as focal active colitis) and to provide a differential diagnosis. Appropriate clinical and genetic workup, and subsequent biopsies, usually resolve the diagnostic dilemma.

2. **Ulcerative colitis** classically involves the entire colon but not the small bowel and has a tendency to be more severe distally. In some cases, the disease involves only the rectum (ulcerative proctitis) or presents as left-sided colitis with discontinuous involvement of the cecum (cecal patch), ascending colon, and/or appendix. Grossly, the affected colon often has a thin and flaccid wall that flattens upon opening. The mucosa loses its normal folds and is granular, friable, erythematous, and ulcerated (e-**Fig. 14.35**). Microscopically, the disease is characterized by diffuse crypt architectural distortion and inflammation. In contrast to Crohn's colitis, crypt architectural distortion is more dramatic, and inflammation is usually limited to the mucosa and immediate submucosa. In severe active disease with broad-based ulcers, the inflammatory infiltrate extends into the submucosa and the muscularis propria in the ulcerated areas. Interestingly, in children with UC, the disease may be inhomogeneous at initial presentation. Treated UC may also

TABLE 14.11 Gross and Histologic Features Distinguishing Ulcerative Colitis from Crohn's Disease

Feature	Ulcerative colitis	Crohn's disease
Distribution	Diffuse, continuous	Focal (skip), segmental
Depth of involvement	Mucosa, submucosa	Transmural
Mucosal appearance	Irregular ulcers, friable, atrophy	Cobblestoning
Bowel wall	Thin	Thickened or normal
Creeping mesenteric fat	Absent	Common
Stricture	Usually absent	Maybe
Fistula	Usually absent	Maybe
Fissuring	Usually absent	Common
Ileal involvement	<10% (backwash)	Common
Upper GI involvement	Usually no	Maybe
Rectal involvement	100%	~15%
Anal involvement	5–10%	~75%
Well-formed granuloma	Absent	Common
Transmural lymphoid aggregates	Absent	Common

GI, gastrointestinal.

show inhomogeneous involvement with rectal sparing, or completely normal mucosa, which may potentially be confused with Crohn's disease.

Fulminant colitis is more commonly seen in UC. Usually the patients have pancolitis with extensive infiltration of the mucosa with inflammatory cells, mucosal denudation, and granulation tissue. The inflammation may extend to involve the muscularis propria and can cause necrosis.

Backwash ileitis may be seen in severe pancolitis, presumably due to reflux of colonic contents. It is characterized by mild but active inflammation in the distal few centimeters of the terminal ileum with relative preservation of the normal villous architecture (e-Figs. 14.36 and 14.37). Table 14.11 summarizes the gross and histologic features that help distinguish UC from Crohn's disease.

3. **Indeterminate colitis** is not a distinct entity, and the diagnosis should be applied only to cases that are truly difficult to classify histologically and clinically. Most cases will eventually evolve into UC or Crohn's disease. The diagnosis is usually rendered because of insufficient clinical, radiologic, or endoscopic data, and because of prominent overlapping pathologic features. Fulminant colitis that lacks specific diagnostic features may also belong to this category.

4. **Dysplasia** is associated with the extent and duration of IBD and is a recognized precursor of adenocarcinoma. In surveillance biopsies for IBD, the presence of dysplasia should be reported as either negative or graded as indefinite, low grade, or high grade. Grade is based on architectural complexity of the crypts, as well as surface epithelial cytologic atypia and maturation defects. Conventional low-grade dysplasia simulates a tubular adenoma, whereas high-grade dysplasia (HGD) is identical to adenocarcinoma in situ or intraepithelial carcinoma (e-Fig. 14.38). However, in some cases where there is abundant inflammation and ulceration, it may be challenging to separate inflammatory or reactive atypia from dysplasia, either in the crypts or the surface epithelium, and these cases usually fall in the category of indefinite for dysplasia.

IBD-associated dysplasia can be flat or polypoid, but distinguishing polypoid dysplasia, or a dysplasia-associated lesion or mass (DALM), from

TABLE 14.12 Distinction Between Polypoid Colitis-Associated Dysplasia and Sporadic Adenomas Arising in Inflammatory Disease Patients

Feature	Adenoma	Colitis-associated dysplasia
Patient age	Older (>50)	Younger (<50)
Disease activity	Active or inactive	Usually active
Disease duration	Shorter, usually <10 years	Longer, usually >10 years
Endoscopic appearance	Well marginated	Irregular
Glands	Regular configuration	Irregular configuration
Surface	Homogenous	Mixture of nonneoplastic and neoplastic glands
Distribution of mucin	Often near luminal surface	Irregular
Dystrophic goblet cells	Rare	Frequent
Nuclei	Stratified, same level	Stratified, various levels
Demarcation from surrounding mucosa	Sharp	Gradual transition
Appearance of surrounding mucosa	Mildly distorted	Prominent architectural distortion
Prominent lamina propria mononuclear cells	No	Yes
Prominent lamina propria neutrophils	±	+
Prominent p53 by immunohistochemistry	No	Yes (nuclear)
Beta-catenin	Yes (nuclear)	No

From: Montogomery E. *Biopsy Interpretation of the Gastrointestinal Tract Mucosa*, p. 303; 2006. Used with permission.

a sporadic adenoma may be difficult. In some cases the distinction may be unnecessary since a DALM can be adequately treated by simple polypectomy and continued surveillance, as with a sporadic adenoma. However, because the clinical consequences of the diagnosis of dysplasia can include increased surveillance or even colectomy, verification of the diagnosis by an experienced GI pathologist is strongly recommended. Immunohistochemical markers in aid for differential diagnosis of dysplasia versus sporadic adenoma are being developed and are in use in some centers (e-**Figs. 14.39** and **14.40**). Table 14.12 summarizes some of the potential differentiating features currently recommended.

   5. **Pouchitis** refers to inflammation of the ileal pouch created after a total colectomy, usually for UC. Active pouchitis shows mixed neutrophilic and lymphoplasmacytic infiltrates in the ileal mucosa, and erosions or ulcerations in more severe cases. Chronic changes, such as villous architectural distortion, villous atrophy, and pyloric metaplasia, may be seen in long-term disease. An important differential diagnosis is recurrent Crohn's disease in a case previously diagnosed as UC. Re-evaluation of a previous colectomy specimen may be necessary if granulomas, a fistula, a sinus tract, or a fissuring ulcer is detected in a pouch.

   D. **Diversion colitis** refers to an inflammatory response in the blind segment, usually the rectum (Hartmann pouch) following ileostomy or colostomy formation. The process is thought to be caused by a deficiency of short-chain fatty acids because the ostomy procedure excludes the rectum from the fecal stream. The classic findings are a granular, friable mucosa with marked lymphoid hyperplasia and cryptitis (e-Fig. 14.41). The features can mimic IBD, and therefore interpretation of the biopsy findings in the clinical context is important.

E. **Microscopic colitis** is a clinical term that includes **lymphocytic colitis** and **collagenous colitis;** these entities share watery diarrhea and normal endoscopic findings clinically, and surface epithelial damage, inflammation, and crypt lymphocytosis microscopically (e-Fig. 14.42). The microscopic findings are nonspecific, in that a focal increase in the number of IELs may be seen in IBD, infectious colitis, gluten-sensitive enteropathy, graft-versus-host disease (GVHD), and human immunodeficiency virus (HIV) infection, as well as in areas adjacent to lymphoid aggregates.

The key feature of collagenous colitis is the additional presence of a thickened collagen layer at the subepithelial region, which can be inhomogeneous (e-Fig. 14.43). The thickness of the collagen layer is variable but should be >10 μm. Small capillaries and scattered inflammatory cells are typically entrapped within the collagen layer. Evaluation requires well-oriented sections; in difficult cases, a trichrome stain may be helpful. The differential diagnosis includes mucosal fibrosis, which involves the full thickness of the mucosa and may be seen in ischemic colitis, a healed ulcer, and radiation colitis.

By definition, a large number of neutrophils should not be present in either form of microscopic colitis. However, neutrophilic cryptitis or crypt abscesses may be seen in some patients but should be far less prominent than the lymphocytic infiltration. In patients with collagenous colitis, focal architectural disarray and Paneth cell metaplasia can be seen, findings that can be misinterpreted as IBD (Table 14.13).

F. **Diverticular disease (diverticulosis),** acquired outpouchings of the mucosa and submucosa through defects in weakened muscularis propria, occurs throughout the colon but is more common in the sigmoid colon (e-Fig. 14.44). Approximately 10% of cases become inflamed (diverticulitis), leading to abscess formation, perforation, and fistula formation. On biopsy, diverticulitis, particularly diverticular disease-associated segmental sigmoiditis, may be difficult to distinguish from IBD due to crypt architectural distortion and active inflammation.

G. **Radiation colitis** occurs as a result of radiation therapy, usually for prostatic or cervical cancer. Biopsies are uncommon in the acute phase but show apoptotic activity, nuclear atypia, mucin depletion, and decreased mitotic activity. Chronic radiation colitis is characterized by telangiectasias of the mucosal capillaries, lamina propria hyalinization, and atypical stromal fibroblasts. Inflammatory cells are sparse (e-Fig. 14.45).

TABLE 14.13	Microscopic Colitis versus Inflammatory Bowel Disease (IBD)	
Feature	**Microscopic**	**IBD**
Cryptitis or crypt abscesses	± (Focal)	Prominent
Crypt distortion	± (Focal)	Prominent
Basal plasmacytosis	+	++
Basal lymphoid aggregates	±	++
Paneth cell metaplasia	+	+
Prominent lymphocytic or plasmacytic inflammation	++	+
Neutrophils in lamina propria	±	++
Prominent eosinophils	+ (cc)	±
Thickened or irregular subepithelial collagen layer	++ (cc)	± (Focal)
Ulcer or erosion	± (Rare)	++ (Common)

H. Infectious colitis is caused by a wide range of microorganisms including bacteria, viruses, parasites, and protozoa.

1. Bacterial infection, for example by *Campylobacter, Shigella,* and *Salmonella,* results in acute self-limited colitis (ASLC) characterized by neutrophilic infiltration of the lamina propria and epithelium with associated cryptitis and crypt abscesses. The inflammation is accentuated in the luminal portion of the mucosa and is accompanied by damage of the surface epithelium with erosion and flattening. The crypt architecture is preserved.

2. Pseudomembranous colitis is a potentially fatal mucosal reaction to toxins produced by *Clostridium difficile.* Most cases are associated with prior antibiotic exposure which results in loss of normal bacterial flora. Pseudomembranous colitis is characterized grossly by adherent yellow-white plaques; microscopically these are parallel arrays of polymorphs within fibrin and mucin. The underlying crypts are ruptured, giving rise to the classic appearance of "volcano" lesions (e-Figs. 14.46 and 14.47). It is important to note that pseudomembranous colitis is a morphologic diagnosis that can occur in *C. difficile* infection or in ischemic colitis; likewise, ischemic colitis can occur as a result of infection such as with *Escherichia coli* O157:H7.

3. Intestinal spirochetosis is not uncommon in HIV-infected patients but can be an incidental finding in immunocompetent individuals. It may also be incidentally detected in appendectomy specimens. It is characterized by a fuzzy, purplish or bluish band of organisms carpeting the mucosal surface (e-Fig. 14.48). The organisms are more easily recognizable on silver stains, such as the Warthin–Starry stain. There is no associated inflammatory response or epithelial damage.

I. Drug-induced colitis presents with a wide spectrum of histologic findings. NSAIDs are the most common medications to induce injury and can be associated with diaphragm disease in small intestines, and lymphocytic infiltrates, apoptosis, and microscopic colitis in the large intestine. Kayexalate, cocaine, and amphetamines are among the agents that are associated with ischemic colitis. Excessive laxative use can cause melanosis coli (*Nat Clin Pract Gastroenterol Hepatol.* 2007;4:442). Agents used for bowel preparation may cause mucosal edema, hemorrhage, surface epithelial detachment, neutrophilic cryptitis, and increased apoptotic activity.

J. So-called **diaphragm disease** in the small intestine is another example of drug-induced injury. It is caused by NSAIDs, and the lesion is characterized by multiple mucosal webs that result in luminal narrowing. Biopsies are rarely obtained in this condition.

K. GVHD commonly affects the skin, liver, and gut. Histologic hallmarks in the intestinal tract include a paucity of inflammatory cells in the lamina propria, apoptosis, and crypt dropout. (e-Figs. 14.49 and 14.50), and the severity of acute colonic GVHD is graded accordingly (Table 14.14). CMV infection shares the finding of "exploding crypt cells" (apoptosis), and thus needs to be excluded. Mycophenolate mofetil toxicity can also result in crypt apoptosis, and thus communication with the clinician is important (e-Fig. 14.51).

L. Miscellaneous conditions. Melanosis coli (pigmented macrophages in the lamina propria) is a common finding in patients due to excessive laxative use (e-Fig. 14.52).

Brown bowel syndrome, in contrast, is a unique condition believed to be caused by vitamin E deficiency, which leads to mitochondrial dysfunction and lipofuscin accumulation in smooth muscle cells.

Irritable bowel syndrome (IBS) is a common cause of abdominal pain and chronic diarrhea. It is a clinical diagnosis, and colonic biopsies from these patients are entirely normal on H&E stain.

TABLE 14.14	Histologic Grading of Colonic Graft-Versus-Host Disease (GVHD)
Grade	Histologic features
1	Individual cell necrosis in a few crypts, sparse lymphocytic infiltrate
2	Apoptotic crypts, crypt abscesses, and mixed lamina propria infiltrate
3	Loss of individual crypts, areas of mucosa devoid of crypts, focal ulceration
4	Widespread loss of crypts, and surface epithelium with mucosal denudation and ulceration

From: Appelbaum FR, Forman SJ, Negrin RS, et al. *Thomas' Hematopoietic Cell Transplantation.* 4th ed., p. 395; 2009.

VI. **DIAGNOSTIC FEATURES OF POLYPS AND NEOPLASMS OF THE LARGE INTESTINE.** (The WHO classification scheme of tumors of the colon and rectum is given in Table 14.15.)

A. **Hyperplastic polyps (HPs)** are typically small (usually <5 mm) and feature a serrated or sawtooth luminal configuration (e-**Fig. 14.53**). The serration is most prominent at the upper portion of the crypts and along the luminal surface, whereas the lower crypt portion remains narrow and proliferative. Thus, there is a progressive maturation as the epithelial cells move toward the surface. There is no cytologic atypia, but occasional multinucleated cells may be noted. A thickened basement membrane may be seen. Three morphologic types of HP have been described: microvesicular, goblet cell-rich, and mucin-poor, although there is no known clinical significance of the variants.

B. **Sessile Serrated Adenoma/Polyp (SSA/P)** most commonly arises in the right colon and is usually >5 mm in size. The crypts have a prominent serrated epithelium which extends to their base; the crypts are also dilated, flask-shaped, L-shaped, or branched (e-**Figs. 14.54** and **14.55**). The overall architecture is distorted and the proliferative zone is altered in these polyps; however, SSAs lack the classical dysplastic features of a tubular adenoma. About 80% of SSA/P polyps carry BRAF mutations, and it is possible that SSA/P may be precursors of sporadic carcinomas with microsatellite instability (MSI). "Serrated dysplasia" can arise in these polyps and is characterized by cytologic features that include eosinophilic cytoplasm, vesicular chromatin, and prominent nucleoli, although the cytologic features of conventional adenomatous dysplasia (discussed later) may also be present (e-**Figs. 14.56** and **14.57**). SSA/P that have dysplastic features are referred as SSA/P with cytological dysplasia. The current recommendation for SSA/P (or any other serrated lesion of the colorectum) is complete removal of the lesion; follow-up guidelines are not established.

C. **Traditional Serrated Adenoma (TSA)** tends to be left-sided and mostly located in the distal colon. These polyps are characterized by a villiform architecture, serration, and the presence of so-called ectopic crypt foci within the villi. An ectopic crypt focus is defined as a small abortive crypt with loss of normal relation between the base of the crypt and the muscularis mucosae. The villi are lined by dysplastic tall columnar cells with eosinophilic cytoplasm (e-**Fig. 14.58**). In addition to BRAF mutations, KRAS mutations are present in up to 25% of TSA. As noted earlier, the current recommendation for all serrated lesions of the colorectum is complete removal of the lesion.

Serrated polyposis, previously referred as HPs, should be viewed as a precancerous syndrome and is defined as at least five serrated polyps proximal to the sigmoid colon, two of which are >1 cm in maximal dimension; any number of polyps proximal to the sigmoid colon in a patient with a first-degree relative having HPs; or >20 polyps of any size throughout the colon.

D. **Adenoma** is traditionally categorized as tubular adenoma if the villous component accounts for <25% of the lesion, villous adenoma if >75% is

TABLE 14.15	WHO Histologic Classification of Tumors of the Colon and Rectum

Epithelial tumors
Adenoma
  Tubular
  Villous
  Tubulovillous
Dysplasia (intraepithelial neoplasia), low grade
Dysplasia (intraepithelial neoplasia), high grade
Serrated lesions
  Hyperplastic polyp, three subtypes (see text)
  Sessile serrated adenoma/polyp
  Traditional serrated adenoma
Hamartomatous
  Cowden-associated polyp
  Juvenile polyp
  Peutz–Jeghers polyp
Carcinomas
Adenocarcinoma
  Cribriform comedo-type adenocarcinoma
  Medullary carcinoma
  Micropapillary carcinoma
  Mucinous carcinoma
  Serrated adenocarcinoma
  Signet-ring cell carcinoma
Adenosquamous carcinoma
Spindle cell carcinoma
Squamous cell carcinoma
Undifferentiated carcinoma
Neuroendocrine neoplasms
Neuroendocrine tumor (NET)
  NET G1 (carcinoid)
  NET G2
Neuroendocrine carcinoma (NEC)
  Large cell NEC
  Small cell NEC
Mixed adenoneuroendocrine carcinoma
EC cell, serotonin-producing NET
L cell, glucagon-like peptide and PP/PYY-producing NETs

Mesenchymal tumors
Lipoma
Leiomyoma
Gastrointestinal stromal tumor
Leiomyosarcoma
Angiosarcoma
Kaposi sarcoma

Lymphomas
B-cell lymphoma, unclassifiable, with features intermediate between diffuse large
B-cell lymphoma and Burkitt lymphoma
Burkitt lymphoma
Diffuse large B-cell lymphoma
Mantle cell lymphoma
Marginal zone lymphoma of mucosa-associated lymphoid tissue (MALT
  lymphoma)

Secondary tumors

WHO, World Health Organization; EC, enterochromaffin; PP, pancreatic polypeptide; PYY, polypeptide
YY; MALT, mucosa-associated lymphoid tissue.
From: Bosman FT, Carneiro F, Hruban RH, Theise ND, eds. *World Health Organization Classification of
Tumours of the Digestive System.* Lyon: IARC Press; 2010. Used with permission.

villous, and tubulovillous adenoma if the villous component is between 25% and 75% (e-**Fig. 14.59**). By definition, adenomas contain at least low-grade dysplasia characterized by nuclear stratification; nuclear enlargement, elongation and hyperchromasia; and cytoplasmic mucin depletion. Paneth cells, neuroendocrine cells, and squamous cell clusters may occur in adenomas.

E. **Mixed hyperplastic and adenomatous polyp** is a synonym for SSA/P with cytological dysplasia.

F. **FAP** is an autosomal dominant disorder caused by germline mutations of the *APC* gene located at 5q21. A minimum of 100 colonic adenomas is required for the diagnosis, but an attenuated form with a reduced number is not uncommon. Adenomas of the upper GI tract, particularly in the ampullary region, and fundic gland polyps are also common findings in FAP patients. Progression to colonic adenocarcinoma approaches 100% by midlife if prophylactic colectomy is not performed (e-**Fig. 14.60**).

Gardner and Turcot syndromes are considered variants of FAP. In addition to adenomas of the GI tract, extra-GI tumors are seen in these patients including osteoid osteoma, epidermal cysts, and intraabdominal fibromatosis (desmoid tumor) for the former; and tumors of the central nervous system for the latter.

G. **Lynch syndrome (LS)**, previously known as **hereditary nonpolyposis colorectal cancer (HNPCC) syndrome,** is an autosomal dominant disorder with an increased risk of colorectal cancer as well as an increased risk of extraintestinal epithelial malignancies including of the endometrium, ovary, stomach, small intestine, upper urinary tract (and others). It is caused by defects in DNA mismatch repair (MMR) genes including *MLH1, MSH2, MSH6,* and *PMS2* that lead to MSI. Defects in MMR can be evaluated indirectly by immunohistochemical stains for DNA mismatch repair proteins or by DNA-based molecular analyses for MSI, or directly by DNA sequence analysis of the MMR genes themselves.

Immunohistochemical analysis is used in many centers to identify the most likely mutated MMR genes; the mismatch repair proteins are normally found in human tissues, thus loss of nuclear staining may represent the presence of a genetic abnormality. The commonly tested proteins are MLH1, MSH2, MSH6, and PMS2. MLH1–PMS2 and MSH2–MSH6 form dimers, the latter member of each pair regulating expression of the former. Thus, if there is a mutation in *MSH6*, expression of both MSH2 and MSH6 proteins will be lost, as will nuclear staining by immunohistochemistry. However, the loss of expression has different implications for each protein pair. If there is loss of MSH2 and MSH6, or of MSH6 and PMS2 alone, the patient is more likely to have LS and therefore should be further referred for genetic counseling. On the other hand, loss of MLH1 and PMS2 can be due to sporadic mutations as well as a rare form of LS, so additional testing for *BRAF* mutation is indicated; the presence of a *BRAF* mutation indicates a sporadic mutation rather than LS.

MSI analysis is currently recommended for all patients that fit revised Bethesda criteria (Table 14.16).

H. **Hamartomatous polyps** can occur sporadically or as part of juvenile polyposis syndrome, Peutz–Jeghers syndrome, Cowden syndrome, and Cronkhite–Canada syndrome. All these syndromes have an autosomal dominant inheritance pattern, except for Cronkhite–Canada which is a nonhereditary disorder.

Juvenile polyps feature cystically dilated and tortuous crypts with edematous and inflamed lamina propria (e-**Figs. 14.61** and **14.62**). Dilated crypts often contain neutrophils and/or mucin, hence the name "retention polyp." The surface of the polyp may be eroded or ulcerated, with granulation tissue and epithelial regenerative changes. Juvenile polyps are not restricted to young individuals. The polyps in patients with Cowden and Cronkhite–Canada syndromes closely resemble juvenile polyps.

TABLE 14.16 Revised Bethesda Criteria for HNPCC (Lynch Syndrome)

1. CRC diagnosed in a patient of <50 years of age
2. Presence of synchronous, metasynchronous colorectal or other LS-related tumors, regardless of age[a]
3. CRC with MSI-H[b] phenotype diagnosed at <60 years of age
4. Patient with CRC and a first-degree relative with a LS-related tumor, with one of the cancers diagnosed before the age of 50 years
5. Patient with CRC with two or more first-degree or a second-degree relative with a Lynch syndrome-related tumor, regardless of age

CRC, colorectal cancer.
[a]Lynch-syndrome related tumors include colorectal, endometrial, stomach, ovarian, pancreas, ureter, renal pelvis, biliary tract and brain tumors, sebaceous gland adenomas, keratoacanthomas and carcinoma of the small bowel.
[b]MSI-H, high level of instability
From: Bosman FT, Carneiro F, Hruban RH, Theise ND, eds. *World Health Organization Classification of Tumours of the Digestive System.* Lyon: IARC Press; 2010. Used with permission.

I. **HGD (adenocarcinoma in situ)** is commonly seen in adenomatous polyps and rarely in juvenile polyps. HGD is characterized by a cribriform or back-to-back growth pattern, loss of mucin, rounded nuclei, coarse chromatin, prominent nucleoli, and loss of nuclear polarity (e-**Fig. 14.63**). HGD is usually focal and situated at the surface of the polyp, and thus requires no additional treatment beyond complete polypectomy. **Intramucosal adenocarcinoma,** defined by lamina propria invasion including invasion into (but not through) the muscularis mucosae, belongs within the category of HGD because of its lack of potential for lymph node metastasis.

J. If **invasive adenocarcinoma arising in a polyp** is detected in a polypectomy specimen, the distance of the invasive focus to the polypectomy margin (e-**Fig. 14.64**), histologic grade, and the presence or absence of lymphovascular invasion should be reported, since these data are important in determining whether segmental resection should be performed. A diagnostic pitfall for adenocarcinoma arising in a polyp is pseudoinvasion, in which adenomatous elements are entrapped or herniated into the submucosa usually secondary to torsion; pseudoinvasion is commonly associated with hemosiderin granules (e-**Figs. 14.65** and **14.66**). Features that aid in the distinction of pseudoinvasion from true invasion include lack of overt malignant histology, presence of lamina propria inflammatory cells around entrapped elements, lack of a desmoplastic response, and lack of direct contact with submucosal muscular vessels. When in doubt, deeper levels of the problematic area may help clarify the diagnosis.

K. **Adenocarcinoma** is currently graded as high grade (poorly differentiated, grade 3) or low grade (well or moderately differentiated, grades 1 and 2). Grade is based on the least differentiated component when heterogenous. Prognostic features in addition to traditional tumor, node, metastasis (TNM) staging elements include the presence of tumor deposits (tumor deposits may represent replaced lymph nodes although no residual lymphatic tissue is seen), status of the circumferential margin, presence of perineural invasion, presence of MSI, tumor regression for previously treated rectal carcinoma (for rectal carcinomas that have received presurgical radiation neoadjuvant treatment, the entire lesion and underlying bowel should be examined in full-thickness sections for evidence of residual tumor, which if present is a feature of poor prognosis), and *KRAS* analysis (Table 14.17). Venous and lymphatic invasion are noted separately. Tumor size is primarily used for documentation and is not a prognostic factor by itself.

TABLE 14.17	Tumor, Node, Metastasis (TNM) Staging Scheme for Carcinoma of the Colon and Rectum

Primary tumor (T)

TX	Primary tumor cannot be assessed
T0	No evidence of primary tumor
Tis	Carcinoma in situ: intraepithelial or invasion of lamina propria[a]
T1	Tumor invades submucosa
T2	Tumor invades muscularis propria
T3	Tumor invades through the muscularis propria into pericolorectal tissues
T4a	Tumor penetrates the surface of visceral peritoneum[b]
T4b	Tumor directly invades or is adherent to other organs or structures[c]

Regional lymph nodes (N)

NX	Regional lymph nodes cannot be assessed
N0	No regional lymph node metastasis
N1	Metastasis in 1–3 regional lymph nodes
N1a	Metastasis in 1 regional lymph node
N1b	Metastasis in 2–3 regional lymph nodes
N1c	Tumor deposit(s) in the subserosa, mesentery, or nonperitonealized pericolic or perirectal tissues without regional nodal metastasis
N2	Metastasis in 4 or more regional lymph nodes
N2a	Metastasis in 4–6 regional lymph nodes
N2b	Metastasis in 7 or more regional lymph nodes

Distant metastasis (M)

M0	No distant metastasis
M1	Distant metastasis
M1a	Metastasis confined to one organ or site
M1b	Metastases in more than one organ/site or the peritoneum

Stage grouping

Stage	T	N	M	Stage	T	N	M
Stage 0	Tis	N0	M0	Stage IIIB	T3–T4a	N1/N1c	M0
Stage I	T1	N0	M0		T2–T3	N2a	M0
	T2	N0	M0		T1–T2	N2b	M0
Stage IIA	T3	N0	M0	Stage IIIC	T4a	N2a	M0
Stage IIB	T4a	N0	M0		T3–T4a	N2b	M0
Stage IIC	T4b	N0	M0		T4b	N1–N2	M0
Stage IIIA	T1–T2	N1/N1c	M0	Stage IVA	Any T	Any N	M1a
	T1	N2a	M0	Stage IVB	Any T	Any N	M1b

[a]Tis includes cancer cells confined within the glandular basement membrane (intraepithelial) or mucosal lamina propria (intramucosal) with no extension through the muscularis mucosae into the submucosa.

[b]Direct invasion in T4 includes invasion of other organs or other segments of the colorectum as a result of direct extension through the serosa, as confirmed on microscopic examination (e.g., invasion of the sigmoid colon by a carcinoma of the cecum) or, for cancers in a retroperitoneal or subperitoneal location, direct invasion of other organs or structures by virtue of extension beyond the muscularis propria (i.e., respectively, a tumor on the posterior wall of the descending colon invading left kidney or lateral abdominal wall; or a mid or distal rectal cancer with invasion of prostate, seminal vesicles, cervix, or vagina).

[c]Tumor that is adherent to other organs or structures, grossly, is classified cT4b. However, if no tumor is present in the adhesion, microscopically, the classification should be pT1-4a depending on the anatomical depth of wall invasion. The V and L classifications should be used to identify the presence or absence of vascular or lymphatic invasion whereas the PN site-specific factor should be used for perineural invasion.

Note: A satellite peritumoral nodule in the pericolorectal adipose tissue of primary carcinoma without histologic evidence of residual lymph node in the nodule may represent discontinuous spread, venous invasion with extravascular spread (V1/2), or a totally replaced lymph node (N1/2). Replaced nodes should be counted separately as positive nodes in the N category, whereas discontinuous spread or venous invasion should be classified in the site-specific factor category tumor deposits (TD).

From: Edge SB, Byrd DR, Compton CC, et al., eds. *AJCC Cancer Staging Manual.* 7th ed. New York, NY: Springer; 2010. Used with permission.

TABLE 14.18 Assessment Parameters for Completeness of Mesorectum[a]

Incomplete
Little bulk to the mesorectum
Defects in the mesorectum down to the muscularis propria
After transverse sectioning, the circumferential margin appears very irregular

Nearly complete
Moderate bulk to the mesorectum
Irregularity of the mesorectal surface with defects >5 mm, but none extending to the muscularis propria
No areas of visibility of the muscularis propria except at the insertion site of the levator ani muscles

Complete
Intact bulky mesorectum with a smooth surface
Only minor irregularities of the mesorectal surface
No surface defects >5 mm in depth
No coning toward the distal margin of the specimen
After transverse sectioning, the circumferential margin appears smooth

[a]The entire specimen is scored on the basis of the worst area.
From: Washington K, Berlin J, Branton P. *Cancer Protocols and Checklists, Colon and Rectum.* Washington, DC: CAP (College of American Pathologists), p. 19; 2011. Used with permission.

The radial resection margin may be the single most critical factor in predicting local recurrence, particularly for rectal carcinoma in a TME specimen. The radial resection margin is the surgically dissected nonperitonealized surface including the perirectal soft tissue (adventitia) and the mesenteric pedicle. Before sectioning, notation of completeness of resection should be made according to established guidelines (Table 14.18).

Similar to other sites of the GI tract, mucinous carcinoma and signet-ring cell carcinoma of the colon are defined by >50% of the tumor bulk consisting of a mucinous component or signet-ring cells. In poorly differentiated mucinous carcinoma, signet-ring cells can be numerous (e-Fig. 14.67). Medullary carcinoma consists of sheets of poorly differentiated or undifferentiated tumor cells with a syncytial growth pattern and a pushing border. Characteristically, there is a marked inter- and intratumoral lymphocytic infiltrate, and Crohn-like lymphoid aggregates may be present at the periphery in some cases. These variants of colorectal adenocarcinoma are frequently associated with DNA mismatch repair deficiency leading to MSI and may have more favorable prognoses despite their high-grade appearance. Although MSI tumors tend to be right-sided, mucinous, or poorly differentiated, they cannot be reliably distinguished on histologic features alone. Nonetheless, since MSI tumors respond to different types of treatment and can be associated with genetic syndromes (e.g., LS; Table 14.16), it is important to note the possibility in the report and send tumor tissue for MSI testing. MSI can be evaluated by immunohistochemical stains for loss of expression of DNA mismatch repair enzymes and by DNA-based molecular analyses (discussed earlier).

Several new molecular markers in predicting the survival and response to treatment in colorectal carcinoma are under investigation. MSI-H tumors are associated with better prognosis and lack of response to 5-FU therapy. The presence of a KRAS mutation is associated with lack of response to treatment with EGFR-targeted antibodies. Patients who have allelic loss of either copy of chromosome region 18q carry a worse prognosis. Finally, greater than 10% of p53 nuclear immunohistochemical reactivity in tumor cells is associated

TABLE 14.19	Tumor, Node, Metastasis (TNM) Staging Scheme for Neuroendocrine Tumors of the Colon and Rectum

Primary tumor (T)

TX	Primary tumor cannot be assessed
T0	No evidence of primary tumor
T1	Tumor invades lamina propria or submucosa and size ≤2 cm
T1a	Tumor size <1 cm in greatest dimension
T1b	Tumor size 1–2 cm in greatest dimension
T2	Tumor invades muscularis propria or size >2 cm with invasion of lamina propria or submucosa
T3	Tumor invades through the muscularis propria into subserosa, or into nonperitonealized pericolic or perirectal tissues.
T4	Tumor invades peritoneum or other organs
	For any Y, add (m) for multiple tumors

Regional lymph nodes (N)

NX	Regional lymph nodes cannot be assessed
N0	No regional lymph node metastasis
N1	Regional lymph node metastasis

Distant metastasis (M)

M0	No distant metastasis
M1	Distant metastasis

Stage grouping

Stage 0	Tis[a]	N0	M0
Stage I	T1	N0	M0
Stage IIA	T2	N0	M0
Stage IIB	T3	N0	M0
Stage IIIA	T4	N0	M0
Stage IIIB	Any T	N1	M1
Stage IV	Any T	Any N	M0

[a]Tis applies only to stomach.
AJCC, American Joint Committee on Cancer.
From: Edge SB, Byrd DR, Compton CC, et al., eds. *AJCC Cancer Staging Manual.* 7th ed. New York, NY: Springer; 2010. Used with permission.

with disease recurrence and decreased overall survival (*Nat Rev Clin Oncol.* 2010;7:318).

VII. NONEPITHELIAL NEOPLASMS OF THE COLON

A. **Neuroendocrine neoplasms.** Table 14.19 presents the current staging scheme for neuroendocrine neoplasms of the colon and rectum.

1. **NET (carcinoid)** is most frequently located in rectum, followed by the cecum (e-Fig. 14.68). It is commonly asymptomatic. The presence of >2 mitoses per 10 high-power fields (HPFs), DNA aneuploidy, atypical histology, lymphatic invasion, size >2 cm, and invasion of the muscularis propria are risk factors for malignant behavior. Most tumors are grade 1 (see Table 14.5).

2. **Neuroendocrine carcinoma (NEC)** of the large intestine is most common in the right colon and is frequently associated with overlying adenomatous epithelium. Histologically, it is indistinguishable from small cell carcinoma or large cell NEC at other anatomic sites and can have a component of adenocarcinoma. In general, immunomarkers such as CK20, CK7, and thyroid transcription factor-1 (TTF-1) do not help in the distinction of a primary colonic NEC from a metastasis. Of note, rectal NETs label with prostatic

acid phosphatase, an immunomarker that is also positive in prostatic adenocarcinoma.

3. **Mixed adenoneuroendocrine carcinomas (MANEC)** contain at least 30% of histologically recognizable adenocarcinoma or squamous cell carcinoma, and NEC. Both components should be graded.

B. **GIST** of the colon accounts for about 5% of all GISTs and is most commonly seen in the rectum (e-**Fig. 14.69**). Colonic GISTs tend to have an aggressive biologic behavior, and tumors with mitotic activity can recur and metastasize despite a small size of <2 cm.

C. **Leiomyoma** is the most common mesenchymal tumor of the colon. It arises from the muscularis mucosae and presents as a well-demarcated nodular expansion in the submucosa. It is typically hypocellular, lacks cytologic atypia, and lacks c-kit expression (e-**Fig. 14.70**).

D. **Submucosal lipoma** can be associated with hyperplastic change in the overlying colonic mucosa (e-**Fig. 14.71**).

E. **Inflammatory polyps** are a heterogeneous group of polypoid lesions and include the pseudopolyps seen in IBD. Inflammatory polyp features inflamed lamina propria and damaged or distorted crypts, and granulation tissue may be present. Inflammatory polyps may be microscopically indistinguishable from a juvenile polyp if cystic dilation of the crypts is prominent; the appropriate diagnosis relies on clinical information. Occasionally, pseudosarcomatous stroma is noted, particularly in eroded or ulcerated areas, characterized by bizarre or multinucleated stroma cells simulating sarcoma (e-**Fig. 14.72**).

F. **Mucosal prolapse** occurs most commonly in the rectum but can be seen anywhere in the colon (the alternative term for this entity, solitary rectal ulcer, is a misnomer). The characteristic histologic features include a fibromuscular lamina propria with vertical extension of the muscularis mucosae into the spaces between crypts, and elongated hyperplastic distorted crypts (e-**Fig. 14.73**). However, since lamina propria smooth muscle proliferation can be seen in any polypoid lesion, the diagnosis of mucosal prolapse should not rely solely on this finding. It should also be noted that smooth muscle fibers are normally present in the duodenal mucosa, and thus should not be viewed as evidence of mucosal prolapse when they are present in that location.

G. **Inflammatory cap polyps** are located mostly in the sigmoid and rectum. These lesions are characterized by hyperplastic, tortuous crypts with abundant inflammation in the lamina propria. The "cap" is composed of an exudate.

H. **Colitis cystica profunda** is a benign condition in which cystically dilated crypts are misplaced in the submucosa and/or deeper layers of the bowel wall (e-**Fig. 14.74**). The distinction from well-differentiated adenocarcinoma lies in the lobular arrangement of the displaced crypts, lack of dysplastic features, lack of desmoplasia, presence of surrounding lamina propria components, and presence of hemorrhage or hemosiderin.

I. **Mucosal ganglioneuroma** resembles a neurofibroma and features a bland Schwann cell proliferation with nerve fibers that expands the lamina propria, with individual or nests of ganglion cells embedded in the spindle cell background (e-**Figs. 14.75** and **14.76**). Multiple (ganglioneuromatous polyposis) and diffuse (ganglioneuromatosis) lesions are usually seen in patients with multiple endocrine neoplasia (MEN) 2B or type 1 neurofibromatosis (NF1).

J. **Inflammatory fibroid polyps** are usually sessile lesions. They contain an abundant fibromyxoid stroma and an inflammatory infiltrate rich in eosinophils (e-**Figs. 14.77** and **14.78**). The lesion is usually submucosal but can also involve the mucosa.

K. **Mucosal folds** and **prominent lymphoid follicles** can resemble polyps endoscopically. On biopsy, a mucosal fold consists of completely normal colonic mucosa.

L. **Miscellaneous polypoid lesions. Pneumatosis coli** is characterized by gas accumulation in colonic wall. It most commonly affects the sigmoid colon. Microscopically, cystic spaces surrounded by histiocytes and giant cells are seen (e-Fig. 14.79). **Endometriosis, pseudolipomatosis,** and **xanthomas** can also present as polypoid lesions.

VIII. **DIAGNOSTIC FEATURES OF COMMON NONNEOPLASTIC AND NEOPLASTIC CONDITIONS OF THE APPENDIX**

A. **Acute appendicitis** usually occurs as the result of luminal occlusion (such as by a fecalith, lymphoid hyperplasia, or *Enterobius vermicularis*), followed by bacterial infection. Diverticulosis of the appendix is a rare cause. Microscopically, acute appendicitis is characterized by transmural neutrophilic infiltration (e-Fig. 14.80). Abscess formation, gangrenous necrosis, and perforation may ensue. When inflammation extends into the mesoappendix and the serosa, periappendicitis should be diagnosed.

B. **Cystic fibrosis** involving the appendix is characterized by thick, eosinophilic, inspissated mucoid material in the lumen and in the crypts (e-Fig. 14.81).

C. **HP** of the appendix is histologically similar to that of the colorectum but tends to be sessile. Hyperplasia can also diffusely involve the appendiceal mucosa (mucosal hyperplasia).

D. **SSA/P,** the most common serrated lesion of the appendix, is histologically similar to SSA/P of the colorectum and has an intact underlying lamina propria.

E. **Adenoma** of the appendix is also similar to that of the colorectum. There is no associated mucin in the wall of the appendix.

F. **Adenocarcinoma** of the appendix has recently been reclassified (Table 14.20), and a staging scheme separate from that for colorectal adenocarcinoma has been developed (Table 14.21).

1. **Low-grade appendiceal mucinous neoplasm (LAMN).** The appendix is generally enlarged and filled with mucin. The lining epithelium is villous, serrated, and undulating and comprises a single layer of columnar or cuboidal cells with low-grade dysplasia. In contrast to adenoma, the neoplastic epithelium rests on fibrous tissue with no underlying lamina propria (e-Fig. 14.82), but no definitive invasion or desmoplasia is present. The associated mucin may be acellular, and lesions are mostly associated with low-grade pseudomyxoma peritonei.

2. **Mucinous adenocarcinoma.** These tumors have >50% extracellular mucin as with their colonic counterparts. The tumor cells have high-grade cytologic features. Malignant glands invade the appendiceal wall and a desmoplastic response is present.

3. **Signet-ring cell carcinoma.** These tumors have a >50% signet-ring cell component.

G. **Pseudomyxoma peritonei** is primarily a clinical diagnosis, and its prognosis depends on the associated mucinous neoplasm. Although appendiceal lesions are responsible for the vast majority of the cases, mucinous tumors of other sites such as the ovary can rarely be the cause.

1. **Peritoneal adenomucinosis (low-grade pseudomyxoma peritonei)** is defined by the presence of mucin-containing epithelium that is benign or shows only mild cytologic atypia.

2. **Peritoneal mucinous carcinomatosis (high-grade pseudomyxoma peritonei)** features the presence of frankly malignant epithelium similar to moderately and poorly differentiated adenocarcinoma in a background of mucinous ascites.

H. **Neuroendocrine neoplasms** are the most common neoplasms of the appendix and include a heterogeneous group of lesions with variable biologic behavior.

1. **NETs** are histologically identical to those seen in the other parts of the GI tract and are typically found in the distal third of the appendix. However,

TABLE 14.20	WHO Histologic Classification of Tumors of the Appendix

Epithelial tumors
Premalignant lesions
Adenoma
  Tubular
  Villous
  Tubulovillous
Dysplasia (intraepithelial neoplasia), low grade
Dysplasia (intraepithelial neoplasia), high grade
Serrated lesions
  Hyperplastic polyp
  Sessile serrated adenoma/polyp
  Traditional serrated adenoma
Carcinoma
Adenocarcinoma
  Mucinous adenocarcinoma
  Low-grade appendiceal mucinous neoplasm
  Signet-ring cell carcinoma
Undifferentiated carcinoma
Neuroendocrine neoplasms
Neuroendocrine tumor (NET)
  NET G1 (carcinoid)
  NET G2
Neuroendocrine carcinoma (NEC)
  Large cell NEC
  Small cell NEC
  EC cell, serotonin-producing NET
  Goblet cell carcinoid
  L cell, glucagon-like peptide and PP/PYY-producing NET
Tubular carcinoid

Mesenchymal tumors
Neuroma
Lipoma
Leiomyoma
Leiomyosarcoma
Kaposi sarcoma

Lymphomas
Secondary tumors

WHO, World Health Organization; EC, enterochromaffin; PP, pancreatic polypeptide; PYY, polypeptide YY; MALT, mucosa-associated lymphoid tissue.
From: Bosman FT, Carneiro F, Hruban RH, Theise ND, eds. *World Health Organization Classification of Tumours of the Digestive System.* Lyon: IARC Press; 2010. Used with permission.

they are distinguished from other GI NETs by their relatively benign behavior. Metastasis is almost never seen in tumors <1 cm in greatest dimension. The risk for metastatic disease is higher for tumors >2 cm in greatest dimension, and in tumors that show invasion of the angiolymphatic spaces and periappendiceal tissues.

2. **Goblet cell carcinoid** is a mixed endocrine–exocrine neoplasm, almost exclusively seen in the appendix. The tumor typically diffusely infiltrates the appendiceal wall, with relative sparing of the mucosa. The hallmark of the tumor is the presence of individual glands or small tight clusters of

TABLE 14.21	Tumor, Node, Metastasis (TNM) Staging Scheme for Carcinoma of the Appendix

Primary tumor (T)
Carcinoma

TX	Primary tumor cannot be assessed
T0	No evidence of primary tumor
Tis	Carcinoma in situ: intraepithelial or invasion of lamina propria[a]
T1	Tumor invades submucosa
T2	Tumor invades muscularis propria
T3	Tumor invades through the muscularis propria into pericolorectal tissues
T4	Tumor penetrates to the surface of visceral peritoneum, including mucinous peritoneal tumor within the right lower quadrant and/or directly invades other organs or structures[b,c]
T4a	Tumor penetrates visceral peritoneum, including mucinous peritoneal tumor within the right lower quadrant
T4b	Tumor directly invades or is adherent to other organs or structures

Carcinoid

TX	Primary tumor cannot be assessed
T0	No evidence of primary tumor
T1	Tumor 2 cm or less in greatest dimension
T1a	Tumor ≤ 1 cm in greatest dimension
T1b	Tumor >1 cm but not >2 cm
T2	Tumor >2 cm but no >4 cm or with extension to the cecum
T3	Tumor >4 cm or with extension to the ileum
T4	Tumor directly invades other adjacent organs or structures, e.g., abdominal wall and skeletal muscle[d]

Regional lymph nodes (N)
Carcinoma

NX	Regional lymph nodes cannot be assessed
N0	No regional lymph node metastasis
N1	Metastasis in 1–3 regional lymph nodes
N2	Metastasis in 4 or more regional lymph nodes

Carcinoid

N0	No regional lymph node metastasis
N1	Regional lymph node metastasis

Distant metastasis (M)
Carcinoma

M0	No distant metastasis (no pathologic M0, use clinical M to complete stage group)
M1	Distant metastasis
M1a	Intraperitoneal metastasis beyond right lower quadrant, including pseudomyxoma peritonei
M1b	Nonperitoneal metastases

Carcinoid

M0	No distant metastasis (no pathologic M0, use clinical M to complete stage group)
M1	Distant metastasis

(continued)

TABLE 14.21	Tumor, Node, Metastasis (TNM) Staging Scheme for Carcinoma of the Appendix (*Continued*)		
Carcinoma stage grouping			
Stage 0	Tis	N0	M0
Stage I	T1	N0	M0
	T2	N0	M0
Stage IIA	T3	N0	M0
Stage IIB	T4a	N0	M0
Stage IIC	T4b	N0	M0
Stage IIIA	T1	N1	M0
	T2	N1	M0
Stage IIIB	T3	N1	M0
	T4	N1	M0
Stage IIIC	Any T	N2	M0
Stage IVA	Any T	N0	M1a G1
Stage IVB	Any T	N0	M1a G2,3
	Any T	Any N	M1b Any G
	Any T	N2	M1a Any G
Stage IVC	Any T	Any N	M1b Any G
Carcinoid stage grouping			
Stage I	T1	N0	M0
Stage II	T2, T3	N0	M0
Stage III	T4	N0	M0
	Any T	N1	M0
Stage IV	Any T	Any N	M1

[a]Tis includes cancer cells confined within the glandular basement membrane (intraepithelial) or lamina propria (intramucosal) with no extension through the muscularis mucosae into the submucosa.
[b]Direct invasion in T4 includes invasion of other organs or other segments of the colorectum by way of the serosa, e.g., invasion of ileum.
[c]Tumor that is adherent to other organs or structures, grossly, is classified cT4b. However, if no tumor is present in the adhesion, microscopically, the classification should be pT1-4a depending on the anatomical depth of wall invasion.
[d]Tumor that is adherent to other organs or structures, grossly, is classified cT4. However, if no tumor is present in the adhesion, microscopically, the classification should be pT1-4a depending on the anatomical depth of wall invasion.
From: Edge SB, Byrd DR, Compton CC, et al., eds. *AJCC Cancer Staging Manual*. 7th ed. New York, NY: Springer; 2010. Used with permission.

glands formed by tumor cells exhibiting a goblet or signet-ring morphology with a small compressed nucleus and conspicuous intracytoplasmic mucin (e-**Figs. 14.83** and **14.84**). Small extracellular mucin pools may be seen; Paneth cells or foci resembling Brunner glands can also be present. The cells show a low Ki67 proliferation index, low mitotic count, and only mild to moderate cytologic atypia. Immunohistochemically, tumors display both neuroendocrine and epithelial differentiation.

3. **Tubular carcinoid** arises from the base of the crypts and is characterized by discrete tubules and/or short tubular nests within abundant stroma (e-**Fig. 14.85**). The orderly pattern, lack of cytologic atypia, and absence of mitotic activity helps distinguish the tumor from metastatic adenocarcinoma. Tubular carcinoid behaves in a benign fashion.

4. **Mixed carcinoid–adenocarcinoma (MANEC)** consists of both carcinoid (usually goblet cell carcinoid) and conventional adenocarcinoma.

IX. **DIAGNOSTIC FEATURES OF COMMON NONNEOPLASTIC AND NEOPLASTIC CONDITIONS OF THE ANUS.** The WHO classification of tumors of the anal canal is given in Table 14.22, and the staging scheme is given in Table 14.23.

TABLE 14.22	WHO Histologic Classification of Tumors of the Anal Canal

Epithelial tumors
Premalignant lesions
Anal intraepithelial neoplasia (dysplasia), low grade
Anal intraepithelial neoplasia (dysplasia), high grade
Bowen disease
Perianal squamous intraepithelial neoplasia
Paget disease
Carcinoma
  Squamous cell carcinoma
  Verrucous carcinoma
  Adenocarcinoma
  Mucinous adenocarcinoma
Neuroendocrine neoplasms
Neuroendocrine tumor (NET)
  NET G1 (carcinoid)
  NET G2
Neuroendocrine carcinoma (NEC)
  Large cell NEC
  Small cell NEC
Mixed adenoneuroendocrine carcinoma
Mesenchymal tumors
Secondary tumors

From: Bosman FT, Carneiro F, Hruban RH, Theise ND, eds. *World Health Organization Classification of Tumours of the Digestive System.* Lyon: IARC Press; 2010. Used with permission.

A. **Hemorrhoids** are characterized by dilated thick-walled submucosal veins, often with thrombi.

B. **Anal tag** is a fibroepithelial polyp, histologically identical to a skin tag (acrochordon).

C. **Inflammatory cloacogenic polyp** is a type of mucosal prolapse featuring fibromuscular proliferation of the lamina propria and villous hyperplasia of the mucosa that often contains areas of ATZ (mixed rectal and squamous) epithelium and surface erosion (e-**Fig. 14.86**). The lesion may resemble a villous or tubulovillous adenoma at low-power.

D. **Hidradenoma papilliferum** is a benign sweat gland tumor that can occur in the anal region and histologically identical to its vulvar counterpart.

E. **Condyloma acuminatum,** also known as genital warts, is caused by low-risk serotypes of human papilloma virus (HPV). It features a papillomatous proliferation of the squamous epithelium with parakeratosis and viral cytopathic (koilocytic) changes (e-**Fig. 14.87**).

F. **Anal squamous intraepithelial neoplasia (ASIN),** previously known as anal intraepithelial neoplasia (AIN), refers to a spectrum of squamous dysplasia strongly associated with high-risk serotypes of HPV. ASIN is graded as ASIN-L (low grade) or ASIN-H (high grade). Ki 67 and p16 can be used in aid for grading (e-**Fig. 14.88**). **Perianal squamous intraepithelial neoplasia (PSIN),** previously known as Bowen's disease, is characterized by full-thickness dysplasia of the squamous epithelium.

G. **Squamous cell carcinoma** accounts for about 80% of anal carcinomas and HPV DNA is present in up to about 80% of cases. The majority of the tumors are heterogeneous and include regions with nonkeratinizing, basaloid, and ductal morphology. The current WHO classification scheme recommends the generic term squamous cell carcinoma for diagnosis of these tumors, with

TABLE 14.23	Tumor, Node, Metastasis (TNM) Staging Scheme for Carcinoma of the Anal Canal		
Primary tumor (T)			
TX	Primary tumor cannot be assessed		
T0	No evidence of primary tumor		
Tis	Carcinoma in situ (Bowen's disease, high-grade squamous intraepithelial lesion (HSIL), anal intraepithelial neoplasia II–III (AIN II–III)		
T1	Tumor ≤2 cm in greatest dimension		
T2	Tumor >2 cm but not >5 cm in greatest dimension		
T3	Tumor >5 cm in greatest dimension		
T4	Tumor of any size invades adjacent organ(s), e.g., vagina, urethra, bladder[a]		
Regional lymph nodes (N)			
NX	Regional lymph nodes cannot be assessed		
N0	No regional lymph node metastasis		
N1	Metastasis in perirectal lymph node(s)		
N2	Metastasis in unilateral internal iliac and/or inguinal lymph node(s)		
N3	Metastasis in perirectal and inguinal lymph nodes and/or bilateral iliac and/or inguinal lymph nodes		
Distant metastasis (M)			
M0	No distant metastasis		
M1	Distant metastasis		
Stage grouping			
Stage 0	Tis	N0	M0
Stage I	T1	N0	M0
Stage II	T2	N0	M0
	T3	N0	M0
Stage IIIA	T1	N1	M0
	T2	N1	M0
	T3	N1	M0
	T4	N0	M0
Stage IIIB	T4	N1	M0
	Any T	N2	M0
	Any T	N3	M0
Stage IV	Any T	Any N	M1

[a]Direct invasion of the rectal wall, perirectal skin, subcutaneous tissue, or the sphincter muscle(s) is not classified as T4.
From: Edge SB, Byrd DR, Compton CC, et al., eds. *AJCC Cancer Staging Manual.* 7th ed. New York, NY: Springer; 2010. Used with permission.

description of the presence of basaloid, mucinous, and keratinization (and adjacent intraepithelial neoplasia) as needed.

H. **Extramucosal (perianal) carcinoma** is a unique type of adenocarcinoma which can be associated with fistulae or arise from the anal duct. The neoplastic glands are usually deeply situated without evidence of mucosal surface involvement. This is a slow-growing, well-differentiated tumor with glandular formation, bland cytology, and mucin production (**e-Fig. 14.89**).

I. **Paget's disease** of the anus is histologically identical to that seen in the breast and vulva (**e-Fig. 14.90**).

J. **Melanoma** of the anus is histologically identical to that seen in other cutaneous and mucosal sites (**e-Fig. 14.91**).

X. MISCELLANEOUS LESIONS OF THE MESENTERY

A. Mesenteric fibromatosis is the most common primary tumor of the mesentery and most often occurs in the mesentery of the small intestine. Even though most cases are sporadic, some are associated with FAP/Gardner syndrome; men are affected more commonly than women. Grossly, the lesion is well-circumscribed and usually measures >10 cm.

Histologically, spindle cells are dispersed in a densely collagenous stroma, and myxoid change of the stroma can be present. The borders of the lesion are infiltrative despite the well-circumscribed gross appearance. Immunohisto-chemically, the tumor cells show nuclear beta-catenin positivity. Patients with Gardner syndrome show similar histologic findings, even though the myxoid stroma can be more prominent.

Due to the infiltrative nature of the lesion, complete excision is difficult, and recurrence is common. The clinical course is more aggressive in Gardner syndrome patients; in fact, fibromatosis is the second most common cause of death in this patient group.

Sclerosing in mesenteritis is in the differential diagnosis of mesenteric fibro-matosis. The lesion is usually solitary and most often arises from the mesentery of the small intestine, although in some cases diffuse involvement by multiple masses may occur. Histologically, the lesion contains areas of fibrosis, inflam-mation, and fat necrosis in varying proportions. By immunohistochemistry, the tumor cells are smooth muscle actin-positive but nuclear beta-catenin-negative.

B. Inflammatory myofibroblastic tumor (IMT) involves the mesentery and omentum as the most common nonpulmonary sites. Being the most common in children, IMT is multinodular or lobular with a rubbery, tan-white cut surface. A variety of histologic patterns can be seen in different lesions or within a single tumor. One common pattern resembles nodular fasciitis with spindle to stellate shaped cells embedded in a myxoid stroma. Other tumors show spindle cells arranged in a storiform or a fascicular growth pattern. Prominent lymphoid aggregates, or lymphoplasmacytic infiltrates, are seen in most cases. Immunohistochem-istry is positive for smooth muscle actin and desmin. Since rearrangements of the *ALK* gene are characteristic of the tumor (see Chap. 46), immunostains for the ALK protein are especially helpful.

C. Desmoplastic small round cell tumor is an aggressive malignancy most com-monly seen in young boys and patients present with an abdominal or pelvic mass. The tumor is composed of nests of small round blue cells embedded in a desmoplastic stroma separated by fibrous tissue. Rhabdoid features are commonly seen. The tumor cells are vimentin and desmin positive; perinu-clear keratin positivity is also present. The t(11:22)(p13; q12) translocation characteristic of the tumor results in an *EWS–WT1* fusion (see Chap. 46).

D. Mesenteric inflammatory venoocclusive disease (MIVD) most commonly occurs in men in the pericolonic soft tissue and subserosa. The presenting symptoms are those of ischemia, thus the clinical differential diagnosis is usually quite broad. **Idiopathic myointimal hyperplasia** is a characteristic feature of the dis-ease, consisting of a concentric proliferation of smooth muscle cells within the small- to medium-sized veins of the affected mesenteric segment. Since the involved veins can be mistaken for arteries, an elastic stain can be helpful in diagnosis (**e-Figs. 14.92** and **14.93**). Trauma and phlebitis have been ques-tioned as the underlying etiology of MIVD. The patients follow an indolent course after surgery.

15 The Liver
Ta-Chiang Liu and Elizabeth M. Brunt

I. **NORMAL ANATOMY.** The largest solid organ of the body, the mass of the adult liver is 1200 to 1600 g. The right, left, and caudate lobes are subdivided into segments on the basis of inflow blood supply (e-**Fig. 15.1**).* The liver has dual inflow supply, with approximately two-thirds from the low pressure, low O_2 portal vein, and one-third from the systemic pressure, high O_2 hepatic artery. Pressure equalization occurs in the sinusoids, along with the nutrient and O_2 gradient from portal tracts to terminal hepatic venules. The venous return is via the left, right, and middle hepatic veins which join to form the inferior vena cava as it enters the heart at the right atrium. Bile duct blood supply is entirely from the hepatic artery plexuses.

Microscopically, the hepatic cords are lined by reticulin fibers and separated by sinusoids. The parenchyma is subdivided into acinar units of Rappaport which reflect an oxygen/nutrient gradient from most (zone 1) to least (zone 3), respectively; zone 2 is an ill-defined area in between. The anatomy of Rappaport's units underlies many pathologic processes. The lobule, often used interchangeably with acinus, is a term based on the concept of the hexagon in which hepatic cords radiate from the central vein toward the portal tracts. Each portal tract is a fibrous matrix that contains a branch of the hepatic artery, a portal vein, a bile duct, and a poorly visualized lymphatic (e-**Fig. 15.2**). Larger portal tracts contain autonomic nerve fibers. Inflammatory cells are typically lacking, or are few in number. The parenchyma is separated from the portal tract at the *limiting plate*.

II. **GROSS EXAMINATION AND SPECIMEN HANDLING**

A. **Needle core biopsy.** Specimen handling depends on the reason for liver biopsy. After measuring and description of the number of cores, liver biopsies are wrapped in lens paper and fixed overnight; use of sponge pads is strongly discouraged because of the artifacts created during sectioning. Protocol "special" stains and six additional unstained sections are recommended for medical liver biopsies at initial preparation. Stains include three hematoxylin and eosin (H&E), a stain for collagen (trichrome or picrosirius red), reticulin, periodic acid-Schiff after diastase (PAS-d), and modified Perls' for iron. Additional stains that must be available include copper or copper binding protein (rhodanine, orcein or Victoria blue; orcein is also useful to differentiate passive septa of collapse from active elastic fiber deposition in fibrosis); and Verhoeff van Gieson (VVG) for vessel wall architecture (*Semin Diagn Pathol*. 2006;23:190).

1. **Tumor.** Processing of biopsies for diagnosis of tumors includes three levels for H&E and six unstained for possible additional immunohistochemistry (IHC).

2. **Immunocompromised patients.** Biopsies from immunocompromised patients (typically solid organ or bone marrow transplant patients) may or may not require "rush" processing; clear communication with the submitting clinicians is required in these cases and fixation, grossing, and processing are tailored to the clinical needs.

3. **Medical liver biopsy.** The reason(s) for the liver biopsy, that is, diagnosis or confirmation; grading and staging of hepatitis; or other possible medical questions should be clearly understood prior to sign out.

---

*All e-figures are available online via the Solution Site Image Bank.

4. **Frozen section.** Indications for frozen sections of liver core or wedge biopsies include donor liver evaluations for quantity of steatosis and/or portal inflammation; acute fatty liver of pregnancy (AFLP) for microvesicular steatosis detection by oil red O stain (from sections of liver biopsies at any stage of processing prior to xylene clearing, cut onto charged slides). Evaluation of intraoperatively encountered lesions is done from fresh tissue submitted on saline-moisturized gauze; cores are best sectioned with as little handling as possible, sectioned at 90 degrees to the long axis. Wedge biopsies may require breadloafing before sectioning. Frozen artifact creates spaces that may be challenging to distinguish from fat; thus conservative estimates of the degree of steatosis are recommended from frozen sections. If electron microscopic examination is expected for a potential metabolic disease, additional tissue should be fixed in 3% buffered glutaraldehyde.

5. **Miscellaneous.** Iron and copper tissue quantitation can be performed in reference laboratories directly from tissue in the paraffin block.

B. **Wedge biopsy or excision.** Wedge biopsy is not typically recommended for the evaluation of diffuse liver parenchymal diseases, as the subcapsular parenchyma contains fibrous extensions for 3 to 5 mm that may mimic fibrosis (e-**Fig. 15.3**). The subcapsular regions tend to show parenchymal collapse; elastosis may occur in this location as well as a result of chronic ischemia. Wedge excisions for superficial, circumscribed lesions are managed similarly to resections, as described below.

C. **Segmentectomy, lobectomy, or partial hepatectomy** are performed for large lesions that are not amenable to wedge excision. The surgery may or may not follow anatomic boundaries, and thus before sectioning, it is important to understand the procedure that was done; review of the imaging studies and reports is invaluable. After the type of surgery, mass, and dimensions of the specimen are recorded, the resection margin is inked, the appearance of the capsule noted, and the specimen is sliced in the axial plane at about 0.5 cm increments. Gross examination of the lesion(s) and nonlesional liver parenchyma should include color(s) (nutmeg; tan; bile-stained; hemorrhagic; yellow), viability (necrotic, nonnecrotic), texture (firm; hard; soft; spongy), and presence of nodularity. If a tumor has been preoperatively embolized via transarterial chemo-embolization (TACE), the percentage of tumor necrosis grossly should be assessed; however, only after complete submission and evaluation microscopically can it be adequately reported. Tumor sections (at least three) should demonstrate relationship of lesions to liver parenchyma, grossly visible vessels or ducts, margins (if close), and any variable areas within the tumor. Sections of nonneoplastic liver and inked resection margin(s) are submitted to evaluate underlying liver disease, vascular alterations, and margin status. One nontumor section of normal liver should be submitted and evaluated by routine special stains.

D. **Total hepatectomy (explant)** – performed for end-stage chronic liver disease, fulminant hepatic failure, or metabolic disorders – is followed by orthotopic liver transplantation. Radiology reports must be consulted before processing the specimen to ensure that radiographically detected lesions are sampled. The total weight, dimensions of each lobe, and capsule appearance are recorded. The hilum is completely removed, breadloafed, and submitted in toto proximally to distally without dissection. If a TIPSS stent has been placed, no attempt should be made to remove it as the spring-opened wires are not protected; rather, the hilar tissue should be dissected away. The liver is then placed on the cutting board facing up, and sectioned axially cephalad–caudad in about 0.5 cm increments. Each slice is carefully examined fresh and after fixation (especially in cirrhotic livers) for bulging, large, or discolored nodules (which are all gross features of dysplastic nodules [DNs], or small HCC) that require documentation which includes location, number, size, color, and relation to the capsule or hilum. In their absence, two random sections from both the left and the right lobes are submitted. Only one section is necessary for routine special stains. The native and donor gallbladders are submitted as for routine cholecystectomies.

III. **DIAGNOSTIC FEATURES OF COMMON NONNEOPLASTIC CONDITIONS.** In the approach to liver biopsy, knowledge of the clinical information is essential. The adequacy of the biopsy should be assessed, which must be judged on the basis of the nature of the question(s) being asked. Grading and staging chronic hepatitis ideally involve a 1.5 cm core, and up to 11 portal tracts; <5 portal tracts is not optimal (*Semin Diagn Pathol.* 2006;23:132) (see Figs. 15.1 and 15.2).

Grading and staging schema were initially developed for comparisons of treatment for autoimmune and "nonAnonB hepatitis" trials, but they quickly transitioned to apply to chronic hepatitis (*Hepatology.* 2000;31:241). All systems share the assessment of portal and lobular necroinflammation for grade and fibrosis for stage (e-Figs. 15.1 and 15.2). One published system (*Am J Surg Pathol.* 1995;19:1409) is simple to apply and communicate clinically; this system can be applied for any form of chronic hepatitis, but is not meant for cholestatic or vascular diseases, or alcoholic or nonalcoholic fatty liver diseases (NAFLD).

Patterns of collagen deposition and architectural remodeling are frequently suggestive of the precedent injury: hepatitic, biliary, vascular, alcoholic, etc. Viral hepatitis and alcoholic hepatitis differ as the former is portal-based, and the latter is centered in zone 3, is perisinusoidal initially, and results in nodules the size of the acinus (e.g., micronodular cirrhosis). The portal–portal fibrosis of the chronic biliary diseases often results in cirrhotic remodeling with maintenance of the terminal hepatic venule in its central location; a "jig-saw" pattern is therefore suggestive of biliary disease.

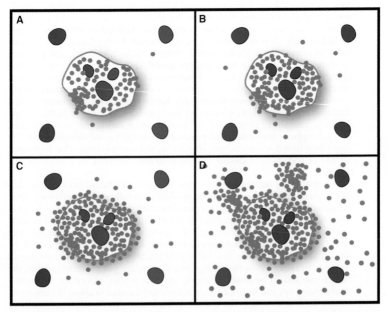

Figure 15.1 Ludwig and Batts Grading of chronic hepatitis. **A:** Stage 1. **B:** Stage 2. **C:** Stage 3. **D:** Stage 4. From: *Am J Surg Pathol.* 1995;19:1409. With permission.

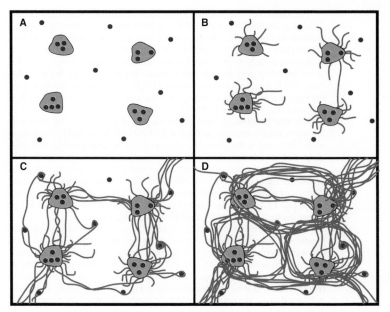

Figure 15.2 Ludwig and Batts Staging of chronic hepatitis. **A:** Grade 1. **B:** Grade 2. **C:** Grade 3. **D:** Grade 4. From: *Am J Surg Pathol.* 1995;19:1409. With permission.

A. Infectious liver diseases

1. **Viral hepatitis** refers to one of the hepatotropic viruses: HAV, HBC, HCV, HDV (with superinfection or coinfection with HBV), and HEV.

   a. **Acute viral hepatitis** is commonly diagnosed clinically by serologic and clinical tests. Pathologists, therefore, have relatively little experience with this form of liver disease. Histopathologically, acute viral hepatitis is characterized by simultaneous hepatocyte injury and regeneration, chronic inflammation, and no fibrosis. The changes include swollen hepatocytes (hydropic degeneration), apoptotic (acidophil) bodies, lobular spotty necrosis, lobular greater than portal inflammation, sinusoidal cell reaction (Kupffer cell and endothelial cell hypertrophy), and bi- and multinucleated hepatocytes. Collectively, these findings result in "lobular unrest" and "disarray" (e-**Fig. 15.4**). The inflammatory infiltrates consist predominantly of mononuclear cells, with occasional plasma cells and eosinophils. In severe cases, confluent perivenular, bridging (zone 3 to zone 3), submassive (panacinar) or massive (multiacinar) hepatic necrosis may occur (e-**Fig. 15.5**). The ductular reaction, a form of regenerative response, may be accompanied by mononuclear or polymorphonuclear cells (e-**Fig. 15.6**). Trichrome and reticulin stains may be confusing as the reticulin collapse may be extensive and the collapsed sinusoids may seemingly react with the stains for collagen. In these cases, the orcein stain for elastic fibers is helpful, as elastic fibers are only found in fibrosis (e-**Fig. 15.7**). Zone 3 canalicular cholestasis may be present; if prominent, a diagnosis of acute cholestatic hepatitis is given (e-**Fig. 15.8**). Careful evaluation of portal tracts will exclude biliary obstruction (see later).

Fulminant hepatic failure or complete resolution may occur in any form of acute viral hepatitis. HAV may have zone 1 confluent or bridging necrosis and numerous plasma cells or may resemble cholestatic obstructive hepatitis. HBV, HCV, and HDV may evolve to chronic hepatitis. It is important to note that the histopathologic differential diagnoses for acute viral hepatitis include autoimmune hepatitis (AIH), Wilson's disease, AFLP, drug-induced liver injury (DILI), and rarely, ischemic hepatitis. Cryptogenic acute hepatitis, for which no clinical cause is found, is reported as such (e-**Fig. 15.9**).

b. **Chronic viral hepatitis,** defined by persistently elevated abnormal liver tests for more than 6 months, is caused by HBV, HCV, or HDV coinfection with HBV, and is histologically characterized by mononuclear cell infiltrates rich in T lymphocytes, greater in the portal tracts than in the lobules. Plasma cells, macrophages, and eosinophils are also present, but in smaller number. The portal inflammation is accompanied by varying degrees of interface activity (previously referred to as piecemeal necrosis) (e-**Fig. 15.10**), lobular activity with acidophil bodies (e-**Fig. 15.11**) or spotty necrosis, and portal-based fibrosis (e-**Fig. 15.12**).

Some features are characteristic of the specific types of chronic viral hepatitis. Chronic HBV is recognized by the presence of ground glass intracytoplasmic inclusions; this is HB S Ag in expanded smooth endoplasmic reticulum (e-**Fig. 15.13**). HB S Ag IHC has three patterns: membranous, cytoplasmic, and inclusion (e-**Fig. 15.14**); intranuclear inclusions require HB C Ag IHC for identification (e-**Fig. 15.15**). In HBV- and HDV-coinfected cases, the necroinflammation tends to be more severe, and delta antigen can be demonstrated in nuclei by immunostaining.

The portal lymphoid aggregates of HCV are not pathognomonic because they may occur in HBV and AIH, but they are common and suggestive (e-**Fig. 15.16**). Steatosis is common: if in zone 1, it is most likely due to HCV; and if in zone 3, it is most likely due to host factors (metabolic or alcoholic). Acidophil bodies, bile duct injury, and sinusoidal lymphocytosis may be seen in HCV; HCV genotype 3 often has marked macrovesicular steatosis. Crystalline material is often present in substances that are abused by intravenous injection, and may be evident as polarizable material within portal macrophages.

c. **Epstein–Barr virus hepatitis** is characterized by a sinusoidal infiltrate of atypical lymphocytes in a "beads on a string" pattern (e-**Fig. 15.17**). The diagnosis can be confirmed by in situ hybridization for viral RNA and serologic tests.

d. **Cytomegalovirus hepatitis** in immunocompromised patients commonly induces microabscesses surrounding infected cells with characteristic intranuclear and intracytoplasmic viral inclusions (e-**Fig. 15.18**). Thus, microabscesses should prompt immunostaining if inclusions are not evident. CMV infection in immunocompetent patients may show microgranulomas; in this setting, viral inclusions are not usually present. Multinucleation of hepatocytes can occur in neonates.

e. **Adenovirus hepatitis,** uncommon in immunocompetent hosts and in adults, causes nonzonal foci of coagulative necrosis with a minimal inflammatory response. Nuclei of infected hepatocytes are hyperchromatic and smudgy, with chromatin margination (e-**Fig. 15.19**). Confirmation is by immunohistochemical staining.

f. **Herpesvirus hepatitis** includes pyknotic debris and nonzonal "punched out" necrosis; nuclear ground glass (Cowdry A) viral inclusions can be found in syncytial nuclei at the periphery of necrosis, or in other cells within the liver (e-**Fig. 15.20**). IHC is confirmatory. HSV is not more common in pregnancy. Rapid diagnosis and treatment may be lifesaving.

2. **Bacterial infections** involve the liver in various ways: space-occupying abscess, toxic cholangitis (e.g., toxic shock syndrome), granulomatous inflammation (*Mycobacterium* spp.), and peliosis (bacillary angiomatosis in AIDS). Sepsis may result in microabscesses, zone 3 canalicular cholestasis, and/or ductular cholestasis (e.g., cholangitis lenta) (e-Fig. 15.21).

3. **Fungal infections** are due to systemic infections such as candidiasis, aspergillosis, and histoplasmosis. The biopsy may show organisms or features of sepsis (see above), or DILI.

4. **Parasitic infections,** including hydatid cyst, amebic abscess, and schistosomiasis, each with characteristic histopathologic features, require a high index of clinical and pathologic suspicion for diagnosis.

B. **Metabolic and toxic liver diseases**

1. **Alcoholic liver disease (ALD)** encompasses a spectrum of fatty liver, alcoholic hepatitis and steatohepatitis, alcoholic foamy degeneration, and alcoholic cirrhosis. Steatosis, steatohepatitis, and cirrhosis may be indistinguishable from NAFLD. Steatosis, reversible with abstinence, is predominantly macrovesicular and initially involves zone 3. The hallmarks of alcoholic hepatitis are hepatocytes with Mallory–Denk bodies (MDBs) and satellitosis (neutrophilic infiltration around hepatocytes containing MDB), commonly embedded in dense pericellular fibrosis (e-Fig. 15.22). The pattern of fibrosis in alcoholic hepatitis/steatohepatitis is characteristic; it begins in zone 3 as perisinusoidal/pericellular collagen deposition and eventually there is dense "chicken-wire" fibrosis that may involve the entire acinus (e-Fig. 15.23). Canalicular cholestasis may be seen. Perivenular fibrosis is common. Obliteration of the terminal hepatic venule occurs in severe alcoholic hepatitis and results in sclerosing hyaline necrosis, a poor prognostic feature (e-Fig. 15.24). Alcoholic cirrhosis is typically micronodular. Obliterated outflow veins may be found, as may copper in periseptal hepatocytes. Steatosis is variably present in ALD.

2. **NAFLD** may resemble some of the histologic findings of milder forms of ALD, and occurs in patients who are not heavy drinkers but who have features of metabolic syndrome (obesity, hypertension, abnormal glucose tolerance, and dyslipidemia) (*Clin Liv Dis.* 2010;14:591). NAFLD may also occur with a variety of medications. Unlike alcoholic hepatitis, however, a diagnosis of nonalcoholic steatohepatitis (NASH) requires the presence of steatosis; NASH does not have cholestasis and has less prominent MDB. Central sclerosing hyaline necrosis has not been reported. Minimum features of adult NASH are zone 3 macrosteatosis and hepatocyte ballooning, and lobular inflammation. Ballooning may be confirmed with K8/18 immunostaining (e-Fig. 15.25). Portal inflammation may be present in all forms of NAFLD, but if disproportionate, should raise concern of a second process such as HCV. Pediatric NAFLD may show greater steatosis, less zone-3 zonality, and more portal inflammation and fibrosis than adult NASH. The pattern of fibrosis in NASH resembles that of ALD, in that it is zone 3 perisinusoidal initially. Advanced fibrosis includes periportal fibrosis, bridging, and cirrhosis. As with ALD, steatosis may be absent in cirrhosis resultant from NASH; "burnt-out" NASH is considered the most likely cause of "cryptogenic" cirrhosis, however, other considerations include AIH and alcoholic cirrhosis (e-Fig. 15.26).

Grading and Staging NAFLD (Table 15.1). The NAFLD Activity Score (NAS) (*Hepatology.* 2005;41:1313), validated and developed for therapeutic trials from the original Brunt proposal for NASH, is the unweighted sum of scores for steatosis, lobular inflammation, and ballooning. The numeric NAS

TABLE 15.1	Grading and Staging of Nonalcoholic Fatty Liver Disease (NAFLD)

Component scores for grading

Steatosis	Lobular inflammation	Hepatocellular ballooning
0: <5%	0: None	0: None
1: 5–33%	1: <2/20× field	1: Mild, few
2: 34–66%	2: 2–4/20× field	2: Moderate-marked, many
3: >66%	3: >4/20 field	

NAFLD activity score: NAS 0–8 (Steatosis + lobular inflammation + ballooning)

Fibrosis scoring: Based on Masson trichrome stain

0: None

1a: Delicate zone 3 perisinusoidal fibrosis, requires trichrome stain

1b: Dense zone 3 perisinusoidal fibrosis, visible on H&E

1c: Portal/periportal fibrosis

 2: Zone 3 perisinusoidal and portal fibrosis

 3: Bridging

 4: Cirrhosis

Modified from Kleiner DE, Brunt EM, Van Natta M, et al. NIDDK sponsored NASH CRN scoring system. *Hepatology.* 2005;41:1313.

and the diagnosis are separately reported, as they reflect different properties. The fibrosis score is based on trichrome stain.

3. **Glycogenic hepatopathy** is an uncommon complication of diabetics due to poor glycemic control; hepatocytes are distended by excess glycogen as in other forms of glycogen storage disease. Steatosis and megamitochondria may be noted (e-**Fig. 15.27**). **Diabetic hepatosclerosis** is manifest by nonzonal dense perisinusoidal fibrosis; steatosis is not present. Alkaline phosphatase may be elevated (e-**Fig. 15.28**).

4. **Iron overload (IO)** is largely due to dysregulated hepcidin, the master iron regulator, which directly controls ferroportin, the macrophage exporter of iron. Production of hepcidin by hepatocytes is complex and at least partially under the control of *Hfe, HJV, Tfr2,* and *HAMP. Hfe* mutation (homozygous C282Y, the most common form of hereditary hemochromatosis [HH]), has midlife onset; *HJV, Tfr2,* and *HAMP* mutations result in younger and more severe onset. ALD, anemia of chronic disease, and the above types of hereditary HH suppress hepatocellular hepcidin with resultant hepatocyte IO.; the so-called secondary forms of IO from aberrant macrophage loading (ferroportin disease, hemophagocytic syndrome) result in macrophage sinusoidal lining cell (SLC) iron accumulation. Hepatocellular iron deposition initially occurs in a gradient from zone 1 hepatocytes, followed by the SLC. In iron-loaded cirrhosis, iron-free foci are dysplastic nodules (DN); hepatocellular carcinoma (HCC) is also iron-free. Ferroportin disease and secondary IO are characterized by preferential panacinar SLC iron loading prior to hepatocellular accumulation.

Many systems exist for iron grading (*Semin Liv Dis.* 2005;25:392) (e-**Fig. 15.29**); however, diagnosis of HH requires mutational analysis as ineffective erythropoiesis also causes hepatocellular iron accumulation. Thus, histologic diagnosis should reflect only the amount of IO and a recommendation for further testing.

HH carries a significant risk of HCC. **Porphyria cutanea tarda** is associated with HH, steatosis, IO, cirrhosis, and also carries a risk of HCC. High ferritin levels are characteristic in NAFLD, and may raise a clinical concern of HH. **Neonatal HH** is a misnomer for a complement-mediated alloimmune maternal-fetal disorder with giant cell hepatitis that may or may not have liver IO (*Hepatology.* 2010;51:2061).

5. **α1-Antitrypsin deficiency,** the most common genetic pediatric liver disease, is characterized by accumulation of intracytoplasmic eosinophilic globules of varying sizes in zone 1 hepatocytes, easily demonstrated by PAS-D (e-**Fig. 15.30**). The diagnosis is confirmed by characteristic peripheral IHC positivity, and serum electrophoresis phenotyping. The hepatocyte globules signify a Z allele, or other rare alleles of M or S; whether or not heterozygosity is causative or enhances liver disease, is an ongoing debate (*Semin Diagn Pathol.* 2006;23:182). In children under 2 years of age, globules may not be present; thus, this disease is included in the differential diagnosis of giant cell or neonatal hepatitis (e-**Fig. 15.31**). Biliary atresia and Alagille syndromes are mimics, and it is important to remember that globules may also occur in benign and malignant liver neoplasms. The differential diagnosis of non-α1AT globules includes polyglucosan inclusions in polypharmacy; Lafora bodies; cyanamide therapy; HB S Ag; adaptation; and fibrinogen inclusions.

6. **Wilson's disease,** which can occur as a result of over 200 mutations of biliary copper transporters and ceruloplasmin formation, results in copper accumulation in the liver, brain, cornea, and kidney, and presents between 5 and 45 years old. Hepatic histology is as protean as the clinical disease. Wilson's disease can be queried for otherwise unexplained macro or microsteatosis, chronic hepatitis, cirrhosis, or submassive necrosis in a young adult. Periportal glycogenated nuclei and MDBs are common. Excessive copper may not be visible by staining as it largely remains intracytosolic; diagnostic testing requires quantitation from the paraffin block (>250 μg/g dry weight). Chronic cholestatic diseases also result in copper deposits in the eyes (Kayser–Fleischer rings) and periportal/periseptal hepatocytes, but the increase in copper does not reach the quantitative levels of Wilson's disease (*Semin Diagn Pathol.* 2006;23:182).

7. **Glycogen storage diseases,** or **glycogenoses,** are characterized by abnormal accumulation of glycogen in hepatocytes giving rise to a pale, distended, and mosaic appearance. PAS stains and electron microscopy may help confirm the diagnosis.

8. **Lysosomal storage diseases,** the most common of which is Gaucher's disease, are characterized by distended Kupffer cells. The cytoplasm of "Gaucher cells" is finely striated as with "wrinkled tissue paper."

9. **Hematologic disorders: Lymphoma, leukemia, hemophagocytic syndrome,** and sickle cell disease. Lymphoma and leukemia are discussed further below. Macrophage activation syndrome (e-**Fig. 15.32**), characterized by Kupffer cell erythrophagocytosis, reflects systemic malignancy, viral infection, or collagen vascular disease. Serum ferritin levels are extremely elevated. Portal and parenchymal CD8+ lymphocytes are common. The sickled cells in sickle cell disease cause microthrombi, erythrophagocytosis, and increased hepatocellular iron (e-**Fig. 15.33**).

10. **Reye's syndrome** (e-**Fig. 15.34**) and other mitochondriopathies are more common in children than adults. The liver shows pauci-inflammatory microvesicular steatosis. Ultrastructural examination highlights mitochondrial alterations. Similar changes occur in alcoholic foamy degeneration.

11. **Total parenteral nutrition (TPN)** results in steatosis or steatohepatitis in adults and cholestasis with a ductular reaction and fibrosis in children. In both, bridging fibrosis and cirrhosis may occur.

12. **Amyloidosis** commonly involves portal tract arteries and may be inconsequential, and can occur as the result of several disease entities (*Clin Liver Dis* 2004;8:915). However, hepatic involvement is considered terminal when amyloid replaces the sinusoids and results in compression and atrophy of the hepatocytes (e-**Fig. 15.35**). Trichrome stain shows the characteristic gray color of amyloid, and polarized Congo red shows the apple-green birefringence of amyloid.

13. **Cystic fibrosis** has hepatic manifestations in about 20% of patients. CF may present as a mimic of biliary atresia or neonatal hepatitis, or later as portal hypertension, due to bile duct mucus plugging and fibrosis. The histologic hallmarks are dense eosinophilic inspissated mucous in dilated ducts, cholangitis, ductular reaction, chronic inflammation, and fibrosis (e-**Fig. 15.36**). Focal biliary fibrosis occurs in up to 70% of adults and may warrant liver transplant.

14. **Drug- and toxin-induced liver injury (DILI)**, commonly in the differential for unexplained liver test elevations, can be direct (predictable, intrinsic) or indirect (unpredictable, idiosyncratic). Direct toxicity involves agents known to produce liver damage in a dose-dependent manner; methotrexate, antibiotics, and chemotherapeutic agents are examples. Indirect toxicity is immune-mediated and dose-independent; granulomatous and eosinophilic inflammation typifies this type of injury. Acute injury may lead to cholestatic hepatitis, bland cholestasis, interlobular duct damage, acute hepatitis, and massive necrosis. Chronic injury may assume the form of chronic hepatitis, granulomatous hepatitis, steatosis, steatohepatitis, vascular injury, fibrosis, cirrhosis, or neoplasia. Oxaliplatin injury is discussed below in sinusoidal obstruction syndrome (SOS).

C. AIH and bile duct disorders of the liver

1. **Autoimmune hepatitis (AIH)** can present in adolescent or postmenopausal females, and is associated with hypergammaglobulinemia (IgG) and high titers of antinuclear and antismooth muscle antibodies in adults, and anti-liver-kidney microsomal type 1 antibodies in girls. The diagnosis should only be made after other metabolic diseases have been excluded, and after negative viral serologies have been demonstrated (*Hepatology.* 2008;48:169). In classic cases, there is a dense portal and lobular mononuclear cell infiltrate enriched in plasma cells (e-**Fig. 15.37**). Marked interface hepatitis, centrilobular confluent or bridging necrosis, and hepatitic rosetting are present. Advanced fibrosis may be found at presentation. Cholestasis is rare but signifies severity. AIH may rarely present as fulminant hepatic failure. Likewise, mild chronic hepatitis and/or cirrhosis may be the initial findings.

2. **Primary biliary cirrhosis (PBC)**, a progressive cholestatic disease of middle-aged women, results in the destruction of intrahepatic bile ducts. IgM and serum cholesterol are elevated. The early stage (Table 15.2) has mixed portal inflammatory infiltrates and the pathognomonic *florid duct lesion* consisting of granulomatous or lymphocytic infiltration of duct epithelium (e-**Fig. 15.38**). The granulomas in PBC are epithelioid, may be portal or lobular, and present in any stage of disease. Stains for fungal and acid-fast organisms are appropriate at the time of initial diagnosis. The disease is inhomogenous, but ductular reaction, interface hepatitis, chronic cholestasis, and biliary piecemeal necrosis develop with progression, with eventual bridging necrosis, septal fibrosis, and biliary cirrhosis. Chronic cholestasis (cholate stasis) is characterized by periportal edema, ductular reaction, MDBs, lobular foam cells, copper (e-**Fig. 15.39**), and cholestatic rosettes. Nodular regenerative hyperplasia (NRH)-like parenchymal features may occur in any stage of PBC and may explain the clinical findings of noncirrhotic variceal bleeding.

   Autoimmune cholangiopathy and anti-mitochondrial antibody (AMA) negative PBC are synonymous terms for seronegative PBC that is otherwise clinically and histologically identical to PBC (and is distinct from *overlap syndrome* as discussed below). ANA testing is often positive in this setting.

3. **Primary sclerosing cholangitis (PSC)**, a progressive fibro-obliterative disorder primarily of young men, is of unknown etiology. PSC affects the extra- and intrahepatic biliary tree leading to biliary strictures and ectasias, and cirrhosis. PSC is strongly associated with ulcerative colitis. The definitive diagnosis

TABLE 15.2 Grading and Staging

Grading and staging of primary biliary cirrhosis[a]

Stage	Scheuer	Ludwig
1	Florid duct lesion	Portal stage
	Bile duct damage	Portal inflammation
	Portal inflammation	
2	Ductular proliferation (reaction)	Periportal stage
	Expanded portal tracts	Periportal inflammation ± piecemeal necrosis
	Proliferated ductules	
	Piecemeal necrosis	
3	Scarring	Septal stage
	Fibrosis	Fibrous septa
	Loss of ducts	Bridging necrosis
4	Nodular cirrhosis	Cirrhosis

Grading and staging primary sclerosing cholangitis[b]

Stage 1	Portal stage	Portal inflammation or bile duct abnormalities
Stage 2	Periportal stage	Periportal fibrosis or enlargement of portal tract
Stage 3	Septal stage	Fibrous septal or bridging necrosis
Stage 4	Cirrhotic stage	Cirrhosis

[a]Modified from Lee R., ed. *Diagnostic Liver Pathology.* 1994, p. 117.
[b]Modified from Lee R., ed. *Diagnostic Liver Pathology.* 1994, p. 127.

of PSC rests on imaging by MRCP or ERCP; liver biopsy may be suggestive (features of chronic cholestasis) or confirmatory (periductal fibrosis), but is not the diagnostic test (see later). Fibrous cholangitis (the so-called onion-skin fibrosis) involving large and/or small bile ducts, duct damage, ductular reaction, and chronic cholestasis are typical findings (e-**Fig. 15.40**). PSC inhomogenously progresses to cirrhosis and is staged according to portal changes (Table 15.2). Cholangiocarcinoma occurs in up to 10% of cases of PSC. Currently, carefully selected and protocolized patients with PSC and cholangiocarcinoma undergo neoadjuvant therapy and months of surveillance prior to transplant.

    Small duct PSC involves only the small intrahepatic ducts, and may be the same disease as idiopathic adulthood ductopenia (IAD). Small duct PSC does not carry a risk of cholangiocarcinoma unless evolution to large duct PSC occurs.

4. **Overlap syndrome** refers to cases of clinical and/or histopathologic AIH with the simultaneous presence of diagnostic features of PBC or PSC, or less often, viral hepatitis. Correlation with clinical and serologic findings is essential as treatment is based on the dominant finding.

5. **Secondary biliary cirrhosis** results from any cause of mechanical obstruction of the biliary tree. The common causes in adults are lithiasis, tumors, external compression from nodes, and stenosis; in children, the common causes are biliary atresia and choledochal cysts. Infiltrative disorders (e.g., amyloidosis and lymphomas) less often result in changes of secondary biliary cirrhosis.

    Histologically, large duct obstruction causes both portal and lobular changes. Initially, there is rounding of portal tracts due to edema; later, pericholangitis (ductular reaction with neutrophils), with or without ascending cholangitis is found, occasionally with bile plugs in dilated ducts. In zone 3, feathery degeneration and canalicular cholestasis are noted. With increased pressure, intraparenchymal bile infarcts occur (e-**Fig. 15.41**); these nonzonal pink-tan clusters are due to membrane saponification by cholate salts. Long-standing obstruction leads to portal and periductal fibrosis or cirrhosis indistinguishable from PSC. Biliary atresia with extensive lobular injury may simulate neonatal or giant-cell hepatitis.

6. **Idiopathic adulthood ductopenia (IAD)** is, by definition, paucity of intrahepatic bile ducts as defined by a ratio of <0.5 interlobular ducts to portal tracts (the normal range is 0.9 to 1.8). This poorly understood condition is pauci-inflammatory, insidious in presentation and progression, and rarely is familial. Immunostains for keratins 7 or 19 aid in identifying hypoplastic or absent ducts and progenitor cells. Unlike extrahepatic biliary atresia or obstruction, ductular reaction (i.e., proliferation of the progenitor cell compartment) is absent in IAD. In pediatric patients, paucity may be syndromic (Alagille syndrome) or nonsyndromic; the latter is associated with other causes of neonatal hepatitis. In adults, the diagnosis requires exclusion of PBC, PSC, chronic allograft rejection, GVHD, sarcoidosis, and untreated Hodgkin's disease.

D. **Major vascular disorders of the liver**

1. **Venous outflow obstruction** can result from cardiac disease (congestive heart failure) or large vessel disease (occlusion of large hepatic veins or the IVC, i.e., Budd–Chiari syndrome). Both involve zone 3 sinusoidal dilatation (congestion) and may show red cell extravasation into the space of Disse with hepatocyte loss. With chronicity, cord atrophy, and withering occur, and fibrous replacement results. Ductular reaction may be prominent. Cardiac sclerosis/cirrhosis with reverse lobulation has become an uncommon finding. Caudate lobe hypertrophy is a feature of Budd–Chiari syndrome due to separate venous drainage.

2. **Sinusoidal obstruction syndrome (SOS)** occurs unpredictably following preconditioning for bone marrow transplant, and following chemotherapy regimens containing oxaliplatin for colorectal metastases. Grossly, the disease is characterized by a "blue liver." Formerly referred to as veno-occlusive disease, the process has been renamed to reflect the fact that the location of initial injury is the sinusoids, which are denuded. Downstream, debris is deposited in the outflow vein branches, which results in subendothelial fibrosis of outflow veins. In the bone marrow transplant (BMT) setting, the onset is soon after BMT; acute abdominal swelling and elevated bilirubin herald SOS, and hepatocyte necrosis in zone 3 is a recognized feature in this setting. VVG is helpful in visualization of affected veins in the area of necrotic hepatocytes (e-**Fig. 15.42**). In oxaliplatin-related SOS, seemingly randomly scattered foci of ectatic sinusoids, some nearly peliotic, may be seen. Hepatocyte anisonucleosis in H&E-stained sections is a diagnostic clue (e-**Fig. 15.43**).

3. **Noncirrhotic portal hypertension** (idiopathic portal hypertension), usually the result of presinusoidal causes, may also be due to hepatic causes such as schistosomiasis, sarcoidosis, or congenital hepatic fibrosis. Clinically, normal liver synthetic function is maintained in IPH.

   a. **Nodular regenerative hyperplasia (NRH)** is a condition related to aberrant flow that commonly results in noncirrhotic portal hypertension. The parenchyma is diffusely nodular, but without fibrosis. The nodularity is appreciated at low magnification and by reticulin stains (e-**Fig. 15.44**), which highlight the regenerative cords outlined by atrophic cords.

   b. **Hepatoportal sclerosis** is due to intrahepatic portal vein injury and scarring. The extrahepatic portal vein is patent, at least initially. The parenchyma shows a variety of alterations: abnormally approximated portal tracts, periportal enlarged vessels in direct contact with hepatic cords, and multiple ectatic sinusoidal structures that resemble angiomatoid structures. Portal and/or sinusoidal fibrosis may be present. Portal veins may be inapparent or show marked wall thickening with luminal narrowing (e-**Fig. 15.45**).

4. **Portal vein thrombosis (PVT)** may result in subtle or gross parenchymal atrophy characterized by approximation of vascular structures (i.e., the infarct of Zahn). Biliopathy may also result from PVT.

5. **Osler–Weber–Rendu syndrome (hereditary hemorrhagic telangiectasia; HHT)** is an autosomal dominant disorder that results in multisystem angiodysplasias. Of the four known genetic subtypes, liver lesions are in the HHT 2 group of *alk1* gene mutations on chromosome 12; final diagnosis rests with fulfillment of three of five Curacao criteria, which include hepatic AVMs as well as family history (*J Med Genet.* 2011;48:73). Nosebleeds are common. The hepatic malformations may be insidious and range from ischemic biliopathy, to focal nodular hyperplasia (FNH) with high output cardiac failure, to noncirrhotic portal hypertension. Hepatic lesions include intraparenchymal thick-walled veins with adherent arteries, scattered dilated sinusoids, and abnormally sized portal tracts with extruded dilated vascular channels. Commonly, grossly observed subcapsular enlarged vessels are present.

E. **Miscellaneous**

1. **Granulomas** of various sizes occur in the liver. Underlying etiologies are as variable as the morphology of the granulomas. Stains for infection organisms and evaluation under polarized light are useful in the evaluation of true epithelioid types. Considerations specific to liver include PBC, sarcoidosis, DILI, HCV, fungal or mycobacterial infections, foreign bodies, and hepatocellular adenoma (HCA); rarely, granulomatous hepatitis is a bona fide clinico-pathologic diagnosis.

2. **Pregnancy** is associated with various mitochondrial alterations. **AFLP** occurs in the late third trimester and is potentially fatal to both mother and fetus; emergent delivery is the treatment. While the histologic hallmark is zone 3 or diffuse microvesicular steatosis, oil red O stain on a frozen section may be required since hepatitic features and extramedullary hematopoiesis may be present. Endophlebitis is common. The affected hepatocytes appear swollen, and the microsteatosis gives an appearance of cytoplasmic reticulation (e-**Fig. 15.46**). Preeclampsia/eclampsia and **HELLP syndrome** (hemolysis, elevated liver enzymes, and low platelets) may cause zone 1 hemorrhage, necrosis, and fibrin deposition.

3. **Ductal plate malformation (DPM)** results from developmental arrest with persistence of the embryologic ductal plate, which assumes an anastomosing ring-like structure lining the periphery of the portal tracts (e-**Fig. 15.47**). DPM may manifest as von Meyenburg complexes, congenital hepatic fibrosis, Caroli's syndrome or disease, or polycystic liver disease.

   a. **Congenital hepatic fibrosis** (e-**Figs. 15.48** and **15.49**) is a significant cause of noncirrhotic portal hypertension. The abnormal portal tracts are expanded, have an increased number of aberrant duct profiles, show hypoplastic or absent portal veins, and numerous hypertrophic hepatic artery branches. Bridging is noted but portal–central relationships are maintained, as is synthetic function. Inspissated bile may be noted in ectatic ducts.

   b. **Caroli's disease** is characterized by segmental cystic dilatation of the larger intrahepatic ducts, usually accompanied by recurrent bacterial cholangitis and biliary lithiasis. When associated with congenital hepatic fibrosis, it is termed Caroli's syndrome.

   c. **Polycystic liver disease** is a debilitating process due to massive enlargement with cystic replacement of the parenchyma (e-**Fig. 15.50**). Liver function is maintained, but transplantation may be needed for quality of life. Berry aneurysm of the middle cerebral artery is a significant complication.

4. **Ascending cholangitis** is diagnosed clinically. Histologically, intraluminal neutrophils are present within the interlobular bile ducts. Other features of biliary obstruction are usually noted (e-**Fig. 15.51**).

IV. TRANSPLANTATION PATHOLOGY

A. Donor liver evaluation is performed on frozen sections to evaluate steatosis, or portal inflammation and fibrosis in an HCV donor. For the former, percentages of the core involved by large droplet steatosis are estimated; the presence of >30% macrovesicular steatosis is commonly accepted as a cut-off potentially associated with poor graft function in the immediate posttransplant period, whereas >50% is unacceptable. Pitfalls of frozen artifacts include the tiny spaces in hepatocytes and sinusoidal spaces that may be misinterpreted as large fat vacuoles. The use of oil red O stain is discouraged as it results in an overestimation of steatosis due to small droplet fat that is not associated with graft dysfunction. For HCV positive donors, portal inflammation, lobular activity, and fibrosis as seen in H&E-stained sections are documented. Coagulative necrosis is a worrisome finding in donor biopsies, and is worth both verbal communication and written documentation.

B. Preservation/reperfusion injury is related to harvesting, transportation, and reperfusion of the graft. The relevant findings are located in zone 3; specifically, hepatocyte ballooning and cholestasis. Frank necrosis may occur in more severe cases. Resolution is expected within 2 weeks.

C. Humoral (hyperacute) rejection rarely occurs with current patient management paradigms. Historically, humoral rejection was associated with changes in the liver, including coagulative and hemorrhagic necrosis or portal/periportal edema, neutrophilic portal infiltrates, and prominent ductular reaction.

D. Acute (cellular) rejection is directed primarily at antigens on duct epithelium and venous endothelium. It can occur anytime immunosuppression is reduced or discontinued, but is most common between 5 and 30 days after transplantation. The classic histologic triad consists of mixed portal chronic inflammation, bile duct damage, and endotheliitis. The portal infiltrates consist of lymphocytes admixed with eosinophils, histiocytes, plasma cells, and occasional neutrophils. Bile duct damage is characterized by inflammatory intercalation into ductal epithelium; it may be accompanied by cytoplasmic vacuolization and other cytologic alterations. Nuclear pyknosis and cytoplasmic eosinophilia are signs of ischemic injury, however (**e-Fig. 15.52**). Endotheliitis is defined as subendothelial lymphocytic infiltration with lifting, detachment, and sloughing of endothelial cells; attachment of lymphocytes to the luminal aspect of the endothelium is insufficient for diagnosis (**e-Fig. 15.53**). Endotheliitis most frequently involves portal veins, but central veins can be similarly affected. Centrilobular necrosis is sufficient for a diagnosis of severe rejection.

Centers differ for treatment thresholds, thus, careful description and standard evaluation is recommended for optimal clinical communication. Acute rejection may be graded using the Banff schema recommended by an international panel (Table 15.3).

E. Chronic rejection (CR) is a misleading moniker as the characteristic feature, specifically loss of bile ducts, may occur any time after transplantation. The diagnostic criteria are: (i) bile duct loss affecting >50% portal tracts, or (ii) obliterative arteriopathy by foamy histiocytes. Biliary epithelial senescence with eosinophilic cytoplasm and nuclear hyperchromasia is considered an early feature of CR. The arterial lesions mainly involve large and medium size vessels and are rarely seen in small vessels sampled by percutaneous biopsy. Therefore, the diagnosis of CR (Table 15.4) is primarily based on the evaluation of bile ducts and has been divided into early and late stages (*Hepatology*. 2000;31:792). The early stage typically shows perivenular hepatocyte dropout and central perivenulitis (**e-Fig. 15.54**); the late stage features duct loss in ≥50% of portal tracts with variable perivenular fibrosis (**e-Fig. 15.55**). Portal inflammation and ductular reaction are typically insignificant in the late stage as the progenitor cell compartment

TABLE 15.3 Banff Scheme for Grading Acute Liver Allograft Rejection

Global assessment	Criteria
Indeterminate	Portal inflammatory infiltrate that fails to meet the criteria for the diagnosis of acute rejection
Mild	Rejection infiltrate in a minority of the triads that is generally mild and confined within the portal spaces
Moderate	Rejection infiltrate expanding most or all of the triads
Severe	As above for moderate, with spillover into periportal areas and moderate to severe perivenular inflammation that extends into the hepatic parenchyma and is associated with perivenular hepatocyte necrosis

is lost along with the ducts, a useful feature that can be used to distinguish CR from recurrent HCV.

F. **Late complications of allograft livers.** The so-called de novo AIH (DNAIH) is a plasma-cell rich portal and lobular hepatitis, frequently accompanied by central necrosis; the mechanism, nomenclature, and outcome of this form of steroid-responsive damage is debated (see later). **Idiopathic posttransplant chronic hepatitis (IPTH)** has been described in 10% to 50% of long-term liver allograft survivors, and is a diagnosis of exclusion. It shows predominantly mononuclear portal inflammation with interface hepatitis, although features resembling central perivenulitis can also be seen. Bile duct damage and endothelial inflammation are absent to minimal. Progression to bridging fibrosis or cirrhosis has been reported, especially in pediatric patients. Current thought is that both DNAIH and ITPH may be forms of alloimmune-mediated rejection.

TABLE 15.4 Banff Criteria for Chronic Liver Allograft Rejection (CR)

Structure	Early CR	Late CR
Small bile ducts	Degenerative changes involving a majority of ducts: Eosinophilic transformation of the cytoplasm; increased nuclear to cytoplasmic (N/C) ratio; nuclear hyperchromasia; uneven nuclear spacing; ducts only partially lined by biliary epithelial cells. Bile duct loss in <50% of portal tracts	Degenerative changes in remaining bile ducts. Loss in ≥50% of portal tracts
Terminal hepatic venules and zone 3 hepatocytes	Intimal/luminal inflammation. Lytic zone 3 necrosis and inflammation. Mild perivenular fibrosis	Focal obliteration. Variable inflammation. Severe (bridging) fibrosis
Portal tract hepatic arterioles	Occasional loss involving <25% of portal tracts	Loss involving >25% of portal tracts
Other	So-called transition hepatitis with spotty necrosis of hepatocytes	Sinusoidal foam cell accumulation; marked cholestasis
Larger perihilar hepatic artery branches	Intimal inflammation, focal foam cell deposition without luminal compromise	Luminal narrowing by subintimal foam cells. Fibrointimal proliferation
Large perihilar bile ducts	Inflammation damage and focal foam cell deposition	Mural fibrosis

G. Technical complications usually occur during the first few months after transplantation. Hepatic artery or PVT or stricture may cause zone 3 hepatocyte necrosis, but infarction is rare. Ischemic damage of the biliary tree is a sign of hepatic artery complication, with protean manifestations including abscess, cholestasis, obstructive changes, stricture, or loss of the bile ducts. Thus, CR cannot be diagnosed without demonstration of a patent hepatic artery. Hepatic vein thrombosis or stricture results in changes of venous outflow obstruction. Stenosis or obstruction of the bile duct anastomosis causes morphologic changes similar to those of biliary obstruction or biliary cirrhosis.

H. Recurrent diseases. Most diseases recur in the transplanted liver but the timeframe and severity vary; diagnosis is complicated by the fact that recurrent diseases share histopathologic features with rejection or technical complications.

Histologic evidence of recurrent HCV initially is acidophil bodies; portal and lobular chronic inflammation occur later. Overlapping features with mild acute rejection include bile duct damage, endotheliitis, and mixed infiltrates; thus, a final diagnosis should include, if possible, description of the balance of damage due to hepatitis versus rejection. HBV recurrence is documented by protocol evaluation of HB S and C Ag testing on every follow-up allograft biopsy (e-Fig. 15.56).

Fibrosing cholestatic hepatitis (FCH) (e-Fig. 15.57) is a rare but progressive disease seen in both recurrent hepatitis B and C, with rapidly rising bilirubin that may result in graft loss. FCH's histologic features include marked portal and periportal perisinusoidal fibrosis with ductular reaction, canalicular cholestasis, and nonzonal hepatocyte ballooning; the latter may be the earliest clue to diagnosis. Inflammatory changes are generally mild. In FCH-B, HB S and C Ag are highly expressed in reinfected hepatocytes.

PBC and PSC may recur several years after transplantation. Even with granulomatous duct lesions, recurrent PBC is difficult to diagnose. Recurrent PSC needs to be distinguished from technical complications due to hepatic artery or biliary stricture, or biliary obstruction. Recurrent steatosis and steatohepatitis are a challenge to distinguish from de novo occurrence due to persistence of the patient's metabolic syndrome and/or the medications utilized for allografts. Recurrent HCC or cholangiocarcinoma are typically rapidly lethal complications.

I. Acute GVHD (e-Fig. 15.58) following bone marrow or stem cell transplantation shows duct damage, and less frequently endotheliitis. Hepatitic forms of GVHD may coexist. The differential diagnosis includes viral infection and DILI. **Chronic GVHD** typically occurs after 100 days and simulates ischemia or ductopenic CR. Skin and GI GVHD are commonly concurrent.

V. DIAGNOSTIC FEATURES OF COMMON NEOPLASTIC AND TUMOR-LIKE CONDITIONS. The current World Health Organization (WHO) histologic classification of tumors of the liver and intrahepatic bile ducts is given in Table 15.5. The 2010 American Joint Committee on Cancer (AJCC) tumor, node, metastasis (TNM) staging is in Table 15.6.

The most common tumor type in noncirrhotic livers is **metastatic**; neoplasms that commonly metastasize to the liver include carcinomas of colorectal, pancreatic, renal, pulmonary, and breast; melanoma; and neuroendocrine tumors. Metastases usually present as multiple nodules, in contrast to the single nodules of primary liver tumors. Metastases to a cirrhotic liver are very uncommon.

A. Epithelial tumors

    1. Benign hepatocellular tumors

        a. Focal nodular hyperplasia (FNH) is a common non-neoplastic lesion. It is not caused by oral contraceptive use, but instead is a polyclonal regenerative response to a local vascular injury. FNH has no malignant potential. The nodularity of the lesion underlies the original moniker of

TABLE 15.5 WHO Histologic Classification of Tumors of the Liver and Intrahepatic Bile Ducts

Epithelial tumors: hepatocellular

Benign

  Hepatocellular adenoma

    HNF1α Mutated

    β-Catenin activating

    Inflammatory, gp130 mutated

    Unclassified

  Focal nodular hyperplasia

Malignancy-associated and premalignant lesions

  Large cell change (formerly "dysplasia")

  Small cell change (formerly "dysplasia")

  Dysplastic nodules

    Low grade

    High grade

Malignant

  Hepatocellular carcinoma

    Early hepatocellular carcinoma

  Hepatocellular carcinoma, fibrolamellar

  Hepatocellular carcinoma, scirrhous

  Hepatocellular carcinoma, sarcomatoid

  Lymphoepithelial-like carcinoma

  Hepatoblastoma, epithelial variant

  Undifferentiated carcinoma

Epithelial tumors: biliary

Benign

  Bile duct adenoma (peribiliary gland hamartoma and others)

  Microcystic adenoma

  Biliary adenofibroma

Premalignant lesions

  Biliary intraepithelial neoplasia, grade 3 (BilIN-3)

  Intraductal papillary neoplasm with low- or intermediate-grade intraepithelial neoplasia

  Intraductal papillary neoplasm with high-grade intraepithelial neoplasia

  Mucinous cystic neoplasm with low- or intermediate-grade intraepithelial neoplasia

  Mucinous cystic neoplasm with high-grade intraepithelial neoplasia

Malignant

  Intrahepatic cholangiocarcinoma

  Intraductal papillary neoplasm with an associated invasive carcinoma

  Mucinous cystic neoplasm with an associated invasive carcinoma

Malignancies of mixed or uncertain origin

Calcifying nested epithelial stromal tumor

Carcinosarcoma

Combined hepatocellular-cholangiocarcinoma

Hepatoblastoma, mixed epithelial-mesenchymal

Malignant rhabdoid tumor

(continued)

TABLE 15.5	WHO Histologic Classification of Tumors of the Liver and Intrahepatic Bile Ducts (*Continued*)

Mesenchymal tumors
Benign
   Angiomyolipoma (PEComa)
   Cavernous hemangioma
   Infantile hemangioma
   Inflammatory pseudotumor
   Lymphangioma
   Lymphangiomatosis
   Mesenchymal hamartoma
   Solitary fibrous tumor
Malignant
   Angiosarcoma
   Embryonal sarcoma (undifferentiated sarcoma)
   Epithelioid hemangioendothelioma
   Kaposi sarcoma
   Leiomyosarcoma
   Rhabdomyosarcoma
   Synovial sarcoma

Germ cell tumors
   Teratoma
   Yolk sac tumor (endodermal sinus tumor)

Lymphomas

Secondary tumors

From: Bosman FT, Carneiro F, Hruban RH, Theise ND, eds. *World Health Organization Classification of Tumours of the Digestive System*. Lyon: IARC Press; 2010. Used with permission.

focal cirrhosis. Rarely larger than 5 to 7 cm, FNH is well-demarcated, nonencapsulated, and characterized by a central stellate scar (**e-Fig. 15.59**), the stalk of which contains large, thick-walled vessels. Ductular reaction and copper are present in periseptal parenchyma; bile ducts are absent. The architecture may be a challenge to appreciate on biopsy of the periphery of the lesion. The hepatocytes of the lesion resemble those of the surrounding parenchyma, or may be steatotic. Altered TGFβ signaling results in a characteristic map-like pattern of glutamine synthetase by IHC; this may also be challenging to discern on a sample in a needle biopsy (**e-Fig. 15.60**). FNH may occur within cirrhosis; FNH can also be syndromic, multiple, and/or associated with hemangiomas, hepatocellular adenomas (HCAs), hereditary hemorrhagic telangiectasia, and CNS vascular lesions.

b. **Hepatocellular adenoma (HCA)** is a rare benign neoplasm only in noncirrhotic livers. HCA is significantly more common in women of reproductive age than in children or men, and occurs in a "stimulated" liver; associations include prolonged use of oral contraceptives, anabolic/androgenic steroid use, and metabolic disorders including GSD types 1 and 3, galactosemia, tyrosinemia, and obesity (with or without diabetes). HCA arising in the setting of metabolic disorders has an increased risk of transformation into HCC. HCA is usually solitary; when >10 adenomas are present, the condition is referred to as adenomatosis. HCA consists solely of bland hepatocytes 1 to 3 cells thick, with minimal nuclear pleomorphism. Small unaccompanied arteries and sinusoidal vessels are present, but portal tracts and bile ducts are absent. Granulomas, steatosis, steatohepatitis with MDB may be present. Mitoses are virtually never seen.

TABLE 15.6	Tumor, Node, Metastasis (TNM) Staging Scheme for Carcinoma of the Liver (Excluding Intrahepatic Bile Ducts; Sarcomas and Tumors Metastatic to the Liver Are Not Included)		
Primary tumor (T)			
TX	Primary tumor cannot be assessed		
T0	No evidence of primary tumor		
T1	Solitary tumor without vascular invasion		
T2	Solitary tumor with vascular invasion or multiple tumors none >5 cm		
T3a	Multiple tumors >5 cm		
T3b	Single tumor or multiple tumors of any size involving a major branch of the portal vein or hepatic vein		
T4	Tumor(s) with direct invasion of adjacent organs other than the gallbladder or with perforation of visceral peritoneum		
Regional lymph nodes (N)			
NX	Regional lymph nodes cannot be assessed		
N0	No regional lymph node metastasis		
N1	Regional lymph node metastasis		
Distant metastasis (M)			
MX	Distant metastasis cannot be assessed		
M0	No distant metastasis		
M1	Distant metastasis		
Stage grouping			
Stage I	T1	N0	M0
Stage II	T2	N0	M0
Stage IIIA	T3a	N0	M0
Stage IIIB	T3b	N0	M0
Stage IIIC	T4	N0	M0
Stage IVA	Any T	N1	M0
Stage IVB	Any T	Any N	M1

From: Edge SB, Byrd DR, Compton CC, et al., eds. *AJCC Cancer Staging Manual.* 7th ed. New York, NY: Springer; 2010. Used with permission.

The tumor may or may not be encapsulated, but variably sized blood vessels, some of which may show fibromyxoid intimal thickening, are often present at the boundary with nontumor liver. Recent multicenter genotype–phenotype studies have classified HCAs into four types on the basis of genetic studies.

i. **HNF1α mutation (35% to 40% of adenomas)** are due to genomic or somatic bi-allelic inactivating mutation of this tumor suppressor gene that results in loss of liver fatty acid binding protein (LFABP-1) expression. By IHC normal liver is positive for LFABP, but the steatotic HCA tumor is negative (e-**Fig. 15.61** and e-**Fig. 15.62**). HNF1α mutated adenomas are characterized by steatosis, are more likely to be multiple than the other subcategories, and have a low risk of malignant progression.

ii. **β-catenin-activated adenomas (10% to 15%)** show nuclear and cytoplasmic β-catenin as well as diffuse expression of upregulated glutamine synthetase by IHC. β-catenin-activated adenomas may be characterized by borderline histology including pseudoacinar architecture, are more common in men than the other types of HCA, and are associated with a higher risk of progression to HCC.

iii. **Inflammatory adenoma (IA),** also known as **telangiectatic adenoma (45%
to 60%),** due to mutation of gp130 in the majority of cases, have overexpression of the inflammatory markers SAA and CRP by IHC. Formerly termed "telangiectatic FNH," IA have been shown to be true

adenomas by a variety of assays, and are associated with obesity and alcohol use. IA are often hemorrhagic, have foci of sinusoidal dilatation and peliosis, and have abnormal vessels; chronic inflammatory infiltrates are common along fibrovascular septa with periseptal ductular reaction (e-**Fig. 15.63**). IA may be confused with FNH by imaging and initial gross and microscopic evaluation, but glutamine synthetase is not "map-like."

   iv. **Unclassified adenoma (10%),** which is without specific genotypic or phenotypic features.

2. **Premalignant.** DN, a well-defined premalignant lesion arising in the background of cirrhosis (*Semin Liver Dis.* 2005;25:133; *Gastroenterol Clin N Am.* 2007;36:867), is diagnosed by the presence of a nodule with abnormal architecture, clonal hepatocytes with an increased N/C ratio, and nuclear atypia. DNs are usually multiple in livers with chronic liver disease or cirrhosis. Additional features include gross differences from surrounding nodules including bulging above the background, expansile growth with pushing borders, small cell change (nuclear crowding and sinusoidal alignment), resistance to iron accumulation in an otherwise iron-loaded cirrhosis (e-**Fig. 15.64**), clear cell change or deep eosinophilia, and the presence of isolated artery branches. Unlike HCC, DNs do not have cords >3 nuclei thick or stromal invasion. Macroregenerative nodules with intralesional portal tracts are considered low-grade DN. DN may contain small foci of nonencapsulated HCC within them, referred to as "nodule-in-nodule" (N-I-N).

   DNs are rarely >2 cm in size. When the lesion is <0.1 cm, it is termed a dysplastic focus. Large cell change, although associated with the presence of HCC, is not itself considered premalignant. Large cell change (LCC) is characterized by cellular and nuclear enlargement with nuclear atypia, but a normal N/C ratio. Small cell change (SCC), on the other hand, is strongly associated with progression to HCC.

3. **Malignant epithelial neoplasms**
   a. **HCC,** more common in middle aged and older men, usually but not exclusively occurs in chronic liver disease with a cirrhotic background. Chronic viral infection accounts for up to 85% of HCC; alcohol abuse is the most significant nonviral cause. Hereditary hemochromatosis (HH) carries a significant risk. Tobacco use is an additive factor. Obesity and the associated complications of diabetes and steatohepatitis are also recognized risks, and multiple risk factors increase the overall risk.

   HCC is usually encapsulated in cirrhotic livers, but not in noncirrhotics. Prior to the advent of advanced imaging for surveillance, several grossly observable types of HCC were documented: the single nodular type, the multifocal/multicentric type, the diffuse (cirrhotomimetic) type, and the uncommon pedunculated type. Tumor nodules are soft, fatty (yellow) or green (bile) stained, and bulge above the cut surface. Central necrosis is not rare, particularly in TACE or radio frequency ablation (RFA) treated HCC. With advanced surveillance in known cirrhotics, detected tumor nodules are often small (<1 to 2 cm) and subtle.

   Microscopically, HCC assumes a variety of patterns: trabecular, pseudoglandular, acinar, compact, or scirrhous. Unattached trabeculae are referred to as "floating trabeculae" and are characteristic of HCC. Mixed patterns are common, particularly with increased tumor size. Cell plates are >3 nuclei wide, a feature of importance in distinguishing DNs from early HCC (discussed later). Isolated arteries noted within the tumor can be detected with trichrome, αSMA, and CD34 IHC. HCC receives blood solely from systemic arteries, thus CD34 positive tumor sinusoidal endothelium differs from CD34 negative endothelium of nontumor liver. Reticulin stain highlights widened cell plates and shows reduction or loss of normal reticulin fibers (e-**Fig. 15.65**). Tumor cells share many characteristics of nonneoplastic liver cells, for example, intranuclear inclusions, eosinophilic or basophilic cytoplasm; small droplet, large droplet, or microvesicular steatosis; clear cell change; MDBs; PASd inclusions; fibrinogen inclusions; and HB S Ag. Bile production by tumor cells must be distinguished from trapped hepatocytes, but can be useful to identify the tumor as hepatocellular; polyclonal CEA and CD10 react with canaliculi and are equally specific, as hepatocytes are the only cells that contain these structures and secrete bile (e-**Fig. 15.66**). Arginase-1, another marker of hepatocellular origin, may be useful in selected cases. The presence of stromal invasion is diagnostic, but uncommon; vascular invasion is an important parameter for tumor staging.

Small HCC (<2 cm) may or may not be well differentiated; most HCC are moderately or poorly differentiated. Well differentiated HCC can be difficult to distinguish from adenoma in noncirrhotic liver or from DNs in cirrhosis; if present, stromal invasion and vascular invasion are diagnostic of HCC. Loss of K7 or K19 positive ductular reaction at the periphery of an encapsulated lesion may signify stromal invasion, and thus malignancy. The oncofetal protein glypican-3 (GPC-3) may be useful when positive; the reactivity is inhomogeneous in a cytoplasmic, membranous, and/or canalicular pattern in up to 70% to 80% of HCCs, but is negative in HCA, although a small fraction of dysplastic and cirrhotic nodules have been reported as immunopositive for GPC-3. Glutamine synthetase, positive only around central veins normally, is commonly diffusely positive in HCC (e-**Fig. 15.67**), and heat shock protein 70 (HSP70) is positive in the majority of HCC. Some investigators advocate the use of a panel of GPC-3, glutamine synthetase, and HSP70 as diagnostic tools in difficult cases (*J Hepatol.* 2009;50:746). The presence of >2% positive K19 tumor cells has been proposed as a poor prognostic marker in HCC, although the specificity of the finding remains unsettled.

Other variants of HCC are listed in Table 15.5. By international consensus, **early HCC** is a low-grade, low-stage, small HCC (*Hepatology.* 2009;49:658) that has grossly and microscopically indistinct borders from the surrounding cirrhotic liver, and may be difficult to distinguish from a high-grade DN. Early HCC may be fatty. Nodules of encapsulated HCC that are distinct from the background are not categorized as independent early HCC since they represent biologically advanced tumors.

b. **Fibrolamellar HCC (FL-HCC)** occurs in noncirrhotic livers and is characterized by large eosinophilic polygonal tumor cells with prominent nuclei and nucleoli in a background of paucicellular lamellar fibrous bands. FL-HCC may bear resemblance to FNH by imaging and grossly. Some of the tumor cells may contain cytoplasmic pale bodies due to the presence of fibrinogen (e-**Fig. 15.68**). The slightly better prognosis of FL-HCC likely is a result of occurrence in nondiseased, noncirrhotic livers in patients younger than is common for HCC. The primary distinction in biopsy is with the scirrhous variant of HCC; the morphology of the hepatocytes is key. Clinical information and serum markers may be helpful. In contrast to HCC, serum AFP is rarely elevated in FL-HCC; however, vitamin B12, vitamin B12 binding capacity, and serum carcinoembryonic antigen may be elevated in FL-HCC.

B. **Malignancies of mixed cellular origin**

1. **Combined hepatocellular-cholangiocarcinoma (HCC-CCa).** According to the 2010 WHO classification, combined HCC-CCa is distinguished from

collision tumors which contain typical HCC and typical CCa separately in the same liver. In contrast, in combined HCC-CCa, the elements are admixed within a single tumor. Combined HCC-CCa is further subdivided into a "classical type," in which all elements are typical by light microscopy and IHC, and subtypes with stem-cell features including "typical," "intermediate," and "cholangiocellular." Notably, in the "typical" HCC-CCa, either intermediate cells (with features of both hepatocellular and biliary differentiation) or stem-like cells may be found at interfaces of the two components of the HCC-CCa. The greater the biliary differentiation of HCC-CCa, the more abundant the sclerotic stroma. The outcome of combined HCC-CCa is worse than traditional HCC, but lack of uniform terminology has prohibited large and comparative series.

2. **Hepatoblastoma,** a primary malignant blastomatous neoplasm of several cell lineages, is rare but is nonetheless the most common liver tumor of children. Up to 80% to 90% of cases present by 5 years, and prematurity and low birth weight are associations. Most present as symptomatic masses in the right lobe.

   a. The **wholly epithelial type** consists of four subtypes: fetal, mixed fetal and embryonal, macrotrabecular, and small cell undifferentiated (SCUD). Fetal cells, resembling adult hepatocytes but smaller in size, contain variable amounts of cytoplasmic fat and glycogen, giving rise to an alternating light-and-dark pattern (e-**Fig. 15.69**). Embryonal cells have a higher N/C ratio and may form nests, rosettes, or small tubules. The macrotrabecular has a growth pattern reminiscent of HCC.

   b. The **mixed epithelial–mesenchymal (MEM) type,** with or without teratoid features, contains malignant mesenchymal components such as cartilage and osteoid in addition to the epithelial elements.

   c. **Hepatoblastoma, NOS,** is the final category.

      The outcome of hepatoblastoma has improved significantly with the improved ability to shrink tumors prior to surgical extirpation. Chemotherapy induces a variety of predictable tumoral alterations. Hepatoblastoma staging systems are based on pretreatment features and postresection findings.

C. **Tumors of the biliary origin**
   1. **Benign**
      a. **Biliary cysts,** whether solitary or as components of the ductal plate malformation (DPM) (described previously), are lined by a single layer of benign, flattened, cuboidal or columnar biliary-type epithelium, surrounded by a variable amount of fibrous tissue.

      b. The **von Meyenburg complex** (e-**Fig. 15.70**) represents persistence of the ductal plate; it is a common finding in normal livers, and may dilate to be the origin of solitary cysts or cysts of polycystic livers. The VMC is usually adjacent to a portal tract and appears as dilated duct-like structures within mature fibrous stroma.

      c. **Ciliated foregut cyst** (e-**Fig. 15.71**), while rare, may be found by imaging or incidentally during surgery. It is subcapsular and often in segment 4. The lining is composed of ciliated pseudostratified columnar epithelium lying on a basement membrane.

      d. **Bile duct adenoma/peribiliary gland hamartoma** is composed of closely packed, well-formed, and relatively uniform small ducts that form a 1 to 20 mm diameter, sharply demarcated nodule (e-**Fig. 15.72**). Careful microscopic examination is necessary to exclude the angulated architecture, desmoplastic stroma, cytologic atypia, mitotic activity, and evidence of invasive growth that are indicative of cholangiocarcinoma or metastatic adenocarcinoma.

2. Premalignant

a. **Biliary intraepithelial neoplasia, grade 3 (BILIN3)** is a precursor of intra-hepatic cholangiocarcinoma (ICC) characterized as flat dysplasia with multilayering of nuclei and micropapillary intraluminal projections. The morphologic findings are identical to of extrahepatic ducts.

b. **Intraductal papillary neoplasm** (IPN) is another precursor of ICC. This category of neoplasms has replaced lesion previously known as biliary papilloma and papillomatosis (e-Fig. 15.73). Synchronous or metachronous IPNs may develop throughout the biliary system. IPNs are classified as low, intermediate, or high grade on the basis of cellular and nuclear features; the parallels with pancreatic intraductal lesions are many, and up to one-third are mucin producing. Most of the intrahepatic papillary neoplasms are lined by biliary epithelium, although intestinal, oncocytic, or gastric type may also be present. Ducts may be massively expanded by the villous growth and distinction with MCN requires thorough evaluation of the stroma (e-Fig. 15.74). Invasive carcinoma may be found in association with IPN; perineural invasion is common. Colloid carcinoma is the type of malignancy that occurs with intestinal-type IPN.

c. **Mucinous cystic neoplasm,** formerly known as biliary cystadenoma as in the gallbladder and pancreas, occurs in women, does not communicate with the biliary tree, and consists of cystic dilated structures lined by a layer of mucin-producing columnar cells on a spindled-type mesenchymal stroma (e-Fig. 15.75). It may additionally show low- or high-grade intraepithelial neoplasia and is graded on the basis of the highest component; thus, numerous sections need to be evaluated. Cases associated with an invasive carcinoma occur in older patients.

3. Malignant Intrahepatic biliary neoplasms

a. **Intrahepatic cholangiocarcinoma (ICC)** is a nonencapsulated mucin-secreting adenocarcinoma usually arising in noncirrhotic livers. Cirrhosis or chronic liver disease cannot be used as evidence to exclude the diagnosis, however. The tumor is characterized by three growth patterns that may coexist: mass-forming, periductal, and intraductal; it is the mass-forming pattern that results in the prominent desmoplastic background with the characteristic firm, white or gray gross appearance.

The tumor is an adenocarcinoma with a variety of architectural patterns resembling canals of Hering, cholangioles, bile ducts of varying sizes, or peribiliary glands. In larger ICC, the central areas may be mostly stroma and paucicellular, while the peripheral regions may show a growth pattern that replaces and incorporates portal tracts. Greater than 90% express keratins 7 and 19, and about 40% also express keratin 20; most cases are also positive for expression of CEA (using a monoclonal antibody) and CA19-9. ICC may be indistinguishable from metastatic ductal adenocarcinoma of the pancreas by histologic and immunohistochemical evaluation. ICC involving only the peribiliary glands may be challenging to distinguish from reactive atypia.

The prognosis of ICC is dismal due to the lack of effective treatments. The exceptions are small peripheral ICCs found incidentally, the mucinous intraductal growth ICC that are completely resected, and the highly selected cases of perihilar cholangiocarcinoma arising in PSC treated with protocolized neoadjuvant chemotherapy and liver transplantation. The 2010 AJCC TNM Staging for carcinomas of the intrahepatic bile ducts is in Table 15.7.

b. **Cystadenocarcinoma** occurs in men as commonly as in women, and no spindled stroma is present. These tumors likely arise from IPN within a

TABLE 15.7	Tumor, Node, Metastasis (TNM) Staging Scheme for Carcinoma of the Intrahepatic Bile Ducts		
Primary tumor (T)			
TX	Primary tumor cannot be assessed		
T0	No evidence of primary tumor		
Tis	Carcinoma in situ (intraductal tumor)		
T1	Solitary tumor without vascular invasion		
T2a	Solitary tumor with vascular invasion		
T2b	Multiple tumors, with or without vascular invasion		
T3	Tumor perforating the visceral peritoneum or involving the local extra hepatic		
T3b	structures by direct extension		
T4	Tumor with periductal invasion		
Regional lymph nodes (N)			
NX	Regional lymph nodes cannot be assessed		
N0	No regional lymph node metastasis		
N1	Regional lymph node metastasis present		
Distant metastasis (M)			
M0	No distant metastasis		
M1	Distant metastasis		
Stage grouping			
Stage 0	Tis	N0	M0
Stage I	T1	N0	M0
Stage II	T2	N0	M0
Stage III	T3	N0	M0
Stage IIIB	T3b	N0	M0
Stage IVA	T4	N0	M0
Stage IVB	Any T	N1	M0
	Any T	Any N	M1

From: Edge SB, Byrd DR, Compton CC, et al., eds. *AJCC Cancer Staging Manual.* 7th ed. New York, NY: Springer; 2010. Used with permission.

markedly dilated duct rather than from MCN. Current data support a prognosis superior to that of ICC.

D. Tumors of mesenchymal origin

1. **Mesenchymal hamartoma** is an uncommon childhood tumor, usually of the right lobe, characterized by a gelatinous mass of bile ducts in a ductal plate pattern; mesenchymal cells; vessels; cystic spaces in a loose, edematous, or myxoid stroma with admixed clusters of liver cells; and extramedullary hematopoiesis (e-Fig. 15.76). MH may result in cardiopulmonary complications if not resected. Transition into embryonal (undifferentiated) sarcoma (UES) occurs, but is very rare.

2. **Cavernous hemangioma** (e-Fig. 15.77), the most common benign tumor of the liver, becomes clinically relevant when >4 cm in maximal dimension. Hemangiomas may increase or rupture during pregnancy. Grossly, tumors are sponge-like and appear well-circumscribed. Microscopically, parenchymal extensions are not uncommon. Organization and fibrosis with time are common but malignant transformation does not occur.

3. **Infantile hemangioma (IH)** is the most common benign mesenchymal liver tumor of infants and children. Girls are more commonly affected than boys; symptoms may include heart failure or hemangiomas of other organs. IH

is characterized by small vascular channels lined by a single layer of plump endothelial cells (**e-Fig. 15.78**) in scant stroma with trapped ducts.

4. **Epithelioid hemangioendothelioma** is a low- or intermediate-grade malignancy. The epithelioid tumor cells have abundant eosinophilic cytoplasm, and may be difficult to discern initially as they are arranged as single cells or small clusters of cells in a dense or myxoid fibrous stroma, and may occasionally be dendritic or spindled. Some tumor cells contain an intracytoplasmic vascular lumen simulating signet-ring-cell carcinoma (**e-Fig. 15.79**). Sinusoidal growth of the tumor cells at the periphery of the lesion is characteristic, often accompanied by hepatocyte atrophy. The tumor may grow into and occlude outflow veins. The tumor cells express at least one endothelial marker such as CD34, CD31, or factor VIII-related antigen.

5. **Angiosarcoma,** a highly aggressive tumor, is the most common mesenchymal malignancy of the liver. The characteristic feature of the tumor is a sinusoidal growth pattern by hyperchromatic, plump, malignant endothelial cells with little associated stromal response (**e-Fig. 15.80**). Solid growth patterns may pose diagnostic challenges, but immunostains demonstrate the vascular nature of the tumor.

6. **Kaposi sarcoma** consists of a pure spindle-cell proliferation with slit-like spaces containing extravasated red cells, and is restricted to patients with human immunodeficiency virus (HIV).

Cytopathology of the Liver

Julie Elizabeth Kunkel and Hannah R. Krigman

I. **INTRODUCTION.** Fine needle aspiration of the liver is typically prompted by the presence of a mass and can be achieved via percutaneous ultrasound or CT-guided fine needle aspiration; lesions in the left lobe can be aspirated by endoscopic ultrasound-guided FNA (EUS-FNA) (*Gastrointest Endosc.* 2002;55:859). Hepatic FNA is a very safe procedure; fatal complications are rare, hemorrhage being the most common which occurs at a rate of 0.006% to 0.031% (*Radiology.* 1991;178:253). The sensitivity for malignancy ranges from 76% to 95%, with a specificity close to 100% (*Diagn Cytopathol.* 2002;26:283; *Diagn Cytopathol.* 2000;23:326).

As with all aspirates, during interpretation it is critical to bear in mind the intervening tissue the needle must pass through, which may be a source of confusion and misdiagnosis. Examples complicating hepatic FNA interpretation include benign or malignant cells originating from the pleura, peritoneum, and lung. Familiarity with and recognition of normal hepatic elements, including bile ductular cells, Kupffer cells, and endothelial cells, are also crucial to avoid a false-positive diagnosis of malignancy (*World J Surg Oncol.* 2004;2:1). Reactive hepatocytes in particular may pose a diagnostic challenge in the distinction from a well-differentiated hepatocellular carcinoma (HCC) (*Arch Pathol Lab Med.* 2002;126:670).

II. **BENIGN NON-NEOPLASTIC MASSES.** Hydatid cysts, abscesses, granulomas, bile duct adenoma/von Meyenburg complexes, focal nodular hyperplasia (FNH), and regenerative nodules are examples of benign non-neoplastic masses.

A. The aspirate of an **abscess** shows abundant neutrophils and necrotic debris (**e-Fig. 15.81**). Amebic abscesses contain more necrotic debris and fewer inflammatory cells. Culture and special stains are usually necessary to identify microorganisms (**e-Fig. 15.82**).

For cases of suspected abscess, it is always necessary to rule out the presence of a necrotic or infected neoplasm by extensive sampling and careful cytologic evaluation for the presence of viable tumor cells which may be obscured by the inflammation. In the instance of suspected tumoral necrosis or well-differentiated HCC, re-biopsy with attention toward the periphery of the lesion should be recommended, such that the interface of the lesion and surrounding normal parenchyma may be examined (*Radiology.* 1997;203:1).

B. In the case of **hydatid cyst**, the aspirated fluid may be clear or turbid. Laminated cyst walls, scolices, and hooklets are observed; a neutrophilic background is sometimes present. Although aspiration of a hydatid cyst poses a risk of anaphylactic reaction, successful procedures are the norm (*Diagn Cytopathol.* 1995;12:173).

III. VASCULAR LESIONS

A. The aspirate of a **hemangioma** usually shows abundant blood. Scattered stromal fragments with bland elongated spindle cells are characteristic (*Diagn Cytopathol.* 1998;19:250). Cell block preparations are helpful to identify the vascular channels.

B. Aspirates of **epithelioid hemangioendothelioma** are paucicellular, containing single cells and small tissue fragments, and display a spectrum of cytomorphology from small bland-appearing epithelioid and spindle cells, to malignant large tumor cells. The epithelioid cells have abundant cytoplasm and may contain characteristic intracytoplasmic lumina or sharply defined intranuclear cytoplasmic inclusions (*Acta Cytol.* 1997;41:5).

C. In **angiosarcoma**, the aspirate shows abundant blood in which there are isolated cells and loose clusters of cells. The malignant cells are spindle-shaped to epithelioid, and have hyperchromatic nuclei and abundant but ill-defined cytoplasm. Necrosis is present. Scattered malignant cells may show hemosiderin-laden cytoplasm or erythrophagocytosis (*Diagn Cytopathol.* 1988;18:208). Vasoformative structures such as intracytoplasmic lumina, microacinar lumen formation, and vascular channels are identified inconsistently (*Anat Pathol.* 2000;114:210).

IV. FNH AND HCA.
These entities typically occur in distinct clinical scenarios as a solitary nodule and as such require clinical, pathologic, and radiologic correlation for the correct diagnosis. In both cases, the diagnosis rests on evaluation of the presence or absence of cytologically benign liver elements; it is therefore critical that only lesional tissue is sampled (*World J Surg Oncol.* 2004;2).

A. **FNH.** Aspirates of **FNH** show both abundant benign hepatocytes and benign biliary epithelial cells (*Acta Cytol.* 1989;33:857).

B. **HCA** aspirates consist of benign hepatocytes *without* biliary epithelial cells (*Acta Cytol.* 1989;33:857).

V. HEPATOCELLULAR CARCINOMA (HCC).
The most characteristic and specific features are thickened hepatocyte trabeculae rimmed by spindle-shaped endothelial cells (e-**Fig. 15.83**), hepatocyte tissue fragments with well-defined traversing capillaries (e-**Fig. 15.84**), increased nuclear to cytoplasmic ratio (e-**Fig. 15.85**), and frequent atypical naked nuclei (e-**Fig. 15.86**) (*Diagn Cytopathol.* 1999;21:370; *Cancer.* 1999;87:270). Poorly differentiated HCC demonstrates loose nests, three dimensional fragments, and occasional gland-like structures of malignant hepatocytes with marked pleomorphism, macronucleoli, necrosis, and numerous mitoses (*Cancer.* 2004;102:247). Features that favor hepatocytic origin include polygonal shaped cells with centrally placed nuclei, abundant granular cytoplasm, and bile pigment (e-**Fig. 15.86**); however, the distinction from cholangiocarcinoma and metastatic adenocarcinoma is challenging and may require immunostains (*Arch Pathol Lab Med.* 2007;131).

The **fibrolamellar variant** of HCC has a distinct cytomorphology which includes poorly cohesive clusters of cells and singly dispersed large monotonous cells with abundant granular cytoplasm, a low nuclear to cytoplasmic ratio, prominent nucleoli, and intracytoplasmic hyaline globules. Fragments of lamellar collagen bands with benign spindle-shaped cells are present. The thickened trabeculae typical of classic HCC are not identified (*Diagn Cytopathol.* 1999;21:180).

VI. CHOLANGIOCARCINOMA. The aspirate is composed of cells arranged in crowded sheets, three-dimensional clusters, acinar structures, or as singly dispersed cells. The malignant cells (e-**Figs. 15.87** and **15.88**) show a high nuclear to cytoplasmic ratio, irregular nuclear membranes, prominent nucleoli, and occasional intracytoplasmic mucin (*Cancer.* 2005;105:220). Poorly differentiated carcinoma displays marked nuclear pleomorphism and necrosis.

 Combined hepatocellular-cholangiocarcinoma is a bi-phenotypic tumor arising from the canal of Hering cells with features of HCC and cholangiocarcinoma. The tumor bridges these two entities both morphologically and by immunohistochemistry. These tumors (e-**Fig. 15.89**) are cytologically malignant but usually require immunostains for correct categorization as the malignant cells exhibit of spectrum of differentiation from hepatoid to glandular (*Acta Cytol.* 1997;41:1269).

VII. METASTATIC MALIGNANCY. Metastasis from an extrahepatic primary tumor is the most common malignancy of the liver (*Diagn Cytopathol.* 2000;23:326). The most common primary tumors that metastasize to the liver are adenocarcinomas arising from the colon (e-**Fig. 15.90**), lung, pancreas, breast, and kidney. Comparison with the primary malignancy in cases of metastases is essential for diagnosis, as is appropriate immunohistochemical characterization. Carcinomas with polygonal cell morphology, such as neuroendocrine tumors, renal cell carcinoma, adrenocortical carcinoma, and others must be differentiated from HCC on the basis of their immunoprofile (*Arch Pathol Lab Med.* 2007;131:1648).

16 The Gallbladder and Extrahepatic Biliary Tree

Ta-Chiang Liu and Elizabeth M. Brunt

I. **NORMAL ANATOMY.** The gallbladder, comprised by the fundus, body, and neck, is covered by serosa, except the portion in the liver fossa which merges with liver parenchyma. The lining mucosa, a layer of folded columnar epithelium and lamina propria of loose connective tissue, directly rests on muscularis propria which consists of longitudinally oriented, to irregularly arranged bundles of smooth muscle with overlying subserosa and serosa. No muscularis mucosae or submucosa are present. Secretory mucous glands in the neck and extrahepatic bile ducts are arranged in a lobular pattern (**e-Fig. 16.1**).*

The extrahepatic ducts include the right and left hepatic ducts, which join to form the common hepatic duct in the porta hepatis; when the common hepatic duct is joined by the cystic duct, the common bile duct is formed. A single layer of columnar cells lines the ducts and rests directly on dense connective tissue; from proximal to distal, there is a variable periductal smooth muscle fiber investment, intermingled with collagen bundles.

II. **GROSS EXAMINATION**

A. **Cholecystectomy** is most commonly performed for cholelithiasis. After the gallbladder is measured and opened longitudinally, the following should be described: serosal, mural, and mucosal appearances; cystic duct integrity; and consistency, quantity, and color of stones. Full-thickness sections should be submitted from the fundus, body, neck, and duct; the cystic duct margin should also be submitted, as well as any lymph nodes. For a suspicious lesion, the overlying serosal surface or hepatic bed should be inked, the lesion breadloafed, and sections taken to demonstrate relevant anatomic relationships.

The gross finding that the gallbladder wall is uniformly firm with an associated flattened mucosal surface suggests the diagnosis of a so-called porcelain gallbladder. After the specimen is photographed, at least one section per cm should be submitted (if not the entire specimen) to exclude adenocarcinoma (**e-Figs. 16.2** and **16.3**).

B. **Biopsy** of the common bile duct is performed for stricture or overt neoplasm during endoscopic retrograde cholangiopancreatography (ERCP). The number and dimensions of specimens should be recorded to ensure that the biopsy fragments are adequately represented; inking is not needed. At the time of initial histologic sectioning, preparation of three hematoxylin and eosin (H&E) stained slides together with six additional unstained slides avoids resurfacing the block if subsequent deeper levels or special stains are required for diagnosis.

C. **Frozen section.** Evaluation of bile duct margins by frozen section during pancreatoduodenectomy, or liver resections for bile duct adenocarcinoma, is often performed. The tissue should be frozen in its entirety, oriented in the frozen section block to obtain enface sections, and cut deeply to obtain sections that

---

*All e-figures are available online via the Solution Site Image Bank.

represent the entire margin so that small foci of tumor are not missed by inadequate sampling. The tissue that remains after frozen section should be submitted for evaluation by permanent sections, which helps assure adequate sampling.

III. DIAGNOSTIC FEATURES OF COMMON NONNEOPLASTIC CONDITIONS

A. **Cholecystitis** is associated with cholelithiasis in >90% of the cases. Acute cholecystitis is characterized by full thickness edema, congestion, and an associated fibrinopurulent serosal exudate. Hemorrhage, transmural necrosis (gangrenous cholecystitis), and/or perforation may occur (e-**Figs. 16.4** and **16.5**).

Chronic cholecystitis is variably characterized by mural hypertrophy or atrophy with fibrosis and chronic inflammation (e-**Fig. 16.6**). Intestinal, pyloric, or foveolar surface metaplasia may occur. Rokitansky–Aschoff sinuses, which are herniations of the lining mucosa into the muscle layers, are common. Adenomyoma represents exaggerated herniations in the fundus accompanied by muscular hypertrophy and may appear as a gross deformity (e-**Figs. 16.7** to **16.9**). Both xanthogranulomatous cholecystitis (due to rupture of Rokitansky–Aschoff sinuses) or mucosal ulceration from stones may be transmural with associated bile extravasation and accumulation of foamy macrophages. Acalculous cholecystitis may be acute or chronic. Follicular cholecystitis may be associated with primary sclerosing cholangitis (PSC) (e-**Fig. 16.10**).

B. **Cholesterolosis** (strawberry gallbladder) is characterized by yellow mucosal specks grossly and lipid-laden macrophages in the lamina propria microscopically (e-**Fig. 16.11**). It is an incidental finding of no clinical significance.

C. **Choledochal cyst,** a form of fibropolycystic disease, results in fusiform or spherical dilatation of the common bile duct. Following photographic documentation, the entire lesion should be submitted for microscopic examination to exclude biliary intraepithelial neoplasia (BilIN) or adenocarcinoma (e-**Fig. 16.12**).

D. **Biliary atresia** is a congenital process in which the extrahepatic ducts and gallbladder may be completely absent, or replaced by fibrous cords with no or only a very small lumen.

E. **PSC** involving the extrahepatic biliary system is an idiopathic disease diagnosed by cholangiography (discussed in more detail in Chap. 15).

F. **Secondary sclerosing cholangitis,** histologically indistinguishable from PSC, has a variety of obstructive and nonobstructive etiologies, including tumors, toxins, ischemia, and infections (including AIDS cholangiopathy).

IV. DIAGNOSTIC FEATURES OF COMMON NEOPLASMS AND PRECURSOR LESIONS (Table 16.1)

A. **Adenoma** is a single, small, and incidentally found polypoid lesion, and is characterized by a tubular, papillary, or tubulopapillary architecture. A pyloric or intestinal type epithelium is more common than a biliary type epithelium; squamous morules, Paneth cells, and neuroendocrine cells may be present. By definition, all adenomas are low grade, but larger adenomas may harbor foci of high-grade intraepithelial neoplasia or invasive carcinoma and thus should be entirely submitted for microscopic examination.

B. **Biliary intraepithelial neoplasia** (BilIN) is a classification nomenclature introduced in 2010 by the World Health Organization (WHO). BilIN-1 and BilIN-2 (low and intermediate grade lesions) are incidental and without established clinical significance. BilIN-3 may be associated with invasive carcinoma, and thus if present in the gallbladder, thorough sampling (including of the cystic duct and margin of excision) is necessary to exclude invasive carcinoma. If no invasive carcinoma is present, and the surgical margin of the cystic duct is not involved, cholecystectomy is considered curative. A distinguishing characteristic between BilIN-3 and reparative atypia is the abrupt transition noted in the former (e-**Fig. 16.13**) compared with the gradual alterations and heterogenous, widespread

TABLE 16.1	WHO Histologic Classification of Tumors of the Gallbladder and Extrahepatic Bile Ducts

Epithelial tumors

Premalignant lesions

Adenoma
    Tubular
    Papillary
    Tubulopapillary

Biliary intraepithelial neoplasia, grade 3 (BilIN-3)

Intracystic (gallbladder) or intraductal (bile ducts) papillary neoplasm with low- or intermediate-grade intraepithelial neoplasia

Intracystic (gallbladder) or intraductal (bile ducts) papillary neoplasm with high-grade intraepithelial neoplasia

Mucinous cystic neoplasm with low- or intermediate-grade intraepithelial neoplasia

Mucinous cystic neoplasm with high-grade intraepithelial neoplasia

Carcinoma

Adenocarcinoma
    Adenocarcinoma, biliary type
    Adenocarcinoma, gastric foveolar type
    Adenocarcinoma, intestinal type
    Clear cell adenocarcinoma
    Mucinous adenocarcinoma
    Signet-ring cell carcinoma

Adenosquamous carcinoma

Intracystic (gallbladder) or intraductal (bile ducts) papillary neoplasm with an associated invasive carcinoma

Mucinous cystic neoplasm with an associated invasive carcinoma

Squamous cell carcinoma

Undifferentiated carcinoma

Neuroendocrine neoplasms

Neuroendocrine tumor (NET)
    NET G1 (carcinoid)
    NET G2

Neuroendocrine carcinoma (NEC)
    Large-cell NEC
    Small-cell NEC

Mixed adenoneuroendocrine carcinoma

Goblet cell carcinoid

Tubular carcinoid

Mesenchymal tumors

Granular cell tumor

Leiomyoma

Kaposi sarcoma

Leiomyosarcoma

Rhabdomyosarcoma

Lymphomas

Secondary tumors

From: Bosman FT, Carneiro F, Hruban RH, Theise ND, eds. *World Health Organization Classification of Tumours of the Digestive System.* Lyon: IARC Press; 2010. Used with permission.

epithelial involvement of the latter. In addition, p53 expression is more extensive in BilIN than in reactive atypia.

C. Intraluminal papillary neoplasms of the gallbladder and extrahepatic bile ducts are currently termed as **intracystic papillary neoplasms** and **intraductal papillary neoplasms (IPMNs)**, respectively.

1. **Intracystic papillary neoplasms** have a biliary rather than pyloric lining, architectural complexity and atypia, and frequent mitoses. These lesions are stratified into low and high grade; the latter may be associated with adenocarcinoma, most commonly tubular. In the gallbladder, the differential diagnosis is adenoma.

TABLE 16.2	The 2010 AJCC TNM Schema for Gallbladder (and Cystic Duct) Carcinoma		
Primary tumor (T)			
TX	Primary tumor cannot be assessed		
T0	No evidence of primary tumor		
Tis	Carcinoma in situ		
T1	Tumor invades lamina propria or muscular layer		
T1a	Tumor invades lamina propria		
T1b	Tumor invades muscular layer		
T2	Tumor invades perimuscular connective tissue; no extension beyond serosa or into liver		
T3	Tumor perforates the serosa (visceral peritoneum) and/or directly invades the liver and/or another adjacent organ or structure, such as the stomach, duodenum, colon, or pancreas, omentum, or extrahepatic bile ducts		
T4	Tumor invades main portal vein or hepatic artery or invades two or more extrahepatic organs or structures		
Regional lymph nodes (N)			
NX	Regional lymph nodes cannot be assessed		
N0	No regional lymph node metastasis		
N1	Metastases to nodes along the cystic duct, common bile duct, hepatic artery, and/or portal vein		
N2	Metastases to periaortic, pericaval, superior mesenteric artery, and/or celiac artery lymph nodes		
Distant metastasis (M)			
M0	No distant metastasis		
M1	Distant metastasis		
Stage grouping			
Stage 0	Tis	N0	M0
Stage I	T1	N0	M0
Stage II	T2	N0	M0
Stage IIIA	T3	N0	M0
Stage IIIB	T1–3	N1	M0
Stage IVA	T4	N0–1	M0
Stage IVB	Any T	N2	M0
	Any T	Any N	M1

From: Edge SB, Byrd DR, Compton CC, et al., eds. *AJCC Cancer Staging Manual.* 7th ed. New York, NY: Springer; 2010. Used with permission.

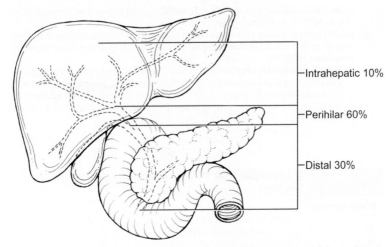

Figure 16.1 Anatomic boundaries for AJCC classification of adenocarcinomas of the extrahepatic bile ducts.

2. **IPMNs of the extrahepatic bile ducts** share the epithelial types characteristic of pancreatic IPMNs, including pancreatobiliary, intestinal, oncocytic, or gastric. **Papillomatosis,** a recurrent and potentially multicentric condition of the entire biliary tree, is considered a subset of IPMN.

3. **Mucinous cystic neoplasm (MCN)** has replaced the term cystadenoma. More common in the extrahepatic ducts than gallbladder, MCN may grow to 20 cm in maximal dimension. As in its hepatic counterpart, the lesion contains estrogen receptor and progesterone receptor positive mesenchymal stroma. As with papillary neoplasms, MCN lesions may be associated with invasive adenocarcinoma.

D. The classification of **adenocarcinomas of the gallbladder and cystic duct** is shown in Table 16.1. Tumors of both sites have similar staging schemes (Table 16.2).

1. **Adenocarcinoma** of the gallbladder may grossly result in mural induration and mimic chronic cholecystitis, or grow as an intraluminal polypoid lesion (e-**Fig. 16.14**). In order of decreasing frequency, the common subtypes are biliary, intestinal (tubular or goblet), and gastric foveolar (e-**Fig. 16.15**).

2. **Biliary adenocarcinomas** may contain mixed cell types including intestinal, goblet, and neuroendocrine cells. The tumors composed of intestinal type cells are usually K20 and CDX2 immunopositive; the goblet cell variant may also have Paneth and neuroendocrine cells. The gastric foveolar type is usually well-differentiated (e-**Figs. 16.16** and **16.17**).

E. **Adenocarcinomas of extrahepatic bile ducts** have been reclassified by the AJCC as perihilar or distal (Fig. 16.1), and each has its own staging scheme (Tables 16.3 and 16.4). Perihilar tumors arise proximal to cystic duct and account for 60% of the adenocarcinomas; the distal tumors arise between the junction of the cystic duct and common bile duct and the ampulla of Vater, and account for 30% of the adenocarcinomas (e-**Fig. 16.18**). Grossly, there may be only subtle thickening of the duct wall, and thorough sampling is required to evaluate margins and local extension.

TABLE 16.3	TNM Stating Scheme for Carcinoma of the Perihilar Bile Ducts		

Primary tumor (T)

TX	Primary tumor cannot be assessed
T0	No evidence of primary tumor
Tis	Carcinoma in situ
T1	Tumor confined to the bile duct, with extension up to the muscle layer or fibrous tissue
T2a	Tumor invades beyond the wall of the bile duct to surrounding adipose tissue
T2b	Tumor invades adjacent hepatic parenchyma
T3	Tumor invades the unilateral branches of the portal vein or hepatic artery
T4	Tumor invades main portal vein or its branches bilaterally; or the common hepatic artery; or the second-order biliary radicals bilaterally; or unilateral second-order biliary radicals with contralateral portal vein or hepatic artery involvement

Regional lymph nodes (N)

NX	Regional lymph nodes cannot be assessed
N0	No regional lymph node metastasis
N1	Regional lymph node metastasis (includes nodes along the cystic duct, common bile duct, hepatic artery, and portal vein)
N2	Metastasis to periaortic, pericaval, superior mesenteric artery, and/or celiac artery lymph nodes

Distant metastasis (M)

M0	No distant metastasis
M1	Distant metastasis

Stage grouping

Stage 0	Tis	N0	M0
Stage I	T1	N0	M0
Stage II	T2a–b	N0	M0
Stage IIIA	T3	N0	M0
Stage IIIB	T1–3	N1	M0
Stage IVA	T4	N0–1	M0
Stage IVB	Any T	N2	M0
	Any T	Any N	M1

From: Edge SB, Byrd DR, Compton CC, et al., eds. *AJCC Cancer Staging Manual.* 7th ed. New York, NY: Springer; 2010. Used with permission.

Cytopathology of the Gallbladder and Extrahepatic Biliary Tree

Brian Collins and Julie Elizabeth Kunkel

I. GALLBLADDER

A. **Inflammatory lesions.** In instances where acute cholecystitis develops into a localized abscess, aspirates typically show numerous acute inflammatory cells with intermixed necroinflammatory debris. Even when an abscess arises within a necrotic neoplasm, aspirates often show only generic features and thus it can

TABLE 16.4 TNM Staging Scheme for Carcinoma of the Distal Bile Ducts

Primary tumor (T)

TX	Primary tumor cannot be assessed
T0	No evidence of primary tumor
Tis	Carcinoma in situ
T1	Tumor confined to the bile duct histologically
T2	Tumor invades beyond the wall of the bile duct
T3	Tumor invades the gallbladder, pancreas, duodenum, or other adjacent organs without involvement of the celiac axis, or the superior mesenteric artery
T4	Tumor involves the celiac axis, or the superior mesenteric artery

Regional lymph nodes (N)

NX	Regional lymph nodes cannot be assessed
N0	No regional lymph node metastasis
N1	Regional lymph node metastasis

Distant metastasis (M)

M0	No distant metastasis
M1	Distant metastasis

Stage grouping

Stage 0	Tis	N0	M0
Stage IA	T1	N0	M0
Stage IB	T2	N0	M0
Stage IIA	T3	N0	M0
Stage IIB	T1–3	N1	M0
Stage III	T4	Any N	M0
Stage IV	Any T	Any N	M1

From: Edge SB, Byrd DR, Compton CC, et al., eds. *AJCC Cancer Staging Manual*. 7th ed. New York, NY: Springer; 2010. Used with permission.

be challenging to recognize that an underlying neoplasm is present based on the cytopathologic findings alone.

B. **Neoplasms.** Adenocarcinoma is the most common type of malignancy encountered. On aspiration smears it shows groups and syncytial fragments of cells that have round to oval nuclei, vesicular chromatin, nucleoli, and nuclear membrane irregularities. The overall findings impart an appearance of adenocarcinoma without any particular distinct features (e-**Fig. 16.19**) (*Cytopathology.* 2006;1:42).

II. **EXTRAHEPATIC BILIARY TREE.** A variety of inflammatory and neoplastic conditions occur in the extrahepatic biliary tree, all of which typically present as strictures with or without an associated mass. Cytopathology can be a valuable method of diagnosis because ERCP provides access to areas involved by a mass or stricture for sampling by brushing (*Cytopathology.* 2004;15:74). The specificity of brushing is high; however, the sensitivity is more variable (*Arch Pathol Lab Med.* 2000;124:387). Ultrasound, CT, and endoscopic ultrasound (EUS) are all used to guide FNA (*Acta Cytol.* 2008;52:24).

A. **Inflammatory.** A variety of inflammatory processes can lead to reactive and inflammatory damage, some of which (primary biliary sclerosis [PSC]) have an underlying associated risk for malignancy. Cytopathology has been shown to be helpful for clarifying the nature of an associated stricture or abnormality (*Cancer.* 2006;108:231).

1. **Reactive.** Lithiasis is a common occurrence in the biliary tract and can lead to localized inflammation and/or stricture formation. Bile duct brushing of

a benign/inflammatory stricture shows flat sheets of ductal epithelium with minimal crowding and overlap. The nuclei are round to oval with fine chromatin, nucleoli, and minimal pleomorphism (e-Fig. 16.20). The background can show granular debris of a postobstructive process. Single atypical cells are not seen. It is important to know if a stent is in place since stents can cause significant reactive atypia which can be confused with neoplasia.

2. **PSC.** Patients with PSC can have multiple strictures throughout the biliary tree that are sampled and followed by bile duct brushing (*Clin Liver Dis.* 2010;14:349). When the strictures are inflammatory in nature, they typically show a florid repair appearance consisting of nuclear enlargement, prominent nucleoli, and cellular crowding and overlap with some loss of polarity. Intraepithelial neutrophils can be present (e-Figs. **16.21** and **16.22**). A spectrum of reactive atypia is present without a distinct second population. Overall, the findings do not meet the criteria required for the diagnosis of carcinoma as detailed below. However, the epithelial atypia present cannot always be clearly categorized, and in these instances a descriptive diagnosis of "epithelial atypia" can be appropriate.

B. **Neoplastic.** Cholangiocarcinoma is most commonly encountered in bile duct brushings, but the advent of endoscopic ultrasound-guided fine needle aspiration (EUS-FNA) is providing more access and better sampling of this neoplasm in the biliary tree. Nonetheless, the lesion's underlying sclerotic nature can present a challenge in obtaining sufficient diagnostic cellular elements (*J Clin Oncol.* 2005;23:4561). By bile duct brushing, there is typically a mixed population of benign/reactive ductal epithelial cells and a second population of ductal carcinoma cells. The ductal carcinoma component shows small syncytial groups and sheets of cells with crowding and overlap, and single cells. The nuclei are enlarged with granular chromatin, nuclear membrane irregularities, anisonucleosis, and nucleoli (e-Figs. **16.23** and **16.24**). The application of UroVysion FISH to bile duct brushing specimens can assist in the diagnosis (e-Fig. **16.25**). By FNA, the aspirate smears can be variably cellular and show small to intermediate groups arranged as syncytial fragments and flat sheets. The nuclei possess nuclear membrane irregularities, coarse chromatin, nucleoli, and show anisonucleosis.

17 The Pancreas

Dengfeng Cao and Hanlin L. Wang

I. **NORMAL ANATOMY.** The pancreas is located in the retroperitoneum. In adults, the pancreas measures 15 to 20 cm in length and weighs 85 to 120 g. The pancreas is divided into four parts: the head (including the uncinate process), neck, body, and tail. The vascular supply to pancreas is from branches of celiac trunk and superior mesenteric arteries. The lymph nodes draining the pancreas consist of two major systems: those ringing the pancreas, and those near the aorta from the level of celiac trunk to the origin of the superior mesenteric artery. Microscopically, the pancreas consists of lobules that include both exocrine and endocrine components.

The vast majority of the exocrine component is the acinar epithelium. The acinar cells are large and polarized, with basally situated nuclei; the apical cytoplasm is eosinophilic due to the presence of abundant zymogen granules, whereas the basal portion is basophilic and contains abundant rough endoplasmic reticulum. The second component of the exocrine pancreas is the duct system that begins with the centroacinar cells. The centroacinar cells then drain into intercalated ducts, intralobular ducts, interlobular ducts, and then into the main pancreatic duct of Wirsung and the accessory duct of Santorini. The duct system is lined by cuboidal to low columnar cells with no visible cytoplasmic mucin by hematoxylin and eosin (H&E) staining.

The endocrine component, constituting 1% to 2% of the pancreas in adults, is composed of islets of Langerhans and extrainsular endocrine cells scattered among the acini and ducts. The islets of Langerhans contain four major cell types: insulin-secreting β cells (60% to 70%), glucagon-secreting α cells (15% to 20%), somatostatin-secreting δ cells, and pancreatic polypeptide-secreting PP cells.

II. **GROSS EXAMINATION AND TISSUE HANDLING**

A. **Biopsy, fine needle aspiration**, and **brushing cytology** specimens may be obtained percutaneously, intraoperatively, or via endoscopic retrograde cholangiopancreatography (ERCP). Needle core biopsies should be immediately fixed in 10% formalin. The number and the length, or length range, of the biopsies should be recorded. Documentation of the number and length is important to ensure that the biopsies are adequately represented on the slides. Three H&E-stained slides from each block are prepared for microscopic examination. Aspiration smears are processed with alcohol fixation for Papanicolaou staining or air dried for Diff-Quik staining. Brushings are handled by routine liquid-based cytology methods.

B. **Distal pancreatectomy** specimens consist of the pancreatic tail (usually with attached spleen) and a portion of the pancreatic body. After orientation, each organ should be measured separately. An externally visible mass or lesion should be documented for its size, extent, and location. The proximal and peripancreatic margins should be inked. Before sectioning through the pancreas, the proximal margin is typically taken either as a shave margin or as a series of perpendicular sections, depending on the location of tumor. The method of sectioning the pancreas depends on personal preference. One method is to bivalve the pancreas using a probe in the main duct as a guide; another method is to section the pancreas in a breadloaf fashion. The size and characteristics of any lesions (masses or cysts), along with their relationship to the main duct, spleen, and peripancreatic soft tissue resection margins should be documented. If the lesion is cystic, the cyst contents and the cysts relationship to the main duct should be also documented.

Sections from the lesion should include samples that demonstrate the relation of the lesion to margins and uninvolved pancreas. If the pancreatic lesion is cystic and small, it should be submitted in its entirety. For large lesions (e.g., >5 cm), at least one section per centimeter is recommended, which should focus on thickened, solid, or irregular areas. One or more perpendicular sections from the inked posterior (retroperitoneal) soft tissue margin should be submitted. One to two representative sections from the spleen are sufficient unless gross abnormalities are detected. Finally, the peripancreatic and splenic hilar soft tissue is searched for lymph nodes; all identified lymph nodes should be submitted in their entirety for microscopic examination.

C. **The Whipple procedure,** performed for tumors of the pancreatic head, common bile duct, ampullary, or periampullary region, involves excision of a composite specimen usually consisting of the pancreatic head, a portion of the common bile duct, the duodenum, the distal stomach, and the gallbladder. After orientation, the dimension of each organ should be measured. The various surgical margins of the pancreas (pancreatic neck, posterior, portal vein groove, and uncinate) should be inked with different colors in the operating room with the surgeon's aid; frozen section evaluation of the pancreatic neck and bile duct margins is almost always requested intraoperatively. The stomach is opened along the greater curvature and the duodenum is opened along the aspect opposite the pancreas to avoid the ampulla. The pancreas can be sectioned along the plane defined by the pancreatic duct and bile duct using probes as a guide, or cut perpendicularly. The size, location, and nature of the tumor are recorded, as is the relation of the tumor to the margins. If the tumor is cystic, the cyst contents and the relationship of the cyst to the main duct should be documented. The specimen is then pinned out and fixed in 10% formalin before grossing. In general, one section per centimeter of the tumor is submitted; if the tumor is an intraductal papillary mucinous neoplasm (IPMN) or mucinous cystic neoplasm (MCN), and is noninvasive in the initial sections, it is necessary to return to the gross specimen and submit the entire lesion to ensure that invasive tumor is not missed. Additional sections should demonstrate the relation of the tumor to the various margins of excision, uninvolved pancreas, ducts, ampulla, duodenum, and soft tissue; one section from the proximal gastric resection margin, and one from distal duodenal resection margin should also be submitted. One section from the uninvolved pancreas and one from uninvolved ampulla are also submitted if not already sampled in the tumor sections. All identified lymph nodes in the soft tissue should be submitted for microscopic examination; there is no need to separate the nodes into groups because they are all considered regional. Microscopic examination of a minimum of 10 to 15 nodes has been recommended for Whipple specimens.

III. **DIAGNOSTIC FEATURES OF PANCREATITIS**

A. **Acute pancreatitis** is an inflammatory process in which pancreatic enzymes autodigest the gland. It is most commonly associated with biliary tract disease (such as gallstones) and alcohol abuse. The pancreas is swollen and edematous, and hemorrhagic in more severe cases. Chalky white fat necrosis may be evident. Histologically, mild pancreatitis is characterized by interstitial edema and leukocytic infiltration; the pancreatic parenchyma may be well preserved, with only limited necrosis. In severe cases, extensive necrosis and hemorrhage are seen (e-**Fig. 17.1**).* Calcification and secondary infection may occur.

---

*All e-figures are available online via the Solution Site Image Bank.

B. Chronic pancreatitis is an inflammatory process characterized by irreversible destruction of the exocrine component with acinar atrophy, mixed inflammatory cell infiltrates, and fibrosis with relative sparing of the islets of Langerhans (e-**Fig. 17.2**). Dilatation of the pancreatic ducts with proteinaceous, often calcified, secretions is characteristic. In later stages, the endocrine component may also be destroyed.

1. **Etiology.** Most cases are associated with chronic alcohol abuse. Other etiologies include bile duct and pancreatic duct obstruction (due to lithiasis), hyperlipidemia, hyperparathyroidism, autoimmune disorders, and hereditary chronic pancreatitis [due to germline mutations in cationic trypsinogen (*PRSS1*), cystic fibrosis transmembrane conductance regulator (*CFTR*), chymotrypsin C, calcium-sensing receptor, and anionic trypsin (*PRSS2*)] (*Dig Dis.* 2010;28:324).

2. **Autoimmune pancreatitis (AIP)** is a distinct type of chronic pancreatitis frequently associated with systemic autoimmune diseases, including inflammatory bowel disease and primary sclerosing cholangitis. AIP may mimic pancreatic cancer radiographically and endoscopically when it presents as a mass lesion in the pancreatic head and/or with strictures of the pancreatic and common bile ducts. Histologically, AIP shares many features of conventional chronic pancreatitis, but is distinguished by a dense lymphoplasmacytic infiltrate, particularly in the periductal region (e-**Fig. 17.3**), and obliterative phlebitis (e-**Fig. 17.4**). In addition to various autoantibodies, selective elevation of serum immunoglobulin G4 (IgG4) level helps establish the diagnosis (*Arch Pathol Lab Med.* 2005;129:1148; *J Gastroenterol.* 2006;41:613). The number of IgG4 plasma cells in the pancreas is typically >10 per high-power field (HPF), and >50 per HPF is highly specific for the diagnosis (*Adv Anat Pathol.* 2010;17:303). Patients often respond well to steroid therapy.

   A recent study has suggested that AIP can be further divided into type 1 and type 2 diseases (*Am J Surg Pathol.* 2011;35:26). Type 1 AIP is the pancreatic manifestation of IgG4-related systemic disease, whereas type 2 is confined to the pancreas; the serum IgG4 level is higher in patients with type 1 disease than in patients with type 2 disease. Pathologically, type 1 and type 2 AIPs share periductal inflammation, however, interlobular inflammation and fibrosis is unique to type 1, and obliterative phlebitis is much more common in type 1 than type 2 (91% vs. 6%). The number of IgG4-positive plasma cells in the pancreas is much higher in type 1 disease than type 2 disease (>50 per HPF in 88% and 7% of type 1 and 2 diseases, respectively; >10 in 100% type 1 and 50% type 2 diseases, respectively). On the other hand, ductular/lobular abscesses and ductal ulceration are much more common in type 2 than type 1 AIP.

IV. **CYSTIC LESIONS AND TUMORS OF THE PANCREAS.** Cystic lesions of the pancreas include non-neoplastic and neoplastic types. The former mainly include pseudocyst, lymphoepithelial cyst, ductal retention cyst, mucinous non-neoplastic cyst, and paraampullary duodenal wall cyst (groove pancreatitis). Neoplastic cystic lesions include serous cystic neoplasm, MCN, IPMN, intraductal tubulopapillary neoplasm (ITPN), solid pseudopapillary neoplasm, and cystic acinar neoplasm. Pancreatic neuroendocrine tumors (islet cell tumors) can also be cystic.

A. Nonneoplastic cystic lesions

1. **Pseudocyst** is the most common cystic lesion of the pancreas and usually develops as a result of pancreatitis or trauma. About two-third of pseudocysts are located in the tail. The cyst is lined by granulation or fibrous tissue without an epithelial lining, with a wall thickness ranging from several millimeters to several centimeters (e-**Fig. 17.5**).

2. **Lymphoepithelial cyst** is usually lined by squamous epithelium, typically keratinized, with abundant underlying lymphocytes that occasionally form germinal centers (e-**Fig. 17.6**). The lining epithelium may be of other types such as flat, cuboidal, or transitional. Rarely sebaceous and mucinous cells may be also seen in the wall, but skin adnexal structures are not found.

3. **Ductal retention cyst** (also named simple cyst) is caused by obstruction. Microscopically, it is a unilocular cyst lined by a layer of simple epithelium. When the lining epithelium becomes mucinous, it is termed a mucinous nonneoplastic cyst.

4. **Paraampullary duodenal wall cyst** (groove pancreatitis, cystic dystrophy of the duodenal wall, paraduodenal pancreatitis) is located within the "groove" between the head of the organ, the duodenum, and the common bile duct (*Hepatogastroenterology*. 1982;29:198). It most likely arises from the submucosal pancreatic tissue associated with remnants of the minor papilla, and is caused by obstruction of the minor papilla. It causes segmental chronic pancreatitis affecting the groove area (hence the name groove pancreatitis). Microscopically, it consists of dilated ductal structures within the duodenal wall; the lining of the ducts is often partially denuded and may contain mucinous epithelium and reactive changes (e-**Fig. 17.7**). The cyst wall is composed of inflamed fibrous tissue containing lymphocytes, plasma cells, and neutrophils, and the adjacent pancreatic tissue shows atrophy, fat necrosis, and fibrosis.

B. Neoplastic cystic lesions

1. **Serous cystadenoma** is a benign cystic neoplasm usually found in the body or tail of the pancreas in elderly patients. The vast majority is sporadic but the lesion can be associated with the von Hippel–Lindau syndrome. It is usually multilocular (microcystic cystadenoma), but occasionally unilocular, oligocystic (macrocystic), or even solid. Grossly, the tumor has a spongy appearance with a stellate central scar (e-**Fig. 17.8**) with cysts that are filled with clear serous fluid. Microscopically, the individual cysts are lined by a single layer of flat to cuboidal epithelial cells, with pale to clear glycogen-rich cytoplasm (e-**Fig. 17.9**). Focally papillary structures lined with clear cells may be seen. Immunohistochemically, the lining cells are positive for cytokeratin and in most cases are also positive for α-inhibin and MUC6 (*Am J Surg Pathol*. 2004;28:339). The solid variant can mimic metastatic clear-cell renal cell carcinoma (e-**Fig. 17.10**).

    Serous cystadenocarcinoma is exceedingly rare in the pancreas and is morphologically indistinguishable from serous cystadenoma. The diagnosis is established by the presence of distal metastasis, but vascular invasion and invasion into adjacent structures have been observed.

2. **MCN** tends to occur in the tail or body of the pancreas, predominantly in women about 50 years of age with a female to male ratio of 20:1. The neoplasm is a solitary, multilocular (rarely unilocular) cystic mass filled with mucin (e-**Fig. 17.11**) or mucin admixed with necrotic material. The cysts do not communicate with the ductal system. The cyst lining, which may be partially denuded, consists of tall columnar mucin-producing cells with characteristic underlying ovarian-type stroma (e-**Fig. 17.12**). The ovarian-type stroma surrounding the cysts is the defining feature of MCN and is useful for distinguishing MCN from IPMN (Table 17.1). The stromal cells are frequently positive for estrogen and progesterone receptors and inhibin, and can be luteinized.

    On the basis of the cytologic and architectural features of the lining epithelium, noninvasive MCN can be divided into three categories: MCN with low-grade dysplasia (mucinous cystadenoma) (e-**Fig. 17.13**), MCN with moderate or intermediate grade dysplasia (borderline MCN) (e-**Fig. 17.14**), and MCN

TABLE 17.1 Distinction Between Intraductal Papillary Mucinous Neoplasm (IPMN) and Mucinous Cystic Neoplasm (MCN)

Features	IPMN	MCN
Patient population	Older women and men	Predominantly middle-aged women
Location in pancreas	Head	Tail or body
Communication with ductal system	Yes	No
Ovarian-type stroma	No	Yes

with high-grade or severe dysplasia (carcinoma in situ, noninvasive mucinous cystic adenocarcinoma). Severe dysplasia is characterized by papillary, cribriform, branching, and budding growth patterns; marked nuclear stratification and atypia; mucin depletion; and frequent mitosis (e-**Fig. 17.15**). Up to one-third of MCNs have an associated invasive carcinoma that commonly is of ductal type and forms tubules and duct-like structures (e-**Fig. 17.16**). Other rare types of invasive carcinoma arising in association with MCN have also been reported including adenosquamous carcinoma, undifferentiated carcinoma, and undifferentiated carcinoma with osteoclast-like giant cells. The prognosis for noninvasive MCN is excellent and surgical resection is curative for almost all patients. The prognosis for those lesions with an invasive component is determined by the extent of invasive carcinoma, stage, and resectability (*Am J Surg Pathol.* 1999;23:410).

3. **IPMN** is defined as a grossly visible (≥ 1 cm) epithelial tumor arising in the main pancreatic duct (main duct IPMN) or its branches (branch-duct-type IPMN). IPMN is typically seen in the head of the pancreas but it may diffusely involve the whole organ. Branch-duct-type IPMN tends to involve the uncinate process. Symptomatic patients often have a main-duct-type IPMN, whereas most of the branch-duct-type IPMNs are detected incidentally. Histologically, the neoplastic epithelium typically forms papillary fronds lined by mucin-producing columnar cells (e-**Fig. 17.17**). On the basis of the degree of architectural and cytologic atypia, IPMN can be divided into four categories: IPMN with low-grade dysplasia, IPMN with intermediate-grade dysplasia, IPMN with high-grade dysplasia, and IPMN with an associated invasive carcinoma. Four types of mucinous epithelium can be seen: gastric type, intestinal type, pancreatobiliary, and oncocytic (intraductal oncocytic papillary neoplasm, e-**Fig. 17.18**). These four types of epithelium show distinct mucin profiles by immunohistochemical staining (gastric-type MUC1+ variable/MUC2–/MUC6+ variable; intestinal-type MUC1–/MUC2+/MUC6 –; pancreatobiliary MUC1+/MUC2–/MUC6+ weak; oncocytic-type MUC1– variable/MUC2–/MUC6+) (*Am J Surg Pathol.* 2010;34:364).

The major determining prognostic factor for surgically resected IPMNs is whether there is an associated invasive carcinoma, which is seen in approximately one-third of cases, since IPMNs without an associated invasive carcinoma are often cured by surgery. Two types of invasive carcinomas are seen: colloid (e-**Fig. 17.19**) and conventional ductal (e-**Fig. 17.20**); the former typically arises in association with intestinal-type IPMNs, whereas the latter is associated with pancreatobiliary-type, oncocytic-type, or intestinal-type IPMNs. The invasive carcinoma may be focal, and therefore IPMNs should be extensively (or, ideally, completely) submitted for histologic examination. Patients with an invasive carcinoma arising in association with an IPMN, except those with an advanced stage invasive carcinoma, usually do better than those with a ductal carcinoma not associated with IPMN. In addition, patients with an invasive colloid carcinoma arising in association with an IPMN have a better prognosis than those with an invasive conventional ductal carcinoma arising in association with an IPMN (*Ann Surg*. 2001;234:313; *Ann Surg*. 2004;239:400).

4. **ITPN** is a grossly visible solid nodular tumor obstructing the duct system (*Am J Surg Pathol*. 2009;33:1164). Architecturally, the tumor forms tubulopapillary structures composed of cell with little cytoplasmic mucin (e-**Fig. 17.21**). The cells uniformly show high-grade dysplasia, and some cases have associated invasive carcinoma. ITPNs do not harbor *KRAS* or *BRAF* mutations. Expression of DPC4 is retained in most cases.

5. **Intraductal tubular adenoma, pyloric gland type,** is an uncommon tumor consisting of pyloric-type glandular structures with mild to moderate atypia (*Am J Surg Pathol*. 2005;29:607) (e-**Fig. 17.22**). **Intraductal tubular carcinoma** is characterized by high-grade cytology and can have an associated invasive carcinoma component (*Anticancer Res*. 2010;30:4435). Some authors consider intraductal tubular carcinoma as part of the spectrum of ITPN (*Am J Surg Pathol*. 2009;33:1164).

6. **Cystic acinar cell cystadenoma** is an extremely rare unilocular or multilocular cystic mass lined by a single layer of cells cytologically resembling acinar cells. In **acinar cell cystadenocarcinoma,** the cysts are lined by layers of cells that exhibit more cytologic atypia and easily identifiable mitotic figures.

7. **Cystic pancreatic neuroendocrine tumors** are probably more common than previously recognized. In one study, 17% of the pancreatic neuroendocrine tumors were cystic (one-third purely cystic and two-thirds were partially cystic) (*J Am Coll Surg*. 2008;206:1154).

V. **SOLID TUMORS OF THE EXOCRINE PANCREAS.** The current World Health Organization (WHO) histologic classification of tumors of the exocrine pancreas is given in Table 17.2. The 2010 American Joint Committee on Cancer (AJCC) tumor, node, metastasis (TNM) staging schema is given in Table 17.3.

A. Pancreatic **ductal adenocarcinoma** (PDA) accounts for 85% to 90% of pancreatic neoplasms and is most frequently found in the head of the pancreas in patients 60 to 80 years of age. Factors associated with an increased risk include tobacco smoking, chronic pancreatitis, and gastrectomy. Several syndromes are also associated with an increased risk for pancreatic carcinomas including Lynch syndrome, familial atypical multiple mole melanoma syndrome (FAMMM), Peutz–Jeghers syndrome, hereditary pancreatitis, mutations in BRCA2 and other Fanconi anemia component genes, and familial pancreatic cancer syndrome. Common somatic genetic alterations that have been detected include activation of the *KRAS* oncogene (by point mutations) in >90% of cases, Her2/neu overexpression in 70% of cases, and inactivation of the tumor suppressor genes *TP53* in 50% to 70% and *DPC4* in 55% of cases. Recent genomic sequencing revealed an average of 63 genetic alterations in cases of pancreatic adenocarcinoma (*Science*. 2008;321:1801), although most mutations are likely passenger mutations with no role in pathogenesis.

Grossly, ductal adenocarcinoma is usually poorly demarcated, firm, and yellowish gray or white due to its infiltrative growth and associated strong desmoplastic response. On the basis of glandular differentiation, mucin production, mitosis, and nuclear features, PDAs can be divided into well-differentiated, moderately differentiated, and poorly differentiated forms. Most tumors are well to moderately differentiated and characterized by glandular structures haphazardly distributed in a desmoplastic stroma (e-**Fig. 17.23**). In well-differentiated tumors, the neoplastic glands are well formed and usually large or medium sized; however, the neoplastic glands may show rupture or be incomplete, features that are not observed in normal ducts. Mucin production may be evident. The most important histologic features that can be used to distinguish well-differentiated

TABLE 17.2 WHO Classification of Tumors of the Pancreas

Epithelial tumors
Benign
Acinar cell cystadenoma
Serous cystadenoma
Premalignant lesions
Pancreatic intraepithelial neoplasia, grade 3 (PanIN-3)
Intraductal papillary mucinous neoplasm
Intraductal tubulopapillary neoplasm
Mucinous cystic neoplasm
Malignant
  Ductal adenocarcinoma
  Adenosquamous carcinoma
  Colloid carcinoma (mucinous noncystic carcinoma)
  Hepatoid carcinoma
  Medullary carcinoma
  Signet-ring cell carcinoma
  Undifferentiated carcinoma
  Undifferentiated carcinoma with osteoclast-like giant cells
  Acinar cell carcinoma
  Acinar cell cystadenocarcinoma
  Intraductal papillary mucinous neoplasm with an associated invasive carcinoma
  Mucinous cystic neoplasm with an invasive carcinoma
  Mixed acinar-ductal carcinoma
  Mixed acinar-neuroendocrine carcinoma
  Mixed acinar-neuroendocrine-ductal carcinoma
  Mixed ductal-neuroendocrine carcinoma
  Pancreatoblastoma
  Serous cystadenocarcinoma
  Solid-pseudopapillary neoplasm
Neuroendocrine neoplasms
  Pancreatic neuroendocrine microadenoma
  Neuroendocrine tumors, nonfunctional (grade 1, grade 2)
  Neuroendocrine carcinoma (large cell, small cell)
  EC cell, serotonin-producing neuroendocrine tumors
  Gastrinoma
  Glucagonoma
  Insulinoma
  Somatostatinoma
  VIPoma

Mature teratoma
Mesenchymal tumors
Lymphomas
Secondary tumors

From: Bosman FT, Carneiro F, Hruban RH, Theise ND, eds. *World Health Organization Classification of Tumours of the Digestive System*. Lyon: IARC Press; 2010. Used with permission.

adenocarcinoma from chronic pancreatitis are a haphazard growth pattern (Table 17.4), perineural invasion (e-**Fig. 17.24**), vascular invasion, and close approximation to muscular vasculature (e-**Fig. 17.25**). In moderately differentiated adenocarcinoma, there is a mixture of medium-sized duct-like structures and small tubular glands of variable size and shape, including some incompletely formed glands. Cribriform and papillary growth patterns are not uncommon

TABLE 17.3	Tumor, Node, Metastasis (TNM) Staging Scheme for Endocrine and Exocrine Pancreas[a]		
Primary tumor (T)			
TX	Primary tumor cannot be assessed		
T0	No evidence of primary tumor		
Tis	Carcinoma in situ, including PanIN-3		
T1	Tumor limited to the pancreas, 2 cm or less in greatest dimension		
T2	Tumor limited to the pancreas, >2 cm in greatest dimension		
T3	Tumor extends beyond the pancreas but without involvement of the celiac axis or the superior mesenteric artery		
T4	Tumor involves the celiac axis or the superior mesenteric artery (unresectable primary tumor)		
Regional lymph nodes (N)			
NX	Regional lymph nodes cannot be assessed		
N0	No regional lymph node metastasis		
N1	Regional lymph node metastasis		
Distant metastasis (M)			
MX	Distant metastasis cannot be assessed		
M0	No distant metastasis		
M1	Distant metastasis		
Stage grouping			
Stage 0	Tis	N0	M0
Stage IA	T1	N0	M0
Stage IB	T2	N0	M0
Stage IIA	T3	N0	M0
Stage IIB	T1–3	N1	M0
Stage III	T4	Any N	M0
Stage IV	Any T	Any N	M1

From: Edge SB, Byrd DR, Campton CC, et al., eds. *AJCC Cancer Staging Manual.* 7th ed. New York, NY: Springer; 2010. Used with permission.

(e-Fig. 17.26); mitotic activity is more brisk (typically 6 to 10 per 10 HPFs), and nuclear pleomorphism is more prominent with nuclear sizes varying by more than a factor of 4 in the same gland. Mucin production is usually decreased and irregular in distribution. In poorly differentiated adenocarcinoma, the tumor cells form solid sheets or nests, or infiltrate as single individual cells. Mucin production is abortive. Neoplastic glands, if present, are typically small and irregular, and the tumor cells exhibit marked nuclear pleomorphism and a high mitotic count (often >10 per 10HPFs).

Immunohistochemically, PDAs are typically positive for pan-CK, CK7, CK8, CK18, CK19, MUC1, MUC3, MUC4, MUC5AC, CEA, CA125, and CA19.9.

TABLE 17.4	Distinction Between Ductal Adenocarcinoma and Chronic Pancreatitis	
Features	**Ductal adenocarcinoma**	**Chronic pancreatitis**
Histologic pattern	Haphazard	Lobular
Ruptured or incomplete glands	Yes	No
Companion muscular vessel	Yes	No
Nuclear pleomorphism	>4:1 in the same glands	Insignificant
Perineural invasion	Yes	No
Angioinvasion	Yes	No
Mitosis	Frequent	Infrequent

CK20 is typically negative or only focally positive. Other markers that are expressed in PDAs include claudin-4, cyclooxygenase (COX)-2, mesothelin, KOC (K homology domain containing protein overexpressed in cancer), S100P, and maspin. These markers may be useful in distinguishing ductal from nonductal pancreatic neoplasms and from benign pancreatic ducts, but are less useful in distinguishing adenocarcinomas of nonpancreatic origin. Approximately 55% of PDAs harbor mutations in *DPC4,* but this is not specific as loss of DPC4 expression is also observed in cholangiocarcinoma (*Hum Pathol.* 2002;33:877) and colonic adenocarcinoma (*Mutat Res.* 1999;406:71).

PDA is associated with a dismal prognosis, and the overall 5-year survival is only 3% to 5%. Resection improves survival as shown by 10% to 20% 5-year survival in patients treated with curative resection, but only 10% to 20% of tumors are resectable at the time of diagnosis.

B. **Variants of ductal adenocarcinoma**

1. **Adenosquamous carcinoma** consists of neoplastic components with both ductal and squamous differentiation (e-**Fig. 17.27**). Diagnosis requires the presence of a squamous component exceeding 30% of the neoplasm. Patients with adenosquamous carcinoma have a poorer prognosis than those with pure adenocarcinoma.

2. **Colloid carcinoma** (mucinous noncystic adenocarcinoma) is almost always associated with intestinal-type IPMN, and rarely with a MCN. Colloid carcinoma is believed to have a better prognosis than conventional ductal adenocarcinoma. Histologically, the tumor is similar to mucinous carcinoma in other locations and is defined by mucin pools comprising >80% of the tumor.

3. **Hepatoid carcinoma** is an extremely rare tumor in the pancreas. It can have a pure form or be associated with ductal adenocarcinoma (*Am Surg.* 2004;70:1030), acinar cell carcinoma, or a neuroendocrine tumor (*Cancer.* 2000;88:1582; *Am J Surg Pathol.* 2007;31:146; *Gut Liver.* 2010;4:98). Morphologically, hepatoid carcinoma consists of large polygonal cells with abundant cytoplasm (e-**Fig. 17.28**). Immunohistochemically, the tumor cells are positive for hepatocyte-specific antigen (hepar 1); CD10 and pCEA highlight a canalicular pattern, and most cases are also positive for alpha fetoprotein. Data on the prognosis of hepatoid carcinoma are very limited. Hepatoid carcinoma should be distinguished from hepatocellular carcinoma arising in ectopic liver in the pancreas (*Virchows Arch.* 2007;450:225) and metastatic hepatocellular carcinoma from liver.

4. **Medullary carcinoma** is characterized by its distinct morphology that features poor differentiation with limited gland formation, a syncytial growth pattern, and a pushing border (*Am J Pathol.* 1998;152:1501). Some cases are also associated with infiltration by prominent CD3+ T lymphocytes. Medullary carcinoma arises sporadically or in association with Lynch syndrome. Immunohistochemically, medullary carcinoma often shows loss of at least one DNA mismatch repair protein (*Hum Pathol.* 2006;37:1498). Prognostically, patients with medullary carcinoma do better than those with ductal adenocarcinoma.

5. **Signet-ring cell carcinoma** is an extremely rare variant with an extremely poor prognosis. Metastasis from a gastrointestinal tract or breast primary should always be excluded.

6. **Undifferentiated/anaplastic carcinoma** histologically exhibits little epithelial differentiation, although some or most of the tumor cells express cytokeratins by immunohistochemistry. Morphologically, three variants have been described: anaplastic giant cell carcinoma (e-**Fig. 17.29**), sarcomatoid carcinoma, and carcinosarcoma (e-**Fig. 17.30**). The prognosis for this tumor is extremely poor; the average survival is only 5 months.

7. **Undifferentiated carcinoma with osteoclast-like giant cells,** which should be separated from undifferentiated carcinoma, is characterized by the presence of nonneoplastic osteoclast-like giant cells (which are histiocytic in origin) within the tumor (e-**Fig. 17.31**). In most cases, there is an associated in situ or invasive adenocarcinoma or MCN. The prognosis is poor (mean survival 12 months).

C. **Acinar cell carcinoma** accounts for 1% to 2% of adult exocrine pancreatic neoplasms. Most tumors occur in late adulthood, but 6% occur in children. Approximately 10% to 15% of the patients develop a lipase hypersecretion syndrome characterized by extrapancreatic fat necrosis, polyarthralgia, and peripheral eosinophilia.

Acinar cell carcinoma frequently presents as a well-circumscribed mass with or without necrosis and cystic degeneration. Microscopically, acinar and solid patterns are most common, although the tumor may grow in a trabecular or gyriform pattern. Intraductal, papillary, or papillocystic variants of acinar cell carcinoma have also been reported (*Am J Surg Pathol.* 2007;31:363; *J Oncol.* 2010;242016). The tumor usually lacks a desmoplastic stroma. The individual tumor cells typically have basally located nuclei, single prominent nucleoli, and moderate amounts of amphophilic or eosinophilic granular cytoplasm (e-**Fig. 17.32**). Mitotic activity and nuclear pleomorphism are variable. Most acinar cell carcinomas are composed of cells that contain zymogen granules in their cytoplasm, which can be demonstrated by periodic acid-Schiff (PAS) stain with diastase or by electron microscopy. The tumor cells also exhibit abundant rough endoplasmic reticulum by electron microscopy.

Immunohistochemically, the tumor cells are reactive with antibodies against trypsin (>95% cases) (e-**Fig. 17.33**), chymotrypsin (>95% cases) (e-**Fig. 17.34**), and lipase (~70% of cases). In more than one third of acinar cell carcinomas, there are scattered tumor cells immunohistochemically positive for chromogranin A or synaptophysin. If >25% of the tumor cells show neuroendocrine differentiation by immunostains, the tumor should be designated as a mixed acinar–endocrine carcinoma.

Acinar cell carcinomas are aggressive tumors but their outcome is generally better than stage-matched ductal adenocarcinomas. Available data suggest that the prognosis of acinar cell carcinomas in children is better than that in adults.

D. **Pancreatoblastoma** is the most common pancreatic neoplasm of childhood, usually occurring in the first decade of life (mean age: 4 years), although the neoplasm also rarely occurs in adults. Approximately 25% of patients have associated elevated serum α-fetoprotein. Pancreatoblastoma is a highly cellular tumor composed of sheets or islands of small monotonous cells divided by cellular stromal bands. The tumor cells may exhibit acinar differentiation and form small acinar lumina, although little endocrine and ductal differentiation may be also seen. A histologic hallmark of pancreatoblastoma is the presence of squamoid corpuscles, which are present in virtually every case (e-**Fig. 17.35**); they serve as a useful feature to distinguish the tumor from other pancreatic neoplasms, particularly acinar cell carcinoma. Squamoid corpuscles consist of an aggregate of plump epithelioid cells, a whorled nest of spindle cells, or a cluster of frankly keratinized squamous cells, and are usually located in the center of the tumor lobules; the cells forming the squamoid corpuscle are usually larger than surrounding tumor cells. The stroma in pancreatoblastoma can also be neoplastic, and may contain heterologous elements such as bone and cartilage. The stroma in adult patients, however, is often less abundant and less cellular than that in pediatric patients. The prognosis of pancreatoblastoma is better in pediatric patients than that in adults, likely due to an increased frequency of localized and encapsulated tumors in children.

E. **Solid-pseudopapillary neoplasm** is most commonly seen in adolescent girls and young women (mean age 28 years, 90% in women). This tumor can be quite large at the time of diagnosis but is typically well demarcated and may be encapsulated. Grossly, it exhibits variable solid and cystic areas with hemorrhage and necrosis. Microscopically, solid-pseudopapillary neoplasm is a cellular neoplasm consisting of sheets of small relatively uniform tumor cells, sometimes surrounding delicate, often hyalinized fibrovascular cores to form pseudopapillae (e-Fig. 17.36). The tumor cells have eosinophilic or clear vacuolated cytoplasm, indented or grooved nuclei, and inconspicuous nucleoli (e-Fig. 17.37). Intra- and extracellular eosinophilic, diastase-resistant PAS-positive hyaline globules may be evident. Foamy cells, cells with cholesterol crystals, and foreign body giant cells may be present within the tumor. In necrotic areas, the tumor cells lose their cohesiveness and may undergo cystic degeneration. Mitotic figures are rare.

The most frequently positive immunomarkers in solid-pseudopapillary neoplasm are vimentin, neuron-specific enolase, α_1-antitrypsin, α_1-antichymotrypsin, progesterone receptor, claudins 5 and 7, galectin 3, cyclin D1, CD10 (e-Fig. 17.38), and nuclear β-catenin (e-Fig. 17.39). Synaptophysin may be positive in tumor cells but chromogranin A is always negative. Positive CD10 and nuclear β-catenin stains are useful in the distinction from pancreatic endocrine neoplasms (PENs). Approximately 50% of solid pseudopapillary neoplasms show c-kit expression by immunohistochemistry without an associated mutation in the *KIT* gene (*Mod Pathol.* 2006;19:1157).

Patients with solid-pseudopapillary neoplasm usually have an excellent prognosis if the tumor is completely excised, as occurs in 85% to 95% of cases. Approximately 5% to 15% of cases show metastasis, usually to the liver and peritoneum, but metastasis is lethal in only a subset of patients. Rarely, solid pseudopapillary neoplasms have an undifferentiated or sarcomatoid component (*Am J Surg Pathol.* 2005;29:512). Biologically aggressive tumors typically show deep extrapancreatic extension, vascular or perineural invasion, significant cellular pleomorphism, nuclear atypia, and increased mitotic activity. In general, solid-pseudopapillary neoplasm is considered a low-grade malignancy.

F. **Pancreatic intraepithelial neoplasia (PanIN)** is considered a precursor to invasive pancreatic ductal adenocarcinoma. Morphologically, PanIN is a microscopic (typically <5 mm in size) papillary or flat epithelial neoplasm confined to the pancreatic duct system. On the basis of the cytologic and architectural atypia, PanINs are further divided into three categories: PanIN-1 (PanIN-1A, PanIN-1B), PanIN-2, and PanIN-3 (*Am J Surg Pathol.* 2004;28:977) (Table 17.5).

TABLE 17.5	Pancreatic Intraepithelial Neoplasias (PanIN) and Corresponding Older Synonyms

Squamous metaplasia: Epidermoid metaplasia, multilayered metaplasia
PanIN-1A: Pyloric gland metaplasia, goblet cell metaplasia, mucinous hypertrophy, mucinous ductal hyperplasia, mucinous cell hyperplasia, mucoid transformation, simple hyperplasia, flat duct lesion without atypia, flat ductal hyperplasia, ductal hyperplasia grade 1, nonpapillary epithelial hypertrophy, nonpapillary ductal hyperplasia
PanIN-1B: Papillary hyperplasia, papillary ductal hyperplasia, papillary ductal lesion without atypia, ductal hyperplasia grade 2, adenomatous ductal hyperplasia, adenomatoid hyperplasia
PanIN-2: Atypical hyperplasia, papillary duct lesion with atypia, low-grade dysplasia, any PanIN lesions with moderate dysplasia
PanIN-3: Carcinoma in situ, intraductal carcinoma, severe ductal dysplasia, high-grade dysplasia, ductal hyperplasia grade 3, atypical hyperplasia

TABLE 17.6	Distinction Between Pancreatic Intraepithelial Neoplasias (PanIN) and Intraductal Papillary Mucinous Neoplasm (IPMN)	
Features	PanIN	IPMN
Radiographically detectable	No	Yes
Grossly visible	No	Yes
Grossly visible mucin	No	Yes
Size of involved duct	Usually <5 mm	Usually >10 mm
Well-formed papillae	No	Yes
Association with colloid carcinoma	No	Yes

PanIN-1A comprises flat epithelial lesions without atypia. It is composed of tall columnar cells with small and round to oval, basal located nuclei and abundant supranuclear mucin (e-Fig. 17.40). The neoplastic nature of many cases of PanIN-1A has not been unambiguously established. PanIN-1B is an intraductal epithelial lesion that has a papillary, micropapillary, or basally pseudostratified architecture, but is otherwise identical to PanIN-1A (e-Fig. 17.41).

PanIN-2 may be flat but is usually papillary. By definition, the lesion must have some degree of architectural and cytologic atypia, such as nuclear crowding, enlargement, pseudostratification, hyperchromasia, and loss of polarity (e-Fig. 17.42). Mitotic figures are rare and not atypical. This category represents low-grade dysplasia, and the degree of atypia is insufficient for a diagnosis of PanIN-3.

PanIN-3 is usually papillary or micropapillary, and is only rarely flat. It is a high-grade intraductal lesion and synonymous with carcinoma in situ. True cribriforming, budding or tufting of small clusters of epithelial cells into the lumen, and luminal necroses should all suggest the diagnosis of PanIN-3. Cytologically, these lesions are characterized by loss of nuclear polarity, the presence of prominent nucleoli, nuclear membrane irregularities, dystrophic goblet cells, and abnormal mitoses (e-Fig. 17.43).

PanIN should not be confused with IPMN, particularly when IPMN extends into small duct branches (Table 17.6). PanIN is a microscopic lesion that is typically <5 mm in size; in contrast, IPMN is a grossly visible lesion usually >10 mm in size (*Am J Surg Pathol*. 2004;28:977). For lesions between 5 and 10 mm in size, it is sometimes difficult to distinguish the entities, but PanINs tend to have short stubby papillary structures whereas the papillae in IPMNs are often long and finger-like. The cytoplasmic mucin in IPMNs is typically more abundant than that in PanIN. In addition, expression of MUC2 favors IPMNs (*Mod Pathol*. 2002;15:1087).

On frozen section of pancreatic margins, PanIN-3 lesions should be reported, but the significance of lower grade PanIN in this context has not been established. However, if the preoperative diagnosis or intraoperative findings suggest IPMN, the presence of PanIN-1, and PanIN-2 lesions should be reported because of the difficulty in differentiating low-grade PanIN from small duct extension by IPMN on frozen sections.

VI. **PANCREATIC NEUROENDOCRINE NEOPLASMS** include well-differentiated (low to intermediate grade) neuroendocrine tumors and poorly differentiated (high grade) neuroendocrine carcinomas. The latter account for <1% of pancreatic neuroendocrine neoplasms and are characterized by >20 mitotic figures per 10 HPFs. Poorly differentiated neuroendocrine carcinomas are further divided into small cell carcinoma and large cell neuroendocrine carcinoma. In the most recent AJCC staging manual, pancreatic neuroendocrine neoplasms are staged with the same system as exocrine tumors (Table 17.2).

A. **Well-differentiated neuroendocrine tumors.** Approximately 30% to 40% of well-differentiated neuroendocrine tumors are nonfunctional (no clinical hormonal syndrome although serum hormone levels can be elevated). Functional tumors produce clinical symptoms corresponding to the hormones they produce, allowing clinical diagnosis even when they are quite small. Among the functional tumors, insulinoma is the most common type, and is benign in 90% to 95% of the cases. In contrast, gastrinoma, glucagonoma, somatostatinoma, and VIPoma tend to be malignant. By definition, pancreatic neuroendocrine microadenomas (<0.5 cm in size) are nonfunctional.

Well-differentiated endocrine tumors are often well circumscribed, soft, homogeneous, and yellow to pink lesions. Cystic spaces may be present in some cases. Histologically, they often grow in an organoid fashion including solid, nesting, trabecular, glandular, tubuloacinar, gyriform, and pseudoglandular patterns. Hyalinized fibrovascular stroma, sometimes with amyloid deposition, is characteristic (**e-Fig. 17.44**). The tumor cells are relatively uniform with finely granular amphophilic to eosinophilic cytoplasm and a centrally located round to oval nucleus with characteristic salt-and-pepper chromatin pattern. Other types of cells described include clear cells (**e-Fig. 17.45**), lipid-rich cells (**e-Fig. 17.46**), oncocytes, and rhabdoid cells (**e-Fig. 17.47**). Sometimes the tumor cells may be pleomorphic. By definition, well-differentiated tumors have no more than 20 mitoses per 10 HPFs (typically no more than 10 per 10 HPFs). Necrosis may be present but it is typically focal. Well-differentiated neuroendocrine tumors are sometimes part of the multiple endocrine neoplasia type I (MEN I) syndrome.

The vast majority of well-differentiated neuroendocrine tumors are immunohistochemically positive for synaptophysin and chromogranin A. Other markers that are expressed include protein gene product 9.5, CD56, islet-1, and PAX8 (*Am J Surg Pathol*. 2010;34:723).

Stage and grade are the most important prognostic factors. On the basis of mitotic figures, well-differentiated neuroendocrine tumors are further divided into low grade (0 to 1 mitotic figures per 10 HPFs) and intermediate grade (2 to 20 mitotic figures per 10 HPFs) (*J Clin Oncol*. 2002;20:2633). Ki-67 proliferation index is also a prognostic factor; tumors with a Ki-67 proliferation index <2% (low grade) do much better than tumors with an index of ≥2% but <20% (intermediate grade) (*Clin Cancer Res*. 2008;14:7798). Recently, KIT and CK19 expression have also been shown to be of prognostic value for well-differentiated endocrine tumors (*Am J Surg Pathol*. 2009;33:1562; *Am J Surg Pathol*. 2006;30:1588).

B. **Poorly differentiated neuroendocrine carcinomas** typically show ill-defined borders. The tumor cells are often arranged in tightly packed nests or diffuse sheets. There is often extensive necrosis. Using similar criteria as in the lung, poorly differentiated neuroendocrine carcinomas are further divided into small cell carcinomas and large cells neuroendocrine carcinomas. By definition, mitotic figures numbering >20 per 10 HPFs and/or the Ki-67 proliferation index is >20%. Given their rarity, a metastasis should be always ruled out before rendering a diagnosis of primary pancreatic poorly differentiated neuroendocrine carcinoma.

Cytopathology of the Pancreas

Brian Collins and Julie Elizabeth Kunkel

I. **INTRODUCTION.** Cytopathology has an important role in the evaluation of pancreatic lesions. In fact, due to a variety of factors, the cytopathologic sample will frequently be the only diagnostic tissue sample obtained. The advent of endoscopic ultrasound-guided fine needle aspiration (EUS-FNA) has greatly expanded the number and type of cases seen. When an abnormality is identified or suspected, EUS makes it possible to visualize the pancreas by ultrasound, directly visualize the lesion, and then perform an FNA.

By imaging, pancreatic lesions can be broadly categorized into two main categories, solid and cystic. However, heterogeneous lesions with mixed solid-cystic imaging features and other confounding factors that obscure a clear classification also occur. The clinical approach and differential diagnostic considerations vary significantly between these broad categories, and thus it is important to ascertain the imaging characteristics of a pancreatic lesion in order to appropriately evaluate and diagnose EUS-FNA specimens from the pancreas.

II. SOLID LESIONS

A. Inflammatory

1. **Chronic pancreatitis** can present a significant clinical and pathologic challenge. Aspirate smears will usually be scant to minimally cellular, show dense fragments of connective tissue with bland spindle cells, and fragments of bland ductal and acinar epithelial elements which typically have only minimal reactive cellular changes (e-Fig. 17.48). The presence of underlying chronic pancreatitis does not alter the cytomorphologic findings required for a diagnosis of malignancy (*Diagn Cytopathol.* 2005;32:65).

B. Neoplasms

1. **Adenocarcinoma** accounts for the vast majority of pancreatic neoplasms. The majority of patients have disease at clinical presentation that is not resectable and thus EUS-FNA provides the definitive diagnosis. The cytopathologic features of adenocarcinoma vary on the basis of the degree of differentiation; individual cases that have a spectrum of differentiation are also encountered.

   a. **Poorly differentiated adenocarcinoma** is less cohesive with single cells and small groups of cells with overlap and crowding. Nuclei are round to oval with evidence of pleomorphism, and have large nucleoli. The cells usually have a moderate amount of granular cytoplasm with only few intracytoplasmic vacuoles (e-Fig. 17.49).

   b. **Moderately differentiated adenocarcinoma** shows more cohesion and flat sheets of cells, with fewer single cells. The sheets frequently show a disordered "honeycomb" pattern. The cells possess nuclei with size and shape variation as well as prominent nucleoli. The cytoplasm is more voluminous with intracytoplasmic vacuoles (e-Fig. 17.50).

   c. **Well-differentiated adenocarcinoma** accounts for roughly 20% of aspirates and can be diagnostically challenging. Aspirates show large cohesive fragments with very few background single cells. The main diagnostic features are nuclear enlargement, nuclear membrane irregularities, anisonucleosis (at least 4× size variation), and cellular crowding and overlap (e-Fig. 17.51 and 17.52). However, these features can vary within aspirate smears (*Cancer.* 2003;99:44).

   d. **Mucinous noncystic carcinoma** shows abundant extracellular mucin with single cells and groups of epithelial cells that have the typical cytomorphology of moderately differentiated adenocarcinoma, but they can be scantily represented (e-Fig. 17.53).

   e. **Signet-ring adenocarcinoma** presents a predominance of single cells and small groups of cells that have a large intracytoplasmic vacuole compressing the nucleus (e-Fig. 17.54).

   f. **Undifferentiated (anaplastic) carcinoma** is cellular with numerous dispersed single cells that are epithelioid and show marked pleomorphism, with scattered intermixed giant tumor cells (e-Fig. 17.55).

g. **Undifferentiated carcinoma with osteoclast-like giant cells** shows an undifferentiated pattern with intermixed benign multinucleated giant cells (e-**Fig. 17.56**).

2. **PEN** presents as a solid mass usually in the body or tail. On aspiration, PEN is very cellular and characteristically shows a loosely cohesive aspirate with single cells and loose clusters of cells (e-**Fig. 17.57**). The individual cells have round to oval nuclei with variable nucleoli, eccentric nuclear placement imparting a plasmacytoid appearance, are often bi- and tri-nucleated, and show neuroendocrine-type chromatin (*Diagn Cytopathol.* 1996; 1:37).

3. **Solid-pseudopapillary neoplasm** is typically seen in young women and is often solid by imaging. On aspiration, the smears are typically cellular, although the predominant cystic component can make the diagnosis difficult. Along with a variable cystic background of histiocytes and granular debris, the epithelial elements consist of large tissue fragments with a papillary pattern. The cells are round to oval, small, uniform, and have a moderate amount of cytoplasm (e-**Fig. 17.58**). Nuclei are eccentrically located and can have grooves and pseudoinclusions (*Am J Clin Pathol.* 2004;121:654).

4. **Acinar cell carcinomas** are most often solid but can have a cystic component. On aspiration, these tumors are cellular with a variable pattern that ranges from cohesive fragments to more dispersed single cells. The cohesive fragments tend to be arranged as monolayers with a sheet-like pattern with varying degrees of vascularity. The cells show monomorphic round to oval nuclei, with nucleoli and an even chromatin distribution (e-**Fig. 17.59**). There is typically a moderate amount of granular cytoplasm imparting an acinar appearance, and small groups of cells can be arranged in acinar-like configurations (*Diagn Cytopathol.* 2006;34:367).

III. **CYSTIC LESIONS.** EUS-FNA is only one factor in the overall assessment of a cystic pancreatic lesion; a variety of clinical features (age, sex, size, shape, duct findings) and concomitantly measured fluid properties (CEA, enzyme levels) also contribute to the evaluation. The variable cellularity obtained by EUS-FNA can significantly limit classification based on the cytomorphologic findings alone (*Surg Clin N Am.* 2010;90:399).

A. **Pseudocysts** can be present in the background of known acute or chronic pancreatitis, although the clinical history and imaging findings are not always definitive. On aspiration, a variable to abundant amount of green-brown bile-tinged thick material is obtained which consists of granular debris with variable amounts of intermixed bile pigment, macrophages, neutrophils (usually a more acute phase component), and scant benign ductal and acinar tissue fragments (e-**Fig. 17.60**). The epithelial elements can show a reactive appearance, however, the atypia does not approach the quantitative and qualitative features of adenocarcinoma (e-**Fig. 17.61**).

B. **Serous cystadenoma.** By aspiration, these lesions are predominantly hypocellular. The lining cells that are present are usually grouped as small to intermediate sized cohesive flat sheets, and have round nuclei and a moderate amount of cytoplasm which tends to be nondescript. The aspirate alone is often not sufficient for diagnosis (*Cancer.* 2008;114:102).

C. **MCN** and **IPMN.** Cytologically, the neoplasms of this category share a variable amount of extracellular mucin, sheets of glandular epithelial cells with varying degrees of cellularity, and a spectrum of cytologic atypia. These tumors can have varying degrees of complexity of cell groups; papillary configurations can be present in IPMN (e-**Figs. 17.62** and **17.63**). Invasion cannot be reliably determined on the basis of aspiration smears (*Cancer.* 2004;102:92).

SUGGESTED READINGS

Ali SZ, Erozan YS, Hruban RH. *Atlas of Pancreatic Cytopathology with Histopathologic Correlations*. New York: Demos Medical Publishing, LLC; 2009.

Bosman FT, Carneiro F, Hruban RH, et al., eds. Tumors of the pancreas. In: *Pathology and Genetics of Tumors of Endocrine Organs (WHO Classification of Tumors)*. Lyon, France: IACR Press; 2010:279–334.

Centeno BA, Pitman MB. *Fine Needle Aspiration Biopsy of the Pancreas*. Woburn, MA: Butterworth-Heinemann; 1998.

Chhieng DC, Stelow EB. *Pancreatic Cytopathology*. New York: Springer Science + Business Media, LLC; 1997.

Hruban RH, Pitman MB, Klimstra DS, eds. Tumors of the pancreas In: *Atlas of Tumor Pathology, Fourth Series*. Washington, DC: American Registry of Pathology; 2007.

Thompson LD, Heffess CS. Pancreas. In: Mills SE, ed. *Steinberg's Diagnostic Surgical Pathology*. 5th ed. Philadelphia: Lippincott Williams & Wilkins; 2009:1432–1491.

Breast

Breast Pathology
Souzan Sanati, Omar Hameed, Joshua I. Warrick, and Craig Allred

I. **INTRODUCTION.** This chapter provides a systematic approach to breast pathology, which enables pathologists to effectively play their role in today's interdisciplinary care of patients with breast disease, especially cancer. It is not intended to be a compendium of histologic alterations occurring in the breast, which is enormous and covered in many excellent textbooks on the subject (see Suggested Readings). Instead, it is based on a template addressing the most common alterations, in order of clinical importance, ranging from potentially lethal cancers to common benign changes (**e-Appendix 18.1**).* Diagnoses are conveyed in a concise, standardized manner addressing specific issues important to other specialists—such as correlating histologic with mammographic findings for radiologists, status of surgical margins for surgeons, tumor, node, and metastasis (TNM) staging [essential elements of which include: tumor size (T), nodal status (N), and distant metastasis (M)] for oncologists, and so on. Although templates cannot be all inclusive, and must be updated to stay current, their advantages far outweigh their limitations.

This chapter begins with a discussion of the methods used in grossing breast specimens. A discussion of normal breast follows, because a comprehensive understanding of normal is necessary to appreciate what is abnormal. This is followed by discussions of invasive carcinomas, noninvasive carcinomas, prognostic and predictive biomarkers, common benign lesions, and reporting results.

II. **SPECIMEN PROCESSING**

A. **General approach.** The primary goals of grossing in breast pathology are to (i) identify the specimen, determine its orientation, and dimensions; (ii) identify the presence, location, and dimensions of lesions (masses, calcifications, etc.); (iii) estimate the distance of lesions from surgical margins; and (iv) take small samples for more precise microscopic evaluation. Secondary goals include taking samples from various other locations depending on the type of specimen (e.g., nipple, all quadrants, and lymph nodes associated with mastectomies).

There are many methods of grossing breast surgical specimens; all acceptable methods adequately address the goals listed above even if their specific strategies vary. This section provides a basic grossing strategy to manage most surgical breast specimens, followed by more detailed discussion of the most common types of samples. More detailed information on grossing can be

*Online availability

found in specialized texts (*Manual of Surgical Pathology*, 2nd ed. Philadelphia: Elsevier Churchill Livingston; 2006).

The central element of the basic strategy is a generic grossing template (e-**Appendix 18.2**), which can accommodate specimens of almost any size, ranging from small lumpectomies to large mastectomies. Utilization of the template creates a permanent record (diagram) of the most important features of a specimen (e.g., size, orientation, location of samples, location of mass lesions, and distance of lesions from margins); the small amount of extra time required to create the diagram has several additional benefits, including (i) providing relatively precise information on the size and distribution of lesions that are not apparent grossly; (ii) enabling better control of margins; (iii) assistance in taking additional samples if necessary; and (iv) facilitating succinct, comprehensive, and standardized gross dictations.

The main steps of grossing a surgical breast specimen are as follows:

1. Identification
2. Orientation
3. Dimensions
4. Inking of margins
5. Sectioning into thin slices to facilitate fixation. Small specimens are usually cut (from 2 to 4 mm in thickness) into a few slices and entirely submitted in a corresponding number of cassettes for formalin fixation. Larger specimens are usually cut into slices (5 mm thick and hinged at the bottom to maintain intact orientation), and allowed to fix before submitting samples in cassettes.
6. Fixation in 10% neutral buffered formalin (NBF) for a minimum of 8 to 12 hours. The recommended maximum fixation time is 72 hours.
7. Production of a diagram of the specimen on the template. Diagrams are more informative and useful than gross dictations alone.

B. **Ancillary information.** Most patients with breast pathology present with a clinically or radiologically detected mass and/or a mammographically detected abnormality, most often in the form of microcalcification. The manner of presentation often dictates the approach to specimen processing. Because most breast specimens lack natural anatomical landmarks, careful specimen processing—especially margin assessment—is crucial for accurate pathologic interpretation. In addition, evaluation of specimen radiographs represents an integral part of examination of breast specimens, and should be reviewed whenever available. Review provides valuable information as to the nature of the lesion (ill-defined vs. well-defined mass; microcalcification); location of the lesion(s); and assists planning of the sectioning of the specimen.

C. **Specimen types.** Most breast specimens received for pathologic evaluation are in one of the following forms.

1. **Needle core biopsies** have almost totally replaced fine needle aspiration (FNA) biopsy specimens for the initial pathologic evaluation of localized breast lesions in most centers. They are obtained to diagnose palpable breast masses or nonpalpable breast lesions detected by screening mammography, such as stellate densities or suspicious microcalcifications. For nonpalpable lesions, biopsy is usually obtained using image guidance (ultrasound guided, stereotactic, or MRI guided). Vacuum-assisted biopsies increase the volume of tissue obtained for microscopic examination. If biopsy is performed for calcifications, a radiograph of the specimen is often obtained to confirm that the calcifications have been adequately sampled. After describing the shape, size, and color of the tissue cores, they should be aligned in parallel and placed in the cassette between two sponges (preferable) or wrapped in tissue paper; similar to biopsies from other organs, overstuffing of cassettes should be avoided. Formalin fixation time is absolutely critical,

as underfixation and overfixation both may result in altered biomarker results by immunohistochemistry. Current College of American Pathologists/American Society of Clinical Oncology (CAP/ASCO) guidelines recommend that core needle biopsy samples be fixed in formalin for 6 to 48 hours prior to processing. At least three histologic levels should be obtained from each paraffin block to ensure adequate representation of the lesion(s). For all other breast specimens, the histologic findings should always be correlated with the clinical and radiologic findings, and, if discrepant (such as when microcalcifications are not seen in original sections of a biopsy performed for microcalcifications) additional deeper sections from the block, and/or radiographic images of the paraffin block need to be examined to resolve the discrepancy.

2. **Excisional biopsy/lumpectomy** specimens are either oriented or nonoriented. Nonoriented specimens are those in which evaluation of the status of specific margins is not required by the surgeon (such as excisions of benign lesions or malignant lesions with separate margin specimens); nonetheless, these specimens should be inked. Oriented specimens need to be inked differentially to facilitate specific margin orientation. A four-ink color approach is useful to orient the margins (the superior, inferior, anterior, and posterior margins will be inked by four different colors); the medial and lateral margins are amputated, sliced, and completely submitted in separate cassettes. Another acceptable approach is to use six ink colors to orient all the margins.

   For these specimens, the gross dimensions and weight should be recorded. Then, the specimen should be serially sectioned as soon as possible to allow for adequate penetration of fixative. Such sectioning is usually performed perpendicular to the long axis of the specimen; however, sectioning may be influenced by the shape and proximity of the lesion(s) to particular margins. Gauze should be placed between the sections, and the specimen should be fixed in formalin for 6 to 48 hours before submitting samples in cassettes.

   a. **If excision is performed for mass lesions.** The size of the mass (accurate to nearest millimeter), consistency (gelatinous, rubbery, firm, or hard), growth pattern (well circumscribed, infiltrative, pushing), and distance from margins should all be described. The presence and size of a biopsy cavity should also be noted. For well-circumscribed lesions thought to be benign (such as fibroadenomas), one section per centimeter of the lesion is usually sufficient. Ill-defined and suspicious lesions need to be entirely submitted if possible. If the mass is too large to be completely submitted, at least one section per centimeter of the mass should be submitted. Margins are microscopically examined by submitting a perpendicular section of the mass with each margin (superior, inferior, anterior, posterior). If the margins are distant from the mass, representative-shave sections suffice. Medial and lateral margins are usually amputated, sliced, and completely submitted in labeled cassettes (Fig. 18.1). Representative sections of grossly noninvolved breast should additionally be submitted with particular attention to fibrous areas of the breast.

   b. **If excision is performed for imaging-detected microcalcifications.** Most of these specimens show no significant gross pathology. These specimens are usually oriented (by two perpendicular sutures or clips), contain a guiding wire, and are accompanied by a specimen radiograph. Similarly, a surgical clip may have been placed at the area of previous core biopsy. The guiding wire, which is placed at the site of imaging-detected abnormality, should be used in conjunction with the specimen radiograph to preferentially sample areas of abnormality, immediately adjacent areas, as well as the margins. For smaller specimens, it is preferable to entirely

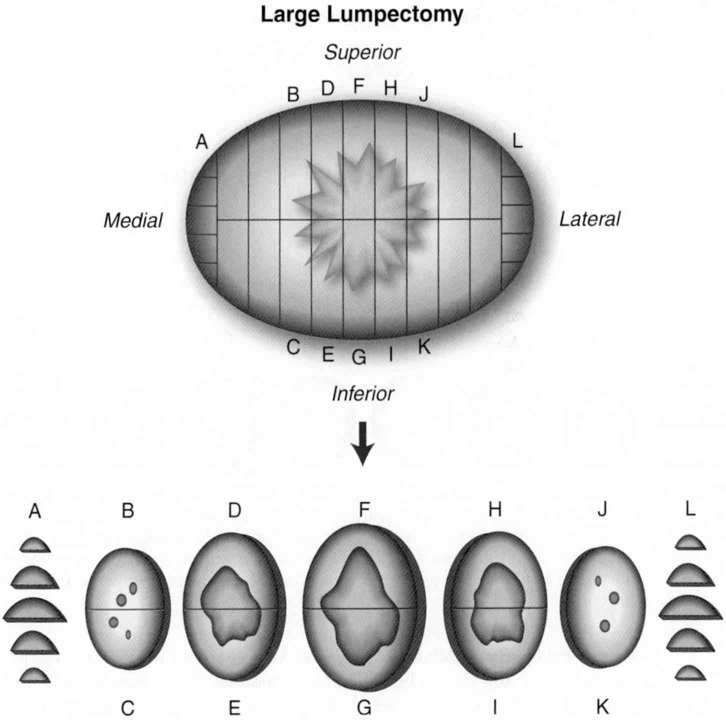

Large Lumpectomy

Figure 18.1 Schematic representation of "bread-loafing" and sampling of mass lesions. **A:** Specimen was serially sectioned perpendicular to its long axis, and an irregular mass was identified in the center of the specimen. Sections A and L would be submitted as medial and lateral margins, respectively, that are perpendicularly sectioned and entirely submitted. Given the size of the specimen and the mass, submission of sections B through K would appear to adequately represent the entire mass, as well as the immediately adjacent superior, inferior, anterior, and posterior (deep) margins.

submit the specimen in consecutive sections, as this facilitates accurate estimation of the extent of disease. In larger specimens, wide sampling of the area of the wire tip and adjacent tissue is advised. If possible, the specimen should be sectioned in a way that facilitates some inference of the three-dimensional aspects of the lesion when histologic sections are evaluated. This can be achieved by labeling the cassette numbers on a generic diagram that can be used to determine the relationship of tissue blocks containing abnormalities with each other (see e-Appendix 18.2). If there are multiple lesions, their location and relationship to each other should be documented; in addition to sampling each lesion individually, sections from normal-appearing areas in between the lesions can be used to determine whether they are individual or multiple masses. Representative sections from grossly noninvolved breast with attention to fibrous areas should also be submitted (Fig. 18.2). In situations where gross examination and initial set of sections do not show a histologic abnormality, the entire specimen, or at least all the fibrous parts of the specimen, should be submitted for microscopic examination.

Small Lumpectomy

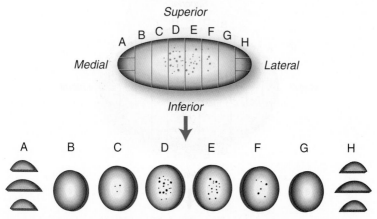

Figure 18.2 Schematic representation of "bread-loafing" and sampling of a specimen excised for microcalcifications. Especially, given the scattered widespread distribution of the microcalcifications and their proximity to several margins, the specimen should be entirely submitted for histologic examination. The medial and lateral margins are amputated, perpendicularly sectioned, and entirely submitted. The remaining tissue is serially sectioned and entirely submitted as marked on the diagram.

3. **Margin and biopsy reexcisions.** These cases range from unorientated flat portions of tissue that should be laid flat in a cassette (shave margin), where the presence of any malignancy seen histologically would thus be indicative of a positive margin; to larger, variably oriented specimens that should be inked preferentially, bread-loafed perpendicular to the new margin (oriented), and submitted in a manner to examine the new margin. For reexcisions following invasive carcinoma, the status of gross residual disease should be evaluated as well as its relationship to different excision margins; in the absence of gross disease, the specimen need only to be representatively sampled. For reexcisions following a diagnosis of in situ carcinoma, the specimen may need to be more widely sampled to detect residual disease and/or associated invasive carcinoma. Complete reexcision of the cavity created by a prior lumpectomy may also be performed; these specimens should be inked with respect to orientation, and serially sectioned as in a lumpectomy. The blood-filled biopsy cavity should be entirely submitted, in particular with respect to new margins to evaluate the residual disease and status of surgical margins.

4. **Mastectomy specimens** range from simple skin-sparing mastectomy (which removes the breast only covered by the nipple–areola complex and a narrow rim of surrounding skin), to simple mastectomy (mastectomy without axillary tissue), to modified radical mastectomy (mastectomy with axillary lymph nodes). Radical mastectomy (modified radical mastectomy with pectoral muscles), is rarely performed in current practice. Mastectomies may be prophylactic or therapeutic. When the specimen is received for pathologic examination, it should first be measured and weighed. Then, the specimen should be oriented and the surgical margins inked; it should then be serially sectioned perpendicular to the skin at 5 mm intervals from the posterior aspect, packed with gauze, and fixed in formalin overnight. The size of any

masses, including their growth pattern, location, and distance from all surgical margins, should be recorded; the same principles discussed above (for excisional biopsy/lumpectomy specimens also apply to grossing mastectomy specimens. Masses should be entirely submitted if small, in a manner that demonstrates the relationship to the surgical margin. If a mass is predominantly composed of ductal carcinoma in situ (DCIS) with focal microinvasion, submitting the entire mass is required to exclude a larger size of invasive carcinoma. In addition, at least one section of nipple, grossly normal tissue from each of the four quadrants of the breast, skin, and dermal scars from previous biopsies should be submitted for microscopic examination. If the specimen is a modified-radical mastectomy, the axillary tail should be removed and dissected for lymph nodes, which should all be submitted for microscopic evaluation (see below). A search for lymph nodes should always be performed even in simple mastectomies and if lymph nodes are found, they should be sampled accordingly. It is important to correlate the gross and microscopic findings with imaging studies to optimize patient care; for nonpalpable lesions, radiographing the specimen with submission of the entire area of radiologic abnormality is recommended.

5. **Mammary implants** should be documented, photographed, and inspected grossly for any evidence of leakage. One or two sections are usually sufficient to evaluate the surrounding fibrous "capsule" that is usually submitted with the implant(s).

6. **Sentinel lymph nodes.** The sentinel lymph node(s) is (are) the first lymph node or group of lymph nodes that drain the breast into the axilla and in most cases they are the first lymph node(s) involved in metastatic carcinoma. Only rarely does cancer "skip" the sentinel node and metastasize to a nonsentinel lymph node. As such, specimens designated as sentinel lymph nodes should be dissected carefully. Intraoperative evaluation (frozen sections and/or touch preparations) is usually limited to lymph nodes grossly suspicious for malignancy; in these situations, intraoperative imprint cytology of the lymph node can provide results at the time of surgery. For permanent sections, each node is serially cut at 2 mm intervals and, in the absence of gross evidence of metastatic carcinoma, entirely submitted for histologic examination. There are many different protocols for microscopic evaluation of sentinel lymph node, but one common approach involves examination of three hematoxylin and eosin (H&E)-stained sections from each paraffin block. The use of cytokeratin-stained sections—if initial H&E sections are negative—is optimal, but not required. In the event of a positive sentinel lymph node, axillary dissection is indicated.

7. **Nonsentinel (axillary) lymph nodes.** Axillary lymph node dissection may be performed in conjunction with lumpectomy in a patient with a positive sentinel lymph node, or may be performed as part of a modified radical mastectomy (see above). After carefully dissecting grossly benign appearing nodes from the fat, nodes <0.4 cm can be submitted intact, whereas larger nodes need to be bisected or trisected and submitted in a manner that permits accurate enumeration (either by submitting them in individual cassettes or by differential inking). If possible, the size of the largest grossly positive node or metastatic deposit should be measured, and the presence of extranodal extension sampled in one section. It is recommended that a minimum of 10 lymph nodes should be identified in an axillary dissection (although this number is dependent on the surgical technique and the extent of axillary lymph node dissection during surgery). Attention should also be directed to identification of possible intramammary lymph nodes, which are usually identified in the upper outer quadrant of the breast.

D. Examples of reporting template. To demonstrate the organization of a pathology report on breast samples using the discussed diagnostic template (see e-Appendix 18.1), a few examples are shown in e-**Appendix 18.3**.

III. **NORMAL BREAST.** An understanding of normal breast histology is essential for accurate histologic evaluation of breast specimens. It should be noted that what constitutes normal varies based on gender, age, menstrual phase, pregnancy, lactation, and menopausal status.

The breast represents a modified skin adnexal structure composed of major lactiferous ducts that originate from the nipple, progressively branching, until eventually inducing grape-like clusters of secretory glands as lobules. Breast development starts during the fifth week of gestation, at which time thickenings of ectoderm appear on the ventral surface of the fetus extending from axilla to the groin (mammary ridges or milk lines). The majority of this thickening regresses as the fetus develops, except an area in the pectoral region. Failure of this regression results in ectopic mammary tissue or accessory nipple. The most common location for accessory nipple is axilla.

The adult female breast consists of a series of branching ducts, ductules, and lobulated acinar units embedded within a fibroadipose stroma. Terminal duct lobular units (TDLUs) are composed of lobules, which are groups of alveolar glands, embedded in loose intralobular connective tissue that connect to a single terminal ductule. These are the structural and functional units of the breast and most pathologic processes arise within them (e-**Figs. 18.1 and 18.2**). The lining throughout the duct/lobular system of the breast is composed of two distinct layers: an inner (luminal) epithelial layer with a cuboidal to columnar appearance, and an outer (basal) myoepithelial layer (e-**Fig. 18.3**). The myoepithelial cells have variable morphologies ranging from flattened, to epithelioid with clear cytoplasm, to a myoid appearance. Identification of these two cell layers is very important in the assessment of breast lesions as they are almost always preserved in benign lesions, as well as in noninvasive malignant lesions, but are absent in invasive carcinomas. Immunohistochemistry can also be used to identify myoepithelial cells, as myoepithelial cells are usually positive for calponin, p63, CD10, and smooth muscle myosin heavy chain, among other markers (e-**Fig. 18.4**). A panel-based approach of two or more markers is recommended (*Arch Pathol Lab Med.* 2011;135:422). In addition, a proportion of luminal epithelial cells almost always expresses estrogen and/or progesterone receptors. The intralobular stroma is usually sharply demarcated from a denser, collagenized, paucicellular interlobular stroma. The proportion of dense stroma to adipose tissue is variable, with younger women having denser connective tissue (which partially explains why mammography is less sensitive in younger individuals). Breast lobules can be classified on the basis of their morphology into three major types. Type 1 lobules are the most primitive and rudimentary, and are usually seen in prepubertal and nulliparous women. Type 3 lobules are the most developed, and are usually seen in parous and premenopausal women. The progression from type 1 to type 3 is accompanied by additional branching and increased number of alveolar buds. Type 1 lobules also predominate in postmenopausal women and premenopausal women with breast cancer (*Dev Biol.* 1989;25:643; *Cancer Epidemiol Biomark Prev.* 1994;3:219; *Breast J.* 2001;7:278).

After birth and in the premenstrual period, breast development starts with puberty and cyclic secretions of estrogen and progesterone. The ducts elongate and branch primarily due to estrogen stimulus and lobulocentric growth advances primarily under the influence of progesterone. In addition, the breast undergoes various physiologic changes during menstruation, pregnancy, and lactation. It is prudent to be aware of these physiologic changes since they can be mistaken for pathologic processes by an inexperienced observer. Cyclic menstrual changes in the breast tissue are subtle in comparison with other sites such as endometrium. The follicular phase of the menstrual cycle is characterized by simple acini and collagenized stroma, while the luteal phase is characterized by apical snouting of the epithelial cells, prominent vacuolization of myoepithelial cells, and loose edematous stroma. The epithelial cells show peak mitotic activity in the late luteal phase. During pregnancy, there is progressive epithelial cell proliferation resulting in an increase in both the number and the size of TDLUs. By late pregnancy, lobular myoepithelial cells become inconspicuous while the cytoplasm of the luminal epithelium becomes vacuolated as secretions accumulate in the expanded lobules. After parturition, florid changes including the frequent presence of luminal cells with atypical nuclei protruding into the lumen (hobnail cells) can be seen, which can be alarming to the inexperienced observer (e-**Fig. 18.5**). Gradually and slowly, the lobules involute to their resting appearance.

In postmenopausal women, the lobules undergo involution and atrophy characterized by reduction in size and complexity with an increase in fat (type 1 lobules) (e-**Figs. 18.6 to 18.8**).

In contrast to women, due to lack of hormonal stimulation, TDLUs do not develop to a significant extent in men, and male breast consists of branching ducts within a fibroadipose stroma.

IV. **INVASIVE BREAST CARCINOMA.** Establishing the diagnosis of invasive breast cancer (IBC) is the first and most critical responsibility of pathologists (Table 18.1). Most invasive carcinomas present as a palpable mass and/or as a mammographic abnormality. However, in some cases the primary tumor is occult, and the patient may present with lymph node or distant metastasis. The purpose of the pathology report is to communicate all the diagnostic, prognostic, and predictive findings to a multidisciplinary team of surgeons, oncologists, and other specialists; some findings are strong prognostic factors (histologic type, histologic grade, lymph node status), some determine the likelihood of response to specific treatment (hormonal therapy, Trastuzumab), and some determine the need for additional surgical procedures (margin status). Determination of pathologic stage (Table 18.2) is vital to determine prognosis and to guide the therapy. In addition to pathologic stage, the prognosis of breast carcinoma is greatly dependent on additional prognostic and predictive factors that are mandatory and should be evaluated and reported for all breast carcinomas (15), and are most significant in lymph node—negative breast carcinoma.

A. **Prognostic and predictive factors**

1. **Histologic subtype.** Histologic typing remains the gold standard for classification of breast carcinoma and provides useful prognostic information. Five major types of IBC are currently recognized. Four are characterized by relatively unique/uniform histologic features and, thus, they are referred to as "special" histologic types. Collectively, the special types account for about 25% of all the IBCs, and include the so-called invasive lobular, tubular, mucinous, and medullary carcinomas (approximately 15%, 5%, 2% to 3%, and 1% to 2%, respectively) (*Breast Cancer Res.* 2008;10:S4). The remaining ~75% of the breast carcinomas are histologically and prognostically very heterogeneous and are referred to as invasive ductal carcinomas (IDCs), no special type, or, not otherwise specified. Except, perhaps, invasive lobular carcinoma (ILC), all the special type carcinomas have more favorable prognosis compared with IDC, although the degree of improved outcome is variable for different types. In addition, some pathologists recognize other less common special types of invasive carcinoma that have a favorable prognosis. These include invasive cribriform (1%), papillary (<1%), and adenoid cystic (0.1%) carcinomas. Different experts have used variable criteria for diagnosing special type carcinomas, which is partially

TABLE 18.1 World Health Organization Classification of Breast Tumors

Epithelial tumors

Invasive ductal carcinoma, not otherwise specified
Invasive lobular carcinoma
Tubular carcinoma
Invasive cribriform carcinoma
Medullary carcinoma
Mucinous carcinoma and related tumors
Neuroendocrine tumors
Invasive papillary carcinoma
Invasive micropapillary carcinoma
Apocrine carcinoma
Metaplastic carcinomas
Lipid-rich carcinoma
Secretory carcinoma
Oncocytic carcinoma
Adenoid cystic carcinoma
Acinic cell carcinoma
Glycogen-rich clear cell carcinoma
Sebaceous carcinoma
Inflammatory carcinoma
Lobular neoplasia
    Lobular carcinoma in situ
Intraductal proliferative lesions
    Usual ductal hyperplasia
    Flat epithelial atypia
    Atypical ductal hyperplasia
    DCIS
Microinvasive carcinoma
Intraductal papillary neoplasms
    Papilloma
    Atypical papilloma
    Intraductal/intracystic papillary carcinoma
Adenomas
    Tubular adenoma
    Lactating adenoma
    Apocrine adenoma
    Pleomorphic adenoma
    Ductal adenoma

Myoepithelial lesions

Myoepitheliosis
Adenomyoepithelial adenosis
Adenomyoepithelioma
Malignant myoepithelioma

Mesenchymal tumors

Hemangioma
Angiomatosis
Hemangiopericytoma
Pseudoangiomatous stromal hyperplasia
Myofibroblastoma
Fibromatosis (aggressive)
Inflammatory myofibroblastic tumor
Lipoma and angiolipoma
Granular cell tumor
Neurofibroma
Schwannoma
Angiosarcoma
Liposarcoma
Rhabdomyosarcoma
Osteosarcoma
Leiomyoma
Leiomyosarcoma

Fibroepithelial tumors

Fibroadenoma
Phyllodes tumor
Periductal stromal sarcoma, low grade
Mammary hamartoma

Tumors of the nipple

Nipple adenoma
Syringomatous adenoma
Paget's disease of the nipple

Malignant lymphoma

Metastatic tumors

Condensed from: Tavassoli FA, Devilee P. *Pathology and Genetics of Tumours of the Breast and Female Genital Organs.* Lyon: IARC Press; 2003. Used with permission

responsible for the variable prevalence reported in different studies. For practical purposes, a carcinoma is considered "special type" if >90% of the tumor shows special type differentiation. For a carcinoma to be considered "no special type," >50% of the tumor should lack special type differentiation. Tumors with special type differentiation in 50% to 90% of the tumor are considered variants or mixed types. Some experts believe that variant/mixed type carcinomas have an outcome intermediate between no special type carcinomas and the pure special type carcinomas (*Am J Surg Pathol.* 1991;15:334; *Breast Cancer Res.* 2008;10:S4). The diagnostic

TABLE 18.2	Tumor, Node, Metastasis (TNM) Staging Scheme for Breast Carcinoma

Primary tumor(T)

TX	Primary tumor cannot be assessed
T0	No evidence of primary tumor
Tis	Carcinoma in situ
Tis (DCIS)	Ductal carcinoma in situ
Tis (LCIS)	Lobular carcinoma in situ
Tis (Paget)	Paget's disease of the nipple not associated with invasive or in situ carcinoma
T1	Tumor ≤ 2 cm in greatest dimension
T1mic	Microinvasion ≤ 0.1 cm in greatest dimension
T1a	Tumor >0.1 cm but ≤ 0.5 cm in greatest dimension
T1b	Tumor >0.5 cm but ≤ 1 cm in greatest dimension
T1c	Tumor >1 cm but ≤ 2 cm in greatest dimension
T2	Tumor >2 cm but ≤ 5 cm in greatest dimension
T3	Tumor >5 cm in greatest dimension
T4	Tumor of any size with direct extension to chest wall and/or skin, only as described below
T4a	Extension to chest wall, not including only pectoralis muscle
T4b	Edema (including *peau d'orange*) or ulceration of the skin of the breast, or satellite skin nodules confined to the same breast that does not meet the criteria for inflammatory carcinoma
T4c	Both T4a and T4b
T4d	Inflammatory carcinoma

Regional lymph nodes (pN)[a]

pNX	Regional lymph nodes cannot be assessed
pN0	No regional lymph node metastasis or lymph node metastasis <0.2 mm. pN0 can be further classified as
	pN0(i+): ITCs (<0.2 mm, or <200 nonconfluent cells on one single histologic section) detected by H&E or immunohistochemistry
	pN0(mol+): Tumor cells detected only by positive molecular findings (reverse transcription–polymerase chain reaction)
pN1	Metastasis in 1–3 axillary lymph nodes, and/or in internal mammary nodes with microscopic disease detected by sentinel lymph node biopsy but not clinically apparent (not detected clinically or by noninvasive imaging techniques)
pN1mi	Micrometastasis (>0.2 mm and <2.0 mm)
pN1a	Metastasis in 1–3 axillary lymph nodes (at least one metastasis >2.0 mm)
pN1b	Metastasis in internal mammary nodes (micro or macrometastasis)
pN1c	Metastasis in 1–3 axillary lymph nodes and in internal mammary lymph nodes detected by sentinel lymph node biopsy but not clinically apparent. If associated with >3 positive axillary lymph nodes, the internal mammary nodes are classified as pN3b to reflect increased tumor burden
pN2	Metastasis in 4–9 axillary lymph nodes or in clinically apparent internal mammary lymph nodes in the absence of axillary lymph node metastasis
pN2a	Metastasis in 4–9 axillary lymph nodes (at least one deposit >2 mm)
pN2b	Metastasis in clinically apparent internal mammary lymph nodes in the absence of axillary lymph node metastasis
pN3	Metastasis in ≥ 10 axillary lymph nodes, or in infraclavicular lymph nodes, or in clinically apparent ipsilateral internal mammary lymph nodes in the presence of ≥ 1 positive axillary lymph nodes; or in >3 axillary lymph nodes with clinically negative microscopic metastasis in internal mammary lymph nodes; or in ipsilateral supraclavicular lymph nodes

(continued)

TABLE 18.2	Tumor, Node, Metastasis (TNM) Staging Scheme for Breast Carcinoma (*Continued*)
pN3a	Metastasis in $\geq$10 axillary lymph nodes (at least one deposit >2 mm), or metastasis to the infraclavicular lymph nodes
pN3b	Metastasis in clinically apparent ipsilateral internal mammary lymph nodes in the presence of $\geq$1 positive axillary lymph nodes; or in >3 axillary lymph nodes and in internal mammary lymph nodes with microscopic disease detected by sentinel lymph node dissection but not clinically apparent
pN3c	Metastasis in ipsilateral supraclavicular lymph nodes

Distant metastasis (M)

MX	Distant metastasis cannot be assessed
M0	No distant metastasis
M0 (i+)	Deposits of molecularly or microscopically detected tumor cells in circulating blood, bone marrow, or other nonregional nodal tissue $\leq$0.2 mm in a patient with no clinical or radiologic evidence of distant metastasis[b]
M1	Distant metastasis, determined by clinical and radiologic means, or histologically proven >0.2 mm

AJCC stage groupings

Stage 0	Tis	N0	M0
Stage IA	T1	N0	M0
Stage IB	T0	N1mi	M0
	T1	N1mi	M0
Stage IIA	T0	N1[c]	M0
	T1	N1[c]	M0
	T2	N0	M0
Stage IIB	T2	N1	M0
	T3	N0	M0
Stage IIIA	T0	N2	M0
	T1	N2	M0
	T2	N2	M0
	T3	N1	M0
	T3	N2	M0
Stage IIIB	T4	N0	M0
	T4	N1	M0
	T4	N2	M0
Stage IIIC	Any T	N3	M0
Stage IV	Any T	Any N	M1

[a]Sentinel nodes (when they are <5 in number) are indicated by adding (sn) to the designation.
[b]This category does not change stage grouping.
[c]T0 and T1 tumors with micrometastases only are classified as Stage IB.
From: Edge SB, Byrd DR, Compton CC, et al., eds. *AJCC Cancer Staging Manual.* 7th ed. New York, NY: Springer; 2010. Used with permission.

features of major histologic subtypes of breast carcinoma are summarized in Table 18.3 and are discussed in more detail below.

a. **Tumor size** is one of the most powerful prognostic factors for clinical outcome. The prognostic value of tumor size is independent of axillary lymph node status and is an especially significant determinant in node negative disease. It is usually determined by taking into consideration the gross findings correlated with the microscopic examination. In some cases, it may also be helpful to include information about tumor size from imaging studies. In small tumors where the bulk of tumor has been excised by previous core needle, it may be best to use the core biopsy in conjunction with radiologic findings to estimate the maximum size

TABLE 18.3 Diagnostic Features of Major Histopathologic Types of IBC

Histologic type	Incidence (%)	Clinical/gross findings	Microscopic features	Favorable prognosis	Typical biomarkers
ILC	5–15	Architectural distortion, density (no distinct mass), multifocal/bilateral	Uniform noncohesive cells, eccentric nuclei, intracytoplasmic lumina, Indian filing, targetoid pattern		ER (+), PgR (+), HER2 (−)
Invasive tubular carcinoma	5	Spiculated mass, small size	Angulated tubules with tapered ends, open lumina, dense stroma	Yes	ER (+), PgR (+), HER2 (−)
Invasive mucinous carcinoma	2–3	Well-circumscribed lobulated mass, gelatinous cut surface	Tumor cells floating in pools of extracellular mucin	Yes	ER (+), PgR (+), HER2 (−)
Invasive medullary carcinoma	1–2	Young women, well-circumscribed mass, no calcifications	Syncytial growth, pushing borders, lymphoplasmacytic infiltrate, high nuclear grade	Yes (if pure)	ER (−), PgR (−), HER2 (−); (triple negative)
Invasive micropapillary carcinoma	1–2	Similar to IDC, NST	Tumor clusters within empty spaces, reverse polarity, no fibrovascular cores	Higher rate of LN metastasis	Variable
IDC, NST	70–75	Spiculated mass, variable	Variable, devoid of special type histologic features	Variable	Variable
Metaplastic carcinoma	<1	Larger size	Tumor transformation to nonglandular (squamous) or mesenchymal elements	Lower LN metastasis, poor overall prognosis	ER (−), PgR (−), HER2 (−); (triple negative) ER and PgR can be positive in glandular elements

IDC, invasive ductal carcinoma; NST, no special type.

TABLE 18.4	Elston–Ellis Modification of Scarff–Bloom–Richardson Grading System for Breast Carcinoma			
Tubule formation				**Score**
	Majority (>75%) of tumor			1
	Moderate (10–75%) of tumor			2
	Little or none (<10%) of tumor			3
Nuclear pleomorphism				
	Small, regular, uniform nuclei			1
	Moderate increase in size and variability			2
	Marked variation			3
Mitotic activity				
Field diameter (mm)	0.44	0.59	0.63	
Field area (mm^2)	0.152	0.274	0.312	
Mitotic count				
	0–5	0–9	0–11	1
	6–10	10–19	12–22	2
	>11	>20	>23	3

Add up the score to reach the total points:

3–5 points: Grade 1 (well-differentiated).
6–7 points: Grade 2 (moderately differentiated).
8–9 points: Grade 3 (poorly differentiated).

of the invasive carcinoma. Although the aggregate volume of multifocal tumors may better correlate with the risk of lymph node metastasis than the size of the largest focus (*Cancer.* 2004;100:20), multiple foci of invasive carcinoma are not currently added together and the diameters of the different foci should be individually reported, and only the largest focus of contiguous area of invasion should be used for staging purposes. Only the size of invasive carcinoma (best measured by microscopic assessment), which does not include adjacent DCIS outside the invasive carcinoma, should be used for staging purposes (http://www.cap.org/apps/docs/committees/cancer/cancer_protocols/2009/InvasiveBreast_09 protocol.pdf).

b. **Histologic grade** is used to convey the degree of differentiation of tumors. The most widely accepted grading system for IBC is the Elston–Ellis modification of the Scarff–Bloom–Richardson (ESBR) grading system. This grading system is based on three characteristics of the tumor: the degree of gland/tubule formation, nuclear pleomorphism, and mitotic activity (e-**Figs. 18.9 to 18.11**). Variation in these three elements is the basis for this universally accepted grading scheme (*Histopathology.* 1991;19:403; *J Clin Oncol.* 2008;26:3153) (Table 18.4). A numerical scoring system on a scale of 1 to 3 is given to each variable to ensure that each factor has been assessed individually. The histologic grade is of particular importance for ductal carcinomas of no special type. However, given the strength of histologic grade as a prognostic marker (second only to axillary lymph node status), it should be reported for all carcinomas (*Histopathology.* 1991;19:403; *J Clin Oncol.* 2008;26:3153). Within each TNM stage grouping, there is a correlation between histologic grade and patient outcome. A combination of factors, such as combination of histologic type and grade (*J Clin Oncol.* 2008;26:3153), or tumor size, nodal status, and histologic grade (Nottingham Prognostic Index [NPI]) is a better tool to assess the prognosis in any given tumor (*Pathol Oncol Res.* 2008;14:113).

c. **Surgical margin.** The distance of tumor from the margin of surgical excision is also important because it is inversely related to the likelihood of local recurrence, especially in tumors removed by lumpectomy. Wide margins with grossly distinct tumors can be adequately measured with a ruler, whereas close margins require microscopic measurement. A margin is considered positive only if the ink that was applied to the margin at the time of gross examination transects tumor cells. The distance of the closest margin, as well as its location, should be reported. The extent of margin involvement can be relayed as unifocal (<4 mm), multifocal (more than one focus), or extensive (5 mm or greater).

d. **Others**

i. (MI) is a measure of the capability of the tumor cells to divide and replicate and is determined by calculating the average number of mitotic figures in a minimum of 10 consecutive high-power fields (HPFs) in the most mitotically active part of the tumor, usually at the periphery of the tumor. Only the clearly identifiable mitotic figures should be counted.

ii. The presence of **lymphvascular space invasion** (e-**Fig. 18.12**) is an important and independent prognostic factor, particularly in node-negative patients with IBC. The presence of lymphatic channel invasion recognizes a subgroup of node-negative patients who are at increased risk of lymph node metastasis or distant metastasis (*Ann Oncol.* 2005;16:1569; *Diagn Pathol.* 2011;13:18). There is a high degree of interobserver variability in diagnosing lymphvascular invasion (LVI); therefore, adherence to strict criteria is recommended in order to reduce this interobserver variability. It is recommended that the focus of LVI should be outside the borders of invasive carcinoma. In addition, identification of an endothelial lining, and lack of conformation of tumor emboli to the shape of vascular space, help to differentiate a vascular space from artifactual stromal clefting. LVI present within lymphatic spaces in the dermis is often correlated with the clinical features of inflammatory carcinoma (diffuse erythema and edema involving one-third or more of the breast). In the absence of the clinical features of inflammatory carcinoma, this finding remains a poor prognostic factor but is insufficient to classify a cancer as inflammatory carcinoma.

iii. **Skin and nipple involvement.** Skin can directly be involved by underlying invasive carcinoma (with or without ulceration). This usually is seen in association with large tumors, or in tumors that are small but very superficial. In addition, tumor cells from underlying lactiferous ducts of the nipple that are involved by DCIS can percolate through the epidermis without breaking through the basement membrane (Paget's disease).

Recently, gene expression profiling studies have classified breast tumors on the basis of their gene transcription patterns into different types or classes with different prognostic implications (*Nature.* 2000;406:747). These new technologies provide important information that can be integrated into routine patient care (see below), but histologic typing of breast tumors still remains the gold standard for classification of breast carcinoma and provides useful prognostic information.

B. **IDC, no special type** is the most common subtype of breast cancer, comprising 70% to 75% of the IBCs. This subtype is composed of a heterogeneous mixture of tumors with different morphologies, clinical findings, and patient outcomes. These tumors are predominantly devoid of histologic features that would allow categorization of these tumors in a special type category, and usually present as a spiculated mass, with or without calcifications, or as a mammographic abnormality. Grossly, the tumors usually form a hard mass, with tan-white to gray, gritty cut surface that is a manifestation of dense stromal desmoplasia. The morphology of these tumors is quite heterogeneous with regard to growth pattern, cytologic features, mitotic activity, and extent of associated in situ carcinoma. The growth pattern can be solid, trabecular, in cords, in tubules, or as single cells (e-Figs. 18.13 to 18.25). Most often, heterogeneity can also be noted within different parts of the same tumor. As mentioned earlier, the ESBR grading system is an important prognostic tool for categorizing these tumors into groups with good versus poor outcome.

C. **Special subtypes**

1. **Invasive lobular carcinoma (ILC)** is the second most common type of IBC, and comprises about 15% of all the invasive carcinomas with a reportedly increased incidence in patients receiving postmenopausal combined hormone replacement therapy (*Breast Cancer Res.* 2004;6:R149). These tumors are associated with a higher rate of multifocality in the ipsilateral breast, and are also more often bilateral than other subtypes. They may present as a palpable mass, but more commonly they present with an area of density or architectural distortion on mammogram. Some tumors do not show any mammographic abnormalities. Grossly, either they may form a mass, which is indistinguishable from a mass of IDC, or they may show only an area of firm, rubbery breast tissue. Sometimes, carcinoma is only revealed upon microscopic examination. Histologically, ILC has a distinct morphology and pattern of infiltration within the stroma. The **classical form** is characterized by small, uniform, noncohesive tumor cells infiltrating in a single "Indian" file pattern and forming linear strands (e-Figs. 18.26 to 18.28) that may concentrically surround benign epithelial elements (targetoid pattern of growth) (e-Fig. 18.29). Typically, the tumor cells infiltrate without provoking a stromal reaction and without destroying normal architecture. Cytologically, the nuclei are small and uniform, and located eccentrically within a cytoplasm that occasionally shows intracytoplasmic lumina (an intracytoplasmic vacuole containing an eosinophilic mucin droplet). Mitotic activity is sparse. Variant forms of ILC differ from the classical type with regards to architecture or cytology. While occasional signet-ring cells can be seen in classical lobular carcinoma, in the **signet-ring cell variant** the tumor shows a prominent population of signet-ring cells (e-Fig. 18.30). In the **solid** and **trabecular variants,** tumor cells are cytologically similar to the classical form; however, they have a different growth pattern of either large sheets (e-Figs. 18.31 and 18.32) or nests of 20 cells or more, which are separated from each other by stroma (e-Fig. 18.33), respectively. In the **pleomorphic variant,** the tumor cells are larger, and show more significant pleomorphism increased mitoses (e-Fig. 18.34). Most cases of ILC show reduced or no expression of E-cadherin by immunohistochemistry. As suggested by their higher grade, pleomorphic ILCs do not share the somewhat better outcome (compared to IDC-NST) that characterizes classic ILC. Other differences from IDC-NST include a lower incidence of parenchymal metastasis, and isolated tumor cell (ITC) metastatic patterns in minimally involved axillary lymph nodes (as opposed to the usual finding of tumor cell clusters in the subcapsular sinuses). ILCs have characteristic metastatic spread to certain organs such as the ovary and stomach (where the metastases can resemble primary signet-ring cell carcinoma). Up to 95% of the ILCs are immunopositive for ER and PgR expression. ILCs typically do

not overexpress the HER2 gene product, except the pleomorphic variant, which may show HER2 overexpression.

2. **Tubular carcinoma.** This tumor type constitutes 5% of the invasive carcinomas, even higher on screening detected tumors (*J Clin Oncol.* 1999;17:1442), and is associated with limited metastatic potential and an excellent prognosis. As a result of increased use of screening mammography, these tumors present as a nonpalpable mammographic abnormality, or are incidentally found on biopsies for other abnormalities. Grossly, they form a spiculated mass. Microscopically, these tumors are characterized by a haphazard arrangement of angulated tubules with tapering ends and open lumens. The tubules are lined by a single layer of epithelial cells that often display eosinophilic to amphophilic cytoplasm with apical snouts and oval nuclei, with only mild to moderate nuclear pleomorphism (e-**Figs. 18.35 and 18.36**). A cellular, often, fibroelastotic stroma is characteristic. The lack of a myoepithelial layer is a helpful feature in distinguishing this tumor from benign sclerosing lesions of the breast (sclerosing adenosis, radial scar, complex sclerosing lesions). Estrogen and progesterone receptors are expressed in >90% of these tumors (*J Clin Oncol.* 1999;17:1442), but they rarely, if ever, overexpress HER2. Axillary lymph node metastasis is uncommon, and if present, occurs only with larger tumors and is limited to the low-axillary lymph nodes; axillary lymph node is not associated with the same adverse outcome as IDC, NST tumors (*J Clin Oncol.* 1999;17:1442).

3. **Mucinous carcinoma.** Depending on the series and stringency of diagnostic criteria, this variant comprises 1% to 6% of all the invasive carcinomas. This tumor is also associated with a favorable outcome. Grossly, the tumor is well circumscribed and lobulated, with a soft gelatinous consistency, and a glistening cut surface. Microscopically, the tumor is composed of tumor cell clusters and trabeculae floating within lakes of extracellular mucin (e-**Fig. 18.37**). Nuclear grade characteristically is low to intermediate. These tumors typically are immunopositive for ER (>90% of the tumors) and PgR biomarkers, and negative for HER2 overexpression (*J Clin Oncol.* 1999;17:1442). A significant proportion of mucinous carcinomas show neuroendocrine differentiation (*Mod Pathol.* 2004;17:568).

Mucinous carcinoma should be differentiated from other mucin-producing lesions of the breast. Mucocele-like lesions are characterized by mucin filled benign ducts and cysts that often rupture and result in extravasation of mucin into surrounding stroma. Sometimes, the ducts show proliferative changes, and portions of ductal epithelium may become detached and float within the mucin pool. However, the linear configuration of epithelial cells and presence of myoepithelial cells favor a diagnosis of mucocele-like lesion. Whenever the distinction between the two is not possible, especially in core needle biopsies, excision should be recommended for definitive evaluation (*J Clin Pathol.* 2008;61:11).

4. **Medullary carcinoma.** This tumor comprises 1% to 2% of all the invasive carcinomas. There is an association between medullary carcinomas and carcinomas with medullary features with familial mutations in the BRCA1 DNA repair gene. Medullary carcinoma is usually diagnosed in younger women and presents with a palpable mass. On mammogram, the tumor is seen as a well-circumscribed mass usually without calcifications. On gross examination, the tumor is a well-circumscribed, soft, tan-brown to gray masses, with a bulging cut surface. Hemorrhage, necrosis, or cystic change may be noted. Microscopically, these tumors are characterized by a syncytial growth pattern in >75% of the tumor, an intense lymphoplasmacytic infiltrate, pushing borders, highly pleomorphic nuclei (nuclear grade 2 to 3), and a lack of glandular differentiation (e-**Fig. 18.38**). Tumors that show

most but not all of the above criteria are recognized as variant medullary carcinomas. Medullary carcinomas are generally are negative for all biomarkers (triple-negative tumors). Pure medullary carcinomas have a favorable outcome, however, variant types do not share this prognostic advantage.

5. **Other rare, but clinically significant subtypes**

a. **Invasive papillary (predominantly micropapillary) carcinoma.** In a "pure" form (>75% of the tumor), invasive micropapillary carcinoma accounts for <1% of the invasive carcinoma; however, it is much more frequently a minor component of IDC, NST tumors. Histologically, this variant is composed of small solid clusters of malignant cells floating within clear stromal spaces (e-**Fig. 18.39**). These cell clusters lack true fibrovascular cores and show reverse polarity (the apical surfaces of the cells are polarized to the outside) (e-**Fig. 18.40**). The importance of recognizing this variant of invasive carcinoma (as well as mixed tumors with a micropapillary component) is the associated high incidence of axillary lymph node metastasis. It should be noted, however, that when matched for stage, this variant does not necessarily have a worse prognosis than IDC-NST (*Mod Pathol.* 1993;6:660; *Am J Surg Pathol.* 2009;33:202; *Breast.* 2010;19:231).

b. **Metaplastic carcinomas** are rare and comprise <1% of the breast carcinomas. They include a heterogeneous group of tumors in which a portion of the malignant cells have undergone transformation into a different cell type: nonglandular epithelial (squamous), or mesenchymal cell (chondroid, osseous, muscle, spindle cell) types. These tumors are similar to IDCs of no special type with regard to clinical presentation except that they are usually larger at the time of presentation.

   Tumors with squamous differentiation show a spectrum of differentiation from well to poorly differentiated. **Low-grade adenosquamous carcinoma,** frequently associated with papillary and sclerosing lesions, is characterized by angulated glands embedded in a cellular stroma composed of cells with low-grade cytologic atypia and focal squamous differentiation (e-**Fig. 18.41**). In contrast to higher-grade tumors that resemble adenosquamous carcinoma elsewhere, low-grade adenosquamous carcinomas rarely metastasize. **Metaplastic spindle cell carcinoma** includes carcinomas with abundant spindle cell transformation (e-**Fig. 18.42**). The diagnosis is relatively straightforward when glandular elements are evident, but when absent, diagnosis may only be made by demonstrating cytokeratin immunoreactivity in the spindle cells. It should be noted that spindle cell carcinoma can be histologically bland and show minimal cytologic atypia (such as in the so-called fibromatosis-like spindle cell carcinoma). The key to correct diagnosis is wide sampling of the tumor to identify areas with clear glandular elements, and/or the use of a panel of immunohistochemical markers, particularly high-molecular weight/basal cytokeratins, myoepithelial markers, and p63 to demonstrate the epithelial nature of the tumor (e-**Fig. 18.43**) (*Histopathology.* 2008;52:45). **Metaplastic carcinomas with heterologous differentiation** are most commonly composed of foci of chondroid or osseous differentiation; however, other types of mesenchymal differentiation such as fibrosarcoma, rhabdomyosarcoma, and other sarcomas can also be seen (e-**Figs. 18.44 to 18.46**). Despite the lower relative rate of lymph node metastasis (considering their larger size at the time of diagnosis), metaplastic nonetheless carcinomas have a high rate of LVI and a poor prognosis overall. ER, PgR, and HER2 are usually negative, but can be focally expressed in the glandular component.

c. **Inflammatory carcinoma** is a clinical-pathologic entity characterized by diffuse erythema, induration, and tenderness of breast skin associated with nonpitting edema (*peu d'orange*) involving one-third or more of the skin of breast. A breast mass may or may not be evident. Histologically, there is extensive dermal lymphatic invasion by tumor emboli, which is believed to be the underlying mechanism for the clinical picture. A tissue diagnosis is necessary to demonstrate invasive carcinoma in the underlying breast tissue. The presence of dermal lymphatic tumor emboli without the skin changes does not qualify as inflammatory carcinoma. These tumors are classified as T4d by the TNM staging system.

d. **Microinvasive carcinoma** is defined as extension of cancer cells beyond the basement membrane of terminal duct-lobular units to an extent ≤1 mm. Microinvasion is usually seen in association with high-grade DCIS. In this setting, the presence of a dense periductal stromal reaction and periductal lymphoplasmacytic infiltration should prompt the pathologist to search for foci of microinvasion that occurs as single cells or small clusters infiltrating outside the confines of TDLUs (e-Figs. 18.47 and 18.48). The focus of invasion should be obvious and care should be taken to avoid interpretation of DCIS involving the lobules (a so-called cancerization of lobules), or DCIS involving sclerosing lesions, as microinvasion. In this setting, immunostains for myoepithelial markers and examination of deeper levels of the block can be extremely helpful. Of note, if there are multiple foci of microinvasion, the number of foci and the size of the largest focus should be noted; separate individual foci of microinvasion should not be added together (http://www.cap.org/apps/docs/committees/cancer/cancer_protocols/2009/InvasiveBreast_09protocol.pdf).

e. **Other rare types of carcinoma** include, among others, adenoid cystic carcinoma, invasive cribriform carcinoma, apocrine carcinoma, myoepithelial carcinoma, sebaceous carcinoma, lipid-rich carcinoma, clear cell/glycogen-rich carcinoma, acinic cell carcinoma, and oncocytic carcinoma.

V. **PATHOLOGY OF TREATED INVASIVE BREAST CANCER.** Neoadjuvant chemotherapy and radiation are increasingly being used in the management of breast cancer, and so it is important to be familiar with radiation-induced changes in normal breast to avoid interpreting them as malignant or premalignant disease. Likewise, familiarity with chemotherapy/radiation-induced changes in tumors is required to evaluate response to treatment.

Posttreatment changes in normal breast tissue usually include lobular atrophy, hyalinization, and nuclear atypia with degenerative changes, both nuclear and cytoplasmic. Response to treatment is often categorized clinically as complete, partial, or no response, and is a strong prognostic factor for disease-free and overall survival. During gross examination, careful attention to identifying and evaluating the tumor bed is necessary. In addition, exhaustive sampling of the tumor bed region is necessary before making a diagnosis of complete treatment response. Treatment may affect the morphology of the primary tumor and lymph nodes involved by metastatic disease producing various histologic changes in tumor morphology including necrosis, chronic inflammation, foamy histiocytic collections, decreased cellularity, cytoplasmic eosinophilia, nuclear alterations, fibrosis, and hemosiderin deposition (e-Figs. 18.49 to 18.51). Invasive carcinomas with a minor response may show little change in size; with greater degrees of response, the carcinoma shows decreased cellularity or may show multiple foci of invasion scattered over a larger tumor bed. When evaluating treated carcinomas, the size of the tumor is determined by the largest focus of contiguous tumor and/or the number of foci involved over the tumor bed, not by the area of tumor bed. Most carcinomas are of the same grade after treatment, but in some cases a change in the grade of tumor occurs. Changes in biomarker status rarely occur after treatment. Many systems have been developed for grading of pathological response to treatment (*Breast.* 2003;12:320; *J Clin Oncol.* 2007;25:4414).

Lymph nodes with treatment response usually show fibrous scarring and foamy histiocytic aggregates in the place of previous tumor (complete response), or may show small tumor deposits within an area of fibrosis. A lymph node with complete response should not be reported as "positive" for carcinoma.

VI. **NONINVASIVE CARCINOMA.** Noninvasive carcinomas have historically been divided into two major categories: ductal and lobular, on the basis of the misconception that they arise from ducts versus lobules, respectively. However, now it is recognized that both of these lesions arise from TDLUs.

A. **Ductal carcinoma in situ (DCIS)** encompasses a heterogeneous group of lesions with highly variable clinical presentations, histologic findings, biomarker profiles, genetic abnormalities, and clinical potential. They have in common a monoclonal proliferation of neoplastic epithelial cells confined to the ductal–lobular system, typically in a segmental distribution, without extension through the basement membrane. DCIS is a nonobligate precursor of invasive cancer. It expands and unfolds TDLUs, and may grow into larger ducts or into adjacent lobules, giving an appearance referred to as cancerization of lobules, or may even grow further and expand into spheres, a source of the misnomer "ductal" carcinoma. The most common clinical presentation of DCIS is as calcifications seen on mammogram (e-**Figs. 18.52 and 18.53**) although up to 30% of the detected DCIS is not associated with calcifications; in this latter scenario, DCIS is seen as densities and architectural distortions on mammogram. Less commonly, DCIS may present as a mass.

Grossly, most cases of DCIS are not visible. If palpable, they may form a mass with cords of tissue extruding a paste-like material from their cut surfaces (a gross correlation to the material seen on histologic sections as comedo necrosis, see below). Morphologically, DCIS is seen as proliferation of neoplastic cells with variable nuclear cytology, and in a variety of growth patterns, which usually grow over and obliterate the luminal space of the ducts and TDLUs. High-grade DCIS may incite a desmoplastic stromal response mixed with chronic inflammation which raises the concern for IBC (e-**Fig. 18.54**). Myoepithelial markers may be useful in such cases as they highlight the myoepithelial layer, thus providing evidence that proliferation has not yet breached the ductal–lobular system. DCIS may become displaced during previous needle biopsy, leading to carcinoma within a biopsy tract that may be confused with IBC in the subsequent excisional specimen. DCIS may show a variety of morphologies including apocrine (e-**Figs. 18.55 and 18.56**) and clear cell (e-**Fig. 18.57**) differentiation. While familiarity with these morphologic patterns is helpful in recognizing the lesion, most of these morphologic variants do not bear clinical significance independent of their nuclear grade.

For clinical purposes, a few prognostic and/or diagnostic characteristics of in situ carcinomas should be reported in a pathology report. This information may affect the clinical decision making.

1. **Size/extent.** If the lesion is only present on one slide, microscopic measurement of the focus of DCIS will be the most accurate measurement. If the lesion is present on multiple slides, the most accurate measurement is achieved by correlating the microscopic sections containing DCIS with the gross diagram of the breast specimen showing location and relationship of different sections within the specimen (see e-**Appendix 18.2**). By correlating the two, an estimate size of the lesion can be provided. In rare cases where an accurate size estimate cannot be given, extent of the lesion can be reported as the fraction of slides involved by DCIS.

2. **Nuclear grade.** On the basis of nuclear features, DCIS is classified into three grades by SBR criteria: low, intermediate, or high grade (Table 18.5). Low-grade DCIS consists of a proliferation of small, monomorphic, and evenly spaced luminal epithelial cells with homogeneous chromatin distribution

TABLE 18.5 The Criteria for Nuclear Grading of DCIS

	Grade 1 (low)	Grade 2 (intermediate)	Grade 3 (high)
Nuclear pleomorphism	Monotonous	Intermediate	Markedly pleomorphic
Nuclear size	1.5–2 times the size of a red blood cell or normal ductal epithelial nucleus	Intermediate	2.5 times the size of red blood cell or normal ductal epithelial nuclei
Chromatin distribution	Diffuse, finely dispersed	Intermediate	Vesicular, irregular chromatin distribution
Nucleoli	Occasional	Intermediate	Prominent, multiple
Mitoses	Occasional	Intermediate	May be frequent
Orientation	Polarized toward the luminal spaces	Intermediate	Not polarized toward luminal spaces

and inconspicuous nucleoli. Mitotic counts are usually low (e-**Fig. 18.58**). In contrast, high-grade DCIS consists of a proliferation of highly pleomorphic, less organized epithelial cells with vesicular or coarse chromatin and prominent/multiple nucleoli. Mitotic counts are high, apoptotic cells are frequent, and comedo necrosis (defined as calcified necrosis in the center of the proliferation) is common (e-**Figs. 18.54 and 18.59**). Intermediate grade carcinomas are lesions with features that fall in between high-grade and low-grade carcinomas (e-**Fig. 18.60**). However, as with invasive carcinomas, DCIS commonly contain areas of multiple histologic grades (*Clin Cancer Res.* 2008;14:370).

3. **Growth pattern.** DCIS is extremely diverse histologically, with respect to nuclear grade and architecture. A variety of different growth patterns can be recognized, although commonly more than one growth pattern is present within a given lesion (e-**Figs. 18.61 and 18.62**). Familiarity with these growth patterns is necessary for recognition of DCIS. The most common growth patterns include solid, papillary, micropapillary, and cribriform (sieve-like) architectural patterns.

   a. In the **cribriform growth pattern,** the neoplastic cells form punched out spaces with round and rigid extracellular lumens formed by neoplastic cells polarizing around the spaces (e-**Figs. 18.63 and 18.64**).

   b. The **micropapillary growth pattern** is manifested by a proliferation of tufts of neoplastic cells projecting into the lumen of TDLUs. These tufts are characterized by a lack of fibrovascular cores, a club-shaped end, and proliferation of a monomorphic, evenly distributed, cell population (e-**Figs. 18.65 to 18.67**).

   c. The **solid growth pattern** is characterized by a proliferation of sheets of monomorphic, cohesive cells that fill the lumen of TDLUs. These cells may form pseudorosettes or microacini with polarization of surrounding cells (e-**Figs. 18.68 and 18.69**).

   d. The **clinging growth pattern** is recognized by some experts as a distinct growth pattern. It is characterized by a duct lined by a few layers of highly atypical neoplastic cells at the periphery and filled by abundant comedonecrosis (e-**Fig. 18.70**). Some experts consider this growth pattern as a variation of the solid growth pattern with extensive necrosis.

   e. **Papillary DCIS** consists of a papillary proliferation characterized by branching fibrovascular cores covered by a monotonous epithelial proliferation showing mild to moderate nuclear atypia (e-**Figs. 18.71 and 18.72**). In contrast to benign papillomas, papillary DCIS has no invested myoepithelial layer (**e-Figs. 18.73 to 18.75**), which can be demonstrated by a lack of staining with myoepithelial markers such as p63 and calponin. Some markers such as smooth muscle actin (SMA) not only highlight the myoepithelial cells, but also stain the vascular walls within the fibrovascular cores of papillary DCIS, which should not be overinterpreted as evidence of a myoepithelial layer.

 f. Intracystic papillary carcinoma (IPC) is considered by most experts as a variant of DCIS that consists of proliferation of monomorphic neoplastic cells within an expanded enlarged cystic space with an outer fibrotic wall (**e-Figs. 18.76 and 18.77**). The intracystic tumor usually shows scattered fibrovascular cores lined by atypical epithelial cells that are not supported by a myoepithelial layer (**e-Figs. 18.78 to 18.80**). Various architectural growth patterns of DCIS, including micropapillary, cribriform, and solid, may be present within the lesion. Care must be taken to avoid overinterpretation of malignant cells in the fibrous wall as a result of distortion of the wall secondary to fibrosis, or at the site of previous core biopsy, as the criteria for invasive carcinoma require the cells to be outside of the fibrous wall (**e-Fig. 18.81**). The presence of adjacent hemorrhage or hemosiderin-laden macrophages can be a helpful clue to the presence of displaced tumor cells secondary to previous biopsy.

4. Extent of comedo necrosis. Comedo necrosis can be seen in any grade DCIS but is more commonly seen in high-grade lesions, and is characterized by calcified necrosis within the center of a duct which is involved by DCIS (**e-Fig. 18.54**). This can be conveyed as an estimate of the percentage of surface area of the ducts involved by DCIS, which contain comedonecrosis. Some studies have shown that abundant comedonecrosis is associated with increased local recurrence following lumpectomy for DCIS.

5. Skin involvement (Paget's disease). Paget's disease of the nipple can be seen when neoplastic cells percolate through the underlying lactiferous ducts to the epithelium without breaching the basement membrane. It is usually associated with underlying high-grade DCIS (**e-Fig. 18.82**). It is important to distinguish the Paget cells within nipple squamous epithelium from other clear cells that occasionally can be seen within the nipple, mainly Toker cells. Toker cells are incidentally found clear cells within the nipple, which are smaller in size compared to Paget cells and do not show significant atypia. A HER2 immunohistochemical stain can be useful in difficult cases, as the cells of Paget's disease are positive for HER2 while Toker cells are negative (*Histopathology*. 2009;24:367).

6. Surgical margin status is of particular importance and has an inverse relationship with the incidence of local recurrence. Since DCIS usually is not grossly visible, margins should be microscopically examined, and the location of the closest margin and its distance from DCIS should be mentioned in the report. As with invasive carcinoma, a margin is considered positive only if carcinoma is present at the inked margin. The extent of involved margin (focal, multifocal, extensive) should be reported. If in situ carcinoma is mixed with invasive carcinoma, the volume of in situ carcinoma in the tumor (reported as the fraction of total tumor) should be mentioned, as extensive DCIS mixed with invasive carcinoma has a higher rate of local recurrence, particularly when DCIS is close to or present at the margins.

7. Presence of associated microcalcifications should be noted, as DCIS that is first detected by microcalcifications will frequently recur as calcifications.

8. Biomarker status. Assessment of ER/PR status is an essential factor in the evaluation of DCIS for adjuvant hormonal therapy. Although ER/PR status can provide prognostic information, their major clinical value is to assess the likelihood of response to hormonal therapy (see below).

B. **Lobular neoplasia.** This term refers to the entire spectrum of atypical epithelial proliferations arising in TDLUs composed of loosely cohesive uniform cells with small nuclei and indistinct nucleoli, which expand TDLUs and grow in a Pagetoid fashion underneath the epithelial layer. Traditionally, LCIS and atypical lobular hyperplasia only differ in the degree of involvement and expansion of the lobules; however, most authorities now consider such lobular proliferations under the rubric of "lobular neoplasia" or "lobular intraepithelial neoplasia." Many studies show that there is a direct relationship between the extent of the disease and risk of developing IBC.

1. **Lobular carcinoma in situ (LCIS)** is characterized by a neoplastic proliferation of small, loosely cohesive, uniform cells, with homogeneous chromatin and inconspicuous nucleoli. The cells may contain intracytoplasmic vacuoles containing eosinophilic mucin globules (e-**Figs. 18.83 and 18.84**). The proliferating cells fill (and often distend) most of the lobules (>50%) in the involved TDLUs. Although Pagetoid extension of neoplastic cells into the major ductal system is usually seen with LCIS, it can also be seen in association with DCIS; such extension undermines the normal epithelial layer and produces a clover leaf-like appearance (e-**Figs. 18.85 and 18.86**). Differentiating LCIS from intermediate and high-grade DCIS is usually straightforward. However, distinguishing LCIS from low-grade DCIS—particularly with a solid growth pattern—can be challenging. In contrast to solid LG-DCIS, the cells of LCIS are usually small and discohesive, and often display intracytoplasmic lumina. The loss of membranous expression of E-cadherin protein by immunohistochemistry has been recognized to be characteristic of lobular carcinoma (cytoplasmic expression may still be evident) (e-**Fig. 18.87**), and retention of expression is characteristic of ductal carcinoma. However, about 10% to 15% of the cases of lobular carcinomas retain E-cadherin expression and a minority of ductal carcinomas lose E-cadherin expression; therefore, the two should be distinguished mainly on histologic grounds (*Am J Surg Pathol.* 2010;34:1472). Most cases of classic LCIS are managed by steroid hormone receptor antagonists, and most data in the literature do not support reexcision for LCIS present at the surgical margins.

2. **Pleomorphic LCIS** is a morphologically distinct type of LCIS which shares with classic LCIS distension of the TDLUs by discohesive malignant cells; however, as the name indicates, it is composed of poorly differentiated cells with significant pleomorphism that show two- to threefold nuclear size variation, nuclear membrane irregularity, and prominent nucleoli. Central comedo necrosis and calcifications may be observed (e-**Fig. 18.88**). The main differential diagnosis for pleomorphic LCIS is intermediate- or high-grade DCIS, a differential confounded by the not infrequent presence of central comedo-like necrosis in all these lesions. The discohesive nature of neoplastic cells can be very useful in confirming the diagnosis. Similar to classic LCIS, pleomorphic LCIS can also spread along the duct system in a Pagetoid fashion. Given the clinical, radiologic, and pathologic similarities of pleomorphic LCIS to DCIS, including the frequent extension into larger ducts, it is managed in a manner similar to DCIS; nevertheless, it is still important to correctly identify pleomorphic LCIS due to the occasional coexistence of ILC that can be focal and quite subtle (e-**Fig. 18.28**), especially on needle biopsy. In such difficult cases, the use of E-cadherin can be potentially useful (*Future Oncol.* 2009;5:233). Intraepithelial macrophages can mimic lobular neoplasia; however, microscopic examination at higher magnification can resolve these issues (e-**Fig. 18.89**).

VII. **THE ROLE OF BIOMARKERS IN BREAST CANCER.** The role of biomarkers in establishing the prognosis and the management of patients with breast cancer cannot be overemphasized. Established biomarkers such as estrogen (ER) and progesterone (PgR) receptors have been used both as prognostic factors and as predictors of response to endocrine therapy in patients with breast cancer. More recently, human epidermal growth factor receptor 2 (HER2) was added to this list as a prognostic factor (marker of poor outcome), and as a predictor of response to certain chemotherapeutic regimens including trastuzumab (a monoclonal antibody against the HER2 receptor). Currently, evaluation of these biomarkers in patients with invasive carcinoma is considered standard of care. Additional biomarkers have changed breast cancer treatment in the past decade and have the potential of enabling individualized therapies to different molecular subgroups. The shift toward an earlier diagnosis of breast cancer due to improved imaging methods and screening programs highlights the need for biomarker discovery to quantify the residual risk of patients to indicate the potential value of novel treatment strategies. With the introduction of high-throughput technologies, numerous multigene signatures have been identified that have the potential to outperform traditional markers (*Endocr Relat Cancer.* 2010;17:R245).

A. Estrogen and progesterone receptors. The estrogen receptor belongs to a family of nuclear hormone receptors that function as transcription factors when they are bound to their respective ligands. Estrogen and progesterone receptors are parts of complex signaling pathways, which interact with multiple survival and proliferation pathways in the cell and play a critical role in the development and progression of breast cancer. They have proven usefulness as prognostic factors, and more importantly as predictive factors, in the clinical management of breast cancer. There is growing evidence that patients with endocrine-responsive breast cancers benefit less from adjuvant chemotherapy.

Assessment of ER and PgR status is an important task in the evaluation of breast cancer and is mandated in every primary carcinoma, as well as metastatic tumors if the result could influence decision making. Approximately 70% to 80% of the breast carcinomas are ER/PgR positive. Immunohistochemistry is the first-line attempt in evaluating hormone–receptor status, although it can be highly affected by a variety of preanalytic factors, including time of tissue fixation and the antigen retrieval method (*J Clin Oncol.* 2010;28:2784). The expression of PgR is strongly dependent on the presence of ER and is reflective of a functioning ER pathway. Tumors expressing PgR but not the ER are uncommon and represent <1% of all the breast cancer cases in some large series; therefore, retesting of the ER status in this setting is recommended to eliminate false ER negativity. In rare cases of solely PgR-positive tumors, the patients still benefit from endocrine therapy. Recently, quantitative methods for RNA-based assays (21-gene assay) have been established for ER and PgR quantification. These quantitative assays have potential advantages compared to IHC methods and may become the assays of choice in the future.

Several studies have shown excellent concordance rate between evaluation of biomarkers on needle core tissue and excisional specimen (*Acta Oncol.* 2008;47:38; *Ann Oncol.* 2009;20:1948; *Clin Breast Cancer.* 2010;10:154; *Cancer Sci.* 2010;101:2074). Because of better fixation of the needle core tissue, and the potential for guiding subsequent therapy, immunohistochemical assessment of hormone receptors and HER2 status is best performed on needle biopsy material if available. In cases of negative hormone receptors on core biopsy material, reevaluation of the excisional specimen may be warranted to exclude a negative result due to tumor heterogeneity. To minimize the effect of preanalytic variables on test results, the ASCO/CAP recommended using only 10% NBF as a fixative and controlling the formalin fixation time between 6 and 48 hours.

The ASCO/CAP has recommended an algorithmic approach to assess hormonal status. To standardize immunohistochemical evaluation of breast carcinoma, several scoring systems incorporating both intensity and percentage of staining have been established. In general, to obtain benefit from hormonal treatment, a sample should demonstrate nuclear staining in at least 1% of the tumor cells (e-**Fig. 18.90**) (*J Clin Oncol.* 2010;28:2784).

B. **Human epidermal growth factor receptor 2 (HER2).** ERBB2 protein is a receptor thyrosine kinase, which is a member of the epidermal growth factor receptor (EGFR) family of thyrosine kinase proteins. It is a membranous protein that is expressed in all epithelial cells at low levels. The HER2/neu oncogene is involved in the regulation of cell proliferation, survival, motility, and invasion, and is overexpressed in about 20% of the breast cancers. ERBB2 amplification is an independent prognostic marker of poor outcome in the absence of adjuvant treatment and has been associated with an increased rate of metastasis, decreased time to recurrence, and decreased overall survival. As a predictive marker, it has been associated with responsiveness to anthracycline-based therapy and trastuzumab. Immunohistochemistry and in situ hybridization are the most common methods to evaluate HER2 status; they determine protein overexpression and gene amplification, respectively. Immunohistochemistry is a simple, rapid, and inexpensive method to assess HER2 protein overexpression on formalin-fixed tissues, and the ASCO/CAP has recommended an algorithmic approach whereby cases are initially tested by immunohistochemistry. Positive for overexpression (3+) is characterized by a uniform, intense membranous staining of >30% of the invasive tumor cells (e-**Fig. 18.91**). A negative result is an IHC staining of 0, defined by lack of any membranous staining, or 1+, weak partial membranous staining (e-**Fig. 18.92**). Equivocal results (2+) are defined as complete membranous staining that is either nonuniform or weak in intensity but with obvious circumferential distribution in at least 10% of the invasive tumor cells (e-**Fig. 18.93**), or intense, complete membranous staining of 30% or fewer of tumor cells. As with hormone receptors, tissue handling, fixation, and processing can greatly affect immunoreactivity of tissue samples. However, well-calibrated immunohistochemistry can identify the majority of cases as positive or negative. According to this algorithmic approach, indeterminate IHC results (2+) are evaluated by fluorescence in situ hybridization (FISH) to determine gene amplification status (e-**Fig. 18.94**) (*Arch Pathol Lab Med.* 2007;131:18; *Arch Pathol Lab Med.* 2009;133:775) (since the initial guidelines were published, chromogenic in situ hybridization (CISH) has also been approved by the Food and Drug Administration (FDA) for the same purpose). There should be a high concordance rate (>95%) between ERBB2 protein overexpression by immunohistochemistry and gene amplification by FISH/CISH.

C. **Other immunohistochemical prognostic markers.** Among other markers, proliferation markers such as Ki67/MIB1 have been used as markers of poor outcome. Ki-67 is reported as the percentage of tumor cell nuclei that are positive, however, the lack of standardized methodology and specific cutoff values limits its value. TP53 tumor suppressor gene mutation has also been associated with a worse outcome. Neither test has been recommended as a prognostic marker for routine use.

D. **Multiparameter-based markers.** Recent expression profiling studies of breast cancer have indicated the existence of at least four molecularly distinct types of breast cancer, which may originate from different cell types (*Nature.* 2000;406:747). These subtypes differ in regards to their patterns of gene expression, clinical features, response to treatment, and outcome, and are termed luminal A, luminal B, HER2, and basal-like, respectively.

Luminal A and B cancers (accounting for approximately 70% of the breast cancers) are characterized by expression of ER. They also express cytokeratin 8 and 18, typical of the mammary gland. Luminal A tumors are mostly histologically low grade, while luminal B tumors tend to be of higher grade; in general, compared with other subtypes, they have a better prognosis. Some of the luminal B cancers may overexpress HER2. Both luminal A and B cancers tend to respond to hormonal therapy, but luminal B cancers show a better response to chemotherapeutic agents than luminal A.

HER2-associated cancers (accounting for 15% of the breast cancers) show high expression of HER2 and low expression of ER and ER-regulated genes. They are usually ER and PgR-negative and are more likely to be high grade and involve axillary lymph nodes.

Basal-like cancers show high expression of basal epithelial genes (basal cytokeratins such as CK 5/6 and CK 17) and low expression of ER, PgR, and HER2 genes, the reason for calling these tumors triple-negative carcinomas. This subtype is especially common in African-American women, has a poor prognosis, and is the most common phenotype in BRCA1-associated breast cancers. These tumors are not amenable to treatment by endocrine therapy or trastuzumab (*Nature.* 2000;406:747).

These results are significant in the sense that they show, although breast cancer shows significant heterogeneity, from a biologic point of view many tumors can be classified into particular groups on the basis of genetic similarities, with gene signatures that correlate with clinical outcome and response to chemotherapy. On the basis of genomic profiling data, several genomic tests have been developed with the intent of providing even stronger prognostic information. A 70-gene signature has been developed to predict the risk of recurrence within 5 years in node-negative, ER-positive, or negative patients; this test is able to accurately classify tumors into good or poor prognostic categories (*Nature.* 2002;415:530; *N Engl J Med.* 2002;347:1999), is performed on fresh frozen tissue, and has FDA approval for clinical use as a prognostic test. Similarly, a 21-gene signature assay has been designed to predict the risk of distant recurrence in patients with ER-positive early breast cancer (stage I and II) who are receiving tamoxifen; it also predicts the benefit from chemotherapy treatment in node-negative, ER-positive patients. This test is done on formalin-fixed paraffin-embedded tissue and is based on real-time polymerase chain reaction (PCR) measurement of the expression of 16 genes with known significance in breast cancer; the results are used to calculate a recurrence score (RS) that is predictive of overall survival independent of age and tumor size, which classifies patients into groups with a low (<10%), intermediate (10% to 30%), or high (>30%) risk of 10-year distant recurrence. Another 76-gene assay has been developed for use on node-negative breast cancers (*PNAS.* 2003;100:10393; *Expert Rev Mol Diagn.* 2004;4:169; *N Eng J Med.* 2009;360:790) the 76 genes used in the assay do not overlap with the genes used in 70-gene or 21-gene assays.

The above assays can only be performed by specific companies that have patented the test, and quality assurance must be maintained within the company. Nonetheless, in current practice, histologic typing of breast tumors still remains the gold standard for classification of breast carcinoma.

VIII. **INTRADUCTAL PROLIFERATIVE LESIONS.** Intraductal proliferative lesions that **carry an increased risk** include atypical ductal hyperplasia (ADH) and atypical lobule hyperplasia.

    A.

       1. **Atypical ductal hyperplasia (ADH)** is a term used to describe an intraductal proliferation with some of the cytologic and/or architectural features of low-grade DCIS, which qualitatively or quantitatively falls short of diagnosis of DCIS. Examples of ADH include a duct partially involved by a uniform cell population resembling LG-DCIS (e-**Figs. 18.95 and 18.96**), or a duct that is focally expanded by a uniform cell population with geometric

spaces (e-Figs. 18.97 and 18.98). Quantitatively, there are a variety of arbitrary criteria for distinction of ADH from LG-DCIS (<2 mm or <2 duct spaces) (*Am J Surg Pathol.* 1992;16:1133; *Hum Pathol.* 1992;23:1095). While there is agreement on the importance of the extent of the lesion for this distinction, there is no widely accepted size cutoff (e-Fig. 18.99). While a diagnosis of DCIS confers a 10-fold risk of later developing IBC, and ADH confers a four- to fivefold risk, they are both on a continuum of the same neoplastic process. A diagnosis of ADH made on a core needle biopsy is usually followed by excision, as studies have shown that depending on the technique of the biopsy and size of the needle, a follow-up excision is associated with an in situ or invasive carcinoma in 20% to 40% of these cases (*Adv Anat Pathol.* 2003;10:113; *Breast.* 2011;20:50). It should be noted that a diagnosis of ADH is only conferred to lesions with low-grade nuclear cytology; intermediate and high-grade DCIS should be diagnosed as such regardless of their size.

2. **Aypical lobular hyperplasia (ALH)** differs from LCIS with regard to the degree of lobular involvement and expansion (e-Figs. 18.100 to 18.102). ALH and LCIS are also on a continuum of the same neoplastic process. While ALH is associated with sixfold increased risk of invasive carcinoma, LCIS is associated with 12-fold increase in risk.

B. Several intraductal proliferative lesions do not carry an increased risk.

1. **Usual ductal hyperplasia** (UDH) is characterized by proliferation of a heterogeneous epithelial cell population with a tendency to bridge across, fill, and distend duct lumens. Haphazard placement of cells of variable size and shape (both epithelial and myoepithelial), variable spacing of the cells often with prominent streaming and/or swirling, indistinct cell borders, and irregular and usually peripheral secondary spaces are all features of UDH that distinguish it from low-grade DCIS (e-Fig. 18.103). Bridges formed in UDH are usually not rigid, and show stretching with a central attenuation. Immunohistochemically, UDH is usually positive for high molecular weight keratin (e-Fig. 18.104) unlike most examples of DCIS. UDH is not a direct precursor of breast cancer; however, if florid, it is a marker of low increased risk of breast cancer (1.5- to 2-fold), and it is usually not acted upon clinically.

2. **Columnar cell hyperplasia (CCH).** The enlargement of normal TDLUs by hyperplastic epithelial cells is one of the most common abnormalities of growth in the adult female human breast (*Adv Anat Pathol.* 2003;10:113; *Semin Diagn Pathol.* 2004;21:18; *Am J Pathol.* 2007;171:252; *Histopathology.* 2008;52:11). These lesions have been called by many names over the years (*Semin Diagn Pathol.* 2004;21:18), but currently they are most commonly referred to as columnar cell lesions (CCLs) or CCH. CCHs are often multifocal, bilateral, and up to 100-fold larger than the TDLUs they evolve from. The majority of CCH are lined by one or two layers of monotonous, crowded columnar epithelial cells (e-Figs. 18.105 to 18.107), but many exhibit more diverse histologic features contributing to the complex terminology that has evolved to describe them.

It is currently unknown whether the cytologic atypia occasionally observed in CCH is associated with significantly higher risk for developing breast cancer than the majority of cases that are without atypia, although in some preliminary studies up to 20% of the cases with atypia identified on core biopsies are associated with cancer in follow-up excisions, a worrisome association that has lead some authors to advocate follow-up excisions in this setting (*Am J Surg Pathol.* 2005;29:734; *Histopathology.* 2008;52:11). However, not all studies find a significant relationship between CCH with atypia and cancer. It seems likely that some CCH may indeed represent relatively high-risk lesions, but it is possible that histologic features alone may not always be sufficient to identify them.

IX. **COMMON BENIGN ABNORMALITIES.** The breast can be involved in a large number of benign abnormalities. While these findings do not harbor clinical importance in terms of breast cancer risk, familiarity with their morphologic features is important to distinguish them from more clinically significant abnormalities. Only the most common findings are briefly discussed.

A. **Fat necrosis.** Although fat necrosis can result from trauma, most cases are idiopathic, or are secondary prior to surgery or radiotherapy. It clinically and mammographically can mimic invasive carcinoma. Histologically, a cellular inflammatory response composed of foamy macrophages and foreign body giant cells is seen infiltrating the fat (e-**Figs. 18.108 and 18.109**). In later stages, fibrosis and dystrophic calcification may be seen.

B. **Duct ectasia** usually presents in middle-aged women as pain and nipple discharge, with or without an associated mass lesion. It is characterized by dilation of the major duct system, often with luminal amorphous material and complete filling and distention by intraepithelial foamy macrophages (e-**Fig. 18.110**). There is usually associated fibrosis and periductal chronic inflammation.

C. **Microcysts and apocrine changes.** Cystic dilation of the breast TDLUs (as opposed to the major duct system in duct ectasia) is quite common and can produce marked expansion and, especially when associated with microcalcification or fibrosis, can result in mammographically detectable and/or palpable lesions. Histologically, these cysts are usually lined by flat nonatypical epithelium (e-**Fig. 18.111**). Apocrine metaplasia is a very common change that occurs in these cystic lesions (as well as normal TDLUs), usually as an incidental finding; it is usually found in premenopausal women and is often part of the so-called fibrocystic changes. Histologically, apocrine change is characterized by eosinophilic cells with abundant finely granular cytoplasm and rounded nuclei, often with a prominent nucleoli (e-**Fig. 18.112**). A papillary architecture is sometimes evident.

D. **Fibroadenoma** is a very common benign lesion of the breast that presents as a mass or radiographic abnormality, more commonly in younger women. On mammogram, it usually presents as a round, well-circumscribed mass. Grossly, fibroadenomas are grayish-white, firm, well-circumscribed, lobulated masses. Histologically, they are composed of a biphasic growth of variably cellular spindle cell stroma, with cleft-like (intracanalicular) (e-**Fig. 18.113**) or tubular glandular (pericanalicular) (e-**Fig. 18.114**) growth patterns. The glandular elements are composed of two cell layers, an inner epithelial layer and an outer myoepithelial cell layer (e-**Figs. 18.115 and 18.116**). Some fibroadenomas, especially those arising in the second decade of life, can grow rapidly and appear quite cellular (an appearance that overlaps with benign phyllodes tumor); such lesions have been termed cellular fibroadenomas. Myxoid fibroadenomas display prominent myxoid changes in the stroma and rarely may be a component of Carney syndrome (primary adrenocortical hypercortisolism, skin hyperpigmentation, and a variety of nonendocrine and endocrine tumors). Fibroadenomas may undergo secondary changes such as infarction or prominent hyalinization of the stroma (e-**Fig. 18.117**), with or without calcification (the former is usually seen with pregnancy, whereas the latter is more often seen in elderly patients with a longstanding lesion). In addition, almost all of the epithelial changes that arise in the breast can secondarily develop in fibroadenomas including various metaplasias, epithelial hyperplasia, sclerosing adenosis, DCIS, LCIS, and invasive carcinoma (e-**Figs. 18.118 and 18.119**). Fibroadenomas with significant epithelial proliferation have been termed complex fibroadenomas. The main differential diagnosis of fibroadenoma is a benign phyllodes tumor.

Phyllodes tumor is much less common than fibroadenoma, accounting for <3% of the fibroepithelial lesions. As mentioned above, the main feature distinguishing phyllodes tumor from fibroadenoma is the presence of the characteristic leaf-like architectural pattern produced by extensive branching of the epithelial component. Stromal hypercellularity is the rule, often with accentuation near the epithelial clefts. Phyllodes tumor can be divided into benign (e-**Fig. 18.120**), borderline (e-**Fig. 18.121**), and malignant (e-**Fig. 18.122**) categories; the first two are only distinguished by the degree of cellular atypia and mitotic activity. A focally infiltrative border can be seen in borderline phyllodes tumor. Malignant phyllodes tumor shows a prominent infiltrative border, unequivocal sarcomatous areas, and stromal overgrowth (areas of stroma devoid of epithelium). Heterologous sarcomatous elements may also be occasionally present in malignant tumors. Overall, about 20% of the phyllodes tumors recur (ranging from 17% for benign tumors to 27% in malignant tumors) and 10% metastasize (0%, 4%, and 22% of benign, borderline, and malignant tumors, respectively). Recurrences can be associated with grade progression. Phyllodes tumors are extremely rare and their comprehensive diagnostic features can be found in more specialized texts.

E. **Intraductal papillomas** usually show an arborizing growth pattern of fibrovascular cores covered by two layers of cells, one layer of myoepithelial cells overlying a layer of nonatypical epithelial cells (e-**Figs. 18.123 to 18.125**). Intraductal papillomas are generally categorized into two groups: central papillomas, which are usually solitary papillomas, which involve large lactiferous ducts of the nipple; and peripheral papillomas, which are smaller papillomas that involve TDLUs and are usually multiple. Central papillomas generally present as a mass or with nipple discharge. Peripheral papillomas present as incidental findings or sometimes as a mammographic abnormality. Secondary hemorrhagic infarction, squamous or apocrine metaplasia, and extensive sclerosis (sclerosing papilloma) can sometimes be seen (e-**Figs. 18.126 and 18.127**). Intraductal papillomas and related lesions can secondarily be involved by other different intraepithelial proliferations including UDH, ADH, DCIS, and LCIS. In the absence of any secondary neoplastic proliferation, primary excision is an adequate treatment for papillomas.

F. **Sclerosing adenosis.** This relatively common lesion is often incidental and admixed with proliferative lesions. However, it can present mammographically with calcification and/or architectural distortion, or clinically as a mass termed "adenosis tumor" or "nodular sclerosing adenosis." Sclerosing adenosis is characterized by a lobulocentric proliferation of tubular glands (adenosis) accompanied by a fibrotic (sclerosing) stromal proliferation (e-**Fig. 18.128**). The fact that the glands/tubules are markedly compressed and often obliterated renders identification of a dual cell layer sometimes difficult (e-**Fig. 18.129**). Accordingly, the main differential diagnosis is invasive (usually tubular) carcinoma, which may be difficult to exclude on small biopsies, especially in areas in which sclerosing adenosis has a pattern mimicking perineural invasion, or is secondarily involved by a neoplastic intraepithelial proliferation such as ADH, DCIS (e-**Figs. 18.130 and 18.131**), or LCIS. Elongated and compressed (as opposed to angulated) tubules, lack of a cellular desmoplastic stroma, and a lobulocentric pattern of growth are useful diagnostic features. If in doubt, immunohistochemical demonstration of myoepithelial cells can additionally exclude an invasive process.

G. **Radial scar/complex sclerosing lesions** are characterized by a central fibrous/fibroelastotic scar from which a stellate arrangement of benign ducts/lobules radiates (e-**Figs. 18.132 to 18.134**). Associated hyperplastic or neoplastic epithelial proliferations are often identified. In addition to their microscopic pseudoinfiltrative nature, these lesions may also be clinically, radiologically, or grossly confused with invasive carcinoma due to their fibrotic nature and their characteristic stellate/spiculated appearance. Nevertheless, excisional biopsy is still recommended after a diagnosis of radial scar of needle biopsy because of the occasional presence of associated unsampled DCIS or invasive carcinoma at the periphery of the lesions.

X. **LYMPH NODE STATUS.** The presence of metastatic tumor deposits in axillary lymph nodes as determined microscopically is a highly unfavorable prognostic feature, as are a high number of involved nodes and (to a lesser degree) large size of the deposits. Nodal status (N) is so powerful prognostically that it plays a major role in determining therapy.

The pathology report should include the total number of examined lymph nodes, the number of positive lymph nodes, size of metastasis, and the presence or absence of extranodal extension by tumor deposits (the presence of extranodal extension is an indicator of tumor recurrence and its presence may dictate additional radiation therapy). According to the TNM staging system, assessment of the size of metastasis is important in determining the stage: ITCs are clusters of tumor cells <0.2 mm or <200 cells (e-**Fig. 18.135**); micrometastasis is defined as metastatic deposits that measure between 0.2 and 2.0 mm, or >200 cells in one cross section; macrometastasis is defined as a metastatic focus >2.0 mm (Table 18.2). For staging purposes, lymph nodes with a micrometastasis are counted towards total number of positive nodes if at least one lymph node with macrometastasis is present; nodes that only show ITCs should not be counted in the total number of positive nodes. Cancer nodules in axillary tissue without histologic evidence of classical lymph node are classified as regional lymph node metastasis unless they are surrounded by breast tissue or DCIS to imply a separate focus of invasive carcinoma.

Histologically, involvement of axillary lymph nodes by metastatic carcinoma is most frequently manifested within the subcapsular sinuses with or without sinusoidal involvement (e-**Figs. 18.136 and 18.137**). However, metastases in ILC most commonly appear as scattered individual tumor cells within the parenchyma and sinusoids. In all of these situations, the size of the largest deposit should be measured and reported.

There are a few pitfalls in the evaluation of axillary lymph nodes for metastatic carcinoma. Awareness of these pitfalls will minimize the risk of overdiagnosis. **Heterotopic epithelial elements** including heterotopic breast tissue are rare findings that can occasionally be seen in axillary lymph nodes (e-**Fig. 18.138**). The heterotopic tissue is subject to all changes that can occur in breast tissue in the mammary gland itself. The presence of myoepithelial cells and sometimes specialized stroma can be helpful diagnostic features. **Nevus cell aggregates** are capsular aggregates of nevus cells that are infrequently identified in axillary lymph nodes (e-**Fig. 18.139**); they usually present as nests of epithelioid cells within the lymph node capsule. The diagnosis of nevus aggregates can easily be substantiated by a combination of S-100 and/or HMB45 immunoreactivity and a negative reaction with cytokeratin antibodies.

Cytopathology of the Breast

Lourdes R. Ylagan

I. METHODS OF SPECIMEN PROCUREMENT
A. **FNA** of palpable and nonpalpable breast lesions through mammographic guidance is currently accepted as a cost-effective, reliable, and accurate tool in the

evaluation of breast lesions. The combination of mammographic features, clinical findings, and cytologic evaluation of breast FNA specimens (the so-called triple test) has considerably decreased the false diagnosis rate of breast cancer.

B. **Ductal lavage** has recently been employed as a screening method in women with a personal history of breast cancer, but the sensitivity and accuracy of the approach for detecting premalignant lesions of the breast ductal epithelium is still under investigation (*Clin Lab Med*. 2005;25:787; *Am J Surg*. 2006;191:57).

II. **SPECIMEN ADEQUACY.** There is no uniform criterion on which specimen adequacy can be determined, even in the presence of well-preserved and well-visualized breast epithelium (e-**Fig. 18.140**), without taking into consideration the experience of the aspirator and/or interpreter, clinical presentation, and mammographic findings of the individual mass.

III. **DIAGNOSTIC CATEGORIES**

A. **Negative for malignancy.** This diagnosis is generally rendered for benign breast lesions, including inflammatory or infectious lesions, that are without clinical or mammographic findings suspicious for malignancy.

B. **Atypical cytology.** This diagnosis is rendered on cellular lesions showing some degree of nuclear atypia; the cells generally maintain a well-organized pattern (e-**Fig. 18.141**).

C. **Suspicious for malignancy.** This diagnosis is rendered when the aspirate shows cells with worrisome cytologic features that fall short of those required for a diagnosis of malignancy.

D. **Positive for malignancy.** This diagnosis is rendered when both the quality of the cytologic changes and the quantity of the malignant cells are sufficient for an unequivocal diagnosis of malignancy.

IV. **CYTOLOGIC FEATURES OF COMMON BREAST LESIONS**

A. **Fibroadenoma** is a clinically well-circumscribed nodule with a homogeneous mammographic appearance. Cytologically, it is composed of benign ductal cells arranged in a staghorn pattern with abundant myoepithelial cells (e-**Fig. 18.142**). Abundant stromal fragments may be seen.

B. **Gynecomastia** is clinically a well-circumscribed and often painful subareolar lesion in a man. The lesion has mammographic and cytologic findings that are similar to those of a fibroadenoma (e-**Fig. 18.142**).

C. **Fibrocystic changes** typically present as a palpable, ill-defined lesion, which may have mammographically detectable microcalcifications. Cytologically, the lesion is composed of apocrine, ductal cells, mucus, and muciphages in varying amounts (e-**Fig. 18.143**).

D. **Subareolar abscess** is a clinically painful, palpable subareolar mass typically associated with lactation. Cytologically, it consists of neutrophils and benign anucleate squamous epithelium (e-**Fig. 18.144**).

E. **Ductal adenocarcinoma** usually presents as a clinically palpable, mammographically suspicious mass, which cytologically shows a cellular smear containing large ductal cells, which maybe poorly cohesive, without a myoepithelial component. The cells have pleomorphic nuclei, vesicular chromatin, and prominent nucleoli. Individual cells may have intracytoplasmic vacuoles containing inspissated material (e-**Fig. 18.145**).

F. **Lobular adenocarcinoma** may not be clinically palpable, but presents mammographically as an ill-defined mass lesion. Cytologic preparations show singly dispersed small plasmacytoid cells with vacuolated cytoplasm often containing inspissated material. The nuclei are uniformly small, round-to-oval, and not much bigger than a neutrophil (e-**Fig. 18.146**).

V. **SPECIAL STUDIES.** Immunocytologic evaluation of estrogen and progesterone receptor studies can be performed on cytospin slide preparations. Immunocytologic evaluation of HER2 on cytospin slide preparations is limited due to the requirement of an intact cell membrane for proper assessment. Immunohistochemical evaluation of these markers can also be performed on paraffin-embedded cell block samples prepared from fine needle aspirates. FISH for HER2 gene amplification can be performed on cytospin slide preparations or paraffin-embedded cell blocks.

SUGGESTED READINGS

Dabbs DJ. *Breast Pathology*. Philadelphia: Elsevier; 2012.

Mckee GT. *Cytopathology of the Breast with Imaging and Histologic Correlation*. Oxford: Oxford University Press; 2002.

O'Malley FP, Pinder SE, Mulligan AM. *Breast Pathology: A Volume in the Foundations in Diagnostic Pathology series*. 2nd ed. Philadelphia: Elsevier Saunders; 2011.

Page DL, Anderson TJ. *Diagnostic Histopathology of the Breast*. Edinburg: Churchill Livingstone; 1987.

Rosen PP. *Rosen's Breast Pathology*. 3rd ed. Philadelphia: Lippincott Williams & Wilkins; 2009.

Schnitt SJ, Collins LC. *Biopsy Interpretation of the Breast*. Philadelphia: Lippincott Williams & Wilkins; 2009.

Tavassoli FA. *Pathology of the Breast*. 2nd ed. Chicago: McGraw-Hill; 1999.

Tavassoli FA, Devilee P. *World Health Organization Classification of Tumors: Tumors of Breast and Female Genital Organs*. Lyon: IARC press; 2003.

Tavassoli FA, Eusebi V. *AFIP Atlas of Tumor Pathology, Series 4, Tumors of the Mammary Gland*. Silver Spring, MD: ARP press; 2009.

Zakhou H, Wells C, Perry NM. *Diagnostic Cytopathology of the Breast*. London: Churchill Livingstone; 1999.

19 Medical Diseases of the Kidney

Joseph P. Gaut and Helen Liapis

I. **MEDICAL RENAL BIOPSY HANDLING AND PROCESSING.** This chapter covers medical renal biopsies; biopsy for diagnosis of renal masses is covered in Chapter 20. Renal allograft biopsy pathology is added at the end of this chapter. Renal biopsies are usually received in transport media, allowing distribution of tissue for light microscopy (LM), immunofluorescence (IF), and electron microscopy (EM).

A. **Light microscopy.** A minimum of three hematoxylin and eosin (H&E), one trichrome, two periodic acid-Schiff (PAS) stains, and one Jones silver-stained section is required. A minimum of seven glomeruli and one artery is required for adequate LM evaluation.

B. **Immunofluorescence.** A minimum of two glomeruli is required. A direct IF method is routinely used employing a panel of antibodies, including anti-IgG, IgA, IgM, C3, C1q, fibrinogen, albumin, and kappa and lambda light chains. It is important to document the staining pattern (linear vs. granular) and distribution (mesangial, loop, or combined).

C. **Electron microscopy.** Ultrastructural evaluation of two glomeruli is recommended. EM allows for evaluation of cellular and extracellular abnormalities in the glomeruli, tubules, interstitium, and vessels. EM is very useful in confirming the presence and distribution of electron-dense deposits, which can be located in the mesangium or the glomerular capillary basement membrane. In the basement membrane, electron-dense deposits can be subepithelial, subendothelial, or intramembranous (surrounded by basement membrane).

II. **GLOMERULAR DISEASES.** Glomerular diseases may be primary or secondary (associated with systemic diseases). Patients can be grouped into those that present with nephrotic syndrome (>3 g urine protein/day), nephritic syndrome (proteinuria + hematuria), or isolated hematuria. It is important for the pathologist to have access to patient's clinical and laboratory data. For example, minimal change disease (MCD), focal segmental glomerulosclerosis, and membranous glomerulonephritis (GN) usually present with nephrotic syndrome. In contrast, postinfectious GN usually presents with nephritic syndrome.

A. **MCD/focal segmental glomerulosclerosis (FSGS).** MCD and FSGS are the most common causes of nephrotic syndrome in children and are also common in adults, affecting about 10% to 20% of patients with kidney disease. Primary

FSGS may be idiopathic, secondary, or familial (*Am J Nephrol*. 2003;23:353). Less than nephrotic range proteinuria may be present in advanced cases. Some patients have concurrent hematuria and hypertension (HTN).

The classic findings in MCD (Table 19.1) are as follows:

LM: Normal-appearing glomeruli

IF: Negative

EM: Extensive foot process effacement (**e-Fig. 19.1**).*

The diagnostic features of FSGS are as follows:

LM: Segmental sclerosis in some but not all glomeruli. Accurate diagnosis of FSGS depends on the extent of the disease and the number of glomeruli present in the biopsy. Diagnosis may be missed because of sampling error, particularly with the smaller needles currently used. It has been estimated that in a biopsy containing 10 glomeruli, there is a 35% chance of missing FSGS. Notably, even one glomerulus with FSGS is sufficient for diagnosis. The corticomedullary glomeruli are the first to be sclerosed; therefore, needle biopsies should opt to sample this region.

IF: Is either entirely negative or has focal and weak mesangial C3 or IgM immunoglobulin deposits.

EM: Shows focal foot process effacement (**e-Fig. 19.2**), the degree of which may depend on the degree of proteinuria. Other EM findings in MCD/FSGS include microvillus transformation of foot processes, endothelial cell edema, podocyte detachment, and glomerular basement membrane (GBM) wrinkling (see **e-Fig. 19.2F**).

Beyond this classic presentation, light and electron microscopic findings may be similar in MCD and FSGS. For example, glomeruli may appear normal in FSGS and focal foot process effacement may be present in MCD.

Glomerular hypercellularity and enlargement (glomerulomegaly) is thought to represent an early lesion of FSGS. A recent FSGS classification scheme describes various histologic patterns with significantly different prognosis (*Kidney Int*. 1990;38:115). Glomerulomegaly is rare (seen in only about 3% of FSGS), but the following variants are more frequent: perihilar FSGS (26%), tip lesion (17%), usual type not otherwise specified (NOS) (42%), and collapsing FSGS (11%) (see **e-Fig. 19.2A–E**) (*Am J Kidney Dis*. 2004;43:368). The tip and cellular lesions have the best prognosis and collapsing FSGS the worst (*Kidney Int*. 2006;69:920). Tubulointerstitial damage and vascular thickening indicate chronic disease. Pathologic similarities between MCD and FSGS initially suggested that they were one disease with a spectrum of findings, but recent clinical and molecular studies have demonstrated that FSGS has worse prognosis and different pathogenesis.

B. Collapsing FSGS is a distinct FSGS variant considered by some to be an entirely different disease.

LM: Characterized by segmental glomerular capillary collapse and podocyte hypertrophy, often accompanied by microcystic tubular dilatation and interstitial inflammation (see **e-Fig. 19.2E**). The main difference from usual FSGS is the collapse of the loops versus sclerosis, and podocyte proliferation versus podocyte loss.

IF: Nonspecific.

EM: Shows proliferating podocytes and wrinkled/collapsed capillary loops. Clinically, it is characterized by black racial predominance, a high incidence of nephrotic syndrome, and rapidly progressive renal failure. First identified in HIV patients, collapsing FSGS was later recognized in association with viruses such as Parvovirus 19 and hepatitis B and C, and with pamidronate chemotherapy

---

*All e-figures are available online via the Solution Site Image Bank.

TABLE 19.1 Major Glomerular Patterns and Differential Diagnosis on Light Microscopy

Minimal changes	FSGS	Mesangial hypercellularity	Thick loops	Tram-track	Proliferative	Crescents	Nodular pattern
Minimal change disease	Primary NOS	IgA-HSP, MCD/FSGS	Membranous	MPGN	Postinfectious GN	>50% = crescentic	Diabetes
Thin membrane disease	Secondary NOS	Lupus	Diabetes	HSP	Lupus	<50% = other GN	MPGN
Early lupus	Cellular type	IgM nephropathy	Alport	Lupus	HSP		Amyloidosis
Early/mild IgA	Perihilar	C1q nephropathy	Amyloidosis				MIDD
Early diabetes	Tip lesion	C₃/IgG glomerulopathy					
	Collapsing						

FSGS, focal segmental glomerulonephritis; GN, glomerulonephritis; NOS, not otherwise specified, IG, immunoglobulin; HSP, Henoch-Schönlein purpura; MCD, minimal change disease; MPGN, membranoproliferative glomerulonephritis; MIDD, monoclonal immunoglobulin deposition disease.

(*Semin Diagn Pathol.* 2002;19:106). It is an aggressive and difficult to treat disease (*Semin Nephrol.* 2003;23:209), and may also involve the allograft kidney. Pathogenesis involves podocyte cell cycle dysregulation resulting in proliferation.

C. **Mesangial proliferative glomerulonephritis (IGA, IgM, IgG and C3).** Mesangial hypercellularity is defined as more than three mesangial cells per glomerular segment; many glomerular diseases may have increased mesangial cells (Table 19.1) including variants of MCD and FSGS. Mesangial hypercellularity indicates mesangial immune deposits and/or reactive proliferation. The most common disease is IgA nephropathy, clinically characterized by micro or macrohematuria and varying proteinuria (rarely nephrotic syndrome or crescentic GN) (*Nephrol Dial Transplant.* 2001;16 Suppl 6:77).

LM: Mesangial hypercellularity varies from focal to diffuse.

IF: Diagnosis is made by the presence of predominant or co-dominant IgA mesangial deposits (e-**Fig. 19.3**). Mild IgG and IgM deposits may also be present, particularly in Henoch–Schönlein purpura (HSP), which is thought of as the systemic form of IgA.

EM: Shows mesangial/paramesangial deposits and occasionally capillary loop, subendothelial deposits that may extend to the GBM and cause splitting (more common in HSP), or "humps."

Histological parameters which negatively affect prognosis in IgA disease include glomerular sclerosis, capillary wall IgA deposits, and vascular and tubulointerstitial fibrosis. Glomerular sclerosis is the best independent predictor of adverse outcome and renal failure. HSP mimics IgA pathologically, but clinically is a systemic disease that presents with skin rash, arthritis, and abdominal pain in addition to nephritis. IgA is the most common glomerular disease worldwide with variable prognosis (~30% develop end-stage renal disease [ESRD]). HSP tends to be self-limiting with only about 18% of patients progressing to ESRD. Both may recur in transplant kidneys, but clinical symptoms are mild despite IgA deposition.

Mesangial hypercellularity not infrequently accompanies various types of GN. For example, MCD and/or FSGS with mesangial hypercellularity are generally thought to have a worse prognosis. Focal IgM deposits are seen in some such cases. Rarely, diffuse IgM deposits are detected (which have raised considerable debate whether they represent a separate entity named IgM nephropathy).

An entity known as *C1q nephropathy* is characterized by predominant C1q deposits and is considered a variant of MCD/FSGS (*Am J Clin Pathol.* 1985:83:415). C1q nephropathy is primarily a disease of children and young adults. Other glomerulopathies characterized by isolated C3 or IgG mesangial deposits in patients without lupus stigmata were described recently and named accordingly. IgG glomerulopathy is a pediatric disease that may be an aberrant manifestation of lupus nephritis (LN), and it has been proposed that it should be treated as such (JASN 2002;13:379).

Recent studies have clarified the entity known as C3 glomerulopathy, which may present with mesangial hypercellularity or minimal changes. Immunofluorescene demonstrates isolated, granular, mesangial C3 deposits without IgG or C1q staining (e-**Fig. 19.4**). Interestingly, the disease is associated with dysregulation of the alternative complement pathway secondary to defects in complement factor H (*Nat Rev Nephrol.* 2010;6:494; *Kidney Int.* 2009;75:1230).

D. **Membranous GN** is the most common cause of nephrotic syndrome in adults (30% to 50% of cases). It may occur at any age, but accounts for <5% of childhood nephrotic syndrome. Most cases are idiopathic, but ~10% are associated with identifiable causes such as malignancy, autoimmune diseases (e.g., systematic lupus erythematosus), drugs, and infections (hepatitis B, syphilis). Glomerular lesions resemble those seen in Heymann nephritis, an animal model in which antibodies react with the Heymann antigen, a complex of *megalin* and the *receptor-associated protein,* expressed in the tubular brush border and the basal surface of the visceral epithelial cells.

LM: Membranous GN is a diffuse process in which the glomeruli are not hypercellular but usually exhibit thickening of the capillary basement membrane while maintaining luminal patency. In Jones silver-stained sections, the basement membrane can show "spikes" projecting from the epithelial side of the basement membrane. Spikes result from the presence of subepithelial electron-dense deposits (silver stain negative) and deposition of basement membrane-like material on the sides of the deposits (**e-Fig. 19.5**). Glomeruli appear essentially normal in early cases.

IF: Diffuse, granular staining for IgG and C3 is present along the glomerular capillary loops by IF. Other immunoglobulins can be present but have lower intensity staining.

EM: At early stages, the electron-dense deposits are subepithelial. As the disease progresses, deposition of basement membrane-like material at the sides of the electron- dense deposits occurs so that with time, the electron-dense deposits are surrounded by basement membrane and thus becomes intramembranous. The deposits eventually become electron-lucent, suggesting resolution (**e-Fig. 19.5**).

E. Postinfectious glomerulonephritis (PIGN). PIGN is a classic complication of streptococcal pharyngitis and presents acutely with nephritic syndrome. However, classic PIGN is currently infrequent; most cases follow staphylococcal skin infections and other bacterial, viral, fungal, or parasitic infections, and are more frequently chronic or atypical (*Hum Pathol.* 2003;34:3).

LM: The pathology is unique, characterized by white cells in the glomeruli (predominantly neutrophils in the acute phase), and lymphocytes or macrophages in chronic cases.

IF: There are large granular IgG and C3 deposits along capillary loops (**e-Fig. 19.6**). Occasionally, deposits are located predominantly in the mesangium (instead of in the loops) and are C3 or IgA/IgM instead of IgG (*Semin Diagn Pathol.* 2002;19:146).

EM: Shows characteristic bell-shaped deposits (humps). Erythrogenic toxin type B is thought to be the target antigen for immune complexes that are implanted in the GBM.

F. Membranoproliferative glomerulonephritis (MPGN). Patients with MPGN can present with features of nephrotic and/or nephritic syndrome, and most patients have a low serum C3 level. Although MPGN can affect patients of all ages, it is more common in children. Three types of MPGN have been described; because all types can have similar histologic findings, EM is used to differentiate them. Type I is the most common type, followed by types II and III. It is important to note that MPGN type I can be associated with other diseases such as viral hepatitis, so patients should be worked up for secondary causes of MPGN when the pathologic diagnosis is established.

LM: MPGN is a diffuse glomerulopathy with endocapillary proliferation that results in lobular accentuation (**e-Fig. 19.7**). The GBMs are thick, and the capillary lumens are not evident. The Jones silver stain reveals double GBM contours, also known as "tram-tracking." These findings are more commonly seen in MPGN type I. MPGN type II tends to have a less consistent histologic pattern.

IF: A strong and diffuse granular staining for C3 is observed along the glomerular capillary walls and the mesangium. Approximately 60% of type I MPGN also exhibit IgG and/or C1q immunostain. Negative immunostains for immunoglobulins and C1q are usually observed in MPGN type II.

EM: This is the most useful tool for differentiating MPGN types. MPGN type I shows mesangial interposition (extension of mesangial cell cytoplasm into the capillary wall) and subendothelial electron-dense deposits. When the mesangial cell cytoplasm extends into the glomerular capillary wall, basement membrane-like material is laid down by the mesangial and endothelial cells, creating a second "new" basement membrane. This process results in the "tramtracking" observed by LM. MPGN type II is also known as dense deposit disease because it has ribbon-like electron-dense deposits along the capillary walls, often replacing the lamina densa. These deposits are not necessarily present in all capillary loops and may only be present in some segments and the mesangium. The composition of these electron-dense deposits remains uncertain. The ultrastructural findings of MPGN type III are similar to those of MPGN type I, but with subendothelial and subepithelial electron-dense deposits (e-**Fig. 19.7**).

G. **Crescentic glomerulonephritis (crescentic GN).** The term "crescentic GN" refers to the presence of cellular crescents in >50% of glomeruli available in a renal biopsy. Its usual clinical presentation is that of rapidly progressive GN. Patients can have a renal limited or systemic disease.

LM: Cellular crescents are identified in >50% of glomeruli (e-**Fig. 19.8**). Necrotizing glomerular lesions are commonly seen. Additional morphologic findings are dependent on the type of renal limited or systemic disease. Immunofluorescence is used to further classify crescentic GN.

IF: In anti-GBM disease or Goodpasture's disease, glomeruli exhibit smooth linear IgG staining along the capillary basement membrane. Immune-complex GN has a granular staining pattern for one or more immunoglobulins. Pauciimmune GN has negative immunostain for all immunoglobulins.

EM: The smooth linear IgG staining of anti-GMB or Goodpasture's disease does not have a morphologic correlation that can be detected by EM. The glomerular changes noted by EM correspond to the necrosis, disruption of the GBM, and crescents that are seen in all crescentic GN. Similar findings are also identified in pauci-immune GN. Cases of immune-complex GN will show electron-dense deposits (e-**Fig. 19.8**).

H. **Lupus nephritis (LN).** Systemic lupus erythematosus (SLE) is a multisystemic autoimmune disorder with a peak incidence in the second and third decades of life and a female predominance (male-to-female ratio of 1:9). It is more common in African-Americans. The clinical diagnosis of lupus is based on clinical and laboratory criteria established by the American Rheumatism Association. Renal involvement by the disease is relatively common; approximately half of lupus patients develop lupus nephritis during the first year of the disease. Although this chapter emphasizes the glomerular findings of (LN), interstitial, tubular, and vascular lesions can also accompany the glomerular changes. Use of the ISN/RPS classification of LN, which is a modification of the WHO classification (*Kidney Int.* 2004;65:521), is recommended.

LM: LN can present with various light microscopic patterns (Tables 19.2 and 19.3). With time and/or treatment, the renal lesion can evolve into a different class. Membranous LN can occur in combination with Class III or IV. The following are considered glomerular active lesions: endocapillary hypercellularity with/without leukocyte infiltration and with substantial luminal reduction; karyorrhexis; fibrinoid necrosis; rupture of the GBM; cellular or fibrocellular crescents; wire loops; hyaline thrombi (e-**Fig. 19.9**). The glomerular chronic lesions are segmental or global glomerulosclerosis, fibrous adhesions, and fibrous crescents.

IF: A glomerular IgG-positive immunostain is almost universal in LN; the term "full house" is used when IgG, IgA, and IgM immunostains are positive. C3 and C1q are usually present.

I. **Diabetes mellitus (DM).** DM is a disorder of carbohydrate metabolism that affects multiple organ systems. In the kidney, it increases the propensity to pyelonephritis, papillary necrosis, arteriosclerosis, and glomerular disease. Hyperglycemia in these patients induces biochemical changes in the GBM, nonenzymatic glycosylation of proteins, and hemodynamic changes with glomerular hypertrophy.

TABLE 19.2   ISN/RPS Classification of Lupus Nephritis

Class I	Minimal mesangial LN	
Class II	Mesangial proliferative LN	
Class III	Focal LN (involvement of <50% glomeruli)	
	III(A)	Focal proliferative LN (purely active lesions)
	III(A/C)	Focal proliferative and sclerosing LN (active and chronic lesions)
	III(C)	Focal sclerosing LN (chronic inactive with glomerular scars)
Class IV	Diffuse LN (Active or inactive diffuse, segmental and/or global endocapillary and/or extracapillary GN involving 50% or more glomeruli)	
	IV-S (A) or IV-G (A)	Diffuse segmental or global proliferative LN
	IV-S(A/C) or IV-G(A/C)	Diffuse segmental or global proliferative and sclerosing LN
	IV-S(C) or IV-G(C)	Diffuse segmental or global sclerosing LN
Class V	Membranous LN	
Class VI	Advanced sclerosing LN (90% or more glomeruli globally sclerosed)	

ISN/RPS, International Society of Nephrology/Renal Pathology Society; S, segmental; G, global; A, active lesions; C, chronic lesions.

Diabetic glomerulosclerosis is unlikely to develop in the absence of vascular changes in the eye fundus.

LM: GBM thickening develops in early stages. Increased mesangial matrix eventually results in diffuse glomerulosclerosis and nodular diabetic glomerulosclerosis, also known as Kimmelstiel–Wilson nodules (e-Fig. 19.10).

IF: IF studies of the renal biopsy are essentially negative. However, glomeruli exhibit a nonspecific IgG linear staining that has the same or less intensity than that observed in the albumin immunostain.

EM: This shows thickening of the GBM and various degrees of mesangial expansion. Electron-dense deposits are not identified by EM.

J. **Amyloidosis.** Renal amyloidosis can be primary or secondary. Patients often present with nephrotic syndrome (~50%), peripheral neuropathy (Carpal tunnel syndrome), heart failure, and/or liver disease due to amyloid deposits. There are many different proteins that form amyloid, including AA, AL amyloid, transthyretin (ATTR) and familial types, which confer a different prognosis (e.g., worse for AL amyloid compared with ATTR). Amyloid is composed of

TABLE 19.3   Summary of Pathologic Findings of Lupus Nephritis

Class	Light microscopy	Immunofluorescence	Electron microscopy
I	Minimal mesangial hypercellularity	Mesangial +	Mesangial deposits
II	Mesangial hypercellularity and increased matrix	Mesangial +	Mesangial deposits
III	Endocapillary and/or extracapillary proliferation in <50% of glomeruli	Mesangial and loop +	Mesangial and subendothelial deposits
IV	Endocapillary and/or extracapillary proliferation in 50% or more of glomeruli	Mesangial and loop +	Mesangial and subendothelial deposits
V	Thick loops and mesangial hypercellularity	Mesangial and loop +	Numerous subepithelial and scattered mesangial deposits

polymerized proteins forming beta-pleated sheets and stains red with Congo red.

LM: Varies from GBM thickening to nodular or segmental sclerosis. Amorphous material is often apparent in the mesangium or the capillary loops. A Congo red stain is diagnostic revealing apple green fluorescence under polarizable filters (e-**Fig. 19.11**).

EM: This shows characteristic randomly arranged fibrils of 4 to 12 nm (e-**Fig. 19.11**C). It shows either finely granular or filamentous deposits in the mesangium or the GBM (*Semin Diagn Pathol.* 2002;19:116).

IF: May show κ or λ chains. Some deposits of fragments of IgG, IgM, or IgA immunoglobulin heavy chains or light chains do not form amyloid; in these cases, a Congo red stain is negative and the term "congo red negative amyloidosis" is used, or the equivalent term "monoclonal immunoglobulin deposition disease" (MIDD).

The differential diagnosis of MIDD includes other nodular GN such as diabetes and fibrillary and immunotactoid glomerulopathy. The latter may have overlapping IF, but EM findings are distinct from amyloid (*Kidney Int.* 2002;62:1764). The other pathologic findings in MIDD are as follows:

LM: In MIDD, glomeruli may appear nodular or have nonspecific changes. Diagnosis is usually (but not always) made by IF.

IF: Identifies the specific type of immunoglobulin fragment as either heavy or light chain (*J Am Soc Nephrol.* 2001;12:1482) (e-**Fig. 19.12**).

K. **Alport syndrome/thin basement membrane disease.** Classic X-linked (X-L) Alport syndrome presents with microscopic or gross hematuria and deafness. Deafness and/or proteinuria are indications of severe disease. Such symptoms are usually absent in young children. Mutations in *COLIVA5* cause X-L Alport; *COLIVA4* mutations cause autosomal dominant (AD) and *COLIVA3* mutations cause autosomal recessive (AR) Alport. As many as 15% of X-L Alport patients have no family history and are thought to represent a new mutation. Patients with AR Alport are clinically similar to X-L Alport; however, AD Alport is rare. The involved organs in Alport syndrome reflect the sites where these collagen IVα chains are normally expressed (α3, α4, and α5 are exclusively found in the kidney, eye, and ear). Renal biopsy is performed for diagnosis as well as assessment of disease progression.

LM: This is not specific; it varies from unremarkable glomeruli, to FSGS, to chronic scarring. Foamy interstitial cells were once thought characteristic of Alport, but they are in fact seen in many types of proteinuria.

IF: Routine stains are negative. Diagnosis of Alport is facilitated by collagen α3–5 chain immunostaining. The α5 chain of collagen IV is distinctly absent in X-L Alport, and it is accompanied by the absence of α3 and α4 chains in glomeruli. (Collagen IV monomers are incorporated into basement membrane as triple helices to form the structural meshwork [*Kidney Int.* 2004;65:1109]; when one chain is mutated, all three chains may degenerate because they become susceptible to enzymatic proteolysis.) Typically, women with X-L Alport have mosaic linear staining with collagen IVα5 in the glomeruli or skin (e-**Fig. 19.13**) (*Hum Pathol.* 2002;33:836). However, some women may have positive staining, making it difficult to distinguish from thin membrane disease (TMD). A screening test for families with potential X-L Alport is skin biopsy (IVα5 is the only chain found in skin); the diagnostic pattern is absence of collagen IVα5 in men and mosaic staining (linear interrupted positivity) in X-L women carriers (e-**Fig. 19.13**B–D).

EM: The cardinal pathologic findings of X-L Alport are seen on EM and consist of abnormal splitting, widening, or thinning of the GBM with degeneration of collagen IV in the lamina densa known as "bread crumbs" (e-**Fig. 19.13**). The lesions may involve tubular basement membranes as well. However, the specificity of the EM findings is moderate (*Kidney Int.* 1999;56:760); for example, young children and women with Alport nephritis may only manifest uniformly thin GBM and thus be indistinguishable from TMD (*Semin Nephrol* 2005;25:149). About 30% of Alport heterozygotes have uniformly thin GBM, but have collagen IVα3–5 mutations by genetic testing. Others show only GBM lamellation in thin segments. Routine genetic testing is not only technically difficult (several different genes must be evaluated and mutational hot spots do not exist), but also does not strictly correlate with pathology or prognosis. A good family history of close relatives is very helpful.

TMD is defined as GBM thinning <200 nm. It is debated as to whether GBM thinning must be diffuse or focal, though most cases have focal GBM thinning involving <50% of loops.

LM: Usually unremarkable.

IF: Routine stains are negative. Collagen IVα3–5 immunostains are positive.

EM: Shows GBM diffuse or segmental thinning without lamellation (e-**Fig. 19.13F**).

III. TUBULOINTERSTITIAL DISEASES

A. Infectious processes. Infectious agents can result in tubulointerstitial nephritis by colonizing the renal parenchyma, or by triggering a systemic immunologic response that will target the renal tubules and interstitium. Bacterial agents are responsible for most cases of *acute pyelonephritis*. Most cases of acute pyelonephritis are ascending infections caused by gram-negative bacteria, particularly *Escherichia coli*. When bacteria reach the kidney using a hematogenous route, *Staphylococcus aureus* is usually the responsible agent. Acute pyelonephritis is characterized by an abundance of neutrophils in the lumen of tubules and the interstitium. Neutrophils are usually accompanied by other inflammatory cells.

Viral agents are also associated with tubulointerstitial nephritis. *Polyoma virus and cytomegalovirus* (*CMV*) are particularly important in renal allografts. The polyoma BK virus is a DNA virus with high prevalence during childhood, causing respiratory infections. Respiratory infection follows hematogenous spread, reaching organs like the kidney, where it remains dormant; when the patient later becomes immunosuppressed, the virus reactivates. Kidneys with either of these viral infections show a chronic interstitial inflammation, sometimes associated with tubulitis, a pattern that is difficult to distinguish from acute cellular rejection. Both viruses elicit cytopathic changes that are seen in endothelial and tubular epithelial cells; polyoma virus forms an intranuclear basophilic inclusion, and CMV forms cytoplasmic and intranuclear basophilic inclusions with a perinuclear halo. It is useful to confirm the morphologic findings of viral infection using antibodies against the specific microorganism.

A granulomatous inflammatory response is usually seen with mycobacterial or some fungal infections. Histochemical stains like acid-fast bacillus (AFB), PAS, and silver stains are needed to visualize the microorganisms.

B. Acute tubular necrosis (ATN). ATN is the most common cause of acute renal failure and can be caused by toxins or ischemia. The histologic changes are mainly confined to the tubules with necrosis of the lining epithelium. Regardless of the cause, the proximal tubule is the main target in ATN. Epithelial necrosis is more extensive and confluent in the toxic type of ATN, but tends to be patchy in the ischemic type. Since necrotic tubular epithelium will exfoliate into the tubular lumen, focal denudation of the tubular basement membrane is common (e-**Fig. 19.14**). Epithelial cells can also exhibit regenerative changes with nuclear enlargement, prominent nucleoli, and mitotic activity. Interstitial edema is usually present in ATN.

C. **Allergic interstitial nephritis.** Most cases of allergic interstitial nephritis are drug related; renal manifestations develop ~2 weeks after drug exposure. The typical presentation includes fever, skin rash, and eosinophilia, but this triad is only present in approximately one-third of the patients. Interstitial eosinophils are the most important histologic clue for diagnosis. Eosinophils are accompanied by other inflammatory cells, mainly lymphocytes, and may only be seen focally (e-**Fig. 19.15**). Tubulitis and tubular injury usually accompany the interstitial changes. Nonsteroidal anti-inflammatory drugs (NSAIDs) can also cause allergic interstitial nephritis, but interstitial eosinophils are usually rare. Moreover, patients taking NSAID can also develop nephrotic syndrome, and their glomeruli exhibit changes indistinguishable from MCD.

D. **Cast nephropathy.** Cast nephropathy is a renal complication of multiple myeloma. Casts are usually located in the collecting ducts, but due to retrograde filling, casts can even be seen in the proximal tubules. Casts are composed of light chains and Tamm–Horsfall protein, and tend to have a fractured appearance. A granulomatous response with multinucleated macrophages and reactive epithelial cells is typically found at the periphery of myeloma casts (e-**Fig. 19.16**); other inflammatory cells, such as neutrophils and lymphocytes, can also be part of the inflammatory process. Nonspecific changes such as tubular atrophy and interstitial fibrosis are commonly present. IF studies exhibit a monoclonal light chain in the casts in most cases.

IV. VASCULAR DISEASES

A. **Vasculitides.** The kidney has a dense arterial, venous, and lymphatic network. Vasculitides affect all these vessels, but most commonly the arteries. They are usually classified as large, medium, and small vessel vasculitides on the basis of the predominant vessel size affected, but although the classification is convenient, it is controversial because there is variability in the size of affected vessels. Vasculitides are also classified by the underlying pathogenetic mechanism as either immune-complex mediated or pauci-immune (absence of immune deposits). The following are the most common vasculitides affecting the kidney, grouped by size:

1. **Takayasu's aortitis** affects large branches of the abdominal aorta and the renal arteries. Mural inflammation with giant cells is the distinct feature.

2. **Polyarteritis nodosa, scleroderma, lupus, rheumatoid arthritis,** and **Wegener's granulomatosis** affect medium- to small-sized vessels. These are systemic diseases and, with the exception of lupus, are pauci-immune systemic vasculitis. Kidney pathology is variable and includes interstitial granulomas, arterial acute inflammation, fibrinoid necrosis, and thrombotic occlusion. The inflammation can lead to aneurysm formation or fibrous wall thickening. Involvement of glomerular capillaries leads to crescentic GN. The diagnosis largely depends on the clinical syndrome, not the pathological findings. For example, Wegener's granulomatosis is associated with serum autoantibodies against components of neutrophils known as circulating antineutrophil cytoplasmic antibodies (ANCA). These antibodies correlate with disease activity and underscore the pathogenesis of vascular injury (see Chap. 9).

3. Of the small vessel systemic vasculitides, some are referred to as *thrombotic microangiopathies*(TMA). A typical presentation is with hemolytic anemia and thrombocytopenia, known as *hemolytic uremic syndrome* (HUS). Entities included under TMA are diarrhea associated (classic HUS), thrombotic thrombocytopenic purpura, eclampsia, pre-eclampsia, thrombosis due to drugs (oral contraceptives, chemotherapy drugs such as bleomycin), cryoglobulinemia, idiopathic hypereosinophilia, antiphospholipid syndrome, hereditary deficiency of blood clotting factors, and malignant HTN (*J Am Soc Nephrol.* 2003;14:1072). Renal biopsy shows arterial intimal thickening (called mucoid degeneration) and luminal fibrin thrombi (e-**Fig. 19.17A**).

All of these entities may also show characteristic arteriolar thickening (also known as onion skinning, e-**Fig. 19.17**B), endothelial swelling, and/or luminal thrombosis.

B. **Systemic HTN.** Vascular diseases of the kidney are often associated with systemic HTN. The most common cause of HTN is idiopathic, which, despite modern pharmacologic therapies, remains a primary cause of renal failure. High blood pressure damages parenchymal arteries causing wall thickening; the arterioles show characteristic acellular eosinophilic material due to increased intravascular pressure and endothelial injury that allows leaking and deposition of plasma proteins. Glomeruli beyond damaged arterioles undergo sclerosis (e-**Fig. 19.17**B).

  1. **Malignant HTN,** defined as diastolic pressure >120 mmHg, complicates ~10% of patients with benign HTN, presents acutely with papilledema, nausea, vomiting, convulsions, and coma. Renal function declines rapidly and patients develop gross hematuria, albuminuria, and hemolytic anemia. Onion skinning is characteristic (e-**Fig. 19.17**C).

  2. A small fraction (5% to 10%) of benign HTN is secondary to specific causes, some of which may be amenable to surgical therapy, that together are known as *renovascular HTN*. Most common is renal artery stenosis due to atherosclerotic aneurysms in older mostly diabetic men. Patients with abdominal or renal artery atherosclerosis may present with acute renal failure or proteinuria due to cholesterol embolism in parenchymal arteries (e-**Fig. 19.17**D). Fibromuscular dysplasia, an idiopathic mural thickening of the renal artery, is seen in young women (*Am J Kidney Dis.* 1997;29:167).

V. **PATHOLOGY OF THE ALLOGRAFT KIDNEY**

  A. **Processing of renal allograft biopsies.** Renal biopsy is a key component of managing transplant recipients since clinical diagnosis is changed in ~40%, and therapy in ~60% of cases following biopsy (*Am J Kidney Dis.* 1998;31:S15). Transplant biopsies in most centers are performed when clinically indicated (indication biopsies) or at standardized time intervals (protocol biopsies). Criteria for indication biopsies include proteinuria, acute renal failure, and increased creatinine levels, among others. Adequacy criteria of the renal allograft biopsy were established at the BANFF 1997 Consensus Conference (*Kidney Int.* 1999:55:713).

  It is recommended that two 16- or 18-gauge needle core biopsies are submitted for pathologic evaluation: one for LM and the other divided for IF and EM. The core for LM is submitted in 10% buffered formalin; the IF core should be submitted in refrigerated transport media; and a small fragment from cortex should be submitted for EM fixed in 2% glutaraldehyde. For LM, 10 glomeruli and 2 arteries are required for definitive diagnosis; 7 to 10 glomeruli and 1 artery are considered marginal, while <7 glomeruli and no arteries are an inadequate sample. The paraffin blocks should be sectioned at 3 to 4 μm thickness; seven slides including three H&E stains, three PAS or silver stains, and one trichrome stain should be prepared (*Kidney Int.* 1999;55:713). For IF, a minimum of two glomeruli is required for the evaluation of glomerular disease; however, IF evaluation for IgG, IgA, IgM, C3, fibrinogen, albumin, and C4d is standard. For electron microscopic evaluation, at least one glomerulus is recommended. See Table 19.4 for BANFF diagnostic categories for renal allograft biopsies.

  B. **Transplant rejection.** Major complications with specific pathologic findings in the allograft biopsy are acute and chronic rejection (which are subdivided into cellular and humoral rejection), and recurrent and de novo disease (see Table 19.2).

  1. **Acute T-cell-mediated rejection.** Tubules, arteries, and the interstitium are the principle targets of acute T-cell-mediated rejection. The BANFF 2005-updated classification of renal allograft rejection (see Table 19.2) is based on

TABLE 19.4	Banff '97 Diagnostic Categories for Renal Allograft Biopsies-Banff '09 Update

1. Normal
2. Antibody-mediated rejection
   Due to documented anti-donor antibody, C4d, and allograft pathology
   Acute antibody-mediated rejection
   Type (grade)
      I. ATN-like minimal inflammation, C4d+ in peritubular capillaries (PTC)
      II. Capillary and/or glomerular inflammation and/or thromboses, C4d+ in PTC
      III. Arterial – v3, C4d+ in PTC
   Chronic antibody-mediated rejection
      C4d+, presence of circulating anti-donor antibodies, glomerular double contours and/or
      peritubular capillary basement membrane multilayering and/or interstitial fibrosis/tubular
      atrophy and/or fibrous intimal thickening in arteries
3. Borderline changes: "suspicious" for acute T-cell-mediated rejection
   This category is used when no intimal arteritis is present, but there are foci of tubulitis (t1, t2, or
   t3) with minor interstitial inflammation (i0 or i1) or interstitial inflammation with mild tubulitis
   (t1). t1 < 4, t2 = 4–10, t3 ≥ 10 intraepithelial lymphocytes per tubular cross section
4. Acute T-cell-mediated rejection
   Type (grade)
      IA. Significant interstitial infiltration (>25% parenchyma, i2 or i3) and foci of moderate
         tubulitis (t2)
      IB. Significant interstitial infiltration (>25% parenchyma, i2 or i3) and foci of severe tubulitis
         (t3)
      IIA. Mild to moderate intimal arteritis (v1)
      IIB. Severe intimal arteritis comprising >25% of the luminal area (v2)
      III. Transmural arteritis and/or arterial fibrinoid change and necrosis of medial smooth muscle
         cells with accompanying lymphocytic inflammation (v3)
   Chronic T-cell-mediated rejection
      Chronic allograft arteriopathy (arterial intimal fibrosis with mononuclear cell infiltration in
      fibrosis, formation of neo-intima)
5. Interstitial fibrosis and tubular atrophy (IFTA), no evidence of specific etiology
   III. Severe IFTA (>50% of cortical area)
6. Other: changes not considered to be due to rejection-acute and/or chronic

Modified from Sis B, et al. Banff '09 Meeting Report: Antibody mediated graft deterioration and implementation of Banff working groups. *Am J Transplant.* 10:464–471, 2010.

histological scoring of tubular, interstitial, and arterial inflammation (*Am J Transplant.* 2007;7:518). Higher-grade rejection correlates with worse outcome and requires more aggressive therapy.

Tubulitis is scored in non-atrophic tubules. The degree of infiltrating mononuclear cells, lymphocytes, and macrophages is graded as mild (t1; <4 cells/tubular cross section), moderate (t2; 4 to 10 cells/tubular cross section), or severe (t3; >10 cells/tubular cross section, **e-Fig. 19.18**).

Interstitial inflammation is typically pleomorphic, consisting predominantly of CD4+ and CD8+ T cells, and macrophages. Involvement of >25% of the parenchyma is required for the diagnosis of acute cellular rejection. If foci of t2 or t3 tubulitis are present with <25% interstitial inflammation, then the specimen is considered borderline or "suspicious" for acute cellular rejection.

Arteritis, or endotheliitis, is the presence of subendothelial or mural mononuclear cell infiltration in the wall of renal parenchymal arteries (**e-Fig. 19.19**). Any size artery may be affected. Arterial inflammation is scored based on the degree of intimal inflammation as follows: mild (v1; <25% luminal diameter), moderate (v2; >25% luminal diameter), and severe (v3; transmural ± fibrinoid necrosis). The presence of even mild endotheliitis is significant and warrants a diagnosis of at least grade IIA rejection (see Table 19.2).

2. **Acute humoral (antibody-mediated) rejection** may occur shortly after implantation, or months to years following transplantation. At present, the diagnosis requires at least two of the following: circulating anti-donor specific antibodies, diffuse C4d+ immunostaining of peritubular capillaries, and morphologic evidence of acute tissue injury (ATN, peritubular capillaritis, glomerulitis, thromboses, and/or arteritis) (*Am J Transplant.* 2010;10:464). The earliest feature of acute antibody-mediated rejection (AMR) may be ATN, but as the lesions develop, peritubular capillaritis becomes prominent. Peritubular capillaritis is defined by the BANFF 2007 working group as dilation of peritubular capillaries by marginating inflammatory cells (*Am J Transplant.* 2008;8:753). A minimum of 10% of peritubular capillaries must be involved (normally, peritubular capillaries contain no more than two mononuclear cells), and the composition (neutrophils, monocytes, etc.) and the extent (focal [<50%] vs. diffuse [>50%]) of peritubular capillaritis should be mentioned in the pathology report (e-**Fig. 19.21**).

   C4d immunostaining is another important feature of acute AMR. Deposition of C4d in peritubular capillaries is used as a surrogate marker for anti-donor antibody activity within the allograft, and IF is considered the gold standard for C4d evaluation (*Kidney Int.* 1993;44:411). Normal kidneys show diffuse glomerular C4d+, acting as an internal control. Diffuse C4d staining is defined as bright, linear peritubular capillary wall staining involving >50% of either cortical or medullary capillaries (e-**Fig. 19.20**). Focal (10% to 50%) C4d+ is also clinically significant (*Am J Transplant.* 2009;9:812).

3. **Chronic rejection.** Repeated graft injury from episodes of cellular rejection may manifest as nonspecific tubulointerstitial fibrosis (IFTA) or glomerular fibrosis (BANFF category 5). The only histological lesion highly suspicious of chronic cellular rejection is transplant arteriopathy (e-**Fig. 19.22**), defined as fibrointimal hyperplasia (thickening of the intima) (*Kidney Int.* 1999;55:713). Elastin staining may help to distinguish transplant arteriopathy from arterial thickening due to HTN since the stain will highlight intimal proliferation with multilamination in HTN, a finding absent in transplant arteriopathy.

4. **Chronic antibody-mediated rejection.** GBM duplication, interstitial fibrosis, tubular atrophy, arterial intimal thickening, serum donor-specific antibodies, and peritubular capillary C4d reactivity are all features of chronic AMR. At least two of these features are required for the diagnosis (*Am J Transplant.* 2010;10:464). GBM duplication is believed to be the most specific indicator of chronic AMR, although this finding may be seen in other chronic kidney diseases such as lupus. EM is a valuable aid in diagnosing chronic rejection; GBM and/or peritubular capillary basement membrane multi-lamellation is highly characteristic.

C. **Recurrent glomerular disease** occurs in up to 36% of cases with a mean interval of 5 years, and is currently the third leading cause of graft loss. The most common recurrent glomerular diseases are focal segmental glomerulosclerosis (10% to 50%), IgA nephropathy (13% to 46%), MPGN type II (80% to 100%), MPGN type I (20% to 25%), membranous GN (10% to 30%), anti-neutrophil cytoplasmic antibody (ANCA) vasculitis (17%), diabetes (8% to 30%), and amyloid (5% to 30%). MPGN type II and FSGS have the highest rates of graft loss at 15% to 30% and 13% to 20%, respectively.

D. **De novo disease** includes glomerular, malignant, tubulointerstitial, and infectious diseases. Combined de novo and recurrent glomerular disease accounts for over 15% of diagnoses in transplant biopsies.

1. **De novo glomerular disease.** Transplant glomerulopathy (TGP) is the most common de novo glomerular disease in the posttransplant setting, accounting for 20% to 30% of cases. Histologically, TGP is characterized by glomerular hypercellularity and a lobular appearance resembling MPGN (e-**Fig. 19.23**). Double contours are characteristic (e-**Fig. 19.24**). Subendothelial edema, GBM multi-lamellation, and endothelial fenestrae closure are typical electron microscopic findings (e-**Fig. 19.25** and e-**Fig. 19.26**). TGP is considered to lie within the spectrum of changes characteristic of chronic rejection, and is commonly associated with class II anti-HLA antibodies. The prognosis of TGP is poor. Other glomerular diseases including FSGS (11%), IgA (2.9%), membranous GN (0.7%), and anti-GBM (0.7%) may occur de novo posttrenal transplant (Table 19.5).

2. **Posttransplant lymphoproliferative disease (PTLD)** is a rare de novo disease following renal transplant. Both kidneys are typically enlarged. Monoclonal or polyclonal B-lymphocyte proliferations can occur, and in most cases are associated with Epstein–Barr virus.

TABLE 19.5	Major Histopathological Findings in Renal Transplant Biopsies	
Rejection	**Recurrent disease**	**De novo disease**
Acute cell mediated	**Glomerular**	**Glomerular**
Tubulitis	FSGS	Transplant glomerulopathy
Arteritis (endotheliitis)	Diabetes	FSGS
Glomerulitis	Lupus	Diabetes
Interstitial inflammation	IgA	Anti-GBM
	MPGN	Postinfectious
	Membranous	Membranous
	Vasculitis (ANCA, anti-GBM)	other
	Amyloidosis/light chain deposition disease	
Chronic cell mediated	**Tubulointerstitial**	
Interstitial inflammation	Myeloma cast nephropathy	**Vascular**
Intimal fibroplasia		Thrombotic microangiopathy (drug induced)
Interstitial fibrosis		Cholesterol embolism
		Renal artery thrombosis
		Renal vein thrombosis
		Antibody-mediated rejection
Antibody mediated (AMR)	**Vascular**	**Tubulointerstitial**
Acute	Recurrent HUS	Acute interstitial nephritis usually drug reaction (e-**Fig. 19.29**)
Chronic		Oxalate crystals
		Calcium phosphate crystals
		ATN
		Malignancy
		Malignant lymphoma
		PTLD

Modified from: Liapis H, Wang H, eds. *Pathology of Solid Organ Transplantation*, 1st ed. Heidelberg: Springer; 2011. Used with permission.

3. Calcineurin inhibitor (CNI) toxicity. The CNI (e.g., cyclosporine, tacrolimus) has markedly improved short-term allograft survival but are, however, nephrotoxic.

  a. Patients with **acute CNI toxicity** typically present with signs of acute renal failure, which manifests on renal biopsy as isometric vacuolization of the proximal tubular epithelial cells and/or ATN. The changes are reversible with decreased exposure to the offending agent. Importantly, isometric vacuolization and ATN are nonspecific findings requiring clinical correlation. Osmotic nephrosis, for instance, may also produce isometric vacuolization.

  b. Chronic CNI toxicity, in contrast to acute CNI toxicity, is irreversible (*Transplantation* 1989;48:965). Biopsy findings include stripe or skip interstitial fibrosis and arteriolar hyalinosis (**e-Fig. 19.27**). Subendothelial beaded arteriolar hyalinosis is particularly characteristic, but since arteriolar hyalinosis may also occur secondary to HTN or diabetes, clinical correlation is warranted. Tubulointerstitial calcium deposits are also part of CNI toxicity.

4. Infection. Infectious agents may be encountered, albeit rarely, in the transplant renal biopsy. The opportunistic fungi *Candida, Aspergillus, Cryptococcus,* and *Zygomyces* account for ∼5% of all renal transplant infections (*Transpl Infect Dis.* 2001;3:203). White blood cell casts, granulomatous inflammation, and crescentic GN are all seen in association with fungal infections, typically occurring within 6 months posttransplantation.

  Viral infections, most commonly polyoma virus (BK and JC) infections, may also be encountered. Polyoma virus typically infects distal tubules and collecting ducts, manifesting histologically with homogenous intranuclear inclusions, clumped nuclear chromatin, or bubbly inclusions (**e-Fig. 19.28**). Cells with these features in urine cytology specimens are known as decoy cells because of their similarity to malignant cells. CMV infects the renal allograft but is currently rare due to CMV prophylactic therapy applied as a standard of practice.

Surgical Diseases of the Kidney

NORMAL ANATOMY

In the adult, the normal kidney weighs about 115 to 155 g in women and 125 to 170 g in men. Anatomically, the kidneys are composed of an outer cortex and an inner medulla that has 8 to 18 pyramids. The base of each pyramid is at the corticomedullary junction, and the apex forms a papilla where the collecting ducts open into the renal pelvis. The minor calyces receive the papillae and in turn join to form the major calyces that are the dilated upper portion of the ureter in the renal pelvis. Histologically, the components of the kidney include glomeruli, tubules, blood vessels, and interstitium.

Maldevelopment and Nonneoplastic Cystic Diseases

Johann D. Hertel, Peter A. Humphrey, and Helen Liapis

The developmental abnormalities and benign cystic diseases of the kidney that are most likely to be seen by the surgical pathologist are presented here.

I. DEVELOPMENT ABNORMALITIES

A. **Renal dysplasia** is seen in malformed kidneys where there is abnormal differentiation of metanephric elements. Most cases are unilateral and sporadic, but a wide variety of genetic diseases, malformation syndromes, and chromosomal disorders have been linked to renal dysplasia (Stocker JT, Dehner LP, Husain AN, eds. *Stocker and Dehner's Pediatric Pathology*, 3rd ed. Philadelphia: Wolters Kluwer/Lippincott Williams and Wilkins, 2011). Bilateral renal dysplasia is less frequent and is associated with renal failure at birth. Renal dysplasia is a common cause of an abdominal mass mimicking neoplasia in children <1 year of age but can also be diagnosed in older children and adults. There is an association with congenital urinary tract obstruction in about 50% of cases.

B. Grossly, *multicystic dysplasia* is characterized by a slightly enlarged kidney, or a small and irregularly cystic kidney (e-**Fig. 20.1**)* Aplastic dysplasia is typified by a small, solid remnant of the kidney. Segmental dysplasia occurs when the collecting system is duplicated; microscopically, there are immature tubules or ducts surrounded by collarettes of condensed mesenchyme (e-**Fig. 20.2**), and islands of immature-appearing cartilage (e-**Fig. 20.3**), cysts of varying sizes that have a flattened epithelial lining, and islands of normal glomeruli and renal tubules between the dysplastic areas. Rare cases of Wilms tumor and renal cell carcinoma (RCC) have been reported in multicystic dysplastic kidneys.

---

*All e-figures are available online via the Solution Site Image Bank.

II. NONNEOPLASTIC CYSTIC DISEASES

A. **Autosomal dominant polycystic kidney disease (ADPKD)** is an autosomal dominant disease with complete penetrance but highly variable expressivity. The disease results from a defective copy of the *PKD1* gene in 85% to 90% of cases (on chromosome 16p13.3) or *PKD2* gene in 10% to 15% of cases (on chromosome 4q22.1). The genes encode polycystin-1 and polycystin-2, respectively, the loss of which causes failure to appropriately assemble cilia in the renal tubules. While the defect is present in utero and initiates cyst formation, a second mutation is required for cyst enlargement (*J Am Soc Nephrol.* 2007;18:1374). The disease typically manifests in adulthood (mean age of onset 30 years), although there are ADPKD cases manifesting in the neonatal period which usually present with glomerular cysts (*Arch Pathol Lab Med.* 2010;134:583). Clinically, ADPKD presents with renal failure, hypertension, hematuria, and flank pain. ADPKD is a systemic disease; the connective tissue abnormality is also associated with liver and pancreatic cysts, intracranial aneurysms, and mitral or aortic insufficiency.

Macroscopically, the involved kidney is dramatically enlarged with loss of its reniform structure (**e-Fig. 20.4**). About 1% to 3% of nephrons are affected by cysts which are usually large and oval in shape, distributed throughout the medulla and cortex, and involve any part of the nephron. The cysts are typically sac-like structures containing fluid ranging from clear and yellow to brown and turbid. The cysts vary in size from a few millimeters to several centimeters in maximal dimension. Microscopically, the cysts are lined by columnar, cuboidal, or flattened epithelium (**e-Fig. 20.5**) surrounded by a thickened basement membrane layer, and micropapillary hyperplasia (**e-Fig. 20.6**) and small intracystic polyps may be present. Some studies have suggested an association between ADPKD and RCC but none has shown a definitive increased risk of malignancy (*Clin J Am Soc Nephrol.* 2009;4:1998). In the end stage, the kidney is hugely enlarged and shows severe interstitial fibrosis, chronic inflammation, and severely thickened vessels, although the glomeruli appear relatively unaffected.

B. **Autosomal recessive polycystic kidney disease (ARPKD)** is an autosomal recessive disease with complete penetrance due to mutations in both copies of the *PKHD1* gene encoding for fibrocystin. Fibrocystin is a transmembrane protein expressed in cilia in many organs including the kidney, liver, and pancreas; how precisely fibrocystin mutations cause ciliary dysfunction and subsequently cyst formation is still under investigation (since the mutant proteins causing cyst formation in ADPKD and ARPKD are localized to cilia, the proposal to classify cystic kidney diseases as ciliopathies is currently favored by some investigators). ARPKD usually develops in utero causing oligohydramnios and in utero renal failure, but it may present later in childhood or adulthood (*Clin J Am Soc Nephrol.* 2010;5:972); in any event, progressive renal failure leads to end-stage renal disease during the first decade of life. Pulmonary hypoplasia secondary to oligohydramnios is a common cause of mortality in the perinatal period. ARPKD is also associated with congenital hepatic fibrosis, and the pancreas can also be involved resulting in pancreatic failure. Macroscopically (**e-Fig. 20.7**), the kidneys are symmetrically enlarged and generally maintain their reniform appearance. The kidney has a sponge appearance caused by innumerable small, smooth lined cysts throughout the cortex and medulla. The cysts are typically cylindrical (as opposed to the spherical cysts seen in ADPKD) and about 1 mm to 2 mm in size; fusiform dilatations of the collecting ducts run radially through the cortex and medulla. Microscopically, the kidneys show ectatic dilated collecting ducts (**e-Fig. 20.8**). The cysts are generally lined by a single cell layer of cuboidal epithelium, although areas of hyperplasia may be seen.

C. **Medullary sponge kidney** is usually asymptomatic unless complicated by urinary tract infection, nephrolithiasis, or hematuria. The condition is typically detected radiologically during examination of an adult for stones. The kidney is not enlarged. Microscopically, there is ectasia of the papillary collecting ducts in the renal medulla, with intraluminal microliths commonly observed.

D. **Medullary cystic kidney disease (MCKD)** complex is an autosomal dominant adult onset kidney disease. The specific gene abnormality has not been identified but has been mapped to 1q22 for MCD type I and to 16p13 for MCD type II by gene linkage analysis. Both types have a similar phenotype, although MCD type II has an earlier age of onset (fourth decade) than MCD type I (seventh decade). Both MCD I and II present as progressive nephropathy and progress to end-stage renal disease. Macroscopically, the kidneys appear normal to shrunken but maintain their reniform appearance. On sectioning, numerous small corticomedullary cysts are seen. Microscopically, the kidney shows focal tubular atrophy and dilatation with cyst formation caused by disintegration of the tubular basement membrane. The cysts are typically at the corticomedullary junction, few in number, small, and lined by columnar, transitional, or metaplastic squamous epithelium. The renal parenchyma reveals a modest interstitial lymphocytic infiltrate and fibrosis indistinguishable from other tubulointerstitial processes.

E. **Nephronophthisis** is a hereditary disease of childhood and early adulthood with gross and microscopic pathology indistinguishable from MCD. Some investigators view juvenile nephronophthisis and MCD as part of the same disease complex. The disease is caused by mutations in at least 12 different nephrocystins—a mutation in any of which leads to a loss of cilia function and development of cystic renal disease. Grossly and microscopically, the findings are nonspecific and similar to those found in MCD.

F. **Simple renal cysts,** or retention cysts, are asymptomatic incidental findings seen on abdominal imaging. Simple renal cysts affect approximately 7% to 10% of the general population and are increasingly common with advancing age. Surgical pathologists typically see tissue only if there is suspicion of malignancy or if there are symptoms (such as pain, hematuria, or infection). On imaging and by gross examination, the cysts are usually unilateral, and unilocular, but can be bilateral and multiple. The size of the cysts can vary dramatically. Microscopically, the cysts have a flattened epithelial lining.

G. **Acquired cystic kidney disease** occurs in the setting of chronic hemodialysis. The cysts are generally asymptomatic and are seen as incidental findings on abdominal imaging. On gross examination the kidney is normal to shrunken and shows multiple smooth-lined cysts filled with clear fluid. Microscopically, the cysts are generally lined by flattened cuboidal epithelium (**e-Fig. 20.9**), although hyperplastic and even dysplastic epithelium has been reported; in this setting, however, no criteria presently exist for separating a region of hyperplastic epithelium from a microscopic papillary RCC.

H. Cysts can be associated with *malformation syndromes* including tuberous sclerosis and von Hippel–Lindau (VHL) disease (see section on renal cell carcinoma). Tuberous sclerosis complex is autosomal dominant and caused by mutations in *TSC1* (on chromosome 9q; encodes for hamartin) or *TSC2* (on chromosome 16p; encodes for tuberin). Renal angiomyolipomas (discussed later) and cortical cysts are common. These distinctive cysts vary in size and are lined by hyperplastic epithelium with eosinophilic cytoplasm, with multilayering and papillary growth seen.

SUGGESTED READINGS

Agarwal MM, Hemal AK. Surgical management of renal cystic disease. *Curr Urol Rep.* 2011;12: 3–10.

Bonsib SM. The classification of renal cystic diseases and other congenital malformations of the kidney and urinary tract. *Arch Pathol Lab Med.* 2010;134:554–568.

Eknoyan G. A clinical view of simple and complex renal cysts. *J Am Soc Nephrol.* 2009;20:1874–1876.

Gascue C, Katsanis N, Badano JL. Cystic diseases of the kidney: Ciliary dysfunction and cystogenic mechanisms. *Pediatr Nephrol.* 2010;26(8):1181–1195.

Gunay-Aygun M, et al. Correlation of kidney function, volume and imaging findings, and PKHD1 mutations in 73 patients with autosomal recessive kidney disease. *Clin J Am Soc Nephrol.* 2010;5:972–984.

Lennarz JK, Spence DC, Iskandar SS, Dehner LP, Liapis H. Glomerulocystic kidney one hundred-year perspective. *Arch Pathol Lab Med.* 2010;135:583–605.

Rosetti S, Harris PC. Genotype–phenotype correlations in autosomal dominant and autosomal recessive polycystic kidney disease. *J Am Soc Nephrol.* 2007;18:1374–1280.

Wilson PD, Goilav B. Cystic disease of the kidney. *Annu Rev Pathol.* 2007;2:341–368.

Pediatric Renal Neoplasms

Jason A. Jarzembowski and Frances V. White

I. **INTRODUCTION.** There are approximately 500 pediatric renal neoplasms diagnosed each year in the United States, the majority of which are unique to children or occur only rarely in adults (Table 20.1). Protocols for specimen processing, the staging system, and differential diagnosis differ from that of adult tumors. At present, the majority of pediatric renal tumors in the United States are centrally reviewed by the Children's Oncology Group (COG), and procurement of snap-frozen tumor for molecular studies has become important for placement of patients in specific treatment protocols (*Pediatr Dev Pathol.* 2005;8:320).

II. **GROSS EXAMINATION AND TISSUE SAMPLING.** A radical nephrectomy is the usual specimen. In cases of bilateral nephroblastoma, partial resections (kidney-sparing procedures) are performed. Pretreatment biopsies may be obtained for unresectable

TABLE 20.1	Pediatric Renal Neoplasms: Percentages and Age Distribution		
Tumor	**Mean age**	**Pediatric renal neoplasms (%)**	**Age distribution (y)**
Classic mesoblastic nephroma	7 d	1	0–2
Cellular mesoblastic nephroma	4 mo	3	0–2
Malignant rhabdoid tumor	18 mo	2	0–3
CCSK	2 y	4	0–9; rare after 9 y of age
Nephroblastoma	36.5 mo (boys) 42.5 mo (girls)	85	0–10; rare in first 3 mo and after 10 y of age
Metanephric stromal tumor	2 y	Rare	0–15
Ewing sarcoma / PNET	28 y	Rare	0–18+
Papillary RCC	10 y	<5	1–18+
Translocation carcinomas	Wide range	<5	1–18+
Metanephric adenoma	41 y	Rare	5–18+
Renal medullary carcinoma	22 y	Rare	11–18+
Angiomyolipoma	50 y	Rare	17–18+
Synovial sarcoma	37 y	Rare	18

PNET, primitive neuroectodermal tumor; RCC, renal cell carcinoma; CCSK, clear cell sarcoma of kidney.
Compiled from References in Suggested Readings

tumors; however, intraoperative biopsies are discouraged due to the risk of tumor spillage unless the diagnosis will alter operative management.

Pediatric renal tumors are often large, friable tumors that bulge beyond the normal renal contour. The capsule should be carefully examined for sites of rupture and inked before incised. The initial plane of section is taken to demonstrate the relationship of tumor to the capsule and renal sinus. At this point, fresh tissue from each tumor nodule, nephrogenic rests, and normal kidney is snap frozen for protocol studies. Tissue may also be taken for cytogenetics, flow cytometry, and electron microscopy, depending on clinical history. Following initial cuts to facilitate fixation, overnight fixation is recommended before histologic sampling to decrease tumor friability and capsule retraction. Tissue for histology should be mainly taken from the tumor's periphery, as histology of the interface between tumor and renal parenchyma is often important in identifying the type of tumor. Each separate tumor nodule should be sampled, with at least one section per centimeter of tumor diameter. Sections should also demonstrate the relationship of tumor to the capsule and the renal sinus. The hilum is a common route of tumor spread, necessitating adequate sampling of this area as well. Ureteral and vascular margins, hilar lymph nodes, nephrogenic rests, and normal kidney are also sampled. Tumor sections are mapped, using either a diagram or photograph of the specimen; mapping is necessary for nephroblastoma, as the presence of diffuse versus focal anaplasia alters type of treatment (*Arch Pathol Lab Med.* 2003;127:1280).

III. **DIAGNOSTIC FEATURES OF PEDIATRIC RENAL TUMORS.** Pediatric renal neoplasms are notorious for their variable histologic patterns, which often show overlap between the various entities; thus, there should be careful examination of the tumor–kidney interface for pattern of infiltration, which is characteristic for each tumor type. Correct diagnosis depends on knowledge of both classic and variant histology, along with adequate sampling and correlation of the microscopic findings with patient age and other clinical information. While immunohistochemical studies may be useful for establishing the diagnosis (e.g., for INI1 in rhabdoid tumor) or for excluding a diagnosis in specific cases, immunohistochemical stains are usually not needed. Molecular studies can also be used to confirm specific diagnoses (Table 20.2).

A. **Nephroblastoma (Wilms tumor) and nephrogenic rests.** Nephroblastoma (Wilms tumor) accounts for 85% of pediatric renal tumors. Most patients present before 10 years of age, with a peak between 2 and 5 years. Rare examples have been reported in adults (*J Clin Oncol.* 2004;22:4500). The tumor is more common in children of African descent than of other races and is slightly more common in girls than boys.

Although genetic abnormalities have been identified in only a minority of nephroblastomas, multiple genetic abnormalities and syndromes are associated with the tumor. Abnormalities of *WT1* on chromosome 11p13, a gene involved in renal and gonadal development, occurs in aniridia and genital anomalies syndrome (WAGR), Denys–Drash, and Frasier syndromes, all associated with a high risk for nephroblastoma. Molecular alterations of imprinted genes at the *WT2* locus on chromosome 11p15 are associated with Beckwith–Wiedemann syndrome, which has an increased risk for nephroblastoma. Both *WT1* and *WT2* locus gene alterations are found in a minority of sporadic tumors. About 1% of patients with nephroblastoma have a family history of nephroblastoma; two familial genes, *FWT1* and *FWT2*, have been identified in this setting in which the disease shows autosomal dominant transmission with variable penetrance (*Curr Opin Pediatr.* 2002;14:5). Other molecular alterations that are associated with tumor progression or aggressiveness have been identified; *TP53* is implicated in progression to anaplastic nephroblastoma, and loss of heterozygosity of 1p and 16q is associated with poor prognosis in favorable histology nephroblastoma (*J Clin Oncol.* 2005;23:7312 and *J Clin Oncol.* 2006;24:2352).

TABLE 20.2 Common Molecular Derangements in Pediatric Renal Neoplasms

Tumor	Cytogenetic abnormality	Implicated genes	Protein role	Related assay(s)
Nephroblastoma	Deletions or mutations involving 11p13, 11p15, or Xq11.1	WT1, WT2, WT3, WTX	Zinc-finger DNA-binding protein; tumor suppressor genes	IPOX for WT1
Cellular mesoblastic nephroma	t(12;15)(p13;q25)	ETV6-NTRK3	Receptor tyrosine kinase	RT-PCR, FISH
Ewing sarcoma/PNET	Translocations of 22q11, usually t(11;22) (q24;q12)	EWS-FLI1	Transcriptional activator	RT-PCR, FISH; IPOX for CD99 or FLI-1
Synovial sarcoma	t(X;18)(p11;q11)	SYT and SSX1, 2, or 4	Chromatin remodeling, transcriptional regulation, β-catenin signaling pathways	RT-PCR, FISH
CCSK	t(10;17), del 14q	Undetermined	Undetermined	Karyotyping
Malignant rhabdoid tumor	Deletions or mutations involving 22q11.2	hSNF5/INI1	Chromatin remodeling and transcriptional regulation	IPOX for INI1 and cytokeratin
Translocation carcinomas	t(X;1)(p11.2;q34) t(X;1)(p11.2;q25) t(X;1)(p11.2;q21) t(6;11)(p21;q12)	ASPL-TFE3 PSF-TFE3 PRCC-TFE3 Alpha-TFEB	Transcriptional activators	Karyotyping, IPOX for TFE and cathepsin K
Renal medullary carcinoma	Constitutional 11p15.5 mutation; possible 22q11.2 involvement	HBB hSNF5/INI1	Hemoglobin S Chromatin remodeling and transcriptional regulation	IPOX for INI1
Angiomyolipoma	9q34, 16p13.3, 5q mutations	TSC1, TSC2	Tumor suppressor genes	Constitutional karyotype

IPOX, immunoperoxidase; RT-PCR, reverse transcription-polymerase chain reaction; FISH, fluorescence in situ hybridization; PNET, primitive neuroectodermal tumor; CCSK, clear cell sarcoma of kidney. Compiled from References in Suggested Readings.

Nephroblastomas are usually solitary masses; however, 10% are multicentric and 5% are bilateral at presentation (e-Fig. 20.10). The cut surface is typically pale gray and friable and may be hemorrhagic or cystic. Stromal-predominant tumors often have a myomatous appearance. The tumor is derived from nephrogenic blastema and is composed of varying proportions of blastemal, epithelial, and stromal elements (e-Fig. 20.11). Nephroblastomas have a pushing border surrounded by a fibrous pseudocapsule; one exception, however, is the diffuse blastemal type, which infiltrates adjacent renal parenchyma. Other blastemal types include serpentine, nodular, and basaloid patterns. Epithelial differentiation includes tubular, papillary, and glomeruloid patterns; squamous cell, mucinous, and neural differentiation can also occur. The stroma may be primitive mesenchyme or show differentiation into skeletal muscle or, less frequently, smooth muscle, adipose tissue, and cartilage. Tumors with prominent heterologous elements are sometimes referred to as *teratoid Wilms tumor.*

Nephroblastomas are designated favorable or unfavorable on the basis of the presence and distribution of anaplasia rather than type of differentiation. *Anaplasia* is defined by the presence of bizarre or multipolar mitotic figures and large hyperchromatic nuclei (three times the size of other tumor nuclei) (e-Fig. 20.11F). *Focal anaplasia* is defined as one or more focal areas of anaplasia surrounded by nonanaplastic tumor and limited to the kidney. Anaplasia that does not meet the definition of focal is considered *diffuse anaplasia.* Anaplasia in a biopsy is also considered diffuse. Approximately 5% of tumors have diffuse anaplasia, which is the sole criterion for unfavorable histology. The incidence of anaplasia is higher in posttreatment nephrectomies (*J Clin Oncol.* 2006;24:2352).

Nephrogenic rests are the precursor lesions of nephroblastoma (e-Fig. 20.10B and e-Fig. 20.12). *Perilobar nephrogenic rests* are located at the periphery of the renal lobule, are well demarcated from adjacent renal parenchyma, and have predominantly blastemal and epithelial elements. The cells in hyperplastic perilobar rests are cytologically identical to malignant tumor cells; however, rests tend to be ovoid in shape rather than spherical, and they are not surrounded by a tumor pseudocapsule. *Intralobar nephrogenic rests* can occur anywhere in the kidney and have a prominent stromal component that intermixes with normal renal parenchyma. The presence of multiple nephrogenic rests or nephroblastomas is consistent with *nephroblastomatosis* and increases the risk for tumor in the contralateral kidney, especially in infants. In *diffuse hyperplastic perilobar nephroblastomatosis,* the renal parenchyma is extensively replaced by nephrogenic tissue (e-Fig. 20.10C). The diagnosis is made by imaging studies and is treated without biopsy. Tumors that grow despite chemotherapy are removed with kidney-sparing surgical procedures (*Pediatr Develop Pathol.* 2009;12:237). Ectopic nephrogenic rests occur rarely (usually in the inguinal canal or intrapelvic sacrococcygeal regions) and can be associated with extrarenal nephroblastoma (*J Pediatr Surg.* 2009;44:e13).

Nephroblastomas with prominent cysts are designated *cystic nephroblastomas.* Multiloculated renal cysts with microscopic areas of nephroblastoma in the cyst walls, without any expansile septal mass, are designated *partially differentiated cystic nephroblastomas* (e-Fig. 20.10D). Multilocular cysts with only mature elements and no expansile nodules are designated *cystic nephroma* (CN) and, in children, are thought to represent end-stage differentiation of nephroblastoma (*Semin Diagn Pathol.* 1998;15:2, and *Cancer.* 1989;64:466). Familial and bilateral CN are associated with DICER1 mutations and pleuropulmonary blastoma (*J Med Genet.* 2010;47:863).

Following chemotherapy, biopsied or partially resected (usually bilateral) nephroblastomas are categorized according to histologically observed treatment effect (*Pediatr Dev Pathol.* 2005;8:320) (summarized in Table 20.3).

TABLE 20.3	Pathologic Staging of Nephroblastoma and Other Pediatric Renal Neoplasms

Stage	Pathologic criteria
I	Tumor limited to the kidney and completely resected
	Intact renal capsule
	No rupture or previous biopsy
	Renal sinus vessels not involved
	No evidence of tumor at or beyond margins of resection
II	Tumor completely resected
	Tumor extends beyond the kidney, due to one of the following:
	Penetration of the renal capsule
	Extensive invasion of the soft tissue of the renal sinus
	Tumor within blood vessels outside the renal parenchyma, including those of the renal sinus
	No evidence of tumor at or beyond the margins of resection
III	Residual nonhematogenous tumor confined to the abdomen, as evidenced by:
	Involvement of lymph nodes within the abdomen or pelvis
	Penetration through the peritoneal surface
	Tumor implants on the peritoneal surface
	Tumor present at the margin of surgical resection
	Tumor not resectable because of local infiltration into vital structures
	Tumor spillage of any degree or disruption occurring before or during surgery
	Tumor removed in more than one piece
	Biopsy by any method prior to removal
IV	Hematogenous metastases (lung, liver, bone, brain, etc.)
	Lymph node metastases outside the abdomen or pelvis
V	Bilateral renal involvement at diagnosis
	Stage each side separately using above criteria

Modified from *Pediatr Dev Pathol.* 2005;8:320.

Most tumors will fall into the "intermediate" grade with subtotal necrosis and classic triphasic elements observed in the remaining viable tumor; under current protocols, these patients receive an additional 6 weeks of chemotherapy. Less frequently, tumors may show complete necrosis, in which case surgical resection can be performed without additional chemotherapy. Biopsy specimens demonstrating worrisome histologic features such as predominance of blastemal elements or anaplasia after initial treatment are switched to more aggressive chemotherapeutic regimens.

B. **Metanephric tumors** are well-differentiated nephroblastic tumors containing varying proportions of epithelial and stromal cells. Metanephric tumors are benign; however, both nephroblastoma and papillary RCC have been reported in tumors with epithelial elements.

1. **Metanephric stromal tumors (MSTs)** occur throughout childhood, but most commonly in infancy (e-**Fig. 20.13**). Historically, these tumors were considered to be mesoblastic nephromas (MN) (discussed later) but are now considered a distinct entity. MST is usually solitary and extends out from the renal medulla as an unencapsulated mass that may be solid or cystic. The cut surface is firm and myomatous. Microscopically, the tumor is composed of spindled to stellate cells with indistinct cytoplasm. Under low-power microscopy, the tumor has a distinct nodular appearance due to alternating areas of hypocellularity and hypercellularity. The tumor is unencapsulated, and bands of tumor cells extend outward to entrap adjacent glomeruli and tubules, resulting in cysts and epithelial embryonal and juxtaglomerular

hyperplasia. Distinguishing features include concentric cuffs of spindled cells around blood vessels and renal tubules ("collarettes") and angiodysplasia of arterioles with epithelioid transformation of smooth muscle. Heterologous elements such as cartilage and glial tissue are infrequently present (*Am J Surg Pathol.* 2000;24:917).

2. **Metanephric adenofibromas (MAFs)** occur in both children and adults. In children, the tumor has been reported as early as 5 months of age. MAFs are centrally located and contain varying proportions of stroma resembling MST as well as the epithelial nodules of metanephric adenoma. The peripheral stromal component merges with normal renal parenchyma in a manner similar to intralobar nephrogenic rests (see section on adult tumors) (*Am J Surg Pathol.* 2001;25:433).

3. **Metanephric adenoma** occurs most frequently in adults, although the tumor has been reported in children as young as 5 years of age (see section on adult tumors). In children, the main differential diagnosis is epithelial nephroblastoma. Unlike nephroblastoma, however, mitoses are rare, and there is no pseudocapsule, blastemal component, or vascular invasion. Immunohistochemical stains are helpful in distinguishing metanephric adenoma from papillary RCC, but not for distinguishing metanephric adenoma from epithelial nephroblastoma.

C. **Mesoblastic nephroma (MN)** is a distinct neoplasm of infancy which may present antenatally as fetal hydrops (e-**Fig. 20.14**). Tumors diagnosed in a child >2 years most likely represent MST, clear cell sarcoma of the kidney (CCSK), or other tumor. The tumors are unencapsulated, solitary, and they tend to infiltrate the renal sinus. Microscopically, they are characterized as cellular, classic, or mixed histology. *Classic MN* consists of intersecting fascicles of spindled cells resembling infantile fibromatosis. Long fascicles of tumor cells extend into the adjacent renal parenchyma, entrapping tubules and glomeruli and resulting in cysts and epithelial embryonal metaplasia. Dysplastic change with cartilage may be present in adjacent parenchyma. Consistent molecular abnormalities have not been identified with classic histology tumors. *Cellular MN* is composed of plump cells with vesicular nuclei, variable amounts of cytoplasm, and increased mitoses. The tumor has a well-demarcated interface with adjacent renal parenchyma, although it lacks a pseudocapsule. Cellular MN is histologically similar to infantile fibrosarcoma, both of which have the t(12;15)(p13;q25) chromosomal translocation that produces the fusion gene *ETV6–NTRK3*. *Mixed MN* contains both cellular and classic areas. MNs are treated by complete surgical resection, with adjuvant chemotherapy for positive margins. The recurrence rate is 5% to 10%, and the tumor rarely metastasizes, usually to lung (*Adv Anat Pathol.* 2003;10:243).

D. **Clear cell sarcoma of kidney (CCSK)** represents 4% of pediatric renal tumors. It is a primitive mesenchymal neoplasm not associated with any consistent chromosomal or genetic abnormality, although t(10;17) and del(14q) are frequently seen (*Arch Pathol Lab Medi.* 2007;131:446). CCSK occurs usually from 1 to 4 years of age but is also seen in infants (including stillborns) and rarely in adults. It is a high-risk neoplasm, with a tendency for metastases (lung, bone, brain, and soft tissue) and late recurrence. Boys are affected more often than girls. The tumor is unilateral, solitary, well-circumscribed, and located in the renal medulla. Its cut surface is typically tan-gray and mucoid, although the surface may have a firm, whorled appearance (e-**Fig. 20.15**). Cysts are often present. Microscopically, areas with classic histology contain nests and cords of uniform polygonal to spindled cells that have ovoid nuclei with finely granular to vesicular chromatin, inconspicuous nucleoli, and indistinct cytoplasm, in a background of clear extracellular matrix. A delicate, arborizing fibrovascular network separates groups of tumor cells. The tumor interface is well circumscribed under low-power microscopy; however, a pseudocapsule is not present, and tumor extends a short distance into adjacent parenchyma, entrapping tubules that may be cystic or have epithelial metaplasia. Almost all tumors have at least focal classic histology; however, numerous variant histologies including myxoid, sclerosing, cellular, epithelioid, palisading, spindle cell, pericytomatous, storiform, and anaplastic patterns may also be present and may predominate (e-**Fig. 20.15**). CCSK tumor cells are positive for vimentin and negative for epithelial markers. Although immunohistochemical stains may be useful in ruling out other tumors on an individual basis, there are no specific markers for CCSK (*Am J Surg Pathol.* 2004;24:4 and *Virchows Arch.* 2005;446:566).

E. Rhabdoid tumor of the kidney (RTK) is a highly aggressive malignant neoplasm of infancy, accounting for 2% of pediatric renal tumors (e-**Fig. 20.16**). Most patients present at <1 year of age with metastatic disease, and almost all patients present by 3 years. ~10% to 15% of RTKs are associated with rhabdoid tumors of the central nervous system. Both renal and extrarenal infantile rhabdoid tumors contain molecular alterations of the *hSNF5/INI1* gene at chromosome 22q11. Grossly, the renal tumor is pale tan, unencapsulated, and arises from the renal medulla. Multicentric or bilateral tumors are considered metastatic lesions. In areas of classic histology, there are sheets of discohesive tumor cells with large vesicular nuclei, prominent nucleoli, and abundant eccentric cytoplasm containing large eosinophilic inclusions. Ultrastructurally, these inclusions consist of whorls of intermediate filaments that are characteristic but not specific for the tumor. Cells with smaller nuclei and less cytoplasm may sometimes predominate. Variant histology includes sclerosing, epithelioid, spindled, and lymphomatoid patterns. Tumor cells have a polyphenotypic immunostaining pattern, with diffuse vimentin positivity and patchy positivity for other markers, including epithelial markers. There is absent nuclear staining for INI1 (*Adv Anat Pathol.* 2003;10:243, *Am J Surg Pathol.* 1989;1313:439, *Am J Surg Pathol.* 2004;28:1485).

F. Pediatric renal cell carcinoma (RCCs). Although pediatric RCCs bear a strong morphologic resemblance to their adult counterparts, they often possess unique clinical, pathologic, and genetic features that distinguish them from the adult versions (*Adv Anat Pathol.* 2003;10:243). The mean age at presentation is between 9 and 10 years, and the sentinel symptoms include a palpable mass, flank and/or abdominal pain, hematuria, polycythemia, and hypertension. Children tend to have a slightly better prognosis than adults, primarily due to their presentation at earlier stages; metastatic disease has a poor prognosis (<10% 5 year survival) in both groups.

   1. In adults, *clear cell RCC* is the most common malignant epithelial renal neoplasm, but in children this tumor is less common and probably occurs only in patients with von Hippel–Lindau syndrome or another predisposing genetic background. The histopathologic features are identical to those in adult clear cell RCC (see section on adult neoplasms). Many previously reported/diagnosed cases of pediatric clear cell RCC are now thought to be associated with Xp11.2 translocations and therefore likely represent different entities (discussed later).

   2. In children, *papillary RCC* is the most common malignant epithelial neoplasm of the kidney (*Am J Surg Pathol.* 1999;23:795). The histologic, molecular, and genetic findings are identical to those of the adult tumors. The tumor is microscopically composed of a single layer of columnar cells lining a papillary stalk, often with clusters of foamy macrophages, hemosiderin, and necrosis in the surrounding background. The neoplasm is often surrounded by a pseudocapsule with an associated lymphoid infiltrate. The tumor cells are strongly positive for CK7 and EMA expression, which can help differentiate papillary RCC from Wilms tumor and metanephric adenoma.

3. Recently, the category of *translocation RCCs* has been developed to describe a group of neoplasms that, despite diversity in their histologic features, share common molecular and genetic abnormalities (*Pediatr Dev Pathol.* 2005;8:168, *Proc Natl Acad Sci USA.* 1996;93:15294, *Am J Clin Pathol.* 2006;126:349, *Med Pediatr Oncol.* 1998;31:153). Although a variety of chromosomal alterations underlie these tumors, the common end result is a chimeric fusion gene involving a member of the *TFE3/MiT* gene family, a group of basic helix–loop–helix transcription factors. Histologically, these translocation carcinomas exhibit voluminous cells with clear to eosinophilic cytoplasm arranged in papilla or nests with thin intervening fibrous septa (e-**Fig. 20.17**). Psammoma bodies and hyaline nodules are frequently seen. The tumor cells show variable immunopositivity for cytokeratins and EMA, as well as CD10, α-methylacyl-coenzyme A racemase (AMACAR), and RCC marker antigen (*Am J Surg Pathol.* 2008;32:656). The most common mimicker, epithelioid angiomyolipoma, shows positivity for HMB-45 and Melan-A, which is absent or weakly expressed in the translocation carcinomas.

The most consistent and specific finding in translocation carcinomas is nuclear positivity for the rearranged TFE/MiT protein. Xp11.2 *translocation RCCs* express TFE3, which can be detected by antibodies directed toward the C-terminal end of the protein, which is retained in the various gene fusion products. The morphologic similarity of these renal tumors to alveolar soft part sarcoma (ASPS) is not surprising as the latter entity also has a characteristic translocation involving *TFE3*. In fact, the *ASPL-TFE3* rearranged renal carcinomas (which harbor the t(X;1)(p11.2;p34) translocation) bear the greatest resemblance to ASPS (*Am J Pathol.* 1997;21:621). Other *TFE3* fusion partners in this group of carcinomas include *PRCC* (in which t(X;1)(p11.2;q21) is present) and *PSF* (in which t(X;1)(p11.2;q25) is present).

Recently, *melanotic Xp11.2 translocation tumors* bearing the *PSF–TFE3* translocation have been described with melanin-containing epithelioid cells arrayed in nests and sheets separated by prominent vascularized septa; the tumor cells are immunopositive for HMB45, Melan A, and TFE3 expression, but immunonegative for expression of S100 protein, cytokeratins, and renal tubular markers (*Am J Surg Pathol.* 2009;33:609, *Am J Surg Pathol.* 2009;33:1894). These melanotic Xp11.2 translocation tumors share morphologic features of melanomas, PEComas, and translocation RCCs, but appear to be molecularly and immunophenotypically distinct, and may carry a worse prognosis.

Another subset of tumors in this category are *renal tumors with* t(6;11) *translocations* that involve the *TFEB* gene, and that have similar morphology including large polygonal clear and eosinophilic cells, in nests and acini, with intervening hyaline material (*Am J Surg Pathol.* 2005;29:230). The other members of the *TFE/MiT* gene family, namely *TFEC* and *MiTF,* have not been implicated in the pathogenesis of translocation RCCs, although *TFEC* is preferentially expressed in kidney and small intestine, and *MiTF* is involved in melanoma and other neural crest disorders (*Nucl Acids Res.* 2004;32:2315).

The translocation carcinomas appear to be unique among renal neoplasms in expressing not only TFE3 or TFEB, but also cathepsin K, a cysteine protease upregulated by TFE proteins. Immunohistochemical stains for these markers appear to be highly specific, but variably sensitive (*Am J Surg Pathol.* 2010;34:1295, *Mod Pathol.* 2009;22:1016).

Overall, children with translocation carcinomas appear to have a better prognosis than adults, and translocation-positive tumors behave more aggressively than translocation-negative ones. However, the best predictors of outcome and the true prognosis for pediatric patients are yet to be determined. Interestingly, all the translocation carcinomas have also been reported as secondary malignancies in patients with a history of receiving chemotherapy for other tumors.

4. **Renal medullary carcinoma** is an extremely rare, highly malignant neoplasm which occurs only in patients with sickle-cell hemoglobin trait (e-**Fig. 20.18**) (*Mod Pathol.* 2007;20;914). The etiologic relationship between medullary carcinoma and sickle cell trait is unknown. Patients typically present as teenagers or young adults, usually at late stages with widely disseminated disease; survival is measured in weeks or months.

   Renal medullary carcinoma grows in an aggressive, infiltrative, and often sarcomatoid pattern, often entrapping native structures. Intrarenal spread occurs hematogenously and gives the appearance of multifocal lesions. Necrosis and hemorrhage are prominent. The tumor can be morphologically heterogeneous with yolk sac-like, cribriform, microcystic, and solid patterns; it often has rhabdoid cytology. Common mimics include *collecting duct carcinoma* (CDC), *endodermal sinus tumor* (EST), and RTK; however, CDC typically occurs in older patients, and EST has a distinguishing immunoprofile. Like RTK, renal medullary carcinoma shows loss of nuclear hSNF5/INI1 staining, but the immunoprofile of renal medullary carcinoma is otherwise nonspecific in that the tumor cells usually express cytokeratin and are variably reactive for carcinoembryonic antigen (CEA) and EMA.

5. **Postneuroblastoma RCC** is exceedingly rare, occurring in children and teenagers 3 to 12 years old who have previously been diagnosed with neuroblastoma (*Pathology.* 2003;35:499 and *Am J Surg Pathol.* 1999;23:772). Interestingly, postneuroblastoma RCC does not appear to be secondary to treatment; no common chemotherapeutic or radiotherapeutic regimen has been implicated, and at least two cases have been reported in patients with previously untreated, spontaneously resolving stage IVS neuroblastoma. The pathogenesis of this neoplasm therefore remains unclear.

   These tumors exhibit morphologic diversity including solid and papillary growth patterns, a characteristic oncocytic cytology, and areas resembling clear cell RCC with occasional psammoma bodies and/or collections of foamy histiocytes. Immunohistochemically, the tumors are positive for vimentin, EMA, and cytokeratin CAM 5.2 expression. No specific genetic aberrations have been identified. Invasive and metastatic behavior is common.

6. The other renal epithelial neoplasms of adulthood—*oncocytoma, chromophobe RCC,* and others—have all been rarely reported in children (*Pediatr Develop Pathol.* 2007;10:125). In addition, clear cell RCC and CDC have been reported in renal adult allografts in pediatric transplant patients (*Pediatr Transplant.* 2008;12:6000, *Int J Urol.* 2008;15:175). Although the histopathologic features are identical to those in adults, these entities occur too infrequently in the pediatric population to ascertain whether the clinical course is also similar.

G. **Other small round cell tumors.** Small round cell tumors that are usually extrarenal but can occur as a primary renal tumor include neuroblastoma, Ewing sarcoma/primitive neuroectodermal tumor (EWS/PNET), synovial sarcoma, desmoplastic small round cell tumor (DSRCT), rhabdomyosarcoma (RMS), and lymphoma. All can be mistaken for one of the relatively more common pediatric renal tumors.

1. **Undifferentiated neuroblastoma** and **EWS/PNET** can mimic blastemal predominant nephroblastoma, and neural pseudorosettes may resemble primitive tubule formation in nephroblastoma (e-**Fig. 20.19**). Features favoring neuroblastoma over nephroblastoma include diffuse infiltration, hemorrhage, calcification, and nonoverlapping nuclei with "salt and pepper"

chromatin (*Lab Invest.* 2003;83:4P). EWS/PNET is distinguished from nephroblastoma by diffuse infiltration; immunoreactivity for CD99 and FLI1, but nonreactivity for WT1; and by chromosomal translocations involving the *EWS* gene detected by fluorescence in situ hybridization (FISH) or reverse transcription–polymerase chain reaction (RT–PCR) (*Am J Surg Pathol.* 2001;25:133, *Am J Surg Pathol.* 2002;26:320). A novel *FUS–ERG* fusion transcript has also been reported in renal EWS/PNET (*Cancer Genet Cytogenet.* 2009;194:53).

2. **Synovial sarcomas** present in older adolescents. In the kidney, they are usually monophasic and may resemble blastemal nephroblastoma or PNET. Synovial sarcomas have the t(X;18) translocation resulting in a *SYT–SSX* fusion transcript (*Am J Surg Pathol.* 2000;24:1087, *Urology.* 2008;72:716).

3. **Desmoplastic small round cell tumor (DSRCT)** has been reported as a rare primary renal tumor in both older children and adults. Primary renal DSRCT may lack the characteristic desmoplastic reaction and can be confused with other small round cell tumors. The tumor cells have nuclear positivity for WT1, perinuclear dot-like positivity for vimentin, and variable perinuclear dot-like positivity for desmin and cytokeratin. DSRCTs have the t(11;22)(p13;q12) translocation resulting in the *EWS–WT1* fusion transcript.

4. **Rhabdomyosarcoma (RMS)** and *undifferentiated sarcoma* are rare primary renal neoplasms that can occur from early to late childhood. In a recent Children's Oncology Group Report, all renal RMS were classified as embryonal subtype, the majority with anaplastic features. (*Pediatr Blood Cancer.* 2008;51:339).

5. **Non-Hodgkin lymphoma** rarely presents in the kidney as bilateral or multicentric masses. Both B- and T-cell lymphomas have been reported in children. Immunohistochemical markers for lymphoma are used for diagnosis (*Pediatr Blood Cancer.* 2007;48:711).

H. **Miscellaneous tumors**

1. **Angiomyolipomas** can occur in children, almost always in association with tuberous sclerosis. Epithelioid angiomyolipoma (pure epithelioid PEComa) with metastases has been reported in older children and adolescents (*Am J Surg Pathol.* 2011;35:161). The main differential diagnosis of epithelioid angiomyolipoma in children is translocation carcinoma (see section on adult renal neoplasms).

2. **Juxtaglomerular cell tumors** have been reported in older children and adolescents (*Pediatr Blood Cancer.* 2008;50:406) (see section on Adult Renal Neoplasms).

3. **Ossifying renal tumor of infancy** is an extremely rare tumor that typically presents as a calcified abdominal mass in male infants with hematuria. The tumor is attached to the renal papilla and protrudes into the calyceal lumen and pelvis. Microscopically, it consists of spindled cells surrounding a partially mineralized osteoid matrix. The tumor is benign, and recurrences have not been reported (*Pediatr Pathol Lab Med.* 1995;15:745).

4. Other rare pediatric renal tumors include *teratoma* (*J Pediatr Surg.* 2010;45:255) and *myofibroma* (*Virchows Arch.* 2007;450:231). Renal *glomus tumor* (*J Pediatr Surg.* 2010;45:e23) and *gastrinoma* (*The Scientific World J.* 2009;9:501) in adolescents have also been described.

IV. **PATHOLOGIC STAGING.** Most pediatric renal tumors are pathologically staged using the National Wilms Tumor Study Group (NWTS) staging system. This system has been recently modified by the COG (Table 20.4). In the current system, any pretreatment biopsy or intraoperative tumor spillage automatically upstages the tumor to stage III. Lymph node sampling and triaging of tumor for molecular studies is required for specific treatment protocols. Pediatric RCCs are best staged using the tumor, node, metastasis (TNM) system (see Table 20.8).

TABLE 20.4		Classification of Post-chemotherapy Nephroblastoma
Category	**%**	**Pathologic features**
Completely necrotic tumors	10	Less than 1% viable tumor tissue (the presence of scattered mature tubules is allowed) Multiple blocks available taken from different areas of a well-sampled tumor (at least 1 block per cm of greatest tumor dimension)
Intermediate tumors	70	Tumors may contain a variety of histologic features, including epithelial, stromal, and blastemal differentiation A spectrum of proliferative changes may be present, and a spectrum of necrosis and regressive changes may likewise be present but fall short of complete necrosis Less than 66% of the viable tumor should be blastemal if the tumor is >1/3 viable grossly
Blastema-predominant tumors	10	Viable tumor must comprise >1/3 of the tumor mass At least 2/3 of the viable tumor consists of blastema Other components of nephroblastoma may be present in varying proportions
Anaplastic tumors	10	Tumors demonstrating the usual criteria of focal or diffuse anaplasia

Modified from *Pediatr Dev Pathol.* 8:320, 2005.

V. REPORTING PEDIATRIC RENAL NEOPLASMS. The histologic type should be reported for resections, along with pathologic stage and margin status. For nephroblastoma, presence of multicentric tumors, presence and extent of anaplasia, presence and type of adjacent nephrogenic rests, and grade of treatment effect postchemotherapy should be reported. For pediatric RCC, Fuhrman nuclear grade should be reported.

SUGGESTED READINGS

Argani P, Beckwith JB. Renal neoplasms of childhood. In: Mills SE, ed. Sternberg's Diagnostic Surgical Pathology. 4th ed. New York: Lippincott, Williams & Wilkins; 2004;2001–2033.

Argani P, Ladanyi M. Recent advances in pediatric renal neoplasia. *Adv Anat Pathol.* 2003;10:243–260.

Murphy WM, Grignon DJ, Perlman EJ. AFIP Atlas of Tumor Pathology, Fourth Series, Fascicle 1: Tumors of the Kidney, Bladder, and Related Urinary Structures. Washington, D.C.: American Registry of Pathology; 2004.

Perlman EJ. Pediatric renal tumors: Practical updates for the pathologist. *Pediatr Dev Pathol.* 2005;8:320–338.

Ramphal R, Pappo A, Zielenska M, Grant R, Ngan BY. Pediatric renal cell carcinoma: Clinical, pathologic, and molecular abnormalities associated with the members of the mit transcription factor family. *Am J Clin Pathol.* 2006;126:349–364.

Adult Renal Neoplasms

Maria F. Serrano and Peter A. Humphrey

I. GROSS EXAMINATION AND TISSUE SAMPLING. Renal tissue sampling for tumor includes partial and radical nephrectomies and, less commonly, needle biopsies and fine needle aspirates.

A. Needle core biopsy is performed in some centers, particularly prior to use of percutaneous ablative therapies such as radiofrequency heat ablation or cryosurgery. It can also be performed if there is a clinical concern for lymphoma or metastatic disease. The cores can usually be submitted in 10% formalin, with generation of H&E-stained slides. If lymphoma is in the differential diagnosis, additional core(s) should be submitted fresh for lymphoma workup. Histopathologic diagnosis of needle core biopsy tissue from renal masses is highly accurate in establishing a malignant diagnosis (*J Urol.* 2008;180:2333) and in renal tumor typing. FISH (*BJU Int.* 2007;99:290), cytogenetics, comparative genomic hybridization, and/or immunohistochemistry (*Arch Pathol Lab Med.* 2011;135:92) may aid in typing. RCC Fuhrman grade in needle core tissue is often lower than grade in the whole tumor (*Urology.* 2010;76:610).

B. Partial nephrectomy. The surgical resection margin is inked, the specimen is serially sectioned, and the distance to the resection margin is recorded. Sections demonstrating the relationship of the mass to the surgical resection margin and perirenal fat are taken. Intraoperative consultation for gross or frozen section examination of the margin is often requested (*Arch Pathol Lab Med.* 2005;129:1505).

C. Radical nephrectomy. A radical nephrectomy includes the kidney; a portion of the ureter, renal vein, and artery; perinephric fat; and Gerota's fascia. The adrenal gland may also be present. Intraoperative consultation is most commonly requested to grossly confirm presence of a renal or pelvic mass in the nephrectomy specimen (*Arch Pathol Lab Med.* 2005;129:1586).

After weighing the entire specimen, the renal hilum is examined to identify the ureter, renal vein, and artery, and cross sections of these margins are taken (Fig. 20.1). The renal vein and ureter are opened longitudinally. Areas suspicious

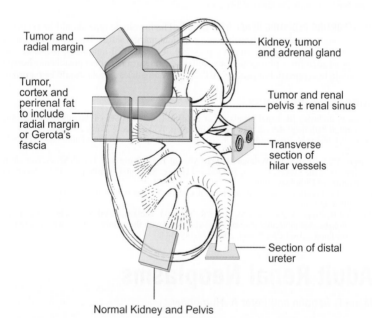

Tumor and radial margin

Kidney, tumor and adrenal gland

Tumor, cortex and perirenal fat to include radial margin or Gerota's fascia

Tumor and renal pelvis ± renal sinus

Transverse section of hilar vessels

Section of distal ureter

Normal Kidney and Pelvis

Figure 20.1 Sampling of radical nephrectomy specimen for adult renal tumors. Sections through renal masses should demonstrate relationship of mass to capsule, peripheral fat, renal parenchyma, and renal pelvis. (Modified from: Schmidt WA. *Principles and Techniques of Surgical Pathology.* Menlo Park, CA: Addison-Wesley; 1983.)

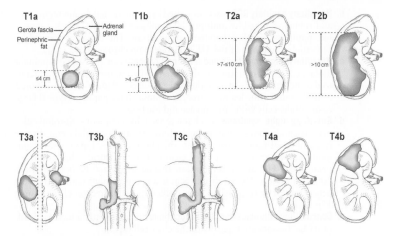

Figure 20.2 RCC pathologic primary tumor (pT) stages. (Modified from: Edge SB, Byrd DR, Compton CC, Fritz AG, Greene FL, Trotti A, eds. *AJCC Cancer Staging Manual*. 7th ed. New York, NY: Springer; 2010.)

for tumor involvement of the perirenal soft tissue are inked selectively. Occasionally, lymph nodes are found in the hilar region.

The kidney is then sectioned sagittally. Tumor size, location (upper or lower pole, cortex, or medulla), involvement of calyceal or pelvic mucosa, invasion of the capsule or perirenal soft tissue, and involvement of the adrenal gland are recorded. The uninvolved parenchyma is also examined: color, cortical thickness, additional focal lesions, and renal pelvis are described. One section per centimeter of tumor, demonstrating its relationship to adjacent capsule, renal parenchyma, and pelvis are submitted, as well as sections of any additional lesions, uninvolved renal parenchyma, and adrenal gland (Fig. 20.2). Nephroureterectomy for urothelial carcinomas is described in Chapter 21.

II. DIAGNOSTIC FEATURES OF COMMON TUMORS OF THE ADULT KIDNEY

A. Carcinoma.
RCC arises from the epithelium of the renal tubules and represents ~90% of all renal malignancies in adults.

1. **Risk factors.** The most important risk factor is tobacco smoking. Additional risk factors include obesity, hypertension, unopposed estrogens, and exposure to arsenic, asbestos, cadmium, organic solvents, pesticides, and fungal toxins. Patients with tuberous sclerosis, chronic renal failure, and acquired cystic disease of the kidney have an increased incidence of RCC. About 5% of patients with acquired cystic disease of the kidney develop renal cell tumors (see section on Acquired Cystic Disease-associated Renal Cell Carcinoma). Most RCCs are sporadic, although there are several inherited cancer syndromes that affect the kidney (*N Eng J Med*. 2005;353:2477), as follows.

a. **Von Hippel–Lindau (VHL) disease** is inherited in an autosomal dominant manner and is characterized by hemangioblastomas of the cerebellum and retina, clear cell RCC, pheochromocytoma, pancreatic cysts, and inner ear tumors. Typically, renal tumors are multiple and bilateral (**e-Fig. 20.20**). Numerous renal cysts, lined by neoplastic clear cells (**e-Fig. 20.21**), are also characteristic. This disease is caused by germline mutations of the *VHL* tumor suppressor gene on chromosome 3p25.3.

b. **Hereditary papillary RCC** is also inherited in an autosomal dominant manner and is characterized by multiple, bilateral papillary RCCs with a type I-like papillary or tubulopapillary architecture. The disease is caused by activating mutations of the *MET* oncogene on chromosome 7q31.

c. **Hereditary leiomyomatosis and renal cell cancer** is an autosomal dominant disease caused by mutations in the fumarate hydratase gene. It is characterized by benign leiomyomas of the skin and uterus. Patients are predisposed to RCC and uterine leiomyosarcoma. Tumors have papillary type II large eosinophilic cells with large nuclei and nucleoli.

d. **Birt–Hogg–Dubé syndrome** is characterized by cutaneous fibrofolliculomas, trichodiscomas, and acrochordons. Multiple and bilateral diverse types of renal tumors are present; the chromophobe type is most common, but oncocytoma, papillary, clear cell, and "hybrid" chromophobe-oncocytic (e-Fig. 20.22) tumors can also be seen (*Arch Pathol Lab Med.* 2006;130:1867). The syndrome is autosomal dominant with incomplete penetrance. The responsible gene, folliculin, is located on chromosome 17p 11.2.

e. **Constitutional chromosome 3 translocations** are related to an increased risk of RCC. Tumors are typically of the clear cell type.

f. **Succinate dehydrogenase germline mutations** in the gene encoding the B subunit (*SDHB*) result in a 15% lifetime risk of RCC development. Several tumor types have been seen, including clear cell carcinoma, papillary carcinoma, and oncocytoma.

2. **Clinical diagnosis.** Hematuria, pain, and a flank mass is the classical triad of presenting symptoms, but in North America most renal tumors are now detected as incidental findings by radiological studies. Other presentations include weight loss, anorexia, fever, hypercalcemia, erythrocytosis, hypertension, gynecomastia, anemia, and hepatosplenomegaly. Radiological studies, especially ultrasound and computed tomography (CT), are useful for detection and characterization of renal masses, but up to 15% of renal masses thought to be malignant by radiology are histologically benign, typically oncocytomas or angiomyolipomas.

3. **Histologic typing and diagnosis of renal epithelial malignancies.** The 2004 World Health Organization (WHO) classification of neoplasms of the kidney is given in Table 20.5. Recently recognized additional renal carcinoma types also exist (*Mod Pathol.* 2009;22:S2), including tubulocystic carcinoma, acquired cystic disease-associated RCC, clear cell papillary RCC, and thyroid-like follicular carcinoma. Most renal neoplasms can be typed on the basis of examination of H&E-stained slides; immunohistochemistry is most often used to confirm a diagnosis of metastatic RCC, although in a minority of cases, it can be useful in typing (Table 20.6).

a. **Clear cell RCC** is the most common histologic type. Grossly, these tumors often have a variegated appearance (e-Fig. 20.23). Bright yellow areas (e-Fig. 20.24) are due to the high lipid content of the cells, whereas red and white-yellow regions are due to hemorrhage, fibrosis, and necrosis. Calcification and cystic change are fairly common. The cysts can be multilocular (e-Fig. 20.25) or secondary to necrosis. Histologic sections show round or polygonal cells with clear or eosinophilic cytoplasm and centrally located nuclei. The cells are arranged in nests within a fine vascular network (e-Fig. 20.26). Tumor cells react with antibodies to low-molecular-weight keratins, RCC marker (RCC Ma), vimentin, epithelial membrane antigen, carbonic anhydrase IX, and CD10. They are usually negative for expression of CD117, kidney-specific cadherin, and parvalbumin (*Arch Pathol Lab Med.* 2011;135:92). Clear cell RCCs are associated with 3p

TABLE 20.5 WHO Histologic Classification of Tumors of the Kidney

Renal cell tumors
Clear cell renal cell carcinoma
Multilocular clear cell renal cell carcinoma
Papillary renal cell carcinoma
Chromophobe renal cell carcinoma
Carcinoma of the collecting ducts of Bellini
Renal medullary carcinoma
Xp11 translocation carcinomas
Carcinoma associated with neuroblastoma
Mucinous tubular and spindle cell carcinoma
Renal cell carcinoma, unclassified
Papillary adenoma
Oncocytoma

Metanephric tumors
Metanephric adenoma
Metanephric adenofibroma
Metanephric stromal tumor

Nephroblastic tumors
Nephrogenic rests
Nephroblastoma
　Cystic partially differentiated nephroblastoma

Mesenchymal tumors
Occurring mainly in children
　Clear cell sarcoma
　Rhabdoid tumor
　Congenital mesoblastic nephroma
　Ossifying renal tumor of infants
Occurring mainly in adults
　Leiomyosarcoma (including renal vein)
　Angiosarcoma
　Rhabdomyosarcoma

Malignant fibrous histiocytoma
Hemangiopericytoma
Osteosarcoma
Angiomyolipoma
Epithelioid angiomyolipoma
Leiomyoma
Hemangioma
Lymphangioma
Juxtaglomerular cell tumor
Renomedullary interstitial cell tumor
Schwannoma
Solitary fibrous tumor

Mixed mesenchymal and epithelial tumors
Cystic nephroma
Mixed epithelial and stromal tumor
Synovial sarcoma

Neuroendocrine tumors
Carcinoid
Neuroendocrine carcinoma
Primitive neuroectodermal tumors
Pheochromocytoma

Hematopoietic and lymphoid tumors
Lymphoma
Leukemia
Plasmacytoma

Germ cell tumors
Teratoma
Choriocarcinoma

Metastatic tumors

From: Eble JN, Sauter G, Epstein JI, Sesterhenn IA, eds. *World Health Organization Classification of Tumours. Pathology and Genetics. Tumours of the Urinary System and Male Genital Organs.* Lyon: IARC Press; 2004. Used with permission.

deletions, and *VHL* gene mutations are found in up to 60% of sporadic cases.

Fuhrman nuclear grading is the most important prognostic factor after staging (Table 20.7). Grade 1 cells have small, round, uniform nuclei without visible nucleoli. Grade 2 cells have larger nuclei with irregular outlines and nucleoli seen only at 400× magnification. Grade 3 cells have recognizable nucleoli at 100×, and grade 4 cells exhibit nuclear pleomorphism and hyperchromasia, with bizarre often multilobed nuclei. Tumors should be graded according to the highest grade present even if focal (defined as occupying at least one 400× high-power field) (e-**Figs. 20.27** to **20.30**).

Clear cell RCC spreads locally into the renal sinus or perinephric fat by direct extension, and by venous invasion into the renal vein and vena cava. Lymphatic spread to lymph nodes can occur. Hematogenous spread to lungs, liver, and bone is most frequent, although spread to unusual

TABLE 20.6	Immunophenotype of Renal Tumors						
Marker	Clear cell RCC	Papillary RCC	Chromo-phobe RCC	Oncocy-toma	Xp11	MTSCC	CCP RCC
RCC Ma	+	+	−/+	−	+	+/−	N/A
PAX2	+	+	−/+	+	−	+	N/A
CD10	+	+	−/+	−	+	−	−
KS- cadherin	−/+	−/+	+	+	−/+	−	N/A
CK7	−	+	+	−	−	+	+
AE1/AE3	+	+	+	+	−	+	+
Vimentin	+	+	−	−	+/−	+/−	+
C-Kit (CD117)	−	−/+	+	+	N/A	−	N/A
AMACR	−	+	−	N/A	+	+	−
CAIX	+	−/+	−/+	−	−/+	N/A	+

RCC, renal cell carcinoma; +, most studies show positive results; −, most studies show negative results; +/−, more studies show positive, some studies show negative; −/+, more studies show negative, some studies show positive; N/A, data not found in used references; Xp11, Xp11 translocation carcinoma; MTSCC, mucinous tubular and spindle cell carcinoma; RCC Ma, renal cell carcinoma marker; KS, kidney-specific; CK7, cytokeratin 7; CCP RCC, clear cell papillary RCC; AMACR, α-methylacyl CoA racemase; CAIX, carbonic anhydrase IX.
Modified from Al-Ghani et al, *Pathol Case Rev.* 2010;15:25.

sites is a well-known characteristic. Metastasis can develop many years after primary diagnosis. Useful immunostains potentially supporting the diagnosis of metastatic RCC include PAX2 or PAX8, and RCC Ma or CD10. These markers are, however, not specific for RCC; PAX2 may be the best marker and has moderate sensitivity (50%–85%) for metastatic clear cell renal carcinoma and high specificity (of at least 90%) but is nonetheless found in other carcinomas, especially müllerian carcinomas (*Adv Anat Pathol.* 2010;17:377). As always, the panel of immunomarkers should be interpreted in the context of the histologic, radiologic, and clinical findings.

Prognostic models predicting clear cell RCC patient survival after radical nephrectomy have been developed (*Urol Int.* 2008;80:113). One such model incorporates tumor size, pT stage, Fuhrman grade, necrosis, and vascular invasion, and mode of clinical presentation (*J Urol.* 2005;173:48).

b. **Multilocular cystic RCC** is composed of multiple cysts separated by thin septa (e-Fig. 20.31) with a neoplastic clear cell epithelial lining, with clear tumor cells in the septa (e-Fig. 20.32). Grossly, this tumor is well circumscribed and contains cysts of variable size filled with clear or hemorrhagic fluid. Calcification is frequent. Tumor cells are reactive with antibodies to cytokeratins and epithelial membrane antigen; these immunostains can be especially useful in the distinction of tumor cells from macrophages in the septa. This tumor type is separate from RCC with multilocular features (e-Fig. 20.25), where expansile mass formation is detected. Chromosome 3p deletion has been detected in about three-quarters of cases, and it

TABLE 20.7	Fuhrman Nuclear Grading of Renal Cell Carcinoma
Grade 1	Small, round and uniform nuclei. No evident nucleoli
Grade 2	Nuclei with irregular outlines. Inconspicuous nucleoli
Grade 3	Irregular nuclei with identifiable nucleoli at 100 × magnification
Grade 4	Large, hyperchromatic, pleomorphic nuclei. Single or multiple nucleoli

has been proposed that multilocular cystic RCC is a subtype of clear cell RCC (*Mod Pathol.* 2010;23:931). No recurrences or metastasis have been reported for this tumor type.

c. **Papillary RCC** comprises about 10% of RCCs. Grossly, the tumor can be cystic, hemorrhagic, and necrotic, with a fibrous pseudocapsule (e-**Fig. 20.33**). Multifocality and bilaterality are more common than for other RCCs. Microscopically, there is a papillary or tubulopapillary architecture composed of papillae with thin fibrovascular cores which may harbor aggregates of foamy macrophages (e-**Fig. 20.34**) and cholesterol crystals.

There are two types of papillary RCC. Type I tumors have papillae lined by a single layer of cuboidal cells with scant cytoplasm (e-**Fig. 20.34**) that has a basophilic quality. Type II tumors have taller cells with more abundant eosinophilic cytoplasm, higher nuclear grade, and pseudostratified nuclei (e-**Fig. 20.35**). Fuhrman grading may be applied (*Am J Clin Pathol.* 2002;118:877), but nucleolar grading may also be useful (*Am J Surg Pathol.* 2006;30:1091). Type I papillary RCC is often positive for vimentin, keratins detected by AE1/AE3 antibodies, CK7, AMACR, and RCC Ma; immunostains that are usually negative include CD117, kidney-specific cadherin, and parvalbumin. Type II RCCs have a variable immunophenotype (*Arch Pathol Lab Med.* 2011;135:92). Genetically, there is characteristic trisomy of chromosomes 7 and 17, with loss of chromosome 4, but chromosomal analysis is not used diagnostically. Papillary RCC, especially type I, has a better outcome than clear cell RCC.

d. **Chromophobe RCC** accounts for ~5% of RCCs. Grossly, chromophobe RCCs are well circumscribed, solid, and beige to light brown (e-**Fig. 20.36**). Tumors are composed of pale polygonal cells with prominent cell borders, often wrinkled nuclear membranes, and perinuclear halos (e-**Fig. 20.37**). The cytoplasm can be finely granular or flocculent (e-**Fig. 20.38**) to eosinophilic (e-**Fig. 20.39**). The use of Fuhrman grading is controversial (*Am J Surg Pathol.* 2007;31:957; *Mod Pathol.* 2009;22:S24). Diffuse cytoplasmic positivity with Hale's colloidal iron is characteristic, and these tumors show extensive aneusomy with loss of chromosomes 1, 2, 6, 10, 13, 17, and 21 which can be detected by FISH (*Mod Pathol.* 2005;18:320).

Hale's colloidal iron and FISH can be used to address the differential diagnosis of the eosinophilic variant of chromophobe RCC versus oncocytoma. For the differential diagnosis with clear cell and papillary RCC, immunostains can be helpful, although H&E slides are typically diagnostic; immunopositivity for kidney-specific cadherin, parvalbumin, CD117, EMA, keratins (detected by AE1/AE3 antibodies), and CK7 is typical, with negative immunostains for vimentin, carbonic anhydrase IX, and AMACR (*Arch Pathol Lab Med.* 2011;135:92). Chromophobe RCC has a much better prognosis than clear cell RCC.

e. **Collecting duct carcinoma (CDC)** is thought to arise from the collecting ducts of Bellini. It accounts for <1% of renal cell tumors. These tumors are centered in the medulla, have tubular or tubulopapillary architecture, and have a surrounding desmoplastic reaction (e-**Fig. 20.40**). The tumor cells are typically of high nuclear grade and can have hobnail cytology. Use of immunostains in diagnosis has limitations; when needed, α-methylacyl coenzyme A racemase (AMACR), CD10, and RCC Ma negativity would favor CDC over papillary RCC, which figures prominently in the differential diagnosis, and which would usually be positive for these three markers (*Semin Diag Pathol.* 2005;22:51). Immunopositivity for PAX2 and PAX8, with negative immunostains for p63 and uroplakin III, would favor CDC over urothelial carcinoma. Most tumors present at an advanced stage with metastatic disease. The prognosis is poor.

f. **Renal medullary carcinoma** is very rare. Tumors in adults are identical to those in the pediatric age group as discussed earlier.

g. **Renal carcinomas associated with Xp11.2 translocations** are defined by various translocations affecting chromosome Xp11.2, resulting in gene fusions involving the *TFE3* gene. Although rare in adults, they are histologically identical to those in the pediatric age group as discussed earlier.

h. **RCC associated with neuroblastoma** is exceedingly rare and occurs in long-term survivors of childhood neuroblastoma, as discussed earlier.

i. **Mucinous tubular and spindle cell carcinoma** is an uncommon, predominantly low-grade renal epithelial neoplasm that is grossly well circumscribed with gray or light tan, uniform cut surfaces (e-**Fig. 20.41**). Microscopically, elongated tubules are separated by a mucinous stroma (e-**Fig. 20.42**). The tumor cells are cuboidal or spindle shaped with low-grade nuclear features. Uncommonly, necrosis, clear cells papillations, foamy macrophages, and inflammation can be present (*Am J Surg Pathol.* 2006;30:1554). Sarcomatoid or high-grade epithelial components are also uncommon. The immunophenotype shows significant overlap with papillary RCC. Loss of chromosomes 1, 4, 6, 8, 13, and 14 and gains of chromosomes 7, 11, 16, and 17 are characteristic of these tumors, but molecular analysis is not currently used diagnostically. This tumor type generally has a good prognosis.

j. **Unclassified RCC** is a diagnosis that should be reserved for those tumors that do not fit into other categories. It is a diagnosis rendered in about 5% of RCC cases. Features that place tumors in this group include the following: a combination of different histologic types, mucin production, sarcomatoid appearance, presence of epithelial and stromal elements, and nonidentifiable patterns. This designation is linked to a worse prognosis than clear cell RCC (*BJU Int.* 2007;100:802).

Sarcomatoid change (e-**Fig. 20.43**, e-**Fig. 20.44**) can be associated with a specific type of carcinoma or can overgrow the preexisting carcinoma type and exist in pure form. The percentage of the tumor that is sarcomatoid should be specified as being less than or greater than 50%. Heterologous malignant bone, cartilage, fat, and skeletal muscle or homologous undifferentiated malignant spindle cells can be seen. Rhabdoid cells (e-**Fig. 20.45**) can be found in about 5% of RCC cases, usually clear cell carcinoma (*Am J Surg Pathol.* 2000;24:1329–1338). Both sarcomatoid and rhabdoid features are associated with a poor prognosis.

k. **Tubulocystic carcinoma** is very uncommon and is of low malignant potential (*Am J Surg Pathol.* 2009;33:384). Grossly, the tumor is usually solitary and circumscribed with a spongy "bubblewrap"-like cut surface. Microscopically, sections show tightly packed tubules and cysts up to a few millimeters in diameter (e-**Fig. 20.46**), separated by fibrous stroma; the lining epithelium has eosinophilic or amphophilic cytoplasm and large prominent nucleoli, and hobnail type cells may be seen. Most cases are positive for CK7, CK19, parvalbumin, CD10, AMACR, and kidney-specific cadherin by immunohistochemistry. Gene expression profiling shows a distinctive signature similar to but not identical to papillary RCC, with no overlap with CDC. Most cases are pT1 and only a few patients have developed metastatic disease.

l. **Acquired cystic disease-associated RCC** can be seen in patients with end-stage renal disease, especially after long-term dialysis (*Am J Surg Pathol.* 2006;30:141). Many RCCs that develop in end-stage renal disease kidneys are clear cell, papillary, and chromophobe RCCs of usual type. However, a unique carcinoma, termed acquired cystic disease-associated RCC, is observed only in end-stage renal disease and acquired cystic disease, and is characterized by microcystic and cribriform/sieve-like architecture (e-**Fig. 20.47**), eosinophilic cytoplasm with Fuhrman grade 3 nucleoli, and frequent intratumoral oxalate crystals. Additional architectural patterns include solid acinar, solid sheet-like, papillary, and macrocystic. Immunostains show positivity for AMACR, vinculin, and parvalbumin, with no reactivity for CK7. Another histologic type of carcinoma found in end-stage kidneys is clear cell papillary RCC (discussed later). Clinically, acquired cystic disease-associated RCC appears to be more aggressive than other tumor types in end-stage renal disease.

m. **Clear cell papillary RCC** can arise in end-stage renal disease but also in kidneys without end stage features. One group, also called clear cell tubulopapillary RCC (*Am J Surg Pathol.* 2010;34:1608) or clear cell papillary and cystic RCC (*Mod Pathol.* 2009;22:S2), is typically cystic with a fibrous capsule and is composed of cells with low nuclear grade (Fuhrman 2) and a cystic, tubuloacinar, and/or papillary architecture (e-**Fig. 20.48**). The papillae are prominent and lined by cells with variable amounts of cleared cytoplasm. A characteristic finding is linear arrangement of the nuclei in the center or apical portions of the cytoplasm. The immunophenotype and molecular genetic profiles are distinct from papillary and clear cell RCC: CK7 and carbonic anhydrase 9 immunostains are positive, and immunostains for AMACR, TFE3, and CD10 are negative. Gains of chromosomes 7 and 17 (typical of papillary RCC) and 3p loss (seen in clear cell RCC) are not present. Most tumors are low stage at presentation and limited outcome data suggest an extremely favorable prognosis.

A second group of clear cell papillary RCCs, identified on the basis of CK7 and AMACR positivity, is termed papillary RCC with clear cell features (*J Urol.* 2011;185:30). A substantial percentage of these cases has high nuclear grade, and in this group of tumors the presence of clear cells is an adverse prognostic indicator compared with conventional clear cell tubulopapillary RCC.

n. **Thyroid-like follicular carcinoma of the kidney** is rare, with less than ten cases reported (*Am J Surg Pathol.* 2009;33:393). Microscopically, macrofollicles and microfollicles with intraluminal colloid-like secretion are present (e-**Fig. 20.49**). A negative TTF-1 immunostain and clinical history are useful in excluding metastatic thyroid carcinoma.

B. **Benign epithelial tumors**

1. **Papillary adenoma of the kidney** is the most common benign epithelial neoplasm of renal cells. Grossly, the tumor consists of single or multiple well-defined white nodules in the renal cortex. The tumors have papillary, tubular, or tubulopapillary architecture (e-**Fig. 20.50**), low nuclear grade (e-**Fig. 20.51**), and measure ≤5 mm in diameter. The cytoplasm is scant and non-cleared, and nuclear grooves can be present. Psammoma bodies and foamy macrophages are common.

2. **Oncocytoma** is a benign epithelial neoplasm that comprises ~5% of all neoplasms of the renal tubular epithelium. The lesion is more frequent in men, and the peak incidence is during the seventh decade of life. Grossly, the tumors are well circumscribed and the cut-surface is typically mahogany-brown (e-**Fig. 20.52**). A central scar (e-**Fig. 20.52** and e-**Fig. 20.53**) is seen in up to 33% of cases, generally with larger tumors; such scarring, although characteristic, is not specific for oncocytoma. Hemorrhage is frequent, but necrosis is almost always absent.

Microscopically, these tumors are composed of nests and tubules of round or polygonal cells with granular eosinophilic cytoplasm, round nuclei, and single central nucleoli (e-**Fig. 20.54**). Scattered larger cells with a higher nuclear/cytoplasmic ratio and hyperchromatic nuclei can be seen (e-**Fig. 20.55**). Smaller cells with scant cytoplasm (known as oncoblasts) can also be noted in some cases (e-**Fig. 20.56**). A hyalinized or edematous stromal background is frequent. Microscopic (but not gross) extension into perirenal fat and vessels has been described. Rare cases of numerous oncocytic tumors (oncocytosis) have been described. Chromosomal abnormalities in oncocytoma include t(5;11) and loss of chromosomes 1 and 14, but assessment for these abnormalities is not usually necessary. No cases of death due to metastatic disease have been reported.

C. **Metanephric tumors** (see also the section on pediatric renal neoplasm)
1. **Metanephric adenoma** occurs in children, and in adults during the fifth and sixth decades. It is more frequent in women. About 50% of cases are incidental. Tumors are usually well circumscribed, gray to tan to yellow, and firm or soft. Hemorrhage, necrosis, calcification, and cyst formation are common. Microscopically, metanephric adenomas are composed of small, uniform round acini with small lumens (e-**Fig. 20.57**). The cells are uniform with small nuclei and inconspicuous nucleoli. Branching and tubular configurations are common, as well as a papillary architecture with numerous psammoma bodies. In the differential diagnosis with papillary RCC, immunostains that are positive for WT1, negative for EMA, and focally positive for CK7 favor metanephric adenoma.
2. **Metanephric adenofibroma** is more common in men. Grossly, it is solitary and partially cystic. Histologically, its cells are similar to those of a metanephric adenoma but are embedded in a stroma of fibroblast-like spindle cells. Psammoma bodies are also common.

D. **Mesenchymal tumors**
1. **Leiomyosarcoma** is the most common renal sarcoma; it occurs mainly in adults and affects women and men equally. They can arise from the renal capsule, parenchyma, pelvis muscularis, or the renal vein. They are solid, gray-white, and focally necrotic. Histologically, these tumors are composed of spindle cells with a fascicular growth pattern (e-**Fig. 20.58**). Necrosis, nuclear pleomorphism, and numerous mitotic figures indicate malignancy. Leiomyosarcoma is an aggressive tumor with a 5-year survival rate of 29% to 36%, and most patients die within 1 year of diagnosis. Sites of metastasis include lung, liver, and bone. Sarcomatoid RCC is in the differential diagnosis and is more common, and so must be excluded; diffuse desmin and smooth muscle actin immunoreactivity would favor leiomyosarcoma.
2. **Rare primary sarcomas** include RMS, angiosarcoma, malignant fibrous histiocytoma, chondrosarcoma, low-grade fibromyxoid sarcoma, malignant mesenchymoma, and osteosarcoma.
3. **Angiomyolipoma** is a benign clonal mesenchymal neoplasm tumor composed of thick-walled blood vessels, smooth muscle cells, and adipose tissue (e-**Fig. 20.59**). This tumor belongs to the perivascular epithelioid cell tumor (PEComa) family. The mean age at presentation is 45 to 55 years for patients without tuberous sclerosis, and 25 to 35 years for patients with tuberous sclerosis. Patients with tuberous sclerosis tend to have multiple, bilateral renal tumors and can have associated pulmonary lymphangioleiomyomatosis. Tumors are nonencapsulated, yellow to pink masses (e-**Fig. 20.60**) depending on the content of the tissue components. Rarely, angiomyolipomas can extend into the renal vein or the vena cava. Vascular invasion and lymph node involvement can be present; however, these features are considered to be evidence of direct extension and multifocality, respectively, rather than metastatic disease.

Microscopically, the limits between the tumor and the kidney are well defined. The smooth muscle cells are generally spindled (e-**Fig. 20.61**) but can appear round or epithelioid in some cases (e-**Fig. 20.62**). The smooth muscle cells often appear to radiate from the outer aspect of the thick-walled, hyalinized blood vessels (e-**Fig. 20.63**). Nuclear atypia can be present (e-**Fig. 20.64**). The amount of fat is variable and can be very focal (e-**Fig. 20.62**). Uncommon to rare histologic variants include fat-predominant, smooth muscle-predominant, lymphangioleiomyomatous (e-**Fig. 20.65**), oncocytoma-like, sclerosing type, and angiomyolipoma with epithelial cysts (e-**Fig. 20.66**). Characteristically, angiomyolipomas coexpress melanocytic markers such as HMB45 and smooth muscle markers such as smooth muscle actin and muscle-specific actin. Epithelial markers including cytokeratin are always negative. Angiomyolipomas can be diagnosed in needle biopsy tissue (e-**Fig. 20.67**). Classic angiomyolipomas are benign.

4. **Epithelioid angiomyolipoma** is a potentially malignant mesenchymal neoplasm that presents more commonly in patients with tuberous sclerosis. It is much less common than usual angiomyolipoma. Grossly, these tumors are usually large with tan-gray or hemorrhagic cut surfaces and necrosis. The cells are epithelioid with abundant granular cytoplasm. Multinucleated cells, nuclear pleomorphism, mitotic activity, vascular invasion, necrosis (e-**Fig. 20.68**), and involvement of perinephric fat can be present. These tumors express melanocytic markers with variable expression of smooth muscle markers. These tumors can metastasize to lymph nodes, liver, lungs, and spine.

5. **Leiomyoma** is a benign smooth muscle neoplasm that can arise from the renal capsule, the muscularis of the renal pelvis, or from cortical vascular smooth muscle. Most are found incidentally. Grossly, they are firm well-defined masses, although calcification and cysts can be present. Necrosis should be absent. Leiomyomas are composed of spindled cells arranged in fascicles, with minimal nuclear pleomorphism and no mitotic activity. They demonstrate a smooth muscle immunophenotype, with actin and desmin immunopositivity. So-called capsulomas that look like leiomyomas originating from the capsule that are HMB-45 positive are thought to be monophasic leiomyomatous angiomyolipomas.

6. **Hemangioma** is a benign vascular tumor that presents in young and middle-aged adults. The tumor is usually unilateral and single, with a red spongy gross appearance. Microscopically, the lesion is characterized by irregular blood-filled spaces lined by a single layer of endothelial cells. No mitoses or nuclear pleomorphism is present.

7. **Lymphangiomas** are more common in adults and can represent a lymphatic malformation or can develop secondary to urinary tract infections. Grossly, they are cystic, encapsulated lesions that can overgrow the entire renal parenchyma. The cysts are filled with clear fluid and lined by a single layer of flat endothelium.

8. **Juxtaglomerular cell tumors** are benign renin-secreting tumors that occur in younger individuals and are more common in women. Clinically, the tumor manifests with severe hypertension and hypokalemia. The tumors are solid, well circumscribed, and composed of sheets of polygonal or spindled cells with central regular nuclei, well-defined borders, and granular eosinophilic cytoplasm. Mast cells, hyalinized vessels, and tubular elements are common. The tumor cells are immunoreactive for renin, actin, vimentin, and CD34.

9. **Renomedullary interstitial cell tumors** are commonly found during autopsy. They are present in about 50% of men and women, and frequently they are multifocal. They are 1 to 5 mm in diameter, white or gray, and located within the renal pyramids. Histologically, they contain small polygonal cells

in a basophilic background. Renal tubules can be entrapped within the tumor nodules (e-**Fig. 20.69**).

E. Mixed mesenchymal and epithelial tumors

1. **Cystic nephroma** is a benign neoplasm that presents after age 30, more commonly in women. It is associated with pleuropulmonary blastoma in the patient or other family members. Grossly, the tumor is well defined, encapsulated, and entirely composed of cysts. Solid areas and necrosis are not present. The cystic change is multiloculated (e-**Fig. 20.70**), with the fibrous septa lined by cuboidal epithelium that often assumes a hobnail appearance (e-**Fig. 20.71**). The fibrous septa may contain tubules but not blastema or clear neoplastic cells.

2. **Mixed epithelial and stromal tumor** predominates in adult perimenopausal women. A history of estrogen therapy is common. Grossly, the tumor is composed of solid and cystic areas. Microscopically, the tumor shows tubules and cysts lined by flattened, to cuboidal, to columnar epithelium. The stromal component is variably cellular and may exhibit myxoid, smooth muscle, ovarian stromal-like, or collagenous features. Fat can be present. The tumor's behavior is benign. Since it is possible that cystic nephroma and mixed epithelial and stromal tumor are related, the unifying term renal epithelial stromal tumor (REST) has been proposed (*Am J Surg Pathol.* 2007; 31:489).

F. Neuroendocrine tumors

1. **Renal carcinoid tumors** are very rare and present between the fourth and seventh decades. There is a tendency for occurrence in horseshoe kidneys, and there is an association with renal teratomas. Renal carcinoid tumors are solid, lobulated, and well circumscribed and are histologically similar to carcinoids in other organs (e-**Fig. 20.72**) (*Am J Surg Pathol.* 2007;31: 1539).

2. **Neuroendocrine carcinoma,** including small cell carcinoma, can rarely arise within the adult kidney. A primary tumor elsewhere should be clinically and radiologically excluded. Grossly, the tumor is usually a white, friable, and necrotic mass. Microscopically, the tumor is composed of small round cells with hyperchromatic nuclei and inconspicuous nucleoli, arranged in sheets and trabeculae. Centrally located tumors can be admixed with urothelial carcinoma. The tumor cells show dotlike cytoplasmic immunostaining with cytokeratin antibodies and are variably positive for synaptophysin and chromogranin. The prognosis is poor.

3. **PNETs** are rare primary renal tumors and are discussed in the section on pediatric renal neoplasm.

4. Primary **renal neuroblastoma** and **paragangliomas/pheochromocytomas** are very rare.

G. Hematopoietic and lymphoid tumors.
Primary renal lymphomas usually arise in transplanted kidneys and are Epstein–Barr virus (EBV)-associated B-cell lymphoproliferations. Secondary involvement of the kidney by lymphoma is more common (e-**Fig. 20.73 and e-Fig. 20.74**). Plasmacytoma can occur as a manifestation of disseminated multiple myeloma. Diffuse infiltration of the kidney secondary to acute leukemias has also been reported.

H. Germ cell tumors
include choriocarcinomas and teratomas and are very rare.

I. Metastatic tumors
to the kidney include tumors of lung, breast, gastrointestinal tract, pancreas, ovary, and testis and malignant melanoma. Involvement is usually in the setting of known, widely metastatic disease. Only infrequently does metastatic tumor mimic a primary renal tumor. Most metastatic masses are multiple and bilateral.

III. HISTOLOGIC GRADING OF RCC
should be reported for all RCCs of clear cell and papillary types, as described earlier and in Table 20.7.

TABLE 20.8	Tumor, Node, Metastasis (TNM) Staging Scheme for Renal Cell Carcinoma (RCC)

Primary tumor (T)

TX	Primary tumor cannot be assessed
T0	No evidence of primary tumor
T1	Tumor ≤7 cm in greatest dimension, limited to the kidney
T1a	Tumor ≤4 cm in greatest dimension, limited to the kidney
T1b	Tumor >4 cm but not >7 cm in greatest dimension, limited to the kidney
T2	Tumor >7 cm in greatest dimension, limited to the kidney
T2a	Tumor >7 cm but ≤10 cm in greatest dimension, limited to the kidney
T2b	Tumor >10 cm, limited to the kidney
T3	Tumor extends into major veins or perinephric tissues but not into ipsilateral adrenal gland and not beyond Gerota's fascia
T3a	Tumor grossly extends into the renal vein or its segmental (muscle containing) branches, or tumor invades perirenal and/or renal sinus fat but not beyond Gerota's fascia
T3b	Tumor grossly extends into vena cava below the diaphragm
T3c	Tumor grossly extends into vena cava above the diaphragm or invades the wall of the vena cava
T4	Tumor invades beyond Gerota's fascia (including contiguous extension into the ipsilateral adrenal gland)

Regional lymph nodes (N)

NX	Regional lymph nodes cannot be assessed
N0	No regional lymph node metastasis
N1	Regional lymph node metastasis

Distant metastasis (M)

MX	Distant metastasis cannot be assessed
M0	No distant metastasis
M1	Distant metastasis

Anatomic stage prognostic groups

Group I	T1	N0	M0
Group II	T2	N0	M0
Group III	T1	N1	M0
	T2	N1	M0
	T3	N0	M0
	T3	N1	M0
Group IV	T4	N0	M0
	T4	N1	M0
	Any T	Any N	M1

From: Edge SB, Byrd DR, Compton CC, et al., eds. *AJCC Cancer Staging Manual*. 7th ed. New York, NY: Springer; 2010. Used with permission.

IV. **PATHOLOGIC STAGING** applies only to RCCs. The 2010 TNM American Joint Committee on Cancer (AJCC)/International Union Against Cancer (UICC) staging classification is given in Table 20.8.

V. **REPORTING OF ADULT KIDNEY CARCINOMA** should follow suggested guidelines (College of American Pathologists kidney, cancer protocol and checklists at http://www.cap.org and *Arch Pathol Lab Med*. 2010;134:e25).

   A. For a *FNA biopsy*, report the presence or absence of a neoplasm, and the type of neoplasm (by WHO classification).

B. For a *core needle biopsy,* report the histologic type, histologic grade (Fuhrman nuclear grade), and any additional pathologic findings (such as inflammation and glomerular disease).

C. For a *nephrectomy,* partial or radical, report the tumor site (upper pole, middle pole, lower pole), focality (unifocal or multifocal), tumor size (largest, if multiple) in greatest dimension, macroscopic extent of tumor (tumor limited to kidney, tumor extension into perinephric tissues, tumor extension into renal sinus, tumor extension beyond Gerota's fascia, tumor extension into adrenal gland, tumor extension into major veins [intraluminal, with or without vein wall invasion], tumor extension into pelvicaliceal system, histologic type, sarcomatoid features [and percentage if present], histologic grade [Fuhrman nuclear grade], pathologic TNM stage, and margin status [cannot be assessed, margins uninvolved by invasive carcinoma, margins involved by invasive carcinoma]). The site(s) of margin positivity should be specified. For partial nephrectomy specimens, the renal parenchymal margin, renal capsular margin, and perinephric fat margin should be assessed. For radical nephrectomy specimens, Gerota's fascial margin, renal vein margin, and ureteral margin should be addressed. The adrenal gland, if present, should be reported as uninvolved by tumor, involved by direct invasion, or involved by metastasis. Lymph-vascular invasion should be designated as absent, present, or indeterminate. Additional pathologic findings in nonneoplastic tissue 5 mm or greater from the mass should be recorded, including glomerular disease (type), tubulointerstitial disease (type), and vascular disease (type). Optional reporting includes cyst(s) and tubulopapillary adenoma(s).

VI. **NONNEOPLASTIC TUMOROUS CONDITIONS** include the maldevelopment and nonneoplastic cystic diseases discussed earlier. Another important pseudoneoplastic category is inflammatory masses such as xanthogranulomatous pyelonephritis (XGP), renal malakoplakia, and tuberculosis (TB).

A. **Xanthogranulomatous pyelonephritis** (XGP) is a subacute to chronic, unilateral inflammatory process that can form a mass in the kidney mimicking RCC clinically, radiographically, grossly, and histologically. This disease most commonly occurs in women from the fourth to the sixth decades of life. XGP typically presents with fever, flank pain, or a tender flank mass and is frequently complicated by nephrolithiasis. Urine cultures show common urinary tract pathogens, such as *Escherichia coli* and *Proteus mirabilis,* in up to 70% of cases. If the kidney itself is cultured, an organism can be isolated in 95% of cases.

Macroscopically, XGP can either be confined to the kidney or extend into the surrounding soft tissue. XGP is typically composed of yellow nodules of varying size replacing the normal renal parenchyma (e-Fig. 20.75); the nodules can range in size from a few millimeters to several centimeters. Microscopically, the nodules are composed of lipid-laden macrophages (e-Fig. 20.76) that can mimic low-grade clear cell RCC, especially in small tissue samples such as needle biopsy specimens. The lesion may also contain reactive and even multinucleated fibroblasts that can mimic a sarcomatoid component in RCC. However, XGP lacks the vascularity typically seen in RCC, and moreover, XGP often exhibits neutrophils, lymphocytes, foreign body giant cells, plasma cells, cholesterol clefts, and microabscesses. If there is concern for RCC, a panel of immunohistochemical stains can be helpful: the clear cells in XGP will be positive for CD68 and vimentin, and negative for epithelial markers such as EMA and pan-cytokeratins.

B. **Renal malakoplakia** is uncommon but can form masses simulating a primary renal neoplasm. Most patients are women who often have extrarenal malakoplakia in the urinary bladder, ureter, or retroperitoneum. The lesion is bilateral in about one-quarter of cases. Grossly, there may be diffuse multinodular cortical enlargement or a large yellow mass. Abscesses and cystic spaces may also be seen. Microscopically, the hallmark, as in the urinary bladder, is sheets of macrophages (von Hansemann histiocytes) with intracellular or extracellular Michaelis–Gutmann bodies (e-**Fig. 20.77**). Lymphocytes and plasma cells may also be present, and with time, fibrosis may develop.

C. **Renal tuberculosis.** The kidney is the most common site of TB in the genitourinary tract. Grossly, miliary TB in the kidney is remarkable for numerous very small white nodules, mainly in the cortex. In the ulcerative form of renal TB, caseating necrosis can involve multiple renal pyramids, with papillary necrosis, cavitation, and extension of the necrosis into the renal pelvis. In advanced disease, necrotic nodules can also efface the renal cortex.

Cytopathology of Renal Neoplasms

Souzan Sanati

I. **INTRODUCTION.** The role of fine needle aspiration (FNA) in diagnosis of renal masses is limited in comparison with many other deep-seated organs, due in part to the success of imaging techniques in correct classification of most renal masses as benign or malignant. FNA is therefore usually considered only when imaging studies show equivocal results. Since most renal cysts with equivocal radiologic findings usually require extensive tissue sampling, the role of FNA of renal cysts is limited and often renders negative results; while FNA can be useful when malignant cellular features are identified, cytologically negative cyst fluid does not exclude a malignant process and thus it has been recommended that these specimens should be reported as nondiagnostic. FNA sampling of pediatric renal masses has not been advocated.

Despite these limitations, FNA of renal masses, under radiologic guidance, can be used as an alternative to core biopsy and can be useful in evaluating metastatic tumors, benign masses (eliminating the need for a surgical procedure), masses diagnosed in patients who are poor surgical candidates, and in masses occurring in candidates for a tumor ablation procedure.

When the renal pelvis is involved by tumor, cytologic sampling can be performed endoscopically. Since the endoscopic biopsies are usually small, cell block processing is advocated, particularly in low-grade lesions where the architectural features are of diagnostic importance. Cytologic evaluation of ureteral catheterization samples is also useful for detecting high-grade urothelial lesion of the upper urinary tract (*J Urol.* 2000;164:1901). In the case of renal abscesses, FNA can have a therapeutic as well as diagnostic role.

II. **CYTOPATHOLOGY OF RENAL NEOPLASMS**
   A. **Benign neoplasms**
      1. **Angiomyolipoma.** Mature adipose tissue, smooth muscle, and blood vessels are the main components of this tumor (e-**Fig. 20.78**). Identification of adipose tissue in the FNA biopsy is an important clue for diagnosis; however, most angiomyolipomas subject to cytological sampling have a low fat content. The smooth muscle component may have an epithelioid appearance with significant nuclear atypia, and it is important not to misinterpret this finding as a malignant process. Immunostains for HMB45 and smooth muscle actin are used to differentiate angiomyolipoma from RCC (*Acta Cytol.* 2006;50:466).
      2. **Oncocytoma** can be solitary or multifocal and usually has a characteristic radiologic appearance that includes good demarcation, a central scar, and

a density similar to the uninvolved renal parenchyma. Cytologic samples are cellular and show numerous singly dispersed large cells and round nests (usually seen on cell blocks) with abundant granular cytoplasm, round nuclei, and distinct cell borders. The nucleolus can be prominent (similar to nucleoli in Fuhrman nuclear grade 2 clear cell RCC), but no necrosis or mitoses are present (e-**Fig. 20.79**). Binucleation and/or multinucleation are common (e-**Fig. 20.80**). The morphology of this tumor has overlapping features with chromophobe RCC and granular variant of clear cell RCC; it is therefore prudent to diagnose these lesions as oncocytic neoplasm on cytologic samples if the round nested architecture is not seen (*Cancer.* 2001;93:390).

B. Malignant neoplasms

1. **Clear cell RCC** is the most common renal malignancy. FNA samples are usually richly cellular and bloody. The neoplastic cells have abundant vacuolated cytoplasm that may be more noticeable in air-dried, Diff Quik-stained slides (e-**Fig. 20.81**). It is not unusual to see naked nuclei from disrupted tumor cells in the background. When tumor microfragments are available, a rich capillary network is seen (e-**Fig. 20.82**). The degree of nuclear abnormality and the presence of prominent nucleoli are dependent on the nuclear grade of the tumor. Application of Fuhrman nuclear grade to cytology samples is appropriate.

   The most common pitfalls which result in a false-positive diagnosis include XGP, in which macrophages can be mistaken for the malignant cells of clear cell RCC, and contamination with benign cellular elements such as benign hepatocytes and adrenal cortical cells. Caution when making a diagnosis of malignancy on sparsely cellular samples will prevent an over-diagnosis in these situations.

2. **Papillary RCC** is characterized by papillary structures, foamy macrophages which usually distend fibrovascular cores on sections of cell block (e-**Fig. 20.83**), and psammoma bodies. Some tumors may show higher degree of cytologic atypia (e-**Figs. 20.84** and **20.85**). Additionally, nuclear pseudoinclusions, nuclear grooves, and cytoplasmic hemosiderin can be identified (*Diagn Cytopathol.* 2006;334:797).

3. **Chromophobe renal cell carcinoma** consists of cells with abundant cytoplasm, well-defined cell borders, and a perinuclear halo. The nuclei show significant size variation, irregular contours, and hyperchromasia resulting in a raisinoid appearance—nuclear features that allow for differentiation from oncocytoma. Nuclear grooves and/or pseudoinclusions and necrotic debris can also be present. The cell block can be quite helpful when it demonstrates a trabecular growth pattern; a cell block also provides material for appropriate stains (such as Hale's colloidal iron).

4. **Urothelial carcinoma** is the most common tumor arising in the renal pelvis. It is morphologically similar to urothelial carcinomas arising at other sites. The tumor consists of large elongated cells with dense cytoplasm and occasionally "cercariform" cells. The cytologic findings vary according to the grade; cells from low-grade tumors lack nuclear atypia and may have a spindle shape (e-**Fig. 20.86**).

5. **Metastatic tumors.** The kidney is a common site for metastatic tumors. The most common origin of metastatic tumors to the kidney is lung. Knowledge of a history of malignancy in another organ and appropriate use of immunohistochemistry (ideally on sections of cell block) are keys to correct diagnosis.

21 Renal Pelvis and Ureter

Souzan Sanati, Frances V. White, and
Peter A. Humphrey

I. **NORMAL ANATOMY.** The upper tract of the urinary collecting system is composed of the renal calyces, pelves, and ureters. Renal papillae protrude into the minor calyces, which expand into two or three major calyces, which in turn are outpouchings of the renal pelvis, a sac-like expansion of the upper ureter.

The mucosa is normally arranged in folds. The urothelium of the renal pelvis is three to five cell layers thick, and five to seven cell layers thick in the ureter. The lamina propria is composed of highly vascularized connective tissue without a muscularis mucosa; it is absent beneath the urothelium lining the renal papillae and is thinned along the minor calyces. The thickness and amount of muscularis propria in the collecting system within the renal sinus fat can be variable; ureteral muscularis propria is composed of interlacing bundles of smooth muscle, without inner or outer layers (Mills SE, ed. *Histology for Pathologists.* 2nd ed. Philadelphia: Lippincott Williams and Wilkins; 2007:839–907).

II. **GROSS EXAMINATION AND TISSUE SAMPLING.** Tissue samples include ureteroscopic biopsies, needle biopsies, pyeloplasty specimens, segmental ureterectomy specimens, radical cystectomy/cystoprostatectomy specimens, and radical nephroureterectomy with urinary bladder cuff resection specimens.

A. **Ureteroscopic biopsies** are entirely submitted. Because these are often minute in size, one approach to processing is to submit the biopsy sample for cytology cell block preparation (*Urology.* 1997;50:117).

B. **Needle core biopsies** of renal masses, including urothelial carcinoma involving the kidney, should be completely submitted. For microscopic examination, it is recommended that three levels on each of three hematoxylin and eosin (H&E)-stained slides be produced.

C. **Pyeloplasty specimens** for ureteropelvic junction obstruction consist of a portion of distal pelvis with a short segment of ureter attached to it. If the specimen is intact, it will be funnel-shaped, and narrowing, and/or angulation of the ureter may be evident. Usually, however, the specimen is longitudinally splayed open by the surgeon and consists of a flat, fan-shaped pelvis with nub of opened ureter at the "handle" of the fan. The mucosa should be examined to rule out rare mass lesions. Measurements include mural thickness of the pelvis and ureter, and both external and internal diameter of the ureter (the latter at its narrowest point). If present, narrowing and angulation of the ureter should be noted. Sections include serial cross sections of ureter and distal pelvis.

D. **Segmental ureterectomy** is performed for tumors of the proximal or mid-ureter. The length and diameter of the intact ureter is recorded, with a search for a mass by palpation and visual inspection. Proximal and distal cross-sectional margins are taken, and the outer aspect of the ureter is inked. The ureter is then opened longitudinally and assessed for mucosal abnormalities. After overnight fixation in 10% formalin, sections are taken to demonstrate the deepest invasion of any lesion(s). At least one section of uninvolved ureter should also be submitted.

E. **Radical cystectomy/cystoprostatectomy with segment of ureters.** Ureteral margin(s) may be submitted for frozen section for evaluation of carcinoma (and particularly carcinoma in situ). These are shaved margins and should be submitted as cross sections.

F. **Radical nephroureterectomy with bladder cuff.** Gross examination and sampling should document the relationship of tumor to adjacent renal parenchyma, peripelvic fat, nearest soft tissue margin, and ureter. Sections of grossly unremarkable kidney, pelvis, and ureter should be submitted. The important urothelial margin is the urinary bladder cuff, which can be sampled as shave sections.

III. DIAGNOSTIC FEATURES OF COMMON DISEASES

A. **Benign conditions** that involve the urothelium in the upper tract have an appearance similar to those in the urinary bladder. Examples are ureteritis (**e-Fig. 21.1**),* pyelitis cystica and glandularis, malakoplakia, nephrogenic adenoma, and squamous metaplasia (**e-Fig. 21.2**).

B. **Ureteropelvic junction (UPJ) abnormalities** can be seen in biopsies done for UPJ obstruction (UPJO), which is the most common cause of pediatric hydronephrosis and is usually diagnosed by fetal ultrasound. UPJO can also be seen in adults. Although in a minority of cases ureteropelvic junction obstruction is due to extrinsic compression by aberrant vessels, most cases are thought to be due to an "intrinsic" abnormality of the UPJ itself. The pathogenesis of intrinsic UPJO is not well established. Proposed etiologies include abnormal recanalization of the proximal ureter during embryogenesis, persistence of fetal mucosal folds, abnormalities of smooth muscle including disorientation and discontinuity, and abnormal innervation. UPJO initially results in pelvic and calyceal dilatation, followed by progressive obstructive renal damage which results in features of renal dysplasia in patients with end-stage disease. Gross and histopathologic findings reported in UPJO specimens include increased mural thickness, abnormal mucosal folds/fibroepithelial polyps, smooth muscle hypertrophy and disarray (**e-Fig. 21.3**), attenuation of smooth muscle with increased collagen to smooth muscle ratio, and chronic inflammation. Prognosis is based on concurrent renal biopsy and renal function rather than UPJ findings (*Pediatr Nephrol.* 2000;14:820, *Pediatr Develop Pathol.* 2006;9:72, *Histopathology* 2007;51: 709). Malignancy should also be excluded.

C. **Benign epithelial neoplasms** are rare and include urothelial papilloma, inverted papilloma, villous adenoma, and squamous papilloma.

D. **Benign nonepithelial neoplasms** include the distinctive fibroepithelial polyp, which is most frequently seen in the proximal ureter of young males. Microscopically, these are exophytic intraluminal projections of a variably inflamed fibrovascular stroma lined by a normal urothelium. Benign mesenchymal neoplasms such as leiomyoma, hemangioma, neurofibroma, and fibrous histiocytoma are rare.

E. **Urothelial dysplasia** in isolated form is rare and displays the same features as in the urinary bladder, where it is defined as low-grade intraurothelial neoplasia.

F. **Renal pelvic and ureteral cancers** are in the vast majority of cases, as in the urinary bladder, of urothelial type (*Am J Surg Pathol.* 2004;28:1545, *Mod Pathol.* 2006;19:494, *Adv Anat Pathol.* 2008;15:127).

Upper tract tumors differ from those in the urinary bladder in the following ways. Upper tract tumors are found at a lower frequency; have a stronger association with long-term analgesic (such as phenacetin) abuse and urinary tract obstruction; are associated with an increased frequency (in up to 65% of patients) of synchronous or metachronous urothelial neoplasms elsewhere in the urinary tract (Murphy WM, Grignon DJ, Perlman EJ. *Tumors of the Kidney, Bladder, and Related Urinary Structures.* Washington, DC: American Registry

---

*All e-figures are available online via the Solution Site Image Bank.

of Pathology; 2004); and tend to present with higher histologic grade and at higher stage. Also, biopsy of upper tract tumors is more difficult than lower tract tumors. In about one of four cases, small ureteroscopic biopsies of the upper tract will be nondiagnostic due to inadequate tissue (*Am J Surg Pathol.* 2009;33:1540).

1. **Risk factors.** The main risk factor, as for urinary bladder malignancies, is smoking. Other risk factors are analgesics (as noted earlier); occupation in chemical, petrochemical, or plastics industries; exposure to tar, coal, or asphalt; papillary necrosis; Balkan nephropathy; thorium contrast exposure; hereditary nonpolyposis colorectal cancer (HNPCC) syndrome (Lynch syndrome II) (*J Urol.* 2011;185:1627); and urinary tract infections or stones (Eble JN, Sauter G, Epstein JI, Sesterhenn IA, eds. *Tumours of the urinary system and male genital organs.* Lyon: IARC Press; 2004).

2. **Clinical features.** Most patients are around 70 years of age, and the chief presenting symptoms are hematuria and flank pain. In the majority of patients, there is a prior history of a bladder cancer, which means that many upper tract tumors are detected during the course of clinical surveillance after diagnosis of a bladder tumor.

3. **Histologic typing and diagnosis of upper tract tumors** are accomplished by examination of H&E-stained sections. Typing of upper tract urothelial neoplasia is the same as that for the urinary bladder as defined in the 2004 World Health Organization (WHO) classification of neoplasms (see Table 22.1).

4. **Urothelial carcinoma** is by far the most common type of upper tract tumor.

   a. **Gross diagnosis** is possible in resection specimens. Patterns of growth include papillary, polypoid, nodular, ulcerative, and infiltrative. Exophytic tumors can fill and distend the pelvis (e-**Fig. 21.4**), with or without associated hydronephrosis and stones. High-grade invasive tumors can grossly involve soft tissue and/or renal parenchyma (e-**Fig. 21.5**). Extensive renal parenchymal involvement can mimic a primary renal parenchymal neoplasm; in these cases there is often a request for an intraoperative consultation to determine whether the mass is a urothelial carcinoma or a renal cell carcinoma (RCC) because the distinction alters the extent of surgery. The correct diagnosis can usually be determined by straightforward gross examination alone, but in some cases a frozen section may be required. The average size of renal pelvic tumors is just under 4 cm, with a range of 0.3 to 9 cm (*Am J Surg Pathol.* 2004;28:1545). Multifocality in the pelvis and ureter is seen in about one-quarter of cases. In the ureter, the tumor may be associated with a stricture and hydroureter.

   b. **Microscopically,** the full range of urothelial carcinoma may be seen from flat intraepithelial neoplasia, including carcinoma in situ (e-**Fig. 21.6**); to noninvasive papillary neoplasia, including papillary urothelial neoplasm of low malignant potential; to low-grade papillary urothelial carcinoma (e-**Fig. 21.7A and B**); to high-grade papillary urothelial carcinoma (e-**Fig. 21.8A and B**; e-**Fig. 21.9**). The full spectrum of invasive urothelial carcinoma and its variants as found in the urinary bladder can also be found in the upper tract. Of note, unusual histomorphological variants seem to be more common in the upper tract (*Mod Pathol.* 2006;19:494), including carcinomas with micropapillary, lymphoepithelioma-like, sarcomatoid, squamous, clear cell, glandular, rhabdoid, signet-ring, and plasmacytoid features or areas.

   Primary resections performed for renal pelvic urothelial carcinoma show high-grade carcinoma in >70% of cases, with deep invasion (pT2 or greater) in 45% of cases and with lymph node metastases in one-quarter of patients. Cancerization of the distal renal collecting ducts is common in high-grade urothelial carcinoma (e-Fig. 21.10). Levels of invasion include lamina propria invasion (e-Fig. 21.11); extension into muscularis propria (e-Fig. 21.12), renal sinus and hilar fat, and peri-ureteral fat (e-Fig. 21.13); and renal parenchymal infiltration. Metastatic sites include lymph nodes, peritoneum, and liver. When the differential diagnosis of a centrally located high-grade carcinoma centers on urothelial carcinoma versus RCC, extensive mucosal sampling is important because identification of urothelial carcinoma in situ (CIS) is in keeping with a urothelial primary.

    c. **Immunohistochemical studies** are not usually needed but can be useful in the differential diagnosis of urothelial carcinoma versus RCC when the diagnosis is not clear by standard gross and microscopic examination. A useful marker panel includes cytokeratin CK7, CK20, p63, thrombomodulin, uroplakin III, RCC marker (RCC Ma), CD10, PAX2, and PAX8. Positivity for the first five favors urothelial carcinoma, whereas immunoreactivity for the last four suggests RCC rather than urothelial carcinoma (*Semin Diagn Pathol.* 2005;22:51; *Pathol Case Rev.* 2010; 15:25).

    d. **Molecular studies.** The most promising test is fluorescence in situ hybridization (FISH) performed on cells in urine from the upper tract. In this test (UroVysion/Vysis/Abbott), a mixture of fluorescent probes to chromosomes 3, 7, 17, and 9p21 locus is used to detect numerical chromosomal abnormalities associated with urothelial carcinoma (*Expert Rev Mol Diagn.* 2007;7:11). The precise clinical indications for its use for upper tract tumors are not yet established.

  5. Squamous cell carcinoma is rare, is more common in the pelvis, is frequently associated with nephrolithiasis and/or infection, and often presents with high-stage and high-grade disease (e-Fig. 21.14A and B). Pure squamous cell carcinomas should be distinguished from urothelial carcinoma with squamous differentiation.

  6. Adenocarcinoma is rare and may display enteric, mucinous, and/or signet-ring features. Pure adenocarcinomas should be separated from urothelial carcinoma with glandular differentiation. Intestinal metaplasia, nephrolithiasis, and infection are predisposing factors.

  7. Small cell carcinomas in very rare cases arise from the renal pelvis. There may be admixed urothelial carcinoma.

  8. Malignant mesenchymal neoplasms are rare. The most common is leiomyosarcoma. Other exceedingly rare mesenchymal tumor types include osteosarcoma, rhabdomyosarcoma, fibrosarcoma, angiosarcoma, and Ewing sarcoma.

  9. Hematolymphoid neoplasms in the ureter and renal pelvis typically are due to secondary involvement.

  10. Miscellaneous neoplasms rarely encountered include paraganglioma, carcinoid tumor, Wilms tumor, malignant melanoma, and choriocarcinoma.

  11. Secondary (metastatic) malignancies include carcinomas of the cervix, prostate, colon, breast, and urinary bladder.

IV. HISTOLOGIC GRADING should be performed for all carcinomas, with urothelial carcinoma grade being assigned as low grade or high grade, as for the urinary bladder. Pure squamous cell carcinoma and adenocarcinoma may be graded as well-differentiated, moderately differentiated, or poorly differentiated.

V. PATHOLOGIC STAGING applies only to carcinomas of the ureter and renal pelvis. Stage is the most important prognostic factor for upper tract carcinoma. The 2010 Tumor, Node, Metastasis (TNM) American Joint Committee on Cancer/International Union Against Cancer (AJCC/UICC) staging classification is given in Table 21.1.;

TABLE 21.1	Tumor, Node, Metastasis (TNM) Staging Scheme for Carcinoma of Renal Pelvis and Ureter

Primary tumor (T)

TX	Primary tumor cannot be assessed
T0	No evidence of primary tumor
Ta	Noninvasive papillary carcinoma
Tis	Carcinoma in situ
T1	Tumor invades subepithelial connective tissue
T2	Tumor invades muscularis
T3	Renal pelvis tumors: Tumor invades beyond muscularis into peripelvic fat or renal parenchyma
	Ureteral tumors: Tumor invades beyond muscularis into periureteric fat
T4	Tumor invades adjacent organs or through the kidney into perinephric fat

Regional lymph nodes (N)

NX	Regional lymph nodes cannot be assessed
N0	No regional lymph node metastasis
N1	Metastasis to a single lymph node ≤ 2 cm in greatest dimension
N2	Metastasis in a single lymph node 2–5 cm in greatest dimension
N3	Metastasis in a lymph node >5 cm in greatest dimension

Distant metastasis (M)

MX	Distant metastasis cannot be assessed
M0	No distant metastasis
M1	Distant metastasis

Stage grouping

Stage 0a	Ta	N0	M0
Stage 0is	Tis	N0	M0
Stage I	T1	N0	M0
Stage II	T2	N0	M0
Stage III	T3	N0	M0
Stage IV	T4	N0	M0
	Any T	N1–3	M0
	Any T	Any N	M1

From: Edge SB, Byrd DR, Compton CC, et al., eds. *AJCC Cancer Staging Manual.* 7th ed. New York, NY: Springer; 2010. Used with permission.

Figure 21.1 illustrates pT stages pTa through pT3; one important note is that renal pelvic carcinoma extending into the renal collecting ducts does not represent renal parenchymal invasion, which is pT3 disease. It is also important to note that clinical staging should be distinguished from pathologic staging.

VI. **REPORTING CARCINOMA OF THE URETER AND RENAL PELVIS** should follow recommended guidelines (College of American Pathologists Protocol for the Examination of Specimens from Patients with Carcinoma of the Ureter and Renal Pelvis, and checklists at http://www.cap.org). In addition to typing, grading, staging, and assessing size and margins, pertinent pathologic features that should be reported include the following. For ureteroscopic biopsies, the amount of sampled stroma available to allow for evaluation of invasion should be specified (*Arch Path Lab Med.* 2003;127:1263). For nephroureterectomy or ureterectomy specimens, gross characteristics such as tumor location, focality (unifocal vs. multifocal), gross appearance (papillary, solid/nodule, flat, ulcerated), gross depth of invasion, and distance to margins should be given. Additional gross abnormalities such

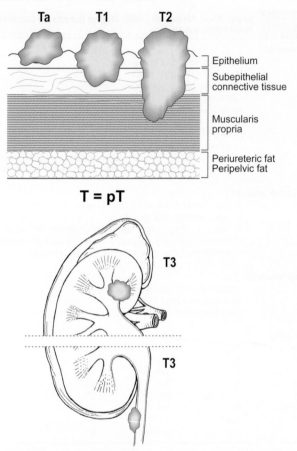

Figure 21.1 Depiction of pT stages pTa, pT1, pT2, and pT3. (Modified from: Greene FL, Compton CC, Fritz AG, et al., eds. *AJCC Cancer Staging Atlas*. New York, NY: Springer; 2006.)

as other mucosal lesions, renal parenchymal lesions, stones, hydronephrosis, and hydroureter should be documented when present. Microscopically, additional relevant pathologic findings, if present, include lymphovascular space invasion by carcinoma, flat urothelial carcinoma in situ (focal vs. multifocal), inflammation, renal epithelial neoplasia or medical renal disease (glomerulopathy), and metaplasias of the urothelium, including keratinizing squamous metaplasia and intestinal metaplasia. A nomogram predicting cancer-specific survival after nephroureterectomy for upper tract urothelial carcinoma uses age, tumor grade, pT stage, and pN stage (*Cancer.* 2010;116:3774).

22 The Urinary Bladder

Omar Hameed and Peter A. Humphrey

I. **INORMAL MICROSCOPIC ANATOMY.** The wall of the urinary bladder is formed by four layers (**e-Fig. 22.1**).* The thickness of the innermost layer, the urothelium, depends on the degree of bladder distension, and the shape of its constituent urothelial cells ranges from smaller cuboidal cells at the base to larger polyhedral cells toward the surface. Umbrella cells, the most superficial cells, have abundant eosinophilic cytoplasm and are often binucleated. The underlying lamina propria is separated from the urothelium by a thin basement membrane and is composed of loose connective tissue with blood vessels, nerves, adipose tissue, and a variable number of smooth muscle fibers forming a discontinuous muscularis mucosae. Aggregates of urothelium termed von Brunn nests (**e-Fig. 22.2**) are often seen as invaginations or separate clusters in the lamina propria. The term cystitis cystica is used when these nests become prominent and undergo cystic change (**e-Fig. 22.3**). Cystitis glandularis is similar to cystitis cystica except that the cells lining the cysts are mucin-secreting cuboidal or columnar cells, or true goblet cells, in which case the term cystitis glandularis with intestinal metaplasia is used (**e-Fig. 22.4**). These proliferative lesions, although sometimes seen associated with local inflammation, represent variants of normal histology. Their main importance lies in the fact that they can occasionally cause visible lesions simulating a bladder neoplasm. The third layer, the muscularis propria or detrusor muscle, is composed of large bundles of muscle fibers and is covered by the outermost adventitial layer, including perivesical adipose tissue. It is important to note that adipose tissue can also be found in the lamina propria and wall (**e-Fig. 22.5**), so identification of fat does not equate to a specific layer of the bladder wall.

II. **GROSS EXAMINATION AND TISSUE SAMPLING OF THE BLADDER.** The most common samples submitted for surgical pathology examination include small biopsies, larger transurethral resection specimens, and partial and radical (complete) cystectomies.

   A. **Biopsy specimens.** These are usually obtained without cautery ("cold-cup") and should be immediately immersed in formalin. If multiple biopsies are submitted separately, as in mapping procedures, they should be processed separately. After gross examination, bladder biopsies should be marked with ink or hematoxylin, then placed in a cassette after being put in a fine mesh envelope, wrapped in lens paper, or sandwiched between sponge pads. After processing, three hematoxylin and eosin (H&E)-stained slides should be prepared, each with a strip of three to four levels.

   B. **Transurethral resection of bladder specimens.** These specimens are usually obtained with the aid of thermal cautery, often for the transurethral resection of bladder tumors (TURBT). Because of the significant prognostic and therapeutic implications for the presence of muscularis propria invasion by the bladder neoplasms, it is often necessary to process all of the submitted tissue to ensure that such foci of invasion are not overlooked.

   C. **Partial cystectomy specimens.** Partial or segmental cystectomy is indicated in only a minority of bladder cancer patients, typically those who suffer a first time tumor recurrence with a solitary tumor, and tumor location that allows for a 1- to 2-cm margin of resection, such as at the dome. Urachal carcinomas at the

---

*All e-figures are available online via the Solution Site Image Bank.

dome and above, with extension toward the umbilicus, may also be treated by partial cystectomy, as can carcinoma in a bladder diverticulum. Carcinoma in situ elsewhere in the bladder (or multifocal tumors) is an absolute contraindication. The specimens usually consist of a sheet-like portion of tissue that should be pinned down and fixed overnight. In addition to describing and sampling any gross tumor(s) as described for cystectomy specimens, the status of the margins is very important; these can be shaved off or sampled by perpendicular sections, depending on their relationship and proximity to the tumor(s). Frozen section of the mucosal margin may be requested.

D. **Total cystectomy and cystoprostatectomy specimens.** Radical cystoprostatectomy in men and anterior exenteration in women, along with pelvic lymphadenectomy, are standard surgical approaches for muscle wall-invasive bladder carcinoma in the absence of metastatic disease. Cystectomy may be performed in some cases for nonmuscle wall-invasive bladder carcinoma, if the bladder is nonfunctional, or for high-grade pT1 carcinoma that is not responsive to intravesical therapy. If not sampled separately, a request to perform frozen sections on the ureteric and urethral margins may be received (*Arch Pathol Lab Med.* 2005;129: 1585–1601). After orientation and inking, one of two methods can be used to fix the specimen. The first entails filling the bladder with formalin (through the urethra, or by using a large bore needle through the dome) and fixing overnight; the second entails opening the bladder (usually through the urethra extending upward on the anterior surface) and pinning it flat, then fixing overnight. After opening the bladder (in the fresh or fixed state), the mucosa is examined for tumors(s) and, if present, the size, location, pattern of growth (exophytic, endophytic, and/or ulcerated), and depth of invasion are recorded. The mucosa of the adjacent bladder should also be examined for areas of hemorrhage and discoloration that may represent areas of carcinoma in situ. In addition to sampling of any tumor(s) (three to four sections of each), representative sections need to be submitted from the different areas of the bladder including the trigone; posterior, lateral, and anterior walls; and the dome (Fig. 22.1). If ureteric and urethral shave margins were not submitted for frozen section examination, they should be sampled for permanent sections, as should any possible lymph nodes identified in the perivesical fat. In cystoprostatectomy specimens, additional blocks from the prostate and seminal vesicles should be submitted, the extent of which depends on whether a preoperative diagnosis or suspicion of prostatic carcinoma exists (see Chap. 29). When the bladder (with or without the prostate) is removed as part of larger pelvic exenteration specimens (that may include portions of the rectum and/or the gynecological tract in females), it then becomes imperative to document the presence or absence of involvement of these additional organs by preferentially sampling suspicious areas, as well as by sampling the resection margins of these organs.

III. **DIAGNOSTIC FEATURES OF COMMON DISEASES OF THE BLADDER**
   A. **Congenital malformations**
   1. **Urachal abnormalities.** The urachus is a vestigial structure that connects the dome of the bladder to the umbilicus; it normally closes by the fourth month of fetal life. Persistence or malformations of the urachus can present in childhood and occasionally in adulthood; they include urachal remnants (e-**Fig. 22.6**), patent urachus, urachal cysts, and urachal sinuses, all of which can result in secondary infection or development of secondary tumors, most frequently adenocarcinoma (e-**Fig. 22.7**).
   2. **Exstrophy.** This is a rare congenital anomaly characterized by failure of development of the anterior wall of the bladder and abdominal wall, usually resulting in severe secondary infection if left untreated.
   B. **Inflammatory conditions.** Cystitis most frequently has an infectious etiology. There are, however, specific variants of cystitis that produce somewhat

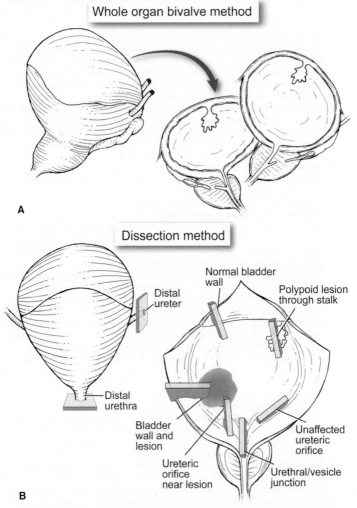

Whole organ bivalve method

A

Dissection method

Distal ureter

Normal bladder wall

Polypoid lesion through stalk

Distal urethra

Bladder wall and lesion

Unaffected ureteric orifice

Ureteric orifice near lesion

Urethral/vesicle junction

B

Figure 22.1 Gross dissection of radical cystectomy specimens by whole organ bivalve method (**A**) and by opening along urethra and anterior wall, with demonstration of sections to be taken (**B**). Three to four sections, or complete embedding, of masses should be performed. (Modified from Schmidt WA. *Principles and Techniques of Surgical Pathology*. Menlo Park, CA: Addison-Wesley Publishing Co.; 1983:525.)

characteristic cystoscopic and/or microscopic appearances. The latter include hemorrhagic, granulomatous, eosinophilic, and interstitial variants, as well as malakoplakia.

1. **Infectious cystitis.** Acute and chronic cystitis is most frequently secondary to bacterial infection (usually by enteric organisms). The incidence is higher in females, and when intermittent urinary obstruction or stasis is present. Biopsy

during active infection is contraindicated, but biopsy may be performed in cases of chronic cystitis to rule out neoplasia, especially carcinoma in situ. The histopathologic features include a nonspecific acute and/or chronic inflammatory infiltrate occasionally with lymphoid aggregates/follicles (follicular cystitis) (e-**Fig. 22.8**), and a variable degree of lamina propria edema. Of note, similar findings may be seen in the absence of infection such as following radiation or cytotoxic chemotherapy. Other infections can produce specific histologic findings such as viral inclusions (polyoma and herpesviruses) or granulomas (tuberculosis, fungal infections, and schistosomiasis).

2. **Granulomatous cystitis.** As noted above, bacterial, fungal, or parasitic infections can lead to granuloma formation. The most frequent cause, however, is iatrogenic, either secondary to intravesical Bacille Calmette-Guerin (BCG) immunotherapy for urothelial CIS and superficially invasive carcinoma (e-**Fig. 22.9**), or following TURBT (e-**Fig. 22.10**).

3. **Hemorrhagic cystitis.** This is an uncommon side effect of cyclophosphamide therapy that results in extensive ulceration and hemorrhage that, if severe, may require cystectomy. Adenovirus infection (in immunocompromised individuals) may also produce the same pattern.

4. **Papillary and polypoid (bullous) cystitis.** These related forms of cystitis are characterized by finger-like (papillary) or broad (polypoid) projections of edematous, variably inflamed lamina propria covered by reactive nonneoplastic urothelium (e-**Fig. 22.11**). These forms of cystitis are most frequently seen with prolonged indwelling catheter use. The presence of such an inflammatory component in papillary cystitis can help in making the occasionally difficult distinction from a low-grade papillary urothelial neoplasm.

5. **Eosinophilic cystitis.** This is characterized by dense infiltration of eosinophils in the bladder lamina propria (e-**Fig. 22.12**) and/or wall. Such infiltrates are most frequently seen adjacent to invasive urothelial carcinoma, but they also occur in patients with allergic conditions and in patients with parasitic infections, both often in association with peripheral eosinophilia.

6. **Interstitial cystitis.** This is an uncommon inflammatory disorder that predominantly affects middle-aged and elderly women and results in severe intractable symptoms of culture-negative cystitis. Petechial submucosal hemorrhages or ulcers (termed Hunner ulcers) are usually evident cystoscopically. The microscopic features are nonspecific and include a mixed inflammatory infiltrate in the lamina propria, often with an increased number of mast cells that can also involve the muscularis propria (e-**Fig. 22.13**) and nerves. Clinical correlation is required in these cases because the histological findings are, at most, consistent with the clinical impression of interstitial cystitis.

7. **Malakoplakia.** This is an uncommon form of cystitis characterized by the presence of soft yellowish mucosal plaques composed of inflammatory cells including abundant epithelioid histiocytes (known as von Hansemann histiocytes) (e-**Fig. 22.14**) that have granular eosinophilic cytoplasm, and characteristic 3- to 10-micron rounded basophilic intracytoplasmic inclusions (Michaelis–Gutmann bodies) that contain iron and calcium, best demonstrated by Prussian blue and von Kossa special stains, respectively. The condition is thought to result from a defect in the ability of histiocytes to degrade phagocytosized bacteria. Control of urinary tract infection can help control the disease.

C. **Reactive and metaplastic urothelial lesions**

1. **Squamous metaplasia.** This can be of two types, nonkeratinizing and keratinizing. The former is considered a normal finding in the trigone and bladder neck of females but can rarely be seen in males receiving estrogen treatment for prostate cancer. In contrast, keratinizing squamous metaplasia is more common in males in association with chronic irritation and is considered

a significant risk factor for the subsequent development of carcinoma (*Eur Urol.* 2002;42:469 and *Am J Surg Pathol.* 2006;20:883).

2. **Intestinal metaplasia.** In addition to the intestinal metaplasia occasionally seen in cystitis glandularis, intestinal metaplasia in the presence of a chronically irritated bladder can involve the bladder mucosa and lamina propria in a focal or diffuse manner, resulting in an appearance almost indistinguishable from colonic mucosa.

3. **Nephrogenic metaplasia (adenoma).** This is a benign epithelial proliferation composed of cells resembling renal tubular epithelium (hence the name), which usually arises in the setting of chronic irritation or injury such as infection or calculi (*Adv Anat Pathol.* 2006;13:247). The lesion was believed to be metaplastic, but more recent evidence has demonstrated that, at least in renal transplant recipients, nephrogenic metaplasia is derived from shed renal tubular epithelial cells that may attach to areas of prior injury. Although most frequently seen in the bladder, it is also quite common in the urethra, and less so in the ureters and renal pelvis. Nephrogenic metaplasia is usually an incidental finding, but it may also present as a mass lesion simulating cancer. Histologically, papillae (e-**Fig. 22.15**), small tubules (e-**Fig. 22.16**), or cystically dilated tubules (e-**Fig. 22.17**) lined by cuboidal, low-columnar, or flattened hobnail cells are seen. The importance of nephrogenic metaplasia lies in the fact that in the bladder it can be confused with adenocarcinoma (especially clear-cell adenocarcinoma) and glandular variants of urothelial carcinoma (*Mod Pathol.* 2009;22:S37–S52); in the urethra it can be confused with prostatic adenocarcinoma. The immunohistochemical reactivity of nephrogenic metaplasia with cytokeratin 7, α-methylacyl coenzyme A racemase (AMACR), PAX2, and PAX8 antibodies and the lack of reactivity with high-molecular-weight cytokeratin (e.g., 34βE12) and prostate-specific antigen (PSA) antibodies help in distinguishing it from its mimics.

4. **Urothelial hyperplasia.** An increase in the thickness of the urothelium (>7 layers) is usually reactive and most frequently seen secondary to chronic inflammatory conditions. Flat urothelial hyperplasia (e-**Fig. 22.18**) is more common than papillary urothelial hyperplasia, which some authors have also found to be associated with papillary urothelial neoplasms.

5. **Pseudocarcinomatous epithelial hyperplasia.** This change may be seen after radiation therapy, chemotherapy, or unassociated with either therapy (*Arch Pathol Lab Med.* 2010;134:427). The light microscopic appearance is of pseudoinfiltrative nests of urothelium in the lamina propria (e-**Fig. 22.19**), sometimes with squamous metaplasia. Nuclear atypia may be detected, secondary to therapy or irritation/ischemia. The irregular nests and aggregates may appear to wrap around ecstatic vessels with fibrin thrombi, which is a useful diagnostic finding.

6. **Reactive urothelial atypia.** Usually seen in a setting of acute and/or chronic inflammation, reactive atypia may be associated with hyperplastic or thin urothelium. Nuclear enlargement, often with vesicular chromatin and a single prominent nucleolus, is the most prominent finding (e-**Fig. 22.20**). Mitotic figures may be increased and cell crowding may be observed; however, polarity, cell uniformity, and maturation are usually well preserved. Acute or chronic inflammation is often identified.

D. **Miscellaneous nonneoplastic conditions**

1. **Endometriosis.** Most frequently seen on the serosal aspect of the bladder in women with a previous history of pelvic surgery, foci of endometriosis can also involve the lamina propria or muscularis propria and may be visible cystoscopically. As elsewhere, at least two of the three histologic features of endometriosis—endometrial glands, endometrial stroma, and hemosiderin-laden macrophages—are required for the diagnosis (e-**Fig. 22.21**).

2. **Endocervicosis and endosalpingiosis.** These are characterized by the presence of glands within the bladder wall lined by columnar endocervical-type mucinous cells or ciliated tubal epithelial cells, respectively. When both are present with endometriosis, the term "Müllerianosis" has been used. Lack of significant nuclear atypia, mitoses, and a stromal tissue reaction help distinguish these benign lesions from invasive adenocarcinoma.

3. **Diverticula.** These outpouchings of mucosa through the muscularis propria are mostly due to increased pressure. Diverticula are frequently complicated by secondary inflammation, squamous metaplasia, and lithiasis, and in <10% of cases by secondary neoplastic development.

4. **Amyloidosis.** The bladder may rarely be involved by systemic amyloidosis, or by a primary localized form of amyloidosis limited to the bladder.

5. **Ectopic prostatic tissue.** These are usually small polypoid projections most frequently seen in the trigone area. They are composed of benign prostatic

---

TABLE 22.1   WHO Histologic Classification of Tumors of the Urinary Tract (Including Bladder)

Urothelial tumors
Infiltrating urothelial carcinoma
  With squamous differentiation
  With glandular differentiation
  With trophoblastic differentiation
  Nested
  Microcystic
  Micropapillary
  Lymphoepithelioma-like
  Lymphoma-like
  Plasmacytoid
  Sarcomatoid
  Giant cell
  Undifferentiated
Noninvasive urothelial neoplasias
  Urothelial carcinoma in situ
  Noninvasive papillary urothelial carcinoma, high grade
  Noninvasive papillary urothelial carcinoma, low grade
  Noninvasive papillary urothelial neoplasm of low malignant potential
  Urothelial papilloma
  Inverted urothelial papilloma

Squamous neoplasms
Squamous cell carcinoma
Verrucous carcinoma
Squamous cell papilloma

Glandular neoplasms
Adenocarcinoma
  Enteric
  Mucinous
  Signet-ring cell
  Clear cell
  Villous adenoma

Neuroendocrine tumors
Small cell carcinoma
Paraganglioma
Carcinoid

Melanocytic tumors
Malignant melanoma
Nevus

Mesenchymal tumors
Rhabdomyosarcoma
Leiomyosarcoma
Angiosarcoma
Osteosarcoma
Malignant fibrous histiocytoma
Leiomyoma
Hemangioma
Other

Hematopoietic and lymphoid tumors
Lymphoma
Plasmacytoma

Miscellaneous tumors
Carcinoma of Skene, Cowper, and Littre glands
Metastatic tumors and tumors extending from other organs

From: Eble JN, Sauter G, Epstein JL, et al., eds. *World Health Organization Classification of Tumors. Pathology and Genetics. Tumours of the Urinary System and Male Genital Organs.* Lyon: IARC Press; 2004. Used with permission.

epithelium (very similar to so-called "prostatic urethral polyps" of the urethra).

6. **Fibroepithelial polyp.** These rare polyps are considered nonneoplastic. They may be acquired or congenital. About one-half are found in neonates and children. Histologically, there is a polypoid configuration, often with club-like or finger-like projections (e-**Fig. 22.22**) (*Am J Surg Pathol.* 2005;29:460). The surface urothelial lining is normal and there may be tubular or anastomosing urothelium in the dense fibrous tissue of the polyp fibrovascular core. Degenerative-type stromal cell atypia, without mitotic activity, may be present. These polyps have a broader fibrovascular core than urothelial papillomas and lack the edema and inflammation of polypoid cystitis.

E. **Neoplastic urothelial lesions.** Urothelial neoplasms are the most common neoplasms that involve the bladder. Histologic typing and diagnosis of urothelial abnormalities are accomplished by examination of H&E-stained sections. The 2004 World Health Organization (WHO) classification of tumors of the urinary tract is given in Table 22.1.

1. **Flat urothelial lesions with atypia.** In addition to reactive atypia discussed earlier, such lesions include urothelial dysplasia and urothelial carcinoma in situ.

   a. **Urothelial dysplasia.** Dysplasia is an intraepithelial neoplastic urothelial proliferation characterized by variable degrees of loss of polarity, nuclear enlargement, and chromatin clumping (e-**Fig. 22.23**), all of which fall short of the degree seen in carcinoma in situ. Dysplasia is often identified in patients with urothelial neoplasms. Occasionally, it may be difficult to distinguish urothelial dysplasia from reactive atypia; in such situations a diagnosis of atypia of unknown significance may be warranted. Isolated urothelial dysplasia progresses to bladder carcinoma in about 15% of cases (*Cancer.* 2000;88:625).

   b. **Urothelial carcinoma in situ.** This is a high-grade, often multifocal intraurothelial neoplastic proliferation characterized by the presence of unequivocal malignant urothelial cells within the bladder epithelial lining (**Fig. 22.2**, e-**Fig. 22.24**). The urothelial proliferation need not involve the entire thickness of the urothelium, and pagetoid and undermining patterns of growth are not uncommon. Another common feature is the discohesive

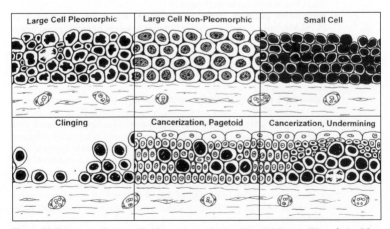

Figure 22.2 Patterns of urinary bladder carcinoma in situ. (From McKenney JK, et al. *Am J Surg Pathol.* 2001;25:356, with permission.)

nature of the neoplastic cells that often leads to denudation and a "cling-ing" pattern of growth in which only scarce malignant cells remain attached to the bladder wall (e-**Fig. 22.25**). Surface carcinoma in situ cells can also extend into and "cancerize" von Brunn nests (e-**Fig. 22.26**). In uncommon cases, glandular differentiation, in the form of more colum-nar cells with apical cytoplasm, can be noted in urothelial carcinoma in situ (*Am J Surg Pathol.* 2009;33:1241). In difficult cases where the differential diagnosis includes reactive urothelial atypia, immunostains for cytokeratin 20, p53, CD44, and Ki-67 can be useful (*Semin Diagn Pathol.* 2005;22:69). Urothelial carcinoma in situ is often associated with invasive urothelial carcinoma and carries a significant risk of death from bladder carcinoma (*Cancer.* 1999;85:2469).

2. **Papillary urothelial neoplasms**
   a. **Urothelial papilloma.** This uncommon benign neoplasm is composed of delicate papillary urothelial fronds with no or minimal branching or fusion. The constituent cells are identical to normal urothelial cells, and no mitoses are present (e-**Fig. 22.27**). The classic cystoscopic finding is a solitary lesion in a younger patient with hematuria. Papillomas may recur (in up to 80% of cases) or progress to higher grade disease (in 2% of cases).
   b. **Inverted papilloma.** Another uncommon neoplasm, an inverted papilloma has a polypoid or sessile appearance cystoscopically. It is composed of anastomosing islands and cords of bland urothelial cells that invaginate and grow downward in the lamina propria with peripheral palisading, no to rare mitoses, and no to minimal cytological atypia (e-**Fig. 22.28**) (*Am J Surg Pathol.* 2004;28:1615, *Cancer.* 2006;107:2622). These latter two features help distinguish this lesion from other papillary neoplasms that may also occasionally have an inverted growth pattern. Inverted papillo-mas rarely recur.
   c. **Papillary urothelial neoplasm of low malignant potential (PUNLMP).** This neoplasm shares the clinical and endoscopic features of papilloma but is characterized histologically by occasionally fused papillae and ordered, yet larger, nuclei than are seen in papillomas (e-**Fig. 22.29A** and **B**). Mitotic figures are rare and basal. Compared with papillomas, PUNLMP has higher recurrence (25% to 35%) and progression rates (up to 4%), and thus close follow-up is warranted.
   d. **Noninvasive papillary urothelial carcinoma, low grade.** In contrast to PUNLMP, this urothelial neoplasm shows frequent branching and fusion of papillae and variations in nuclear size, shape, and contour (e-**Fig. 22.30**). Mitoses are occasional and may be found at any level. These tumors tend to be larger than papillomas and PUNLMPs and are more likely to be multiple. They are also more likely to recur (64% to 71%) and progress (2% to 10%).
   e. **Noninvasive papillary urothelial carcinoma, high grade.** These are uncom-mon noninvasive papillary neoplasms; more frequently there is associated invasion. They are characterized by frequent branching and fusion with moderate to marked cytoarchitectural disorder and nuclear pleomorphism (e-**Fig. 22.31**). Mitoses are frequent. Similar to low-grade tumors, these tumors frequently recur (56%) and progress to invasive carcinoma (18%).

3. **Invasive urothelial neoplasms.** Invasive urothelial carcinomas can have papil-lary, polypoid, nodular, or ulcerative configurations. Most are cytologically high-grade tumors. Determination of anatomic depth of invasion by carci-noma is vital, because pathological stage is the single most important prog-nostic feature.

   Recognition of diagnostic patterns of lamina propria invasion can facili-tate pT1 stage assignment (Table 22.2). There are several different patterns,

TABLE 22.2	Tumor, Node, Metastasis (TNM) Staging Scheme for Bladder Carcinoma

Primary tumor (T)

TX	Primary tumor cannot be assessed
T0	No evidence of primary tumor
Ta	Noninvasive papillary carcinoma
Tis	Carcinoma in situ (i.e., flat tumor)
T1	Tumor invades subepithelial connective tissue
T2	Tumor invades muscle
pT2a	Tumor invades superficial muscle (inner half)
pT2b	Tumor invades deep muscle (outer half)
T3	Tumor invades perivesical tissue
pT3a	Microscopically
pT3b	Macroscopically (extravesical mass)
T4	Tumor invades any of the following: prostatic stroma, seminal vesicles, uterus, vagina, pelvic wall, or abdominal wall
T4a	Tumor invades the prostatic stroma, uterus, vagina
T4b	Tumor invades the pelvic wall, abdominal wall

Note: The suffix "m" should be added to the appropriate T category to indicate multiple lesions. The suffix "is" may be added to any T to indicate the presence of associated carcinoma in situ.

Regional lymph nodes (N)

NX	Regional lymph nodes cannot be assessed
N0	No regional lymph node metastasis
N1	Single lymph node metastasis in the true pelvis (hypogastric, obturator, external iliac or presacral lymph node)
N2	Multiple regional lymph node metastasis in the true pelvis (hypogastric, obturator, external iliac or presacral lymph node)
N3	Lymph node metastasis to the common iliac lymph nodes

Distant metastasis (M)

M0	No distant metastasis (no pathologic M0; use clinical M to complete stage group)
M1	Distant metastasis

AJCC pathologic stage groups

Stage 0a	Ta	N0	M0
Stage 0is	Tis	N0	M0
Stage I	T1	N0	M0
Stage II	T2a	N0	M0
	T2b	N0	M0
Stage III	T3a	N0	M0
	T3b	N0	M0
	T4a	N0	M0
Stage IV	T4b	N0	M0
	Any T	N1	M0
	Any T	N2	M0
	Any T	N3	M0
	Any T	Any N	M1

From: Edge SB, Byrd DR, Compton CC, et al., eds. *AJCC Cancer Staging Manual.* 7th ed. New York, NY: Springer; 2010. Used with permission.

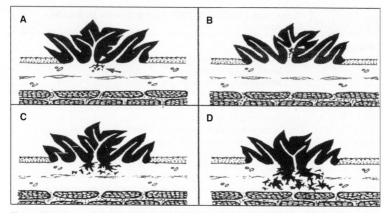

Figure 22.3 Patterns of invasion from papillary carcinoma. **A:** Microinvasive carcinoma at base. **B:** Stalk invasion. **C:** Lamina propria invasion up to muscularis mucosae. **D:** Lamina propria invasion beyond muscularis mucosae. (From Amin MB, et al. *Am J Surg Pathol.* 1997;21:1057, with permission.)

including those seen with papillary urothelial carcinoma (Fig. 22.3, e-**Figs. 22.32** and **22.33**), carcinoma in situ (CIS) (e-**Fig. 22.34**), nested carcinoma, and inverted pattern carcinoma (Fig. 22.4) (*Am J Surg Pathol.* 1997;21:1057). Recently emphasized pitfalls in the diagnosis of lamina propria invasive urothelial carcinoma include tangential sectioning, thermal artifact, obscuring inflammation, carcinoma in situ involving von Brunn nests, deceptively bland urothelial carcinoma, invasion into indeterminate type of muscle, and invasion into adipose tissue within lamina propria (Epstein JI, Amin MB, Reuter VE. *Bladder Biopsy Interpretation.* 2nd ed. Philadelphia: Lippincott Williams & Wilkins; 2010).

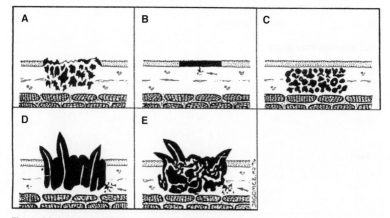

Figure 22.4 Patterns of lamina propria invasion. **A and B:** From carcinoma in situ. **C:** Nested variant. **D:** Endophytic growth and invasion. **E:** Inverted growth and invasion. (From Amin MB, et al. *Am J Surg Pathol.* 1997;21:1057, with permission.)

The level of invasion of carcinoma in pT1 disease is related to patient outcome, with a worse prognosis for patients with tumors that invade the muscularis mucosae (pT1b) or deeply into the subepithelial connective tissue, as quantitated using an ocular micrometer. The WHO 2004 group recommended that some estimate of extent of lamina propria invasion (e.g., pT1a [invasion above muscularis mucosae] vs. pT1b tumors) be provided, but this is currently not a formal part of the 2010 TNM system because there is no established method for estimation that is consistently applicable and reproducible.

Invasion by bladder carcinoma into muscularis propria (muscle wall, detrusor muscle) (e-**Fig. 22.35**) is an ominous finding that makes the patient a candidate for aggressive surgical therapy (radical cystectomy) or radiation therapy, with or without adjuvant chemotherapy.

Determination of the type of muscle (muscularis mucosae vs. muscularis propria) invaded by carcinoma can occasionally be difficult because of small tissue sample size, tissue distortion, cautery artifact, poor orientation, fibrosis, inflammation elicited by destructive growth of invasive tumor, or even hypertrophy of the normally thin, wispy, and discontinuous muscularis mucosae. The designation of "muscle type indeterminate" is a viable description in some cases. Smoothelin immunohistochemistry has potential for distinction of muscularis mucosae from muscularis propria, with the latter showing strong and diffuse immunostaining, with relatively high sensitivity and specificity (*Am J Surg Pathol.* 2010;34:792).

Substaging of pT2 (pT2a, invasion of "superficial" muscle = inner half vs. pT2b, invasion of "deep" muscle = outer half) and distinction of pT2 versus pT3 can be performed only on radical cystectomy specimens and not samples from transurethral resections of bladder tumor. Even in cystectomy specimens, it can be a challenge at times to determine extravesical (pT3) spread because the boundary between muscularis propria and its fat is not well demarcated from perivesical fat. Moreover, this boundary can be distorted, obscured, or obliterated by fibrosis and inflammation associated with infiltrating tumor.

Numerous **histologic variants of urothelial carcinoma with divergent differentiation** have been described (*Mod Pathol.* 2009;22:S96), including the following.

a. **Invasive urothelial carcinoma with squamous differentiation.** Focal squamous differentiation, to be distinguished from pure squamous cell carcinoma, is seen in up to 20% of invasive urothelial carcinomas, with an increased likelihood of squamous features in high-grade urothelial carcinomas. Squamous differentiation may predict a poor response to radiotherapy and systemic chemotherapy, although this has not been definitely established.

b. **Invasive urothelial carcinoma with glandular differentiation.** True glandular spaces with or without mucin production and/or signet cells is seen in approximately 6% of invasive urothelial carcinomas (e-**Fig. 22.36**). Although this variant needs to be distinguished from adenocarcinoma, it is not clear whether it behaves any different from classic invasive urothelial carcinoma.

c. **Urothelial carcinoma with trophoblastic differentiation.** Trophoblastic differentiation can be manifested by the presence of any of the following: syncytiotrophoblastic giant cells, immunoreactivity for human chorionic gonadotropin (hCG), or choriocarcinoma. hCG immunoreactivity can be found in about one-third of high-grade urothelial carcinomas and can be associated with serum elevations of hCG, but because such immunoreactivity is not of prognostic significance hCG immunostains should not be performed; a very few cases of urothelial carcinoma with hCG-positive syncytiotrophoblasts (e-Fig. 22.37) have been reported. True syncytiotrophoblasts should be distinguished from the tumoral giant cells of giant cell carcinoma and from osteoclast-like giant cells, and it is important to recognize that true syncytiotrophoblasts represent examples of divergent differentiation and not a primary germ cell tumor of the urinary bladder. Nonetheless, this variant should be reported because the prognosis is extremely poor, with most patients dead of disease within 1 year. Very rare cases of pure choriocarcinoma of the urinary bladder have been described, but most likely represent urothelial carcinoma with trophoblasts.

d. Sarcomatoid variant (previously known as carcinosarcoma). This is a biphasic neoplasm displaying histomorphologic and/or immunophenotypic evidence of both epithelial and mesenchymal differentiation (*Am J Surg Pathol.* 1994;18:241). Because both components share the same clonal origin, this tumor is another example of a neoplasm with divergent differentiation. This variant accounts for <1% of bladder malignancies. Previous radiation and cyclophosphamide treatment are predisposing factors. Grossly, the tumor is often exophytic, polypoid, and deeply invasive into muscularis propria. Microscopically, the growth is typified by a biphasic population of neoplastic cells with the epithelial and mesenchymal-like components often in continuity (e-Fig. 22.38A and B). The carcinomatous component is usually urothelial (85%) but can be adenocarcinoma, squamous cell carcinoma, or small cell carcinoma. The amount of the malignant epithelial element varies and in some cases is only represented by carcinoma in situ; consequently, apparently pure malignant spindle cell tumors of the bladder should be sampled extensively in an attempt to find epithelial areas. The sarcomatous component is usually an undifferentiated high-grade spindle cell proliferation arranged in fascicles, a storiform pattern, or as a patternless confluence. The most common heterologous element is osteosarcoma, followed by chondrosarcoma (e-Fig. 22.39), rhabdomyosarcoma, leiomyosarcoma, liposarcoma, angiosarcoma, or mixtures thereof. The sarcomatous regions are almost always high-grade. Immunohistochemical staining of the sarcomatoid variant shows strong, diffuse immunopositivity for pan-cytokeratin (e-Fig. 22.38B), although epithelial membrane antigen (EMA) immunostaining is characteristically weak; note, however, that epithelial markers can be negative and focal immunoreactivity for desmin and smooth muscle actin may be present. The opposite pattern of staining favors a leiomyosarcoma, in the correct histopathologic context. Anaplastic lymphoma kinase (ALK)-1 immunostaining, which typifies inflammatory myofibroblastic tumor, is negative in sarcomatoid carcinoma. For cases of sarcomatoid carcinoma, the pathology report should include whether the sarcomatoid carcinoma is homologous or heterologous, although to date this does not appear to be of prognostic importance. Surgery and radiation result in 25% survival at 2 years.

Histologic variants of urothelial carcinoma with unusual growth patterns:

e. Nested variant. This variant is characterized by the presence of infiltrating small nests and tubules of urothelial carcinoma (e-Fig. 22.40). Despite its relatively bland low-grade cytological features, this variant is often aggressive. Because of its cytoarchitectural features, florid von Brunn nests, cystitis cystica and glandularis, inverted papilloma, nephrogenic adenoma, and paraganglioma are all in the differential diagnosis. Clues that are of aid in establishing the diagnosis are the high density, nearly confluent nests that can anastomose and invade muscularis propria. Nuclear atypia may be only focally present and is often found in the deeper aspects of the prolif-eration. Although the nested variant of urothelial carcinoma has a higher proliferation index than florid von Brunn nests by MIB-1 immunostaining (8.8% vs. 2.8%), and a higher p53 immunopositivity (4.2% vs. 1.5%), the degree of overlap precludes use of these markers as diagnostic tools (*Am J Surg Pathol.* 2003;27:1243).

f. **Microcystic variant.** This variant is also deceptively bland and somewhat similar to the nested variant, except for characteristic prominent cystic change (e-**Fig. 22.41**). It is uncommon, accounting for only about 1% of bladder carcinomas. Microscopically, there are variable-sized cysts rang-ing up to 1 to 2 mm in diameter. The cysts are round to oval and may contain necrotic material or pink secretions. The layer of lining cells may be flattened or denuded. The differential diagnosis includes cystitis cys-tica, cystitis glandularis, and nephrogenic adenoma. Correct diagnosis is achieved by the detection of an association with usual urothelial carci-noma, haphazard and infiltrative growth, and variability in cyst size and shape. In the largest series, 25% of cases had invasion of muscularis pro-pria and 11 of 12 were high grade (*J Urol.* 1997;74:722).

g. **Micropapillary variant.** This rare pattern of urothelial carcinoma resembles papillary serous carcinoma of the ovary, an important differential diag-nosis in women. It is characterized by the presence of small nests of cells and filiform papillae that have retracted from the surrounding stroma (e-**Fig. 22.42**). Lymphovascular invasion is common. Admixed invasive usual urothelial carcinoma is detected in a majority of cases. Because the proportion of the tumor that is micropapillary seems to be of prognos-tic significance, the percentage of the invasive tumor that is micropap-illary should be reported (*Adv Anat Pathol.* 2010;17:182). This variant is characteristically aggressive. While muscle wall invasion is commonly detected, some cases, especially those with a low percentage (<10%) of micropapillary component and surface micropapillary growth, can be low stage (pTa or pT1). It has been argued that early cystectomy should be offered to patients with such low-stage, nonmuscle-invasive micropapil-lary urothelial carcinoma (*Cancer.* 2007;110:62). Intravesical therapy is ineffective (*Urol Oncol.* 2009;27:3). The 10-year overall survival is 24%.

h. **Lymphoepithelioma-like variant.** This is characterized by sheets and nests of poorly differentiated malignant cells that grow in a syncytial pattern with an admixed dense lymphoplasmacytic infiltrate (e-**Fig. 22.43**) (*Am J Surg Pathol.* 2011;35:474). It may be pure or mixed with usual urothelial carci-noma. There is a tendency for patients to present with muscularis propria-invasive disease. The differential diagnosis centers on large cell lymphoma and severe chronic cystitis, including follicular cystitis; immunostains for pan-cytokeratin and CD45 are confirmatory, and Epstein–Barr virus is not present. These are aggressive carcinomas with a 26% mortality at 3 years. These tumors should be treated as other bladder carcinomas—that is, based on stage—although they do also appear to be chemoresponsive.

Histologic variants of urothelial carcinoma with unusual cytologic fea-tures:

i. **Lymphoma-like and plasmacytoid variants.** These variants are exceedingly rare and are usually admixed with conventional urothelial carcinoma. However, the diagnosis of urothelial carcinoma in small biopsies com-posed solely of such variants (e-**Fig. 22.44**) may be achieved only with the help of immunohistochemistry (positive reactivity to cytokeratin with negative reactivity to CD45 and other lymphoid markers).

j. **Giant cell variant.** This high-grade variant is characterized by numerous pleomorphic and bizarre tumor giant cells (e-**Fig. 22.45**), and needs to be distinguished from urothelial carcinoma with osteoclast-like giant cells, which represents an unusual stromal response to invasive carcinoma. Outcome is poor, with median survival of 11 months (*Br J Urol.* 1995;75:167).

k. Glycogen-rich (clear-cell) and lipid-rich variants. The main importance of these rare variants is the fact that they may be confused with clear-cell adenocarcinoma of the bladder or kidney, and liposarcoma or signet-ring carcinoma, respectively. The lipid-rich (also known as lipoid-cell) variant carries a poor prognosis (*Br J Urol.* 1995;75:167).

l. Urothelial carcinoma with rhabdoid features. Rhabdoid cells may rarely be observed in urothelial carcinoma; < 10 cases have been reported (*Hum Pathol.* 2006;37:16). This variant is a high-grade carcinoma with a poor clinical outcome. Morphologically, the rhabdoid cells have large, eccentric nuclei with prominent nucleoli and eosinophilic cytoplasmic inclusions. In children, primary malignant rhabdoid tumor of the bladder is in the differential diagnosis, a diagnosis which requires molecular evidence of mutations of the *SMARCB1* gene (*Ann Diagn Pathol.* 2011; Jul 18 [Epub ahead of print]).

F. Squamous neoplasms

1. Squamous papilloma. This is a very rare papillary lesion that typically presents in elderly women and, unlike condyloma acuminatum (which can also involve the bladder), has not been associated with human papilloma virus infection or with subsequent development of carcinoma (*Am J Surg Pathol.* 2006;20:883, *Cancer.* 2000;88:1679). Recurrence is rare.

2. Squamous cell carcinoma. In areas of the world where schistosomiasis is endemic (parts of Africa and the Middle East), this type of carcinoma is the most common primary neoplasm of the bladder. Elsewhere, squamous cell carcinoma is relatively rare, representing <5% of bladder carcinomas. Other predisposing conditions include chronic cystitis and chronic irritation due to vesical lithiasis or long-term indwelling catheters. Smoking is also a significant risk factor (as for conventional urothelial carcinoma). Squamous cell carcinomas are represented at a higher percentage in patients with nonfunctioning bladders (50% of carcinomas) or diverticula (20%), and in renal transplant patients (15%). Keratinizing squamous metaplasia is a potential precursor and is a risk factor for subsequent detection of carcinoma; 20% to 42% of patients with keratinizing squamous metaplasia are later diagnosed with carcinoma.

Squamous cell carcinoma typically presents as invasive carcinoma, although in a few cases pure squamous cell carcinoma in situ may be detected (*Am J Surg Pathol.* 2006;20:883). Squamous cell carcinoma in situ is a strong risk factor for subsequent detection of invasive carcinoma and approximately 45% of patients with in situ disease are diagnosed with invasive squamous cell or urothelial carcinoma within 12 months (*Am J Surg Pathol.* 2006;20:883). Grossly, squamous cell carcinomas are often large, solid necrotic masses that can fill the entire bladder lumen (e-**Fig. 22.46**). Some, however, may be flat and infiltrative with ulceration. Microscopically, the carcinoma should be purely squamous, with keratin production and/or intercellular bridges (e-**Fig. 22.47**). Adjacent keratinizing squamous metaplasia strongly supports a diagnosis of squamous cell carcinoma; such metaplasia is seen in 20% to 60% of cases of invasive squamous cell carcinoma. Histologic variants of squamous cell carcinoma of the bladder include the exceptionally rare basaloid variant and the uncommon verrucous variant.

Grading is three tiered (well, moderately, or poorly differentiated), and histologic grade may correlate with stage and outcome. However, stage is the most important determinant of outcome. Many patients with squamous cell carcinoma of the bladder present with muscularis propria-invasive disease, and this accounts for the poor outcome for most patients. No molecular genetic abnormalities are currently used for diagnosis or prognosis. Treatment is radical cystectomy, with or without radiation therapy and chemotherapy.

3. **Verrucous squamous cell carcinoma.** This variant of squamous cell carcinoma is seen almost exclusively in patients with schistosomiasis and appears as an exophytic "warty" mass composed of thickened papillary squamous epithelium with minimal cytoarchitectural atypia and a rounded pushing border. This tumor is considered to be clinically indolent.

G. **Glandular neoplasms**

1. **Villous adenoma.** An uncommon exophytic papillary neoplasm histologically resembling its colonic counterpart, villous adenoma is usually located in the trigone and, unless associated with an invasive component, does not recur following excision.

2. **Adenocarcinoma.** Primary adenocarcinomas are rare, representing 2% of malignant bladder neoplasms, and may be of urachal or nonurachal origin. The latter are more common and usually arise in patients with a nonfunctional bladder or with exstrophy. Urachal adenocarcinomas usually arise from the dome or anterior wall of the bladder but may also involve urachal remnants in the anterior abdominal wall. Characteristics of urachal adenocarcinomas that are helpful in differentiating them from nonurachal adenocarcinomas are that their bulk is in the wall rather than the lumen of the bladder; they lack an associated in situ component or cystitis glandularis; and they are sharply demarcated from surface urothelium. Identification of urachal tumors is important because, unlike nonurachal tumors, surgical management of urachal adenocarcinomas usually includes excision of the median umbilical ligament and umbilicus. Bladder adenocarcinomas (of urachal or nonurachal type) may have different morphologic appearances including enteric (e-**Fig. 22.48A** and **B**), mucinous (e-**Fig. 22.7**), signet-ring cell, clear cell, and mixed. The main differential diagnosis for most of these patterns is the more common metastasis or secondary extension from another primary tumor site, most notably the prostate and the colon. Immunohistochemistry may be helpful in this situation, especially when the clinical findings are not helpful or available. Immunoreactivity with PSA and prostatic acid phosphatase, β-catenin (nuclear), or thrombomodulin supports a diagnosis of prostate, colon, or bladder adenocarcinoma, respectively; cytokeratin 7 and 20 immunostains are not very useful in this context because of significant overlap (*Semin Diagn Pathol.* 2005;22:69). Adenocarcinoma of the bladder has a generally poor prognosis with 5-year survival rates ranging from 18% to 47%.

H. **Neuroendocrine neoplasms**

1. **Paraganglioma.** Derived from bladder paraganglia, paragangliomas are typically found in the muscularis propria and are not infrequently associated with hypertension and/or headaches, palpitations, and sweating that may be precipitated by micturition. The tumor is composed of cells with abundant amphophilic, clear, or eosinophilic cytoplasm arranged in a diffuse or nested (Zellballen) pattern of growth with an associated thin capillary network (e-**Fig. 22.49**). Nuclear atypia can occasionally be prominent. The tumor is frequently immunopositive for neuroendocrine markers and negative for cytokeratin (useful in distinguishing the tumor from nested urothelial carcinoma), whereas the spindle cells surrounding tumor nests (sustentacular cells) are positive for S100 protein. The majority (85% to 90%) of bladder paragangliomas are benign and do not recur following surgical excision.

2. **Small cell carcinoma.** This is a rare neoplasm, which is diagnosed even when mixed with other bladder carcinomas (urothelial, squamous, or

adenocarcinomas) because the presence of any small cell carcinoma component has a significant negative impact on prognosis. As with other bladder carcinomas, hematuria is the most common presentation; however, almost half of the patients present with metastatic disease, with or without a paraneoplastic syndrome. Histologically, the tumor cells are characteristically small with scant cytoplasm, stippled chromatin, and inconspicuous nucleoli with nuclear molding. Admixture with usual urothelial carcinoma is common and is present in about one-half of cases (e-Fig. 22.50). The diagnosis can often be confirmed by immunoreactivity with one or more neuroendocrine markers such as neuron-specific enolase, chromogranin, synaptophysin, and CD56, with or without cytokeratin expression (which is usually seen in a dot-like paranuclear pattern).

3. **Rare neuroendocrine tumors.** Large cell neuroendocrine carcinomas and carcinoid tumors are rare as primary tumors in the urinary bladder.

I. **Mesenchymal lesions and neoplasms**

1. **Myofibroblastic proliferations.** These spindle cell proliferations can develop a few weeks to several months following bladder instrumentation (for which the term "postoperative spindle cell nodule" has been used), or may be unrelated to trauma. They can be quite large (up to 9 cm in diameter). These neoplasms are composed of myofibroblasts and have been variously termed inflammatory myofibroblastic tumor (*Am J Surg Pathol.* 2007;20:592) and pseudosarcomatous myofibroblastic proliferation (*Am J Surg Pathol.* 2006;30:787); it remains unsettled as to whether these are all the same entity or a heterogeneous group of proliferations. Histologically, these lesions are composed of elongated spindle or stellate cells resembling tissue-culture fibroblasts, embedded in a myxoid matrix that contains a variable chronic inflammatory infiltrate and extravasated red blood cells (e-Fig. 22.51). Although enlarged nuclei with prominent nucleoli (as well as prominent mitotic activity) can be observed, the presence of significant nuclear atypia and/or abnormal mitotic figures should suggest an alternative diagnosis such as sarcomatoid carcinoma or leiomyosarcoma. Immunohistochemistry can sometimes be a useful diagnostic tool as the spindle cells are often positive for cytokeratin, actin, and vimentin. In addition, more than two-thirds of cases display expression of ALK, often associated with a translocation involving its locus on the short arm of chromosome 2 (2p23). Recurrences can be seen and the proliferations can be locally aggressive, with deep extension into muscularis propria and even into perivesical adipose tissue. In only one case, there has been metastatic spread and in this case overt sarcomatous features were also present (*Am J Surg Pathol.* 2006;30:1502).

2. **Smooth muscle neoplasms.** Leiomyomas and leiomyosarcomas represent the most common benign and malignant mesenchymal neoplasms of the bladder, respectively. Leiomyomas usually present as well-circumscribed lamina propria (two-thirds of cases), intramural, or subserosal masses and are composed of intersecting fascicles of spindle cells with abundant eosinophilic cytoplasm and oval/elongated nuclei with blunt ends. By definition, there should be no significant nuclear atypia (hyperchromasia, nuclear membrane irregularities, or pleomorphism) or evidence of an infiltrative growth pattern. In contrast, leiomyosarcomas (e-Fig. 22.52) are infiltrative tumors with nuclear atypia, coagulative tumor cell necrosis, and brisk mitotic activity (usually >5 mitoses per 10 high-power fields), the latter being a typical feature of high-grade tumors. In addition to showing immunoreactivity with one or more smooth muscle markers (actins, desmin, and caldesmon), leiomyosarcomas can also be at least focally immunopositive for cytokeratin and EMA. Most patients with leiomyosarcoma develop recurrences and/or metastasis resulting in mortality in almost one-half of cases.

3. **Rhabdomyosarcoma.** Almost a quarter of all childhood rhabdomyosarcomas arise in the genitourinary tract, and a significant proportion are of bladder origin. Almost all genitourinary tract cases are of the embryonal type. Grossly, most embryonal rhabdomyosarcomas of the bladder present as polypoid intraluminal masses (e-**Fig. 22.53**) resembling a cluster of grapes (hence the alternative name botryoid type), with the remainder being deeply invasive tumors. Histologically, they are mostly composed of small round tumor cells with a variable admixture of spindle cells embedded in a myxoid stroma, often with cell condensation under the surface urothelium forming the so-called "cambium layer" (e-**Fig. 22.54**). The latter feature, as well as the identification of rhabdomyoblasts and cross-striations, is particularly useful for diagnosis. Immunohistochemistry can confirm the diagnosis as these tumors are usually positive for myogenin and myoD1, among other muscle markers. The prognosis of embryonal rhabdomyosarcoma has greatly improved with multimodality treatment, although the alveolar type and the rare rhabdomyosarcomas presenting in adulthood are associated with a worse outcome.

4. **Other spindle cell neoplasms.** There are other spindle cell neoplasms that can occasionally involve the bladder including hemangioma, neurofibroma, solitary fibrous tumor, angiosarcoma, osteosarcoma, and malignant fibrous histiocytoma. These tumors are histologically identical to their nonbladder counterparts.

J. **Other miscellaneous neoplasms.** As discussed earlier, the bladder can be involved by metastatic carcinomas and those extending from adjacent organs, where clinical data and immunohistochemical findings can help resolve the diagnosis. Hematolymphoid neoplasms can also involve the bladder, either primarily or secondarily (more common), and may present as mass lesions. Finally, there are a few reported primary bladder melanomas in the literature.

IV. **HISTOLOGIC GRADING OF UROTHELIAL CARCINOMA** is indicated as low grade or high grade, as discussed earlier. Histologic grade of primary adenocarcinoma or squamous cell carcinoma of the urinary bladder can be reported as well-, moderately-, or poorly differentiated.

V. **PATHOLOGIC STAGING OF URINARY BLADDER CANCER** applies to carcinomas only. Pathologic primary tumor (pT) 2010 TNM AJCC stage categories are given in Table 22.2 and illustrated in Figure 22.5. pN and pM groupings are also listed in Table 22.2.

VI. **REPORTING URINARY BLADDER CARCINOMA** should follow suggested guidelines (see the College of American Pathologists urinary bladder cancer protocol and checklists at http://www.cap.org). For urinary bladder biopsy and transurethral resections, the histologic type, grade, and depth of invasion are reported. The presence or absence of muscularis propria should also be noted for each biopsy sample. Carcinoma in situ, when present in flat urothelium adjacent to papillary tumor, should also be reported. If lymphovascular space invasion by carcinoma is seen, it should be reported.

For cystectomy (partial or total), radical cystoprostatectomy, and pelvic exenteration specimens, the following are reported: tumor location, size in three dimensions, gross growth pattern (papillary, nodular/solid, flat, ulcerated), gross depth of invasion, gross involvement of adjacent structures (prostate, vagina, uterus, colon), and relation to surgical margins. Microscopic features that should be reported include histologic type, grade, site(s) of involvement, growth pattern, extent of invasion, involvement of other structures, lymphovascular invasion, and margin status. Important margins include the ureters, distal urethra, perivesical soft tissue (for cystectomy specimens), and pelvic soft tissue (for exenteration specimens). For regional lymph nodes, the total number examined, number positive for carcinoma, presence of extranodal extension, and size of largest metastatic deposit should be documented.

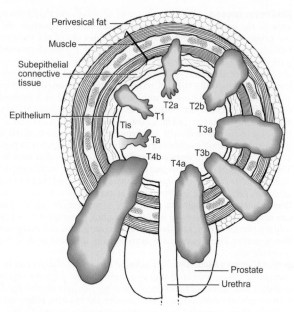

Figure 22.5 Pathologic T staging of carcinoma of the urinary bladder. (Modified from Greene FL, et al., eds. *AJCC Cancer Staging Atlas*. New York, NY: Springer; 2006.)

Cytopathology of the Urinary Bladder

Rosa M. Dávila

I. TYPES OF SPECIMENS

A. **Voided urine** normally has a mixture of benign urothelial cells and squamous cells. Although the squamous cells may be a vaginal or skin contaminant, they can also be derived from areas of squamous metaplasia that often develop in the bladder trigone. When urothelial cells are present in papillary-like clusters, the possibility of a low-grade urothelial neoplasm should be raised. Similar clusters may also be due to recent instrumentation or lithiasis.

B. **Catheterized urine** normally has papillary-like clusters of urothelial cells resulting from the mechanical disruption of the urothelial mucosa. They should not be confused with low-grade urothelial carcinoma.

C. **Bladder washings** are obtained by irrigating the bladder with saline instilled via a catheter, or during cystoscopic evaluation. The cytologic findings in this specimen type are similar to those seen in catheterized urine.

D. **Neobladder or ileal conduit samples** have abundant degenerated cells, some of which are arranged in clusters and have vacuolated cytoplasm. Well-preserved intestinal-type epithelium is rarely present. A variable number of inflammatory cells, macrophages, and bacteria are seen (**e-Fig. 22.55**).

II. INFLAMMATORY/INFECTIOUS PROCESSES

A. **Eosinophils.** Detection of eosinophils may be difficult in Papanicolaou-stained slides because the cytoplasmic granules do not stain prominently. Therefore, identification of eosinophils is based on their bilobed nucleus. Patients with allergic interstitial nephritis or eosinophilic cystitis, or those who have had recent bladder biopsies, can display urinary eosinophils.

B. **Human polyoma virus (BK virus)** is an important cause of morbidity in renal transplant patients. This DNA virus initially infects children and becomes dormant until the patient becomes immunosuppressed. Because it infects the renal tubular epithelial cells and urothelial cells, the cellular changes can be detected by urine cytology. Infected cells are usually arranged singly and have a blackish-blue inclusion that occupies most of the nucleus. The cellular changes can resemble those of high-grade urothelial carcinoma, and therefore infected cells are also known as "decoy cells." In contrast to high-grade urothelial carcinoma, decoy cells have a round nucleus with smooth contours that has dark, homogenous staining (*Am J Transplant.* 2001;1:373).

C. **Acute inflammation** is common in patients with lower urinary tract infections that do not require cytologic evaluation. However, urine samples with acute inflammation may be submitted to cytology when an underlying pathology is clinically suspected. In addition to the acute inflammation, urothelial cells may display reactive changes characterized by cellular and nuclear enlargement, a normal nucleus/cytoplasm ratio, and prominent nucleoli.

D. **Trichomonas** is commonly identified in cervical–vaginal samples, and occasionally it is identified in urine samples from female and male patients. Because men are often asymptomatic carriers, the infection is often initially detected by urine cytology. This protozoan is small (15 to 50 μm) and pear shaped and has a small nucleus, eosinophilic cytoplasmic granules, and flagella. Flagella are often difficult to visualize in cytologic samples (**e-Fig. 22.56**).

III. NEOPLASMS

A. **Urothelial carcinomas** can be divided into the following groups: low-grade neoplasms composed of normal-appearing urothelial cells and high-grade neoplasms composed of overtly abnormal urothelial cells. Urine cytology has a poor sensitivity ($\sim$30%) in diagnosing low-grade urothelial neoplasms (*Acta Cytol.* 1996;40:676). Papillary urothelial clusters in a voided sample, even in the absence of nuclear atypia, can be a manifestation of low-grade papillary neoplasm (**e-Fig. 22.57**). The sensitivity of urinary cytology is approximately from 40% to 80%, and the specificity >80%, with improved performance for high-grade urothelial neoplasms (*Urol Clin North Am.* 2000;27:25). High-grade urothelial carcinoma cells exhibit nuclear enlargement, a high nucleus/cytoplasm ratio, and nuclear hyperchromasia with a coarse chromatin pattern (**e-Fig. 22.58**); in addition, the cells have a tendency to be arranged singly or in small, poorly cohesive clusters.

One particularly promising method as an adjunct to urinary cytology is fluorescence in situ hybridization (FISH) to detect chromosomal abnormalities, specifically the commercially marketed UroVysion FISH test (Abbott Laboratories, Abbott Park, IL). The test uses FISH probes to detect aneuploidy of chromosomes 3, 4, and 17, and loss of 9p21, in voided urine specimens fixed on glass slides. The approach has a sensitivity of 72% and specificity of 83%, and studies with paired data have shown that the UroVysion test has a better performance than cytology (*Urol Oncol.* 2008;26:646), although when superficial cancer cases are excluded the differences between UroVysion and routine cytology almost disappear. Most laboratories employ the FISH-based method in conjunction with cytology, an approach that can likely be used to lengthen the interval between surveillance cystoscopy in evaluation of patients with urothelial carcinoma.

B. **Squamous cell carcinoma** can occur as a primary bladder tumor or can arise in adjacent organs, such as the uterine cervix, and extend into the bladder. A more common scenario is the presence of a squamous component within a conventional urothelial carcinoma. Cytologic features that indicate the presence of squamous differentiation include neoplastic cells with a variable amount of dense and eosinophilic cytoplasm, pyknotic nuclei, and bizarre cell shapes (e-Fig. 22.59). Parakeratotic and/or anucleated cells are often seen in the background. Poorly differentiated squamous cell carcinoma that is nonkeratinizing may be confused with high-grade urothelial carcinoma.

C. **Adenocarcinoma of the bladder** can be primary or metastatic. Although most (87%) of adenocarcinomas of the bladder can be identified as malignant by urine cytology, only 67% will be additionally classified as adenocarcinoma (*Cancer Cytopathol.* 1998;84:335). Columnar or cuboidal cell shapes, with cytoplasmic vacuoles within the neoplastic cells, are cytologic features that support the diagnosis of adenocarcinoma.

23 Urethra

Souzan Sanati and Peter A. Humphrey

I. **NORMAL ANATOMY.** The male urethra is divided into three anatomic regions: prostatic (bladder neck to apex of the prostate), bulbomembranous (apex of the prostate to inferior surface of urogenital diaphragm), and penile (inferior surface of urogenital diaphragm to the urethral meatus). The prostatic portion is lined by urothelium, the bulbomembranous portion is lined by pseudostratified or stratified columnar epithelium, and the penile portion shows a transition from the stratified columnar epithelium at its origin to squamous epithelium at the meatus. The female urethra is lined by urothelium in the proximal one-third and squamous epithelium in the distal two-thirds.

The urethra has associated periurethral glands. Skene glands are present in females and are concentrated distally. Bulbourethral (Cowper glands) and glands of Littre, located in the bulbomembranous portion and along the penile urethra, respectively, are present in males.

II. **GROSS EXAMINATION AND TISSUE SAMPLING**

A. Urethroscopic biopsy tissue samples should be entirely submitted for histologic examination, and three levels should be examined.

B. Surgical excision of urethral carcinoma. For men, the type of surgery is dependent on tumor location and extent and includes transurethral resection (TUR), local segmental excision, partial or radical penectomy, and cystoprostatectomy. TUR chips should be submitted in their entirety. Segmental excision specimens should be sampled to include sections of the proximal and distal margins and area of deepest growth. Urethrectomy (primary or secondary) involves stripping of all or part of the urethra with preservation of the penis and is performed for patients with primary urethral carcinoma or secondary involvement by bladder carcinoma; sampling should include sections of the proximal and distal margins and area of deepest growth. Gross processing of penectomy and cystoprostatectomy specimens is covered in Chapters 30 and 29, respectively.

For women, local excision of the distal urethra and adjacent vaginal wall is often sufficient surgical therapy for carcinoma of the urethra; sections of the mass, and urothelial, radial soft tissue, and vaginal mucosal margins should be submitted. For proximal urethral cancer in women, cystourethrectomy (anterior exenteration, with excision of part or all of the vagina) is often necessary; sections of the mass demonstrating relationships with adjacent structures and depth of invasion, grossly uninvolved urethra and urinary bladder, and ureteral and radial soft tissue margins should be submitted.

III. **DIAGNOSTIC FEATURES OF BENIGN DISEASES**

A. Congenital anomalies

1. **Urethral valves** are mucosal folds lined by normal urothelium that project into the urethral lumen causing obstruction, hematuria, or inflammation. Posterior urethral valves are usually seen in men and are associated with bladder neck hypertrophy.

2. **Diverticula** are invaginations of urethral mucosa usually seen in women as a result of infection, trauma, or obstruction. They are lined by urothelium that may undergo squamous or glandular metaplasia (e-Fig. 23.1).*

---

*All e-figures are available online via the Solution Site Image Bank.

3. **Fibroepithelial polyp** is a congenital anomaly usually involving the posterior urethra of male infants and young boys. It consists of a fibrous connective tissue stalk lined by urothelium.

B. **Inflammation and infection**

1. **Urethritis** is an inflammatory response in the urethra that is usually secondary to sexually transmitted diseases. Diagnosis is made by examination of a ure-thral smear that shows neutrophils. Polypoid urethritis is usually seen in the prostatic urethra near the verumontanum and is the result of inflammation that induces multiple polypoid lesions with edematous stroma, distended blood vessels, and chronic inflammation (e-**Fig. 23.2**).

2. **Caruncle** is a pedunculated or sessile polypoid inflammatory mass in the distal urethra in postmenopausal women showing a mixed inflammatory infiltrate with rich vascularity (e-**Fig. 23.3A and B**).

3. **Malakoplakia** is a rare urethral granulomatous inflammatory process, show-ing histiocytes containing characteristic Michaelis–Gutmann bodies, more commonly seen in women.

4. **Condyloma acuminatum** of the urethra is caused by human papilloma virus (HPV), usually serotypes 6, 11, 16, and 18. It can primarily involve the ure-thra but more commonly arises by direct extension from similar lesions in adjacent sites including the external genitalia, perineum, and anus. Histolog-ically, there is a flat or polypoid proliferation of squamous epithelium (e-**Fig. 23.4**) with koilocytic atypia. Multiplicity and recurrence are common.

C. **Metaplasia**

1. **Squamous metaplasia** can occur as a response to chronic inflammatory insults secondary to infection, diverticula, calculi, or instrumentation.

2. **Urethritis cystica and glandularis** are small cysts lined by urothelial and glan-dular cells, respectively.

3. **Nephrogenic adenoma** (metaplasia) is rare in the urethra. It occurs at the site of previous damage, often related to a previous surgical procedure. Micro-scopically, there is a proliferation of tubular and papillary structures, some-times with cystic change, lined by flattened to cuboidal to hobnail cells with bland nuclear features. Some cases may be due to implantation and growth of tubular epithelial cells shed from the kidney.

D. **Hyperplasia**

1. **Urothelial hyperplasia** is a reactive thickening of cytologically bland urothe-lium and can be flat or papillary. In the papillary form the mucosa can be undulating but still lacks a well-developed fibrovascular core.

2. **Prostatic urethral polyp** is seen in the verumontanum in young men and con-sists of benign prostatic tissue arranged in a polypoid or papillary configu-ration, with projection into the urethral lumen.

IV. **DIAGNOSTIC FEATURES OF NEOPLASTIC DISEASES**

A. **Benign neoplasms** are exceedingly rare and have the same appearance as in the urinary bladder.

1. **Benign epithelial neoplasms** include villous adenoma, squamous papilloma, and urothelial (including inverted) papilloma.

2. **Benign mesenchymal neoplasms** include leiomyoma and hemangioma.

B. **Malignant neoplasms** originating in the urethra are very rare and are carci-nomas in the vast majority of cases (*Semin Diagn Pathol.* 1997;14; *Urol-ogy.* 2006;68:1164). Compared with urinary bladder carcinomas, urethral carcinomas are more often found in women; a much higher percentage are squamous cell carcinomas; there is a greater percentage of high-grade and high-stage tumors; and there is a poorer prognosis. The histologic type of pri-mary urethral carcinomas corresponds to the anatomic site of origin in the urethra. In general, proximal neoplasms (prostatic urethra in men; proximal one-third in females) tend to be urothelial carcinomas, whereas distal tumors (bulbomembranous or penile in men; distal two-thirds in women) are frequently squamous cell carcinomas. Often it is difficult to ascertain the precise site of origin of a urethral carcinoma due to its infiltrative growth and destruction of normal cells. For primary and secondary urothelial neoplasia, the 2004 World Health Organization (WHO) urinary bladder classification is used for typing purposes (Table 22.1).

1. **Squamous cell carcinoma** is the most common urethral carcinoma in both sexes. HPV infection has a significant role in its etiology; 30% of squamous cell carcinomas in men and 60% in women test positive for high-risk HPV, although molecular HPV typing is not necessary for diagnosis. Grossly, squamous cell carcinoma can be verruciform or grayish-white and scirrhous, with necrosis (e-**Fig. 23.5A** and **B**). Microscopically, most are moderately differentiated and deeply invasive. Squamous cell carcinomas of the distal penile urethra frequently invade the corpus cavernosum; more proximal tumors in men may penetrate directly into the urogenital diaphragm, prostate, rectum, and bladder neck. In women, tumors arising in the distal third of the urethra are commonly low-grade squamous cell carcinoma (e-**Fig. 23.6**) or verrucous carcinomas.

2. **Urothelial carcinoma** rarely primarily involves the urethra but more commonly results from secondary involvement by bladder carcinoma; so-called secondary involvement can represent direct extension, multifocal disease, and/or lymphovascular invasion. Grossly, carcinoma in situ (CIS) can be erythematous and/or ulcerative; carcinomas can be papillary, nodular, ulcerative, and/or infiltrative. Histopathologically, primary or secondary urothelial tumors can present as pure CIS, noninvasive papillary neoplasia (e-**Fig. 23.7A** and **B**), or invasive carcinoma, with or without a papillary component. In men there is a propensity for high-grade carcinoma (CIS or invasive) to involve the prostate, which can represent in situ duct/acinar spread and/or stromal-invasive disease. In women, CIS can cancerize suburethral glands, which can mimic invasion.

3. **Adenocarcinoma** is usually seen in the proximal urethra and can originate in a diverticulum. Grossly, the tumor is often infiltrative, with or without an exophytic component, with mucinous, gelatinous, and/or cystic cut surfaces (e-**Fig. 23.8A** and **B**). Microscopically, glandular metaplasia, and urethritis cystica and glandularis, is frequently seen in adjacent epithelium. In women, the most common subtype is clear cell adenocarcinoma (40% of cases). In men, enteric, colloid, or signet-ring histomorphological features are common but the clear cell type is rare.

   a. **Clear cell adenocarcinoma** is a rare tumor that is almost always found in women. Histologically, it is similar to clear cell adenocarcinoma of the vagina or uterus. A distinct feature of this tumor is pattern heterogeneity within the same neoplasm with solid, tubular, tubulocystic, micropapillary, or papillary structures lined by hobnailed cells (e-**Fig. 23.9A** and **B**). Necrosis and mitoses are frequent. The neoplastic cells are uniform and ovoid with well-defined borders and amphophilic, acidophilic, or clear cytoplasm containing glycogen. Nuclei are large and hyperchromatic with prominent nucleoli. Clear cell adenocarcinoma should be differentiated from nephrogenic adenoma (metaplasia) which lacks an infiltrative pattern, sheet-like growth, mitotic figures, necrosis, and significant nuclear atypia (*Hum Pathol.* 2010;41:594).

   b. **Non-clear cell adenocarcinoma** includes enteric, mucinous (e-**Fig. 23.10A** and **B**), signet-ring cell, and not otherwise specified subtypes. Extension of adenocarcinoma from adjacent organs should be excluded.

4. **Paraurethral gland carcinomas** usually develop in paraurethral (Skene glands in females; glands of Littre in males) and bulbourethral (Cowper)

| TABLE 23.1 | TNM Staging Scheme for Urethral Carcinoma |

Primary tumor (T)

TX	Primary tumor cannot be assessed
T0	No evidence of primary tumor

Urethra (male and female)

Ta	Noninvasive papillary, polypoid, or verrucous carcinoma
Tis	Carcinoma in situ
T1	Tumor invades subepithelial connective tissue
T2	Tumor invades any of the following: corpus spongiosum, prostate, periurethral muscle
T3	Tumor invades any of the following: corpus cavernosum, beyond prostatic capsule, anterior vagina, bladder neck
T4	Tumor invades other adjacent organs

Urothelial (transitional cell) carcinoma of prostate

Tis pu	Carcinoma in situ, involvement of prostatic urethra
Tis pd	Carcinoma in situ, involvement of prostatic ducts
T1	Tumor invades subepithelial connective tissue
T2	Tumor invades any of the following: prostatic stroma, corpus spongiosum, periurethral muscle
T3	Tumor invades any of the following: corpus cavernosum, beyond prostatic capsule, bladder neck (extra-prostatic extension)
T4	Tumor invades other adjacent organs (invasion of bladder)

Regional lymph nodes (N)

NX	Regional lymph nodes cannot be assessed
N0	No regional lymph node metastasis
N1	Metastasis in a single lymph node ≤2 cm in greatest dimension
N2	Metastasis in a single lymph node >2 cm in greatest dimension, or multiple lymph nodes

Distant metastasis (M)

M0	No distant metastasis
M1	Distant metastasis

Stage grouping

Stage	T	N	M
Stage 0a	Ta	N0	M0
Stage 0is	Tis	N0	M0
	Tis pu	N0	M0
	Tis pd	N0	M0
Stage I	T1	N0	M0
Stage II	T2	N0	M0
Stage III	T1,	N1	M0
	T2		
	T3	N0, N1	M0
Stage IV	T4	N0, N1	M0
	Any T	N2	M0
	Any T	any N	M1

From: Edge SB, Byrd DR, Compton CC, et al., eds. *AJCC Cancer Staging Manual.* 7th ed. New York, NY: Springer; 2010. Used with permission.

glands. Establishing the origin of adenocarcinoma can be difficult because of mucosal ulceration and obliteration of landmarks by the time of diagnosis.

5. **Other rare carcinomas** include small cell carcinoma, adenosquamous carcinoma, sarcomatoid carcinoma, and lymphoepithelioma-like carcinoma.

6. **Melanoma.** The urethra is the most common site of primary melanoma of the genitourinary tract (*Am J Surg Pathol.* 2000;24:785), but secondary involvement as a result of spread from the glans penis or vulvar lesions is more common. Amelanotic melanoma is commonly seen in this location. Evaluation of margin status and the absence of skip lesions are important in determining the prognosis (e-**Fig. 23.11**).

7. **Hematopoietic neoplasms.** Case reports exist of non-Hodgkin lymphoma, mucosal associated lymphoid tissue (MALT) lymphoma, and plasmacytoma in the urethra.

V. **HISTOLOGIC GRADING OF URETHRAL CARCINOMA.** For squamous cell carcinoma and adenocarcinoma, well, moderately, or poorly differentiated grades may be applied. Urothelial carcinomas are graded as low or high grade.

VI. **PATHOLOGIC STAGING OF URETHRAL CARCINOMA** is presented in Table 23.1. Pathologic stage and tumor location are the most significant pathologic prognostic indicators for urethral carcinoma. Proximal tumors have a worse outcome.

VII. **REPORTING URETHRAL CARCINOMA.** The pathology report of a urethral malignancy should include the histologic type, histologic grade, anatomic location (proximal vs. distal), extent of invasion (depth and involvement of adjacent anatomic structures, if resected), presence or absence of lymphovascular space invasion and perineural invasion, and pathologic tumor, node, metastasis (TNM) staging for resection specimens (*Arch Pathol Lab Med.* 2010;134:345). The status of the margins should also be indicated, if applicable, including identification of the number and location of positive sites. Any additional findings such as inflammation, metaplasia, presence of a diverticulum, or presence of a stricture should also be reported.

Endocrine System

<table>
<tr><td>**24**</td><td>**Thyroid**
Changqing Ma, James S. Lewis Jr.,
and Rebecca D. Chernock</td></tr>
</table>

I. **NORMAL ANATOMY.** The thyroid gland is a bilobed organ in the lower neck surrounding, and in intimate contact with, the trachea. It consists of right and left lobes connected by a small isthmus in the midline (Fig. 24.1). Two functioning cell types, follicular cells and C (calcitonin) cells, comprise the thyroid follicle. The follicular component develops from invaginating tissue from the tongue base (foramen cecum) at 5 to 6 weeks gestation. Through differential embryonic growth and migration, the bilobed gland assumes its definitive location in the neck, and the thyroglossal duct, the structure along the path of its downward migration, undergoes atrophy. The C-cells, which comprise 0.1% or less of the total thyroid cell mass, originate from the ultimobranchial body that develops from the fourth branchial pouches; they are distributed in a density gradient, being most prominent in the upper lobes.

The normal gland has a relatively firm consistency, is light brown, and lacks any obvious nodules. Microscopically, it consists of follicles lined by low cuboidal bland epithelial cells. This follicular epithelium surrounds a central core of eosinophilic colloid. In normal glands, the follicles are relatively consistent and regular in size (e-**Fig. 24.1**).* The C-cells lie within the follicular epithelium and are invested by the basement membrane. They are inconspicuous in normal thyroid.

II. **GROSS EXAMINATION, TISSUE SAMPLING, AND HISTOLOGIC SLIDE PREPARATION**
  A. **Biopsy.** Tissue needle biopsies of the thyroid gland are only very rarely performed because fine needle aspiration is technically easy to perform, has low morbidity, and is effective for triaging lesions for further management (see the section on Cytopathology).
  B. **Resection.** Hemithyroidectomy and total thyroidectomy are common procedures for management of thyroid disease. The specimens from both types of procedure are handled in a similar manner. The gland is oriented, if possible, on the basis of the anatomy alone or on markings provided by the surgeon. It is then measured and weighed. The surface is inspected for any disruptions or attached soft tissue. Small nodules of tissue situated in the adjacent tissues may represent lymph nodes, parathyroid glands, or sequestered thyroid in cases of nodular hyperplasia. The gland should be inked, sectioned in an axial plane (bread loafed) at intervals of 3 to 5 mm, and described, clearly indicating masses and their size(s), color, and consistency. For diffuse or inflammatory lesions, three

---

*All e-figures are available online via the Solution Site Image Bank.

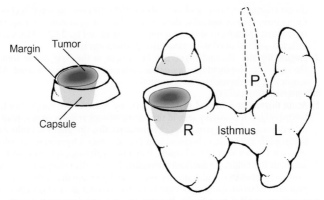

Figure 24.1 Thyroid anatomy/grossing (R, right lobe; L, left lobe; P, pyramidal lobe).

or four sections from each lobe should be submitted for microscopic examination, along with one of the isthmus. For a solitary, encapsulated mass, the entire circumference of the capsule should be sampled, including the surrounding thyroid tissue because the distinction of adenoma from carcinoma relies on features seen in the capsule. For a solitary, nonencapsulated or not completely encapsulated mass, at least one section per centimeter should be submitted, and some sections should demonstrate the closest inked margin (Fig. 24.1). For multinodular glands (nodular hyperplasia), sections of each major nodule should be submitted, including the edge and/or adjacent soft tissue margin. Any attached perithyroidal soft tissue should be removed and sampled. Any lymph nodes or parathyroid glands should be removed and sampled as well, although oftentimes, the parathyroid gland(s) are first detected by microscopic examination (the number of parathyroid glands should be recorded in one of the final diagnostic lines to highlight their presence).

Prophylactic thyroidectomy is currently recommended in infancy, early childhood, adolescence, or early adulthood for patients with a germline *RET* gene mutation. The gross specimen often consists of the thyroid gland with no grossly identifiable lesions. Each lobe should be entirely submitted sequentially from superior to inferior to allow thorough examination for C-cell hyperplasia or medullary microcarcinoma.

III. **DIAGNOSTIC FEATURES OF COMMON DISEASES**
   A. **Developmental.** Residual thyroid tissue can be present anywhere along the path of thyroid migration during development. Carcinomas can rarely develop outside of the thyroid gland in these residual tissue sites.
      1. **Pyramidal lobe.** The most common development remnant is a pyramidal lobe, a linear projection of thyroid tissue from the isthmus pointing cranially (Fig. 24.1).
      2. **Thyroglossal duct cyst.** Failure of closure of the thyroglossal duct commonly results in a midline cyst known as a thyroglossal duct cyst (TDC). Excision specimens generally consist of several nondescript fragments of tissue, and a visible cyst is not always appreciated. Because remnants of the midline tract pass through the hyoid bone, the latter should be identified. Failure to resect the bone often results in persistence of the TDC. If a cyst is identified grossly, it should be sampled in a few sections to document the type of epithelial lining, which is often obscured by acute inflammation. Because TDCs develop from a hollow tube, not all of them have thyroid tissue in their walls (only ~5%

do on routine sections, and only about 40% do even on serial sectioning). Otherwise, microscopically, these lesions have a squamous or respiratory-type lining epithelium without a muscular wall (e-**Fig. 24.2**). TDCs can get infected and inflamed with associated granulation tissue.

3. **Lingual thyroid.** Thyroid tissue can be present at the base of the tongue at the site of developmental invagination, referred to as lingual thyroid. Microscopically, the thyroid tissue is normal.

B. **Inflammation (thyroiditis)**

1. **Acute thyroiditis** is caused predominantly by bacteria but rarely can have a fungal origin. It is usually seen in the setting of neck trauma or as spread from infection of adjacent structures. Microscopically, the gland is infiltrated by neutrophils with microabscesses and necrotic foci. Organisms can often be seen with or without special stains. Patients usually recover with antibiotics.

2. **Subacute thyroiditis: de Quervain thyroiditis.** Technically referred to as granulomatous thyroiditis or subacute thyroiditis, de Quervain thyroiditis is a disease primarily of women and is thought to be due to systemic viral infection. There is linkage to HLA type Bw35. Patients present with fever, malaise, and neck pain. The disease consists of three phases: hyperthyroidism, hypothyroidism, and recovery.

Grossly, the gland is usually asymmetrically enlarged and slightly firm. Microscopically, in the hyperthyroid phase, there is disruption of the follicles, with depletion of colloid and associated acute inflammation with microabscesses. Aggregates of neutrophils in the follicles are a characteristic feature. Multinucleated giant cells are rare. In the hypothyroid phase, the follicular epithelium may be very scarce, and there is a florid mixed inflammatory response with lymphocytes, plasma cells, and multinucleated giant cells. Finally, in recovery, there is regeneration of follicles with fibrosis. Virtually all patients recover thyroid function after a few months without specific treatment.

3. **Chronic thyroiditis**

a. **Focal lymphocytic thyroiditis.** Also termed nonspecific thyroiditis or focal autoimmune thyroiditis, this is a common disorder usually discovered incidentally in surgically excised thyroids, and is found in 25% to 60% of patients in autopsy studies, and is most common in older women. Patients are asymptomatic but often have a low level of antithyroid antibodies.

There are no significant gross findings. Microscopically, focal lymphocytic thyroiditis consists of aggregates of lymphocytes, occasionally with germinal centers, between the follicles (e-**Fig. 24.3**). The lymphocytes can infiltrate follicles, but there is no significant destruction or damage. The disease is not progressive.

b. **Hashimoto thyroiditis.** Hashimoto thyroiditis, or chronic lymphocytic thyroiditis, is an autoimmune disease with thyroid enlargement and circulating antithyroid antibodies. It occurs most often in middle-aged women and is caused by autoantibodies against thyroglobulin (Tg) and thyroid peroxidase (TPO) that lead to inflammation and destruction of the follicles. There is a familial association, and Hashimoto thyroiditis is often associated with other autoimmune diseases. There is also an association with HLA types DR3 and DR5. Patients can present with a hyperthyroidism or hypothyroidism and are typically in their sixth decade. Ultrasound shows an enlarged gland with a hypoechogenic pattern, and anti-Tg and anti-TPO antibodies are present in approximately 60% and 95% of cases, respectively.

Grossly, the thyroid is diffusely enlarged and firm with a mildly nodular surface. On sectioning, lobulation is accentuated due to fibrosis, and the gland is tan-yellow or off-white rather than the usual brown due to the abundant lymphoid tissue. Microscopically, there are sheets of lymphocytes and plasma cells with abundant germinal centers. Florid inflammation often renders the residual follicles and follicular epithelium inconspicuous. The follicles are atrophic with minimal colloid. Characteristic Hürthle cell change is present, consisting of large cells with abundant, granular, eosinophilic cytoplasm and large, round nuclei with vesicular chromatin and prominent nucleoli (e-**Fig. 24.4**). The inflammatory infiltrate may extend into the perithyroidal soft tissue causing adherence of the gland at the time of surgery. Finally, there may be fibrous septa between the lobules, and the follicular epithelium may develop squamous metaplasia.

A number of variants of Hashimoto thyroiditis occur, including fibrous (sclerosing), fibrous atrophy, juvenile, and cystic forms. Both of the fibrous variants show the same histologic findings, namely retention of a lobulated pattern with extensive and severe fibrosis. Atrophic follicular cells are more scattered but show Hürthle cell change, and there is abundant chronic inflammation with germinal centers. In the fibrous variant, the gland is markedly enlarged throughout. In the fibrous atrophy variant, the gland is small and shrunken. Both of the latter variant forms are associated with marked hypothyroidism and high titers of antithyroid antibodies.

The differential diagnosis for Hashimoto thyroiditis includes Riedel thyroiditis and lymphoma. The fibrous variant of Hashimoto thyroiditis may simulate Riedel thyroiditis with an enlarged fibrotic gland. However, the fibrosis is typically limited to the gland itself, whereas in Riedel thyroiditis there is severe adherence of the fibrotic gland to the neck soft tissues. The dense inflammation in Hashimoto thyroiditis can simulate lymphoma, and most thyroid lymphomas do arise in the setting of Hashimoto thyroiditis. The distinction lies in the absence of sheets of atypical lymphocytes, the lack of a strikingly prominent lymphoepithelial pattern, and the lack of clonality of the lymphocytes by flow cytometry or molecular studies.

The issue of whether there is an increased risk of papillary carcinoma in Hashimoto thyroiditis is a controversial topic. Whether this is the case or not, the nuclear features of the epithelium can simulate those of papillary carcinoma (including nuclear crowding, clear chromatin, and occasional nuclear grooves) and develop frequently in the inflamed follicular epithelium. A true carcinoma arising in Hashimoto thyroiditis should stand out sharply from the neighboring follicular epithelium, as in uninflamed thyroid.

c. **Graves disease.** Graves disease is also known as diffuse hyperplasia and is an autoimmune condition resulting in excess thyroid hormone production. It causes the majority of cases of spontaneous hyperthyroidism, occurs most often in the third and fourth decades, and is 5 to 10 times more common in women. Thyroid-specific autoantibodies, specifically thyroid-stimulating immunoglobulin (TSI), are present in Graves disease patients. TSI binds to and stimulates thyrocytes through the thyroid-stimulating hormone (TSH) receptor, resulting in thyrotoxicosis. Patients also develop a characteristic infiltrative ophthalmopathy with proptosis.

Grossly, the thyroid gland is diffusely and symmetrically enlarged. Posttreatment or after long-standing disease, the gland may be somewhat nodular or fibrotic. Microscopically, the gland typically shows a low-power lobular accentuation due to increased septal fibrous tissue. Inflammation varies from none, to patchy lymphocytic, to lymphocytic with formation of germinal centers. The follicular epithelium has increased amounts of cytoplasm, is convoluted and irregular, and often assumes an almost papillary appearance. Colloid is decreased or absent and typically has a "scalloped" appearance from clearing at the interface with the follicular epithelium (e-Figs. 24.5 and 24.6). Treated cases have a variable morphology and often have cellular nodules mimicking adenomas. After radioactive iodine treatment, there can be marked nuclear atypia. The differential diagnosis includes papillary carcinoma when the stellate outlines of follicles resemble papillae. The lack of cytologic changes of papillary carcinoma and the diffuse gland involvement are keys to the correct diagnosis of Graves disease.

d. Riedel thyroiditis. A peculiar form of fibrosing disease, Riedel thyroiditis is a chronic thyroiditis of unknown etiology which is more common in women, occurs most commonly in the fifth decade, and is commonly associated with fibrosing disease at other sites such as the mediastinum, retroperitoneum, and lung. Patients present with firm thyroid enlargement and local symptoms such as dysphagia, stridor, or dyspnea. Recurrent laryngeal nerve or sympathetic trunk involvement can lead to hoarseness or Horner syndrome; compression of the large vessels can lead to superior vena cava syndrome. Most patients are euthyroid at presentation, but many subsequently develop hypothyroidism.

Grossly, the thyroid gland is usually received in irregular pieces because the fibrosis makes it difficult to remove surgically. It is tan to white, firm, and may have attached muscle. Microscopically, the characteristic finding is dense and hypocellular eosinophilic fibrous tissue with scattered and patchy aggregates of lymphocytes, plasma cells, neutrophils, and eosinophils, without germinal centers or granulomas. Rare entrapped and atrophic thyroid follicles are seen without Hürthle cell change. A characteristic finding is small veins with infiltrating lymphocytes and myxoid intimal thickening (features of occlusive vasculitis). Marked fibrosis extends into and involves the surrounding soft tissue as well.

The differential diagnosis includes hypocellular anaplastic thyroid carcinoma and fibrous or sclerosing Hashimoto thyroiditis. The lack of necrosis or markedly atypical cells rules out anaplastic carcinoma. The lack of Hürthle cell change and germinal centers, and the profound degree of perithyroidal fibrosis, rules out fibrous Hashimoto disease.

C. Nodular hyperplasia. Nodular hyperplasia (clinically termed multinodular goiter) is an extremely common disorder of the thyroid gland. It is the enlargement of the gland with varying degrees of nodularity. The pathogenesis is complex but has been classically related to iodine deficiency with impaired thyroid hormone synthesis and subsequent TSH stimulation. With supplementation of iodine in the diet, nodular hyperplasia has also been related either to excess iodine intake with impaired organification or to genetic factors. It is much more common in women than men and typically presents in middle age as asymptomatic enlargement. Large goiters, however, can cause dysphagia, hoarseness, or stridor and can extend into the upper mediastinum. A small percentage of patients present with hyperthyroidism (toxic multinodular goiter).

Grossly, the thyroid gland is diffusely but irregularly enlarged. Some glands can attain a weight of several hundred grams. Parasitic nodules that have only a tenuous connection to the gland can develop. On sectioning, the nodules may be semitranslucent, glistening, fleshy, red-brown, tan, and solid or, more commonly, show varying degrees of degeneration with cystic change, hemorrhage, fibrosis, and calcification. Heterogeneity of the nodules is typical (e-Fig. 24.7).

Microscopically, nodular hyperplasia is also heterogeneous. The common appearance is nodules composed of variably sized follicles (e-Fig. 24.8). The nodules may be quite cellular with tightly packed follicular epithelium and little colloid, resembling follicular adenomas or carcinomas. Around cystic areas there is often fibrosis with variably sized foci of dystrophic calcification and

| TABLE 24.1 | WHO Histological Classification of Thyroid Tumors |

Thyroid carcinomas
Papillary carcinoma
Follicular carcinoma
Poorly differentiated carcinoma
Undifferentiated (anaplastic) carcinoma
Squamous cell carcinoma
Mucoepidermoid carcinoma
Sclerosing mucoepidermoid carcinoma with eosinophilia
Mucinous carcinoma
Medullary carcinoma
Mixed medullary and follicular carcinoma
Spindle cell tumor with thymus-like differentiation
Carcinoma showing thymus-like differentiation

Thyroid adenoma and related tumors
Follicular adenoma
Hyalinizing trabecular tumor

Other thyroid tumors
Teratoma
Primary lymphoma and plasmacytoma
Ectopic thymoma
Angiosarcoma
Smooth muscle tumors
Peripheral nerve sheath tumors
Paraganglioma
Solitary fibrous tumor
Follicular dendritic cell tumor
Langerhans cell histiocytosis
Secondary tumors

From: DeLellis RA, Lloyd RV, Heitz P, et al., eds. *World Health Organization Classification of Tumours. Pathology and Genetics. Tumours of Endocrine Organs.* Lyon, France: IARC Press; 2004. Used with permission.

hemorrhage, with abundant hemosiderin-laden macrophages. Hürthle cell change is common. Pseudopapillary and truly papillary structures (Sanderson polsters) can project into the cystic areas. The surrounding grossly normal thyroid tissue usually demonstrates microscopic nodularity as well.

The differential diagnosis for cellular nodules includes follicular adenoma or carcinoma. Hyperplastic nodules have a fibrous capsule that is not as well developed or continuous as the capsule of adenomas and carcinomas. Follicular adenomas are discrete and well-encapsulated lesions, are microscopically different from the surrounding thyroid tissue, do not show cystic change or degeneration, and have a monotonous cell population—all features that are not characteristic of hyperplastic nodules. Papillary areas in nodular hyperplasia show basally oriented nuclei without the crowding or other features of papillary carcinoma.

D. **Neoplasms.** The World Health Organization (WHO) classification of tumors of the thyroid gland is listed in Table 24.1.

1. **Adenoma.** Follicular adenomas are benign, encapsulated tumors that are clonal. They are seen mostly in young to middle-aged adults and are more common in women than men. There is a relationship with previous irradiation or radiation exposure, just as with follicular carcinoma. There is also an association with inherited diseases including Cowden disease and Carney

TABLE 24.2	Histologic Features Differentiating the Solitary Benign from the Malignant Follicular Lesion

Benign	Malignant
Complete but delicate capsule	Dense, circumferential fibrosis
Entrapped or sequestered thyroid in/near capsule	Transcapsular "mushrooming" invasion
Juxtaposed or prolapsed thyroid tissue near vessels, but with intact endothelium	Adherence of thyroid tissue to endothelium with associated thrombus

complex. Most follicular adenomas are asymptomatic and are detected by careful physical examination or incidentally by imaging performed for other reasons.

Grossly, follicular adenomas are very well-defined, round to oval lesions with a complete capsule. They are typically very soft and homogeneous with a color ranging from gray-white to tan or dark brown depending on the amount of colloid (e-Fig. 24.9). Cystic change and hemorrhage are uncommon. Microscopically, they are encapsulated without, by definition, capsular or vascular invasion. They show a monotonous follicular or trabecular arrangement. The microfollicular pattern features trabeculae with only scattered small follicles with colloid. The macrofollicular pattern has prominent, large follicles with abundant colloid. The cells typically have small amounts of eosinophilic cytoplasm and are quite regular with uniform, round nuclei with condensed chromatin and inconspicuous nucleoli. There is a well developed and moderately thick capsule (e-Fig. 24.10). As with all endocrine organ tumors, there may be a marked degree of nuclear pleomorphism which is not necessarily an indication of malignancy or aggressive behavior. Mitotic figures are rare.

A number of adenoma variants, most notably the oncocytic or Hürthle cell adenoma, which have cells with abundant granular eosinophilic cytoplasm (due to the accumulation of abundant mitochondria) and vesicular nuclei with nucleoli and pleomorphism (e-Fig. 24.11) are recognized. Lipoadenoma (with intratumoral fat; e-Fig. 24.12), signet-ring-cell adenoma, and follicular adenoma with papillary hyperplasia are other adenoma variants.

Follicular adenomas are benign, so surgical removal is curative. The differential diagnosis includes hyperplastic nodules of nodular hyperplasia, follicular variant of papillary thyroid carcinoma (PTC), and minimally invasive follicular carcinoma. Consequently, it is critical to thoroughly sample the lesions, including sectioning of the entire capsule to look for microscopic capsular penetration or vascular invasion (see Table 24.2). The follicular variant of papillary carcinoma can present as an encapsulated mass but will manifest at least some of the cellular, nuclear, and colloid features of papillary carcinoma.

2. **Follicular carcinoma.** Follicular carcinomas account for approximately 10% to 15% of thyroid malignancies and are best thought of as occurring in two types that have vastly different clinical behavior: minimally invasive and widely invasive. Follicular carcinomas are more common in women than men, occur in middle-aged adults, and usually present as asymptomatic masses. There is some association with iodine deficiency and prior irradiation.

Minimally invasive and widely invasive follicular carcinomas are distinguished primarily on the gross appearance. Minimally invasive follicular carcinomas are well encapsulated and, thus, are grossly indistinguishable from follicular adenomas (microscopic evidence of capsular or vascular invasion is necessary to render a diagnosis of carcinoma, as discussed below) In contrast, widely invasive follicular carcinomas are not encapsulated and show extensive invasion of the surrounding gland and/or soft tissue beyond the thyroid (e-**Fig. 24.13**). Follicular carcinomas are almost always unifocal and have tan to brown, solid cut surfaces.

Microscopically, the growth pattern ranges from well-formed follicles throughout, to solid, to trabecular. The nuclei of follicular carcinoma tend to be round to oval with granular chromatin (e-**Fig. 24.14**). Mitotic activity is present, but rarely brisk, and necrosis is lacking. The oncocytic variant (Hürthle cell) is the main histopathologic variant and compromises 20% to 25% of all follicular carcinomas. To be classified as oncocytic variant, a tumor should be composed of at least 75% oncocytic cells. These cells have voluminous eosinophilic and granular cytoplasm and nuclei that are characteristically vesicular with prominent, single nucleoli (e-**Fig. 24.15A**).

By immunohistochemistry, follicular carcinomas are positive for thyroglobulin, thyroid transcription factor-1 (TTF-1), and low-molecular-weight cytokeratins, but these are rarely necessary or useful for diagnosis except occasionally to assess distant metastases as thyroid in origin. In addition, molecular rearrangements in the *PPARγ* gene, most commonly with fusion to the *PAX8* gene, have been detected in 25% to 50% of cases, but this finding is not currently useful in diagnosis or management.

The differential diagnosis includes follicular adenoma, medullary thyroid carcinoma (MTC), and poorly differentiated (insular) carcinoma. The distinction of minimally invasive follicular carcinoma from adenoma lies in capsular and/or vascular penetration alone (Table 24.2). Capsular invasion is defined by the WHO as tumor penetration through the capsule not caused by previous fine-needle aspiration. This invasion needs to be definitive and classically takes the form of "mushrooming" of the tumor outward (e-**Fig. 24.14**). Vascular invasion is defined by the WHO as the presence of intravascular tumor cells either covered by endothelium or associated with thrombus (e-**Fig. 24.15B**). Strict adherence to these criteria is necessary to assure that the diagnosis of carcinoma is correct.

The distinction of follicular carcinoma from MTC is based on morphology (MTCs are rarely follicular in their growth patterns and their nuclei tend to be more spindle shaped) and immunohistochemical findings (neuroendocrine markers, carcinoembryonic antigen [CEA], and calcitonin are positive in MTC but negative in follicular carcinomas, whereas immunohistochemistry for thyroglobulin is positive in follicular carcinoma and negative in MTC). Finally, poorly differentiated (insular) carcinomas can be similar to widely invasive follicular carcinomas, but the former have cells with less cytoplasm, minimal follicular architecture, marked mitotic activity, and necrosis.

Unlike PTC, follicular carcinomas only uncommonly involve regional lymph nodes. Instead, metastasis is via a hematogenous route to lung and bone. In general, minimally invasive follicular carcinomas have an excellent prognosis with an approximately 15% long-term mortality. There is evidence that the presence and extent of vascular invasion may provide further prognostic information for patients with minimally invasive follicular carcinomas. Carcinomas that lack vascular invasion have a better outcome (<5% long-term mortality), while the presence of four or more foci of vascular invasion has been shown to correlate with increased tumor-related mortality. Widely invasive follicular carcinomas have a poorer long-term mortality approaching 50%.

3. **Poorly differentiated (insular) carcinoma.** This type of thyroid carcinoma shows evidence of follicular differentiation but fits morphologically and

biologically between well-differentiated and undifferentiated thyroid carcinomas (UTCs). Some prefer to group this variant under the follicular carcinoma heading, but the WHO recognizes it as a separate entity.

Because the classification of poorly differentiated carcinoma is somewhat controversial, epidemiologic data are difficult to obtain. In general, however, it represents much <5% of thyroid carcinomas in the United States, but between 4% and 7% in Italy and some Latin American countries. It is more common in women, particularly after age 50. Most cases present as sizable asymptomatic masses, with or without pathologically enlarged regional lymph nodes. There is occasionally a history of a long-standing mass with recent, rapid growth.

Grossly, most tumors are large with solid gray to white nodules. Necrosis is common. Extrathyroidal extension is present in some cases but is much less common than in undifferentiated carcinomas (e-Fig. 24.16). The Turin criteria for the histologic diagnosis of poorly differentiated carcinoma include (i) a solid, trabecular or insular growth pattern, (ii) lack of well-developed nuclear features of papillary carcinoma, and (iii) one of the following: convoluted nuclei, tumor necrosis, or three or more mitoses per high power field (e-Figs. 24.17 to 24.20). Most cells have only a small amount of cytoplasm giving the tumor a decidedly neuroendocrine look, although the tumor nuclei typically do not have "salt and pepper" chromatin and often have prominent nucleoli as well as convoluted nuclei (e-Figs. 24.17 to 24.20). Occasional follicles with colloid can be seen. It is not uncommon for well-formed capsules to be present around some of the nodules. Vascular invasion is often a prominent feature. Although rarely useful for routine diagnosis, by immunohistochemistry the tumors are positive for thyroglobulin and TTF-1, although the thyroglobulin reactivity may be focal.

The differential diagnosis includes MTC, the solid variant of papillary carcinoma, and metastasis (particularly from a carcinoid tumor). The mean 5-year survival is approximately 50%.

4. **Papillary carcinoma.** PTC is defined by the WHO as a carcinoma showing evidence of follicular differentiation and characterized by distinct nuclear features. The terminology has become somewhat confusing because papillary architecture, although very commonly present, is not necessary for diagnosis. PTC is the most common malignant thyroid tumor (representing 85% to 90% of differentiated thyroid carcinomas) and has been increasing in incidence, but its prognosis is excellent (discussed later). The commonality of the tumor relative to its indolent behavior makes the appropriate management of PTC controversial. PTC occurs across all ages, and women are affected four times more commonly than men. There is a close link with previous radiation exposure, particularly in younger patients.

Grossly, most tumors are tan or white with infiltrative borders and a firm, often gritty cut surface (e-Fig. 24.21). Cystic change is relatively common, particularly in lymph node metastases, and the bulk of nodal metastatic disease may far outstrip the volume of tumor in the thyroid gland. Microscopically, PTC is diagnosed on the basis of a constellation of architectural and cytologic features (Table 24.3). Architectural patterns include papillary, trabecular, micro- and macrofollicular, solid, and cystic. The stroma around the tumor is often fibrotic or sclerotic. In tumors with follicles, the colloid is typically described as "bright" or dark red relative to the normal thyroid. Another very typical feature is the presence of psammoma bodies (small, round, laminated calcifications; e-Fig. 24.22). Psammoma bodies are not pathognomonic of PTC but are an extremely typical feature. Distinct nuclear features include marked crowding with overlapping of adjacent nuclei, pale

TABLE 24.3	Diagnostic Histologic Features of Papillary Thyroid Carcinoma

True papillae
Psammoma bodies
Dark red colloid
Crowded nuclei
Optically clear ("Orphan Annie") chromatin
Irregular nuclear contours
Nuclear grooves
Intranuclear cytoplasmic inclusions

or clear chromatin, irregular nuclear contours, grooves (e-**Fig. 24.23**), and intranuclear cytoplasmic inclusions where round nodules of cytoplasm overlap the nucleus. Grading is not important because PTC is, by definition, well differentiated, although some authors have found that PTC with necrosis and/or mitotic activity higher than 4 per 10 high power fields is more clinically aggressive. PTC is very frequently multifocal (in up to 50% of cases), which often can be appreciated grossly.

Although rarely needed for diagnosis, immunohistochemistry in PTC is positive for pancytokeratin, cytokeratin 7, thyroglobulin, and TTF-1 but negative for cytokeratin 20, calcitonin, CEA, and neuroendocrine markers. Other markers that have been reported to be useful for differentiating the follicular variant of PTC from follicular adenoma include HBME-1, CK19, and galectin 3; however, these markers have not gained widespread acceptance, and the diagnosis ultimately rests on hematoxylin and eosin (H&E) morphology.

A number of morphologic variants of PTC have been described, with the diagnosis of those without a papillary architecture based on the typical nuclear features. The follicular variant (e-**Fig. 24.24**) is often encapsulated and is composed of follicles throughout without papillae. The oncocytic variant has lining cells with abundant eosinophilic and granular cytoplasm akin to Hürthle cells. So-called papillary microcarcinoma is a focus (or foci) of PTC <1 cm in maximal diameter (e-**Fig. 24.25**); papillary microcarcinoma is an extremely common incidental finding and, although capable of metastasizing, the vast majority of these tumors pursue a benign course. The cells of the clear cell variant have a partially or completely clear cytoplasm, often admixed with oncocytic features. Both a tall cell (tumor cells at least three times as tall as they are wide; e-**Fig. 24.26**) and columnar cell variant of PTC also exist, both of which have been reported to be more aggressive than classic PTC. Finally, the diffuse sclerosing variant tends to occur in younger patients, shows diffuse involvement of one or both lobes without a dominant mass, and has numerous psammoma bodies, dense lymphocytic infiltration, and stromal fibrosis. Because there is an element of subjectivity in the assessment of the morphologic variants of PTC, disagreement often arises in the diagnosis among different observers.

The prognosis for PTC is excellent, with a 10-year survival approaching 100% for younger patients, and >90% overall. Patients older than 45 years typically have more aggressive tumors. The American Joint Committee on Cancer (AJCC) staging system strongly reflects this age-related difference (see Table 24.4).

Recently, molecular analysis has demonstrated translocations, inversions, or other chromosomal rearrangements involving the receptor tyrosine kinase

TABLE 24.4	Tumor, Node, Metastasis (TNM) Staging Scheme for Tumors of the Thyroid

Primary tumor (T)

TX	Primary tumor cannot be assessed
T0	No evidence of primary tumor
T1	Tumor ≤2 cm in greatest dimension, limited to the thyroid
T1a	Tumor ≤ 1 cm, limited to the thyroid
T1b	Tumor >1 cm but not >2 cm in greatest dimension, limited to the thyroid
T2	Tumor >2 cm but not >4 cm, limited to the thyroid
T3	Tumor >4 cm in greatest dimension limited to the thyroid or any tumor with minimal extrathyroid extension (e.g., extension to sternothyroid muscle or perithyroid soft tissues)
T4a	Tumor of any size extending beyond the thyroid capsule to invade subcutaneous soft tissues, larynx, trachea, esophagus, or recurrent laryngeal nerve
T4b	Tumor invading prevertebral fascia or encasing carotid artery or mediastinal vessels

All anaplastic carcinomas are considered T4 tumors

T4a	Intrathyroidal anaplastic carcinoma
T4b	Anaplastic carcinoma with gross extrathyroidal extension

Regional lymph nodes (N)

NX	Regional lymph nodes cannot be assessed
N0	No regional lymph node metastasis
N1a	Metastasis to Level VI (pretracheal, paratracheal, and prelaryngeal/Delphian lymph nodes)
N1b	Metastasis to unilateral, bilateral, or contralateral cervical (levels I, II, II, IV, or V) or retropharyngeal or superior mediastinal lymph nodes (level VII)

Distant metastasis (M)

MX	Distant metastasis cannot be assessed
M0	No distant metastasis
M1	Distant metastasis

Stage grouping

Separate stage groupings are recommended for papillary or follicular (differentiated), medullary, and anaplastic (undifferentiated) carcinoma.

Papillary or Follicular (differentiated), <45 years

Stage I	Any T	Any N	M0
Stage II	Any T	Any N	M1

Papillary or Follicular (differentiated), 45 years and older

Stage I	T1	N0	M0
Stage II	T2	N0	M0
Stage III	T3	N0	M0
Stage III	T1	N1a	M0
Stage III	T2	N1a	M0
Stage III	T3	N1a	M0
Stage IVA	T4a	N0	M0
Stage IVA	T4a	N1a	M0
Stage IVA	T1	N1b	M0
Stage IVA	T2	N1b	M0
Stage IVA	T3	N1b	M0
Stage IVA	T4a	N1b	M0
Stage IVB	T4b	Any N	M0
Stage IVC	Any T	Any N	M1

(*continued*)

TABLE 24.4	Tumor, Node, Metastasis (TNM) Staging Scheme for Tumors of the Thyroid (*Continued*)		
Medullary Carcinoma (all age groups)			
Stage I	T1	N0	M0
Stage II	T2	N0	M0
Stage II	T3	N0	M0
Stage III	T1	N1a	M0
Stage III	T2	N1a	M0
Stage III	T3	N1a	M0
Stage IVA	T4a	N0	M0
Stage IVA	T4a	N1a	M0
Stage IVA	T1	N1b	M0
Stage IVA	T2	N1b	M0
Stage IVA	T3	N1b	M0
Stage IVA	T4a	N1b	M0
Stage IVB	T4b	Any N	M0
Stage IVC	Any T	Any N	M1
Anaplastic Carcinoma			
All anaplastic carcinomas are considered Stage IV			
Stage IVA	T4a	Any N	M0
Stage IVB	T4b	Any N	M0
Stage IVC	Any T	Any N	M1

From: Edge SB, Byrd DR, Compton CC, et al., eds. *AJCC Cancer Staging Manual.* 7th ed. New York, NY: Springer; 2010. Used with permission.

gene *RET* in approximately 20% to 30% of PTCs. In addition, approximately half of PTCs have activating point mutations in *BRAF* (substitution of valine to glutamate at residue 600 [V600E], and 10% of cases harbor chromosomal rearrangements of the *TRK* gene.

Of these genetic changes, *BRAF* mutation analysis may prove to be the most clinically relevant. *BRAF* activating mutations are not found in other well-differentiated thyroid tumors and in PTC are associated with aggressive tumor behavior including extrathyroidal extension, tumor recurrence, and a higher rate of tumor-related mortality. *BRAF* mutations are more commonly found in classical PTC, the tall cell variant, and approximately 10% of cases of the follicular variant. *BRAF* mutations are also detected in approximately 25% of undifferentiated (anaplastic) carcinomas. Therapeutic agents targeted against *BRAF* are in development and may have clinical utility in the treatment of PTC in the future, especially for radioiodine-refractory, unresectable tumors.

5. **Undifferentiated (anaplastic) carcinoma.** Undifferentiated thyroid carcinomas (UTCs) are extremely aggressive malignant tumors composed, at least in part, of pleomorphic cells that show evidence of epithelial differentiation either by light microscopy, immunohistochemistry, or ultrastructural analysis. UTC is rare and compromises 2% or less of all thyroid carcinoma in the US. UTC is a tumor of the elderly, with 75% of cases occurring in patients older than 60 years. There is a slight female preponderance. Etiologic factors include iodine deficiency, radiation exposure, and preexisting thyroid disease. Long-standing goiter is a well-known risk factor for UTC. Patients classically present with a rapidly growing neck mass with local signs and symptoms such as hoarseness, dysphagia, pain, vocal cord paralysis, and/or dyspnea.

At surgery, the tumor is usually large, ill-defined, and difficult to excise due to extensive surrounding soft tissue invasion. Grossly, UTC is usually fleshy and tan-white with areas of hemorrhage and necrosis. Microscopically, it is typically composed of a variable admixture of spindle cells, epithelioid cells, and giant cells. The cells have a moderate amount of eosinophilic cytoplasm and almost always show brisk mitotic activity with abundant apoptosis (e-**Fig. 24.27**). There is often geographic necrosis, and typically the remaining thyroid gland is obliterated by tumor. On thorough examination, a residual, well-differentiated carcinoma, either papillary or follicular, is sometimes identified. Predominantly spindled tumors often mimic true sarcomas. The prognosis for UTC is very poor with a median survival of <6 months despite aggressive surgery, radiation, and chemotherapy.

Immunohistochemistry for cytokeratin is positive in approximately 80% of cases, and for epithelial membrane antigen in 30% to 50%. These stains are useful for diagnosis of tumors in which no obvious carcinomatous differentiation is present on H&E in order to confirm that the neoplasm is a carcinoma rather than a high-grade sarcoma. However, lack of staining with epithelial markers does not completely exclude the diagnosis of UTC. TTF-1 and thyroglobulin are typically negative in UTC. Nuclear reactivity for PAX8 has recently been reported in approximately 80% of UTC and may be useful for diagnosis.

6. **Medullary thyroid carcinoma.** MTC is a carcinoma with C-cell differentiation and represents a neuroendocrine neoplasm of the thyroid. C-cells secrete calcitonin, a peptide that causes increased renal excretion of calcium and inhibits osteoclasts to prevent calcium liberation from bone.

MTC represents approximately 5% to 10% of thyroid tumors. Although the majority of cases are sporadic, up to 20% may be familial and there is a strong association with multiple endocrine neoplasia (MEN) type 2, which must always be considered in the work-up of patients with MTC. The clinical presentation of MTC strongly depends on the familial or nonfamilial nature of the tumor. Sporadic and non-MEN familial MTCs present in fifth or sixth decades of life as a unilateral thyroid mass. A high percentage of patients have associated cervical lymphadenopathy. As an index case, familial MTCs associated with MEN type 2A are frequently detected at a younger age (mean, third decade) and are multicentric and bilateral. When associated with MEN type 2B, MTC usually occurs in even younger patients (i.e., in childhood or adolescence). Virtually all patients with MTC have an elevated serum calcitonin level.

Grossly, MTC is circumscribed but unencapsulated and is tan-yellow to white. Sporadic tumors are solitary, whereas familial tumors are often multifocal and bilateral. Microscopically, MTC shows great variability. The typical features are sheets, nests, or trabeculae of polygonal, round to oval cells with moderate to generous amounts of eosinophilic to amphophilic cytoplasm. The nuclei are round to oval with a coarse and somewhat granular neuroendocrine chromatin. Nucleoli are usually not prominent (e-**Fig. 24.28**). A great number of variants have been described including papillary or pseudopapillary (e-**Fig. 24.29**), plasmacytoid, glandular, giant cell, spindle cell (e-**Fig. 24.30**), small cell or neuroblastoma-like, paraganglioma-like, and oncocytic. Another characteristic feature of MTC is the presence of amyloid, which is formed from the deposition of calcitonin in the peritumoral stroma (e-**Fig. 24.28**). The amyloid is positive by Congo red staining.

Reactive, or nonneoplastic, C-cell hyperplasia occurs in aging and a number of other thyroid diseases, most notably hyperparathyroidism and lymphocytic thyroiditis. Although the histology of C-cell hyperplasia is somewhat controversial, a few generalities apply. First, reactive C-cell hyperplasia is usually unilateral and is not identifiable by H&E examination alone. Second, if there are aggregates of C cells >50 in number, in nodules, bilaterally, or diffusely, neoplastic C-cell hyperplasia is diagnosed.

Neoplastic C-cell hyperplasia, a precursor lesion to MTC that is more commonly seen in hereditary cases, is identified in the middle third to upper third of the thyroid lobes where C-cells are preferentially located; it is characterized by groups of enlarged, intrafollicular atypical C-cells that may begin to obliterate the normal follicular epithelium (e-Figs. 24.31 and 24.32). Neoplastic C-cell hyperplasia progresses to medullary carcinoma when C-cells extend through the follicular basement membrane into the stroma. Distinction between neoplastic C-cell hyperplasia and medullary microcarcinoma (a focus of MTC <1 cm in greatest dimension) can be difficult. Helpful histologic features of microcarcinoma include: (i) nuclear pleomorphism, (ii) expansile growth pattern with C-cell clusters spilling out of follicles, (iii) sclerotic stroma, and (iv) amyloid deposition.

Immunohistochemistry is useful for diagnosis of MTC. C-cells and MTC tumor cells are usually strongly positive for calcitonin, synaptophysin, chromogranin-A, and CEA, but negative for thyroglobulin. Although the differential diagnosis of MTC includes thyroid paraganglioma, intrathyroidal parathyroid adenoma, follicular adenoma, follicular carcinoma, poorly differentiated (insular) carcinoma, and oncocytic tumors, all of these tumors can be differentiated from MTC by histology and immunohistochemistry.

MTC (whether sporadic, non-MEN familial, or in the context of MEN type 2A or 2B) is strongly associated with activating point mutations of the *RET* proto-oncogene. Thirty percent to 66% of sporadic MTCs are associated with somatic *RET* gene mutations; 2% to 9% of sporadic MTCs are associated with de novo *RET* germline mutations. All cases of hereditary MTC have germline *RET* mutations. Recent studies show that each specific germline mutation of the *RET* proto-oncogene correlates with/predicts the age of onset and aggressiveness of the MTC that occurs in that kindred. In addition, clinical trials of tyrosine kinase inhibitors targeting the RET kinase have shown promise in reducing tumor burden in metastatic disease.

The behavior of MTC is highly stage dependent. Patients who do not have metastatic disease are usually cured by total thyroidectomy, and their 10-year survival approaches 100%. Lymph node metastases are very common, and common distant metastatic sites include the lungs, liver, and bone. The overall 10-year survival for patients with cervical lymph node metastases is approximately 70% to 80%, and for patients with distant metastases 40% to 50%. Because C-cell hyperplasia and MTC occur early in life in hereditary cases, prophylactic thyroidectomy and central lymph node dissection should be performed as early as possible in MEN type 2B, although it may be delayed somewhat in MEN type 2A and familial non-MEN MTC. Among the different clinical settings in which it arises, the prognosis is best for MTC in patients with non-MEN familial inheritance, slightly worse for those with MEN type 2A or sporadic tumors, and worst for those patients with MEN type 2B.

IV. **PATHOLOGIC REPORTING OF THYROID CARCINOMA.** American Joint Committee on Cancer (AJCC) staging of thyroid carcinomas is quite different than for other organ sites because the histologic type and age of the patient are critical for prognosis (Table 24.4). Patients with papillary carcinoma that has not metastasized distantly have an excellent prognosis, particularly those younger than 45 years of age, in whom survival approaches baseline. Any nonepithelial tumor type is excluded from staging.

Cytopathology of the Thyroid

Michael E. Hull and Julie Elizabeth Kunkel

I. **INTRODUCTION.** The advent of widespread use of thyroid FNA has dramatically decreased surgical excision of abnormal clinical lesions for diagnostic purposes. The sensitivity for the detection of lesions requiring surgical management is up to 98%, but specificity lags. The recent introduction of the Bethesda System for Reporting Thyroid Cytopathology (*Am J Clin Pathol.* 2009;132:658) has made possible a more probabilistic approach to the cytology of the thyroid, on the basis of cellularity, colloidal composition, architectural patterns, and nuclear morphology.

II. **NONDIAGNOSTIC/UNSATISFACTORY**

A. Six groups of well-visualized follicular cells, with each group containing ten or more cells, preferably on one slide, constitute the minimal adequacy criteria for thyroid FNA. Exceptions include paucicellular samples with marked cytologic atypia; solid nodules with inflammation (i.e., Hashimoto thyroiditis, abscess, or granulomatous inflammation) in which inflammatory cells predominate over a very scant epithelial population; and colloid nodule, in which abundant thick colloid is readily identified in the near-absence of follicular cells. Failure to meet the above criteria makes an aspirate nondiagnostic/unsatisfactory (e-Fig. 24.33).

B. **"Cyst fluid only"** is an important subset of the nondiagnostic category. If only macrophages and noncolloidal cyst fluid are present, and there is a solid clinical/sonographic lesion, the assumption should be made that the lesion has not been adequately sampled. In more reassuring clinical/sonographic cases, cyst fluid only may be consistent with a benign process. It should be clear that "cyst fluid only" requires careful contextual interpretation.

III. **BENIGN.** This is a category with high negative predictive value (0% to 3% malignancy rate on follow-up). Smears generally show significant amounts of colloid and variable degrees of cellularity. Benign follicular nodule is the most common pathologic correlate, but the presence of inflammatory cells or fibrous stroma may indicate a thyroiditis.

A. **Benign follicular nodules,** the most common diagnosis in thyroid aspirates, are characterized by benign follicular cells and colloid in variable proportions, variably sized follicular groups, Hürthle cells, and macrophages. Abundant colloid and relatively low cellularity are reassuring features of benignity (e-Figs. 24.34 and 24.35). However, since the pattern is seen in a constellation of benign proliferations, the underlying process can be diagnosed definitively only upon resection: nodular goiter, hyperplastic nodules, colloid nodules, and nodules in the setting of Graves disease.

B. **Thyroiditis**

1. **Acute thyroiditis** is rarely sampled given its typical clinical presentation. The aspirate shows predominantly neutrophils and necrotic debris with scattered histiocytes and scant reactive follicular cells. Special stains and culture are required for the identification of microorganisms.

2. **Chronic lymphocytic (Hashimoto) thyroiditis.** The aspirate is usually cellular and consists of two major components: (i) a large population of polymorphous lymphocytes, plasma cells, tingible body macrophages; and (ii) scattered, two-dimensional clusters of Hürthle cells with variable nuclear atypia (e-Fig. 24.36). Occasional multinucleated giant cells can be identified. Normal follicular cells and colloid are scant (*Diagn Cytopathol.* 1994;11:141).

3. **Subacute granulomatous (de Quervain) thyroiditis.** The aspirate can be hypocellular due to fibrosis. Granulomas consisting of cohesive

aggregates of epithelioid histiocytes with elongated and kidney-shaped nuclei, granular chromatin, small nucleoli, and abundant pale cytoplasm with ill-defined borders (e-Fig. 24.37) are the key diagnostic features. Multinucleated giant cells and lymphocytes are usually present (*Diagn Cytopathol.* 1997;16:214).

4. **Riedel thyroiditis.** The aspirate is markedly hypocellular, containing microfragments of stroma with bland spindle-shaped cells. Other cellular components are absent.

IV. **ATYPIA OF UNDETERMINED SIGNIFICANCE/FOLLICULAR LESION OF UNDETERMINED SIGNIFICANCE (AUS/FLUS).** AUS/FLUS is an equivocal category created in recognition of the fact that the cytologic pattern does not always allow discrimination between a benign nodule and a more serious lesion such as a follicular neoplasm or papillary carcinoma. The features in these aspirates are variable but generally consist of only rare cytologically or architecturally abnormal follicular groups in a background of scant colloid (e-Fig. 24.38). The architectural arrangement of the follicular cells in the lesion is the key to correct classification (*Cancer.* 1993;71:2598). This designation should generally comprise 7% to 8% of a cytology laboratory's thyroid interpretations and carries a 5% to 15% risk of malignancy upon rebiopsy/resection. The recommended follow-up is reaspiration in 6 months; too-early reaspiration may lead to diagnostic difficulty due to resolving hemorrhage and reparative changes (*CytoJournal.* 2008;5:6).

V. **FOLLICULAR NEOPLASM/SUSPICIOUS FOR FOLLICULAR NEOPLASM (FN/SFN).** FN/SFN yields richly cellular smears with both architectural and cytologic abnormalities, consisting of nuclear crowding, overlap, microfollicle formation, and dispersed single cells (e-Fig. 24.39). However, definitive features of papillary carcinoma are not seen. Such a pattern brings follicular adenoma, follicular carcinoma, and the follicular variant of papillary carcinoma into the differential diagnosis, thus the lesion requires excision; the nonspecificity of the diagnosis underlies use of the phrase "suspicious for follicular neoplasm" although FN and SFN are equivalent monikers in the Bethesda system.

Most patients with this diagnosis will undergo lobectomy or complete thyroidectomy, although only 20% to 30% of lesions will be malignant upon resection (*CytoJournal.* 2008;5:6). This lack of specificity is the impetus for investigation of ancillary techniques for the prediction of malignancy in these lesions, in particular determination of the mutational status of the four genetic aberrations present in the majority of cases of papillary and follicular carcinoma: point mutations of *BRAF* and *RAS*, and rearrangements of *RET–PTC* and *PAX8–PPARγ* (*Mol Cell Endocrinol.* 2010;322:29). These investigations may eventually lead to dual cytologic-genetic triage of patients for surgery and aid in pre- and postoperative planning (hemithyroidectomy vs. total thyroidectomy, necessity of node dissection, radiation treatment, etc.).

VI. **FOLLICULAR NEOPLASM, HÜRTHLE CELL TYPE/SUSPICIOUS FOR FOLLICULAR NEOPLASM, HÜRTHLE CELL TYPE (FNHCT/SFNHCT).** Hürthle cells are present in both neoplastic and nonneoplastic processes (*Am J Clin Pathol.* 1993;100:231). Hürthle cell neoplasms are cytologically distinct in that they yield hypercellular specimens composed of an almost pure population of Hürthle cells (e-Figs. 24.40 and 24.41). The Hürthle cells are often dyshesive single cells with prominent nucleoli, and the background contains an insignificant number of normal follicular cells, lymphocytes, and colloid. As is the case in other follicular neoplasms, the diagnosis of Hürthle cell carcinoma is based on assessment of capsular and vascular invasion, which cannot be evaluated in cytology specimens. It should also be noted, in further similarity to FN/SFN, that papillary carcinoma is in the differential diagnosis of FNHCT/SFNHCT.

VII. **SUSPICIOUS FOR MALIGNANCY (SFM).** SFM describes malignant appearing features similar to those in the "malignant" category (discussed later) but in an insufficient quantity to allow a confident diagnosis of malignancy. Use of this diagnosis is at the discretion of the pathologist and will certainly vary between laboratories and pathologists on the basis of a number of factors including patient population, cytologic preparations, aspiration technique, and so on. About 50% to 75% of the lesions in this cytologic category are proven malignant at resection.

VIII. **MALIGNANT.** This category encompasses cytologic features diagnostic of any of the malignant primary or metastatic tumors that may be seen in the thyroid. When the criteria are appropriately applied, there are very few false positives.

  A. **Papillary thyroid carcinoma (PTC).** The specimen is richly cellular, consisting of large sheets with occasional papillary structures (e-**Figs. 24.42** and **24.43**). The follicular cells are slightly enlarged and have crowded nuclei. The characteristic nuclear features are fine open chromatin with nuclear membrane prominence, small and peripherally located nucleoli, intranuclear cytoplasmic inclusions, and longitudinal nuclear grooves (e-**Fig. 24.44**). Other associated features include dense cytoplasm, "bubble gum"-like dense colloid, psammoma bodies (e-**Fig. 24.45**), and multinucleated giant cells (*Diagn Cytopathol.* 1991;7:462).

  B. **Hyalinizing trabecular adenoma** is a controversial entity with great similarity to PTC, including the characteristic nuclear features and *RET–PTC* rearrangements. Definitive diagnosis rests upon histologic examination (*Am J Clin Pathol.* 1989;91:115).

  C. **Poorly differentiated (insular) carcinoma.** The aspirate is richly cellular and composed of monomorphic follicular cells with scant colloid. The follicular cells are present predominantly as single cells, with only occasional crowded clusters and microfollicles (e-**Fig. 24.46**). The necrosis and mitosis seen in tissue biopsy specimens are rare in smears. There are no distinct cytological features to render definitive diagnosis (*Diagn Cytopathol.* 2001;25:325).

  D. **Anaplastic carcinoma.** The aspirate is highly cellular and contains single cells exhibiting marked nuclear atypia. Necrosis is common. The malignant cells show diverse morphology, including epithelioid (e-**Fig. 24.47**), spindle-shaped, and giant pleomorphic cells (*Acta Cytol.* 1996;40:953).

  E. **Medullary carcinoma** typically generates highly cellular specimens, predominantly consisting of single cells and loose clusters of cells. The cell morphology is variable, ranging from monotonous with little atypia, to highly atypical. The characteristic features are mixtures of plasmacytoid and spindle-shaped cells with characteristic salt-and-pepper chromatin (e-**Fig. 24.48**). Amyloid is usually present, but its distinction from colloid is impossible without a Congo red stain (*Pathologica* 1998;90:5).

  F. **Lymphoma.** Most primary thyroid lymphomas develop in the background of Hashimoto thyroiditis. Diffuse large B-cell lymphoma (DLBCL) is the major type, followed by extranodal marginal zone B-cell lymphoma of mucosa-associated lymphoid tissue (*Am J Surg Pathol.* 2000;24:623). DLBCL exhibits monotonous large atypical lymphoid cells with irregular nuclear contours, vesicular chromatin, and single prominent nucleoli (immunoblast-like cells) or multiple nucleoli (centroblast-like cells) (e-**Fig 24.49**). Marginal zone B-cell lymphoma shows a heterogeneous population of lymphoid cells with a predominance of small lymphoid cells, and intermixed plasmacytoid cells and immunoblasts; monocytoid cells with abundant pale cytoplasm are frequently seen. Demonstration of light chain restriction by flow cytometry is critical for diagnosis.

  G. **Metastatic malignancy.** Metastasis to the thyroid is uncommon. The kidney is the most common primary site of metastatic tumors, followed by lung and breast. In a patient with a history of malignancy, the differential diagnosis for a new thyroid nodule should include metastasis. Comparison of the aspirate with the slides of the primary malignancy, together with immunostains, is critical for diagnosis.

SUGGESTED READINGS

Adair C. Non-neoplastic lesions of the thyroid gland. In: Thompson LDR, ed. *Endocrine Pathology*. New York: Churchill Livingstone; 2006.

DeLellis RA, Nikiforov YE. Thyroid and parathyroid glands. In: Gnepp DR, ed. *Diagnostic Surgical Pathology of the Head and Neck*. Philadelphia: W.B. Saunders Elsevier Publishers; 2009.

Lloyd RV, Douglas BR, Young WF. Thyroid gland. In: King DW, ed. *Fascicle #1—Endocrine Diseases, First Series. Armed Forces Institute of Pathology Atlas of Non-Tumor Pathology*. Washington, DC: American Registry of Pathology; 2002.

Nikiforov YE, Biddinger PW, Thompson LDR. *Diagnostic Pathology and Molecular Genetics of the Thyroid*. Baltimore, MD: Wolters Kluwer Health/Lippincott William & Wilkins; 2009.

Thompson LDR. Benign neoplasms of the thyroid gland. In: Thompson LDR, ed. *Endocrine Pathology*. New York: Churchill Livingstone; 2006.

Thompson LDR. Malignant neoplasms of the thyroid gland. In: Thompson LDR, ed. *Endocrine Pathology*. New York: Churchill Livingstone; 2006.

25 Parathyroid Glands

James S. Lewis Jr.

I. **NORMAL ANATOMY.** The endodermally derived parathyroid glands develop from the third (inferior parathyroids) and fourth (superior parathyroids) pharyngeal pouches. They produce parathyroid hormone (PTH) which acts to increase serum calcium. They are normally found along the posterior surface of the thyroid gland, but given their complex embryologic development, normal variations in location range from within the substance of the thyroid gland, superiorly to the hyoid bone, inferiorly into the mediastinum, within the thymus gland, or within the pericardium. Furthermore, 2% to 7% of individuals have more than the usual four glands.

Most normal parathyroid glands are from 0.3 to 0.6 cm in largest dimension, and the normal aggregate weight of all glands is 120 to 140 mg. They are brown to yellow-brown, oval, and have a thin capsule. Histologically, they consist of chief (or principal) cells and oxyphil cells. The former have round nuclei with granular chromatin and slightly eosinophilic to clear cytoplasm, and the latter have round nuclei and more abundant brightly eosinophilic and granular cytoplasm (e-**Fig. 25.1**).* Both types of cells are arranged in sheets, nests, and cords. Occasional pseudoglandular or pseudoacinar foci with central eosinophilic proteinaceous material can also be seen in the normal parathyroid. Oxyphil cells may also form small nodules in adults. Intraparenchymal adipose tissue is a normal feature of the parathyroid glands. It is usually scant in children but progressively increases with age to constitute about 50% of the gland by the fifth decade, and plateaus beyond that time (e-**Fig. 25.2**).

Parathyroid cells, both chief and oxyphil, are positive by immunohistochemistry for PTH, chromogranin-A, and cytokeratins, and this immunoprofile is maintained in virtually all pathologic processes. Parathyroid cells are negative for thyroglobulin and thyroid transcription factor-1 (TTF-1).

II. **GROSS EXAMINATION, TISSUE SAMPLING, AND HISTOLOGIC SLIDE PREPARATION**

A. **Fine needle aspiration.** Fine needle aspiration of parathyroid lesions is rarely performed. The two exceptions are, first, when an adenoma arises within the substance of the parathyroid gland and thus a biopsy is taken as part of the evaluation of a presumed thyroid lesion, and second, when parathyroid carcinoma presents as a large neck mass.

B. **Biopsy.** Intraoperative biopsies (frozen sections) are frequently performed to confirm that the excised tissue is parathyroid because lymph nodes, thymus, thyroid, and fat may all be mistaken surgically for parathyroid tissue. The tissue should be weighed, but no other special handling is required.

C. **Excision.** The initial step in the gross examination of parathyroid glands is recording their weight and measurements in three dimensions. The glands should be closely examined and if firm, ragged, or irregular, should be inked around their periphery. They should then be sectioned and their color and consistency described. One section should be taken for histologic examination or, if the gland is 2 cm or larger, two to three sections should be taken.

---

*All e-figures are available online via the Solution Site Image Bank.

III. DIAGNOSTIC FEATURES OF COMMON DISEASES

A. Nonneoplastic

1. **Abnormal development** of the parathyroid glands sometimes occurs. The classic example is DiGeorge syndrome, in which there is failure in the development of several of the branchial pouches with resulting absence of the thymus and parathyroid glands. Neonates develop hypocalcemia due to lack of parathyroid hormone. Albright's hereditary osteodystrophy is due to pseudohypoparathyroidism as a result of target organ unresponsiveness to PTH, and neonates present with hypocalcemia, hyperphosphatemia, and blunted responses to PTH.

2. **Parathyroiditis** is a rare and poorly understood condition thought to be autoimmune in nature. It is characterized by extensive infiltration of the glands by lymphocytes. It is usually idiopathic and isolated but may be associated with a rare autoimmune polyglandular syndrome in which two or more endocrine glands are affected. Between one quarter and three quarters of patients will have circulating antiparathyroid tissue antibodies. Most patients have hypoparathyroidism, but parathyroiditis is sometimes associated with parathyroid hyperplasia. Histologically, the glands are infiltrated by clusters of lymphocytes, often with germinal center formation (e-Fig. 25.3). Plasma cells and fibrosis with clear parenchymal destruction are sometimes seen.

3. **Cysts** of the parathyroid glands are relatively uncommon. They occur in the neck and less commonly in the mediastinum. Most patients do not have clinical hyperparathyroidism. Grossly, they are often loosely attached to the thyroid gland, range from microscopic up to as large as 10 cm, have thin walls, and contain watery fluid. Microscopically, they are lined by a cuboidal layer of parathyroid cells with round, hyperchromatic nuclei (e-Figs. 25.4 and 25.5). The cyst wall consists of fibrous tissue with entrapped islands of parathyroid chief cells.

4. **Hyperplasia** is an increase in the overall mass of parathyroid cells and accounts for approximately 15% of all cases of primary hyperparathyroidism. Hyperplasia is divided into primary (where there is no known clinical stimulus), secondary (usually due to renal failure or another known metabolic cause), and tertiary (where there is an autonomously increased parathyroid mass in patients who have had secondary hyperparathyroidism and now are on dialysis or have had a renal transplant) (Table 25.1). A significant minority of cases of primary hyperparathyroidism (up to 40%) have been shown to have cells which are monoclonal, indicating that some cases represent true neoplasia. However, the clinical and pathophysiologic importance of this finding is unclear.

   Approximately 75% of patients are women, and 20% present with familial disease (most commonly multiple endocrine neoplasia [MEN] types 1 or 2A). Many patients are asymptomatic and are identified only indirectly through clinical evaluation for other reasons. The symptoms and signs of hyperparathyroidism can be vague such as fatigue, lethargy, nausea, constipation, arthralgia, or anorexia. The classic "bones, stones, and abdominal

TABLE 25.1	Classification of Parathyroid Hyperplasia
Primary hyperparathyroidism	No known stimulus
Secondary hyperparathyroidism	Known stimulus such as chronic renal failure, malabsorption, or vitamin D metabolism abnormality
Tertiary hyperparathyroidism	After longstanding renal failure with development of autonomous parathyroid hyperfunction

moans" (osteitis fibrosa cystica, kidney stones, and peptic ulcer disease) presentation is rare, and patients rarely present with a neck mass. Psychological disorders such as depression, psychosis, emotional instability, and confusion are sometimes the presenting symptoms. Patients frequently have osteopenia on clinical evaluation.

In hyperplasia, all of the glands are involved but to varying degrees, leading to asymmetric findings. Grossly, the glands are usually enlarged and are soft and brown, but they may also be nodular or cystic. The total weight is above normal but is still usually <1 g. Microscopically, all of the glands show similar findings, but to different degrees, including increased parenchymal cells and a commensurate decrease in fat (e-Fig. 25.6). Both chief and oxyphil cells are usually increased, although chief cells usually predominate in a nodular, multinodular, or diffuse pattern. Sometimes a follicular (pseudoglandular) pattern is present. Cytologic atypia can be seen but is rarely widespread. There is minimal mitotic activity. A rare type of hyperplasia termed "water-clear cell hyperplasia" is sometimes encountered, in which all the cells have abundant, perfectly clear cytoplasm and no adipose tissue is present (e-Fig. 25.7).

The differential diagnosis of hyperplasia includes parathyroid adenoma. Because the histologic features of an adenoma are not consistently different than those of hyperplasia, examination of more than one gland is necessary, as is correlation with the clinical findings, to distinguish between the two entities. Water-clear cell hyperplasia must be distinguished from metastatic renal cell carcinoma (RCC). RCC will show diffuse nuclear atypia and will be negative for PTH and neuroendocrine marker expression by immunohistochemistry.

a. **Autotransplantation.** A common surgical approach to hyperplasia is to remove three glands entirely and then a portion of the fourth. Alternatively, all four glands are excised, and a portion of one gland is implanted (usually in the skeletal muscle of the forearm or neck) to facilitate further surgery in case of recurrent hyperparathyroidism. Because the cells of a hyperplastic autotransplanted gland can be mitotically active and infiltrate the skeletal muscle imitating a malignant process, clinical history is required for correct diagnosis.

b. **Parathyromatosis** is a rare condition that presents as a primary or, more commonly, secondary disease in which numerous nests of parathyroid tissue are present throughout the neck and/or mediastinum. When it is a primary condition, it is commonly associated with an MEN syndrome. Secondary parathyromatosis is thought to occur after parathyroid surgery as a result of spillage of cells into the soft tissues which then become hyperplastic. The morphology of the nodules in parathyromatosis is similar to that of the glands in hyperplasia (e-Fig. 25.8).

B. **Neoplasms.** The World Health Organization (WHO) classification of tumors of the parathyroid gland is listed in Table 25.2.

TABLE 25.2	WHO Histological Classification of Parathyroid Tumors
Parathyroid carcinoma	
Parathyroid adenoma	
Secondary tumors	

From: DeLellis RA, Lloyd RV, Heitz P, et al., eds. *World Health Organization Classification of Tumours. Pathology and Genetics. Tumours of Endocrine Organs.* Lyon, France: IARC Press; 2004. Used with permission.

1. **Adenoma.** Parathyroid adenomas are benign neoplasms composed of chief cells, oxyphil cells, or a mixture of both. They occur in approximately 0.1% of the population and account for approximately 80% of cases of hyperparathyroidism. They are more common in women and have a peak incidence in the sixth and seventh decades of life. Adenomas are sometimes (albeit rarely) familial. These cases are usually associated with MEN types 1 or 2, or the uncommon hyperparathyroidism-jaw tumor syndrome. Adenomas involve a single gland (it is controversial as to whether patients with more than one adenoma actually suffer from asymmetrical hyperplasia). Patients present with signs and symptoms related to hypercalcemia (as detailed in Section III.A.4 on parathyroid hyperplasia). Technetium is concentrated in parathyroid tissue, so technetium sestamibi scans are often used to detect and localize the abnormal gland.

   Grossly, adenomas are rounded, encapsulated, and tan to reddish-brown, with an average weight of 1 g (e-**Fig. 25.9**). On sectioning, they are soft and homogeneous, although degeneration and cystic change may occur. Microscopically, adenomas are well-circumscribed, thinly or nonencapsulated masses with little stroma and no, or very minimal, fat, often with a rim of normal appearing parathyroid gland. The cell population is usually uniform and predominantly of one cell type, chief or oxyphil (e-**Figs. 25.10** and **25.11**). The cells are usually arranged in solid sheets, although pseudoglandular (pseudoacinar or follicular) areas may be seen (e-**Fig. 25.12**), sometimes containing central eosinophilic material mimicking thyroid follicles. The nuclei in chief cell adenomas are small, round, regular, and hyperchromatic. The nuclei in oxyphilic adenomas are round and may have prominent eosinophilic nucleoli. Nuclear pleomorphism can be seen although it is usually very localized (e-**Fig. 25.13**). Mitotic figures are scarce (1 or fewer per 10 high-power fields).

   The differential diagnosis of an adenoma includes parathyroid hyperplasia. Adenomas simply cannot be distinguished from hyperplasia without sampling more than a single gland because the morphologic features of adenomas overlap those of large hyperplastic glands. If only one gland is provided for evaluation, it is best to diagnose "hypercellular parathyroid consistent with adenoma" to reflect the fact that only one gland was excised, implying that the other glands were not clinically abnormal and that intraoperative PTH monitoring likely confirmed a sufficient drop after the single gland was excised. Adenomas can be distinguished from cellular nodules of thyroid tissue (particularly from patients with nodular hyperplasia of the thyroid) by finding convincing colloid in thyroid lesions, finding a rim of definite parathyroid tissue in adenomas, or by immunostaining for thyroglobulin, PTH, and/or TTF-1.

2. **Carcinoma.** Parathyroid carcinoma is rare and is estimated to be the cause of <1% of hyperparathyroidism. The average age of patients is between 45 and 55 years, and the sex distribution is roughly equal. The etiology is unknown, and there is no significant association with any of the familial syndromes that cause other parathyroid disease. Most patients present with profound hyperparathyroidism and hypercalcemia (with serum calcium levels often >16 mg per dL with secondary nephrolithiasis, renal insufficiency, and bone involvement with osteopenia and/or "brown tumors"), and most have nonspecific symptoms such as weakness, fatigue, nausea, and depression.

   Grossly, parathyroid carcinomas are usually large, poorly circumscribed, and adherent to surrounding tissues, particularly the thyroid gland (e-**Fig** 25.14). They range from 1.5 to 6.0 cm or larger, and average 6.7 g. Their cut surface is usually gray-white and firm. Microscopically, they usually have a

TABLE 25.3	Pathologic Features of Parathyroid Carcinoma	
Thick capsule	Vascular invasion[a]
Fibrous bands	Perineural invasion[a]
Capsular penetration[a]	Marked cytologic atypia
Soft tissue extension[a]	Mitotic activity
Necrosis	Tumor cell spindling

[a] Most useful and specific features.

thick, hypocellular, and collagenous capsule with intratumoral fibrous bands (e-Fig 25.15). Capsular invasion by the tumor is common, and invasion through the capsule as tongue-like or mushroom-like extensions is typical (e-Fig. 25.16). Carcinoma often extensively invades soft tissue and nearby structures, but vascular and perineural invasion are relatively uncommon. The growth pattern is usually solid, occasionally with areas of necrosis. The individual cells may have clear cytoplasm or be exclusively oxyphilic, but most often they have an intermediate eosinophilic color. Most carcinomas have nuclei that show mild to moderate variability, but occasional tumors will show marked nuclear pleomorphism (e-Fig. 25.17). Mitotic activity can be quite low, but most tumors have >5 mitoses per 50 high-power fields.

The differential diagnosis of parathyroid carcinoma is primarily with parathyroid adenoma. Although there is no single diagnostic feature other than metastasis that is considered completely diagnostic of carcinoma, the overall constellation of findings is usually definitive. Vascular invasion, capsular penetration, invasion of the thyroid gland, and/or perineural invasion are indicative of carcinoma (Table 25.3). Primary thyroid neoplasms, as well as metastases from RCC or thyroid medullary carcinoma, can be excluded by morphology and immunohistochemistry. Rare non-functioning parathyroid carcinomas present as large neck masses with no associated hyperparathyroidism. Immunohistochemistry is usually necessary to confirm the diagnosis.

Surgery is the mainstay of treatment, and complete surgical excision at presentation offers the best chance for cure. The 5-year survival is approximately 85%, and 10-year survival is 50%. Patients frequently develop local recurrence and less commonly develop metastases to neck lymph nodes, lung, liver, and bone. Severe hypercalcemia is a cause of significant morbidity and frequently is the cause of death.

3. **Metastatic tumors.** The parathyroid glands are an uncommon site for metastases, although they are sometimes involved by direct extension from thyroid or laryngeal tumors. The rare metastases from distant sites most commonly arise from breast, kidney, and lung carcinomas or melanoma.

IV. **HISTOLOGIC GRADING, STAGING, AND REPORTING OF PARATHYROID CARCINOMA.** Grading of parathyroid carcinoma based on cytologic features or degree of differentiation has not been found to predict behavior. Similarly, there is no durable staging system for parathyroid carcinoma, so no American Joint Committee on Cancer (AJCC) guidelines are available in this regard. Neither tumor size nor lymph node status at presentation is predictive of outcome.

For resection specimens, the surgical pathology report should include tumor size in three dimensions, growth pattern, involvement of adjacent structures, and relation to surgical margins. Although lymph node status is not predictive of outcome, the number of regional lymph nodes examined and the number positive for carcinoma should also be reported.

Cytopathology of the Parathyroid Glands

Hannah R. Krigman

I. **INTRODUCTION.** The parathyroid glands are sampled infrequently by fine needle aspiration (FNA) for diagnostic purposes since adjunct testing (including serum calcium levels), radiolabeled imaging studies (sestamibi scans), and assessment of aspirated fluid for parathyroid hormone levels generally obviate presurgical analysis of parathyroid masses. However, FNA may be used to evaluate the presence of parathyroid tissue in unusual locations, or to evaluate persistent hypercalcemia following excision of parathyroid glands. In addition, parathyroid glands may be incidentally sampled during assessment of thyroid nodules. Rarely, unanticipated parathyroid adenomas are aspirated as thyroid or neck nodules.

II. **CYTOLOGIC FINDINGS.** Direct smears show predominantly two dimensional groups of 50 to 100 relatively evenly sized cells with granular cytoplasm. Three dimensional groups, papillary fragments, and microacinar structures may also be seen (**e-Fig 25.18**). Oxyphilic epithelial change may be seen rarely. Nuclei are predominantly round, with finely mottled chromatin (**e-Fig 25.19**); sometimes nuclear molding and overlap are present. Modest variation in nuclear size may be seen, but this feature has no prognostic importance; mitotic activity is uncommon. The background often contains stripped nuclei and single cells, macrophages, and colloid-like material. Diff-Quik stained fresh smears may show fat vacuoles which are a helpful clue since they are not typically seen in aspirates of thyroid tissue.

Cytologic features do not reliably discriminate among normal parathyroid tissue, hyperplasia, adenoma, or carcinoma.

Differentiation of parathyroid from thyroid in FNA specimens can be problematic. Microacinar groupings of parathyroid cells are an occasional source of error in that they may be misinterpreted as follicular neoplasm/suspicious for follicular neoplasm, especially in the setting of parathyroid adenomas. Follicular groups of parathyroid cells can also be misinterpreted as thyroid follicular cells, although intervening fat should suggest the correct diagnosis. In problematic cases, parathyroid origin can be confirmed with an immunostain for parathyroid hormone.

SUGGESTED READINGS

Absher KJ, Truong LD, Khurana KK, et al. Parathyroid cytology: avoiding diagnostic pitfalls. *Head Neck.* 2002;24:157–164.

Agarwal AM, Bentz JS, Hungerford R, et al. Parathyroid fine-needle aspiration cytology in the evaluation of parathyroid adenoma: cytologic findings from 53 patients. *Diagn Cytopathol.* 2009;37:407–410.

DeLellis RA, Nikiforov YE. Thyroid and parathyroid glands. In: Gnepp DR, ed. *Diagnostic Surgical Pathology of the Head and Neck.* 2nd ed. Philadelphia: W.B. Saunders; 2009.

Dimashkieh H., Krishnamurthy S. Ultrasound guided fine needle aspiration biopsy of parathyroid gland and lesions. *CytoJournal.* 2006;3:6

Lloyd RV, Douglas BR, Young WF. Parathyroid gland. In: King DW, ed. *Fascicle #1—Endocrine Diseases, First Series.* Armed Forces Institute of Pathology Atlas of Non-Tumor Pathology. Washington, DC: American Registry of Pathology; 2002.

Thompson LDR, ed. *Endocrine Pathology.* China: Churchill Livingstone; 2006.

26 The Adrenal Gland and Paraganglia

Louis P. Dehner

I. **NORMAL ANATOMY AND HISTOLOGY.** The definitive or adult adrenal glands are located anterior to the upper poles of the kidneys. The glands are pyramidal on the right and crescentic on the left. In adults the normal combined weight should not exceed 6 g. Each adrenal gland is divided into head (most medial), body (middle), and tail (most lateral).

The adrenal gland is composed of an outer cortex and an inner medulla, and as a compound gland is unique to mammals (*Pharmacol Rev.* 1971;23:1971). The gland is derived from two embryologic progenitors: the coelomic epithelium between the urogenital ridge and dorsal root mesentery as the primordial cortex, and migratory neural crest cells as the future medulla as well as the ganglia and paraganglia. Migratory neural crest cells are identified as small dark cells as they pass through the cortex into the center of the gland as individual cells or small aggregates of neuroblasts (*Endocr Pathol.* 2009;20:92; *Folia Histochem Cytochem.* 2010;48:491); however, a definitive medulla does not become apparent until 1 to $1^{1}/_{2}$ years of age.

Microscopically, the cortex consists of three zones: the outer zona glomerulosa (secreting aldosterone), middle zona fasciculata (secreting mainly cortisol and minor amounts of sex steroids), and inner zona reticularis (secreting mainly sex steroids) (e-Fig. 26.1).* The zona glomerulosa is composed of a thin, usually discontinuous layer of cells with ball-like formations; these cells have less cytoplasm than those in other two cortical zones. The zona fasciculata consists of radial cords or columns of cells with abundant lipid-rich cytoplasm. The cells of the zona reticularis have compact, finely eosinophilic cytoplasm with or without lipofuscin pigment. Normally the medulla accounts for 10% of the adrenal volume and grossly has a gray-white color. The predominant cells in the medulla are the mature chromaffin cells, the pheochromocytes, organized in nests and cords (e-Fig. 26.2). The cytoplasm of the chromaffin cells is usually basophilic but may be amphophilic or even eosinophilic. These cells have indistinct cell borders and usually a single nucleus which may show variation in size and hyperchromasia. The chromaffin cells are peripherally surrounded by the sustentacular cells; rare ganglion cells may be identified in the adrenal unlike their prominence in ganglia (e-Fig. 26.3). The major function of adrenal medulla is the synthesis and secretion of catecholamines (epinephrine and norepinephrine).

II. **GROSS EXAMINATION OF ADRENAL GLAND SPECIMEN.** The adrenal gland is removed either as part of a radical nephrectomy or for excision of an adrenal tumor. Biopsies of the adrenal are generally fine needle aspirations or thin needle biopsies to evaluate for the presence of metastatic tumor.

A. **Needle biopsy.** The entire tissue should be submitted for histologic examination.

B. **Adrenal gland removed as part of radical nephrectomy.** After gross examination of the kidney, the gland should be measured and weighed. Then the gland should be serially sectioned at 2- to 3-mm intervals perpendicular to its long axis; the thickness of the cortex and medulla should be noted. Infrequently,

---

*All e-figures are available online via the Solution Site Image Bank.

the adrenal may be invaded directly by renal cell carcinoma or be the site of discontinuous metastases.

C. **Adrenectomy for a primary pathologic process.** The first step is to orient the specimen and examine the contour of the adrenal gland. If it is apparent that the gland has been largely replaced by a mass, the periphery should be inked since the margins may be important (assuming that the mass has not already invaded surrounding structures like the liver). If the cortex and medulla maintain their normal relationship to each other, the thickness of each should be recorded. Serial sectioning should be done at intervals appropriate for the pathology. If the disease process is apparently diffuse hyperplasia, the periadrenal soft tissue should be removed and the gland should be measured and weighed. If the adrenal contains a solitary mass or multiple nodules, three dimensional measurements should be obtained. The cut surface of the lesion and its relationship to any identifiable normal tissue should be described, including color, consistency, presence of hemorrhage or necrosis, degree of circumscription, and degree of encapsulation. If any portions of adjacent organs such as liver, kidney, spleen, or abdominal wall are attached (usually for tumors), their appearance and relationship to the gland should be noted. A large, en bloc resection will require numerous sections from the peripheral margins. For diffuse and/or nodular hyperplasia, representative sections are sufficient.

For a neoplasm, the following sections should be taken: tumor, (including sections demonstrating the relationship of the tumor to the associated soft tissues and adjacent organs, and relationship of the tumor to uninvolved adrenal gland); the tumor capsule, if present; margins; periadrenal fatty tissue overlying a bulging mass; a representative section from uninvolved adrenal, if any; and regional lymph nodes. The gross description should clearly document the site of the sections. For large specimens, a gross photograph is extremely helpful in that it depicts the specimen at a time when landmarks are still maintained with some anatomic orientation.

D. **Neuroblastoma specimens.** Neuroblastic tumors present some special issues regarding acquisition of neoplastic tissue for a variety of special studies to biologically profile the tumor for children enrolled in a Children's Oncology Group (COG) protocol. If the specimen is an adrenal-based neuroblastoma (NB), then generally the amount of available tumor is sufficient for pathologic diagnosis as well as for all other ancillary studies. The difficulties arise in those cases of NB when only biopsies are obtained prior to chemotherapy in cases of nonresectable tumors. Accuracy of tumor grading is based upon a thorough microscopic examination which may be limited by the amount of well-preserved tumor in the specimen.

A resected primary NB of the adrenal, or extraadrenal retroperitoneal mass, should be examined fresh if at all possible as discussed in section C above. The COG reference laboratory requests at least 1 g of snap frozen tumor tissue but will accept any frozen sample of tumor; the snap freezing should occur as soon as the specimen becomes available following resection. Tumor samples should be labeled "primary" or "metastatic"; involved bone marrow is required as well. Storage at $-70°C$ is preferable to $-20°C$.

Fresh tissue should also be collected for local institutional studies including conventional cytogenetic studies. Snap-frozen fresh tissue should be saved for possible molecular studies. Tumor for fluorescent in situ hybridization can be recovered from formalin-fixed, paraffin-embedded tissue without compromising the quality of results.

III. ADRENAL CORTICAL LESIONS

A. **Congenital abnormalities.** The most common congenital anomaly of the adrenal is an incidental finding of heterotopia consisting of microscopic foci of cortical tissue or nodule(s) along the path of descent of the gonads, although rare cases of heterotopia at a wide variety of other anatomic sites have been reported. Heterotopias are identified in 1.5% to 2.7% of groin procedures in males (*BJE Int.* 2005;95:407); the spermatic cord, inguinal hernia sac, or paraepididymal soft tissues are the three most common sites (*Int Surg.* 2006;91:125). Only cortical tissue is identified as a rule (e-**Fig. 26.4**), but cortex and medulla have been seen in heterotopias in the celiac axis. Other congenital abnormalities include adrenal union/fusion, adrenal cytomegaly, intraadrenal heterotopic tissue, and congenital adrenal hyperplasia. Adrenal cytomegaly is characterized by the presence of foci of bizarre cells with eosinophilic granular cytoplasm and large hyperchromatic nuclei with pseudoinclusions; this finding is detected in Beckwith–Wiedemann syndrome. Heterotopic tissues within the adrenal gland include liver, thyroid, and ovarian stroma.

B. Incidental adrenal cortical nodules. Nonfunctional cortical nodules are found in 1% to 10% of autopsies, are usually multiple and bilateral, and can protrude into adjacent fat. These variably sized nodules have a yellow appearance on cut surface. Circumscribed but nonencapsulated nodules consist of fasciculata-type cells with various patterns. Myelolipomatous metaplasia, osseous metaplasia, and secondary changes (hyalinization, calcification, or hemorrhage) may be present. Pigmented nodules are composed of zona reticularis-type cells with lipofuscin or neuromelanin.

C. Adrenal cortical hypofunction (insufficiency) is divided into primary and secondary types.

1. Primary adrenal cortical insufficiency (Addison disease) is due to destruction of the adrenal cortex. In developed countries, over 80% of cases are due to autoimmune adrenalitis as an isolated manifestation of autoimmune polyendocrinopathy (*Lancet.* 2003;361:1881). This T-cell mediated immunologic destructive process of the cortex results in small glands which have a mixed inflammatory infiltrate of lymphocytes, plasma cells, and histiocytes. Lymphoid follicles with germinal centers may be present in a pattern similar to that in Hashimoto thyroiditis (*Endocr Dev.* 2011;20:161). Cortical cells may be difficult to identify, but the medulla remains intact. Various inborn errors of metabolism, hemorrhage, and neoplastic infiltrates or replacement are other etiologies.

Adrenal cortical insufficiency may occur on the basis of infectious etiologies including tuberculosis, other bacterial infections (including *Meningococcus, Pseudomonas, Streptococcus pneumoniae,* and *Haemophilus influenzae*), fungal infections, cytomegalovirus, herpes simplex virus, and toxoplasmosis (in HIV-infected individuals). These infections lead to destruction of the entire gland. Acute adrenal insufficiency with bilateral cortical hemorrhage and necrosis are features of the Waterhouse–Friderichsen syndrome, more commonly seen at autopsy. Adrenoleukodystrophy (X-linked peroxisomal disorder) is also manifested by adrenal insufficiency with cortical nodules composed of enlarged ballooned cells (*J Clin Endocrinol Metab.* 2011;96:E925).

Other causes of primary insufficiency include amyloidosis and drugs. Treatment with mitotane may cause adrenal atrophy with fibrosis.

Congenital adrenal hypoplasia (CAHP) is an uncommon condition that is more likely to be encountered in a fetopsy or perinatal autopsy. Its estimated incidence is 1:12,500 live births, compared to the incidence of anencephaly of 2.23:10,000 live births in the United States. It should be anticipated that 1% to 2% of fetopsies have CAHP as defined as combined adrenal weights of <2 g at term, or more accurately an adrenal weight over body weight of <1:1000. There are three distinct morphologic patterns: cytomegaly type (most common with X-linked inheritance with inactivating deletion mutations at Xp 21.2 in the gene that encodes DAX-1);

anencephalic type (without CNS or pituitary defects but the cortex is attenuated and the fetal cortex is inconspicuous); and a miniature type with a definitive cortex and an attenuated fetal cortex.

2. **Secondary and tertiary adrenal cortical insufficiencies.** These are due to the failure of the pituitary gland to secrete ACTH (secondary) or of the hypothalamus to secrete CRH (tertiary). The gland size is decreased. Histologically, the zona fasciculata is atrophic whereas the zona glomerulosa and medulla are usually relatively normal.

D. **Adrenal cortical hyperplasia** can be divided into congenital and acquired types.

1. **Congenital adrenal hyperplasia** is an autosomal recessive disorder caused by one of five enzymatic defects that result in a failure in cortisol synthesis; 21-hydroxylase deficiency accounts for 90% to 95% of cases (*Lancet.* 2005;365:2125; *Endocr Dev.* 2011;20:80). Marked diffuse hyperplasia of the zona fasciculata results from ACTH stimulation, whereas cells of the zona fasciculata are lipid-depleted due to their conversion into zona reticularis-type cells with compact eosinophilic cytoplasm. Persistent ACTH stimulation may also give rise to adrenal cortical neoplasms. Nodules resembling hyperplastic adrenal cortical tissue in testis can develop into the so-called testicular tumors of the adrenogenital syndrome (*Am J Surg Pathol.* 1988;12:503).

2. **Acquired adrenal cortical hyperplasia** is a nonneoplastic bilateral process characterized by a gland weighing in excess of 6 g. The gland has either a diffuse, nodular, or combined appearance.

   a. **Diffuse hyperplasia** is usually ACTH dependent and caused by a hyperfunctional pituitary (most often pituitary adenoma, less often corticotropin-releasing hormone (CRH) from the hypothalamus) or an ectopic ACTH/CRH-producing tumor. The latter neoplasms include small cell carcinoma (usually from the lung), low grade neuroendocrine carcinoma or carcinoid (usually from the lung or thymus), medullary thyroid carcinoma, pancreatic endocrine neoplasms, and pheochromocytoma (PHEO). Both glands are symmetrically enlarged. The zonae fasciculata and reticularis are expanded with their relative proportions varying from case to case. The zona fasciculata is lipid depleted but markedly expanded by a population of cortical cells with abundant eosinophilic cytoplasm (e-**Fig. 26.5**).

   b. **Nodular cortical hyperplasia** is ACTH-independent in most cases. The glands are markedly enlarged, in excess of 15 to 20 g in some cases. The cortical nodules may constitute a transformation from diffuse hyperplasia in its late stage; these nodules are yellowish and vary from 0.2 to over 4.0 cm. Fasciculata-type clear cells, reticularis-type cells, or a mixture of these two cell types characterize the nodules. Nodular adrenal cortical disease with discrete nodules of hyperplastic zona glomerulosa with intervening cortical atrophy is seen in children with McCune–Albright syndrome (*Am J Surg Pathol.* 2011;35:1311).

   c. **Primary pigmented nodular adrenocortical disease (PPNAD),** an uncommon but specific form of ACTH-independent nodular hyperplasia, is generally diagnosed in the second decade of life with or without the other stigmata of Carney complex (*Orphanet J Rare Dis.* 2006;1:21; *Best Pract Res Clin Endocrinol Metab.* 2010;24:389). A germline heterozygous inactivating mutation of *PRKR1A* is found in the Carney complex (65% to 70% of cases) and may also have a role in primary PPNAD (*Pituitary.* 2006;9:211). The glands are of normal size, but the cut surface has scattered pigmented micronodules, or less often macronodules measuring 1 to 4 mm in size. Uniform compact cells with eosinophilic cytoplasm and some balloon cells are histologic features of the nodules. Pigmentation is

TABLE 26.1	World Health Organization Histologic Classification of Tumors of Adrenal Gland and with Additional Entities

Adrenal cortical tumors	**Extraadrenal paraganglioma**
Adrenal cortical adenoma	Jugulotympanic
Adrenal cortical carcinoma	Vagal
Adrenal medullary tumors	Laryngeal
Benign pheochromocytoma	Orbital nasopharyngeal
Malignant pheochromocytoma	Carotid body
Composite pheochromocytoma	Aorticopulmonary
Other adrenal tumors	Gangliocytic
Adenomatoid tumor	Cauda equine
Sex cord-stroma tumor	Cervical paravertebral
Soft tissue and germ cell tumors	Intrathoracic
Myelolipoma	Intra-abdominal
Teratoma	Superior paraaortic
Schwannoma	Inferior paraaortic
Ganglioneuroma	Urinary bladder
Angiosarcoma	
Leiomyoma	
Wilms tumor (extrarenal)	
Secondary or metastatic tumors	

Modified from: DeLellis RA, Lloyd RV, Heitz P, et al., eds. *World Health Organization Classification of Tumours. Pathology and Genetics. Tumours of Endocrine Organs.* Lyon, France: IARC Press; 2004. Used with permission.

due to intracytoplasmic lipofuscin. The same cells are strongly positive for synaptophysin but nonreactive for chromogranin. The nodules may abut the cortical medullary junction, extend into the periadrenal fat, or involve the entire thickness of the cortex.

    d. Adrenal cortical hyperplasia with hyperaldosteronism (Conn syndrome) occurs in the absence of an adenoma in 30% of cases as bilateral cortical hyperplasia. The size, weight, and appearance of the glands are variable and the size may be within the normal range. The zona glomerulosa has tongue-like projections toward the underlying zona fasciculata. Micronodules may be present with fasciculata-type cells.

E. Adrenal cortical neoplasms are traditionally divided into adenomas and carcinomas (Table 26.1). In terms of functioning adrenal cortical neoplasms, these tumors present with the following: Cushing syndrome (60% to 65% of cases), mineralocorticoids-androgens (20%), combined Cushing-androgens (4%), estrogen (12%), and aldosterone (4%).

  1. Adrenal cortical adenoma is typically unilateral, solitary, rarely larger than 50 g or 5 cm in size, and heterogeneous with or without clinical manifestations due to hyperfunction (e-Fig. 26.6). The hormone-associated syndromes are hyperaldosteronism, Cushing syndrome, and adrenogenital syndrome in descending order of frequency. Most cortical adenomas are nonfunctioning and detected as incidentalomas.

    a. Hyperaldosteronism (Conn syndrome) is associated with an adenoma in 70% of cases; the adenoma is <2 cm in size in most cases (e-Fig. 26.7) (*Orphanet J Rare Dis.* 2010;19(5):9). Histologically, a yellowish, circumscribed, but encapsulated nodule is composed of zona fasciculata-type cells, zona reticularis-type cells, zona glomerulosa-type cells, or cells showing hybrid features (e-Fig. 26.8). Occasionally, the adjacent cortex may show hyperplasia of the zona glomerulosa (paradoxical hyperplasia). If there has been treatment with spirolactone (an aldosterone antagonist), characteristic spirolactone bodies are usually present, consisting of small, intracytoplasmic, 2 to 6 μm round to oval inclusions with a slightly eosinophilic appearance and two to six concentric rings within the tumor cells and the adjacent zona glomerulosa (*Am J Clin Pathol.* 1970;54:22). A halo separates the spirolactone bodies from the surrounding cytoplasm.

b. **Cushing syndrome** is characterized by an adenoma which is sharply demarcated or even capsulated and has a homogeneous yellow to golden-yellow appearance or irregular foci of dark discoloration on cut surface. Solid nests or alveolar-like profiles are present, composed of cells which are usually larger than the normal cortical cells. The cells of the adenoma have features of zona fasciculata-type cells with the occasional presence of foci of smaller zona reticularis-type cells (e-**Fig. 26.9**); both types of tumor cells usually have single, round to oval nuclei with a small nucleolus. In some cases, there are scattered cells with larger, hyperchromatic nuclei with pseudoinclusions; they have no prognostic importance. Mitotic figures are rare. Fibrosis, organizing thrombi within sinusoids, and lipomatous and myelolipomatous metaplasia are other features. The compressed residual cortex is invariably atrophic.

c. **Adrenogenital syndrome with sex hormone production** is infrequently caused by an adenoma, but is more often associated with cortical carcinomas that produce estrogen. Androgen-producing adenomas are generally larger than those in Cushing syndrome and are also sharply demarcated from the adjacent cortex. The tumor cells have the features of zona reticularis cells with compact, eosinophilic cytoplasm.

2. **Other adrenocortical neoplasms** with special microscopic features beyond the usual appearance of adenoma and carcinoma include oncocytic tumor, myxoid adrenal cortical neoplasm, sarcomatoid carcinoma, and the so-called adrenal blastoma.

a. **Black (pigmented) adenoma** is associated with Cushing syndrome, and rarely with Conn syndrome (*Int J Surg Pathol.* 2004;12:57). In most cases the tumor is composed predominantly or entirely of cells resembling zona reticularis cells with a variable amount of intracytoplasmic brown or golden-brown pigment (lipofuscin) (*Endocr Pathol.* 1999;10:353).

b. **Oncocytic neoplasms** include both benign and malignant tumors as in other organs. A cytoplasm rich in mitochondria accounts for the oncocytic appearance of the tumor cells in common with extraadrenal oncocytoma. These tumors are often characterized by large, bizarre cells; despite the presence of these very atypical cells, the histologic criteria to differentiate an adenoma from a carcinoma are applicable (*Int J Surg Pathol.* 2004;12:231; *Ann Diagn Pathol.* 2010;14:204). These tumors may have cytoplasmic globules and inclusions like those seen in pheochromocytoma (*Virchow Arch.* 2008;453:301), which can be problematic since the latter tumor may also have oncocytic features in rare cases (*Am J Surg Pathol.* 2000;24:1552).

c. **Myxoid neoplasms** are rare morphologic variants of a cortical adenoma or carcinoma with a focal or near diffuse background that has a myxoid-mucoid appearance consisting of hyaluronidase digestible Alcian blue positive stromal mucin. The myxoid stroma separates the tumor cells into cords, nests, pseudoglands (e-**Fig. 26.10**), and trabecula (*Ann Diagn Pathol.* 2008;12:344; *Am J Surg Pathol.* 2010;34:973). The individual tumor cells are spindled to epithelioid. The various microscopic features for differentiation of a benign from malignant tumor are applicable to the myxoid variant.

d. **Ectopic adrenal cortical adenoma** has been reported in the kidney and within the spinal canal (*Mod Pathol.* 2009;22:175; *Brain Tumor Pathol.*

2010;27:121). Ectopic adrenal rest or "tumor" has been described in congenital adrenal hyperplasia in the testis (*Eur J Endocrinol.* 2008;159:489).

   e. Sarcomatoid carcinoma, like similar high-grade neoplasms in the lung and kidney, has a pleomorphic spindle cell pattern in addition to focal areas of recognizable but poorly differentiated ACC (*Pathol Res Pract.* 2010;206;59).

   f. Adrenal blastoma has been reported in a single case (*Hum Pathol.* 1992;23:1187). This tumor had a biphasic epithelial and mesenchymal pattern.

3. **Adrenal cortical carcinoma (ACC)** is a rare neoplasm with an incidence of about one per million in the United States. This tumor can occur in any age, but it appears to have a bimodal age distribution with one peak in children <5 years old and another peak in adults in the fourth or fifth decade of life. However, many of the cases of putative ACC in children, especially those diagnosed early in the first decade of life, do not behave clinically as their adult counterparts although the microscopic features associated with ACC in adults are present (discussed later). ACC is a manifestation of several hereditary syndromes including Li–Fraumeni syndrome (*TP53*), Beckwith–Wiedemann syndrome (*CDKN1C/NSD1*), MEN1 (*MEN1*), and Gardner's syndrome (*APC*) (*J Clin Pathol.* 2008;61:787; *Adv Anat Pathol.* 2011;18:206); together hereditary cases represent 5% or less of all ACCs. ACC presents as a functioning neoplasm in 50% to 60% of cases, with Cushing syndrome as the most common presentation (*Nat Rev Endocrinol.* 2011;7:323). Approximately 40% to 45% of ACCs are confined to the adrenal and are completely resectable; only 5% to 10% of tumors are ≤5 cm (T1) whereas 35% to 40% are >5 cm (T2); over 50% of cases have infiltrated beyond the adrenal (T3) or have already metastasized at presentation in 30% to 35% of cases (T4) (*Best Pract Res Clin Endocrinol Metab.* 2009;23:273). The AJCC Staging scheme for adrenal neoplasms is presented in Table 26.2.

   Grossly, hemorrhage and necrosis often provide the background for a soft yellowish to tan neoplasm with or without cystic areas (**e-Fig. 26.11**). However, ACC can have a variety of gross features in terms of coloration and presence or absence of apparent necrosis. Those ACCs <5 cm tend to have a more uniform gross appearance as do adenomas; these are the cases which may prove to be problematic in the differential diagnosis between an ACC and adenoma, a point that is especially pertinent as it relates to adrenocortical neoplasms in children (*Pediatr Dev Pathol.* 2009;12:284).

   Any number of individual microscopic features have been evaluated in primary adrenocortical neoplasms in adults for discrimination between an adenoma and carcinoma. The modified Weiss system requires a score of 3 or more to predict malignant behavior (of the following five microscopic features): mitotic rate (>5 per 50 hpf), cytoplasm (dense eosinophilic cytoplasm in 75% or more of tumor cells since a predominant clear cell pattern is a feature of adenomas); atypical or bizarre mitotic figures; necrosis; and capsular invasion (**e-Fig. 26.12A–D**) (*Hum Pathol.* 2009;40:757). Once an adrenal cortical neoplasm has invaded into adjacent soft tissues or organs, invaded a major vessel, or metastasized to regional lymph nodes or remote site(s), the diagnosis of ACC is beyond dispute.

   Immunohistochemistry to corroborate that a primary neoplasm is cortical in nature is infrequently necessary, with the uncommon exception of a dilemma between a cortical and medullary neoplasm (which is generally obvious in most cases). Another example is metastatic renal cell carcinoma to the adrenal which can mimic a primary cortical neoplasm. A more

TABLE 26.2	Adrenal Gland Staging and Prognostic Groups		

Definition of TNM
Primary tumor (T)

TX	Primary tumor cannot be assessed		
T0	No evidence of primary tumor		
T1	Tumor 5 mm or less in greatest dimension, no extraadrenal invasion		
T2	Tumor >5 mm, no extraadrenal invasion		
T3	Tumor of any size with local invasion, but not invading adjacent organs		
T4	Tumor of any size with invasion of adjacent organs[a]		

Regional lymph nodes (N)

NX	Regional lymph nodes cannot be assessed		
N0	No regional lymph node metastasis		
N1	Metastasis in regional lymph node(s)		

Distant metastasis (M)

M0	No distant metastasis		
M1	Distant metastasis		

Anatomic stage/prognostic groups

Stage 1	T1	N0	M0
Stage II	T2	N0	M0
Stage III	T1	N1	M0
	T2	N1	M0
	T3	N0	M0
Stage IV	T3	N1	M0
	T4	N0	M0
	T4	N1	M0
	Any T	Any N	M1

[a]Adjacent organs include kidney, diaphragm, great vessels, pancreas, spleen, and liver.
From: Edge SB, Byrd DR, Compton CC, et al., eds. *AJCC Cancer Staging Manual*. 7th ed. New York, NY: Springer, 2010. Used with permission.

frequent diagnostic challenge is presented by a needle biopsy of a retroperitoneal mass in which the microscopic features consist of dense cords and nests of eosinophilic, epithelioid appearing cells that raise the differential diagnosis of a hepatic, adrenal, or renal neoplasm, as well as perivascular epithelioid cell tumor (PEComa), angiomyolipoma (AML), epithelioid smooth muscle neoplasm, epithelioid mesothelioma, and epithelioid gastrointestinal stromal tumor (Table 26.3). Most adrenal cortical neoplasms are vimentin (70% to 80% of cases), inhibin (85% to 90%), melan-A (85% to 90%), adrenal cortical antigen SF-1 (85% to 90%), and calretinin (85% to 90%) immunopositive (*Am J Surg Pathol.* 2011;35:678). There is an overlap of the immunophenotype with ovarian and testicular sex-cord stromal neoplasms, which should come as no surprise since these tumors have similar developmental and functional attributes (*Semin Diagn Pathol.* 2005;22:3; *Semin Diagn Pathol.* 2005;22:33).

4. **Adrenocortical neoplasms in children** have been disproportionately diagnosed as ACCs in the past because of the frequent presence of microscopic features that are correlated with malignancy in adrenal cortical neoplasms in adults. However, the predictive value of malignant behavior in the pediatric age group based on these histologic features is poor (*Am J Surg Pathol.* 2003;27:867). For cortical tumors confined to the adrenal gland in children, neoplasms weighing in excess of 400 g are more likely to behave in a malignant fashion (*Pediatr Dev Pathol.* 2009;12:284); few tumors that

TABLE 26.3	Comparative Immunohistochemistry of Adrenal Cortical Tumors and Other Similar Appearing Extraadrenal Neoplasms						
	ACT	**HCT**	**RCT**	**PEComa-AML**	**EGIST**	**ESMT**	**EMESO**
VIM	−	−	+[a]	+	−	+	+
CK (AE1/AE3)	±	±	+	−	−	−	+
CK5/6	−	−	−	−	−	−	+
CK7	−	−	±	−	−	−	+
CK20	−	−	−[b]	−	−	−	−
34βE12	−	+	−	−	−	−	−
EMA	−	−	±	−	−	−	±
HEP-PAR	−	+	−	−	−	−	−
CD10	±[d]	±[d]	+	−	−	−	−
CD34	−	−	−	−	+	−	−
CD117	−	−	−	−	+	−	−
HMB-45	−	−	±[e]	+[e]	−	−	−
MEL-A103	+	−	−[c]	+	−	−	−
INH	+	−	−	−	−	−	−
CAL	−	−	−	−	−	−	+
RCC	−	−	+	−	−	−	−
SMA	−	−	−	+	±	+	−
WT1	−	−	−	−	−	−	+

[a]VIM negative in most chromophobe RCCs and oncocytomas.
[b]CK20 positive in type PAPRCC (*Arch Pathol Lab Med.* 2011;135:92).
[c]MEL-A positive in 90% Xp11 translocation RCCs.
[d]CD10 canalicular staining (*Arch Pathol Lab Med.* 2007;131:1648).
[e]HMB-45 positive in 50% Xp11 translocation RCCs.
ACT, adrenocortical tumor; HCT, hepatocellular tumor; AML, angiomyolipoma; RCT, renal cell tumor; PEC, perivascular epithelioid cell tumor, including angiomyolipoma; EGIST, epithelioid gastrointestinal stromal tumor; ESMT, epithelioid smooth muscle tumor; EMESO, epithelioid mesothelioma; VIM, vimentin; CK, cytokeratin; INH, inhibin; MEL, melanoma; HepPar, hepatocyte antigen; SMA, smooth muscle actin; EMA, epithelial membrane antigen; RCC, renal cell carcinoma antigen; CAL, calretinin; WT1, Wilms tumor.

    weigh <200 g are malignant, but those between 200 and 400 g are less predictable.
IV. ADRENAL MEDULLARY LESIONS. Major categories of adrenal medullary lesions include medullary hyperplasia, pheochromocytoma (PHEO), and neuroblastic tumors.
    A. Adrenal medullary hyperplasia (AMH) is defined as an increase in the mass of medullary cells with expansion of these cells into areas of the gland that normally do not contain pheochromocytes. Multiple endocrine neoplasia (MEN) (type 2A, 2B) is the most common setting of AMH, but it is also seen in association with Beckwith–Wiedemann syndrome, neurofibromatosis, somatostatin-rich duodenal low-grade neuroendocrine carcinoma (carcinoid), cystic fibrosis, and sudden infant death syndrome. Mutation of succinate dehydrogenase subunit B (*SDHB*) is associated with familial paraganglioma and less often familial PHEO, and a germline mutation has also been detected in an individual with AMH (*J Clin Oncol.* 2011;29:e200). Sporadic examples of AMH are rare. Diffuse or nodular hyperplasia with multiple nodules is present in both glands in MEN 2A and 2B; medullary tissue is present in both alae (normally it is present in only 1 ala) or in the tail (normally not present), with increased medullary volume. The microscopic distinction between AMH and normal medulla can be difficult, requiring morphometric evaluation (>10% of adrenal volume is indicative of medullary hyperplasia) or determining that the cortex to medullary ratio is <10:1. Differentiation of medullary

TABLE 26.4	Pheochromocytomas and Paragangliomas as Part of Inherited Tumor Syndromes	
Syndrome	Gene/chromosomal location	Pathology[a]
MEN 2	*RET*/10q11.2	Pheochromocytoma
Neurofibromatosis type 1	*NF1*/17q11	Pheochromocytoma/head and neck paraganglioma
Von Hippel-Lindau disease	*VHL*/3p25–26	Pheochromocytoma/abdominal paraganglioma
Pheochromocytoma-paraganglioma syndrome 1	*SDHD*/11q23	Pheochromocytoma/ head, neck, and abdominal paraganglioma
Pheochromocytoma-paraganglioma syndrome 3	*SDHC*/1q21–23	Head and neck paraganglioma
Pheochromocytoma-paraganglioma syndrome 4	*SDHB*/1p36	Pheochromocytoma/head, neck, thoracic, and abdominal paraganglioma

[a]Both sympathetic and parasympathetic paragangliomas occur in these various syndromes.
From Zhang Y, Nosé V. Endocrine tumors as part of inherited tumor syndromes. *Adv Anat Pathol.* 2011;18:206 with permission.

hyperplasia from PHEO is more important; some investigators have recommended a size distinction with 1 cm as the demarcation, with nodules >1 cm considered PHEOs (as arbitrary as that may be). AMH is often present adjacent to a PHEO.

B. **Pheochromocytoma** arises from chromaffin cells of the adrenal medulla and is derived from neuroblasts from the neural crest. There are rare examples of neoplasms with the combined features of a neuroblastic tumor and PHEO reflecting the common progenitorship; these tumors are generally referred to as composite PHEOs. PHEO refers to the intraadrenal chromaffin neoplasm whereas paraganglioma is the designation for those neural crest neoplasms with similar morphology that present in the various extraadrenal sites of sympathetic and parasympathetic paraganglia (discussed later). Approximately 65% to 70% of PHEOs and paragangliomas are sporadic and the remaining 30% to 35% are manifestations of inherited tumor syndromes (Table 26.4). Germline mutations in genes which encode B, C, and D subunits of succinate dehydrogenase (SDH) are found in three of the PHEO–paraganglioma syndromes (*Best Pract Clin Endocrinol Metab.* 2010;24:943; *Adv Anat Pathol.* 2011;18:206). PHEO has been referred to as the "10% tumor": 10% bilateral, 10% extraadrenal, 10% malignant, and 10% in children. The clinical presentation of a PHEO reflects the tumor's catecholamine synthesis, but Cushing and watery diarrhea (vasoactive intestinal peptide) syndromes are reported in a small minority of cases.

Grossly, PHEOs range from 2 to 10 cm or greater, have a yellow-tan to dark hemorrhagic appearance, appear multinodular, and weigh between 10 and 100 g (e-Fig. 26.13). It is not always clear from the gross examination whether the tumor is arising from the cortex or medulla, especially in those tumors which have largely replaced the entire gland, but remnants of the cortex may be identified microscopically.

Microscopically, a nested/nesting pattern with the formation of so-called zellballen is the classic morphology of PHEO (e-Fig. 26.14A and B), but other patterns include trabecular, mixed alveolar and trabecular, solid, diffuse, and rarely spindle cell formations (which are usually focal). A myxohyaline stroma has been noted in those tumors occurring in the setting of von Hippel–Lindau syndrome (*Ann NY Acad Sci.* 2006;1073:557). The chromaffin cells often have slightly eosinophilic and finely granular cytoplasm, but they may be amphophilic to basophilic or even oncocytic (e-Fig. 26.14). A finely vacuo-lated cytoplasm is present in some cases due to lipid accumulation. Intracy-toplasmic periodic acid-Schiff positive, diastase-resistant hyaline globules are yet another finding (e-Fig. 26.15). Melanin-containing PHEOs are rare but well documented (*Hum Pathol.* 1993;24:420). The polygonal cells can vary in size and nuclear detail, with marked nuclear enlargement and hyperchromasia, although less impressive cytologic atypia is often present. Prominent nucleoli and nuclear pseudoinclusions are additional but inconsistent findings (e-Fig. 26.16). Mitotic figures, if seen, are not an indication of malignancy per se. The stroma may exhibit extensive hyalinization, fibrosis, or rarely amyloid deposition, and the vasculature may be prominent. The periadrenal adipose tissue often has a hibernomatous appearance regardless of the age of the patient (e-Fig. 26.17). The chromaffin cells are positive for chromogranin A, synaptophysin, and cytokeratin in 25% of cases (*Arch Pathol Lab Med.* 1990;114:506); the tumor cells do not express EMA, melan A, or inhibin. S-100 labels sustentacular cells that are usually located at the periphery of the nests.

Prognostic assessment of an individual PHEO which is confined to the gland and without metastasis is an exercise in uncertainty. A number of morphologic features of the tumor have been assessed from the architectural pattern (nested vs. diffuse), presence or absence of confluent necrosis, mitotic rate, Ki-67 index, as well as several others including weight (less than or greater than 10 g), but the conclusion that there are "no absolute histologic criteria for predicting malignant potential" still seems to be true (*Histopathology,* 2011;58:155). Overall, 10% to 25% of PHEOs prove to be malignant as demonstrated by metastasis to bone, lymph nodes, lungs, and liver (e-Fig. 26.18).

Composite or compound PHEO, a rare variant, is defined in most cases as a PHEO with a ganglioneuromatous (80%), ganglioneuroblastomatous (20%), neuroblastomatous (<1%), malignant peripheral nerve sheath tumor, or neu-roendocrine carcinoma (extremely rare) component (e-Fig. 26.19) (*Arch Pathol Lab Med.* 1999;123:1274; *Am J Clin Pathol.* 2009;132:69; *J Clin Pathol.* 2009;62:659). This variant accounts for 1% to 3% of all PHEOs, and these tumors are reported in the clinical settings of neurofibromatosis I and MEN 2A (*Am J Surg Pathol.* 1993;17:837; *Am J Surg Pathol.* 1997;21:102). There is also a case with a cortical adenoma (*Ann Diagn Pathol.* 2011;15:185).

C. **Neuroblastic tumors** (also known as peripheral neuroblastic tumors) are embry-onal tumors arising from the sympathoadrenal neuroendocrine system and are the most common extracranial solid malignancy of childhood (*Nat Rev Can-cer.* 2003;3:203; *N Engl J Med.* 2010;362:2202). About 600 new cases are diagnosed each year in the United States. Approximately 98% of neuroblas-tomas are diagnosed by 10 years of age, and 85% to 90% are detected before 5 years of age. The abdomen and/or retroperitoneum is the site of clinical pre-sentation in 65% of cases; 50% of NBs arise in the adrenal medulla. Though most neuroblastomas have a number of overlapping histopathologic features, they are clinically, pathologically, and molecularly divisible into indolent or aggressive subtypes (*Pediatr Clin North Am.* 2008;55:97; *Curr Probl Cancer.* 2009;33:333; *Oncogene.* 2010;29:1566).

1. **Neuroblastoma (NB)** is best characterized as having a variegated appearance since the gross features are dependent on its morphologic composition and on secondary changes such as hemorrhage, yellowish foci of necrosis and calcification, cystic degeneration, and fibrosis; some or all of these find-ings may be found in any one tumor (e-Fig. 26.20). It is often difficult to judge whether some of the gross changes are spontaneous since resection may be preceded by adjuvant therapy. A well-circumscribed, soft, gray-tan tumor, measuring 2 to 10 cm in dimension, with or without hemorrhage and calcifications, is the common appearance of a poorly differentiated NB

(e-**Fig. 26.21**). Ganglioneuroblastoma (GNB) with intermixed features typically has a uniform grayish-tan mucoid cut surface, which is shared with some poorly differentiated NBs and ganglioneuromas (e-**Fig. 26.22**). A neuroblastic tumor with one or more discrete nodules with variable dimensions in a background of grayish-tan, firm tissue is the gross appearance of nodular GNB (e-**Fig. 26.23**). Some neuroblastic tumors are entirely hemorrhagic and may have undergone near total cystic degeneration (with or without calcifications).

Histologically, the tumor cells are small with hyperchromatic nuclei and scanty cytoplasm and are arranged in sheets or lobules (e-**Fig. 26.24**). The cell borders are indistinct except in the case of undifferentiated NB which is typically devoid of neuropil in the background (e-**Fig. 26.25A** and **B**). A lobular appearance at low power is associated with thin fibrovascular septa between nests of tumor cells. Homer-Wright rosettes or pseudorosettes have a central tangle of neuropil surrounded by a mantle of neuroblasts (e-**Fig. 26.26A** and **B**). Poorly differentiated NBs have neuritic differentiation, and some fraction of tumor cells are larger with a rim of cytoplasm as a feature of differentiation toward ganglion cells; greater or lesser than 5% of gangliocytic differentiation has been the threshold for classifying a NB as differentiating. In differentiating NB, the ganglion cell differentiation is asynchronous (e-**Fig. 26.27**) whereas in ganglioneuroblastoma it tends to be more synchronous with readily identifiable groups of mature ganglion cells (e-**Fig. 26.28**). In all subtypes of NBs, the Schwannian stroma must account for <50% of the tumor (Schwannian stroma-poor); Schwannian stroma is not neuropil but has a spindle cell pattern that is almost fibrous appearing with features resembling those of a Schwannoma (e-**Fig. 26.29**). The absence of a discrete capsule at the periphery may be the initial clue that a posterior mediastinal or paraspinal tumor is a ganglioneuroma.

An undifferentiated NB is composed of a relatively monotonous population of malignant round cells without a fibrillary network. These tumors must be differentiated from other similar appearing round cell neoplasms, especially malignant rhabdoid tumor. Undifferentiated NB expresses vimentin and chromogranin and clinically can be nonfunctioning. There is a large cell variant of undifferentiated NB (*Pathol Oncol Res.* 2007;13:269).

The prognosis of a poorly differentiated NB is based on multiple factors: age, primary site, pathologic subtype, mitosis-karyorrhexis index (MKI), biologic markers, and stage of disease (localization and metastasis) (Table 26.5). Despite all of the pathologic and molecular refinements in the

TABLE 26.5	International NB Staging System
Stage	**Definition**
1	Localized tumor with gross complete excision, with or without microscopic residual disease, negative lymph nodes
2A	Unilateral tumor with incomplete gross excision, negative lymph nodes
2B	Unilateral tumor with complete or incomplete gross excision, positive ipsilateral lymph nodes but negative contralateral lymph nodes
3	Unresectable unilateral tumor infiltrating cross the midline (positive or negative lymph nodes) or localized unilateral tumor with positive contralateral lymph nodes
4	Tumor disseminated to distant lymph node groups, bone, bone marrow, liver, skin and/or other organs (except as defined in 4s)
4s	Stage 1–2 tumor but with dissemination that is limited to skin, bone marrow, and/or liver

TABLE 26.6	International NB Pathology Committee Age-linked Prognostic Classification	
Age group	**Favorable histology**	**Unfavorable histology**
Any age	Ganglioneuroma Ganglioneuroblastoma, intermixed subtype	Neuroblastoma, undifferentiated subtype (any MKI)
<1.5 years old	Neuroblastoma, poorly differentiated with low or intermediate mitosis-karyorrhexis-index (MKI) (≤4% or 200/5000 cells) Ganglioneuroblastoma, nodular, with poorly differentiated nodule(s) or differentiating nodule(s) with low-intermediate MKI	Neuroblastoma, poorly differentiated with high MKI Neuroblastoma, differentiating with high MKI (>4% or 200/5000 cells) Ganglioneuroblastoma, nodular, with undifferentiated nodules (2) or nodules with high MKI
1.5–5 years old	Neuroblastoma, differentiating with low MKI Ganglioneuroblastoma, nodular, with differentiating nodule(s) with low MKI	Neuroblastoma, poorly differentiated (any MKI) Neuroblastoma, differentiating with intermediate or high MKI (>2% or >100/5000 cells) Ganglioneuroblastoma, nodule, with undifferentiated or differentiating nodule(s) or nodule(s) with intermediate-high MKI
> 5 years old		Neuroblastoma, any subtype Ganglioneuroblastoma, nodular type

From *Cancer.* 2003;98:2274; *Arch Pathol Lab Med.* 2005;129:874.

characterization of NBs, age (<1 year old) and pathologic stage remain the most significant determinants of outcome (*Lancet* 2007;369:2106; *Klin Padiatr.* 2008;220:137). Patients with extraadrenal tumors tend to do better than those with adrenal-based NBs, and undifferentiated NBs generally have a poor outcome.

Neuroblastic tumors are categorized into favorable and unfavorable pathologic groups on the basis of features that incorporate age at diagnosis and the MKI (Table 26.6). The latter is calculated on the number of mitotic or karyorrhectic tumor cells based on 5000 cells in random fields; in all practicality, "high" or "low" MKI NB is easily recognized after a high magnification examination of several microscopic fields. Tumors with favorable histopathology on the basis of histologic subtype and low MKI have better outcomes. The molecular genetic markers associated with a poor prognosis are *MYCN* amplification and several chromosomal abnormalities (1p deletion, 14q deletion, 11q deletion, 17q gain) (*Cancer Genet.* 2011;204:113). More recently, multiple somatic and activating mutations of the *ALK* gene have been identified; there is no clear relationship to date between tumor behavior and *ALK* mutations though there is a possible association with *MYCN* amplification (*Oncogene.* 2010;29:1566).

2. **Ganglioneuroblastoma (GNB),** seen in young children, tends to present in the retroperitoneum or mediastinum more often than in the adrenal gland. Intermixed GNB has a uniform grayish-white to tan mucoid appearance, whereas nodular GNB has grossly visible nodules or discrete microscopic foci of poorly differentiated neuroblasts (**e-Fig. 26.30**). The Schwannian stroma accounts for at least 50% of the tumor in both types, and

well-defined microscopic foci of neuroblastic cells show various stages of neuroblastic maturation to ganglionic differentiation in a fibrillary and neuromatous or Schwannian background. The macroscopic nodules are composed of neuroblasts in varying phases of differentiation; these are sharply demarcated from the surrounding stroma that has neuromatous or ganglioneuromatous features. Nodules of poorly differentiated NB with a high MKI connote a worse prognosis than those nodules with a low MKI (e-Fig. 26.31); the parameters used to group NBs into favorable and unfavorable categories also apply to GNB in general (*Cancer.* 2003;98:2274; *Pediatr Blood Cancer.* 2009;53:563). The overall favorable prognosis of GNB is related to the fact that most tumors are localized and have intermixed rather than nodular features.

3. **Ganglioneuroma** (GN) is the most common neoplasm of the sympathetic nervous system in adults and occurs in the posterior mediastinum, retroperitoneum, and rarely in the adrenal gland. Most GNs are discovered incidentally, but some are known to present with VIP manifestations (*Surgery.* 2011;149:99). The tumor is grossly a solid, circumscribed, encapsulated homogenous gray-white mass, measuring 5 to 10 cm (e-Fig. 26.32). Mature GN is characterized by mature scattered single cells or groups of cells in a neuromatous stroma (e-Fig. 26.33). The differential diagnosis of maturing GN is intermixed GNB, but the stroma should constitute >50% of the tumor in the former. There is a definitional fine line between intermixed GNB and the so-called maturing GN, although in terms of a favorable prognosis, the distinction is an unimportant one.

V. LESIONS OF THE EXTRAADRENAL PARAGANGLIOMA

A. **Normal anatomy and histology.** The extraadrenal paraganglia are divided into two broad categories as they relate to the parasympathetic or sympathetic nervous system. The former are concentrated in the head and neck region with a close proximity to cranial nerves IX and XII and associated blood vessels and are further divided into jugulotympanic, vagal, carotid body, laryngeal, and aorticopulmonary paraganglia (*AJR.* 2006;187:492). The aorticopulmonary paraganglia are distributed in parallel with the sympathetic nervous system along the paravertebral and paraaortic axis and are further divided into cervical, intrathoracic, and intra-abdominal groups. Paraganglia are also found in the bladder, prostate, and gallbladder. All paraganglia have a similar composition of chief cells arranged in well-defined nests or zellballen surrounded by peripheral sustentacular cells. Catecholamine concentrations tend to be higher in the sympathetic paraganglia (including the adrenal medulla). A greater proportion of sympathetic derived paragangliomas are functional and noradrenergic (25% to 85% of cases) compared with those of parasympathetic origin (10% or less) (*Histopathology.* 2011;58:155).

B. **Extraadrenal paraganglioma** presents in a sporadic (70% to 75% of cases) or heredofamilial (25% to 30%) clinical setting, but in children it is almost always the latter with or without a PHEO (*J Pediatr Surg.* 2010;48:383). The various hereditary paraganglioma syndromes are summarized in Table 26.4. Not included in this table are the Carney triad (CT) of paragangliomas, gastrointestinal stromal tumor (GIST) of the stomach, and pulmonary chondromas (*J Clin Endocrinol Metab.* 2009;94:3656; *J Int Med.* 2009;266;43). The deletion in CT may be located within the 1p or 1q12–q21 region; there are no mutations in *SDHA, SDHB, SDHC, SDHD, KIT,* or *PDGFRA* genes (*J Int Med.* 2009;266:93).

1. **Parasympathetic paragangliomas** have a predilection for the head and neck with an estimate incidence of 1:30,000 to 100,000; these tumors are found in association with cranial nerves IX and XII (*Head Neck.* 2008;31:381). Though these tumors are rare, the head and neck region is the most common

site (*J Clin Endocrinol Metab.* 2001;86:5210). Almost 60% of cases are carotid body tumors at the bifurcation of the internal and external carotid arteries (*Head Neck Pathol.* 2009;3:303). Other sites in the head and neck in approximate descending order of frequency are the glomus jugulare, glomus tympanicum (both of the latter present in the middle ear), and the glomus vagale (which presents as a neck mass). The glomus jugulare arises in the adventitia of the jugular bulb (a dilated portion of the internal jugular vein at its origin at the jugular foramen) along the auricular branch of cranial nerve X (also known as Arnold's nerve) or the tympanic nerve (a branch of cranial nerve IX, also known as the nerve of Jacobson); the glomus tympanicum is contiguous with the tympanic nerve in the inferior temporal bone. Other less common sites in the head and neck include the larynx, paranasal sinus, salivary gland, orbit, and oral cavity. The thyroid and parathyroid rarely harbor paragangliomas (*Arch Otorhinolaryngol Ital.* 2009;29:97; *Head Neck Pathol.* 2010;4:37).

The carotid body tumor and glomus vagale are usually resected intact to reveal a firm to rubbery well-circumscribed mass with a fibrous pseudocapsule measuring 1 to 6 cm in greatest dimension. A grayish-tan to pale brownish surface is present on sectioning; focal hemorrhage may be seen. Groups of uniform pale staining tumor cells with finely granular nuclear chromatin are surrounded by a prominent and sometimes hemorrhagic fibrovascular network. Compressed spindle-shaped cells at the periphery of the cellular nests are S-100 protein positive sustentacular cells. There is typically more cellular pleomorphism, nuclear atypia, and hyperchromatism in PHEO in contrast to paragangliomas, although individual case exceptions are acknowledged. Vascular invasion and infiltrative growth are unusual findings.

There are some special problems associated with middle ear paragangliomas. These tumors are often submitted in a piecemeal fashion, and artifacts introduced during excision may yield an initial impression of a vascular tumor. Immunohistochemistry is helpful in establishing the diagnosis and shows a phenotype of reactivity for chromogranin, synaptophysin, CD56, and focally for cyclin-D1 (*Otolaryngol Head Neck Surg.* 2010;143: 531).

2. **Sympathetic paragangliomas** are present in the abdomen-retroperitoneum in more than 80% of cases, specifically in the superior paraaortic region (45% of cases), region of the adrenal gland or renal hilum (10%), inferior paraaortic region (30%), and organ of Zuckerkandl or bladder (10%) (e-**Fig. 26.34**). The remaining 5% of cases are collectively reported in the gallbladder, kidney, urethra, prostate, spermatic cord, ovary, and vagina. Were the adrenal gland included in the discussion, it would be the most common site of "sympathetic paraganglioma." Unlike the nonfunctional and infrequently metastasizing parasympathetic paragangliomas, sympathetic paragangliomas are more often malignant (25% to 65% of cases) with a metastatic potential in excess of that seen in PHEOs (*J Clin Endocrinol Metab.* 2011;96:717). In the absence of metastasis, many of the same problems exist in the reliable pathologic identification of the potentially malignant paraganglioma as in the case of a PHEO (e-**Fig. 26.35**). Size (>100 g), confluent necrosis, mitotic and proliferative activity (Ki-67 index), absence of hyaline globules, and small cell morphology are some of the features that have been correlated with malignant behavior (*Histopathology.* 2011;58:155).

3. **Gangliocytic paraganglioma** usually arises in the periampullary portion of the duodenum but is also rarely seen in the nasopharynx, lung, esophagus, mediastinum, pancreas, and appendix (*BMC Cancer 20;11:187*). It occurs

in patients over a wide age range as a solitary, polypoid mass that projects into the lumen of the intestine and measures up to 7 cm in diameter. It is an infiltrative neoplasm composed of three cell types in variable proportions, namely spindle cells, epithelioid cells, and ganglion cells (e-**Fig. 26.36**). The spindle cells are elongated and have wavy nuclei resembling Schwanni cells, with S-100 and neurofilament immunopositivity; these cells can envelope the ganglion and epithelioid cells, analogous to sustentacular cells. The larger epithelioid cells are arranged in solid nests, ribbons, or pseudoglandular or papillary structures and have neuroendocrine features including granular eosinophilic to amphophilic cytoplasm with uniform oval nuclei and finely stippled chromatin (e-**Fig. 26.37**); these cells express cytokeratin, chromogranin, and synaptophysin. The ganglion cells have atypical features, and there may be a morphologic continuum with the epithelioid cell population. Recurrences are rare, but metastatic behavior is restricted to regional lymph nodes or liver (*J Gastrointest Surg.* 2007;11:1351; *Ann Diagn Pathol.* 2011;15:467).

VI. OTHER ADRENAL PARENCHYMAL LESIONS

A. **Myelolipoma** accounts for <5% of primary adrenal tumors and is usually detected incidentally on imaging studies of the abdomen, although hemorrhage with pain is a rare presentation (*Asian J Surg.* 2009;32:172). Several cases have been discovered in individuals with congenital adrenal hyperplasia and Cushing syndrome (*Exp Clin Endocrinol Diabetes.* 2009;117:440; *Endocr Pract.* 2011;17:441). While the tumor can be larger than 20 cm and 2 kg, it measures 3 to 5 cm in most cases. The tumor has a soft yellow to red surface, depending on the fat content and presence of hemorrhage. The usual microscopic appearance includes varying proportions of mature adipose tissue admixed with normal trilineage hematopoiesis (e-**Fig. 26.38**). Clonality has been demonstrated (*Am J Surg Pathol.* 2006;30:838). Lipoma, angiomyolipoma, and liposarcoma are in the differential diagnosis.

B. **Adenomatoid tumor,** like myelolipoma, is usually detected as an incidentaloma (*Am J Surg Pathol.* 2003;27:969). The tumor is a well circumscribed, solid or solid and cystic and measures from 0.5 to 9 cm. Microscopically, the tumor is composed of tubules, cysts, papillary structures, and occasional solid sheets of low cuboidal cells (e-**Fig. 26.39**). The tumor cells may have cytoplasmic vacuoles with signet ring features (e-**Fig. 26.40**) but are mucicarmine-negative for mucin. The tumor cells have the same immunophenotype as mesothelial cells with reactivity for vimentin, CK7, calretinin, and WT-1 (*Pathol Res Int.* 2010;2010:702472). Adenomatoid tumor is believed to arise from mesothelial inclusions within the adrenal gland. The main differential diagnoses include lymphangioma, metastatic carcinoma, and vascular tumors, especially epithelioid angiosarcoma (*Arch Pathol Lab Med.* 2011;135:268).

C. **Mesenchymal tumors** include lipoma, schwannoma, hemangioma, leiomyoma, leiomyosarcoma, angiosarcoma, perivascular epithelioid cell tumor, Ewing sarcoma-primitive neuroectodermal tumor, solitary fibrous tumor, hemangioblastoma, and papillary endothelial hyperplasia.

D. **Lymphoma** is most commonly seen in previously diagnosed cases of non-Hodgkin lymphomas (NHL) and occurs in as many as 25% of cases at some point in the clinical course; bilateral involvement is present in 75% to 80% of cases, and adrenal insufficiency is a known complication. However, rare examples of NHL with a primary presentation in the adrenal have been reported (*Exp Clin Endocrinol Diabetes.* 2011;119:208). Diffuse large B-cell lymphoma is the most common pathologic type (*Mod Pathol.* 2009;22:1210), although Burkitt lymphoma also occurs (*Tumori.* 2007;93:625). Hodgkin lymphoma of the adrenal is rare (*Br J Haematol.* 2010;148:341).

VII. ADRENAL CYSTS are relatively uncommon and are divided into four cate-gories: parasitic cysts (7%), epithelial cysts (9%), pseudocysts (39%), and endothelial cysts (45%) (*Arch Surg.* 1966;92:131; *Endocr Pathol.* 2008;19:274).

   A. Pseudocysts are discovered as another incidentoma on CT imaging. The usual appearance is a well-defined cyst with water-like density and a median size of 6 to 10 cm in diameter. Pseudocysts are unilocular, are filled with yellow-brown to bloody amorphous semi-liquid material, and have a wall thickness of 1 to 5 mm. The densely hyalinized connective tissue of the wall may contain focal calcifications or even metaplastic bone formation, and entrapped cortical tissue may also be present; the smooth muscle in the wall of the cyst is continuous with the smooth muscle of the adrenal vein. An identifiable lining is absent. The differential diagnosis includes a cystic NB or PHEO (*Cancer.* 2004;101:1537).

   B. Vascular cysts are the most common type of adrenal cyst in some series (*Arch Pathol Lab Med.* 2006;130:1722). Endothelial cysts are usually well circum-scribed and multiloculated (e-**Fig. 26.41**). The endothelial cells are immunopos-itive for CD31, and if derived from lymphatic endothelium, then also positive for D2–40 (e-**Fig. 26.42A and B**).

   C. Epithelial cysts are divided into true glandular cysts and embryonal cysts (*World J Surg.* 2006;30:1817), although in some classification schemes cystic adrenal tumors are also considered in the category of epithelial cysts. Mesothelial cysts also occur (*Endocr Pathol.* 2008;19:203).

   D. Parasitic cysts are a manifestation of echinococcal infection in the adrenal and retroperitoneum (*Bull Soc Pathol Exot.* 2010;103:313; *Int Surg.* 2010;95:189). The wall of the cyst is often calcified.

VIII. METASTATIC NEOPLASMS to the adrenal gland are common. Metastatic carcinoma is present in the adrenals in 25% to 30% of carcinoma-related deaths at autopsy (*Cancer.* 1950;3:74). The lung is the most common primary site (adrenal metas-tases are found in 30% to 35% of cases) (e-**Fig. 26.43**) followed by the breast; other malignancies that frequently metastasize to the adrenals include adenocar-cinomas of the kidney, stomach, and colon (e-**Fig. 26.44**); melanoma (10% to 15% or greater of cases) (e-**Fig. 26.45**); hepatocellular carcinoma; and urothe-lial carcinoma (*Clin Endocrinol.* 2002;56:95; *Am J Surg.* 2008;195:363; *Semin Oncol.* 2008;35:172). Renal cell carcinoma (RCC) involves the adrenal by either direct extension from an upper pole tumor or metastasis in 5% to 10% of cases; metastatic RCC should always be differentiated from a primary adrenal cortical carcinoma (*Am J Surg Pathol.* 2011;35:678; *Eur Urol.* 2011;60:458) (Table 26.3). Other types of neoplasms arising in the retroperitoneum or as a metastasis to the adrenal can be differentiated in most cases by immunohistochemistry (see Table 26.3).

IX. ADRENAL GLAND CYTOLOGY

   A. Fine needle aspiration (FNA). FNA is frequently used to evaluate adrenal gland mass lesions and is performed under percutaneous CT and ultrasound guidance, or endoscopic ultrasound guidance for left adrenal lesions (*Diagn Cytopathol.* 2005;33:26). FNA diagnosis of adrenal lesions has an accuracy of 98% and specificity of 100% (*Diagn Cytopathol.* 1999;21:92). FNA biopsy of pheochromocytoma is regarded as a relative contradiction due to possible induction of hypertensive crisis (*Radiology.* 1986;159:733).

   B. Specific Neoplasms

   1. Myelolipoma. The aspirate shows a mixture of mature adipose tissue and hematopoietic elements, including nucleated red blood cells, granulocytes and precursors, and megakaryocytes (*Acta Cytol.* 1991;35:353).

   2. Adrenal cortical neoplasms. The distinction between adrenal cortical hyper-plasia, adrenal cortical adenoma, adrenal cortical carcinoma, and normal adrenal cortical cells is not always possible in cytologic specimens. Radiological correlation is essential.

    a. Adrenal cortical adenoma yields moderately cellular smears that contain poorly cohesive sheets of epithelial cells with ill-defined and vacuolated cytoplasm, and abundant stripped small round uniform nuclei. Bubbly and vacuolated lipid background is prominent (**e-Fig. 26.46**). Scattered cells show nuclear atypia. Some cells may have cytoplasmic lipofuscin (*Acta Cytol.* 1995;39:843; *Acta Cytol.* 1998;42:1352; *Diagn Cytopathol.* 1999;21:92).

    b. Adrenal cortical carcinoma yields richly cellular aspirates. It consists of more frequent single cells that have marked nuclear atypia, intact granular cytoplasm, eccentric nuclei, and necrosis (**e-Fig 26.47**). The cytologic diagnosis of a well-differentiated adrenal cortical carcinoma is difficult (*Acta Cytol.* 1997;41:385).

3. Pheochromocytoma. The cytomorphology shows similarity to that of other neuroendocrine tumors. The aspirate contains abundant isolated and loose clusters of malignant cells with intervening vasculature (**e-Fig. 26.48**). The isolated polygonal or spindle-shaped cells exhibit poorly defined fragile cytoplasm and fine granular salt-and-pepper chromatin (**e-Fig. 26.49**). Red cytoplasmic granules can be seen on Romanowsky-type stains (*Acta Cytol.* 1999;43:207).

4. Metastatic malignancy. The most common malignancies metastatic to the adrenal are adenocarcinoma of the lung or breast (**e-Fig. 26.50**). The confirmation of metastasis is straightforward given a known malignant history. It is important to integrate clinical, laboratory, radiologic, cytologic, and immunocytochemical findings to differentiate primary neoplasms from metastasis (*Acta Cytol.* 1995;39:843).

SUGGESTED READINGS

Chen H, Sippel RS, O'Dorisio SO, et al. The North American Neuroendocrine Tumor Society consensus guideline for the diagnosis and management of neuroendocrine tumors. Pheochromocytomas, paraganglioma, and medullary thyroid carcinoma. *Pancreas.* 2010;39:775–783.

Conran RM, Chung E, Dehner LP, et al. The pineal, pituitary, parathyroid, thyroid and adrenal glands. In: Stocker JT, Dehner LP, Husain AN, eds. Stocker & Dehner's Pediatric Pathology. 3rd ed. Philadelphia, PA: Lippincott Williams & Wilkins; 2011:941–970.

DeLellis RA, Lloyd RV, Heitz PU, et al., eds. World Health Organization Classification of Tumours. Pathology and Genetics of Tumours of Endocrine Organs. Lyon, France: IARC Press; 2004.

Khan A, ed. Surgical Pathology of Endocrine and Neuroendocrine Tumors. Totowa, NJ: Humana Press; 2009.

Lloyd RV, ed. Endocrine Pathology. Differential Diagnosis and Molecular Advances. 2nd ed. New York, NY: Springer; 2010.

McNicol AM. Update of tumours of the adrenal cortex, phaeochromocytoma and extra-adrenal paraganglioma. *Histopathology.* 2011;58:155–168.

Raygada M, Pasini B, Stratakis CA. Hereditary paragangliomas. *Adv Otorhinolaryngol.* 2011;70:99–106.

Thompson LDR, ed. Endocrine Pathology: A Volume on Foundations in Diagnostic Pathology Series. Philadelphia, PA: Churchill Livingstone; 2006.

27 Pituitary Gland

Richard J. Perrin, Sushama Patil, and Arie Perry

I. **NORMAL ANATOMY AND HISTOLOGY.** The pituitary gland (hypophysis or "undergrowth") is located at the base of the brain, beneath the hypothalamus, within the sella turcica of the sphenoid bone. The smaller, posterior lobe of the pituitary contains the neurohypophysis (pars nervosa), which is connected to the hypothalamus via the pituitary stalk, or infundibulum ("little funnel"). Associated with the pituitary stalk is the infundibular portion (pars tuberalis) of the adenohypophysis. The other portions of the adenohypophysis form the anterior lobe (pars distalis) and vestigial intermediate lobe (pars intermedia); the latter contains remnants of Rathke's cleft cyst (glandlike cystic spaces).

Histologically, on H&E-stained sections, normal adenohypophysis (e-Fig. 27.1)* is composed of three different cell types: acidophils (producing growth hormone [GH] or prolactin [PRL]), basophils (producing adrenocorticotrophic hormone [ACTH], thyroid-stimulating hormone [TSH], luteinizing hormone [LH], and follicle-stimulating hormone [FSH]), and chromophobes (hypogranulated acidophils and basophils); all are arranged in an acinar pattern. The acini are demarcated by a delicate fibrovascular stroma best visualized on reticulin stains. Although each acinus contains a mixed population of these cell types, the composition varies regionally. Acidophils dominate the lateral portions, basophils (ACTH and TSH) dominate the medial portions, and basophilic gonadotrophs (LH and FSH) are distributed uniformly. Occasionally with aging, basophils extend into the neurohypophysis; this phenomenon, termed "basophilic invasion," should not be misinterpreted as an infiltrating neoplasm. The posterior pituitary is composed of axons, axon terminals, and sometimes axonal swellings (spheroids) called Herring bodies which contain vasopressin and oxytocin. Specialized glial cells (true "pituicytes") accompany the axons; these are generally considered to be the cells of origin for the rare and related benign tumors pituicytoma and choristoma (granular cell tumor [GCT]). Ectopic pituitary tissue can be found in the nasal cavity, sphenoid sinus, or rarely, within ovarian teratomas.

II. **INTRAOPERATIVE EVALUATION AND TISSUE HANDLING.** Intraoperative evaluations are frequently requested for pituitary neoplasms, most often to confirm the clinical diagnosis of pituitary adenoma. Although frozen sections usually provide adequate information to make an intraoperative diagnosis, a small (1 mm^3) amount of tissue should be used for cytologic examination. Intraoperative cytologic smears or "touch preps" lack freezing artifacts that obscure nuclear details (e-Fig. 27.2) and thus provide extremely valuable complementary information at the time of frozen section. Likewise, ample tissue should be reserved for paraffin embedding, free from freezing artifacts, to preserve antigenicity and morphologic features that might otherwise be compromised. This point is particularly important in the evaluation of a smaller microadenoma, which can easily be exhausted through cavalier intraoperative processing. Finally, a small (1 mm^3) amount of tissue should be reserved for ultrastructural examination; tissue fixed directly in 3% glutaraldehyde and embedded in plastic will retain fine structural features that cannot be recovered from formalin-fixed, paraffin-embedded tissue.

---

*All e-figures are available online via the Solution Site Image Bank.

III. NONNEOPLASTIC LESIONS

A. **Pituitary hyperplasia.** Diffuse expansion of pituitary acini, best evaluated on reticulin stained sections, is the histologic hallmark of pituitary hyperplasia. However, this diagnosis is often difficult to render with certainty. Nodular expansion of acini with one single hormonal cell type is noted in a variety of clinical scenarios, including pregnancy and estrogen therapy. One must also be cognizant of the naturally heterogeneous composition of the anterior pituitary, which favors acidophils laterally and basophils medially.

B. **Pituitary apoplexy (e-Fig. 27.3).** Spontaneous hemorrhage and infarction of non-neoplastic or neoplastic pituitary may represent a surgical emergency (in the setting of increased intracranial pressure, subarachnoid hemorrhage, or visual disturbance). For diagnosis of an underlying tumor in a partially necrotic specimen, a reticulin stain may prove more reliable than immunohistochemistry; immunohistochemistry should usually be performed but is often difficult to interpret in this setting.

C. **Lymphocytic hypophysitis** is a rare autoimmune disorder of the adenohypophysis that progressively destroys the gland, resulting in panhypopituitarism. The posterior hypophysis may also be affected, resulting in diabetes insipidus. Lymphocytic hypophysitis occurs with greater frequency in pregnant or postpartum women. Subsets of patients also have other associated autoimmune disorders. Microscopically, the anterior pituitary demonstrates lymphoplasmacytic infiltrates *without* granuloma formation. The resulting glucocorticoid deficiency is often fatal if untreated.

D. **Granulomatous hypophysitis.** This rare autoimmune disorder expands and selectively destroys the anterior pituitary with well-formed, noncaseating granulomas and a mild lymphocytic infiltrate. Radiologically, this condition may mimic adenoma, but it also often involves the thyroid, adrenal glands, and testes. Unlike lymphocytic hypophysitis, it shows no association with pregnancy.

E. **Rathke's cleft cyst (e-Fig. 27.4)** is a developmental abnormality that arises between the anterior and the posterior lobes or in the infundibular stalk. Smaller examples are often detected incidentally. Lesions > 1 cm are usually symptomatic (e.g., cause hypopituitarism or visual disturbances related to compression of the optic chiasm). The cyst is lined by cuboidal to columnar epithelium that may or may not be ciliated and may or may not contain goblet cells. Focally, the epithelium may show flattening and/or squamous metaplasia. The cyst contents are variably serous or mucoid. Xanthogranulomatous inflammation may be present in cysts that have undergone prior hemorrhage. Surgical resection is curative.

F. **Other.** Rarely, in the setting of hypopituitarism, only xanthogranulomatous inflammation is identified; such a finding may simply represent overwhelming reactive changes within a craniopharyngioma or Rathke's cleft cyst, but the entity "xanthogranuloma of the sellar region" that is generally restricted to the sella has also been described. The pituitary may also become involved by systemic histiocytic disorders, such as Langerhans cell histiocytosis (LCH), Rosai–Dorfman disease, Erdheim–Chester disease, and xanthoma disseminatum. LCH in particular may involve the sellar/suprasellar region more often than is generally considered; diabetes insipidus is a common manifestation.

IV. BENIGN NEOPLASMS

A. **Pituitary adenoma** is by far the most common sellar neoplasm. Tumors <1 cm are typically identified as microadenomas, and those >1 cm are categorized as macroadenomas. Microadenomas are most often functional (hormone producing), which explains why they draw clinical attention before reaching larger sizes. Nonfunctional tumors which account for one-third of all adenomas grow to a large size before drawing clinical attention. Often, large tumors produce so-called "stalk effect," in which mild to moderate elevations of PRL hormone result from compression of the infundibular stalk, which blocks the transport of dopamine (formerly, PRL inhibitory factor) from the hypothalamus. Some macroadenomas may compress the normal pituitary tissue and cause panhypopituitarism. In many cases, macroadenomas are detected only after they compress the optic chiasm, producing bitemporal hemianopsia or other vision disturbance. Approximately half of nonfunctioning adenomas are referred to as null-cell adenomas. These chromophobic (or less commonly, oncocytic) tumors have a negative hormonal immunoprofile despite showing reactivity for synaptophysin and exhibit few if any secretory granules on ultrastructural analysis (oncocytic adenomas show abundant mitochondria). Although some null-cell adenomas appear to express the alpha subunit of the glycoprotein hormones (LH, FSH, TSH) and thus might be considered "silent" gonadotrophic or thyrotrophic adenomas, expression of the alpha subunit has also been documented in somatotroph adenomas (*Neurol Res.* 1999;21:247), so this feature may have limited specificity.

Microscopically, adenomas lack the normal reticulin-rich acinar structure of the adenohypophysis. Instead, they may appear patternless, pseudorosette-rich, papillary, endocrine/organoid, or paraganglioma-like and may focally form glands. In ambiguous cases, a reticulin stain may be useful for accentuating loss of acinar architecture. Adenoma tumor cells are typically larger than their nonneoplastic counterparts and have round-to-oval nuclei, delicate stippled ("salt and pepper") chromatin, and small or inconspicuous nucleoli. Occasionally, adenomas exhibit moderate to marked cytologic atypia, but this feature is not associated with aggressive behavior unless accompanied by elevated mitotic and/or proliferation indices (see section on "atypical pituitary adenoma"). Cytoplasmic quality varies within and among different adenoma (hormonal) subtypes and may even vary among cells within an individual tumor, particularly in some tumors that secrete more than one hormone. Cytologic, histochemical, and ultrastructural features can be used to subtype adenomas. Although immunohistochemical profiles of hormone expression and cell proliferation are now in greater use for this purpose, familiarity with morphologic and histochemical features remains worthwhile.

Indirect histologic clues toward adenoma biology (hormonal secretion patterns) include the presence of calcium and amyloid bodies (rare) in prolactinoma. In prolactinoma treated with dopamine agonists, fibrosis and smaller cells with high nuclear to cytoplasmic (N/C) ratios are common. Perivascular pseudorosettes usually indicate a gonadotrophic or null-cell adenoma (e-Fig. 27.5). Deposits of Crooke's hyaline (ringlike cytoplasmic cytokeratin inclusions) most commonly accumulate in nonneoplastic corticotrophic cells in patients with hypercortisolism of any cause, including, but not limited to, Cushing disease (see section on corticotroph adenoma). Strong PAS staining suggests a corticotroph adenoma, whereas weak PAS positivity is seen in glycoprotein (FSH, LH, TSH expressing) adenomas. Round, weakly eosinophilic, cytokeratin positive, paranuclear "fibrous bodies" in a relatively chromophobic tumor most often indicate a GH-producing adenoma (e-Fig. 27.6).

B. Prolactinoma. Also called lactotrophic adenoma, prolactinoma comes to clinical attention most commonly in women of reproductive age with amenorrhea and galactorrhea. Men with prolactinoma are usually asymptomatic or present with decreased libido. Patients with prolactinomas are often treated medically with a dopamine agonist (e.g., bromocriptine) to impair adenoma cell growth and inhibit PRL production, but such agents are not cytotoxic. Tumors resected post-therapy usually show interstitial fibrosis, reduced cell size, and high N/C ratio and may be reminiscent of small-cell carcinoma (e-Fig. 27.7). However, they are usually at least focally positive for PRL and display a low mitotic/proliferative index.

C. **Corticotroph (ACTH-producing) adenoma.** Corticotroph adenomas most often present as microadenomas and account for 20% of all pituitary adenomas. These tumors, which may be as small as 1 or 2 mm, can be difficult to localize radiographically and intraoperatively. In such cases, a surgeon might employ inferior petrosal sinus sampling to evaluate lateralization and monitor the progress of resection. Even under these circumstances, exhaustive microscopic evaluation of the pathology specimen (examining multiple levels using reticulin and immunohistochemical stains) may yield no diagnostic findings. Fortunately, a postoperative drop in the patient's serum ACTH level may serve as evidence that the tumor was removed. Most ACTH adenomas are amphophilic to basophilic, deeply PAS positive, and arise in the central region of the gland where nonneoplastic corticotrophic cells are concentrated. Crooke's hyaline, appearing as glassy, eosinophilic cytoplasmic inclusions that ring the nucleus, results from hypercortisolism and represents an accumulation of cytokeratin filaments already present in corticotrophs (e-**Fig. 27.8**). Rare ACTH adenomas that themselves exhibit Crooke's hyaline are called Crooke's adenomas. Other ACTH adenomas that show immunoreactivity for ACTH but do not secrete biologically significant amounts of the hormone and do not induce Cushing syndrome are termed silent corticotroph adenomas. Such tumors are more common in men, tend to be invasive, and do not come to clinical attention until they become large (macroadenomas).

D. **Somatotroph (GH cell) adenoma.** This subgroup of pituitary adenomas includes tumors with exclusive GH production (PAS negative), tumors producing GH and PRL (mammosomatotroph adenomas), and plurihormonal adenomas (most positive for GH, PRL, and TSH). Somatotroph adenomas (e-**Fig. 27.9**) usually appear either intensely eosinophilic or rather chromophobic and show correspondingly strong or weak GH immunoreactivity. Aiding diagnosis, these chromophobic somatotroph tumor cells often contain weakly eosinophilic, cytokeratin-reactive paranuclear whorls known as fibrous bodies (e-**Fig. 27.6**). The systemic effects of somatotrophic adenomas (acromegaly in adults, gigantism in adolescents) are mediated by insulin-like growth factor-1 (IGF-1). These tumors may appear in the setting of Carney complex and multiple endocrine neoplasia I (MEN I).

E. **Gonadotroph adenomas.** These adenomas are more common in elderly males, are often nonfunctional, and grow to a very large size before coming to clinical attention by compressing adjacent structures; invasion is relatively less common in this subtype. Histologically, these tumors are usually chromophobic and often feature pseudorosettes, papillary architecture, or organoid features. Immunohistochemically, these tumors exhibit markedly variable reactivity for the beta subunits of LH and FSH and for the common α subunit.

F. **Pituicytoma** (infundibular astrocytoma). This rare benign tumor is thought to arise from the specialized glial cells of the posterior pituitary. Radiographically, it shows strong postcontrast enhancement. Histologically, it exhibits a solid growth pattern and is formed by plump spindled tumor cells arranged in short, interlacing fascicles. Rosenthal fibers and eosinophilic granular bodies are not present. Strong reactivity for vimentin, S100, and TTF-1 (nuclear pattern), patchy reactivity for GFAP, and no reactivity for cytokeratins, synaptophysin and neurofilament have been described (*J Neuropathol Exp Neurol.* 2009;68:482). Mitotic figures are uncommon.

G. **GCT of the neurohypophysis** (choristoma). Like pituicytoma, this tumor is thought to be derived from pituicytes; some consider these two tumors to be phenotypic variants. Although minute asymptomatic examples are quite common, larger symptomatic GCTs are relatively rare; these appear in the fifth or sixth decade with a female predominance and commonly present as an enhancing sellar/suprasellar mass compressing the optic chiasm. Histologically, these tumors are formed by closely apposed polygonal cells with small nuclei and generous granular eosinophilic cytoplasm. Spindled/fascicular areas may also be present. Lymphocytic infiltrates are common and may be robust. Staining with PAS is resistant to diastase digestion. Immunoreactivity is strong for S100 and TTF-1, and variable for the lysosomal marker CD68; reactivity for pituitary hormones, synaptophysin, cytokeratins, neurofilament, and chromogranin A is not observed. Ultrastructurally, these cells show abundant phagolysosomes and no evidence of neurosecretory granules.

H. Craniopharyngiomas (discussed in Chap. 41).

V. LOW-GRADE NEOPLASMS

A. Atypical pituitary adenomas are histologically similar to benign pituitary adenomas except for elevated mitotic and proliferative indices. For this diagnosis, current World Health Organization criteria require nuclear immunoreactivity for the proliferation marker Ki-67/MIB-1 in >3% of tumor cells and extensive nuclear immunoreactivity for p53; others suggest that Ki-67 labeling >10%, regardless of p53 status, correlates with more aggressive behavior and warrants an "atypical" designation (*Neuroendocrinology.* 2006;83:179). Relative to benign adenomas, these tumors are more likely to invade adjacent structures and to recur.

VI. HIGH-GRADE NEOPLASMS

A. Pituitary carcinoma is a very rare neoplasm that cannot be diagnosed by its innate appearance or any known markers; instead, it is diagnosed by the presence of craniospinal or extracranial metastases. The Ki-67/MIB-1 and p53 labeling indices are typically high, but cytologic and histologic features are often benign. These tumors are usually functional, secreting PRL or ACTH. Its designation in this chapter as a high-grade neoplasm may be inappropriate in the truest sense, but the term is applied here to reflect its more aggressive clinical behavior.

28 Testis and Paratestis
Kiran R. Vij and Peter A. Humphrey

I. **NORMAL ANATOMY.** The normal adult testis is an ovoid paired organ, measuring $4.5 \times 2.5 \times 3$ cm^3, and weighing approximately 20 g. The testes are suspended within scrotal sacs by spermatic cords. The testis is covered by a capsule composed of an outer tunica vaginalis lined by mesothelium, the collagenous tunica albuginea, and the inner tunica vasculosa. The tunica vaginalis forms a sac filled with serous fluid. The posterior portion of the testis not covered by a capsule is called the mediastinum and contains blood vessels, nerves, lymphatics, and the extratesticular rete testis.

The testicular parenchyma is subdivided into lobules containing seminiferous tubules separated by fibrous septae. The terminal portions of the seminiferous tubules drain into the tubuli recti that connect to the tubules of the rete testis at the mediastinum. The tubules of the rete testis anastomose with the ductuli efferentes, which form the head of the epididymis and empty into the vas deferens, which traverses the inguinal canal as a component of the spermatic cord. The testicular artery arises from the aorta and is the major source of vascular supply to the testes. The venous drainage occurs through numerous small veins that form a convoluted mass known as the pampiniform plexus that surrounds the testicular artery. These small veins anastomose to form the right testicular vein, which drains into the inferior vena cava, and two left testicular veins, which drain into the left renal vein.

Histologically, prepubertal and postpubertal seminiferous tubules are quite different. Prepubertal tubules are small, with few or no lumina, and contain mostly Sertoli cells with a few primordial germ cells (e-**Fig. 28.1**).* Postpubertal seminiferous tubules are larger and harbor Sertoli cells and germ cells at varying stages of maturation (e-**Fig. 28.2**). The Sertoli cells abut the basement membrane and are aligned perpendicular to the membrane; their nuclei are round to oval with prominent nucleoli, and the cytoplasm has Charcot–Böttcher crystals, which can occasionally be seen by light microscopy. Within the seminiferous tubules, the least mature germ cells—spermatogonia—are present along the basement membrane, with the most mature cells—elongate spermatids—found at the luminal border. Primary and secondary spermatocytes are found in an adluminal position.

The interstitial tissue between the seminiferous tubules contains Leydig cells, vessels, and connective tissue. Leydig cells are arranged singly and in clusters

---

*All e-figures are available online via the Solution Site Image Bank.

(e-**Fig. 28.3**), and can be associated with nerves. They are large and irregularly spherical to polyhedral, with small spherical nuclei and abundant acidophilic cytoplasm. The cytoplasm can exhibit lipofuscin and rod-shaped Reinke crystals.

II. **GROSS EXAMINATION, TISSUE SAMPLING, AND HISTOLOGIC SLIDE PREPARATION.** Tissue samples of the testes received for surgical pathologic examination include testicular biopsies, and unilateral and bilateral orchiectomy specimens. Retroperitoneal lymph node dissection can be performed as part of a staging maneuver for testicular cancer.

A. **Fine needle aspiration biopsy of the testis** in infertile patients (with sperm aspiration and cytopathologic examination) is occasionally performed. Cytologic touch imprints or wet preparations may be made at the time of open testicular biopsy in infertile patients to rapidly identify the presence of sperm. The role of cytology in the evaluation of testicular tumors is limited to diagnosis of lymph node metastases by fine needle aspiration. Although seminomas can usually be differentiated from nonseminomatous tumors, subtyping of nonseminomatous tumors cannot be reliably performed by cytology.

B. **Testicular biopsies,** which can be open or percutaneous, are typically performed for evaluation of infertility. They are usually contraindicated in the evaluation of solid testicular masses, with the possible exception of epidermoid cysts, which can be removed by excisional biopsy. Testicular biopsy specimens are usually received in Bouin's fixative. An accurate documentation of the number and size of the biopsy fragments and exact site(s) of the biopsy for each container should be made during gross dictation. The biopsy fragments should be inked with hematoxylin to facilitate identification during embedding, wrapped in lens paper, placed between sponges, and processed entirely. Three hematoxylin and eosin (H&E)-stained slides, each with three to four serial sections, should be prepared from each block.

C. **Unilateral simple orchiectomy** is performed in cases of testicular torsion. Gross examination of the testis similar to that for tumor cases should be performed. One section of the testicular parenchyma in relation to the capsule, and a section each of the epididymis and spermatic cord, should be submitted with description and sampling of focal lesions.

D. **Radical orchiectomy** is performed for testicular tumors. The specimen consists of the testis and paratesticular organs (surrounding tunica vaginalis, epididymis, soft tissue, and a segment of spermatic cord). In cases of tumor resection, the specimen should ideally be sent fresh and intact to the surgical pathology laboratory for immediate gross examination. Alternatively, when delay is anticipated, the specimen is placed in 10% buffered formalin and sent intact. In such cases, tumor morphology is often suboptimal due to poor fixation. The surgeon may occasionally bisect the specimen to aid fixation; this approach is not recommended as it prevents evaluation of involvement of the tunica by the tumor as well as procurement of fresh tissue for ancillary studies.

The specimen is weighed, and measurements are recorded in three dimensions. The length and diameter of the resected segment of spermatic cord are noted separately. The external surfaces of the testis and spermatic cord are examined for involvement by tumor. The proximal shave resection margin of the spermatic cord is submitted in a separate cassette, and then the cord is serially sectioned and inspected for tumor involvement; representative sections are submitted proximal to distal. The tunica vaginalis is opened anteriorly to show the tunica albuginea; presence of fluid, if any, within the sac is noted. The testis is then bisected anteroposteriorly through the epididymis, and serial sections are made parallel to this plane. Each slice is examined, and the tumor is described in relation to the epididymis and the tunica albuginea. The size, color, and consistency of the tumor should be noted. Foci of hemorrhage, necrosis, and variegation, as well as multifocality, if present, should be described.

Photographs or digital images should be taken and tissue procured for tumor bank and ancillary studies such as flow cytometry and karyotyping, if necessary. The specimen should then be fixed overnight in an adequate amount of 10% buffered formalin prior to submission of one section per centimeter of tumor. Representative sections should include heterogenous areas and sections of tumor in relation to uninvolved parenchyma, epididymis, and tunica albuginea. One section of grossly normal-appearing parenchyma should be included. If correlation of identified histologic tumor type with serum markers (alpha-fetoprotein [AFP] and human chorionic gonadotropin [hCG]) is not achieved, additional sections should be submitted (note that such correlation will not always be perfect because metastatic deposits may harbor different elements than the primary tumor).

E. **Retroperitoneal lymph node dissection** is performed as a separate procedure. The specimen is received in 10% buffered formalin. During gross examination, the tissue fragments should be measured in aggregate and carefully dissected to harvest as many lymph nodes as possible, and the size of the largest and the smallest putative nodes should be noted. Possible foci of tumor encountered during dissection should be measured and sampled. An effort should be made to sample any area(s) suspicious for viable tumor.

F. **Bilateral orchiectomy specimens** may be submitted as part of treatment of carcinoma of the prostate. Gross examination and sectioning are similar to that for unilateral simple orchiectomy. Prostate cancer is rarely encountered within these specimens.

III. DIAGNOSTIC FEATURES OF BENIGN DISEASES OF THE TESTIS

A. Congenital abnormalities

1. **Cryptorchidism** is maldescent of the testis in which the testis is found, after 1 year of age, to be located high in the scrotum, within the inguinal canal, or in an intra-abdominal location. Grossly, the prepubertal undescended testis differs little from normal, but after puberty the undescended testis is smaller. Histologically, there is a progressive loss of germ cells with age, along with decreased size of seminiferous tubules and increased thickness of tubular tunica propria. Sertoli cell nodules (e-Fig. 28.4), which are foci of tubules containing immature Sertoli cells and laminated calcific deposits, are often seen in cryptorchid testes. These are likely hyperplastic foci, although they have also been termed tubular adenoma of Pick. Rarely, Sertoli cell nodules can present as a mass (*Am J Surg Pathol.* 2010;23:1874). The major complications of cryptorchidism are infertility and germ cell neoplasia, ranging from intratubular germ cell neoplasia (IGCN) to invasive germ cell tumors, particularly seminoma, embryonal carcinoma, and embryonal carcinoma/teratoma. For patients >1 year of age, placental-like alkaline phosphatase (PLAP) and CD117 immunostains can be useful in highlighting intratubular germ cell neoplastic cells.

2. **Anorchism and polyorchidism** are absence of testes and more than two testes, respectively.

3. **In testicular–splenic fusion,** encapsulated splenic tissue is found adjacent to the left testis, which can show germ cell aplasia in the seminiferous tubules.

4. **Adrenal cortical rests** are usually incidental, millimeter-sized nodules of adrenal cortical tissue that are detected along the pathway of descent of the testis, including along the spermatic cord and testis.

B. Infertility.
The causes of infertility may be pretesticular, which include endocrine disorders involving the pituitary and adrenal glands; testicular, including genetic disorders; or posttesticular, which are mainly obstructive and include varicocele and cystic fibrosis. The evaluation of the patient includes a detailed clinical history, physical examination, semen analysis, tests of endocrine function, analysis of sperm function, and serology for antisperm antibody. Testicular biopsy

TABLE 28.1	Reporting Infertility Biopsies

1. Method of obtaining sample
   a. Percutaneous testis sperm aspiration
   b. Incisional testis sperm extraction
   c. Orchiectomy/other
2. Presence/absence of testicular tissue
3. Seminiferous tubules
   a. Number
   b. Tunica propria: Normal/thickened
   c. Mean number of spermatozoa/tubule (count 20 tubules)
   d. Most advanced stage of spermatogenesis
   e. Sertoli cells: Present/absent
4. Interstitium
   a. Leydig cells: Present/absent/hyperplastic
   b. Amount of interstitial inflammation
   c. Presence of macrophages and mast cells
5. Extratesticular/other comments
   a. Epididymis: Present/absent
   b. Vas deferens: Present/absent
   c. Immunohistochemical/special stains
6. Histologic diagnoses
   a. The most advanced histologic pattern is:
   b. The predominant histologic pattern is:

(preferably open biopsy) is indicated in cases where an endocrine dysfunction has been ruled out. Biopsies from patients with azoospermia may show germ cell aplasia (Sertoli cell only) (**e-Fig. 28.5**), maturation arrest (**e-Fig. 28.6**), and/or normal spermatogenesis that points to an obstructive etiology (*Arch Pathol Lab Med.* 2010;134:1197). Patients with oligospermia show a combination of one or more of the following: tubular hyalinization, fibrosis, hypospermatogenesis, normal or arrested spermatogenesis, and sloughing or disorganization. Although testicular biopsies are rarely performed in cases of endocrine dysfunction, the findings include small tubules with fibrosis and basement membrane thickening, and Leydig cell aplasia or hyperplasia. Synoptic-style reporting of testicular biopsies for infertility is described in Table 28.1.

C. **Inflammation and infection.**
   1. **Epididymitis** is typically more common and severe than orchitis, and is commonly related to urinary tract infection (from the urinary bladder, urethra, or prostate) by *Chlamydia, Neisseria, Escherichia coli,* or *Pseudomonas.* Tissue sampling is not needed for the diagnosis of orchitis and/or epididymitis.
   2. Most cases of **orchitis** are due to infection that spreads from the vas deferens and epididymis. Infectious agents that can cause orchitis include bacteria, mycobacteria, fungi, viruses, or spirochetes.
      a. **Tuberculous orchitis** always emanates from another site and spreads into the testis from the epididymis or bloodstream. Both testes are usually involved. The testicular inflammatory infiltrate varies from nonspecific to caseating granulomas.
      b. **Mumps orchitis** is caused by a paramyxovirus. Microscopically, there is an initial interstitial lymphocytic inflammatory infiltrate, followed by a mixed infiltrate that can result in tubular atrophy and peritubular fibrosis.

    c. **Syphilitic orchitis** occurs prior to infection of the epididymis. Histologically, peritubular lymphocytes and plasma cells can be seen along with obliterative endarteritis and perivascular plasma cells. Gummas can form an intratesticular mass with central necrosis.

    d. Other types of orchitis include nonspecific granulomatous orchitis and malakoplakia. Before diagnosing nonspecific granulomatous orchitis, a specific infectious orchitis, sarcoidosis, lymphoma, and exuberant granulomatous inflammation associated with a germ cell neoplasm should be excluded.

D. **Vascular disorders**

  1. **Systemic vasculitis** can affect the testis, but isolated vasculitis involving only the testis is rare. Testicular vasculitis can cause infarction that clinically simulates a neoplasm. Most cases of testicular vasculitis are characterized by polyarteritis nodosa-like changes in small- to medium-sized arteries, with transmural necrotizing inflammation (*Urology.* 2011;77:1043).

  2. **Varicocele** is an abnormal dilatation and tortuosity of veins of the pampiniform plexus of the spermatic cord.

  3. **Torsion and infarction** generally occur in young men and in the setting of abnormal testicular descent. Initially, there is congestion, edema, and hemorrhage, followed by hemorrhagic infarction (**e-Fig. 28.7**).

E. **Atrophy** can be caused by many factors, but the morphologic findings are similar. Grossly, the testis is small. Microscopically, the tubules are decreased in size and the tunica propria is thickened and hyalinized. End-stage atrophic tubules are completely hyalinized, without intraluminal cells (**e-Fig. 28.8**).

IV. **TUMORS OF THE TESTIS.** These are of germ cell origin in the vast majority of cases, with sex cord/gonadal stromal tumors occurring in 4% to 6% of cases. The highest incidence is found in Europe and parts of New Zealand. Populations in Africa and Asia show a much lower incidence. The 2004 World Health Organization classification of the neoplasms of the testis is given in Table 28.2.

A. **Germ cell tumors.** Clinical diagnosis is usually made when the patient presents with a painless mass in the testis. Associated symptoms such as a dull ache in the scrotum or lower abdomen may be present. Less commonly, patients present with gynecomastia and thyrotoxicosis. In 10% of cases, metastatic disease may produce presenting signs and symptoms. Patients with cryptorchidism are at an increased risk (about three- to fivefold) of developing germ cell neoplasia both in the cryptorchid and in the normal contralateral testis. Patients with testicular microlithiasis, testicular atrophy, infertility, a family history of germ cell neoplasia, 46,XY or 45,X/46,XY mixed gonadal dysgenesis, testicular dysgenesis syndrome (TDS), or a previous history of IGCN are also at an increased risk. The age of the patient as well as characteristic elevations in the levels of serum tumor markers in different subtypes of germ cell tumors can be very helpful in predicting tumor type. Yolk sac tumor and/or teratoma are seen in infants and children; seminomas and nonseminomatous germ cell neoplasms (including embryonal carcinoma, teratoma, yolk sac tumor, and choriocarcinoma) are found in adolescents and young adults; and spermatocytic seminoma occurs in patients older than 50 years. Serum AFP levels can be elevated in nonseminomatous germ cell tumors, especially those with a yolk sac tumor component, whereas serum beta-hCG levels are increased in choriocarcinoma and tumors with syncytiotrophoblasts, which include about 10% of seminomas. The levels of these tumor markers are monitored posttreatment and are indicators of residual disease.

    Imaging studies such as ultrasound are extremely sensitive and inexpensive in evaluating testicular masses. Localization of the mass, including evaluation of extratesticular versus intratesticular sites of involvement, and presence of

TABLE 28.2 WHO Histologic Classification of Tumors of the Testis and Paratestis

Germ cell tumors
IGCN, unclassified
Other types

Tumors of one histologic type (pure forms)
Seminoma
  Seminoma with syncytiotrophoblastic cells
Spermatocytic seminoma
  Spermatocytic seminoma with sarcoma
Embryonal carcinoma
Yolk sac tumor
Trophoblastic tumors
  Choriocarcinoma
  Trophoblastic neoplasms other than choriocarcinoma
  Monophasic choriocarcinoma
  Placental site trophoblastic tumor
Teratoma
  Dermoid cyst
  Monodermal teratoma
  Teratoma with somatic type malignancies

Tumors of more than one histologic type (mixed forms)
Mixed embryonal carcinoma and teratoma
Mixed teratoma and seminoma
Choriocarcinoma and teratoma/embryonal carcinoma
Others

Sex cord/gonadal stromal tumors
Pure forms
Leydig cell tumor
Malignant Leydig cell tumor
Sertoli cell tumor
  Sertoli cell tumor, lipid-rich variant
  Sclerosing Sertoli cell tumor
  Large cell–calcifying Sertoli cell tumor
Malignant Sertoli cell tumor
Granulosa cell tumor
  Adult-type granulosa cell tumor
  Juvenile-type granulosa cell tumor
Tumors of the thecoma/fibroma group
  Thecoma
  Fibroma
Sex cord/gonadal stromal tumor
Incompletely differentiated
Sex cord/gonadal stromal tumors, mixed forms
Malignant sex cord/gonadal stromal tumors
Tumors containing both germ cell and sex cord/gonadal stromal elements
  Gonadoblastoma
  Germ cell sex cord/gonadal stromal tumor, unclassified

(*continued*)

TABLE 28.2	WHO Histologic Classification of Tumors of the Testis and Paratestis (*Continued*)

Miscellaneous tumors of the testis

Carcinoid tumor

Tumors of ovarian epithelial types

   Serous tumor of borderline malignancy

   Serous carcinoma

   Well-differentiated endometrioid carcinoma

   Mucinous cystadenoma

   Mucinous cystadenocarcinoma

   Brenner tumor

Nephroblastoma

Paraganglioma

Hematopoietic tumors

Tumors of collecting ducts and rete

Adenoma

Carcinoma

Tumors of paratesticular structures

Adenomatoid tumor

Malignant mesothelioma

Benign mesothelioma

   Well-differentiated papillary mesothelioma

   Cystic mesothelioma

Adenocarcinoma of the epididymis

Papillary cystadenoma of the epididymis

Melanotic neuroectodermal tumor

Desmoplastic small round cell tumor

Mesenchymal tumors of the spinal cord and testicular adnexae

Secondary tumors of the testes

From: Eble JN, Sauter G, Epstein JI, et al., eds. *World Health Organization Classification of Tumours. Pathology and Genetics. Tumours of the Urinary System and Male Genital Organs.* Lyon, France: IARC Press; 2004. Used with permission.

heterogeneity within the tumor can be accurately determined. Epididymal lesions cannot be characterized with a similar degree of sensitivity. Computed tomography and magnetic resonance imaging are not used as primary diagnostic tools but can be helpful in tumor staging.

1. **Histologic typing and diagnosis of germ cell tumors** is made by examination of H&E-stained sections (*J Clin Pathol.* 2007;60:866). Gross examination can provide useful diagnostic clues as to tumor type. For instance, a white to gray, solid, homogenous, well-circumscribed appearance is characteristic of classic seminoma. Choriocarcinomas show extensive areas of hemorrhage and necrosis, whereas teratomas are multicystic and nodular, and may have grossly visible cartilage or bone. Embryonal carcinomas are smaller, soft, tan-white, and show hemorrhage and necrosis. Yolk sac tumors may show gelatinous, mucoid, and cystic areas. Lymphomas are fleshy and ill defined and often exhibit extratesticular extension. Scarring may represent a regressed germ cell tumor. Because many germ cell tumors are of mixed type, the importance of adequate sampling of heterogenous areas cannot be overemphasized.

2. **Histopathologic diagnosis** is based on the presence of one (pure) or more (mixed) histologic types.

a. **Intratubular germ cell neoplasia of unclassified type (IGCNU)**, a precursor of invasive germ cell neoplasia, may be found in isolated form or adjacent to invasive germ cell tumors. Patients with infertility, cryptorchidism, intersex syndrome, gonadal dysgenesis, a history of invasive germ cell tumor in the contralateral testis, or a retroperitoneal germ cell tumor have an increased likelihood of development of IGCNU. The high sensitivity of testicular biopsy in detecting IGCNU makes it a useful screening tool in these subgroups of patients. IGCNU is not recognizable grossly. Histologically, the seminiferous tubules show enlarged neoplastic cells with clear cytoplasm and prominent nucleoli, and often a thickened tunica propria (e-**Fig. 28.9**). Mitoses may be seen. Normal spermatogenesis is lacking. The surrounding stroma may show a prominent lymphocytic response. The presence of scattered neoplastic germ cells in the surrounding stroma qualifies as microinvasion (e-**Fig. 28.10**). Occasionally, the neoplastic cells spread along the tubules or the rete testis in a pagetoid fashion (e-**Fig. 28.11**). Periodic acid–Schiff histochemical stains highlight glycogen in the cytoplasm of IGCNU cells; immunohistochemically, PLAP, CD117 (c-kit), and OCT4 (e-**Fig. 28.12**) positivity are observed (*Semin Diagn Pathol.* 2005;22:33). In infants up to 1 year of age, and in patients with delayed germ cell maturation (cryptorchidism or gonadal dysgenesis), intratubular germ cells can resemble IGCNU morphologically and by PLAP or OCT4 staining (*Am J Surg Pathol.* 2006;30:1427), so caution is advised in diagnosing IGCNU in these cases. About 90% of pure IGCNU cases progress to invasive disease within 7 years.

b. **Seminoma** comprises almost 40% to 50% of all testicular germ cell tumors. Grossly, it has a homogeneous white to gray cut surface (e-**Fig. 28.13**). Necrosis may be seen, but hemorrhage and cystic change are uncommon. Histologically, seminoma is composed of a diffuse sheet of uniform cells. The cells may be separated into nests, clusters, or columns by delicate fibrous septae infiltrated by mature lymphocytes (e-**Fig. 28.14**). A parenchymal or intratubular granulomatous reaction may be present (e-**Fig. 28.15**). The granulomatous inflammation can be so extensive, both in the testis and in the draining lymph nodes, that the tumor cells are nearly obscured, resulting in a misdiagnosis of granulomatous orchitis. The tumor may entirely replace the normal testicular parenchyma, and may show an intratubular and less commonly an interstitial growth pattern. Other morphologic patterns include pseudoglandular (e-**Fig. 28.16**), tubular, cribriform, and occasionally microcystic appearances (*Am J Surg Pathol.* 2005;29:500). In these latter cases, membranous PLAP and c-kit positivity, together with a negative staining pattern for AFP, inhibin, pan-cytokeratin, and CD30 can be useful for differentiation from nonseminomatous germ cell tumors (Table 28.3). An OCT4 immunostain will mark seminoma and embryonal carcinoma, but not other germ cell tumor types (*Am J Surg Pathol.* 2004;28:935). Podoplanin immunoreactivity has been reported in seminomas but not embryonal carcinoma (*Ann Diagn Pathol.* 2010;14:331); CD117 (c-kit) (e-**Fig. 28.17**) is likewise immunopositive in seminomas and so can also be useful in separating these two entities in difficult cases. Foci of scarring may indicate a regressed germ cell tumor, and areas of calcification should prompt a search for possible foci of gonadoblastoma. Although brisk mitotic activity (>6 mitoses per high-power field) is observed in some tumors, there is little evidence to support that this denotes a worse prognosis, although it has been hypothesized that this finding may indicate progression to embryonal carcinoma. Marked cytologic atypia and mitoses have been used in the past to define "anaplastic seminoma," but this is not a

TABLE 28.3	Immunophenotype of Testis Neoplasms											
Tumor type	LIN28	SALL4	PLAP	c-kit (CD117)	OCT4	CD30	AFP	AE1/ AE3	CK7	EMA	Inhibin	CD45 (LCA)
Seminoma	+	+	+	+	+	−	−	v	v	−	−	−
Spermatocytic seminoma	−	v	−	v	−	−	−	−	nd	−	nd	−
Embryonal carcinoma	+	+	+	−	+	+	v	+	+	−	−	−
Yolk sac tumor	+	+	+	−	−	v	+	+	−	−	−	−
Sertoli/Leydig cell tumor	−	−	−/v	−	−	nd	nd	−/v	nd	v	v/+	−
Lymphoma	−	−	−	−	−	v	nd	−	nd	−	−	+

+, ≥80% of cases positive; v, variable staining (20–80% of cases); −, ≤20% of cases positive; nd, no data.
Modified from *Semin Diagn Pathol.* 2005;22:33, with additional data on LIN28 and SALL4.

currently recognized subtype of seminoma. Scattered multinucleated syncytiotrophoblasts are seen in up to 10% of seminomas (e-Fig. 28.18); this finding has no prognostic significance, but is important to diagnose such cases as seminoma with syncytiotrophoblastic cells because this may correlate with a mildly elevated serum hCG level. However, seminoma with syncytiotrophoblastic cells does need to be differentiated from choriocarcinoma; the lack of a cytotrophoblastic component is helpful in this regard. Other important entities in the differential diagnosis of seminoma include inflammatory conditions (especially in the presence of a prominent lymphocytic response), spermatocytic seminoma, and sex cord/stromal tumors (*Adv Anat Pathol.* 2008;15:18).

c. **Spermatocytic seminoma** is rare and lacks the associations (i.e., cryptorchidism and IGCNU) commonly seen with classic seminoma (*Arch Pathol Lab Med.* 2009;133:1985). This neoplasm is seen in older patients, and is more often than not unilateral. Extratesticular extension is rare. The tumor cells are noncohesive and arranged in sheets, and are of three types: small lymphocyte-like with dark nuclei and scant cytoplasm, intermediate with round nuclei and moderate eosinophilic cytoplasm, and large with single or multiple nuclei (e-Fig. 28.19). The presence of stromal edema may cause the tumor cells to appear to be nested or pseudoglandular. Mitoses are frequent, but a lymphocytic or granulomatous response is usually not present. The main differential diagnosis is with classic seminoma and lymphoma. Clinicomorphologic features and, if necessary, PLAP and OCT4 immunostains are useful in the distinction from classic seminomas (Table 28.3); lymphomas are more often bilateral and extratesticular, and have a more monomorphic cell population. Only one case of metastatic pure spermatocytic seminoma has been reported, and so radical orchiectomy alone is curative for almost all patients with spermatocytic seminoma. Spermatocytic seminoma with sarcoma is an aggressive variant of spermatocytic seminoma associated with a high-grade sarcomatous component such as rhabdomyosarcoma or chondrosarcoma, and has been described in about a dozen cases; no known etiology or familial predisposition has been reported, and most patients present with metastatic disease.

d. **Embryonal carcinoma** occurs in young adults, most commonly as a component of a mixed germ cell tumor. Grossly, hemorrhage and necrosis are common (e-Fig. 28.20). The tumor cells are large and undifferentiated with an epithelial appearance, and are arranged in a solid, papillary, and/or glandular pattern (e-**Fig. 28.21**). Nuclei are polygonal and vesicular with coarse chromatin. Mitotic activity and necrosis are extensive. IGCNU can be present at the periphery and frequently displays intratubular necrosis. Vascular invasion can be seen (e-**Fig. 28.22**) and should be differentiated from retraction artifact and artificial implantation during sampling. Pan-cytokeratin, SALL4, OCT4, and CD30 positivity is seen in tumor cells; PLAP and AFP are only focally positive in pure tumors. Epithelial membrane antigen (EMA) is negative, which is important in the differential diagnosis with somatic carcinomas (Table 28.3). Evaluation of H&E-stained slides is usually sufficient to establish the diagnosis; in occasional cases, immunohistochemistry is needed to help differentiate embryonal carcinoma from yolk sac tumor, seminoma, anaplastic large-cell lymphoma, and/or choriocarcinoma.

e. **Yolk sac tumor (endodermal sinus tumor)** shows differentiation reminiscent of embryonic yolk sac, allantois, and extraembryonic mesenchyme. In infants and young children, it tends to occur in pure form, whereas in adults it is found as a component of malignant mixed germ cell tumors. The morphologic appearance is varied and includes reticular (most common), microcystic, endodermal sinus-like (with Schiller–Duval bodies), papillary, solid, glandular, alveolar, enteric, polyvesicular vitelline, and hepatoid patterns (e-**Fig. 28.23**). Rarely, a neoplastic spindle cell component has been observed in association with the myxomatous and reticular variants. The immunoprofile reveals AFP, glypican 3, SALL4 (e-**Fig. 28.24**), PLAP, and low-molecular-weight cytokeratin positivity. IGCNU is commonly seen in adult yolk sac tumors but not as frequently in childhood yolk sac tumors. Embryonal carcinoma may, in certain foci, be difficult to distinguish from yolk sac tumor, and indeed the two tumor types can appear to merge; however, embryonal carcinoma nuclei are usually more pleomorphic, and immunostains can help in difficult cases (Table 28.3). Follicle-like areas of granulosa cell tumors in infants may resemble the solid and cystic pattern of yolk sac tumor, and the enteric pattern may appear similar to glandular areas in teratoma; usually, the former problem can be resolved with immunohistochemical stains for AFP and inhibin.

f. **Trophoblastic tumors** are almost always choriocarcinoma. Pure choriocarcinoma is extremely rare; instead, choriocarcinoma most commonly occurs as a component of mixed germ cell tumors. Grossly, necrotic and hemorrhagic nodules can be observed. Microscopically, the more viable peripheral areas show randomly admixed syncytiotrophoblasts, cytotrophoblasts, and intermediate trophoblasts, although one component may predominate giving rise to a monophasic tumor (e-**Fig. 28.25**); the tumor has a propensity for vascular invasion (e-**Fig. 28.25**). Very rare tumors composed of intermediate trophoblastic cells resembling placental site trophoblastic tumor have also been reported. The syncytiotrophoblasts are positive for hCG, the alpha subunit of inhibin, and EMA, and the intermediate trophoblasts are reactive for human placental lactogen (HPL); all cell types are positive for cytokeratin. The differential diagnosis includes syncytiotrophoblast-rich seminoma, and isolated syncytiotrophoblasts found in nonseminomatous germ cell tumors.

g. **Teratomas** include mature and immature teratoma, dermoid cyst, monodermal teratoma, and teratoma with somatic-type malignancies. The age distribution is bimodal. Teratomas occurring in children are benign, whereas those in young adults have significant rates of metastases despite their histologic appearance. Grossly, there are cystic and solid areas, and cartilage (e-**Fig. 28.26**) and bone may be evident. Microscopically, teratomas may show well-differentiated elements derived from one (monodermal) or all three germ layers (ectoderm, mesoderm, and endoderm), or may be immature with fetal-type tissue. Skin and its appendages, respiratory and intestinal-type epithelium, cartilage, and muscular tissue are common (e-**Fig. 28.27A** and **B**); neural-type tissue is less frequent. Immature tissues can resemble renal blastema or embryonic neural tube (**Fig. 28.28**). Foci with the appearance of a primitive neuroectodermal tumor (PNET) have been classified as such if present. Pure teratomas are much less common than the finding of teratoma as an element of a mixed malignant germ cell tumor.

Dermoid cysts, which harbor keratinizing squamous epithelium and skin appendages, are very rare and are benign. Epidermoid cysts lack skin appendages and possibly represent monodermal teratomas; grossly, epidermoid cysts are distinctive with a ringlike "onion-skin" cut surface (e-**Figs. 28.29** and **28.30**).

Several nongerm cell malignant tumors, characterized by expansile growth of at least a 4× field, including adenocarcinoma, squamous cell carcinoma, neuroendocrine tumors, sarcomas, and PNET have been known to arise in primary or metastatic teratomas.

Immunostains are not usually necessary for the diagnosis of teratoma, but it is noteworthy that AFP immunopositivity can be present in intestinal-type areas of teratomas.

h. **Tumors of more than one histologic type** (mixed forms), termed "**mixed malignant germ cell tumor**," are germ cell neoplasms composed of more than one type of tumor. They comprise approximately 30% of all germ cell tumors, and the most frequently encountered components include embryonal carcinoma (in about one half of the cases), yolk sac tumor (one half), and teratoma (about 40%). About 40% of mixed malignant germ cell tumors also contain scattered syncytiotrophoblasts. A rare subtype of mixed germ cell tumor is the polyembryoma with characteristic embryoid bodies with central cores of embryonal carcinoma (forming the dorsal amnion-like cavity) and a surrounding (ventral) yolk sac component. Mixed germ cell tumors with an embryonal component are predictive of a higher stage than tumors with a large seminomatous component, so for mixed tumors it is very important to quantitate, on a percentage basis, the amount of embryonal carcinoma (as well as all other components). Tumors with a yolk sac or teratoma component show a lower incidence of metastatic disease.

i. **Burnt out (regressed) germ cell tumors** are germ cell tumors in which the primary tumor in the testis has undergone necrosis and fibrosis. This most commonly occurs with seminoma (*Am J Surg Pathol.* 2006;30:858) and choriocarcinoma. The most specific histologic finding of a regressed germ cell tumor is a distinct scar (e-**Fig. 28.31**) in association with either IGCNU or coarse intratubular calcifications; however, many cases lack these latter two features (*Am J Surg Pathol.* 2006;30:858). Some patients may present with metastatic disease, the only evidence of the testicular primary being a scar, with or without IGCNU.

j. **New immunophenotypic markers** that are transcription factors involved in the maintenance of stem cell pluripotency have been developed for germ cell tumors. These markers include SALL4, OCT4, NANOG, SOX2, and SOX17, and all demonstrate a nuclear pattern of expression. SALL4 labels all IGCNUs, classic seminomas, embryonal carcinomas, and yolk sac tumors (*Am J Surg Pathol.* 2009;33:1065). Choriocarcinoma, teratoma, and spermatocytic seminoma are also variably positive for SALL4. Both OCT4 and NANOG label IGCNU, classic seminoma, and embryonal carcinoma (*Am J Surg Pathol.* 2004;28:935; *Histopathology.* 2005;47:48).

SOX2 only labels embryonal carcinoma and teratoma (*Am J Surg Pathol.* 2007;31:836; *J Pathol.* 2008;215: 21) and SOX17 labels IGCNU, classic seminoma, and yolk sac tumor (*J Pathol.* 2008;215: 21; *Am J Clin Pathol.* 2009;131:131). Among these markers, SALL4 demonstrates the highest sensitivity and showed particular utility for yolk sac tumors. For yolk sac tumors, SALL4 is much more sensitive than PLAP, AFP, and glypican-3 (*Am J Surg Pathol.* 2009;33:1065). SALL4 is also particularly useful in differentiating metastatic germ cell tumors from metastatic carcinoma of nontesticular origin, a setting in which it has been found to be more sensitive than OCT3/4 (*Cancer.* 2009;115:2640).

More recently, an RNA-binding protein LIN28 has been discovered as a novel sensitive and general germ cell tumor marker, which shows sensitivity similar to SALL4 (*Hum Pathol.* 2010;42:710). A potential diagnostic pitfall that must be kept in mind is that all new markers described above are also expressed in early fetal germ cells. SALL4 is also expressed in spermatogonia in both children and adults (*Am J Surg Pathol.* 2009;33:1065).

  k. Molecular genetics is not currently used in diagnosis. The only exception is detection of isochromosome 12p by fluorescence in situ hybridization to identify metastatic germ cell neoplasms, since gain of material in 12p is the most common structural chromosomal alteration in invasive germ cell tumors (*Mod Pathol.* 2004;17:1309).

B. Sex cord/gonadal stromal tumors comprise 4% to 6% of all testicular tumors in adults and include Leydig cell tumor, Sertoli cell tumor, granulosa cell tumor, thecoma, and fibroma.

  1. Leydig cell tumors are the most common and are known to occur in patients with gynecomastia, Klinefelter syndrome, and cryptorchidism. Grossly, the tumor cut surface is homogeneous, solid, and brown to yellow. The tumor cells are large and polygonal, and have abundant eosinophilic, lipid-laden cytoplasm (**e-Fig. 28.32**). The characteristic Reinke crystals are found in only 30% of cases. The tumor cells are positive for inhibin, calretinin, and Melan-A by immunohistochemistry. The main differential diagnoses are Leydig cell hyperplasia and syndromic adrenogenital tumors. Leydig cell tumors form a nodule without seminiferous tubules, whereas in Leydig cell hyperplasia, the foci are bilateral and multifocal, and wrap around and extend between the tubules (**e-Fig. 28.33**); adrenogenital tumors are bilateral and dark brown, with pigmentation and fibrous stroma. About 90% of Leydig cell tumors are benign, but constellation of features, including size >5 cm, cytologic atypia, increased mitotic activity, necrosis, and vascular invasion, favors malignancy.

  2. Sertoli cell tumors account for only 1% of all testicular tumors. Grossly, the mass is usually well circumscribed, with tan-yellow to white, sometimes hemorrhagic cut surfaces (**e-Fig. 28.34**). The pathologic subtypes are the lipid-rich, large cell calcifying (**e-Fig. 28.35**), and sclerosing variants. The known clinical associations are with Carney syndrome, Peutz–Jeghers syndrome (which can be associated with bilateral tumors), and androgen insensitivity syndrome. Histologically, the cytologically bland cells are arranged in tubules, potentially with retiform, tubular-glandular, and solid nodular areas. The tubules can be closed (solid) (**e-Fig. 28.36**) and are surrounded by a basement membrane. Intratubular growth can be present. Sertoli cell tumors should be distinguished from small incidental Sertoli cell nodules (benign and thought to be nonneoplastic) as can be seen in cryptorchid testes. The tumor cells are cytokeratin and sometimes inhibin and calretinin positive, but PLAP and OCT4 negative, by immunohistochemistry. Malignant Sertoli cell tumors are rare.

  3. Granulosa cell tumors and **thecoma/fibroma tumors** are similar in appearance to those in the ovary, and are rare in the testis. There are two granulosa cell tumor variants in the testis, the adult and juvenile types, as in the ovary.

C. **Mixed germ cell and sex cord/gonadal stromal tumors** include gonadoblastoma, most commonly seen in the setting of mixed gonadal dysgenesis, ambiguous genitalia, and 45X/46XY mosaicism. Microscopic examination shows two cell populations: a germ cell component resembling seminoma and a component resembling immature Sertoli cells (e-**Fig. 28.37**). Round deposits of basement membrane-like material and coarse calcification are common features. A large number of patients develop invasive germ cell tumors, particularly seminoma, and so patients are treated with bilateral orchiectomy.

D. **Miscellaneous tumors** of the testis include carcinoid tumors, tumors of ovarian epithelial types (serous borderline tumor, serous carcinoma, mucinous cystadenomas and cystadenocarcinomas, Brenner tumor, and endometrioid carcinoma), nephroblastoma, and paraganglioma.

E. **Hematolymphoid neoplasms**, of which the most common is malignant lymphoma, comprise 5% of all testicular malignancies. These are the most common bilateral tumors of the testis, and their incidence is higher in elderly men. The most common subtype is diffuse large B-cell lymphoma. The growth pattern is typically intertubular (e-**Fig. 28.38**), and the main differential diagnosis is with seminoma, especially the spermatocytic type. Immunostains can be helpful in establishing the diagnosis (Table 28.3). The prognosis is generally poor. Young age, low stage, and presence of sclerosis are indicators of a good prognosis. Isolated plasmacytoma of the testis is rare.

F. **Tumors of the collecting ducts and rete.** Benign tumors of the rete include adenoma, cystadenoma, and adenofibroma. Adenocarcinomas of the rete are rare, and their diagnosis is subject to strict histologic criteria that include tumor centered on testicular hilum, morphology distinct from any other testicular/paratesticular tumor, solid growth pattern, transition between tumor and normal tissue, and absence of histologically similar extratesticular malignancy (especially lung and prostate). The main histologic patterns are tubular, papillary, and solid. The main differential diagnoses are extratesticular adenocarcinomas and mesothelioma. The tumor shows extensive regional spread and distant metastasis, and the overall prognosis is poor.

G. **Tumors of the paratesticular organs.**

   1. **Benign.** The most common benign neoplasm of the testicular adnexa is **adenomatoid tumor,** representing almost 60% of all cases. These are of mesothelial origin (*Semin Diagn Pathol.* 2000;17:294) and arise in the upper or lower pole of the epididymis as solitary, round to oval nodules invariably <5 cm in size. Histologically, the tumor shows round to oval or slit-like tubules in a fibrous, hyalinized, and/or muscular stroma (e-**Fig. 28.39** and **28.40**). The lining cells are columnar or flat with vacuolated cytoplasm. Adenomatoid tumors show immunoreactivity for cytokeratin, EMA, and mesothelial markers including calretinin and WT-1. The tumor should be differentiated from signet-ring-cell carcinoma and mesothelioma; tumors with a more diffuse growth pattern simulate Sertoli or Leydig cell tumors (inhibin positivity, lipofuscin pigment, and presence of Reinke crystals favor Leydig cell tumor).

   Another benign paratesticular tumor is **papillary cystadenoma of epididymis** (e-**Fig. 28.41**). About two-thirds of cases are seen in patients with von Hippel–Lindau disease, and in this setting, the tumor tends to be bilateral.

   A much rarer entity is the **retinal anlage tumor** or the melanotic neuroectodermal tumor, which is composed of two cell populations: larger melanin-containing cells and smaller neuroblast-like cells.

   2. **Malignant.** Malignant mesothelioma of the testicular adnexa has a microscopic appearance and immunophenotypic profile similar to those of mesothelioma of the pleura. The main differential diagnoses are with adenomatoid tumor, which is better circumscribed, and with carcinoma of the rete testis.

Primary **adenocarcinoma** of the epididymis is rare, and may histologically and cytologically simulate a cystadenoma due to the presence of columnar cells with clear cytoplasm containing glycogen. Metastatic adenocarcinoma from other organs should also be excluded.

Desmoplastic small round cell tumor occurs in the epididymis of young adults. Molecular, genetic, histologic, and immunohistochemical features are similar to those of the tumor when it occurs at more conventional sites such as the peritoneum. The tumor should be differentiated from other small blue cell tumors such as malignant lymphoma and embryonal rhabdomyosarcoma.

Mesenchymal tumors of the scrotum, paratesticular organs, and spermatic cord include benign neoplasms such as lipoma, leiomyoma, neurofibroma, and granular cell tumor and malignant tumors such as liposarcoma, leiomyosarcoma (e-**Fig. 28.42**), malignant fibrous histiocytoma, and rhabdomyosarcoma (e-**Figs. 28.43** and **28.44**).

H. Secondary malignancies include metastatic adenocarcinomas from the prostate (e-**Fig. 28.45**), lung, and colon, and melanoma.

V. PATHOLOGIC STAGING applies only to germ cell neoplasms of the testis (Fig. 28.1). The 2010 Tumor, Node, Metastasis (TNM) American Joint Committee on

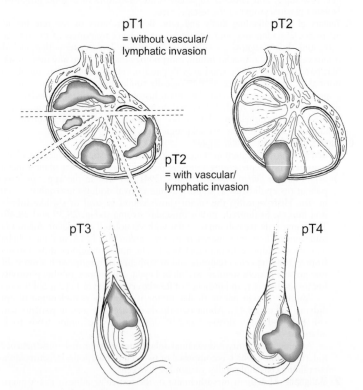

Figure 28.1 Pathologic staging of germ cell tumors of the testis. (Modified from: Greene FL, Compton CC, Fritz AG, et al., eds. *AJCC Cancer Staging Atlas*. New York, NY: Springer; 2006.)

TABLE 28.4	TNM Staging Scheme for Germ Cell Tumors of the Testes

Primary tumor (T)

pTX	Primary tumor cannot be assessed
pT0	No evidence of primary tumor (e.g., histologic scar in the testes)
pTis	IGCN (carcinoma in situ)
pT1	Tumor limited to the testis and epididymis without vascular/lymphatic invasion, tumor may invade into the tunica albuginea but not the tunica vaginalis
pT2	Tumor limited to the testis and epididymis with vascular/lymphatic invasion, or tumor extending through the tunica albuginea with the involvement of the tunica vaginalis
pT3	Tumor invades the spermatic cord with or without vascular/lymphatic invasion
pT4	Tumor invades the scrotum with or without vascular/lymphatic invasion

Regional lymph nodes (N)

Clinical

NX	Regional lymph nodes cannot be assessed
N0	No regional lymph node metastasis
N1	Metastasis with a lymph node mass of ≤2 cm in greatest dimension or multiple lymph nodes, none >2 cm in greatest dimension
N2	Metastasis with a lymph node mass of >2 cm but not >5 cm in greatest dimension; or multiple lymph nodes, any one mass >2 cm but not >5 cm in greatest dimension
N3	Metastasis with a lymph node mass >5 cm in greatest dimension

Pathologic (PN)

pNx	Regional lymph nodes cannot be assessed
pN0	No regional lymph node metastasis
pN1	Metastasis with a lymph node mass of ≤2 cm in greatest dimension and ≤5 nodes positive, none >2 cm in greatest dimension
pN2	Metastasis with a lymph node mass of >2 cm but not >5 cm in greatest dimension; or >5 nodes positive, none >5 cm; or evidence of extranodal extension of tumor
pN3	Metastasis with a lymph node mass >5 cm in greatest dimension

Distant metastasis (M)

M0	No distant metastasis
M1	Distant metastasis
M1a	Nonregional nodal or pulmonary metastasis
M1b	Distant metastasis other than nonregional lymph nodes and lungs

Serum tumor markers (S)

SX	Marker studies not available or not performed
S0	Marker study levels within normal limits
S1	LDH <1.5 × N* and hCG (mIu/mL) <5000 and AFP (ng/mL) <1000
S2	LDH 1.5–10 × N or hCG (mIu/mL) 5000–50,000 or AFP (ng/mL) 1000–10,000
S3	LDH >10 × N or hCG (mIu/mL) >50,000 or AFP (ng/mL) >10,000

(continued)

Cancer/International Union Against Cancer (AJCC/UICC) staging classification is given in Table 28.4. Clinical staging should be distinguished from pathologic staging.

VI. **REPORTING OF GERM CELL NEOPLASMS** should follow suggested guidelines (College of American Pathologists testis cancer protocol and checklists at

TABLE 28.4	TNM Staging Scheme for Germ Cell Tumors of the Testes (*Continued*)

Stage grouping

Stage 0	pTis	N0	M0	S0
Stage I	pT1-4	N0	M0	SX
Stage IA	pT1	N0	M0	S0
Stage IB	pT2	N0	M0	S0
	pT3	N0	M0	S0
	pT4	N0	M0	S0
Stage IS	Any pT/Tx	N0	M0	S1–3
Stage II	Any pT/Tx	N1–3	M0	SX
Stage IIA	Any pT/Tx	N1	M0	S0
	Any pT/Tx	N1	M0	S1
Stage IIB	Any pT/Tx	N2	M0	S0
	Any pT/Tx	N2	M0	S1
Stage IIC	Any pT/Tx	N3	M0	S0
	Any pT/Tx	N3	M0	S1
Stage III	Any pT/Tx	Any N	M1	SX
Stage IIIA	Any pT/Tx	Any N	M1a	S0
	Any pT/Tx	Any N	M1a	S1
Stage IIIB	Any pT/Tx	N1–3	M0	S2
	Any pT/Tx	Any N	M1a	S2
Stage IIIC	Any pT/Tx	N1–3	M0	S3
	Any pT/Tx	Any N	M1a	S3
	Any pT/Tx	Any N	M1b	Any S

Except for pTis and pT4, extent of primary tumor is classified by radical orchiectomy. TX may be used for other categories in the absence of radical orchiectomy.
LDH, low-density lipoprotein; hCG, human chorionic gonadotropin; AFP, alpha-fetoprotein; N*, upper limit of normal.
From: Edge SB, Byrd DR, Compton CC, et al., eds. *AJCC Cancer Staging Manual.* 7th ed. New York, NY: Springer; 2010. Used with permission.

http://www.cap.org). The basic elements that need to be included for the primary tumor are size, multifocality, and presence or absence of involvement of extratesticular tissues including the epididymis, tunica vaginalis (via penetration through the tunica albuginea), spermatic cord, and scrotum (if present). Note that the rete testis is not considered to be an extratesticular structure. Histologic typing should follow the WHO classification (Table 28.2) and, for mixed tumors, the percentage of each component should be provided; it is particularly critical to assess for the presence and amount of embryonal carcinoma. It is also vital to report on the presence or absence of lymphovascular invasion. Spermatic cord margin status should be given. For metastatic deposits, the histologic components and tumor viability should be reported. Postchemotherapy, the report should indicate whether the viable tumor is teratoma or another germ cell component.

29 Prostate

Peter A. Humphrey

I. **NORMAL ANATOMY.** The normal weight of the prostate is 20 g for ages 20 to 50, and 30 g for ages 60 to 80. Anatomically, the prostate gland comprises three zones: central zone, transition zone (where benign prostatic hyperplasia [BPH] occurs), and peripheral zone (where most carcinomas originate). (e-Fig. 29.1).* Microscopically, the normal adult prostate is a branching duct-acinar glandular system embedded in a dense fibromuscular stroma (e-Fig. 29.2). The epithelium has two layers: a luminal or secretory cell layer and a basal cell layer. Central zone epithelium can normally have architectural patterns that include cribriform and Roman bridge-like structures (e-Fig. 29.3).

II. **GROSS EXAMINATION, TISSUE SAMPLING, AND HISTOLOGIC SLIDE PREPARATION.** The most common prostatic parenchymal tissue samples examined in surgical pathology laboratories in the United States are, in order, 18-gauge needle cores, transurethral resection of prostate (TURP) chips, radical prostatectomy specimens, and fine needle aspirates.

A. **Needle cores.** Needle core biopsy sample handling and processing begins in the room where the procedure is performed. The needle biopsy tissue should be immediately placed into a container with fixative, which is usually 10% neutral buffered formalin, although a few laboratories prefer Bouin's solution, Hollande's solution, or IBF fixative. Bouin and Hollande's solutions are picric acid-based fixatives that provide superior nuclear detail, but these strong oxidizing agents can react violently with combustible materials and reducing agents. Fixation in formalin should be for at least 6 hours. The number of cores received per container is highly variable, from 1 to >20. If the urologist and treating physician desire site-specific diagnosis, the core(s) should be placed in separate site-designated containers. Inking of cores to indicate site, with placement of cores marked with different colors into the same container, should not be performed because fragmentation renders site assignment impossible. Gross examination of prostate needle core tissue is not diagnostic, but is important for correlation with amount of tissue seen in the histologic sections and so it is vital to record, for each container, the size and number of tissue cores or fragments. It is recommended that no more than two cores be submitted per cassette for processing and embedding; some laboratories submit one core per cassette. Prostate cores can be marked with ink, which facilitates identification during embedding and the ability to see the cores in the paraffin blocks. Regardless, the cores should be placed into a cassette after being put into a fine mesh envelope, wrapped in lens paper, sandwiched between sponge pads, or double-embedded in agar–paraffin wax. After processing, the cores should be embedded in the same plane, in the same direction, with even spacing. From each paraffin block, three hematoxylin and eosin (H&E)-stained slides should be prepared, with three to four serial sections on each slide. Some laboratories cut interval, unstained sections on coated slides in case special studies such as immunohistochemistry are needed. Clinical requests for frozen section diagnosis of prostate needle cores are rare and should be restricted to patients with clinical evidence of metastatic cancer who are to undergo immediate treatment (usually orchiectomy) for pain relief.

---

*All e-figures are available online via the Solution Site Image Bank.

B. **TURP chips.** The amount of prostate tissue resected in TURP procedures is variable, ranging from 5 to >75 g of tissue, with a mean of about 25 g. The gross description should include the aggregate weight of the chips. Recognizable gross features such as yellow coloration and induration can be recorded, but it has not been proven that chip color, size, or induration is linked to cancer presence, so gross selection of specific chips is not required. Although gross TURP chip sampling procedures are not standardized, one initial approach is to submit 12 g of chips or 6 to 8 blocks of tissue (with 1 to 2 g per cassette). For specimens >12 g, the initial 12 g are submitted, with one cassette for every additional 5 g (*Arch Pathol Lab Med.* 2009;133:1568). If the patient is younger than 60 years, all tissue should be submitted; all chip tissue should also be submitted if microscopic examination of partially submitted chips reveals carcinoma in <5% of tissue, or if high-grade prostatic intraepithelial neoplasia (PIN) or atypical glands (atypical small acinar proliferation [ASAP]) is found in sections of partially submitted chips. One H&E-stained slide, with one or two sections, is typically generated from each paraffin block of TURP chips.

C. **Open suprapubic or retropubic simple prostatectomy (enucleation) tissue.** The prostatic tissue from simple prostatectomies may be submitted to the pathology laboratory as a single mass or as pieces. The prostatectomy tissue should be weighed and sectioned at 3- to 5-mm intervals. The gross description for each piece should include size in three dimensions, weight, firmness, and coloration. Hard nodules should be sampled, and a total of eight cassettes or one cassette of tissue for each 5 g of tissue submitted. Additional tissue should be submitted if carcinoma is histologically detected in initial sections of partially submitted tissue, although no rules or recommendations exist on how many additional sections are required. One H&E-stained slide should be made per block.

D. **Radical prostatectomy.** The entire prostate gland is excised in prostate cancer surgery using open retropubic or perineal approaches, or using laparoscopic (including robotic) approaches. The prostate gland is also resected in toto in radical cystoprostatectomy for bladder cancer.

1. **Pelvic lymph nodes.** Pelvic lymphadenectomy may be performed as a separate procedure, often laparoscopic, or during the radical prostatectomy operation. Sentinel lymph node sampling is not routinely performed.

    Frozen section analysis of the sampled lymph nodes may be requested for patients at risk for nodal metastasis, on the basis of serum prostate-specific antigen (PSA) level, needle biopsy Gleason score, and clinical stage. All grossly recognizable lymph nodes should be examined by frozen section; cytologic touch imprints can be made at the same time. Frozen section diagnosis of metastatic carcinoma in lymph nodes is highly specific, but fairly insensitive. The low sensitivity rate of 58% to 73% is due to sampling error.

    Gross sampling of tissue after frozen section should entail submission of all grossly identifiable lymph node tissue and wide sampling of associated adipose tissue. The gross description of pelvic lymph nodes should include number, location, and size. One H&E-stained slide is made per paraffin block. Special studies to detect occult lymph node metastases, such as immunohistochemistry for cytokeratins or PSA, or reverse transcription–polymerase chain reaction (RT–PCR) for PSA RNA, are currently experimental and not performed in routine practice.

2. **Prostate gland and seminal vesicles.** The prostate gland and seminal vesicles from radical prostatectomy procedures may be received fresh or in fixative. All three dimensions and specimen weight should be recorded. Frozen section requests on fresh specimens are uncommon, and are usually made to evaluate margin status; this procedure has a high false-negative rate and is not standard practice. Fresh specimens are also used for tissue-banking protocols; after inking the entire outside of the specimen, tissue can be harvested from

inside the gland while preserving the inked periphery. Alternatively, after inking, margin sampling, and seminal vesicle amputation (see below), the whole unfixed gland can be sectioned with a large sharp knife from apex to base at 4-mm intervals perpendicular to the prostatic urethra; areas suspicious for carcinoma, as judged by palpation or visual inspection, may be sampled by imprints, scrapes, core biopsy, or small wedge sections.

Fixation of the inked radical prostatectomy specimens (sectioned or unsectioned) is accomplished by at least overnight (or 24 to 48 hour) room temperature immersion in 10% neutral buffered formalin at 10 times the volume of the specimen. For gross examination of unsectioned glands after inking, the seminal vesicles are amputated (including the soft tissue and prostatic tissue at the base of the seminal vesicles) and submitted separately as right and left seminal vesicles. The prostate weight without the seminal vesicles is recorded, and distal apical (urethral) and bladder neck margins are taken if not already submitted separately by the surgeon. The distal apical margin is evaluated by amputating the distal 5 to 10 mm of the gland, dividing it into the right and left sides, and submitting radial sections (as for a cervical cone biopsy). The bladder neck margin can be assessed by a thin 2-mm shave margin or by conization; the latter is recommended. Ink on tumor cells is indicative of a positive margin for cone sections and the peripheral margin, whereas tumor anywhere in shave margin tissue indicates a positive margin. Vasa deferentia stumps may be sampled using *en face* sections, but this is not routine. The prostate gland is serially sectioned in a plane perpendicular to the urethra at 3- to 5-mm intervals using a long knife. The cut surfaces should be evaluated for gross evidence of BPH and carcinoma. Photographs or digital images can be used to document location and gross appearance of tissue in submitted cassettes. Diagrams (Fig. 29.1) or pictorial maps can also be used to indicate location of sections and any gross abnormalities.

Both complete and partial embedding methods are acceptable (*Mod Pathol.* 2011;24:6). Several protocols for partial submission have been published (*Scand J Urol Nephrol Suppl.* 2005;216:34; *Mod Pathol.* 2011;24:6). When there is grossly visible tumor, all lesions grossly suspicious for carcinoma should be submitted, along with distal apical and bladder neck margins and seminal vesicles. For cases with no grossly evident tumor, the posterior aspect of each transverse slice is submitted, as well as a mid-anterior block from each side, distal apical and bladder neck margins, and the seminal vesicles. Sections should be submitted as quarters or halves of the prostate, depending on gland size. Whole-amount sections are rarely made and do not provide additional morphologic information. If no or minimal tumor is seen in initial sections of a partially submitted gland, all remaining tissue should be embedded (including any frozen tissue sent to a tissue bank). If still no tumor is seen, basal cell and AMACR immunostains of atypical foci should be performed, and deeper sections should be obtained from block(s) from the region of the positive needle biopsy and areas of high-grade PIN. If cancer remains undetected, the tissue blocks should be flipped, and histologic sections prepared from the new tissue faces (*Mod Pathol.* 2011;24:6).

E. Cystoprostatectomy. The prostate gland in radical cystoprostatectomies performed for bladder cancer can be sampled by taking several sections of prostatic urethra and surrounding prostate tissue, any gross lesions, one block from the periphery of each side, and both seminal vesicles. The distal urethral shave margin is important in urothelial carcinoma cases.

III. DIAGNOSTIC FEATURES OF COMMON DISEASES OF THE PROSTATE

A. Inflammation and infection. Histopathologic identification of inflammatory cells in the prostate is common, but histologic identification of specific infectious agents is rare.

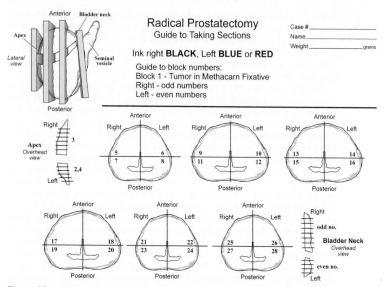

Figure 29.1 Diagram depicting guide to taking sections from a radical prostatectomy specimen. (Modified from: True LD. Surgical pathology examination of the prostate gland. Practice survey by American Society of Clinical Pathologists. *Am J Clin Pathol.* 1995;103:376.)

1. **Asymptomatic inflammatory prostatitis,** including acute neutrophilic inflammation and chronic lymphocytic, lymphoplasmacytic, or lymphohistiocytic inflammation, is common in all prostate tissue samples. Reporting this inflammation is optional; it may be useful to report if the inflammation is extensive or persistent in several needle core samples taken over time, because prostatic inflammation can raise the serum PSA. Inflammation can be associated with prostatic glandular atrophy, and reactive nuclear changes including prominent nucleoli. Inflammation is more commonly associated with benign epithelial conditions, especially atrophy and BPH, compared with high-grade PIN and carcinoma where usually only a small percentage of foci (around 10%) are inflamed.

2. **Granulomatous prostatitis** can clinically elevate the serum PSA and/or present as a palpable abnormality. The most common type is nonspecific granulomatous prostatitis, which is thought to be a response to prostatic secretions released into stroma by duct-acinar rupture. Microscopically, there is a lobulocentric noncaseating granulomatous inflammatory cell infiltrate with giant cells (**e-Fig. 29.4**). Variants include xanthogranulomatous prostatitis and prostatic "xanthoma." Other types of granulomatous prostatitis include infectious and postbiopsy/postresection cases. Infectious granulomatous prostatitis is most often Bacille Calmette–Guérin (BCG)-related in patients treated for bladder urothelial carcinoma (**e-Fig. 29.5**). Fungal prostatitis is rare and usually seen in immunosuppressed patients. Postbiopsy/resection granulomas are most often identified in TURP chip tissue, and are characterized by a fibrinoid central zone surrounded by palisading histiocytes.

B. **Atrophy** of prostatic glands is the benign condition most likely to be misdiagnosed as prostatic carcinoma by light microscopy. It is a common, age-related process that could be related to inflammation, hormones, obstruction, or ischemia. It can also be treatment related, due to radiotherapy or hormonal therapy.

Histologically, atrophy is defined as cytoplasmic volume loss. It is not necessary to subtype atrophy, but it is important to recognize the existence of different histomorphologic patterns including simple atrophy (with or without cystic change) (e-Fig. 29.6), sclerotic atrophy, partial atrophy (e-Fig. 29.7), and postatrophic hyperplasia (or hyperplastic atrophy) (e-Figs. 29.8 and 29.9). Atrophy can be confused with carcinoma because it is usually a small gland lesion that can show a pseudoinfiltrative pattern of growth, stromal sclerosis, nuclear atypia, and closely packed acini (in postatrophic hyperplasia). Atrophy can also be noted in cystically dilated peripheral zone glands (e-Fig. 29.10) and in cystic change in BPH nodules. Another diagnostic pitfall is that atrophic glands can show a fragmented basal cell layer and even loss of basal cells in a few glands by immunohistochemical stains (such as 34betaE12 and p63) (*Semin Diagn Pathol.* 2005;22:88). In addition, the selective but not specific marker for neoplastic epithelial cells alpha-methylacyl coenzyme A racemase (AMACR) can be immunopositive in atrophy, particularly partial atrophy.

C. **Metaplasia** or change in cell type in benign prostatic epithelium can be squamous, transitional cell (urothelial), mucinous, and eosinophilic. These metaplasias are usually secondary to inflammation, therapy, or injury. They are not preneoplastic.

1. **Squamous cell metaplasia** is most often an incidental finding associated with inflammation and infarction in BPH nodules. Microscopically, small, solid nests or partially involved glands with a retained lumen are common (e-Fig. 29.11). Squamoid cytoplasm and intercellular bridges may be evident, but keratin pearls are rare. Nuclear atypia, including prominent nuclei and mitoses, may be present in squamous metaplasia adjacent to infarcts. Squamous metaplasia postradiation or hormonal therapy can be more diffuse and is frequently immature with less cytoplasm and an absence of keratinization.

2. **Transitional cell or urothelial metaplasia** should be distinguished from urothelial cells that normally line the prostatic urethra and central ducts of the prostate. This is usually a focal, incidental finding with small, solid nests or partial gland involvement by cytologically bland and uniform elongated cells, with some cells exhibiting nuclear grooves and cytoplasmic clearing (e-Fig. 29.12).

3. **Mucinous metaplasia** is replacement of benign luminal epithelium by benign mucin-secretory cells. This is a focal, incidental microscopic finding in which the constituent cells have a granular blue cytoplasmic appearance (e-Fig. 29.13). Goblet cells and luminal secretion of the mucin are uncommon.

4. **Eosinophilic metaplasia** is the designation for benign epithelium with large supranuclear eosinophilic granules, which represent exocrine differentiation with lysosome-like granules. This uncommon and typically focal change is more often seen in prostatic ductal epithelium and is associated with variable degrees of chronic inflammation and atrophy. Paneth cell-like change, which is also characterized by large eosinophilic cytoplasmic granules, is usually seen in PIN and carcinoma and reflects neuroendocrine differentiation. Paneth cell-like alteration may be found in nonneoplastic prostatic epithelium after radiation.

D. **Hyperplasia.** BPH is a clinical diagnosis. Histologically, BPH can be diagnosed in TURP chips and simple and radical prostatectomy specimens, but it should not be diagnosed in needle biopsy tissue.

1. **Usual nodular epithelial and stromal hyperplasia** is the most common morphologic presentation of BPH. Grossly, the nodules, which characteristically arise in the transition zone and periurethral area, are multiple and vary from solid white to spongy with cystic change.

   a. **Pure stromal nodules (nodular stromal hyperplasia)** exist. Microscopically, the nodules can appear myxoid (e-Fig. 29.14), hyalinized, or leiomyomatous, with spindled, ovoid, or stellate cells. Prominent thick-walled blood vessels and lymphocytes may be noted.

b. **Mixed epithelial and stromal hyperplasia** is most common, with variable admixtures of spindled stromal cells and complex benign glands with complex papillary and branching architecture (e-**Fig. 29.15**). Cystic change, inflammation, and basal cell hyperplasia are commonly detected in BPH nodules. Fibroadenomatoid features (e-**Fig. 29.16**) can rarely be seen.

c. **Epithelial predominant BPH nodules** (e-**Fig. 29.17**) are unusual.

d. **Infarcts** can be identified in larger BPH nodules and can elevate the serum PSA.

2. **Basal cell hyperplasia** is usually discovered in BPH nodules, but can also be found in peripheral zone needle biopsy tissue, often associated with inflammation. Microscopically, there are two or more layers of basal cells arranged in acinar, cribriform, and solid growth patterns (e-**Fig. 29.18**). In usual basal cell hyperplasia, the basal cells are uniform and cytologically bland, whereas in so-called atypical basal cell hyperplasia prominent nucleoli are discerned. The term "atypical" should be avoided because no form of basal cell hyperplasia is a known risk factor for neoplasia.

3. **Cribriform hyperplasia** (e-**Fig. 29.19**), which is completely benign and not a risk factor for neoplasia, is an infrequently seen variant of BPH. The luminal lining cells are cytologically bland and there is a prominent rim of basal cells.

4. **Mesonephric remnant hyperplasia** is a very rare prostatic proliferation displaying a vaguely lobular or infiltrative pattern of small tubules with cuboidal epithelium and intraluminal, eosinophilic secretions (*Am J Surg Pathol.* 2011;35:1054). Immunostains for high-molecular-weight cytokeratin (34betaE12) and/or p63 can be negative in some cases, and AMACR can be focally positive. These results may raise concern for prostatic adenocarcinoma, but helpful clues are negative PSA and prostate-specific acid phosphatase (PSAP) but positive PAX8 immunostains.

5. **Verumontanum gland hyperplasia** is a benign, small gland proliferation of the verumontanum and adjacent posterior urethra (e-**Fig. 29.20**). The closely packed glands can architecturally be alarming, but the lack of nuclear atypia and the presence of basal cells rules out carcinoma.

E. **Atypical adenomatous hyperplasia (adenosis)** is a nodular proliferation of closely packed small acini (e-**Fig. 29.21**). It is invariably an incidental histologic finding, most often found in transition zone tissue in TURP chips or prostatectomy specimens. The densely packed small pale acini are sometimes intermingled with larger, more complex glands. Nuclear atypia is absent to minimal. The basal cell layer is fragmented, and, on average, 50% of glands completely lack basal cells. Of note, AMACR is diffusely positive in about 8% of cases. Adenosis can be mistaken for well-differentiated Gleason score 2 to 4 adenocarcinoma. It does not have known premalignant potential.

F. **Prostatic intraepithelial neoplasia (PIN)** is a proliferation of atypical epithelial cells in preexisting ducts and acini (synonyms used in the past include atypical hyperplasia and dysplasia). Currently, PIN is graded as low-grade PIN and high-grade PIN (HG-PIN), although only HG-PIN has potential clinical significance and merits reporting. Isolated HG-PIN is diagnosed in about 5% to 10% of needle biopsies (*J Urol.* 2006;175:820). It is found in the vast majority of radical prostatectomy specimens with prostatic carcinoma. Microscopically, there are four major structural patterns of HG-PIN growth: tufting, micropapillary, cribriform, and flat (*Mod Pathol.* 2004;17:360) (Fig. 29.2 and e-**Fig. 29.22**). These patterns are often admixed. At high-power magnification, HG-PIN shows basal cells (which are typically reduced in number) and atypical luminal cells. Nuclear abnormalities that should be present to diagnose HG-PIN include increased nuclear size, increased chromatin clumping and content, and prominent nucleoli.

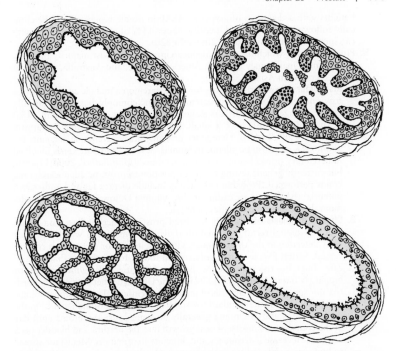

Figure 29.2 Architectural patterns of high-grade PIN. (Reproduced from: Humphrey PA. *Prostate Pathology*. Chicago, IL: ASCP Press; 2003. Used with permission.)

The diagnosis can usually be made on H&E-stained sections. Immunostains for basal cells (34betaE12 and p63) and AMACR can be useful when the differential diagnosis is HG-PIN with outpouching versus HG-PIN with associated invasive adenocarcinoma (*Am J Surg Pathol.* 2005;29:529). Isolated HG-PIN in needle biopsy and TURP chips has been considered a risk factor for subsequent detection of carcinoma on rebiopsy, although the level of risk has decreased with increased 10- to 12-core sampling of the prostate (*Am J Surg Pathol.* 2005;29: 1201; *Urology.* 2005;65: 538), such that not all patients necessarily need to undergo rebiopsy in the first year following diagnosis of isolated HG-PIN (*J Urol.* 2006;175: 820). However, patients with two or more cores with HG-PIN do appear to be at increased risk for subsequent detection of carcinoma and should be considered candidates for rebiopsy (*J Urol.* 2009;182: 485).

G. **Focal glandular atypia (atypical small acinar proliferation or ASAP)** is a descriptive diagnosis for a gland or group of glands with architectural or cytologic atypia that does not allow for a definitive diagnosis of reactive atypia, atypical adenomatous hyperplasia, PIN, or carcinoma. If there is significant concern for malignancy, a diagnosis of focal glandular atypia, suspicious for carcinoma may be rendered. A diagnosis of atypia is applied in about 3% (range 1% to 9%) of needle biopsies (*J Urol.* 2006;175: 820). Distortion artifact, section thickness, and overstaining can contribute to difficulty in interpretation; immunostains for basal cells (34betaE12 and p63) and AMACR can be very useful in establishing a definitive diagnosis when atypia is the initial diagnosis in H&E-stained sections.

Patients with a diagnosis of atypia or ASAP in needle biopsy should be clinically followed and rebiopsied, because about 43% of men are diagnosed with carcinoma on rebiopsy (*J Urol.* 2006;175:820).

H. **Prostate cancer,** which is acinar adenocarcinoma in the vast majority of cases, is a common malignancy in North America, Europe, and Australia, whereas it is less common in Asia.

1. **Risk factors.** Proven risk factors for adenocarcinoma include age, family history, and race. Prostatic adenocarcinoma is uncommonly diagnosed clinically before the age of 50, whereas a significant minority of men (around 31%) in their 30s and 40s have a small adenocarcinoma detectable at autopsy (*In Vivo.* 1994;8:1459). Hereditary prostatic adenocarcinoma accounts for about 10% of prostatic adenocarcinomas. Several candidate genes involved in hereditary transmission have been identified (*Mod Pathol.* 2004;17:380), but currently genetic testing for predisposition to prostatic adenocarcinoma is not performed. Probable risk factors include dietary fat and androgens; potential risk factors are cadmium, low vitamin D, low vitamin E, low selenium, herbicides, and sedentary lifestyle.

2. **Clinical diagnosis** of clinically localized prostate cancer is based on serum PSA and digital rectal examination (DRE). Serum PSA is widely used for early detection in the United States, although its use for screening is controversial. Serum PSA level is clearly related to risk for histologic diagnosis of carcinoma, but risk exists below the most often used 4.0 ng/mL prompt for biopsy (*N Engl J Med.* 2003;347:215). The DRE is neither particularly sensitive nor specific for a diagnosis of prostatic carcinoma. Thus, histopathologic tissue diagnosis is the standard to establish a diagnosis of malignancy in the prostate. Prostatic carcinoma generally does not cause symptoms until late in the course of the disease. Local growth into the urethra and bladder neck can cause increase in frequency and difficulty in urination. Metastatic spread to bone can produce pain in the lower back, chest, hip, legs, and shoulders. Response to treatment is followed by serum PSA determinations, and in some cases, radiologic studies.

3. **Histologic typing and diagnosis.** The 2004 World Health Organization (WHO) classification of neoplasms of the prostate is given in Table 29.1.

4. **Acinar adenocarcinoma** of the prostate is by far the most common type of prostate cancer.

   a. **Gross diagnosis** of prostatic carcinoma is possible in radical prostatectomy tissues but not in needle biopsy or TURP chip tissues. Impalpable prostatic carcinomas detected due to an elevated serum PSA (clinical stage T1c) are difficult to impossible to visualize on cut sections of radical prostatectomy specimens. When visible, the carcinoma can appear nodular and white to irregular and gray or white-yellow (**e-Fig. 29.23**).

   b. **Microscopic diagnosis** is based on a synthesis of a constellation of histologic attributes (Table 29.2) (*J Clin Pathol.* 2007;60:35). Major criteria are architecture (pattern of growth), absence of basal cells, and nuclear atypia.

      The architectural patterns of cellular arrangement are well depicted in the Gleason grading diagram (Fig. 29.3). Well-differentiated prostatic adenocarcinoma of Gleason patterns 1 and 2 displays abnormal glandular arrangements in the form of well-circumscribed nodules of closely packed small acini (**e-Fig. 29.24**). Gleason pattern 3 usually presents as single, small, infiltrating glands, with wide stromal separation (**e-Fig. 29.25**). High-grade Gleason pattern 4 is cribriform (**e-Fig. 29.26**), fused small acinar, or shows poorly formed glands. High-grade Gleason pattern 5 is composed of sheets, cords, single cells, or comedocarcinoma (**e-Fig. 29.27**) (*Am J Surg Pathol.* 2005;29:1228; *J Urol.* 2010;183:433).

TABLE 29.1 WHO Histologic Classification of Tumors of Prostate

Epithelial tumors

Glandular neoplasms

Adenocarcinoma (acinar)
  Atrophic
  Pseudohyperplastic
  Foamy
  Colloid
  Signet ring
  Oncocytic
  Lymphoepithelioma-like
  Carcinoma with spindle cell differentiation
    (carcinosarcoma, sarcomatoid carcinoma)
Prostatic intraepithelial neoplasia (PIN)
Ductal adenocarcinoma
  Cribriform
  Papillary
  Solid

Urothelial tumors

Urothelial carcinoma

Squamous tumors

Adenosquamous carcinoma
Squamous cell carcinoma

Basal cell tumors

Basal cell adenoma
Basal cell carcinoma

Neuroendocrine tumors

Endocrine differentiation within adenocarcinoma
Carcinoid tumor
Small cell carcinoma
Paraganglioma
Neuroblastoma

Prostatic stromal tumors

Stromal tumor of uncertain malignant potential
Stromal sarcoma

Mesenchymal tumors

Leiomyosarcoma
Rhabdomyosarcoma
Chondrosarcoma
Angiosarcoma
Malignant fibrous histiocytoma
Malignant peripheral nerve sheath tumor
Hemangioma
Chondroma
Leiomyoma
Granular cell tumor
Hemangiopericytoma
Solitary fibrous tumor

Hematolymphoid tumors

Lymphoma
Leukemia

Miscellaneous tumors

Cystadenoma
Nephroblastoma (Wilms tumor)
Rhabdoid tumor
Germ cell tumors
  Yolk sac tumor
  Seminoma
  Embryonal carcinoma and teratoma
  Choriocarcinoma
Clear cell adenocarcinoma
Melanoma

Metastatic tumors

Tumors of the seminal vesicles

Epithelial tumors

Adenocarcinoma
Cystadenoma

Mixed epithelial and stromal tumors

Malignant
Benign

Mesenchymal tumors

Leiomyosarcoma
Angiosarcoma
Liposarcoma
Malignant fibrous histiocytoma
Solitary fibrous tumor
Hemangiopericytoma
Leiomyoma

Miscellaneous tumors

Choriocarcinoma
Male adnexal tumor of probably Wolffian
  origin

Metastatic tumors

From: Eble JN, Sauter G, Epstein JI, et al., eds. *World Health Organization Classification of Tumours. Pathology and Genetics. Tumours of the Urinary System and Male Genital Organs.* Lyon, France: IARC Press; 2004. Used with permission.

| TABLE 29.2 | Criteria for Diagnosis of Prostatic Adenocarcinoma |

Major criteria

Architectural: Infiltrative small glands or cribriform glands too large or irregular to represent high-grade PIN

Single cell layer (absence of basal cells)

Nuclear atypia: Nuclear and nucleolar enlargement

Minor criteria

Intraluminal wispy blue mucin (blue-tinged or basophilic mucinous secretions)

Pink amorphous secretions

Mitotic figures

Intraluminal crystalloids

Adjacent high-grade PIN

Amphophilic cytoplasm

Basal cell absence, the second major criterion, can sometimes be difficult to evaluate in H&E-stained sections, so in difficult cases and for small foci of adenocarcinoma (minimal or limited adenocarcinoma), immunohistochemical staining for basal cells using antibodies against high-molecular-weight cytokeratins (such as 34betaE12, also known as CK903) and p63 may be performed (e-**Fig. 29.28**). While a positive basal

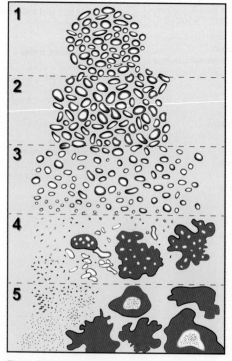

Figure 29.3 Gleason grades 1 to 5.

TABLE 29.3	Immunophenotype of Prostatic Versus Urothelial (Transitional Cell) Carcinoma	
	Prostatic carcinoma	**Urothelial carcinoma**
Marker	**(percentage of cases positive)**	
PSA	94–100	0
PSAP	89–100	0
PSMA	92	0
NXK3.1	95	0
Prostein	100	6
p63	0–3	81–96
Thrombomodulin	0	69–91
Uroplakin III	0	57
High-molecular-weight cytokeratin[a]	0–10[b]	65–100

[a]Detected by antibody 34betaE12.
[b]Mean = 3% prostatic carcinoma cases positive. Up to 20% of cases of metastatic prostatic carcinoma can be positive.
PSAP, prostate-specific acid phosphatase; PSMA, Prostate specific membrane antigen.

cell immunostain effectively rules out invasive adenocarcinoma, benign glands can focally lack a basal cell layer, so basal cell immunostains should be interpreted in the context of the H&E histologic findings (*Semin Diagn Pathol.* 2005;22:88).

Nuclear atypia, the third of the major criteria, takes the form of nuclear enlargement and nucleolar enlargement.

The minor criteria (Table 29.2) tend to be found more often in adenocarcinoma, but are not specific for adenocarcinoma. Features considered specific for a diagnosis of prostatic adenocarcinoma include extraprostatic spread of prostatic glands, collagenous micronodules (e-**Fig. 29.29**), glomeruloid intraglandular projections (e-**Fig. 29.30**), and perineural invasion (e-**Fig. 29.31**). Of note, benign glands can abut intraprostatic nerves (*Am J Surg Pathol.* 2005;29:1159).

c. **Immunohistochemical studies** are helpful in a minority of cases. The most commonly used immunostains are those for basal cells and for a neoplastic cell-selective marker (AMACR or P504S), and are usually used to assess a few atypical glands in a needle biopsy. AMACR is fairly sensitive for neoplastic prostatic epithelial cells (in both PIN and invasive carcinoma), staining 80% to 100% of adenocarcinomas, but is not specific as it can be found focally in benign glands (*Semin Diagn Pathol.* 2005;22:88). Cocktails using p63 and AMACR or p63/34betaE12/AMACR antibodies are useful when a limited amount of tissue is available for staining (e-**Fig. 29.28**) (*Am J Surg Pathol.* 2005;29:579; *Semin Diagn Pathol.* 2005;22:88). PSAP, PSA, thrombomodulin, p63, and high-molecular-weight cytokeratin immunostains should be used for poorly differentiated carcinomas when the differential diagnosis is poorly differentiated prostatic adenocarcinoma versus poorly differentiated urothelial (transitional cell) carcinoma (Table 29.3) (*Semin Diagn Pathol.* 2005;22:88). PSMA, prostein, and NKX3.1 may be used if prostatic carcinoma is suspected but the PSA and PSAP immunostains are negative. PSA, PSAP, and prostein immunostains should always be performed when confronted with a metastatic adenocarcinoma of unknown primary origin in a man.

d. **Molecular studies** are not currently used to diagnose prostatic carcinoma.

5. **Variants of acinar adenocarcinoma** include atrophic, pseudohyperplastic, foamy, colloid (mucinous), signet ring, oncocytic, lymphoepithelioma-like,

and sarcomatoid carcinoma (carcinosarcoma) (Table 29.1). Atrophic pattern adenocarcinoma displays decreased cytoplasm and can thereby mimic benign atrophy (e-**Fig. 29.32**). Such cytoplasmic volume loss can be seen with or without a history of hormonal or radiation therapy. Most cases are Gleason pattern 3. Pseudohyperplastic carcinoma is another malignancy that can resemble benign glands (*Am J Surg Pathol*. 1998;22:1139). Here, the malignant glands simulate BPH glands (e-**Fig. 29.33**) in that they are complex with intraluminal papillary projections, undulating luminal surfaces, branching patterns, and/or cystic dilatation. Gleason grade assignment is pattern 3. Foamy gland carcinoma is characterized by xanthomatous cytoplasm and bland nuclei (e-**Fig. 29.34**); these carcinomas are usually Gleason score 6 or 7, but can be higher grade. Mucinous carcinoma of the prostate is defined as adenocarcinoma with at least 25% of the tumor composed of lakes of extracellular mucin (e-**Fig. 29.35**); this is a rare variant, with a Gleason grade pattern of 4 (usually) or 3. In the past, this variant was thought to be more aggressive than usual acinar adenocarcinoma, but recent reports suggest that it may not be. Signet-ring carcinoma of the prostate is also rare and clinically aggressive; the Gleason grade is 5. Only a few cases of oncocytic and lymphoepithelioma-like carcinoma have been reported. Sarcomatoid carcinoma of the prostate is rare (*Am J Surg Pathol*. 2006;30:1316) and may be a homologous spindle cell malignancy or heterologous, with an osteosarcomatous (e-**Fig. 29.36**), chondrosarcomatous, or rhabdomyosarcomatous component. In one half of the men there is a history of prostatic adenocarcinoma treated by hormonal and/or radiation therapy; the outcome is poor. Variants described since the 2004 WHO classification include microcystic adenocarcinoma (*Am J Surg Pathol*. 2010;34:556), PIN-like adenocarcinoma, and pleomorphic giant cell carcinoma.

6. **Ductal adenocarcinoma** is the second most common subtype of prostatic adenocarcinoma (after acinar). Previously known as endometrioid adenocarcinoma, in pure form it accounts for about 1% of prostatic cancers and, when mixed with acinar adenocarcinoma, roughly 5% of prostatic cancers. Microscopically, these are usually papillary and/or cribriform adenocarcinomas (e-**Fig. 29.37**) that can arise centrally (causing urinary obstruction and hematuria) or peripherally. Cytologically, tall columnar neoplastic cells with cleared or amphophilic cytoplasm may be observed. Most patients present at a more advanced stage, and outcome is worse than that of acinar adenocarcinoma. Gleason grade is typically pattern 4.

7. **Rare types of prostatic carcinoma** include urothelial carcinoma (arising from central prostatic ducts), squamous and adenosquamous carcinoma (e-**Figs. 29.38** and **29.39**), basal cell carcinoma, and neuroendocrine carcinoma, including small cell and large cell neuroendocrine carcinoma (*Mod Pathol*. 2004;17:316). It is important to exclude primary urethral and urinary bladder urothelial carcinoma before diagnosing primary prostatic urothelial carcinoma. An in situ component can be extensive in the prostate, with solid plugs of cytologically pleomorphic tumor cells, often with comedo necrosis and stromal inflammation; prostatic stromal invasion is typified by irregular solid nests and cords. Squamous cell and adenosquamous carcinomas of the prostate comprise <1% of all prostatic carcinomas, and in about two thirds of cases there is a history of hormonal and or radiation treatment (*Am J Surg Pathol*. 2004;28:651). Average survival is 2 years. Basal cell carcinoma of the prostate includes malignant basaloid proliferations (basaloid or basal cell carcinomas) and also neoplasms that resemble, to a certain degree, adenoid cystic carcinomas of the salivary glands (*Am J Surg Pathol*. 2003;27:1523). Basal cell carcinomas have several growth arrangements, including large basaloid nests with peripheral palisading and necrosis, a florid basal cell

hyperplasia-like pattern, and an adenoid basal cell hyperplasia-like pattern (adenoid cystic carcinoma pattern). Small cell carcinoma of the prostate is quite rare and in one half of cases is admixed with adenocarcinoma; the histologic appearance is similar to that of small cell carcinoma of the lung. In one third of cases there is a history of prostatic adenocarcinoma followed by hormonal therapy (e-**Fig. 29.39**). A similar history is obtained in most cases of large cell neuroendocrine carcinoma of the prostate (*Am J Surg Pathol.* 2006;30:684). Outcome is very poor for neuroendocrine carcinomas of the prostate.

8. **Mesenchymal neoplasms** are rare. The most common benign mesenchymal neoplasm is leiomyoma, and the most common malignant mesenchymal neoplasms are rhabdomyosarcoma in children and leiomyosarcoma in adults. Stromal tumors arising from specialized prostatic stroma include stromal tumors of uncertain malignant potential (STUMPs) (e-**Fig. 29.40**) and stromal sarcomas.

9. **Hematolymphoid neoplasms** may involve the prostate, including leukemia, lymphoma, Hodgkin disease, and multiple myeloma. Leukemic infiltrates almost always indicate secondary spread, usually of chronic lymphocytic leukemia. However, about one third of prostatic lymphomas are primary, most commonly diffuse large B cell lymphoma.

10. **Miscellaneous neoplasms** rarely encountered in the prostate include cystadenoma, clear cell carcinoma of the utricle/prostate, paraganglioma, melanocytic neoplasms, and germ cell tumors.

11. **Secondary malignancy** in the prostate is overall uncommon, but can be seen in a substantial minority of patients with urothelial carcinoma of the bladder (e-**Fig. 29.41**), leukemia, and non-Hodgkin lymphoma.

12. **Treatment effects** can substantially alter the morphology of prostatic carcinoma, resulting in difficulty in diagnosis.
    a. **Hormonal androgen deprivation therapy** can cause a decrease in the number of glands, glandular atrophy, single tumor cells, nuclear pyknosis, and cytoplasmic vacuolization (e-**Fig. 29.42**). The carcinoma cells often resemble lymphocytes or histiocytes. PSA and pan-cytokeratin immunostains can be useful.
    b. **Radiation therapy** can induce striking nuclear atypia in benign glands. Positive basal cell and negative AMACR immunostains support a diagnosis of benign atypia. Adenocarcinoma postradiotherapy shows a decrease in number of neoplastic glands, poorly formed glands and single cells, cytoplasmic vacuolization, and nuclear pyknosis (e-**Fig. 29.43**). Immunostains for basal cells and AMACR can be useful in diagnosis in this setting (e-**Fig. 29.44**).

I. **Seminal vesicles** are rarely the site of origin of primary disease, whether inflammatory or neoplastic. Amyloid can be identified in about 10% of seminal vesicles, as a function of aging; its presence does not indicate systemic amyloidosis unless there is also co-existing vascular amyloid deposition, which is rare. Seminal vesicles are usually examined for prostatic carcinoma as a part of pathologic staging.

J. **Prostatic urethra** urothelium is subject to the same diseases as urothelium in the urinary bladder, namely inflammation, metaplasia (squamous metaplasia, urethritis cystica and glandularis, and nephrogenic metaplasia [adenoma]), hyperplasia, and neoplasms such as papilloma and carcinoma. However, primary isolated malignancies of the prostatic urethra are exceedingly rare, and malignancy in the prostatic urethra is most often due to secondary synchronous involvement by urothelial (transitional cell) carcinoma of the urinary bladder.

IV. **HISTOLOGIC GRADING OF PROSTATIC ADENOCARCINOMA.** Gleason grade is critical for patient prognosis and management. It is commonly used clinically, along with serum PSA level and clinical or pathologic stage, in tables (Partin tables) (http://urology.jhu.edu/Partin_tables/index.html) and nomograms (*J Urol.* 2001;165:1562; *Cancer.* 2009;115(Suppl):3107) to predict pathologic stage and response to treatment and outcome.

Grading should be performed using the modified Gleason system (Fig. 29.3). All adenocarcinomas of the prostate should be graded, except those that are posthormonal therapy or postradiotherapy (when radiation effect is evident). Grading is based solely on architecture and does not incorporate cytologic atypia or mitotic counting. At low magnification (40 to $100\times$), the most common pattern and the second most common pattern are summed to yield a score (on a scale of 2 to 10). Recent recommendations in application of the Gleason system include the following (*Am J Surg Pathol.* 2005;29:1228; *J Urol.* 2010;183:433):

A. Do not (or rarely) assign a well-differentiated Gleason score 2 to 4 to carcinoma in needle biopsy. This almost always represents undergrading.

B. When three grades are present, in a needle biopsy give most common grade and worst grade. Thus, if $3 + 4 + 5$ are present, the Gleason grade is $3 + 5 =$ score of 8. In a radical prostatectomy, give the most common and second most common grades, but if there is a minor tertiary high-grade 4 or 5 pattern, this should be noted in a comment.

C. If there is 95% high-grade pattern 4 or 5 and 5% or less of 2 or 3, ignore the lower-grade component. Any high-grade pattern (4 or 5) should be incorporated into a needle biopsy Gleason score; thus, 98% pattern 3 and 2% pattern 4 in a needle biopsy is Gleason grade $3 + 4 =$ score of 7.

D. Variants of prostatic adenocarcinoma can be graded (see above).

E. Cribriform adenocarcinomas are high-grade pattern 4.

F. For needle biopsies, provide grade by clinically submitted container, even if several cores are within the container. Alternatively, provide the Gleason grade for the core with highest Gleason score, if different from the overall Gleason score for cores from that container.

V. **PATHOLOGIC STAGING.** Staging applies only to adenocarcinomas of the prostate, and not to sarcomas or prostatic carcinoma variants that are not adenocarcinomas. The 2010 Tumor, Node, Metastasis (TNM) American Joint Committee on Cancer/International Union Against Cancer (AJCC/UICC) staging classification is given in Table 29.4. Clinical staging should be distinguished from pathologic staging.

A. **Needle biopsy.** Pathologic staging is not performed. However, extraprostatic spread should be diagnosed if carcinoma is seen in fat or in seminal vesicle tissue.

B. **TURP chips and open prostatectomy.** Pathologic staging is not done, but for incidental carcinoma, the amount of carcinoma determined by light microscopic inspection of tissue involved will place the patient into clinical stage Tla or Tlb.

C. Radical prostatectomy and pelvic lymphadenectomy are used for pathologic staging (Table 29.4) (*Arch Pathol Lab Med.* 2009;133:1568).

1. **pT2:** Organ-confined prostatic carcinoma, subdivided into a, b, and c.

2. **pT3:** Extraprostatic extension (EPE) by carcinoma, diagnosed if carcinoma extends into posterolateral periprostatic adipose tissue (e-**Fig. 29.45**), beyond the outer boundary of normal prostatic glands at the anterior or apical prostate, or microscopically into the bladder neck. Note that carcinoma in skeletal muscle at apex does not always mean EPE. Site(s) and extent of EPE should be specified. EPE extent should be given as focal (only a few glands outside the prostate) or nonfocal. Capsular invasion is not part of the staging scheme. pT3b is seminal vesicle wall invasion (e-**Fig. 29.46**).

3. **pT4:** Gross bladder neck or rectal involvement by carcinoma.

4. **pN:** Number of involved and total number of examined lymph nodes should be given.

5. **pM:** At time of radical prostatectomy, patients are clinical M0 (cM0).

TABLE 29.4	Tumor, Node, Metastasis (TNM) Staging Scheme for Prostatic Carcinoma

Primary tumor, clinical (T)

TX	Primary tumor cannot be assessed
T0	No evidence of primary tumor
T1	Clinically inapparent tumor neither palpable nor visible by imaging
T1a	Tumor incidental histologic finding in ≤5% of tissue resected
T1b	Tumor incidental histologic finding in >5% of tissue resected
T1c	Tumor identified by needle biopsy (e.g., because of elevated PSA)
T2	Tumor confined within prostate[a]
T2a	Tumor involves one half of one lobe or less
T2b	Tumor involves more than one half of one lobe but not both lobes
T2c	Tumor involves both lobes
T3	Tumor extends through the prostate capsule[b]
T3a	Extracapsular extension (unilateral or bilateral)
T3b	Tumor invades seminal vesicle(s)
T4	Tumor is fixed or invades adjacent structures other than seminal vesicles; bladder, external sphincter, rectum, levator muscles, and/or pelvic wall

Primary tumor, pathologic (pT)[c,d]

pT2	Organ confined
pT2a	Unilateral, involving one half of one lobe or less
pT2b	Unilateral, involving more than one half of one lobe but not both lobes
pT2c	Bilateral
pT3	Extraprostatic extension
pT3a	Extraprostatic extension or microscopic invasion of bladder neck
pT3b	Seminal vesicle invasion
pT4	Invasion of bladder, rectum

Regional lymph nodes (N)

NX	Regional lymph nodes cannot be assessed
N0	No regional lymph node metastasis
N1	Metastasis in regional lymph node or nodes

Distant metastasis[e] (M)

MX	Distant metastasis cannot be assessed
M0	No distant metastasis
M1	Distant metastasis
M1a	Nonregional lymph node(s)
M1b	Bone(s)
M1c	Other site(s)

(continued)

VI. **REPORTING PROSTATE CANCER** (*Arch Pathol Lab Med.* 2009;133:1568; *Mod Pathol.* 2011;24:1–57)

   A. For fine needle aspiration biopsy samples with carcinoma identified, grade should be given as well, moderately, or poorly differentiated.

   B. For needle core biopsy samples, histologic type, Gleason grade, and amount of tumor should be provided. Amount of tumor can be quantitated as number of positive cores/total number of cores, percentage of tissue involved by carcinoma (by visual inspection), and linear millimeters of carcinoma per total millimeters of tissue. If present, periprostatic fat invasion, seminal vesicle invasion, perineural invasion, and lymphovascular space invasion should be reported.

TABLE 29.4	Tumor, Node, Metastasis (TNM) Staging Scheme for Prostatic Carcinoma (*Continued*)

Anatomic stage/prognostic groups

Group	T	N	M	PSA	Gleason	M	PSA	Gleason
Group I	T1a–c	N0	M0	PSA <10	Gleason ≤6	M0	PSA <20	Gleason 7
	T2a	N0	M0	PSA <10	Gleason ≤6			
	T1–2a	N0	M0	PSA X	Gleason X			
Group IIA	T1a–c	N0	M0	PSA <20	Gleason 7	M0	PSA ≥10 <20	Gleason ≤6
	T1a–c	N0	M0	PSA ≥10 <20	Gleason ≤6			
	T2a	N0	M0	PSA <20	Gleason ≤7			
	T2b	N0	M0	PSA <20	Gleason ≤7			
	T2b	N0	M0	PSA X	Gleason X			
Group IIB	T2c	N0	M0	Any PSA	Any Gleason			
	T1–2	N0	M0	PSA ≥20	Any Gleason			
	T1–2	N0	M0	Any PSA	Gleason ≥8			
Group III	T3a–b	N0	M0	Any PSA	Any Gleason			
Group IV	T4	N0	M0	Any PSA	Any Gleason			
	Any T	N1	M0	Any PSA	Any Gleason			
	Any T	Any N	M1	Any PSA	Any Gleason			

[a]Tumor found in one or both lobes by needle biopsy, but not palpable or reliably visible by imaging, is classified as T1c.
[b]Invasion into the prostatic apex or into (but not beyond) the prostatic capsule is not classified as T3, but as T2.
[c]There is no pathologic T1 classification.
[d] Positive surgical margin should be indicated by an R1 descriptor (residual microscopic disease).
[e]When more than one site of metastasis is present, the most advanced category is used. pM1c is most advanced.
From: Edge SB, Byrd DR, Compton CC, et al., eds. *AJCC Cancer Staging Manual*, 7th ed. New York, NY: Springer; 2010. Used with permission.

C. For TURP and simple (enucleation) prostatectomy specimens, report the histologic type, Gleason grade, and amount of tumor. For Gleason grade, if three patterns are present, use the predominant and worst pattern of the remaining two. The percentage of tissue involved by tumor (by visual inspection) should be indicated; it is also recommended to report the number of positive chips per total number of chips. If present, periprostatic fat invasion, seminal vesicle invasion, perineural invasion, and lymphovascular space invasion should be reported.

D. For radical prostatectomy specimens, report histologic type, Gleason grade, amount of tumor, pathologic stage, and margin status. The amount of tumor can be reported as percentage of tissue involved by carcinoma (by visual inspection); another option is to report the greatest dimension of the dominant nodule (if present). For margins involved by carcinoma, the number and location of positive sites should be specified; the extent of margin positivity can be measured in linear mm (note: if a margin is positive for carcinoma without EPE, it is designated as pT2+). Additional findings worth reporting include lymphovascular space invasion by carcinoma, inflammation, BPH, PIN, and adenosis.

SUGGESTED READING

Epstein JI, Cubilla AL, Humphrey PA. Tumors of the prostate gland, seminal vesicles, penis, and scrotum. In: *Atlas of Tumor Pathology*. 4th Series. Washington, DC: American Registry of Pathology; 2011.

30 Penis and Scrotum

Peter A. Humphrey

I. **NORMAL ANATOMY.** The penis is anatomically composed of three parts: posterior (root); central body or shaft; and anterior portion composed of glans, coronal sulcus, and foreskin (prepuce). In the shaft there are three cylinders of erectile tissues: a ventral corpus spongiosum surrounding the urethra and two corpora cavernosa. Histologically, the erectile tissues are characterized by numerous vascular spaces with surrounding smooth muscle fibers (e-Fig. 30.1).* The tunica albuginea, a sheath of hyalinized collagen, encases the corpora cavernosa. All three corpora are surrounded by Buck's fascia, adipose tissue, dartos muscle, dermis, and a thin epidermis. Distally, the corpus spongiosum forms the conical glans, which is also composed of a stratified squamous epithelium, lamina propria, tunica albuginea, and corpora cavernosa. The coronal sulcus is a cul-de-sac just below the glans corona. The foreskin is a double membrane that has five layers: mucosal epithelium similar to glans epithelium, lamina propria, dartos smooth muscle, dermis, and epidermis.

The scrotum contains the testes and lower spermatic cords. It consists of skin that covers the dartos smooth muscle, fibers of the cremasteric muscle, and several layers of fascia. The skin is pigmented, hair bearing, and loose, with numerous sebaceous and sweat glands. Lymphatic drainage is to the superficial inguinal lymph nodes.

II. **GROSS EXAMINATION AND TISSUE SAMPLING.** Tissue samples include mucosal or skin biopsies, penile urethral biopsies, foreskin resection specimens, and partial and total penectomy specimens.

A. **Punch and shave biopsies** of penile glans and skin should be handled as skin biopsies from other sites (see Chap. 38).

B. **Foreskin resection** is indicated for primary carcinomas of this site. The entire periphery of the mucosal margin should be submitted as a shave resection margin (usually in three to four sections). The foreskin should then be pinned and fixed overnight in 10% formalin. Several full-thickness sections should be examined microscopically to permit evaluation of all five layers.

C. For **partial penectomy specimens,** the surgical division of the penis is made 2 cm proximal to gross tumor extent. Three to four frozen sections are typically necessary to sample the cut surface of this margin. Permanent sections are taken as described below.

D. For **total penectomy specimens,** only proximal urethral and periurethral margin tissues should be submitted for frozen section, unless the mass is grossly close to or involves the skin, which should also then be sampled. For permanent sections of both partial and total penectomy specimens, the foreskin (when present) should be removed and handled as noted previously. A thin 2-mm shave of all the structures of the shaft margin should be taken, if not already sampled by frozen section. One to three additional transverse sections should be taken from the glans. Any mass(es) should be sampled to demonstrate pattern of growth, depth of extension, and relationship to normal anatomic structures.

E. **Lymph nodes.** There may be a clinical request for frozen section(s) of enlarged inguinal lymph nodes; if positive for carcinoma, a more extended ilioinguinal

---

*All e-figures are available online via the Solution Site Image Bank.

lymph node dissection may follow. Bilateral inguinal lymphadenectomy specimens may also be received after removal of the primary tumor and a course of antibiotics, or in patients with T2 tumors, high-grade tumors, or tumors with vascular invasion (*Crit Rev Oncol Hematol.* 2005;53:165).

A nomogram has been developed to predict nodal metastases using the presence of clinically palpable groin lymph nodes and histologic lymphovascular invasion in the primary tumor (*J Urol.* 2006;175:1700). The utility of sentinel lymph node sampling is not yet settled. A prognostic index has also been generated to predict nodal metastasis (*Am J Surg Pathol.* 2009;33:1049); this index incorporates histologic grade, deepest anatomic level involved by cancer, and the presence of perineural invasion by carcinoma.

III. DIAGNOSTIC FEATURES OF COMMON DISEASES OF THE PENIS AND SCROTUM

A. **Inflammation and infection.** Three categories can be defined: inflammatory conditions specific to penis and scrotum, systematic dermatoses (discussed in Chap. 38), and sexually transmitted diseases (*BJU Int.* 2002;90:498).

1. **Phimosis,** the clinical condition in which the foreskin cannot be retracted behind the glans penis, is associated with fibrosis, inflammation, and edema of the prepuce.

2. **Paraphimosis** is diagnosed clinically when the foreskin cannot be advanced back over the glans secondary to fibrosis and inflammation.

3. **Balanoposthitis** is an inflammation of the glans penis and prepuce, usually in uncircumcised men with poor hygiene.

4. **Balanitis,** or inflammation of the glans, occurs in several forms.

   a. **Plasma cell balanitis (Zoon balanitis)** can clinically and grossly mimic carcinoma in situ, with presentation as brown or red patches or plaques. The histologic appearance can vary with time, and the inflammatory cell infiltrate can vary from patchy and lymphoplasmacytic (early) to dense and plasmacytic (later) (*Am J Dermatopathol.* 2002;24:459).

   b. **Balanitis xerotica obliterans** (BXO) is lichen sclerosus of the glans and prepuce that macroscopically appears as a white patch or plaque. Histologically, the squamous epithelium is typically atrophic and hyperkeratotic, with a band of pale homogenous collagen in the upper dermis and an underlying lymphocytic infiltrate (e-**Fig. 30.2**). Complications include meatal stenosis (urethral stricture), and very uncommonly, squamous cell carcinoma.

   c. **Balanitis circinata** microscopically resembles pustular psoriasis and is seen in Reiter syndrome, which includes nongonococcal urethritis, conjunctivitis, and arthritis.

5. **Human papillomavirus (HPV) infection** can lead to condyloma acuminata. The growth is typically papillary or warty, and histologically papillomatosis, acanthosis, parakeratosis, and hyperkeratosis are found; intraepithelial neoplasia may also be present. Koilocytes with wrinkled nuclear membranes, nucleomegaly, cytoplasmic halos, and binucleation may be prominent or inconspicuous. The causal HPV serotypes are usually 6 or 11, but it is not necessary to verify the presence of HPV. **Bowenoid papulosis** is also an HPV-related proliferation that presents with multiple 2 to 10 mm papules than can coalesce to form plaques; it is usually caused by serotypes 16, 18, and/or 35. Microscopically, although the appearance is similar to carcinoma in situ, the clinical course is typically self-limited and benign.

6. **Herpes simplex virus (HSV) infection** of the male genitalia is usually caused by subtype 2, which produces multiple vesicles. The diagnosis may be confirmed by scraping and performance of a Tzanck smear, which reveals multinucleated giant cells with intranuclear inclusions.

7. **Scabies** is an infestation by a mite that burrows into the keratin layer of the epidermis with generation of erythematous papules and nodules. Detection

of the mites may be accomplished via scrapes or biopsy. In tissue sections, the 400 μm mite, eggs, or egg walls, are diagnostic. Dermal eosinophils and epidermal spongiosis are characteristic responses.

8. **Pediculosis pubis** is an infection by *Pediculus pubis*, also known as the crab louse. Biopsy is not necessary; the lice may be seen by a magnifying lens.

9. **Syphilis** is caused by *Treponema pallidum*, a gram-negative spirochete. The primary lesion, the chancre, is a single, round, craterlike painless ulcer most often located on the glans or prepuce. Biopsy is not usually necessary, but if done (e.g., when syphilis is not clinically suspected) it shows a perivascular lymphoplasmacytic infiltrate. The spirochetes may be identified in the epidermis or in dermal perivascular regions by silver stains (Steiner, Dieterle, or Warthin–Starry). The secondary and tertiary stages of syphilis are characterized by condyloma latum and gumma, respectively. Smears from the gray maculopapules of condyloma latum should be examined by dark-field microscopy for spirochetes since biopsy may yield nonspecific findings. The gumma is a necrotic mass with surrounding granulomatous inflammation, and associated obliterative endarteritis with perivascular plasma cells.

10. **Gonorrhea** is caused by *Neisseria gonorrhoeae*, a gram-negative diplococcus. Urethritis with urethral discharge may lead to urethral stricture. Biopsies are hardly ever performed.

11. **Lymphogranuloma venereum** is due to *Chlamydia trachomatis*. Vesicles, then ulcers, develop in the primary genital phase; biopsies are not useful for diagnosis of the primary phase. In the secondary stage, patients develop painful inguinal lymphadenopathy (bubo). Histologically, the lymph nodes demonstrate stellate necrosis surrounded by palisaded histiocytes, a nonspecific picture that can also be seen in cat scratch fever, tularemia, bubonic plague, and fungal and atypical mycobacterial infections.

12. **Granuloma inguinale** is caused by *Calymmatobacterium granulomatis*, a gram-negative intracellular bacillus. Infection results in ulcers. Smears or biopsy sections reveal histiocytes with inclusions (Donovan bodies), best visualized by Warthin–Starry or Giemsa stains.

13. **Chancroid** is caused by *Haemophilus ducreyi*, a gram-negative rod, and is typified by painful nonindurated penile ulcers and lymphadenopathy. The organisms can be found in smears or histologic sections stained with Giemsa, Gram, or methylene blue stains.

14. **Molluscum contagiosum** is caused by a DNA poxvirus and produces multiple small dome-shaped papules with a central umbilication. Biopsy sections show a crater with an acanthotic epidermis and the diagnostic intracytoplasmic viral inclusions (molluscum bodies).

15. **Penile infections in acquired immunodeficiency syndrome (AIDS)** include almost all sexually transmitted infections including gonorrhea, syphilis, herpes, candidiasis, chancroid, molluscum contagiosum, HPV, scabies, and Reiter syndrome.

16. **Lipogranulomas** in the scrotum or penis are secondary to injections of oil-based chemicals. Sections show a foreign body, lymphoplasmacytic, and histiocytic reaction to lipid droplets that appear as cleared spaces.

17. **Hidradenitis suppurativa,** more typical of the sweat glands in the axilla, can also involve the scrotum. Acute and chronic inflammation, fibrosis, and even sinus tract formation can occur.

18. **Gangrene,** as a necroinflammatory process, can involve the scrotum due to a variety of insults. Fournier gangrene is an extreme fulminant infection of the genitals, perineum, or abdominal wall (*Int J Urol.* 2006;13:960).

19. **Idiopathic scrotal calcinosis** can occur due to calcification of dermal connective tissue (idiopathic) or in association with keratinous cysts. Multiple firm nodules are found, measuring several millimeters to several centimeters

in greatest dimension, typically in the scrotum of younger men. Microscopically, calcific material is present with or without granulomatous inflammation and/or cyst wall remnants.

   20. Elephantiasis or massive scrotal lymphedema is usually secondary to filariasis.
B. **Miscellaneous benign nonneoplastic conditions**
   1. **Peyronie disease** presents with a painful bending of the erect penis. Histologically, there is fibrosis or fibromatosis of the tunica albuginea (**e-Fig. 30.3**). Rarely, calcification and ossification may occur in these fibrous plaques.
   2. **Penile cysts**
      a. **Median raphe cyst** is most commonly located in the midline on the ventral aspect of the shaft. It is lined by pseudostratified, columnar, mucinous epithelial cells.
      b. **Mucoid cysts** are thought to arise from ectopic urethral mucosa, can be seen on the prepuce or glans, and are lined by stratified columnar epithelium with mucinous cells.
      c. **Epidermal inclusion cysts** are usually found on the penile shaft. They are also common in scrotal skin. They have the same appearance as they do elsewhere in the skin.
C. **Benign epithelial neoplasms** include squamous papilloma, common condyloma, and the very rare giant condyloma of Buschke–Löwenstein. Most reported giant condylomas likely represent warty or verrucous carcinomas. Grossly, giant condylomas are 5 cm in average diameter, and microscopically resemble a typical condyloma except for exuberant surface papillomatosis and pushing bulbous growth at the base. When carefully defined, they may be locally destructive but do not show malignant cytologic features or metastasize.
D. **Penile intraepithelial neoplasia (PeIN).** Carcinoma in situ (or high-grade squamous intraepithelial lesions) includes erythroplasia of Queyrat (on the glans) and Bowen disease (on the penile shaft or prepuce). These are HPV-related (usually serotypes 16 or 18) intraepithelial proliferations. Grossly, erythroplasia of Queyrat appears as a sharply demarcated patch on the glans, whereas Bowen disease is a solitary, brownish-red plaque on the shaft or foreskin. Microscopically, the two lesions are similar and are composed of a full-thickness proliferation of pleomorphic basaloid cells that exhibit loss of polarity (**e-Fig. 30.4**). Traditionally, these two high-grade intraepithelial proliferations have been assigned grade III, while lower grade intraepithelial lesions have been graded as I or II.

   Recently, a new PeIN classification scheme has been proposed with categories of differentiated, undifferentiated, and mixed differentiated and undifferentiated (*Am J Surg Pathol.* 2010;34:385). Differentiated PeIN is characterized by hyperkeratosis, parakeratosis, hypergranulosis, acanthosis, elongated rete ridges, abnormal maturation, intraepithelial pearl formation, prominent intercellular bridges, and atypical basal or prickle layer cells. In the undifferentiated category are warty, basaloid, and warty-basaloid variants.
E. **Penile cancer**
   1. **Risk factors for penile cancer** are phimosis, chronic inflammation, lichen sclerosus, smoking, ultraviolet (UV) radiation, condyloma, HPV infection (usually type 18, less commonly type 18), and lack of circumcision (*J Am Acad Dermatol.* 2006;54:364). This latter factor is an extremely strong risk factor.
   2. **Clinical diagnosis.** Patients are typically 50 to 70 years of age and present with an exophytic or flat ulcerative mass of the glans, prepuce, or coronal sulcus. Patients with advanced disease may present with pubic or scrotal skin nodules and inguinal lymph node metastasis. Magnetic resonance imaging of primary penile cancer can help define local tumor extent and any shaft involvement (*Radiographics.* 2005;25:1629).
   3. **Histologic typing and diagnosis.** The 2004 World Health Organization (WHO) classification of penile neoplasms is provided in Table 30.1.

TABLE 30.1	WHO Histologic Classification of Tumors of the Penis

Malignant epithelial tumors of the penis
Squamous cell carcinoma
  Basaloid carcinoma
  Warty (condylomatous) carcinoma
  Verrucous carcinoma
  Papillary carcinoma
  Sarcomatous carcinoma
  Mixed carcinoma
  Adenosquamous carcinoma
Merkel cell carcinoma
Small cell carcinoma
Sebaceous carcinoma
Clear cell carcinoma
Basal cell carcinoma

Precursor lesions
Penile intraepithelial neoplasia
Paget disease

Melanocytic tumors
Melanocytic nevus
Melanoma

Mesenchymal tumors

Hematopoietic tumors

Secondary tumors

From: Eble JN, Sauter G, Epstein JI, et al., eds. *World Health Organization Classification of Tumours. Pathology and Genetics. Tumours of the Urinary System and Male Genital Organs.* Lyon, France: IARC Press; 2004. Used with permission.

4. **Squamous cell carcinoma of usual type** accounts for the vast majority of penile cancers.
  a. **Gross diagnosis** is readily performed for penectomy specimens because most masses are several centimeters in diameter, and are usually solitary, firm, and ulcerated (e-**Fig. 30.5**). Multicentric tumors occur more frequently in the foreskin.
  b. **Microscopic diagnosis** is usually straightforward, but small superficial biopsies can be problematic in the differential distinction from pseudoepitheliomatous squamous cell hyperplasia. There are three major prognostically important growth patterns: superficial spreading, with horizontal growth and only superficial invasion; vertical growth, which is deeply invasive (e-**Fig. 30.6**); and multicentric. Histologically, most usual squamous cell carcinomas are moderately differentiated with some keratinization (e-**Fig. 30.7**). Small nests, cords, and single neoplastic cells infiltrate into the lamina propria, corpus spongiosum, and uncommonly, the corpus cavernosum (e-**Fig. 30.8**). Poorly differentiated carcinoma may grow as sheets, with necrosis and a high mitotic rate. Giant cells and sarcomatoid features may be found in these high-grade tumors. Local extension into several anatomic compartments may occur; for example, a carcinoma originating on the glans may spread to the foreskin, to skin of the shaft, and to the urethra. In very advanced cases, direct spread to inguinal, pubic, or scrotal skin can occur.
  c. **Immunohistochemical studies** are useful in the small minority of cases when uncertainty exists after examination of the H&E-stained slides, mainly for

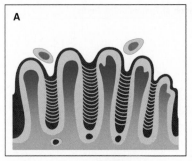
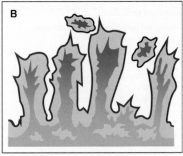
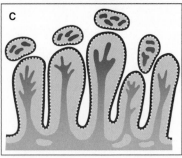
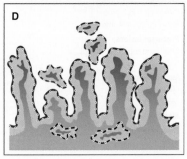

Figure 30.1 Verruciform tumors of the penis. **A:** Verrucous carcinoma with regular papillae, broad pushing base, and hyperkeratosis. **B:** Papillary carcinoma with irregular papillae and cores, and ragged infiltration at base. **C:** Giant condyloma, with branching cores and koilocytosis. **D:** Warty (condylomatous) carcinoma with irregular papillae and koilocytosis. (Modified from: Young RH, Srigley JR, Amin MB, et al., eds. *Tumors of the Prostate Gland, Seminal Vesicles, Male Urethra, and Penis.* Washington DC: Armed Forces Institute of Pathology; 2005:424.)

the distinction of a poorly differentiated squamous cell carcinoma from another malignant neoplasm such as a sarcoma, melanoma, or lymphoma. Immunohistochemical detection of carcinoma cells in lymph nodes is of uncertain significance (*BJU Int.* 2006;98:70).

   d. Molecular studies are not currently used to diagnose penile carcinoma. HPV typing is not necessary.

5. **Variants of squamous cell carcinoma** include basaloid, warty (condylomatous), verrucous, papillary, sarcomatoid, mixed, and adenosquamous (Table 30.1) (*Urology.* 2010;76(suppl 2A):S7). Basaloid carcinoma is an uncommon, aggressive, HPV-related variant that comprises small, uniform, basaloid cells with high-nuclear/cytoplasmic ratios and numerous mitoses (**e-Fig. 30.9**). Warty (condylomatous) carcinoma is one of the verruciform carcinomas (the others being verrucous carcinoma and papillary carcinoma) (Fig. 30.1); microscopically, it is hyperkeratotic and papillomatous with cells of low to intermediate nuclear grade, and koilocytic atypia may be prominent. Verrucous carcinoma is a very well-differentiated papillary neoplasm with hyperkeratosis, papillomatosis, and a broad pushing base. Papillary carcinoma is well differentiated, hyperkeratotic, and has complex papillae and an irregular infiltrative base; it has a favorable prognosis (*Am J Surg Pathol.* 2010;34:223). Sarcomatoid (spindle cell) carcinoma is an aggressive, high

grade, deeply invasive spindle cell malignancy with or without heterologous elements such as muscle, bone, and cartilage; coexisting carcinoma in situ or invasive carcinoma is usually evident (*Am J Surg Pathol.* 2005;29:1152). In adenosquamous carcinoma the glandular component is a minority component. In one quarter of cases the carcinoma can be mixed, such as warty–basaloid, adenocarcinoma–basaloid, and squamous–neuroendocrine.

Rare, recently recognized patterns of squamous cell carcinoma include pseudohyperplastic squamous cell carcinoma (*Am J Surg Pathol.* 2004;28:895), carcinoma cuniculatum (*Am J Surg Pathol.* 2007;31:71), and pseudoglandular (adenoid, acantholytic) squamous cell carcinoma (*Am J Surg Pathol.* 2009;33:551). Pseudohyperplastic squamous cell carcinoma can resemble pseudoepitheliomatous hyperplasia, and carcinoma cuniculatum is another verruciform squamous cell carcinoma that is low grade and has deeply penetrating and burrowing patterns of growth. Pseudoglandular squamous cell carcinoma is often deeply infiltrative and of high histologic grade.

6. **Rare types of primary penile carcinoma** include Merkel cell carcinoma, small cell carcinoma, sebaceous carcinoma, and clear cell carcinoma.

7. **Mesenchymal neoplasms** are rare and comprise only 5% of all penile tumors. The most common benign soft tissue tumors are vascular (hemangioma and lymphangioma), followed by neural, myxoid, and fibrous tumors. The most frequent malignant soft tissue tumors are Kaposi sarcoma and leiomyosarcoma (*Anal Quant Cytol Histol.* 2005;28:193).

8. **Hematolymphoid neoplasms** include very rare primary penile lymphomas and secondary lymphomas.

9. **Miscellaneous neoplasms** rarely encountered include melanoma (*J Urol.* 2005;173:1958).

10. **Secondary malignancies** are rare, with prostatic and urinary bladder carcinomas predominating (*Int J Surg Pathol.* 2010; Jan 14, epub ahead of print). The corpus cavernosum is the most common site of metastasis, but the spongiosum, skin, and glans may also be involved.

F. **Scrotal cancer** is most commonly squamous cell carcinoma.

1. **Squamous cell carcinoma** of the scrotum is usually detected as invasive disease, but some examples of squamous cell carcinoma in situ have been reported. Associations exist with exposure to soot (in chimney sweeps, described in 1775 by Sir Percival Pott), machine oil, psoriasis treated with coal tar, arsenic, psoralens/UV radiation, and HPV infection. Grossly, scrotal squamous cell carcinomas initially appear as a solitary nodule; later in their course they show ulceration and induration. Microscopically, most are well to moderately differentiated (e-**Fig. 30.10**). The tumor typically invades the scrotal wall, and larger cancers can involve the testis, spermatic cord, penis, and perineum. Initial metastatic spread is to ipsilateral inguinal lymph nodes. Outcome is related to tumor size and pathologic stage.

2. **Basal cell carcinomas** of scrotal skin are rare and have the same appearance as they do elsewhere in the skin.

3. **Paget disease** of the scrotum can be associated with underlying carcinoma of the urinary bladder, urethra, prostate, or eccrine sweat glands.

4. **Sarcomas** of the scrotal wall are rare and should be distinguished from paratesticular, intrascrotal sarcomas. By far the most common histologic type of scrotal wall sarcoma is leiomyosarcoma, which likely arises from the dartos muscle.

IV. **HISTOLOGIC GRADING OF PENILE AND SCROTAL SQUAMOUS CELL CARCINOMAS** is done in three tiers as well differentiated, moderately differentiated, or poorly differentiated. Histologic grade of penile squamous cell carcinoma is linked to depth of infiltration, inguinal lymph metastasis, and survival.

TABLE 30.2	**Tumor, Node, Metastasis (TNM) Staging Scheme for Penile Carcinoma**

Primary tumor (T)

TX	Primary tumor cannot be assessed
T0	No evidence of primary tumor
Tis	Carcinoma in situ
Ta	Noninvasive verrucous carcinoma
T1	Tumor invades subepithelial connective tissue
T1a	Tumor invades subepithelial connective tissue without lymphovascular invasion and is not poorly differentiated
T1b	Tumor invades subepithelial connective tissue with lymphovascular invasion or is poorly differentiated
T2	Tumor invades corpus spongiosum or cavernosum
T3	Tumor invades urethra
T4	Tumor invades other adjacent structures

Regional lymph nodes (N): Pathologic stage definition

pNX	Regional lymph nodes cannot be assessed
pN0	No regional lymph node metastasis
pN1	Metastasis in a single inguinal lymph node
pN2	Metastasis in multiple or bilateral inguinal lymph nodes
pN3	Extranodal extension of lymph node metastasis or pelvic lymph node(s) unilateral or bilateral

Distant metastasis (M)

M0	No distant metastasis
M1	Distant metastasis

Additional descriptor

The suffix "m" indicates the presence of multiple primary tumors and is recorded in parentheses, for example, pTa(m)N0M0.

Anatomic stage/prognostic groups

Stage 0	Tis	N0	M0
	Ta	N0	M0
Stage I	T1a	N0	M0
Stage II	T1b	N0	M0
	T2	N0	M0
	T3	N0	M0
Stage IIIa	T1–3	N1	M0
Stage IIIb	T1–3	N2	M0
Stage IV	T4	Any N	M0
	Any T	N3	M0
	Any T	Any N	M1

From: Edge SB, Byrd DR, Compton CC, et al., eds. *AJCC Cancer Staging Manual.* 7th ed. New York, NY: Springer; 2010. Used with permission.

V. **PATHOLOGIC STAGING OF PENILE CANCER** applies to carcinomas only. Pathologic primary tumor (pT) 2010 Tumor, Node, Metastasis (TNM) American Joint Committee on Cancer (AJCC) stage categories are given in Table 30.2 and are illustrated in Fig. 30.2. pN and pM groupings are also indicated in Table 30.2. The AJCC staging scheme for scrotal carcinoma is the same as for cutaneous squamous cell carcinomas.

VI. **REPORTING PENILE CARCINOMA** (*Arch Pathol Lab Med.* 2010;134:923). For circumcision and penectomy specimens, the following should be reported for the primary

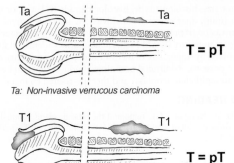

Ta: *Non-invasive verrucous carcinoma*

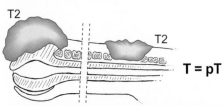

T1: *Tumor invading subepithelial connective tissue*

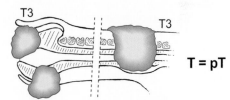

T2: *Tumor invading corpus spongiosum or cavernosum*

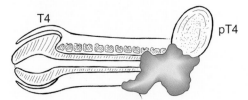

T3: *Tumor invading urethra or prostate*

T4: *Tumor invading other adjacent structures*

Figure 30.2 pT staging of penile carcinoma. (Modified from: Greene FL, Compton CC, Fritz AG, et al., eds. *AJCC Cancer Staging Atlas.* New York, NY: Springer; 2006.)

tumor: tumor size, histologic type, histologic grade (G1, G2, or G3), origin, depth of invasion (mm), anatomic level of invasion, structures involved, vascular and perineural invasion (if present), and status of the margins of resection. For regional lymph nodes, the report should include the number identified and their location, number involved by tumor, size of metastatic deposit (if present), and extracapsular extension (if present). Additional pathologic findings that can be noted (if present) are penile intraepithelial neoplasia and therapy-related changes.

SUGGESTED READING

Epstein JI, Cubilla AL, Humphrey PA. Tumors of the prostate gland, seminal vesicles, penis, and scrotum. In: *Atlas of Tumor Pathology.* 4th Series. Washington, DC: American Registry of Pathology; 2011.

31 The Ovary

Meredith E. Pittman, John D. Pfeifer, and Phyllis C. Huettner

I. **NORMAL GROSS AND MICROSCOPIC ANATOMY.** The ovaries rest on either side of the uterus and are anchored by the broad ligament. Age and reproductive status greatly impact size and weight, which range from 3 to 5 cm and 5 to 8 g, respectively. The outer surface of the ovary is white-tan and smooth during early reproductive years but becomes more bosselated with age due to repeated rupture of ovarian follicles. The cut surface is vaguely organized into three ill-defined zones: an outer cortex, underlying medulla, and inner hilum. The cortex and medulla contain cystic follicles, yellow or orange corpora lutea, and gritty, white corpora albicantia.

Histologic sections of the ovary show a simple cuboidal surface epithelial layer derived from mesothelium. Within the ovarian cortex and medulla, follicular structures composed of an inner layer of granulosa cells and an outer layer of theca cells (e-Fig. 31.1* and e-Fig. 31.2), in varying phases of development, are surrounded by a stroma comprised closely packed S-shaped spindled cells and collagen (e-Fig. 31.3). Centrally hemorrhagic corpora lutea composed of granulosa cells with abundant eosinophilic cytoplasm and smaller theca cells (e-Fig. 31.4 and e-Fig. 31.5), as well as white acellular corpora albicantia (e-Fig. 31.6), may also be seen. The hilus, where the ovary connects to the broad ligament, is composed of abundant blood vessels, nerves, and interspersed eosinophilic hilar cells that are histologically similar to the Leydig cells of the testis (e-Fig. 31.7). Rete ovarii, the developmental analogue of the rete testis that are composed of slit-like spaces lined by nonciliated cuboidal epithelium, are also present in the hilum (e-Fig. 31.8).

II. **GROSS EXAMINATION AND TISSUE SAMPLING.** The most common ovarian specimens encountered in surgical pathology are from oophorectomy (with or without hysterectomy) or cystectomy procedures. The weight and gross measurements of all three dimensions are recorded. The capsule is inspected for areas of rupture, adhesions, tumor involvement, or other abnormalities. In most cases, the ovary is then bivalved along the long axis and any lesions on the cut surface are noted. Solid, cystic, or papillary lesions are thoroughly sampled (one section per cm). If no lesions are identified, one section for every 2 cm is adequate. If cysts are present, the color and consistency of the cyst fluid are noted, and any areas of nodularity or papillary excrescences are sampled. Prophylactic oophorectomy specimens, performed for a personal history of cancer or family history of a hereditary cancer syndrome, are cut perpendicular to the long axis and entirely submitted.

The surgical management of malignant primary ovarian tumors typically includes a staging procedure, and so an ovary excised for a primary malignancy will usually be accompanied by multiple abdominal-peritoneal biopsies, an omentectomy specimen, and regional lymph nodes. The small peritoneal biopsies are submitted entirely. The omentum sample must be serially sectioned. If grossly visible tumor is present, it should be measured and only one section needs to be submitted; when no tumor is identified, from 5 to 10 sections are submitted. All identified lymph nodes are submitted from the lymph node dissections.

III. **DIAGNOSTIC FEATURES OF COMMON BENIGN DESEASES OF THE OVARY**
   A. **Inflammatory Diseases**
      1. **Infection** of the ovary is almost always accompanied by infection of the fallopian tube (e-Fig. 31.9), systemic infection, or the development of a

---

*All e-figures are available online via the Solution Site Image Bank.

tubo-ovarian abscess (e-Fig. 31.10). The most common cause of oophoritis is ascending pelvic inflammatory disease (PID), which typically causes intense pelvic pain and is usually polymicrobial. The ovary contains sheets of neutrophils and often shows paraovarian adhesions or adhesions to an inflamed fallopian tube. Severe PID may require hospitalization and treatment, while mild PID may resolve on its own. The subsequent fibrosis and scarring from PID is a leading cause of infertility (e-Fig. 31.11).

2. **Autoimmune oophoritis** typically presents with oligomenorrhea and infertility and is often associated with other autoimmune disorders. The ovaries are normal in size but filled with a lymphoplasmacytic infiltrate in developing follicles and corpora lutea. Premature ovarian failure and premature menopause is the final sequelae of the disease.

3. **Noninfectious granulomas** may also be seen within the ovary as an incidental finding. These may form secondary to systemic diseases such as sarcoidosis, or represent a foreign body response following a pelvic or abdominal surgery.

B. Cysts

1. **Follicular cysts** are commonly found in prepubescent and reproductive-aged women. Normal follicles measure only up to 1 cm in greatest dimension, while follicular cysts measure 2.5 to 10 cm in diameter and contain serosanguineous fluid. Most cysts are asymptomatic, but women may present with an abdominal mass or rupture. Follicular cysts are typically unilateral with a thin, smooth lining comprised of an inner layer of granulosa cells and an outer layer of theca cells similar to normal follicles. Multiple follicular cysts may be associated with polycystic ovarian syndrome (PCOS) and McCune–Albright syndrome.

2. **Corpus luteum cysts** are also common in women of reproductive age. Like follicular cysts, they may present as a mass or with rupture. On gross examination, corpus luteum cysts are >3 cm, filled with thick hemorrhagic fluid, and rimmed by a yellow lining. Microscopically, the cyst has an undulating wall of luteinized granulosa cells (that have abundant, eosinophilic cytoplasm) with interspersed peripheral theca cells with an overall architecture similar to that of a normal corpus luteum.

3. **Polycystic ovarian syndrome** is an incompletely understood disease characterized by anovulation, infertility, hirsutism, and obesity. It is estimated that up to 10% of American women are affected by this syndrome, which typically presents between the ages of 20 and 30. In general, the ovaries are enlarged with a thickened, collagenized cortical surface; multiple, uniform follicles all in a similar phase of development (typically antral); and an absence of corpora lutea (indicting infrequent ovulation) (e-Fig. 31.12).

4. **Surface epithelial inclusion cysts,** thought to be formed by repeated invaginations of ovarian epithelium secondary to surface rupture with ovulation, are common. By convention, inclusion cysts measure <1 cm in diameter. The cysts are lined by a single layer of bland flat, cuboidal, or ciliated columnar cells (e-Fig. 31.13). Psammoma bodies may be seen. It is hypothesized that benign, borderline, and low-grade serous epithelial neoplasms arise from these inclusions.

5. **Paraovarian or paratubal cysts** are found in the hilar region of the ovary and arise from mesonephric (Wolffian) or paramesonephric (Müllerian) duct remnants. Mesonephric cysts are lined by simple or stratified epithelium and have prominent muscular walls (e-Fig. 31.14). Paramesonephric cysts are lined by columnar epithelium with a mixture of ciliated and nonciliated cells similar to epithelial inclusion cysts (e-Fig. 31.13).

6. **Endometriosis,** characterized by endometrial glands and stroma outside the uterus, is frequently seen within the ovary. Symptomatic patients typically present during the reproductive years with menstrual-associated pain and

infertility. Grossly, the ovary shows a thickened cortex, surface adhesions, and a cyst filled with thick brown fluid resembling chocolate syrup, the so-called chocolate cyst. Histologically, endometrial epithelium or glands and stroma with associated hemosiderin-laden macrophages and fibrosis are diagnostic (e-Fig. 31.15). Endometriotic cysts frequently contain areas with atypical cytologic features associated with acute inflammation, but areas of epithelial tufting, more complex architectural changes, or increased mitotic activity should raise suspicion for malignancy arising in endometriosis.

C. Hyperplastic changes

1. **Stromal hyperplasia,** defined as a proliferation of non-luteinized ovarian stroma in the cortex and medulla, and **hyperthecosis,** luteinized stromal cells in a background of stromal hyperplasia (e-Fig. 31.16), are changes most commonly seen in the sixth to seventh decades of life and in women with PCOS. The ovaries are enlarged bilaterally. While most women are asymptomatic, some present with estrogenic symptoms (endometrial hyperplasia) or androgenic symptoms (acne) due to hormone production by the luteinized cells.

2. **Hilus (Leydig) cell hyperplasia** is most common in postmenopausal women who also have stromal hyperplasia and hyperthecosis. The hilus cell proliferation rarely causes symptoms on its own. Microscopically, eosinophilic cells with hyperchromatic nuclei are arranged in nests or clusters found most often in the hilar region of the ovary. Elongated, eosinophilic intracytoplasmic inclusions, called Reinke's crystals, may be seen (e-Fig. 31.17).

D. Pregnancy changes

1. **Solitary luteinized follicle cysts** are benign, unilocular, unilateral cysts that may grow up to 25 cm in diameter. They have the same lining of inner granulosa cells and outer theca cells as normal follicles.

2. **Hyperreactio luteinalis** is characterized by symmetric, bilateral enlargement of the ovaries with multiple luteinized cysts. The condition is associated with high levels of human chorionic gonadotropin, which also occurs with multiple pregnancies, ovulation induction protocols, and gestational trophoblastic disease. The cysts usually resolve in the months after completion of pregnancy. Microscopically, the follicular cysts are lined by luteinized granulosa and theca cells with stromal edema.

3. **Pregnancy luteoma** is seen in the second half of pregnancy and is most common in multiparous African American women. The lesion consists of hyperplastic proliferations of luteinized cells, likely stromal and theca cells. Most pregnancy luteomas are incidental findings, but 25% of patients will have symptoms of virilization. Grossly, the nodules are multiple (50%), bilateral (33%), yellow-brown, hemorrhagic, and soft. Microscopically, they are well-circumscribed collections of large eosinophilic cells that may have many mitotic figures (e-Fig. 31.18). The nodules regress after pregnancy.

E. Ovarian torsion

is frequently accompanied by torsion of the fallopian tube as well. Torsion is caused by twisting of the adnexa on its fibrovascular pedicle impeding blood flow into and out of the adnexal structures, ultimately resulting in infarction. The ovary is often enlarged and hemorrhagic or dusky. Microscopically, there is extensive interstitial hemorrhage, edema, and necrosis of normal tissue. Frequently there is an associated ovarian mass or neoplasm. Pregnant women and women with adnexal masses are at increased risk, but torsion can occur in children, infants, and occasionally in utero. Patients typically present with acute abdominal pain, nausea, and vomiting, and may have a palpable adnexal mass.

IV. OVARIAN NEOPLASMS.

Table 31.1 presents a simplified version of the World Health Organization (WHO) histologic classification of tumors of the ovary.

TABLE 31.1	Modified WHO Histologic Classification of Tumors of the Ovary

Surface epithelial-stromal tumors
Serous tumors
   Malignant
      Adenocarcinoma
   Borderline tumor
   Benign
      Cystadenoma, adenofibroma, cystadenofibroma
Mucinous tumors
   Malignant
      Adenocarcinoma
   Borderline tumor
   Benign
      Cystadenoma, adenofibroma, cystadenofibroma
   Mucinous cystic tumor with pseudomyxoma peritonei
Endometrioid tumors including variants with squamous differentiation
   Malignant
      Adenocarcinoma
      Malignant mixed Müllerian tumor (carcinosarcoma)
      Endometrioid stromal sarcoma (low grade)
      Undifferentiated ovarian sarcoma
   Borderline tumor
   Benign
      Cystadenoma, adenofibroma, cystadenofibroma
Clear cell tumors
   Malignant
      Adenocarcinofibroma
   Borderline tumor
   Benign
      Cystadenoma, adenofibroma, cystadenofibroma
Transitional cell tumors
   Malignant
      Transitional cell carcinoma (non-Brenner type)
      Malignant Brenner tumor
   Borderline
   Benign
      Brenner tumor
Squamous cell tumors
   Squamous cell carcinoma
Mixed epithelial tumors (specify components)
   Malignant
   Borderline
   Benign
Undifferentiated and unclassified tumors
   Undifferentiated carcinoma
   Adenocarcinoma, not otherwise specified

Sex cord-stromal tumors
Granulosa-stromal cell tumors
   Granulosa cell tumor group
      Adult granulosa cell tumor
      Juvenile granulosa cell tumor

(continued)

TABLE 31.1	Modified WHO Histologic Classification of Tumors of the Ovary (*Continued*)

Thecoma-fibroma group
  Thecoma, not otherwise specified
    Typical
    Luteinized
  Fibroma
  Cellular fibroma
  Fibrosarcoma
  Stromal tumor with minor sex cord elements
  Sclerosing stromal tumor
  Signet-ring stromal tumor
  Unclassified (fibrothecoma)
Sertoli-stromal cell tumors
  Sertoli-Leydig cell tumor group
    Well differentiated
    Of intermediate differentiation
      Variant with heterologous elements (specify type)
    Poorly differentiated (sarcomatoid)
      Variant with heterologous elements (specify type)
    Retriform
      Variant with heterologous elements (specify type)
  Sertoli cell tumor
  Stromal-Leydig cell tumor
Sex cord-stromal tumors of mixed or unclassified cell types
  Sex cord tumor with annular tubules
  Gynandroblastoma (specify components)
  Sex cord-stromal tumor, unclassified
Steroid cell tumors
  Stromal luteoma
  Leydig cell tumor group
    Hilus cell tumor
    Leydig cell tumor, non-hilar type
    Leydig cell tumors, not otherwise specified
  Steroid cell tumor, not otherwise specified
    Well differentiated
    Malignant
Germ cell tumors
Primitive germ cell tumors
  Dysgerminoma
  Yolk sac tumor
  Embryonal carcinoma
  Polyembryoma
  Nongestational choriocarcinoma
  Mixed germ cell tumor (specify components)
Biphasic or triphasic teratoma
  Immature teratoma
  Mature teratoma
    Solid
    Cystic
    Fetiform teratoma (homunculus)
Monodermal teratoma and somatic-type tumors associated with dermoid cysts
  Thyroid tumor group
    Struma ovarii
      Benign
      Malignant (specify type)

(*continued*)

TABLE 31.1	Modified WHO Histologic Classification of Tumors of the Ovary (*Continued*)

Carcinoid group
Neuroectodermal tumor group
Carcinoma group
Melanocytic group
   Malignant melanoma
   Melanocytic nevus
Sarcoma group (specify type)
Sebaceous tumor group
Pituitary-type tumor group
Retinal anlage tumor group
Others

Germ cell sex cord-stromal tumors
Gonadoblastoma
   Variant with malignant germ cell tumor
Mixed germ cell-sex cord-stromal tumor
   Variant with malignant germ cell tumor

Tumors of the rete ovarii
Adenocarcinoma
Adenoma
Cystadenoma
Cystadenofibroma

Miscellaneous tumors
Small cell carcinoma, hypercalcemic type
Small cell carcinoma, pulmonary type
Large cell neuroendocrine carcinoma
Hepatoid carcinoma
Primary ovarian mesothelioma
Wilms tumor
Gestational choriocarcinoma
Hydatidiform mole
Adenoid cystic carcinoma
Basal cell tumor
Ovarian Wolffian tumor
Paraganglioma
Myxoma
Soft tissue tumors not specific to the ovary
Others

Tumor-like conditions
Luteoma of pregnancy
Stromal hyperthecosis
Stromal hyperplasia
Fibromatosis
Massive ovarian edema
Others

Lymphoid and hematopoietic tumors
Malignant lymphoma (specify type)
Leukemia (specify type)
Plasmacytoma

Secondary tumors

From: Tavassoli FA, Devilee P, eds. *World Health Organization Classification of Tumours. Pathology and Genetics. Tumours of the Breast and Female Genital Organs.* Lyon: IARC Press; 2003. Used with permission.

A. **Surface epithelial-stromal tumors.** Tumors of ovarian surface epithelium represent approximately two-thirds of all ovarian neoplasms. Ovarian surface epithelium may differentiate into any Müllerian-type epithelium, accounting for the various subtypes of ovarian epithelial tumors: serous (resembling fallopian tube), endometrioid (resembling endometrium), and mucinous (resembling endocervix). Clear cell and transitional tumors have no normal counterpart in the gynecologic tract. The standard of treatment for these tumors is surgery, with the goal of staging and optimally debulking the tumor, followed by chemotherapy for all but certain stage I tumors.

1. **Serous tumors** are the most common subtype of surface epithelial tumors. The majority of serous tumors are benign and occur in women aged 30 to 40 years. About 15% are borderline (also known as low malignant potential [LMP] or atypical proliferating) tumors. About 25% are malignant. The neoplastic epithelium, particularly in benign and borderline tumors, resembles fallopian tube epithelium and contains ciliated and secretory cells; the cystic spaces contain serous or serosanguineous fluid.

   a. **Serous cystadenoma/cystadenofibroma.** These benign lesions make up over half of all serous tumors, and they are most commonly found in reproductive-aged women. Grossly they are unilocular, smooth-walled cysts with varying amounts of fibrous stroma, usually ranging from 1 to 10 cm. Histologically, the cystadenoma lining is a single layer of columnar and usually ciliated epithelium (e-Fig. 31.19). Cystadenofibromas show broad stromal papillae lined by simple columnar ciliated epithelium (e-Fig. 31.20). The lining may be attenuated in longstanding lesions. Lesions without a cystic component are termed adenofibromas.

   b. **Borderline serous tumors (serous tumors of low malignant potential)** are predominantly cystic and generally present in perimenopausal women. As many as one-third are bilateral. These tumors have papillary excrescences with hierarchically branching stromal cores. The lining alls show mild to moderate cytologic atypica and demonstrate mildly increased mitotic activity, stratification, tufting, and detached buds of epithelium (e-Fig. 31.21). Psammoma bodies are frequently seen. By definition these tumors do not demonstrate stromal invasion.

   Although most borderline serous tumors are confined to the ovary, extraovarian disease such as peritoneal implants may be present at diagnosis. The classification of the tumor is then based on the features found within the primary ovarian tumor, not the extraovarian disease. Peritoneal implants associated with borderline tumors are classified as invasive or noninvasive (*Cancer.* 1988;62:2212). Noninvasive implants have a smooth interface with the surrounding tissue. By convention, a specimen that contains only implant with no surrounding normal tissue is assumed to be a noninvasive implant. Noninvasive implants are subclassified as epithelial if there is an epithelial proliferation with no stromal response, and desmoplastic if there is a stromal response that distorts or compresses the epithelial cells (e-Fig. 31.22). In contrast, invasive implants irregularly infiltrate and efface the underlying tissue (e-Fig. 31.23); some groups have proposed that implants with epithelium exhibiting a micropapillary architecture or solid nests surrounded by a clefted space also represent a form of invasive implant. The presence of invasive implants is associated with a poorer prognosis and is generally treated with chemotherapy.

   Two additional architectural patterns may be seen in serous borderline tumors: micropapillary and cribriform. In the micropapillary pattern, long thin filiform projections (five times as long as they are wide) project directly from stromal cores without hierarchical branching (e-Fig. 31.24). The cribriform pattern is often associated with the micropapillary pattern and shows fusion of the tips of papillae with the formation of cribriform structures (e-**Fig. 31.25**). Both of these patterns are associated with a poorer prognosis due to their association with invasive implants. Some groups classify tumors with these patterns as a form of low-grade serous carcinoma and use the term micropapillary or micro-cribriform serous carcinoma.

c. **Serous borderline tumors with microinvasion.** Occasional serous borderline tumors exhibit microinvasion where individual eosinophilic cells or small nests of cells, often surrounded by a clefted space, invade the stroma (e-**Fig. 31.26**). These microinvasive areas should involve <3 mm in greatest linear extent or <10 mm^2 in area. The prognostic significance of microinvasion is not completely understood, but it may be a risk factor for disease progression (*Am J Surg Pathol.* 2006;30:1209).

d. **Serous adenocarcinoma** most commonly presents as bilateral masses with widespread peritoneal metastases. Grossly, the tumors are large and friable with multiloculated cysts and polypoid growths. Microscopically, the tumors may show a wide variety of architectural patterns including papillary, solid, and nested with slit-like spaces. Nuclear atypia is variable but often marked. By definition, serous carcinomas demonstrate destructive stromal invasion (e-**Fig. 31.27**). Psammoma bodies may be present.

Serous carcinomas should be graded into high grade and low grade. Low-grade tumors (<12 mitoses/10 high power fields and low-grade cytologic atypia) (e-**Fig. 31.28**) are frequently resistant to chemotherapy and are more appropriately treated surgically.

A rare form of serous adenocarcinoma known as psammocarcinoma is characterized by invasive stromal growth, abundant psammoma bodies in at least 75% of the papillae, and no areas of solid growth >15 cells across (*Gynecol Pathol.* 1990;9:110). This tumor generally has a good prognosis.

2. **Mucinous tumors** are the second most common type of surface epithelial tumor. The neoplastic epithelium resembles intestinal (goblet cells with intracytoplasmic mucin), gastric (foveolar), or endocervical (apical mucin with no cilia) epithelium. Eighty percent of these tumors are benign, 10% are borderline, and 10% are malignant. Because mucinous neoplasms are quite heterogeneous and a malignant component may be very focal, it is imperative that all mucinous neoplasms be well sampled (one to two sections per cm).

a. **Mucinous cystadenomas** are usually unilateral, multiloculated, and large (up to 50 cm). They have a smooth external surface and are filled with thick viscous secretions. Microscopically, the cysts are lined by a single layer of tall columnar cells with bland basal nuclei, most often of intestinal type (e-**Fig. 31.29**). If there is a prominent stromal component, the lesion is termed a mucinous cystadenofibroma.

b. **Borderline mucinous tumors (mucinous tumors of low malignant potential)** also present as unilateral, multiloculated masses. They are most common in perimenopausal women. Grossly, these tumors have thick cyst walls sometimes with papillary excrescences. Microscopically, mucinous borderline tumors have a stratified, tufted intestinal-type epithelial lining with mild to moderate nuclear atypia (e-**Fig. 31.30**). By definition, borderline mucinous tumors do not demonstrate destructive stromal invasion.

Borderline tumors with endocervical-type epithelium (15% of mucinous borderline tumors) have the hierarchical branching pattern of serous borderline tumors but the papilla are lined by mucinous epithelium; they are often associated with acute inflammation and frequently with endometriosis and bilaterality (e-**Fig. 31.31**). Some borderline tumors show a mixture of endocervical-type mucinous epithelium, serous epithelium, and even endometrioid epithelium; these tumors also have the hierarchical branching architecture of serous borderline tumor and are also associated with endometriosis and bilaterality.

c. **Mucinous borderline tumors with intraepithelial carcinoma** resemble borderline tumors but contain focal areas that demonstrate increased cytologic atypia with marked pleomorphism and prominent nucleoli (e-**Fig. 31.32**). No destructive stromal invasion is present, and the intraepithelial carcinoma does not appear to portend a worse prognosis (*Ann Surg Oncol.* 2010;18:40).

d. **Mucinous borderline tumors with microinvasion.** These are mucinous borderline tumors with small foci of invasion either as small nests or as individual cells, often with more eosinophilic cytoplasm. These foci should not exceed 3 mm in greatest linear extent or 10 mm^2 in area (e-**Fig. 31.33**).

e. **Mucinous adenocarcinoma** also presents in perimenopausal women as unilateral, multiloculated cystic masses. Frank stromal invasion is present microscopically (e-**Fig. 31.34**), but mucinous carcinomas frequently demonstrate areas of benign and borderline mucinous epithelium as well. Two patterns of invasion are recognized. The expansile pattern shows crowded glands, little stroma, and, sometimes a cribriform architecture. The destructive pattern shows single glands or individual cells invading >3 mm in two linear dimensions or >10 mm^2 in area.

Approximately 5% of women with a mucinous ovarian tumor will present with **pseudomyxoma peritonei,** a condition in which pools of mucin, with or without associated neoplastic epithelium, fill the peritoneal cavity. Although controversial in the past, there is now general consensus that most mucinous tumors in the ovary associated with pseudomyxoma peritonei are metastatic in origin. The appendix is the most common primary site (*Am J Surg Pathol.* 1995;19:1390). Microscopically, the ovary shows pools of mucin dissecting through the stroma (pseudomyxoma ovarii) with or without associated mucinous epithelium (e-**Fig. 31.35**).

When trying to distinguish a primary from a metastatic ovarian mucinous adenocarcinoma, both histologic and immunohistochemical features are helpful. Primary tumors exhibit benign, borderline, and malignant epithelium whereas metastatic tumors are more uniformly malignant. Features seen more commonly in metastatic disease include bilaterality, concomitant extraovarian disease, involvement of the external surface of the ovary, pseudomyxoma ovarii, and extensive lymphovascular space invasion. Metastatic adenocarcinoma from the colorectum will show abundant luminal karyorrhectic debris (dirty necrosis), a garland pattern of glands lining cystic spaces, an abrupt transition between viable and necrotic epithelium, and immunopositivity for CK20 and CEA but immunonegativity for CK7 and CA125 (e-**Fig. 31.36**).

3. **Endometrioid tumors.** The majority of endometrioid tumors of the ovary are carcinomas. From 10% to 20% are associated with endometriosis, and about 15% have a concomitant endometrioid tumor of the endometrium. Squamous differentiation may be seen in all types of endometrioid tumors.

a. **Benign endometrioid tumors** are adenofibromas/cystadenofibromas, with organized endometrial glands arranged in a fibrous stroma. These are quite rare and can be distinguished from endometriosis by a lack of associated endometrial-type stroma and hemosiderin-laden macrophages.

b. **Borderline endometrioid tumors.** Endometrioid tumors that show cytologic atypia and areas of confluent epithelial proliferation without stromal support up to 5 mm in maximal dimension are borderline endometrioid tumors, although there is some controversy as to diagnostic criteria and

TABLE 31.2	FIGO Grading Scheme for Endometrioid Adenocarcinoma
Grade 1 or well differentiated	Well-formed glands resembling villoglandular carcinoma of the uterine corpus[a]
	≤5% solid tumor growth
Grade 2 or moderately differentiated	More complex glandular architecture
	Increased nuclear stratification
	6%–50% solid tumor growth
Grade 3 or poorly differentiated	Poorly formed glands, large sheets of cells
	>50% solid tumor growth

[a]Areas of squamous differentiation are not included when assessing the amount of solid tumor growth.

nomenclature (*Am J Surg Pathol.* 2000;24:1465) (e-**Fig. 31.37**). Criteria for microinvasion within these tumors are not well established.

    c. **Endometrioid adenocarcinomas** may be cystic or solid. Microscopically, they show villoglandular structures and/or tubular glands composed of a stratified layer of epithelial cells with smooth luminal borders (e-**Fig. 31.38**). Squamous metaplasia is common. By definition, destructive stromal invasion is present. These tumors are graded using the International Federation of Gynecology and Obstetrics (FIGO) grading scheme identical to that for endometrial tumors, which is listed in Table 31.2.

4. **Clear cell tumors.** The vast majority of clear cell tumors are frank adenocarcinomas; benign and borderline clear cell tumors are quite rare. Clear cell carcinomas make up 5% of ovarian cancers and are often associated with endometriosis either in the ovary or elsewhere in the pelvis. They are also associated with age >50, nulliparity, and endometriosis. Grossly, clear cell adenocarcinomas are white-tan to yellow, solid, and cystic masses. Histologically, the tumor grows in sheets, tubules, and/or papillae. The large tumor cells have clear cytoplasm that may contain hyaline globules; the nuclei often jut into the lumen, giving the cells a "hobnail" appearance. The stroma is densely hyalinized and eosinophilic (e-**Fig. 31.39**). These tumors are always high grade and carry a poor prognosis.

5. **Brenner and transitional cell tumors**

    a. **Benign Brenner tumors** are usually unilateral and often an incidental finding. Grossly, they have a firm, white to tan whorled cut surface but may show cystic spaces and calcification. Histologic sections show nests of oval epithelial cells with pale cytoplasm, uniform nuclei, and longitudinal nuclear grooves surrounded by abundant fibrous stroma, often with areas of calcification. Cystic spaces may contain eosinophilic material or be lined by mucinous epithelium (e-**Fig. 31.40**). Brenner tumors have an associated benign mucinous cystic component in 25% of cases.

    b. **Borderline Brenner tumors (Brenner tumor of low malignant potential)** are grossly cystic with papillary excrescences. Microscopically, the cysts and broad frond-like papillae jut into cystic spaces and are lined by a stratified lining that resembles the epithelium of low-grade papillary urothelial carcinoma. Stromal invasion is absent (e-**Fig. 31.41**).

    c. **Malignant Brenner tumors** may be solid or cystic. By definition, stromal invasion is present and there is always an identifiable borderline or benign Brenner component (e-**Fig. 31.42**). The invasive component may resemble low-grade or high-grade urothelial carcinoma, or even squamous cell carcinoma or adenocarcinoma.

    d. **Transitional cell carcinomas (TCC)** of the ovary closely resemble TCC of the bladder, and the grading scheme is the same. These tumors are solid and cystic on gross examination. Microscopically, they are composed of papillary cores lined by stratified, cytologically atypical epithelium. By definition, no benign or borderline Brenner tumor component is present.

6. **Carcinosarcoma.** Also known as malignant mixed Müllerian tumor, carcinosarcoma occasionally presents as a primary tumor of the ovary, although the tumor much more commonly arises in the endometrium. The tumor usually occurs in postmenopausal women and has a poor prognosis. As with its endometrial counterparts, ovarian carcinosarcoma contains both malignant epithelial and malignant mesenchymal elements. Numerous genetic studies have demonstrated that both elements are derived from the same precursor, proving that the neoplasm does not represent a collision tumor but rather a poorly differentiated carcinoma with metaplastic sarcomatous elements. The epithelial component is most often a high-grade serous carcinoma but may be endometrioid, mucinous, clear cell, or even squamous carcinoma. The mesenchymal component may be homologous to the female genital tract (e.g., smooth muscle, endometrial stroma) or may be composed of heterologous elements not normally found in the female genital tract (e.g., cartilage, fat) (e-**Fig. 31.43**).

B. **Sex cord-stromal tumors.** These tumors represent approximately 8% of ovarian tumors and comprise the majority of the hormonally active ovarian neoplasms.

1. **Granulosa cell tumors**

a. **Adult granulosa cell tumors** (AGCTs) are low-grade neoplasms that occur most commonly in postmenopausal women but can occur at any age. AGCTs are the most common ovarian tumors with estrogenic manifestations (e.g., endometrial hyperplasia or carcinoma). Hormonal manifestations may alert the clinician to the presence of a granulosa cell tumor, but patients more commonly present with an adnexal mass. In about 10% of cases, patients present with hemoperitoneum from tumor rupture. The tumors are usually large (>10 cm) and unilateral. The cut surface is soft and yellow-tan with cysts and hemorrhage (e-**Fig. 31.44**).

These tumors exhibit a variety of histologic patterns including diffuse (e-**Fig. 31.45**), trabecular (e-**Fig. 31.46**), microfollicular, macrofollicular (e-**Fig. 31.47**), or gyriform (e-**Fig. 31.48**), and often more than one pattern is found within the same tumor. No matter the architecture, the cytology is usually bland with oval nuclei, longitudinal nuclear grooves, and a low mitotic rate (e-**Fig. 31.49**). The microfollicular and diffuse variants often contain characteristic Call-Exner bodies consisting of a small collection of eosinophilic material lined by palisaded granulosa cells (e-**Fig. 31.50**). AGCTs usually exhibit minimal cytologic atypia although areas of "bizarre" nuclei may be seen (e-**Fig. 31.51**).

AGCTs are usually confined to the ovary and spread outside the ovary is a poor prognostic factor. Tumors with high stage, large size, nuclear atypia, high mitotic activity, and a sarcomatoid pattern have a poorer prognosis, although tumors with none of these factors may recur. AGCTs are unusual in that they may recur decades after diagnosis.

b. **Juvenile granulosa cell tumors** (JGCTs) occur in children and young adults, typically under the age of 20. They usually present with a palpable mass and symptoms of hyperestrogenism such as breast development in children or menstrual irregularities in adolescents. The gross findings are similar to those of adult granulosa cell tumors with yellow-tan solid areas and interspersed blood-filled cysts.

Microscopically JGCTs are characterized by solid sheets of cells mixed with small follicle-like spaces with basophilic or eosinophilic secretions lined by more mature-appearing granulosa cells. Luteinization is prominent (e-**Fig. 31.52**). JGCTs exhibit more cytologic atypia and a higher mitotic rate than adult granulosa cell tumors. The nuclei do not have grooves (e-**Fig. 31.53**).

JGCTs are usually confined to the ovary and high stage is a poor prognostic factor. Unlike their adult counterparts, patients with JGCT who recur usually do so within 2 years of diagnosis. Cytologic atypia is not a poor prognostic factor in JGCTs.

2. Fibroma-thecoma

a. Fibromas represent the most common of the sex cord-stromal tumors. They typically occur in perimenopausal women and are not hormonally active. Grossly, fibromas are unilateral, solid, and lobulated with a firm, white-gray cut surface. Cystic degeneration sometimes occurs. Histologically, they are characterized by interlacing bundles and storiform areas of spindle cells that show no atypia and few mitoses (e-**Fig. 31.54**). The tumor cells stain diffusely positive for vimentin and are usually negative for inhibin.

Fibromas may be associated with two syndromes. Meig syndrome (fibroma, ascites, and pleural effusion) and Gorlin syndrome (basal cell nevus syndrome). In Gorlin syndrome, fibromas occur in younger women or even children, are often multiple or bilateral, and are calcified.

b. Thecomas are unilateral solid tumors found most often in postmenopausal women. Hyperestrogenic symptoms are present in 50% to 80% of cases. Grossly, these tumors have a lobulated, yellow-tan cut surface. Histologically, thecomas comprise round to oval, lipid-laden theca cells in a fibromatous stroma with little atypia or mitotic activity (e-**Fig. 31.55**). Immunohistochemically, the tumor is positive for inhibin. Oil Red O fat stains (which require fresh tissue) highlight the intracellular lipid. When clusters of lutein cells (eosinophilic cells with large round nuclei) are present, the tumor is termed a luteinized thecoma (e-**Fig. 31.56**); this variant is more common in younger women.

3. Sertoli and Sertoli-Leydig Cell Tumors

a. Sertoli cell tumors are rare, low-grade, nonfunctioning tumors that occur in women of child-bearing age. Grossly, they are yellow-tan, solid, lobulated tumors. Microscopically, they are composed of closely packed tubules separated by fibrous stroma. The tubules are lined by cuboidal to columnar cells with abundant pale eosinophilic cytoplasm with little atypia or mitotic activity.

b. Sertoli-Leydig cell tumors (SLCT) are rare, unilateral neoplasms that occur in young women and, in 30% of cases, secrete androgenic hormones. Grossly, these tumors average 10 cm in diameter, are yellow-orange to red-brown, and frequently have a nodular appearance with a central scar (e-**Fig. 31.57**). Well-differentiated SLCTs contain tubules (similar to those seen in Sertoli cell tumors) and interspersed clusters of Leydig cells that have abundant eosinophilic cytoplasm (e-**Fig. 31.58**). SLCT of intermediate differentiation contain solid cords of Sertoli cells (e-**Fig. 31.59**), while Leydig cells may be more difficult to find but are typically located at the periphery of cellular nodules. The Leydig cells often show lipidization with foamy rather than eosinophilic cytoplasm (e-**Fig. 31.60**). Poorly differentiated SLCT show densely packed atypical spindled cells resembling a sarcoma (e-**Fig. 31.61**).

Two morphologic variants of SLCT occur, usually in association with tumors of intermediate differentiation or poorly differentiated tumors. About 20% of SLCT harbor heterologous elements that take the form of intestinal type mucinous glands (e-**Fig. 31.62**) or carcinoid tumor, (which have a good prognosis) or rhabdomyoblastic or cartilaginous differentiation (which have a poor prognosis). About 15% of SLCT contain tubules and slit-like glandular structures, or micropapillary structures with dense fibrovascular cores (e-**Fig. 31.63**); these tumors are referred to as retiform variants. Retiform tumors are less likely to be androgen secreting and more common in younger age groups (average age is 15 years).

4. **Steroid cell tumors** are uncommon neoplasms composed of large cells with intracellular lipid that resemble Leydig cells or luteinized stromal cells.

   a. **Stromal luteomas** are benign, hormonally active steroid cell tumors that usually occur in postmenopausal women. Estrogenic manifestations are seen in 60% of cases; androgenic in 10% of cases. These well-circumscribed tumors grow within the ovarian parenchyma and have a yellow-brown cut surface. Microscopically, polygonal cells with eosinophilic cytoplasm grow in sheets, nests, and cords (e-**Fig. 31.64**). Degenerative changes may cause slit-like spaces within the tumor. Crystals of Reinke (slender, eosinophilic, rod-shaped crystals) are absent (e-**Fig. 31.17**). Stromal hyperplasia may occur in the ipsilateral or contralateral ovary.

   b. **Leydig cell tumors** are also benign steroid cell neoplasms found in postmenopausal women, although these tumors are more often androgenic or nonfunctioning. The majority of these tumors arise within the ovarian hilus although they also can occur in the ovarian stroma. The cut surface is yellow-brown with areas of hemorrhage. Microscopically, large polygonal cells with foamy or granular eosinophilic cytoplasm and round nuclei grow in cellular clusters separated by pink acellular areas (e-**Fig. 31.65**). In order to classify a tumor as a Leydig cell tumor Reinke's crystals must be identified.

   c. **Hilus cell tumors** are benign tumors composed of the same cell population but that originate in the hilus of the ovary. Hilus cell tumors are usually associated with androgenic symptoms.

   d. **Steroid cell tumor, not otherwise specified** (NOS) is a steroid cell tumor that does not meet the criteria for any of the types mentioned earlier. These are the most common of the steroid cell tumors and may occur at any age. They are often hormonally active (50% androgenic, 10% estrogenic), and their gross morphology is similar to the other types of steroid cell tumor. Histologically, steroid cell tumor, NOS is composed of large cells with abundant granular cytoplasm separated by a vascular stroma. Reinke's crystals are absent. A poorer prognosis is seen in tumors with necrosis, hemorrhage, an increased mitotic rate, or size >7 cm.

5. **Other sex cord-stromal tumors**

   a. **Sclerosing stromal tumors** are rare benign neoplasms seen most often in girls and women <30 years of age. Grossly the tumor is firm to rubbery and white with areas of cystic degeneration. Histologically, cellular areas, consisting of both spindled cells and round cells with vacuolated cytoplasm, alternate with edematous and collagenized areas giving the tumor a pseudolobular appearance (e-**Fig. 31.66**).

   b. **Sex cord tumors with annular tubules (SCTAT)** occur in women of childbearing age. In some women, the tumor occurs as a component of Peutz–Jeghers syndrome, in which case the SCTATs are small and incidental. Those unassociated with Peutz–Jeghers syndrome form a large, solid, yellow mass. Histologically, the tumor is composed of well-circumscribed, ring-shaped tubules that contain central hyalinized material. The tubules are lined by cells with pale cytoplasm oriented toward the center of the tubule, with peripheral elongated nuclei (e-**Fig. 31.67**).

C. **Germ cell tumors**

1. **Teratomas**

   a. **Mature teratomas** are the most common ovarian germ cell tumor. They occur most often in adult women of reproductive age but may occur at any age. Grossly, they are usually cystic with a single solid nodule that may contain fat, teeth, bone, and many other tissue types. The cysts usually contain hair, soft yellow sebaceous debris. Microscopically, mature tissue from all three germ layers (ectoderm—skin or central nervous system elements; mesoderm—smooth muscle, teeth, bone; endoderm—respiratory epithelium, GI epithelium, thyroid) may be present (e-**Fig. 31.68**). The term dermoid cyst is commonly used to refer to mature cystic teratomas lined by squamous epithelium that containing skin appendages (e-**Fig. 31.69**). Mature cystic teratomas should be thoroughly sampled (one section per cm) in order to exclude an immature component, and to exclude malignant transformation of one of the mature components (a rare occurrence).

   b. **Immature teratomas** are rapidly growing malignant tumors that occur in children and young adults. They are unilateral and typically have solid and cystic components. The solid areas are generally more extensive than in a mature teratoma. Microscopically, they contain immature or primitive tissue (derived from any or all three germ cell layers) that is usually mixed with areas of mature tissue. The most common immature element is neuroectodermal and consists of rosettes, masses, or tubules of primitive neural cells (e-**Fig. 31.70**).

   Immature teratomas are graded based on the relative amount of immature tissue present (*Int J Gynecol Pathol.* 1994;13:283). Tumors with more than one low-power field of immature neuroepithelium on any given slide are considered high grade and require adjuvant chemotherapy.

   c. **Monodermal teratomas** are teratomas in which all the tissue is derived from one germ cell layer. **Struma ovarii** is the most common monodermal teratoma and consists of mature thyroid tissue, including follicles and colloid (e-**Fig. 31.71**). Secondary changes such as hyperplasia, adenoma, and even carcinoma may be seen.

2. **Carcinoid tumors** of the ovary usually arise in a mature cystic teratoma. They most commonly have an insular or trabecular pattern identical to that seen in the gastrointestinal tract. The cells are small and uniform with round nuclei with stippled chromatin. Goblet cell carcinoids are very uncommon. Metastasis from a primary carcinoid tumor outside the ovary must always be excluded; metastatic carcinoid tumors are more likely to be bilateral, larger, unassociated with a teratoma, and more commonly associated with carcinoid syndrome.

3. **Dysgerminoma** is the most common malignant germ cell tumor. It occurs as pure dysgerminoma or as a component of mixed germ cell tumor. Dysgerminoma develops most commonly in adolescents and young women and is frequent in patients with ovarian dysgenesis. Patients with dysgerminomas frequently have elevated LDH levels and occasionally mildly elevated hCG levels. Pure dysgerminomas have an excellent prognosis when treated by current therapeutic regimens.

   Grossly, dysgerminomas are large and solid with a smooth external surface and a lobulated gray-tan cut surface. The tumor should be thoroughly sampled (one section per cm) for microscopic examination to exclude other germ cell tumor types, and special attention should be directed to hemorrhagic and cystic areas.

   Dysgerminomas are analogous to testicular seminomas and have an identical histologic appearance. They are composed of nests and sheets of uniform large round cells with abundant clear cytoplasm, large nuclei, and prominent nucleoli. Tumor cells are separated by a lymphocyte-rich fibrous stroma (e-**Fig. 31.72**). Often a histiocytic or granulomatous infiltrate is present, and multinucleated syncytiotrophoblastic cells may also be identified (sometimes the former component can obscure the dysgerminoma cells).

Dysgerminomas are immunopositive for placental alkaline phosphatase (PLAP), c-kit (CD117), SALL4, and OCT 3/4.

4. **Yolk sac tumors,** also known as endodermal sinus tumors, occur in young women, usually with an associated elevated serum alpha fetoprotein (AFP) level. Yolk sac tumors grow rapidly and have often spread outside the ovary at the time of diagnosis. They are often a component of mixed germ cell tumors. Grossly, yolk sac tumors are unilateral and large, with a smooth external surface and a solid and cystic yellow to tan cut surface. Hemorrhage and necrosis are often present.

   Many different histologic patterns occur, including microcystic, endodermal sinus, macrocystic, solid, polyvesicular-vitelline, papillary, hepatoid, and glandular. The microcystic pattern is the most common variant and is composed of small cystic spaces lined by cuboidal to columnar cells with clear cytoplasm and large hyperchromatic nuclei (e-**Fig. 31.73**). The endodermal sinus pattern is the second most common pattern. This pattern features characteristic Schiller–Duvall bodies (rounded fibrovascular papillae containing a single central vessel and lined by columnar tumor cells) (e-**Fig. 31.74**). The polyvesicular-vitelline pattern is composed of abundant cystic structures lined by tumor cells that are embedded in a dense cellular stroma. Yolk sac tumors are usually immunopositive for expression of keratins, alpha-1-antitrypsin, glypican 3, and AFP; immunostaining shows a lack of expression of EMA.

5. **Embryonal carcinoma** is a rare neoplasm in the ovary and is often a component of mixed germ cell tumors. Half of cases occur in prepubertal girls, and half have elevated beta-HCG levels. Grossly, these tumors are large ($\sim$17 cm) and solid with areas of hemorrhage and necrosis. Morphologically, the tumor is identical to embryonal carcinoma of the testis and is composed of large anaplastic cells with pale eosinophilic vacuolated cytoplasm that grow in sheets and nests. The nuclei are hyperchromatic with prominent nucleoli (e-**Fig. 31.75**). Atypical mitotic figures are common. Embryonal carcinoma is immunopositive for CD30, cytokeratin, PLAP, SALL4, and OCT 3/4.

6. **Polyembryoma** is a very rare, highly malignant neoplasm that usually is a component of a mixed germ cell tumor. Grossly, it presents as a unilateral solid mass with areas of hemorrhage and necrosis. Microscopically, the tumor is composed of embryoid bodies (embryonic disks lined by endoderm on one side, ectoderm on the opposite side, and associated yolk sac and amniotic cavities).

7. **Choriocarcinoma** of the ovary is rare in pure form. It is most often seen as a component of a mixed germ cell tumor, or as a metastasis from gestational trophoblastic disease. Primary choriocarcinoma presents in children and adolescents where elevated hCG levels are invariably present. Grossly, the tumor mass is hemorrhagic, soft, and tan. Microscopically, both cytotrophoblast and syncytiotrophoblast are present. Cytotrophoblasts have centrally located hyperchromatic nuclei, prominent nucleoli, clear cytoplasm, and well-defined cytoplasmic borders. Syncytiotrophoblast are multinucleated and are immunopositive for hCG. While syncytiotrophoblast may be seen as a component of other germ cell tumors, cytotrophoblast is seen only in choriocarcinoma.

8. **Mixed germ cell tumors** make up 10% of germ cell tumors. The most common combination is dysgerminoma and yolk sac tumor, although any combination may occur. The relative composition of the various histologic subtypes should be included in the final report since it can impact therapy and prognosis.

D. Miscellaneous

1. **Gonadoblastoma** is a rare tumor that contains both germ cell and sex cord-stromal components. Most patients have gonadal dysgenesis, and over 90%

have a Y chromosome. Approximately half of all cases harbor a malignant germ cell component, most often dysgerminoma. Gonadoblastoma is benign unless a malignant germ cell component is present.

Grossly, the tumor is usually small with a yellow to gray cut surface and areas of calcification. Histologically, the tumor consists of admixed primitive germ cells and sex cord-stromal derivatives (which resemble immature granulosa cells and Sertoli cells) surrounded by abundant basement membrane-like material, often with calcification.

2. **Hypercalcemic small cell carcinoma** is a highly malignant tumor with a poor prognosis that presents in young women. Approximately two-thirds of patients manifest hypercalcemia. This tumor is generally large and unilateral with a soft, white-tan, lobulated cut surface that shows areas of hemorrhage and necrosis. Histologic examination demonstrates sheets of small cells with scant cytoplasm admixed with follicle-like spaces filled with eosinophilic fluid (e-**Fig. 31.76**). The tumor nuclei are round with coarse chromatin and prominent nucleoli (e-**Fig. 31.77**). Some tumor cells have globular hyaline inclusions producing a vague rhabdoid morphology. The tumor cells are usually immunopositive for CK, EMA, WT-1, calretinin, CD10, and p53 and less commonly positive for vimentin, NSE, and chromogranin.

3. **Primary hematopoietic malignancies** of the ovary are extremely rare; however, secondary ovarian involvement may be seen in up to one-half of all lymphomas. The tumors are generally bilateral with a fleshy cut surface. Microscopically, they resemble their nodal or marrow counterparts. The most common lymphoma with secondary involvement of the ovary is diffuse large B-cell lymphoma containing sheets of large noncohesive cells that have irregular nuclear contours and increased mitotic activity. Immunohistochemical stains such as CD45 (leukocyte common antigen), as well as B and T cell markers, may be used to demonstrate a hematopoietic origin in difficult cases.

4. **Primary ovarian tumors of mesenchymal origin.** A wide variety of these tumors have been described, although they are quite rare.

   a. **Vascular tumors,** including hemangioma, lymphangioma, and low-grade angiosarcoma, have all been reported as primary ovarian neoplasms. The morphologic features are identical to tumors occurring primarily in the soft tissue.

   b. **Tumors of striated muscle origin,** such as rhabdomyoma and rhabdomyosarcoma, also rarely occur in the ovary. Primary osteosarcomas and chondrosarcomas have also been reported. For these neoplasms, generous sampling of the tumor is required to exclude the presence of an epithelial component which would indicate a carcinosarcoma of heterologous type.

   c. **Neural tumors,** including neurofibromas, schwannomas, and ganglioneuromas, have been reported in the ovary and may present in association with neurofibromatosis. The morphologic features are identical to tumors occurring in the peripheral nervous system.

   d. **Primary ovarian myxomas** are rare unilateral tumors composed of stellate and spindled cells in an abundant myxoid stroma. These tumors must be distinguished from pseudomyxoma ovarii, which is characterized by pools of mucin usually with associated strips of mucin-secreting epithelium.

5. **Metastases.** About 8% of ovarian tumors represent metastases, of which most are derived from the gastrointestinal tract (especially the large intestine, stomach, and appendix), breast, uterine corpus, and cervix. In young girls, ovarian metastases may be from neuroblastoma, rhabdomyosarcoma, Ewing sarcoma/peripheral neuroectodermal tumor, and malignant rhabdoid tumor of kidney.

TABLE 31.3 2010 TNM Staging for Ovarian Carcinoma and Primary Peritoneal Carcinoma

TNM categories (T)	FIGO stages	Description
TX		Primary tumor cannot be assessed
T0		No evidence of primary tumor
T1	I	Tumor limited to ovaries (one or both)
T1a	IA	Tumor limited to one ovary; capsule intact, no tumor on ovarian surface. No malignant cells in ascites or peritoneal washings
T1b	IB	Tumor limited to both ovaries; capsules intact, no tumor on ovarian surface. No malignant cells in ascites or peritoneal washings
T1c	IC	Tumor limited to one or both ovaries with any of the following: capsule ruptured, tumor on ovarian surface, malignant cells in ascites or peritoneal washings
T2	II	Tumor involves one or both ovaries with pelvic extension
T2a	IIA	Extension and/or implants on uterus and/or tube(s). No malignant cells in ascites or peritoneal washings
T2b	IIB	Extension to and/or implants on other pelvic tissues. No malignant cells in ascites or peritoneal washings
T2c	IIC	Pelvic extension and/or implants (T2a or T2b) with malignant cells in ascites or peritoneal washings
T3	III	Tumor involves one or both ovaries with microscopically confirmed peritoneal metastasis outside the pelvis
T3a	IIIA	Microscopic peritoneal metastasis beyond pelvis (no macroscopic tumor)
T3b	IIIB	Macroscopic peritoneal metastasis beyond pelvis ≤2 cm in greatest dimension
T3c	IIIC	Peritoneal metastasis beyond pelvis >2 cm in greatest dimension and/or regional lymph node metastasis
Regional lymph nodes (N)		
NX		Regional lymph nodes cannot be assessed
N0		No regional lymph node metastasis
N1	IIIC	Regional lymph node metastasis
Distant metastasis (M)		
M0		No distant metastasis
M1	IV	Distant metastasis (excludes peritoneal metastasis)

Anatomic stage/prognostic groups			
Stage I	T1	N0	M0
Stage IA	T1a	N0	M0
Stage IB	T1b	N0	M0
Stage IC	T1c	N0	M0
Stage II	T2	N0	M0
Stage IIA	T2a	N0	M0
Stage IIB	T2b	N0	M0
Stage IIC	T2c	N0	M0
Stage III	T3	N0	M0
Stage IIIA	T3a	N0	M0
Stage IIIB	T3b	N0	M0
Stage IIIC	T3c/Any T	N0/N1	M0
Stage IV	Any T	Any N	M1

From: Edge SB, Byrd DR, Compton CC, et al., eds. *AJCC Cancer Staging Manual.* 7th ed. New York, NY: Springer; 2010. Used with permission.

V. STAGING OF OVARIAN MALIGNANCIES

A. **Pathologic staging.** Ovarian cancer is staged surgically. The staging procedure includes bilateral salpingo-oophorectomy, hysterectomy, and omentectomy; biopsies of multiple pelvic and abdominal peritoneal surfaces; and regional lymph node dissections (as noted earlier). Cytologic examination of peritoneal washings is also performed. The 2010 AJCC/UICC/FIGO staging classification is given in Table 31.3.

B. **Items to include in the pathology report.** Because tumor histologic subtype and grade have prognostic and therapeutic significance, these items must always be included in the final pathology report. For stage I tumors (confined to the ovary), it is important to note whether tumor involves the surface of the ovary or whether the ovary was ruptured (preoperatively or during the procedure), assessments best made at the time of frozen section.

32 Fallopian Tube

Mitra Mehrad, John D. Pfeifer, and Phyllis C. Huettner

I. **NORMAL ANATOMY.** The fallopian tubes are formed from the Müllerian (paramesonephric duct) system and lie within the broad ligament between the ovary and the uterus. They conduct eggs from the surface of the ovary to the uterine cavity and are the usual site of fertilization. Each fallopian tube is shaped like an elongated funnel and is divided into four parts from lateral to medial: infundibulum, ampulla, isthmus, interstitium; the infundibulum contains the finger-like fimbriae distally.

The fallopian tube mucosa is branched and folded into plicae. The mucosa is lined by a nonstratified epithelium composed of three cell types: ciliated, secretory, and intercalated cells. The most common are the ciliated cells, followed by secretory cells, which together comprise over 90% of the cell population. The intercalated cells are seen as elongated nuclei sporadically present between the ciliated cells. The wall of the fallopian tube contains smooth muscle to aid in moving the fertilized egg into the uterus. The serosa contains abundant blood vessels and is continuous with the broad ligament.

II. **GROSS EXAMINATION, TISSUE SAMPLING, AND HISTOLOGIC SLIDE PREPARATION.** Fallopian tubes are usually received as a portion of a total abdominal hysterectomy–bilateral salpingo-oophorectomy specimen. Short cross sections of fallopian tube are received after tubal ligation procedures. Ectopic pregnancy specimens also usually contain a portion of fallopian tube. Rarely, specimens are received for primary fallopian tube tumors.

At the grossing station, the length and diameter of the fallopian tube should be documented, as well as the presence or absence of a fimbriated end, or evidence of prior ligation. The serosal surface should also be assessed for the presence of adhesions, cysts, exudates, rupture, or metastatic tumor. The tube is then serially sectioned.

A. **Benign specimens.** Three sections are submitted from a normal fallopian tube, specifically from the fimbriated end, ampulla, and isthmus end. Additional sections of any gross lesions are also submitted. Complete cross sections must be identified from a tubal ligation specimen.

When examining an ectopic pregnancy specimen, an embryo and/or placental villi will often be grossly evident. Hemorrhagic areas, including blood clot, along with obvious villous or embryonic tissue, should be submitted for histologic examination.

B. **Neoplastic specimens.** Primary tubal carcinoma specimens will show a dilated lumen filled with a papillary or solid tumor. An ovarian tumor secondarily involving the fallopian tube is more common than a primary fallopian tube tumor, and careful sectioning can help distinguish the two. Grossly, papillary and solid areas should be sampled thoroughly (at least one section per centimeter of tumor), along with uninvolved areas. If possible, a section showing the tumor's relationship to the ovary should be submitted.

C. **Prophylactic excision specimens.** Fallopian tube specimens received as part of a prophylactic hysterectomy–oophorectomy from patients with hereditary cancer syndromes (e.g., *BRCA1* syndrome) should be, together with the ovaries, entirely submitted for histologic examination. For the fallopian tube, the goal is to ensure sectioning and extensive examination of the fimbria (so-called SEE-FIM protocol), since the majority of early serous tumors occur in this area.

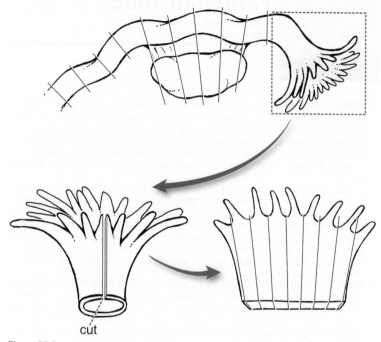

cut

Figure 32.1 Approach to sectioning fallopian tube specimens received as part of a prophylactic hysterectomy–oophorectomy from patients with a hereditary cancer syndrome. Each tube and ovary should be entirely submitted for histologic examination; note that the fimbriated end of the tube should be transected, opened longitudinally, serially sectioned longitudinally, and then entirely submitted for microscopic examination.

The protocol (*Am J Surg Pathol*. 2006;30:230) specifies that the entire tube is fixed for at least 4 hours to minimize loss of epithelium during manipulation, the distal 2 cm of the fimbriated end is transected, the fimbrial mucosa is sectioned longitudinally into four pieces, the remainder of the tube is sectioned transversely every 2 to 3 mm, and that all the sections are submitted in toto (Fig. 32.1).

III. DIAGNOSTIC FEATURES OF COMMON DISEASES

A. Inflammatory and nonneoplastic lesions of the fallopian tube

1. **Cystic lesions.** Embryologic remnants may be found in the fallopian tube wall, usually as an incidental finding (e-**Fig. 32.1**).* Paratubal cysts of Müllerian origin (ciliated lining) or Wolffian origin (stratified transitional lining) may be encountered; if the lining is atrophic secondary to compression, the two can be difficult to differentiate microscopically. Pedunculated paratubal cysts with a Müllerian epithelium present along the fimbriae are termed hydatid of Morgagni.

2. **Inflammatory lesions**

   a. **Acute salpingitis** usually presents in young- to middle-aged women, is generally an ascending infection initiated by *Chlamydia* or *Neisseria*

---

*All e-figures are available online via the Solution Site Image Bank.

gonorrhoeae, and is often followed by polymicrobial infection (pelvic inflammatory disease). The damage to the tube that results from acute salpingitis may lead to infertility and/or ectopic pregnancy. Grossly, the tubal lumen may be distended by pus, blood, or secretions. Histologic sections show marked acute inflammation, with congestion and edema in the plicae and the tubal wall which often severely distorts the normal tubal architecture (e-**Fig. 32.2**).

  b. Chronic salpingitis is usually due to resolving acute salpingitis. Grossly, the tube is often enlarged, fibrotic, distorted, and adherent to the ovary or adjacent structures. Microscopically, a lymphoplasmacytic infiltrate is seen in the plicae. Fusion of the tubal plicae after resolution of acute salpingitis may lead to formation of follicle-like spaces, a histologic pattern known as salpingitis follicularis. Hydrosalpinx may be seen in end-stage chronic salpingitis, microscopically characterized by a dramatically thinned wall with few plicae and a lumen filled with clear fluid. Numerous adhesions are typically present on the serosal surface (e-**Fig. 32.3**).

  c. Granulomatous salpingitis may be caused by tuberculosis, fungal infection, Crohn disease, or sarcoidosis.

  d. Salpingitis isthmica nodosum typically presents in young women. It is associated with ectopic pregnancy and infertility, and has an unclear pathogenesis. Grossly, it presents as 1 to 2 cm diameter nodules in the wall of the fallopian tube isthmus. It is bilateral in 85% of cases. The lesions consist of outpouchings of tubal epithelium surrounded by a thickened wall of smooth muscle (e-**Fig. 32.4**).

3. Other nonneoplastic lesions of the fallopian tube

  a. The fallopian tube is a frequent site of involvement of *endometriosis,* primarily in women of reproductive age, which may be associated with infertility. Grossly, tubal endometriosis consists of dark brown serosal nodules. The microscopic findings include endometrial glands surrounded by a cuff of endometrial stroma with associated hemosiderin-laden macrophages and chronic inflammatory cells (e-**Fig. 32.5**).

  b. Ectopic pregnancy affects 1% to 2% of all conceptions, and the fallopian tube is the most common site; the most commonly involved region of the tube is the ampulla. Risk factors include prior ectopic pregnancy, salpingitis, congenital tubal anomalies, salpingitis isthmica nodosum, and endometriosis. Patients may present with tubal rupture and shock. Grossly, the fallopian tube is dilated and hemorrhagic with identifiable chorionic villi, with or without an identifiable embryo. Histologic sections should show chorionic villi or trophoblast in the tubal mucosa or wall (e-**Fig. 32.6**).

B. Neoplastic lesions of the fallopian tube. The World Health Organization (WHO) histologic classification of tumors of the fallopian tube is presented in Table 32.1.

1. Benign tumors

  a. Adenomatoid tumors are the most common benign tumor of the fallopian tube. They are usually incidental, unilateral, and present grossly as a well-circumscribed, white-tan lesion in the tubal wall. They are derived from mesothelium, and the usual histologic pattern shows slit-like or glandular spaces lined by a single layer of flattened cuboidal cells (e-**Fig. 32.7**). The cells are immunopositive for expression of cytokeratin, calretinin, and vimentin and are immunonegative for expression of factor VIII-related antigen and CD31, a profile that indicates a mesothelial rather than a vascular origin.

  b. Other benign tumors include epithelial papillomas, adenomas, cystadenomas, adenofibromas, and leiomyomas. *Epithelial papillomas* are usually

TABLE 32.1 — WHO Histological Classification of Tumors of the Fallopian Tube

Epithelial tumors
Malignant
  Serous adenocarcinoma
  Mucinous adenocarcinoma
  Endometrioid adenocarcinoma
  Clear cell adenocarcinoma
  Transitional cell carcinoma
  Squamous cell carcinoma
  Undifferentiated carcinoma
  Others
Borderline tumor (of low malignant potential)
  Serous borderline tumor
  Mucinous borderline tumor
  Others
Carcinoma in situ (specify type)
Benign tumors
  Cystadenoma (specify type)
  Adenofibroma
  Cystadenofibroma
  Endometrioid polyp
  Papilloma (specify type)
  Metaplastic papillary tumor
  Others
Tumor-like epithelial lesions
  Tubal epithelial hyperplasia
  Salpingitis isthmica nodosa
  Endosalpingiosis

Mixed epithelial-mesenchymal tumors
Malignant mixed Müllerian tumor (carcinosarcoma)
Adenosarcoma

Soft tissue tumors
Leiomyosarcoma
Leiomyoma
Others

Mesothelial tumors
Adenomatoid tumor

Germ cell tumors
Teratoma
  Mature
  Immature
Others

Trophoblastic disease
Choriocarcinoma
Placental site trophoblastic tumor
Hydatidiform mole
Placental site nodule
Others

Lymphoid and hematopoietic tumors
Malignant lymphoma
Leukemia

Secondary tumors

From: Tavassoli FA, Devilee P, eds. *World Health Organization Classification of Tumours. Pathology and Genetics. Tumours of the Breast and Female Genital Organs.* Lyon, France: IARC Press; 2003. Used with permission.

TABLE 32.2	Tumor, Node, Metastasis (TNM) Staging Scheme and International Federation of Gynecology and Obstetrics (FIGO) Classification of Carcinomas of the Fallopian Tube

Primary tumor (T)

TNM Categories	FIGO Stages	
TX		Primary tumor cannot be assessed
T0		No evidence of primary tumor
Tis	0	Carcinoma in situ (preinvasive carcinoma)
T1	I	Tumor confined to fallopian tube(s)
T1a	IA	Tumor limited to one tube, without penetrating the serosal surface, no ascites
T1b	IB	Tumor limited to both tubes, without penetrating the serosal surface, no ascites
T1c	IC	Tumor limited to one or both tube(s) with extension onto or through the tubal serosa, or with malignant cells in ascites or peritoneal washings
T2	II	Tumor involves one or both fallopian tube(s) with pelvic extension
T2a	IIA	Extension and/or metastasis to uterus and/or ovaries
T2b	IIB	Extension to other pelvic structures
T2c	IIC	Pelvic extension (2a or 2b) with malignant cells in ascites or peritoneal washings
T3 and/or N1	III	Tumor involves one or both fallopian tube(s) with peritoneal implants outside the pelvis and/or positive regional lymph nodes
T3a	IIIA	Microscopic peritoneal metastasis outside the pelvis
T3b	IIIB	Macroscopic peritoneal metastasis outside the pelvis ≤ 2 cm in greatest dimension
T3c and/or N1	IIIC	Peritoneal metastasis >2 cm in greatest dimension and/or positive regional lymph nodes
M1	IV	Distant metastasis (excludes metastasis within the peritoneal cavity)

Note: Liver capsule metastasis is T3/stage III, liver parenchymal metastasis, M1/stage IV. Pleural effusion must have positive cytology for M1/stage IV.

Regional lymph nodes (N)

NX	Regional lymph nodes cannot be assessed
N0	No regional lymph node metastasis
N1	Regional lymph node metastasis

Distant metastasis (M)

MX	Distant metastasis cannot be assessed
M0	No distant metastasis
M1	Distant metastasis

Stage grouping

Stage 0	Tis	N0	M0
Stage IA	T1a	N0	M0
Stage IB	T1b	N0	M0
Stage IC	T1c	N0	M0
Stage IIA	T1c	N0	M0
Stage IIB	T2b	N0	M0
Stage IIC	T2c	N0	M0
Stage IIIA	T3a	N0	M0
Stage IIIB	T3b	N0	M0
Stage IIIC	T3c	N0	M0
	Any T	N1	M0
Stage IV	Any T	Any N	M1

From: Edge SB, Byrd DR, Compton CC, et al., eds. *AJCC Cancer Staging Manual*. 7th ed. New York, NY: Springer; 2010. Used with permission.

incidental and show a branched pattern with a central fibrovascular core lined by a single layer of eosinophilic cells. Adenomas, cystadenomas, adenofibromas, and leiomyomas all resemble their ovarian and uterine counterparts.

2. Malignant tumors

   a. Primary fallopian tube carcinoma is quite rare. Carcinomas typically occur in elderly women and are usually widespread at the time of diagnosis with a correspondingly poor prognosis. Serum CA125 levels may be elevated. Grossly, the fallopian tube is distended by a papillary or solid tumor. Serous adenocarcinoma, which microscopically is identical to ovarian serous adenocarcinoma (e-**Fig. 32.8**), is the most common subtype of carcinoma. Other more uncommon subtypes, such as endometrioid or clear cell carcinoma, resemble their counterparts in the ovary. The pathologic staging of primary fallopian tube malignancies is presented in Table 32.2.

   Carcinoma in situ, also called serous tubal intraepithelial carcinoma (STIC), is characterized by cellular stratification, loss of polarity, high-grade nuclear atypia, increased mitotic activity, and increased apoptosis and is distinguished from carcinoma by the lack of stromal invasion (e-**Fig. 32.9**).

   b. Other primary malignant tumors of the fallopian tube include *leiomyosarcoma*, which may affect the fallopian tube or broad ligament, and *carcinosarcoma* (malignant mixed Müllerian tumor). Both tumors microscopically resemble their ovarian counterparts and are quite rare in the fallopian tube.

   c. Metastatic tumors are the most common category of malignancies involving the fallopian tube. Consequently, metastasis from a primary tumor at another site must always be excluded before making the diagnosis of a primary fallopian tube malignancy. Other primary tumors of the female reproductive tract, especially the ovary and endometrium, are the most frequent sources of metastases. It has recently been proposed that small serous carcinomas of the fallopian tube, particularly in the fimbria in women with *BRCA* mutations, are the primary source for peritoneal, and possibly ovarian, serous carcinomas (*Am J Surg Pathol.* 2007;31:161).

C. Reporting. The final report in any case of malignancy should include the histologic type and grade of the malignancy; the presence or absence of a precursor lesion (carcinoma in situ/STIC); tumor size, including depth and width; whether the malignancy is unifocal or multifocal; and the presence or absence of lymphovascular space invasion. In addition, the report should explicitly include all of the information required for assigning a stage, as well as other information of clinical interest not required for staging.

33 Uterus (Corpus)

Jena Beth Hudson, John D. Pfeifer,
and Phyllis C. Huettner

I. **NORMAL ANATOMY.** The uterus is a pear-shaped hollow organ with a normal weight of between 40 and 80 g in adults. It is divided into the corpus, the lower uterine segment, and the cervix. The uterine cavity is triangular, measuring on average 6 cm in length. It is composed of the inner endometrial lining and the myometrium or muscular wall, with a serosal covering which extends to the peritoneal reflection. The peritoneal reflection is shorter anteriorly than posteriorly and so can be used for orienting hysterectomy specimens.

II. **GROSS EXAMINATION, TISSUE SAMPLING, AND HISTOLOGIC SLIDE PREPARATION**

A. **Endometrial biopsy and curettage specimens.** The most common endometrial tissue samplings examined in surgical pathology are endometrial biopsy and curettage specimens, obtained from cervical dilation and curettage procedures. Endometrial biopsy samples are obtained from a relatively limited office sampling procedure in which no cervical dilation is required. The dimension (size range of the largest tissue fragments, or the dimensions of the tissue in aggregate) and/or volume of the specimen should be documented. The entire specimen should be submitted for microscopic examination and three H&E stained levels prepared for microscopic examination.

B. **Products of conception specimens** are usually obtained by curettage (although the tissue is often spontaneously passed). The dimension (size range of the largest tissue fragments, or the dimensions of the tissue in aggregate) and/or volume of the specimen should be documented. At least three cassettes should be submitted, focused on any villous tissue that is grossly present, to optimize microscopic identification chorionic villi both for confirmation of the presence of an intrauterine pregnancy and to rule out a molar gestation. If the initial three blocks do not contain villi, the remainder of the specimen should be submitted; if villi are still not identified, the possibility of an ectopic pregnancy exists, a result that should be immediately communicated to the clinician.

C. **Hysterectomy specimens.** The type of hysterectomy (abdominal or vaginal, with or without salpingo-oophorectomy) should be determined and the size, weight, and shape of the uterus recorded (the processing of radical hysterectomy specimens, which differs substantially, is discussed in Chap. 34). The uterine serosa should be carefully examined for any abnormalities, which should be sampled. The uterus is next bivalved in the coronal plane to show the endometrial cavity and endocervical canal, which are examined and measured. The maximum thickness of the endometrium and myometrium should also be noted. Both halves of the uterus are then serially sectioned parallel to the long axis of the uterus.

1. For specimens excised for benign disease, sections of the anterior cervix, posterior cervix, anterior endomyometrium, and posterior endomyometrium are submitted. Additional sections of any identified lesions must also be submitted.

2. For specimens excised for malignancies, contiguous sections of both anterior and posterior endomyometrium, lower uterine segment, and cervix should be submitted to assess for tumor involvement of the lower uterine segment and cervix. In addition, at least one full thickness section of the uterine wall containing tumor from both anterior and posterior uterus (including the serosa from the deepest area of myometrial invasion by the

tumor) are submitted to enable calculation of the depth of invasion. Representative sections from any other lesions must also be submitted.

III. ENDOMETRIUM

A. Dating

1. The endometrial mucosa is composed of glands and stroma. It is divided into the functional (luminal) layer and the basal (inner) layer. The basal cell layer acts as a reserve cell layer and is responsible for the regeneration of the endometrium after menses. The stroma is composed of endometrial stromal cells and blood vessels.

2. The menstrual cycle is divided into menstrual phase, proliferative phase, and secretory phase. Menstrual endometrium, present for the first 4 days of the 28-day cycle, is characterized by glandular (karyorrhectic debris in glandular cells) and stromal (dense balls of collapsed stroma with surrounding neutrophils and reactive epithelium) breakdown, glandular secretory exhaustion, and background inflammation (e-Figs. 33.1 and 33.2).*

   Day 1 of menstrual bleeding is defined as day 1 of the cycle; the menstrual phase lasts for 3 to 4 days. Proliferative phase begins on day 4 and in an idealized situation lasts until day 14. Although it usually lasts about 11 days, it may greatly vary. During the early proliferative phase, the endometrium is thin and composed of straight, evenly spaced glands in a loose stroma (e-Fig. 33.3). By day 8 to 10, stromal edema due to estrogen causes increased endometrial thickening, and the glands become more coiled as the gland–stroma growth rate increases (e-Fig. 33.4). Throughout the proliferative phase, the epithelium lining the glands shows nuclear stratification, with a high mitotic rate in both glands and stroma (e-Fig. 33.5).

   The secretory phase begins with ovulation. In an idealized 28-day cycle, secretory phase begins at day 14 and lasts 14 days, although it may range from 11 to 18 days. Following an interval phase from day 14 to day 15 (during which there are no dateable changes), the first dateable feature of early secretory phase is the appearance of subnuclear vacuoles on day 16, which appear as a clear zone between the basement membrane and the nucleus pushing the nucleus toward the glandular lumen. On day 17 the epithelium exhibits uniform subnuclear vacuoles, giving the appearance of "piano keys" (e-Fig. 33.6). The vacuoles then move to the supranuclear position (day 18) and eventually are secreted into the glandular lumen (e-Fig. 33.7). Maximal stromal edema occurs during the mid-secretory phase, around day 22. At day 23, the stroma begins to condense, and the first signs of periarteriolar decidualization (where stromal cells acquire abundant, eosinophilic cytoplasm under the influence of progesterone) become apparent (e-Fig. 33.8). On day 25, this decidualization extends beneath the surface epithelium. Prominent glandular saw-toothing and maximal stromal decidualization occur on days 26 to 27 (e-Fig. 33.9). Numerous granular lymphocytes, marked stromal decidual change, and glandular breakdown are the features of day 28 of late secretory phases.

B. Pregnancy

1. The earliest gestation-related changes occur following the implantation of the blastocyst. These changes are characterized by decidualization of the stroma with edema; the glands exhibit distension with increased secretion and a serrated architecture (e-Fig. 33.10). By 4 to 8 weeks post implantation, the endometrial epithelium often exhibits a physiologic response known as the *Arias-Stella reaction* characterized by glands that have a

---

*All e-figures are available online via the Solution Site Image Bank.

hypersecretory pattern and are lined by cells with enlarged, hyperchromatic nuclei that often jut into the gland lumens (e-**Fig. 33.11**).

2. The placental implantation site, often seen in curettage specimens obtained because of a missed abortion, is characterized by decidualized stroma infiltrated by intermediate trophoblast. Intermediate trophoblast have hyperchromatic, angulated nuclei and amphophilic cytoplasm and are often multinucleated (e-**Fig. 33.12**). Intermediate trophoblast also normally infiltrates maternal spiral arteries causing fibrinoid deposition in the vessel wall which serves to dilate the vessels and increase blood flow to the placenta (e-**Fig. 33.13**). Intermediate trophoblast also normally infiltrates myometrium which can occasionally be present in curettage specimens (e-**Fig. 33.14**).

3. Placental site nodules are incidental, usually microscopic findings that are characterized by small foci of hyalinized material with entrapped intermediate trophoblast cells, often with vacuolated cytoplasm (e-**Fig. 33.15**). They are thought to arise from the chorionic type intermediate trophoblast of the fetal membranes which is also vacuolated. Placental site nodules are occasionally encountered in endometrial biopsies and curettage specimens but may also be seen in cervical specimens.

4. Abnormalities of implantation. Placenta accreta occurs when a layer of decidua is not present between the placental villi and the myometrium at the implantation site (e-**Fig. 33.16**); fibrin and intermediate trophoblast may be present between villi and myometrium in accreta. Cytokeratin, which will be positive in trophoblast and negative in decidua, can be used if the distinction is difficult on H&E. Placenta increta is present when villi invade into the myometrium, and transmural extension of villi with perforation is termed placenta percreta.

   Risk factors for placenta accreta include prior Cesarean section, placenta previa, and prior instrumentation, among others. All forms of accreta may be associated with life-threatening hemorrhage, which may require immediate hysterectomy.

C. **Exogenous hormone therapy**

1. Estrogen causes proliferation of endometrial glands and stroma. Persistent exposure to estrogen (exogenous as well as endogenous estrogen, as occurs with anovulatory cycles, obesity, or an estrogen-secreting tumor) causes endometrial proliferation with subsequent glandular and stromal breakdown, often clinically interpreted as irregular menstrual bleeding. Microscopically, the findings include stromal condensation with formation of so-called exodus bodies or stromal blue-balls, glandular degeneration and apoptosis of the glandular epithelial cells, and fibrin thrombi in stromal vessels (e-**Fig. 33.17**).

2. Prolonged exposure to progestogens results in endometrium with a characteristic pattern that includes underdeveloped, inactive glands in a background of a stroma that shows marked decidual change (e-**Fig. 33.18**).

3. Tamoxifen is primarily used for the treatment of breast cancer. In the endometrium, tamoxifen competitively binds to estrogen receptors and acts as an agonist. It increases the risk of endometrial hyperplasia and adenocarcinomas (*Ann NY Acad Sci*. 2001;949:237), and up to 20% of women on tamoxifen develop endometrial polyps (*Cancer*. 2001;92:1151).

IV. **COMMON BENIGN DISEASES OF THE ENDOMETRIUM**

A. **Endometritis**

1. **Acute endometritis** is defined by the presence of acute neutrophilic inflammation in the stroma of the nonmenstruating endometrium. In severe cases, the neutrophils are present throughout the stroma, the endometrial epithelium, and the glandular lumina (e-**Fig. 33.19**). Acute inflammation present during the menstrual phase of the endometrium should not be misdiagnosed as

active infection. Acute endometritis is uncommon and is usually seen only in postpartum or postabortive endometrium.

2. **Chronic endometritis** is defined by the presence of plasma cells in the endometrial stroma. Associated features include glandular and stromal breakdown, and dyssynchronous glandular and stromal development (e-**Fig. 33.20**). The most common causes of chronic endometritis include *Chlamydia trachomatis, Ureaplasma urealyticum,* cytomegalovirus, and herpes virus infection. Infection by *Actinomyces israelii* or *Neisseria gonorrheae* usually causes a mixed acute and chronic pattern of inflammation. Granulomatous inflammation is rare; common causes include *Mycobacterium tuberculosis* infection, fungal infection, sarcoidosis, and hysteroscopic ablation therapy.

B. **Atrophy** is most commonly seen in postmenopausal women. Premenopausal causes include treatment with oral contraceptives or gonadotropin agonists (Lupron). Patients with premature menopause also show an atrophic pattern. Microscopically, the endometrium is composed of a thin layer of endometrial glands lined by an attenuated layer of inactive epithelial cells surrounded by thin stroma. No mitotic activity is present (e-**Fig. 33.21**).

C. **Metaplasia** is the presence of any type of glandular epithelium other than the normal columnar type. Metaplasia is a common finding in perimenopausal and postmenopausal women and is often associated with abnormal uterine bleeding or recent use of exogenous hormonal therapy.

1. **Tubal metaplasia** consists of foci of normal tubal epithelium within the endometrial glands, including ciliated, nonciliated secretory, and intercalated cells. The ratio of the ciliated to nonciliated cells is cyclical and depends on hormonal influences.

2. **Ciliated cell metaplasia** is the most common form of metaplasia. It is composed of a layer of ciliated columnar cells with round to oval nuclei and abundant pale eosinophilic cytoplasm (e-**Fig. 33.22**). Ciliated cell metaplasia is a normal response of endometrial epithelium to various hormonal exposures. It is most commonly found in perimenopausal endometrium and is associated with endometrial polyps, anovulatory cycles, and exogenous hormonal therapy.

3. **Squamous metaplasia** (e-**Fig. 33.23**) is often caused by chronic irritation and often takes the form of squamous morules or rounded, swirling nests of squamous cells. Squamous metaplasia must not be confused with endometrial hyperplasia or malignancy, although it can occur as a secondary change in both.

4. **Eosinophilic metaplasia** or eosinophilic change refers to glandular epithelium with abundant eosinophilic cytoplasm and a central round to oval nucleus (e-**Fig. 33.24**). It is often associated with a neutrophilic infiltrate, the formation of small epithelial papilla, and mild nuclear atypia.

5. **Mucinous metaplasia** is rare. It is morphologically similar to endocervical mucinous epithelium in that it consists of columnar epithelium with basally located oval nuclei and abundant apical mucin (e-**Fig. 33.25**).

6. **Clear cell metaplasia** is also rare. It is characterized by columnar cells with round nuclei and clear cytoplasm.

D. **Endometrial polyps** are local overgrowths of endometrial glands and stroma that protrude into the endometrial cavity. Polyps are present in about 20% to 25% of women and are frequently found in the perimenopausal and postmenopausal period. Grossly, polyps appear as broad-based to pedunculated lesions; some pedunculated polyps can extend into the endocervical canal, and even through the os. Microscopically, polyps are composed of endometrial glands within a fibrous stroma; the presence of thick-walled blood vessels within the fibrous stroma is the most common key to the diagnosis (e-**Fig. 33.26**). Frequently, the glands are variably shaped and irregularly distributed.

Although endometrial polyps in postmenopausal women usually contain dilated glands lined by one layer of atrophic epithelium, foci of metaplastic or hyperplastic epithelium, as well as frank adenocarcinoma, may be present. Consequently, endometrial polyps should be entirely submitted for microscopic examination.

1. Polyps with stromal smooth muscle are referred to as **adenomyomatous polyps.**

2. **Atypical polypoid adenomyoma** is a polypoid lesion characterized histologically by crowded irregular endometrial glands with a complex architecture and cytologic atypia in stroma that is predominantly composed of smooth muscle (e-**Fig. 33.27**). The lesion has a high rate of recurrence after incomplete surgical removal and mainly occurs in premenopausal, nulliparous women. It is associated with a clinical history of infertility.

E. **Disordered proliferative endometrium** predominantly exhibits a normal proliferative pattern, with mild irregular branching and budding and some cystic dilation. However, the glands to stroma ratio is not increased—the main factor that helps to differentiate a disordered proliferative pattern from simple hyperplasia. The epithelium lining the glands is composed of stratified and columnar cells with no atypia. Mitotic activity is similar to that of normal proliferative endometrium (e-**Fig. 33.28**).

V. **ENDOMETRIAL HYPERPLASIA AND ENDOMETRIAL INTRAEPITHELIAL CARCINOMA.** Endometrial hyperplasia is thought to develop as a result of unopposed estrogenic stimulation. Any disorder that causes an increase in endogenous or exogenous estrogenic stimulation such as polycystic ovarian disease, obesity, or ovarian neoplasms (e.g., thecomas, granulosa cell tumors) can therefore predispose to endometrial hyperplasia. Abnormal bleeding is the major clinical symptom.

A. **Endometrial hyperplasia** is subclassified as simple or complex on the basis of the architectural pattern, and as with or without atypia on the basis of the cytologic features. Numerous studies have demonstrated that the risk of progression to adenocarcinoma (specifically, endometrioid adenocarcinoma and its variants) is more highly correlated with the presence of cytologic atypia than the degree of glandular crowding.

1. **Simple hyperplasia** shows a glands to stroma ratio that is slightly increased (more than 1:1) with prominent variability in size of the glands, glandular budding, and cystic glandular dilatation (e-**Fig. 33.29**).

2. **Complex hyperplasia** is composed of crowded, architecturally complex glands with little intervening stroma. The glands to stroma ratio is elevated (at least 3:1) (e-**Fig. 33.30**).

3. **Cytologic atypia,** which may be a feature of simple or complex hyperplasia, is based on the nuclear cytology of the glandular epithelium. The most reliable indicators of cytologic atypia are an enlarged nucleus that is round rather than oval, that has coarse clumped chromatin, and that has a prominent nucleolus (e-**Fig. 33.31**). A diagnosis of hyperplasia should be made with extreme caution during the secretory phase of the endometrium because of the usual crowding of the glands in this phase of the menstrual cycle. The presence of cytologic atypia must be distinguished from the cellular changes that accompany metaplasias, and from Arias-Stella reaction.

B. **Endometrial intraepithelial neoplasia (EIN)** represents an alternative classification scheme for premalignant endometrial lesions. EIN is defined as a proliferation of islands of endometrial glands which have cytological and architectural abnormalities and are considered to be premalignant. The EIN scheme has been proposed both as an approach to simplify the diagnosis of premalignant changes and as a classification more closely linked to the genetic changes in premalignant endometrial epithelium (*Gynecol Oncol.* 2000;76:287) preceding transformation into endometrial adenocarcinoma. Studies have shown that some of these lesions harbor *PTEN* tumor suppressor gene inactivation, mutations of *k-ras,* and microsatellite instability. EIN is considered to be a monoclonal proliferation composed of cells in early stages of carcinogenesis.

Diagnostic criteria for EIN (http://www.endometrium.org) are based on size of the lesion, nuclear cytology, and glandular architecture (including glandular crowding with an increased glands to stroma ratio, cytologic differences between the neoplastic glands and the adjacent normal glands, and an area of glandular crowding that is >1 mm in greatest dimension). EIN can have squamous, mucinous, or clear cell differentiation. The treatment of these lesions is similar to the clinical management of atypical endometrial hyperplasia.

C. Endometrial intraepithelial carcinoma (EIC) is thought to represent the precursor lesion to serous carcinoma. Microscopically, EIC is composed of glands lined by cells with the same cytologic abnormalities as serous carcinoma, but without evidence of myometrial stromal invasion (**e-Fig. 33.32**). The development of EIC is independent of prior unopposed estrogenic stimulation and typically arises in a setting of atrophic endometrium.

VI. EPITHELIAL MALIGNANCIES. Epithelial malignancies are the most common gynecological malignancy in women in developed countries. Endometrial cancer can be divided into two broad categories which have differences in their clinical and pathologic features, as well as their underlying genetic abnormalities.

A. Type I tumors consist of endometrioid adenocarcinoma and its variants. They account for over 80% of endometrial tumors and usually develop in postmenopausal women in their fifth and sixth decades in the background of long-term estrogen stimulation. Type I tumors are strongly associated with diabetes and obesity and have a relatively good prognosis. The endometrial glands and stroma in Type I tumors are strongly positive for estrogen and progesterone receptors. In addition, the stromal cells show diffuse strong immunopositivity for CD10 (CALLA) antigen. Genetically, they show microsatellite instability, and mutations in the *PTEN* tumor suppressor gene, *k-ras,* and *CTNNB1,* but assessment for these genetic abnormalities is not necessary for diagnosis.

B. Type II tumors, for example serous papillary carcinoma, usually occur in women in their sixth and seventh decades and are not associated with estrogen stimulation, and therefore do not occur in a background of complex atypical hyperplasia but rather in atrophic epithelium. They are more likely than Type I tumors to be at an advanced stage at the time of presentation and so have a relatively poor prognosis. Genetically they are characterized by *TP53* mutations.

The WHO classification of uterine corpus malignancies is presented in Table 33.1, and the pathologic staging of uterine corpus carcinomas is shown in Table 33.2 and Figure 33.1.

1. Endometrioid adenocarcinoma usually arises in the uterine corpus and grossly usually consists of a raised to exophytic, pink tan, hemorrhagic mass that projects into the endometrial cavity.

Microscopically, the tumor consists of irregular, confluent, complex glandular or villoglandular structures lined by pleomorphic stratified columnar cells with pleomorphic nuclei. The presence of areas with definitive cribriform architecture is a microscopic feature that can be used to distinguish well-differentiated endometrioid adenocarcinoma from complex hyperplasia with cytologic atypia. Foci of squamous differentiation, which should not be mistaken as solid component of the tumor, are often encountered.

Myometrial invasion is recognized by the presence of an irregular endometrial–myometrial border or by an associated desmoplastic and inflammatory stromal response (**e-Fig. 33.33**). The depth of myometrial invasion compared with the full thickness of the myometrium and the presence or absence of lymphovascular space invasion should be noted.

TABLE 33.1 WHO Histologic Classification of Tumors of the Uterine Corpus

Epithelial tumors and related lesions
Endometrial carcinoma
  Endometrioid adenocarcinoma
    Variant with squamous differentiation
    Villoglandular variant
    Secretory variant
    Ciliated cell variant
  Mucinous adenocarcinoma
  Serous adenocarcinoma
  Clear cell adenocarcinoma
  Mixed cell adenocarcinoma
  Squamous cell carcinoma
  Transitional cell carcinoma
  Small cell carcinoma
  Undifferentiated carcinoma
  Others
Endometrial hyperplasia
  Nonatypical hyperplasia
    Simple
    Complex
  Atypical hyperplasia
    Simple
    Complex
Endometrial polyp
Tamoxifen-related lesions

Mesenchymal tumors
Endometrial stromal and related tumors
  Endometrial stromal nodule
  Endometrial stromal sarcoma, low grade
  Undifferentiated endometrial sarcoma
Smooth muscle tumors
  Leiomyosarcoma
    Epithelioid variant
    Myxoid variant
  Smooth muscle tumors of uncertain
    malignant potential
  Leiomyoma, not otherwise specified
    Histologic variants
      Mitotically active variant
      Cellular variant
      Hemorrhagic cellular variant
      Epithelioid variant
      Myxoid Variant
      Atypical variant
      Lipoleiomyoma variant

    Growth pattern variants
      Diffuse leiomyomatosis
        Dissecting leiomyoma
        Intravenous leiomyomatosis
        Metastasizing leiomyomatosis
Miscellaneous mesenchymal tumors
  Mixed endometrial stromal and smooth
    muscle tumors
  Perivascular epithelioid cell tumor
  Adenomatoid tumor
  Other malignant mesenchymal tumors
  Other benign mesenchymal tumors

Mixed epithelial and mesenchymal tumors
  Carcinosarcoma (malignant mixed mullerian
    tumor)
  Adenosarcoma
  Carcinofibroma
  Adenofibroma
  Adenomyoma
    Atypical polypoid variant

Gestational trophoblastic disease
Trophoblastic neoplasms
  Choriocarcinoma
  Placental site trophoblastic tumor
  Epithelioid trophoblastic tumor
Molar pregnancies
  Hydatidiform mole
    Complete
    Partial
    Invasive
    Metastatic
Nonneoplastic, nonmolar trophoblastic lesions
  Placental site nodule and plaque
  Exaggerated placental site

Miscellaneous tumors
  Sex cord-like tumors
  Neuroectodermal tumors
  Melanotic paraganglioma
  Tumors of germ cell type
  Others

Lymphoid and hematopoietic tumors
  Malignant lymphoma
  Leukemia

Secondary tumors

From: Tavassoli FA, Devilee P, eds. *World Health Organization Classification of Tumours. Pathology and Genetics. Tumours of the Breast and Female Genital Organs.* Lyon: IARC Press; 2003. Used with permission.

The FIGO grading system for endometrioid adenocarcinoma is based on the degree of differentiation as defined by the percentage of glandular and solid components (areas of squamous differentiation are not considered regions of solid growth). Tumors with 0% to 5% solid growth are

| TABLE 33.2 | TNM and FIGO Staging of Uterine Carcinomas |

TNM and FIGO classification
Primary tumor (T)

TNM Categories	FIGO Stages	
TX		Primary tumor cannot be assessed
T0		No evidence of primary tumor
Tis		Carcinoma in situ (preinvasive carcinoma)
T1	I	Tumor confined to corpus uteri
T1a	IA	Tumor limited to endometrium or invades less than one-half of the myometrium
T1b	IB	Tumor invades one-half or more of the myometrium
T2	II	Tumor invades cervix but does not extend beyond uterus
T3a	IIIA	Tumor involves serosa and/or adnexa (direct extension or metastasis)
T3b	IIIB	Vaginal involvement (direct extension or metastasis)
T4	IVA	Tumor invades bladder mucosa and/or bowel mucosa
M1	IVB	Distant metastasis (excluding metastasis to vagina, pelvic serosa, or adnexa)

Regional lymph nodes (N)

NX		Regional lymph nodes cannot be assessed
N0		No regional lymph node metastasis
N1		Regional lymph node metastasis
N2		Regional lymph node metastasis to paraaortic lymph nodes, with or without positive pelvic lymph nodes

Distant metastasis (M)

MX		Distant metastasis cannot be assessed
M0		No distant metastasis
M1		Distant metastasis (excludes metastasis to paraaortic lymph nodes, vagina, pelvic serosa, or adnexa)

Stage grouping

Stage 0	Tis	N0	M0
Stage IA	T1a	N0	M0
Stage IB	T1b	N0	M0
Stage II	T2	N0	M0
Stage IIIA	T3a	N0	M0
Stage IIIB	T3b	N0	M0
Stage IIIC1	T1–T3	N1	M0
Stage IIIC2	T1–T3	N2	M0
Stage IVA	T4	Any N	M0
Stage IVB	Any T	Any N	M1

From: Edge SB, Byrd DR, Compton CC, et al., eds. *AJCC Cancer Staging Manual.* 7th ed. New York, NY: Springer; 2010. Used with permission.

grade 1, with 6% to 50% solid growth are grade 2, and with >50% solid growth are grade 3 (e-**Figs. 33.34** to **33.38**). Notable nuclear pleomorphism inappropriate for the tumor architecture increases the tumor grade by one degree.

a. Variants of endometrioid adenocarcinoma include villoglandular, secretory, mucinous, and squamous. The *villoglandular pattern* is diagnosed by the presence of a predominantly branching glandular architecture with central fibrovascular cores lined by stratified columnar cells containing elongated pleomorphic nuclei. The *secretory pattern* is

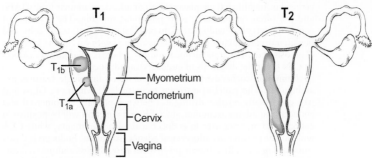

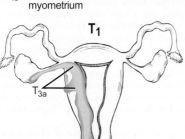

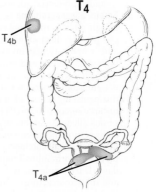

T_{1a} - Tumor limited to endometrium or invades less than one-half of the myometrium

T_{1b} - Tumor invades one-half or more of the myometrium

T_2 - Tumor invades cervix

T_{3a} - Tumor involves the serosa and/or adnexa (direct inv or met)

T_{3b} - Tumor invades vagina or parametrium (direct ext or met)

T_{4a} - Tumor invades bladder or rectum

T_{4b} - Distant metastasis (excluding adnexa, pelv & abd)

Figure 33.1 pT staging of uterine carcinoma

characterized by glands composed of cells with supra or subnuclear vacuoles resembling secretory endometrium. The *mucinous pattern* is defined by the presence of foci of endometrial glands lined by columnar cells with abundant intracytoplasmic mucin, often with a papillary architecture. *Squamous differentiation* (e-**Fig. 33.39**) is defined as the presence of sheets of squamous cells which are usually, but not always, nonkeratinizing.

b. The distinction between endocervical adenocarcinoma and endometrial adenocarcinoma is often difficult, especially on small biopsy specimens or when the tumor involves the lower uterine segment. The distinction has clinical significance, as endometrial adenocarcinomas are treated with simple hysterectomy and endocervical adenocarcinomas are treated with radical hysterectomy or radiation therapy. The clinical history can often be very helpful in the distinction. Woman with endometrial cancer are typically obese and often diabetic; their uteri are often enlarged and they report menometrorrhagia or postmenopausal bleeding. Women with cervical cancer do not necessarily have a history of obesity but are often smokers; they have a history of abnormal Pap smears or prior cervical intraepithelial neoplasia (CIN) or adenocarcinomas in situ (AIS) and are often symptomatic with postcoital spotting. The presence of coexisting atypical endometrial hyperplasia, stromal foam cells and benign morular squamous elements associated with carcinoma favor the diagnosis of endometrial adenocarcinoma, whereas adjacent cervical AIS or CIN favor the diagnosis of endocervical adenocarcinoma.

Immunohistochemistry can be useful when histologic features are ambiguous. The panel of estrogen receptor (ER), vimentin, CEA, and p16 can usually reliably distinguish between primary endometrial and endocervical adenocarcinoma, since ER and vimentin will be positive in endometrial and negative in endocervical adenocarcinoma, while CEA will only be positive in endocervical adenocarcinomas. Endocervical carcinomas are typically diffusely positive for p16 whereas endometrial carcinomas show only patchy positivity. In situ hybridization with HPV may also be helpful; endocervical adenocarcinomas should be positive and endometrial adenocarcinomas negative.

2. **Serous adenocarcinoma** is a high-grade tumor characterized by cells with a high nuclear to cytoplasmic ratio and a high mitotic rate that form a complex papillary architecture (e-**Figs. 33.40 and 33.41**). Deep myometrial and lymphovascular invasion are often present. The distinction between high-grade serous and grade 3 endometrioid tumors is often difficult and has high interobserver variability but is clinically meaningful as the survival is significantly worse for serous adenocarcinoma. Although not useful for distinguishing serous adenocarcinoma from lower grade endometrioid adenocarcinomas, p16 and PTEN stains are sensitive and specific for high-grade serous adenocarcinoma when used to distinguish the tumor from grade 3 endometrioid adenocarcinoma.

3. **Clear cell adenocarcinoma** is a high-grade tumor composed of pleomorphic cells with hobnail nuclei (nuclei that jut into the gland lumen), abundant clear cytoplasm, and distinct cell borders arranged in papillary, solid, and tubular structures, often admixed (e-**Fig. 33.42**). A characteristic feature is the presence of hyalinized stromal cores (e-**Fig. 33.43**). Clear cell adenocarcinoma is often at an advanced clinical stage at the time of presentation.

4. **Mixed adenocarcinoma** is defined as a tumor demonstrating a mixture of endometrioid adenocarcinoma (or its variants) together with serous, mucinous, or clear cell adenocarcinoma. By convention, the minor component must comprise at least 10% of the tumor.

5. **Carcinosarcoma (malignant mixed mullerian tumor or MMMT)** comprises ~10% of all uterine malignancies. The diagnostic criteria are based on the presence of both malignant epithelial and mesenchymal (sarcomatous) elements. Numerous genetic studies have demonstrated that both elements are derived from the same precursor, proving that the neoplasm does not represent a collision tumor. Consequently, the tumor is now considered to represent a poorly differentiated endometrial carcinoma with metaplastic differentiation.

Grossly, carcinosarcomas appear to be larger and fleshier than typical adenocarcinomas and are often described as polypoid. Microscopically, they consist of areas of adenocarcinoma (typically high-grade serous) intermixed with a wide range of malignant mesenchymal elements such as smooth muscle, cartilage, skeletal muscle, or undifferentiated (e-**Fig. 33.44 and 33.45**). Foci of poorly differentiated cells with marked pleomorphism and a high mitotic rate with no distinct pattern are not uncommon. Extensive areas of necrosis are often present. Carcinosarcomas can be divided into homologous or heterologous tumors depending on whether the malignant mesenchymal component is normally found in the uterus or not; this distinction is now recognized to have no clinical significance.

Carcinosarcoma generally has a poor prognosis. Specific adverse prognostic factors include the presence of epithelial component with foci of serous or clear cell differentiation, deep myometrial invasion, cervical involvement, and lymphovascular space involvement. The grade of tumor, type of the mesenchymal element, and mitotic rate have no correlation with the outcome.

6. **Squamous cell carcinoma** of the endometrium is rare and usually occurs in postmenopausal women in association with pyometria and cervical stenosis. Microscopically, it is identical to squamous cell carcinoma of the cervix, and so must be distinguished from a cervical primary that has extended into the endometrium.

7. **Other primary malignant tumors.** *Transitional cell carcinoma* (TCC) is extremely rare and occurs in postmenopausal women. Microscopically, it consists of sheets of urothelial cells admixed with another type of the endometrial adenocarcinoma, and must be distinguished from metastatic TCC from the urinary bladder or ovary. *Small cell carcinoma* of the endometrium is extremely rare and comprises <1% of primary endometrial malignancies. Microscopically, the tumor has the same cytomorphology as high-grade neuroendocrine tumors arising at other sites. *Undifferentiated carcinomas* do not show differentiation toward any defined tumor pattern.

VII. **ENDOMETRIAL STROMAL TUMORS.** These are composed of small cells with scant cytoplasm that morphologically resemble the endometrial stromal cells of proliferative phase endometrium. A subset of tumors exhibit variant morphologic patterns including smooth muscle differentiation, a fibromyxoid component, and sex cord-like/epithelioid patterns. The t(7;17)(p15;q21) translocation which produces a JAZF1–JJAZ1 fusion protein is a recurring feature of all classes of endometrial stromal tumors, but demonstration of its presence is not required for diagnosis.

A. **Endometrial stromal nodules** are grossly tan to yellow, well-circumscribed lesions with a smooth border that range from 0.5 to 12 cm in greatest dimension. They are primarily located in the myometrium, and an obvious connection to the endometrium is not necessary for diagnosis. Histologically, these tumors are composed of sheets of small cells with scant cytoplasm and an accompanying vascular pattern reminiscent of the spiral arterioles present in the stroma of proliferative phase endometrium. These tumors stain strongly and are diffusely positive with CD10 (although a minority of cases may show weak positivity) and are negative with desmin. Since cellular leiomyomas and leiomyosarcomas are usually negative for CD10 but positive for desmin, immunohistochemistry can be helpful in difficult cases. Endometrial stromal nodules are benign and total abdominal hysterectomy is curative.

B. **Endometrial stromal sarcomas** predominantly occur in the middle-aged women and do not share the same risk factors as endometrial carcinoma. On gross examination, endometrial stromal sarcomas exhibit a tan to yellow cut surface with an infiltrative border into the surrounding myometrium, often with foci of hemorrhage and necrosis. Microscopically, the tumor consists of finger-like projections into the myometrium of cells with similar cytomorphology as those seen in endometrial stromal nodules, but with a higher rate of mitosis, greater nuclear pleomorphism, prominent stromal vascularity, and areas of collagenized stroma (**e-Fig. 33.46**). Extensive lymphatic invasion is the hallmark of the tumor. Hysterectomy with salpingo-oophorectomy is the treatment of choice. Radiation therapy has been shown to decrease local recurrence rates but does not have a significant effect on long-term survival. The same chemotherapeutic agents used to treat soft tissue sarcomas have been used to treat endometrial stromal sarcoma with widely variable results. Patients with early stage disease

TABLE 33.3	TNM and FIGO Staging of Leiomyosarcoma and Endometrial Stromal Sarcoma

TNM and FIGO classification
Primary tumor (T)

TNM Categories	FIGO Stages	
TX		Primary tumor cannot be assessed
T0		No evidence of primary tumor
T1	I	Tumor limited to the uterus
T1a	IA	Tumor ≤5 cm in greatest dimension
T1b	IB	Tumor >5 cm
T2	II	Tumor extends beyond the uterus, within the pelvis
T2a	IIA	Tumor involves adnexa
T2b	IIB	Tumor involves other pelvic tissues
T3	III	Tumor infiltrates abdominal tissues
T3a	IIIA	One site
T3b	IIIB	More than one site
T4	IVA	Tumor invades bladder or rectum

Regional lymph nodes (N)

NX		Regional lymph nodes cannot be assessed
N0		No regional lymph node metastasis
N1		Regional lymph node metastasis

Distant metastasis (M)

MX		Distant metastasis cannot be assessed
M0		No distant metastasis
M1		Distant metastasis (excluding adnexa, pelvic and abdominal tissues)

Stage grouping for uterine leiomyosarcoma and endometrial stromal sarcoma

Stage I	T1	N0	M0
Stage IA	T1a	N0	M0
Stage IB	T1b	N0	M0
Stage II	T2	N0	M0
Stage IIIA	T3a	N0	M0
Stage IIIB	T3b	N0	M0
Stage IIIC	T1–T3	N1	M0
Stage IVA	T4	Any N	M0
Stage IVB	Any T	Any N	M1

From: Edge SB, Byrd DR, Compton CC, et al., eds. *AJCC Cancer Staging Manual.* 7th ed. New York, NY: Springer; 2010. Used with permission.

have 5-year survival rates of 90%; recurrence may occur in up to 25% of patients, often several years to a decade or more following primary diagnosis. The pathologic staging of uterine corpus endometrial stromal sarcomas is shown in Table 33.3.

   C. **Undifferentiated endometrial sarcoma** is composed of sheets of pleomorphic undifferentiated cells with a moderate volume of cytoplasm and a high mitotic rate with frequent atypical forms. This tumor lacks the plexiform vasculature reminiscent of proliferative phase endometrium. These tumors have an aggressive course usually resulting in death within 3 years of diagnosis.

VIII. **SMOOTH MUSCLE NEOPLASMS**
   A. **Leiomyoma** is the most common neoplasm of the uterus and can occur as a submucosal, intramural, or subserosal lesion. Leiomyomas predominantly affect

women of reproductive age; they can be found in 20% to 30% of women in their fourth decade, and more than 40% of women in their fifth decade. They tend to enlarge during pregnancy since they express estrogen and progesterone receptors. Grossly, leiomyomas are well-circumscribed lesions; they have a white-tan cut surface and are sharply demarcated from the adjacent myometrium. Microscopically, leiomyomas are composed of interlacing fascicles of closely packed cells with uniform elongated nuclei and eosinophilic cytoplasm (e-Figs. 33.47 and 33.48). Degenerative changes including hyaline change, coagulative necrosis, and hydropic degeneration are often present.

1. **Cellular leiomyomas** have the same gross features as ordinary leiomyomas but microscopically demonstrate an increased cellularity with sheets of spindle cells with hyperchromatic elongated nuclei and a scant amount of eosinophilic cytoplasm (e-Fig. 33.49). There is no pleomorphism or increased mitotic activity. These lesions behave as classic leiomyomas. One important differential diagnosis for this lesion is endometrial stromal sarcoma. Endometrial stromal sarcomas lack a fascicular growth pattern, thick-walled vessels, and a cleft-like space between the lesion and the adjacent myometrium; in addition, endometrial stromal sarcomas often have plaques of collagen and foamy cells which are not seen in leiomyomas. Endometrial stromal sarcomas are typically positive for CD10 and negative for H-caldesmon and CD44v3. Also, the presence of mast cells is a sensitive and specific finding, favoring cellular leiomyoma, when there are usually >7 mast cells per high power field.

2. **Epithelioid leiomyomas** are composed of predominantly epithelioid cells with eosinophilic to clear cytoplasm and fine nuclear chromatin. The cells are arranged in clusters and as single cells, with no pleomorphism. The mitotic rate is not elevated, and necrosis is absent. They behave the same as classic leiomyomas.

3. **Symplastic leiomyoma** contains scattered enlarged, markedly atypical cells, often with multiple nuclei. However, the mitotic count is still <10 mitotic figures per 10 high-power fields (hpf), and no necrosis is present. These lesions have the same benign behavior as classic leiomyoma.

4. **Lipoleiomyoma** refers to a classic leiomyoma which contains islands of mature adipocytes. This variant has no clinical significance.

5. **Myxoid leiomyoma** consists of fascicles of uniform spindle cells surrounded by pools of myxoid edematous stroma. Large vessels are not uncommonly present.

B. **Benign metastasizing leiomyoma.** Many patients who have benign metastasizing leiomyoma have a prior history of hysteroscopy with dilatation and curettage, or other procedures such as myomectomy or hysterectomy. Microscopically, benign metastasizing leiomyomas have the same histologic features as ordinary leiomyomas, although they may extend into adjacent vessels. The tumor cells can migrate to the lung, and lymph node involvement may be present. The differential diagnosis includes low grade leiomyosarcoma, and a smooth muscle tumor of another site (such as gastrointestinal or retroperitoneum) must be excluded. Some cases may respond to hormonal therapy.

C. **Intravascular leiomyomatosis** refers to classic leiomyomas that grow into the lumen of the uterine or pelvic veins. The tumor may migrate or extend into the inferior vena cava, and even into the right heart. The tumor is composed of sheets of spindled to round cells with minimal atypia and rare mitoses, for which the differential diagnosis often includes low grade endometrial stromal sarcoma. With local control, the tumor has an excellent long-term prognosis.

D. **Leiomyosarcoma** is the malignant counterpart of leiomyoma. It is the most common sarcoma of the uterus, with an incidence of 2 to 3 for every 1000 women with leiomyomata. Leiomyosarcoma usually occurs in women over

TABLE 33.4	Strategy for Diagnosis of Uterine Smooth Muscle Tumors

Morphologic features to be evaluated

Degree of cytologic atypia; none to mild (insignificant) or moderate to severe (significant)

Presence or absence of CTCN

Mitotic index

Tumors with usual differentiation

Mitotic index (MI) <20 per 10 hpf, no CTCN, no atypia or no more than mild cytologic atypia – leiomyoma or leiomyoma with increased mitotic index (MI < 5 per 10 hpf – leiomyoma; MI ≥ 5 per 10 hpf – leiomyoma with increased mitotic index)

MI ≥ 20 per hpf, no CTCN, no atypia or no more than mild cytologic atypia-leiomyoma with increased mitotic index, but experience limited

MI < 10 per hpf, no CTCN but with diffuse moderate to severe cytologic atypia – atypical leiomyoma with low risk of recurrence

MI ≥ 10 per 10 hpf, no CTCN but with diffuse moderate to severe cytologic atypia – leiomyosarcoma

MI < 20 per 10 hpf, no CTCN but with focal moderate to severe cytologic atypia – atypical leiomyoma, but experience limited

Any MI, with diffuse moderate to severe atypia and with CTCN – leiomyosarcoma

MI ≥ 10 per 10 hpf, no to mild atypia but with CTCN –leiomyosarcoma

MI < 10, no to mild atypia but with CTCN – smooth muscle tumor of low malignant potential, but experience limited.

Modified from *Am J Surg Pathol.* 1994;18:535.

the age of 50 and has a higher rate of occurrence in African Americans. Some studies have suggested unopposed estrogen exposure as one of the underlying etiologies. The genetics of leiomyosarcomas has confirmed that they do not arise from leiomyomas.

Grossly, leiomyosarcoma consists of an irregular, soft and fleshy mass with a pink-tan cut surface that has obvious foci of hemorrhage and necrosis. The tumor almost always demonstrates an ill-defined and infiltrating border. Microscopically, leiomyosarcoma is composed of sheets of pleomorphic spindle cells with elongated nuclei, high-grade cytologic atypia, and a high mitotic rate with frequent atypical mitotic figures (e-**Fig. 33.50**). A comprehensive study (*Am J Surg Pathol.* 1994;18:535) recommended that the diagnostic approach for leiomyosarcoma includes evaluation of the degree of cytologic atypia (graded as mild, moderate, or severe), assessment of the presence or absence of coagulative tumor cell necrosis (CTCN, defined as an abrupt transition from viable cells to necrotic cells without a transition zone of hyalinized tissue or granulation tissue) (e-**Fig. 33.51**), and determination of the mitotic index (MI), as outlined in Table 33.4.

Leiomyosarcoma has a poor prognosis. The patient's age, tumor mitotic index, and clinical stage of the disease at the time of presentation are among the important prognostic factors. Surgical intervention including total abdominal hysterectomy with bilateral salpingo-oophorectomy is the treatment of choice. Variants include epithelioid (clear cell) leiomyosarcoma and myxoid leiomyosarcoma; both are relatively rare. The pathologic staging of uterine corpus leiomyosarcomas is shown in Table 33.3.

E. **Smooth muscle tumor of uncertain malignant potential (STUMP)** is the nomenclature used to designate problematic uterine smooth muscle neoplasms that fall between benign leiomyoma and leiomyosarcoma. Cases of STUMP represent tumors for which the classification by established criteria is uncertain, and for which the alternative diagnostic possibilities vary in their clinical implications.

IX. OTHER MYOMETRIAL DISEASES

A. **Adenomyosis** is defined as the presence of benign endometrial glands surrounded by endometrial stroma within the myometrium (conventionally at least 2.5 mm below the endomyometrial junction). Grossly, the adjacent myometrium can show a thick trabeculated pattern with punctuate hemorrhage. Microscopically, the glands usually show an inactive pattern, or a pattern that is dyssynchronous with the endometrium (e-Fig. 33.52). In some cases, particularly in postmenopausal women, only the stromal component is present and the glands are sparse or completely absent. Endometrial adenocarcinoma occasionally involves adenomyosis but this occurrence is not considered myometrial invasion for staging purposes.

B. **Postoperative spindle cell nodule** is a benign lesion that usually occurs within a few weeks following endometrial instrumentation or other surgical procedure. It is grossly pink-tan and friable. Microscopically, it consists of granulation tissue with surface ulceration, accompanied by a hypercellular proliferation of spindle cells with elongated nuclei, moderate amounts of pink cytoplasm, and a high mitotic rate arranged in fascicles. Numerous extravasated red blood cells are usually present. Postoperative spindle cell nodule must be distinguished from leiomyosarcoma; the former's distinct fascicular pattern of growth, lack of pleomorphism, and characteristic clinical presentation are clues to the correct diagnosis.

C. **Adenofibroma** is a rare entity that usually occurs in postmenopausal women who present with abnormal bleeding. Microscopically, it is composed of a layer of epithelium with bland nuclear cytology that overlies a cellular fibrous stroma composed of fibroblasts and endometrial stromal cells. Adenofibroma is a benign entity and hysterectomy is curative.

D. **Adenosarcoma** is characteristically a tumor of postmenopausal women. It is a rare neoplasm that arises most commonly from the endometrium and forms a large, polypoid, lobulated mass that may fill the entire endometrial cavity and prolapse through the cervical os. Microscopically, adenosarcomas are composed of benign glandular elements in a malignant stroma that shows increased cellularity, pleomorphism, and a mitotic rate of >2 mitotic figures per 10 hpf (e-Fig. 33.53). The stroma is often condensed and hypercellular in periglandular areas and often juts into gland lumens in a characteristic pattern (e-Fig. 33.54).

Adenosarcoma is best considered a tumor of low malignant potential and has a better outcome compared with other uterine sarcomas. However, recurrence (which occurs in up to 25% of patients) is associated with very poor prognosis. Treatment includes hysterectomy with bilateral salpingo-oophorectomy. The pathologic staging of uterine corpus adenosarcoma is shown in Table 33.5.

X. GESTATIONAL TROPHOBLASTIC DISEASE.
This group of diseases comprises abnormal trophoblastic proliferations that arise from gestational trophoblast. In Western populations, about 0.1% of pregnancies are affected; patients are often at the extremes of reproductive age, and women with previous gestational trophoblastic disease are at higher risk.

A. **Hydatidiform mole**

1. **Complete molar pregnancies** develop from fertilization of an empty ovum. Complete moles are diploid but may be either heterozygous (15% of cases due to fertilization of an empty ovum by two sperm) or homozygous (85% of cases due to fertilization of an empty ovum by a single sperm with subsequent duplication). Complete moles classically present as a larger uterus than expected for gestational age that on ultrasound examination shows a so-called snow storm pattern without fetal parts; the patient's serum hCG is usually elevated for gestational age. Histopathologically, classic complete moles are composed of markedly enlarged villi with central villous

TABLE 33.5	TNM and FIGO Staging of Adenosarcoma	

TNM and FIGO classification
Primary tumor (T)

TNM Categories	FIGO Stages	
TX		Primary tumor cannot be assessed
T0		No evidence of primary tumor
T1	I	Tumor confined to corpus uteri
T1a	IA	Tumor limited to endometrium/endocervix
T1b	IB	Tumor invades less than one-half of myometrium
T1c	1C	Tumor invades one-half or more of myometrium
T2	II	Tumor extends beyond the uterus, within the pelvis
T2a	IIA	Tumor involves adnexa
T2b	IIB	Tumor involves other pelvic tissues
T3	III	Tumor involves abdominal tissues
T3a	IIIA	One site
T3b	IIIB	More than one site
T4	IVA	Tumor invades bladder mucosa and/or bowel mucosa

Regional lymph nodes (N)

NX		Regional lymph nodes cannot be assessed
N0		No regional lymph node metastasis
N1		Regional lymph node metastasis

Distant metastasis (M)

MX		Distant metastasis cannot be assessed
M0		No distant metastasis
M1		Distant metastasis (excluding adnexa, pelvic and abdominal tissues)

Stage grouping for uterine sarcomas

Stage I	T1	N0	M0
Stage IA	T1a	N0	M0
Stage IB	T1b	N0	M0
Stage IC	T1c	N0	M0
Stage II	T2	N0	M0
Stage IIIA	T3a	N0	M0
Stage IIIB	T3b	N0	M0
Stage IIIC	T1–T3	N1	M0
Stage IVA	T4	Any N	M0
Stage IVB	Any T	Any N	M1

From: Edge SB, Byrd DR, Compton CC, et al., eds. *AJCC Cancer Staging Manual.* 7th ed. New York, NY: Springer; 2010. Used with permission.

cavitation and circumferential, markedly atypical trophoblastic proliferation (e-**Fig. 33.55**).

With the advent of early ultrasound and better serum hCG screening, abnormal pregnancies, including molar pregnancies, are evacuated earlier which can complicate diagnosis. Although early complete moles are usually associated with normal ultrasound and hCG levels, microscopically they show "claw-like" or "cauliflower-like" villous shapes, a blue mesenchymal-like stroma, labyrinthine stromal canaliculi, atypical implantation trophoblast, and circumferential trophoblast hyperplasia at least focally (e-**Figs. 33.56** to **33.58**). Both classic and early complete moles carry an increased risk of subsequent development of choriocarcinoma (up to 10% in Asian populations).

2. **Partial molar pregnancies** develop from fertilization of a normal ovum by two sperm, and so have a triploid karyotype. Patients may have a normal, elevated, or even low serum hCG for gestational age; fetal parts are sometimes present by ultrasound imaging. Histologically, partial moles are composed of two populations of villi; one population is essentially normal or small and fibrotic, and the other exhibits enlargement with at least focal cavitation, irregular villous outlines, trophoblast inclusions, and subtle circumferential trophoblast in the form of buds or lacy mounds (**e-Figs. 33.59 and 33.60**). Partial moles also carry a small but increased risk of subsequent development of choriocarcinoma.

3. **Invasive mole** refers to a molar pregnancy (either complete or partial) in which the villi and associated trophoblast invade the myometrium and blood vessels or are exported to extrauterine sites (**e-Fig. 33.61**).

B. **Trophoblastic tumors**
1. **Choriocarcinoma.** Although molar pregnancies have a much increased risk of subsequent development of gestational choriocarcinoma, the tumor can develop following any type of pregnancy, including normal gestations. Microscopically, choriocarcinoma is composed of sheets of highly atypical trophoblast with prominent foci of hemorrhage and necrosis (**e-Fig. 33.62**). The pleomorphic trophoblast consists of admixture of cytotrophoblast, syncytiotrophoblast, and intermediate trophoblast and often forms alternating collections of syncytiotrophoblast and mononucleate trophoblast. Choriocarcinoma spreads hematogenously, and the most common metastatic sites are the lung, pelvis, vagina, liver, and brain. Choriocarcinoma is strongly positive for cytokeratin, hCG, Mel-CAM, human placental lactogen (hPL), and placental alkaline phosphatase expression by immunohistochemistry.

2. **Placental site trophoblastic tumor** is composed of intermediate trophoblast. Characteristic features include abundant eosinophilic fibrinoid deposition and dissection of individual smooth muscle cells by the neoplastic cells (**e-Figs. 33.63 to 33.65**). This tumor typically presents as a mass which may be deeply invasive; serum hCG levels are usually only mildly elevated. About 15% of cases exhibit malignant behavior; unlike most forms of gestational trophoblastic disease, the tumor is not very responsive to chemotherapy.

3. **Epithelioid trophoblastic tumor** is composed of chorionic-type intermediate trophoblast. It is a very rare form of trophoblastic disease that has only recently been recognized as a distinct disease entity. Morphologically, the tumor is composed of a uniform population of atypical mononucleate cells arranged in sheets and nests associated with eosinophilic material and surrounded by necrotic debris (**e-Fig. 33.66**).

XI. **SEROSAL TUMORS**
A. **Endometriosis** affects 5% to 10% of women of childbearing age. Patients usually present with symptoms of pelvic pain, dyspareunia, secondary dysmenorrhea and, in some cases, infertility. Many cases remain asymptomatic. The three most common accepted theories regarding its etiology are retrograde spillage of menstrual tissue into the pelvic cavity, serosal metaplasia, and a developmental abnormality. The most commonly involved sites include the ovary, uterine serosa, fallopian tube, peritoneum, and cul-de-sac. Oral contraceptives have been shown to have a protective role. Histologically, endometriosis is defined as the presence of endometrial glands surrounded by endometrial stroma; associated hemosiderin deposition and chronic inflammation are usually present.

B. **Adenomatoid tumor** is a benign peritoneal tumor that originates from mesothelium. It most commonly involves the serosal surfaces of the uterus and fallopian tubes. Grossly, the tumor usually forms a tan 1- to 2-cm well-circumscribed nodule. Microscopically, the tumor is composed of tubular and slit-like spaces lined by a single layer of flattened cuboidal cells with bland cytology (e-**Fig. 33.67**). The cells are immunopositive for cytokeratin, calretinin, and vimentin expression, but immunonegative for factor VIII-related antigen and CD31 expression—a profile that can be used to distinguish the tumor from metastatic carcinoma and vascular tumors. Adenomatoid tumor is clinically asymptomatic and usually found incidentally.

XII. OTHER MISCELLANEOUS NEOPLASMS

A. **Lymphoid neoplasms** involving the uterine corpus (of which the most frequent is large B cell lymphoma) most commonly represent a manifestation of disseminated disease. Primary disease of the uterus is extremely rare.

B. **Metastatic tumors** only rarely involve the uterus. The most common primary tumors that spread to the uterus are those of breast, lung, stomach, gallbladder, thyroid, and melanoma. In most instances, uterine involvement by primary tumors of the ovary, cervix, bladder, and rectum/colon represents direct extension rather than hematogenous spread.

SUGGESTED READINGS

Mazur MT, Kurman RJ. *Diagnosis of Endometrial Biopsies and Curettings. A Practical Approach.* 2nd ed. New York: Springer; 2005.

Tavassoli FA, Devilee P, Eds. *Tumours of the Breast and Female Genital Organs.* 1st ed. Lyon: International Agency for Research on Cancer; 2003.

34 Uterine Cervix
Michael E. Hull

I. NORMAL GROSS AND MICROSCOPIC ANATOMY

A. Gross. The cervix is the tubular distal portion of the uterus, divided into the ectocervix and endocervix. The smooth ectocervix is covered by a reflection of the vaginal mucosa, and the anterior and posterior fornices are formed by the protrusion of the cervix into the vaginal vault. The posterior fornix is deeper than the anterior fornix. The tan, rugous endocervix is a narrow canal that begins at the external os. The external os is round and small in the nulliparous state and becomes slit-like with parity. An internal os, or isthmus, marks the transition from the endocervix to the endometrium. The parametrial soft tissue, which attaches to the lateral aspects of the cervix, contains the uterine vessels and the ureters. The posterior cervix is the anterior border of the pouch of Douglas, the space between the uterus and the rectum; the anterior cervix is immediately posterior and inferior to the bladder.

B. Microscopic. The ectocervix is generally covered by squamous epithelium in continuity with the vaginal epithelium, while the endocervix is lined by columnar mucinous epithelium. The transition from columnar to squamous epithelium through the process of squamous metaplasia occurs over a region of the cervical epithelium called the transformation zone. In states of low estrogenization, the transition occurs approximately at the external os. With higher levels of estrogen, the transition is observed on the portion of cervix visible in the vaginal vault. The transformation zone is important diagnostically because it is the site of the majority of cervical epithelial neoplasms and their precursors (e-Fig. 34.1).*

1. Squamous epithelium. The squamous epithelium is composed of a basal layer, intermediate layer, and superficial layer. The basal layer is one-cell thick and has a relatively high nuclear/cytoplasmic (N/C) ratio. The N/C ratio decreases progressively from the basal layer to the superficial layer during normal maturation, and the superficial squamous cells tend to align with their longest axis parallel to the basement membrane. Directly sampled normal squamous epithelium in cytologic preparations shows individual and clustered superficial polygonal squamous cells with pyknotic nuclei, intermediate cells with somewhat larger nuclei, and more rounded parabasal cells with the highest N/C ratios. In the estrogenized state, superficial cells predominate.

2. Columnar epithelium. The mucinous columnar epithelium of the endocervix is one cell layer thick, with basal polarization of the cells' nuclei, little, if any, mitotic activity, and an N/C ratio of about 1:4. Mucinous columnar epithelium also lines the endocervical glands, which represent infoldings of the surface epithelium rather than true glands. Directly sampled endocervical columnar epithelium is seen in cytologic preparations as sheets of uniform round nuclei in a "honeycomb" arrangement or as single-layered strips of epithelium with basally oriented nuclei.

2. Squamous metaplastic epithelium. This is an expected finding in the transformation zone of cervical specimens. Histologically, in the immature form, the squamous epithelium underlies a layer of superficial residual columnar

---

*All e-figures are available online via the Solution Site Image Bank.

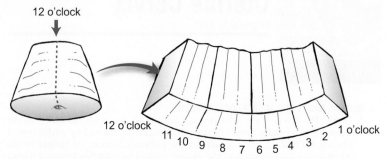

12 o'clock

12 o'clock

11 10 9 8 7 6 5 4 3 2 1 o'clock

Figure 34.1 Gross processing of conization specimens. After the endocervical and stromal margins are inked, the specimen is radially sectioned so that each tissue slice includes the endocervical margin, the mucosal surface of the endocervical canal, and the ectocervix.

epithelium (e-**Fig. 34.1**); with full maturation, it may appear very similar to native squamous epithelium. Metaplastic squamous cells in cytologic smears occur as either singly dispersed cells or small sheets of cells, and they show cyanophilic cytoplasm and nuclear sizes and N/C ratios between those of normal intermediate and basal cells.

II. **GROSS EXAMINATION, TISSUE SAMPLING, AND HISTOLOGIC SLIDE PREPARATION.** Cervical specimens for screening and diagnosis are obtained in several ways.

A. **Exfoliative cytology (Pap test).** See the section below on cytology of the uterine cervix for a discussion of the Pap test.

B. **Biopsy.** Colposcopic cervical biopsy specimens are small pieces of mucosa and superficial stroma that are taken, most often, from acetowhite areas identified visually. Documentation of the number and size of tissue fragments is important to ensure that the biopsy tissue fragments are adequately represented on the slides. If a tissue fragment exceeds 4 mm in maximal dimension, it should be bisected prior to histologic processing. In general, the biopsy tissue should be wrapped in lens paper or placed between sponges to avoid loss during processing, and the tissue should be embedded such that the microscopic sections are perpendicular to the mucosal surface. Three H&E-stained levels are prepared for microscopic examination.

C. **Curettage.** Curettage specimens consist of numerous and often miniscule tissue fragments in mucus, so it is imperative to both filter the contents of the container and collect any tissue that may be adherent to the pad or paper submitted within the specimen container. It is necessary to wrap curettings in lens paper to avoid loss during processing. The specimens obtained from curettage procedures should be submitted in their entirety. Three H&E-stained levels are prepared for microscopic examination.

D. **Conization.** Ideal cold knife cone biopsy specimens consist of a single tube of ectocervix and cervical canal surrounded by stroma. Marking sutures attached by the surgeon enable the sections to be designated using the hours of the clock; by convention, the mid-anterior location is the 12 o'clock position. The endocervical margin must be identified and inked differentially from the ectocervical and stromal margins. After fixation, the specimen should be radially sectioned, with each section encompassing the endocervical margin, the mucosal surface of the endocervical canal with the transformation zone, and ectocervical margin, as shown in Fig. 34.1.

E. **Loop electrosurgical excision procedure (LEEP).** The key to correct processing of these specimens is identification of the endocervical margin (which may be inked by the surgeon to facilitate identification); the ectocervix is smooth and tan-white, whereas the endocervix is tan and more rugous. The endocervical margin should be differentially inked from the ectocervical and stromal margins. Radial sections should be taken perpendicular to the mucosa, encompassing the endocervical margin, transformation zone, and ectocervical margin in the same manner as for conization specimens.

F. **Radical hysterectomy**

1. **Uterus.** Before opening the uterus, the parametrial soft tissue is inked as it represents soft tissue margins of interest. The vaginal margins are also inked. The uterus is then bivalved. If no tumor is visible or the tumor does not appear to extend into the parametrial soft tissue, the parametrial soft tissue is removed, sectioned, and completely submitted. If the vagina appears free of tumor, shave margins are submitted. If tumor appears to extend into the parametrial soft tissue or vagina, radial sections (that include the tumor's relationship to the margin) are submitted. If a cervical mass is present, at least one section per centimeter of tumor, including the deepest extension into the cervical wall, is submitted. If no tumor is visible, the cervix is amputated and processed as a conization specimen.

2. **Lymph nodes.** Separate packets of pelvic and para-aortic lymph nodes are typically submitted with radical hysterectomy specimens. The lymph nodes should be separated from the soft tissue and entirely submitted.

III. **DIAGNOSTIC FEATURES OF COMMON NONNEOPLASTIC DISEASES**

A. **Inflammation and infection.** Acute cervicitis is a pattern of inflammation marked by a stromal and epithelial neutrophilic infiltrate, with associated stromal edema, and, often, reactive epithelial atypia. Reactive epithelium shows enlarged nuclei and prominent nucleoli in a pattern that may be confused with neoplasia. Acute cervicitis is usually a nonspecific diagnosis, as the inciting agent can be any of a wide variety of bacterial, fungal, or protozoan organisms. Chronic cervicitis consists of a lymphoplasmacytic infiltrate that is also nonspecific. Papillary endocervicitis is a term describing inflamed endocervical mucosa forming papillary structures.

1. **Noninfectious cervicitis.** Cervicitis can be due to irritation from chemical exposure, foreign materials (e.g., pessary, tampons), or surgical trauma. The cervix may also be a site of involvement in systemic inflammatory conditions such as collagen vascular disease. The type of inflammatory response may be neutrophilic, lymphoplasmacytic, or granulomatous.

2. **Infectious cervicitis**

   a. **Bacterial cervicitis.** *Neisseria gonorrhoeae* and *Chlamydia trachomatis* both produce a mucopurulent cervicitis that requires additional nonhistologic methods for specific diagnosis. With chronicity, *C. trachomatis* infection can result in follicular cervicitis, a pattern of intense lymphocytic infiltration that characteristically includes lymphoid aggregates with germinal centers (e-Fig. 34.2). Although often associated with *C. trachomatis*, follicular cervicitis is not specific for that infection.

   Actinomyces spp. infection is associated with intrauterine device (IUD) use and is often asymptomatic. The morphologic pattern is distinctive in that clusters of purple-red filamentous organisms are seen in curettings and smears, with associated "sulfur granules" consisting of clusters of neutrophils with a basophilic center.

   Bacterial vaginosis is characterized by "clue cells," squamous cells coated with bacterial organisms. *Gardnerella vaginalis* and *Mobiluncus* spp. are both implicated in the disease.

   b. **Viral cervicitis.** Herpes simplex virus (HSV; primarily HSV type 2) infection is characterized by ulceration with enlarged epithelial nuclei, nuclear molding, multinucleation, and margination of the chromatin in virally infected cells at the edge of the ulcer (e-**Fig. 34.3**). Cytomegalovirus is distinctive for its nuclear and cytoplasmic inclusions. Adenovirus is notable for its smudged nuclear inclusions. The poxvirus *Molluscum contagiosum* generates large, round, intensely eosinophilic cytoplasmic inclusions, as it does in its cutaneous sites. Human papillomavirus (HPV) infection is closely tied to cervical neoplasia; its features are discussed in the sections on preinvasive and invasive squamous neoplasia.

c. **Granulomatous cervicitis.** Infectious causes of granulomatous cervicitis include *Mycobacterium tuberculosis* and *Treponema pallidum* infections. As noted above, noninfectious etiologies are also in the differential diagnosis of granulomatous inflammation.

d. **Fungal.** *Candida* spp. are commonly encountered in smears and are not necessarily always pathogenic. They cannot be speciated reliably on their morphology, in either tissue sections or cervical smears.

e. **Parasitic.** *Trichomonas vaginalis* is one of the most common causative agent of sexually transmitted infections in women. Many infections are asymptomatic. In Papanicolaou-stained smears or liquid-based preparations, an ovoid organism with an eccentric nucleus is observed; in liquid-based preparations, squamous cells may be coated with the organism.

3. **Vasculitis.** Most cases of vasculitis involving the gynecologic tract are incidental, and the vasculitis is often confined to the cervix. However, some cases are associated with known collagen vascular disease, and rare cases represent the first manifestation of a collagen vascular disorder (e-**Fig. 34.4**) (*Int J Gynecol Pathol.* 2000;19:258).

B. **Atrophy.** Epithelial atrophy is seen in the postmenopausal state, when estrogen levels are decreased. As noted in the discussion of normal histology, high estrogen states are associated with large numbers of superficial squamous cells; however, when the epithelium is thinned, the histologic picture is dominated by small cells with increased N/C ratios and nuclei at least as large or larger than those of normal intermediate cells. The overall appearance of a well-organized epithelial architecture and a lack of nuclear atypia distinguish atrophy from a severe squamous dysplasia.

C. **Metaplasia.** Tubal metaplasia occurs most frequently in the upper endocervix. Transitional-cell metaplasia is rare and recapitulates urothelium; it is not associated with a specific insult and must not be confused with neoplasia. Intestinal metaplasia is another uncommon metaplasia; it features columnar epithelium with goblet and Paneth cells.

D. **Hyperplasia**

1. **Squamous hyperplasia** consists of thickening of the epithelium with normal maturation. It occurs in situations of prolapse and chronic irritation.

2. **Squamous papilloma** is a benign squamous proliferation that covers fibrovascular cores. Squamous papilloma may be associated with HPV infection but it does not show classic koilocytic atypia.

3. **Microglandular hyperplasia** is an increase in glandular elements in the cervical stroma. Seen in histologic sections, the exuberant proliferation sometimes has a cribriform architecture that can raise the question of neoplasia. However, microglandular hyperplasia shows no cytologic atypia, does not infiltrate the stroma, and is not associated with a desmoplastic reaction.

4. **Lobular endocervical glandular hyperplasia** is a benign proliferation of bland glands usually surrounding a central dilated gland and forming a well-circumscribed lobule.

5. **Diffuse laminar endocervical glandular hyperplasia.** In this entity, the proliferation is primarily in the very superficial aspects of the stroma and extends in a band-like fashion with an intermingled lymphocytic infiltrate that may be dense.

E. **Nabothian cysts** are pronounced dilatations of endocervical glands. They are extremely common (e-**Fig. 34.5**).

F. **Endocervical tunnel clusters** are superficial collections of endocervical gland ductal spaces.

G. **Mesonephric remnants** are developmental remnants of the mesonephric (Wolffian) duct that are occasionally identified in the deep stroma. Mesonephric remnants must not be confused with adenocarcinoma; helpful distinguishing features include the bland cytology of the lining epithelium, a lack of atypia in the overlying endocervical glands, and the absence of a desmoplastic stromal response (e-**Fig. 34.6**).

H. **Postoperative spindle-cell nodule** is a benign proliferation of fibroblasts that usually occurs following surgical manipulation.

I. **Endocervical polyps** are often identified colposcopically. They consist of an exophytic configuration of benign glands and stroma usually with thick-walled vessels (e-**Fig. 34.7**). They must be carefully examined microscopically to exclude coexisting squamous dysplasia or a glandular neoplasm.

J. **Inclusion cysts** are benign. Microscopically, they are filled with keratin debris and are related to surgical manipulation. Similar inclusions occur in the vagina, following episiotomies.

K. **Endometriosis** can involve any layer of the cervical stroma, as well as the parametrial/paracervical soft tissue.

L. **Decidual change** occurs in the cervical stroma during pregnancy. The nests of cells that show abundant amphophilic cytoplasm, a prominent cell border, and a single, centrally placed nucleus are usually not visible grossly, but sometimes form polyps (e-**Fig. 34.8**).

M. **The Arias-Stella reaction**, characterized by epithelial cells with nuclear enlargement and clear cytoplasm in response to progesterone, is most commonly seen in the uterine corpus in pregnancy but may also occur in the cervix. The significance of the Arias-Stella reaction lies in the fact that it can easily be confused with a glandular neoplasm.

IV. **CERVICAL NEOPLASIA.** The WHO classification of cervical tumors is shown in Table 34.1.

A. **Benign**

1. **Submucosal and stromal neoplasms.** Leiomyomas identical to those of the uterine corpus are also seen in the cervix.

2. **Blue nevus.** This benign melanocytic proliferation is common, noted clinically as a bluish discoloration of the cervical epithelium. Microscopic examination shows hyperpigmented spindle cells infiltrating the stroma in a haphazard pattern (e-**Fig. 34.9**).

3. **Ectopic tissue.** While not neoplastic, several types of ectopic tissue may be seen in the cervix. The most common types of ectopic tissue are cutaneous adnexal structures and mature cartilage. Prostatic ectopia has also been noted to occur on occasion (e-**Fig. 34.10**) and is important to recognize to avoid overdiagnosis of a glandular malignancy.

B. **Malignant and premalignant squamous lesions.** Worldwide, cervical cancer is the third most common malignancy and the fifth most common cause of cancer mortality in women. Effective screening programs have dramatically reduced deaths due to cervical cancer in the developed world, but gains have been more modest elsewhere.

The major risk factor for cervical cancer is sexually transmitted HPV infection. Although there are >40 different HPV serotypes that infect the female genital tract, high-risk serotypes (including 16, 18, 35, 39, 45, 51, 56, and 58) are associated with a markedly increased risk of severe squamous dysplasia and subsequent cervical squamous cell carcinoma. Immunodeficiency may increase the likelihood of persistent infection and may increase the risk of

TABLE 34.1	WHO Histologic Classification of Tumors of the Uterine Cervix

Epithelial tumors
Squamous tumors and precursors
  Squamous cell carcinoma, not otherwise specified
    Keratinizing
    Nonkeratinizing
    Basaloid
    Verrucous
    Warty
    Papillary
    Lymphoepithelioma-like
    Squamotransitional
Early invasive (microinvasive) squamous cell carcinoma
Squamous intraepithelial neoplasia
    Cervical intraepithelial neoplasia (CIN3) squamous cell carcinoma in situ
Benign squamous cell lesions
    Condyloma acuminatum
    Squamous papilloma
    Fibroepithelial polyp
Glandular tumors and precursors
  Adenocarcinoma
    Mucinous adenocarcinoma
      Endocervical
      Intestinal
      Signet-ring cell
      Minimal deviation
      Villoglandular
    Endometrioid adenocarcinoma
    Clear cell adenocarcinoma
    Serous adenocarcinoma
    Mesonephric adenocarcinoma
  Early invasive adenocarcinoma
  Adenocarcinoma in situ
  Glandular dysplasia
  Benign glandular lesions
    Müllerian papilloma
    Endocervical polyp
Other epithelial tumors
  Adenosquamous carcinoma
    Glassy cell carcinoma variant
  Adenoid cystic carcinoma
  Adenoid basal carcinoma
  Neuroendocrine tumors
    Carcinoid
    Atypical carcinoid
    Small cell carcinoma
    Large cell neuroendocrine carcinoma
  Undifferentiated carcinoma
Mesenchymal tumors and tumor-like conditions
Leiomyosarcoma
Endometrioid stromal sarcoma, low grade
Undifferentiated endocervical sarcoma

(continued)

| TABLE 34.1 | WHO Histologic Classification of Tumors of the Uterine Cervix (*Continued*) |

Sarcoma botryoides
Alveolar soft part sarcoma
Angiosarcoma
   Malignant peripheral nerve sheath tumor
   Leiomyoma
   Genital rhabdomyoma
Postoperative spindle cell nodule
Mixed epithelial and mesenchymal tumors
   Carcinosarcoma (malignant mixed Müllerian tumor)
   Adenosarcoma
   Wilms' tumor
   Adenofibroma
   Adenomyoma
Melanocytic tumors
   Malignant melanoma
   Blue nevus
Miscellaneous tumors
Tumors of germ cell type
   Yolk sac tumor
   Dermoid cyst
   Mature cystic teratoma
Lymphoid and hematopoietic tumors
   Malignant lymphoma (specify type)
   Leukemia (specify type)
Secondary tumors

From: Tavassoli FA, Devilee P, eds. *World Health Organization Classification of Tumours. Pathology and Genetics. Tumours of the Breast and Female Genital Organs.* Lyon: IARC Press; 2001. Used with permission.

subsequent epithelial malignant transformation. Host factors such as smoking, concomitant sexually transmitted diseases, high parity, and oral contraceptive use may also increase the risk of malignant transformation among already infected women. For example, among women with HPV infection, smoking doubles to quadruples the odds in favor of malignant transformation (*J Natl Cancer Inst.* 2002;94:1406; *Cancer Causes Control.* 2003;14:805).

1. **HPV infection.** The viral cytopathic effect that results from HPV infection is termed koilocytosis and consists of nuclear enlargement with irregular nuclear borders, condensed chromatin, occasional binucleation or multinucleation, and a perinuclear halo. Flat lesions that exhibit koilocytosis are usually associated with low-risk HPV types 6 and 11. High-risk HPV types such as HPV 16 and 18 encode proteins that have the capacity to immortalize keratinocytes by enhancing the ubiquitin-mediated degradation of the tumor suppressors TP53 and pRb. Malignant transformation is not a committed endpoint of HPV infection, but its likelihood may be enhanced by environmental and host factors as discussed earlier.

2. **Cervical intraepithelial neoplasia-1** (CIN1; also known as mild dysplasia, or low-grade squamous intraepithelial lesion [LSIL]) is defined by disordered maturation and cytologic abnormalities of the lower one-third of the squamous epithelium, often with koilocytic changes in the upper two-thirds of the epithelium (e-**Fig. 34.11**). Most cases of CIN1 regress (*Int J Gynecol Pathol.* 1993;12:186).

3. **Cervical intraepithelial neoplasia-2 and -3** (CIN2 and CIN3; also known as moderate dysplasia and severe dysplasia, respectively, or high-grade

squamous intraepithelial lesion [HSIL]) are defined by cytologic abnormalities of the lower two-thirds and full thickness of the epithelium, respectively (e-Figs. 34.12 and 34.13). Spontaneous regression occurs at lower rates than in CIN1, ranging from 40% for CIN2 to 33% for CIN3. A more aggressive approach to the management of these lesions is warranted, because progression to invasive carcinoma occurs in a higher percentage of these lesions (*Int J Gynecol Pathol.* 1993;12:186).

4. **Invasive squamous cell carcinoma** is recognized by penetration of the epithelial basement membrane by neoplastic squamous cells with an associated desmoplastic stromal response (e-Fig. 34.14). Keratinizing and nonkeratinizing types are encountered. In contrast to the atypical cells characteristic of high-grade squamous dysplasia in which the N/C ration is markedly increased, the invasive tumor cells often exhibit paradoxical maturation evidenced by abundant eosinophilic cytoplasm.

   a. **Microinvasive squamous cell carcinoma** is defined as a tumor that is not recognized as such clinically, that invades ≤ 5 mm from the basement membrane of the adjacent surface epithelium or endocervical gland from which it arises, and that extends ≤ 7 mm in greatest lateral extent (FIGO Stage 1A). When no lymphatic or vascular involvement is present, when the entire lesion is excised, and when no dysplasia is present at the margins of excision, the potential for lymph node metastasis or recurrence is very low. Long-term follow-up studies have shown that the percentage of patients harboring residual invasive carcinoma in a hysterectomy specimen after conization for microinvasive squamous cell carcinoma with maximum invasion of ≤ 1 mm is 0; when invasion is ≤ 3 mm, the recurrence and lymph node metastasis rates are <1 %. For lesions between 3 and 5 mm in depth, the recurrence and lymph node metastasis rates increase to around 2% and 4%, respectively (*Pathol Ann.* 1995;30:103). Most studies find 3 mm of invasion to be a cutoff beyond which recurrence and lymph node metastasis risk become significant.

   b. **Squamous cell carcinoma variants**

      i. **Keratinizing tumors** contain keratin pearls and nests of tumor cells with central keratin; cytoplasmic keratinization and keratohyaline granules are also present. Intercellular bridges can be identified.

      ii. **Nonkeratinizing tumors** show cytoplasmic keratinization of individual cells and intercellular bridges, but keratin pearls and nests of tumor cells with central keratin are not present.

      iii. **Basaloid carcinoma** features cells with scanty cytoplasm that resemble basal type squamous cells. Only rare nests of tumor cells show central keratin. This variant has an aggressive behavior.

      iv. **Verrucous carcinoma** is a very well-differentiated squamous cell carcinoma that betrays its malignant character only in its invasion of the stroma along broad pushing borders. There is minimal cytologic atypia, and viral cytopathic effect is absent. Aggressive local invasion and recurrence after excision are common. Metastasis is uncommon.

      v. **Warty carcinoma** is a rare squamous malignancy that shows definitive stromal invasion but also abundant cytologic features of HPV infection. It may behave less aggressively than other well-differentiated squamous cell carcinomas.

      vi. **Papillary squamous cell carcinoma** is an exophytic tumor in which epithelium resembling CIN2 or CIN3 covers fibrovascular cores. Koilocytosis is not characteristic. Although much of the tumor may have the appearance of a precursor lesion, definitive stromal invasion is present in the deep aspects of the lesion. Therefore, superficial biopsies of papillary lesions should be interpreted with caution.

vii. **Lymphoepithelial-like carcinoma** resembles the nasopharyngeal tumor of the same name. The tumor consists of syncytial sheets and islands of undifferentiated epithelioid cells that have eosinophilic cytoplasm and large vesicular nuclei with prominent nucleoli in a background that contains an intense lymphocytic infiltrate.

C. Glandular neoplasms

1. **Adenocarcinoma in situ (AIS)** is an HPV-associated glandular lesion (most strongly associated with HPV serotypes 16 and 18) that is a precursor to invasive adenocarcinoma. Cytologically, AIS is characterized by loss of cytoplasmic mucin, cellular stratification, cellular crowding, nuclear enlargement and atypia, mitotic activity, and epithelial apoptotic debris (e-**Fig. 34.15**). The various subtypes can mimic endocervical, endometrial, or intestinal epithelium and can have a papillary or cribriform architectural pattern. AIS is often seen in conjunction with CIN.

   In contrast to in situ squamous epithelial lesions, AIS of the cervix is less common than its invasive counterpart. Because of this, follow-up studies are sparse. However, a number of series do show that a positive margin for AIS in a cone biopsy predicts the presence of either an invasive adenocarcinoma or the recurrence of AIS (*Gynecol Oncol.* 2000;79:207), and therefore AIS requires complete excision.

2. **Microinvasive adenocarcinoma.** The FIGO definition of microinvasive adenocarcinoma is the same as that of microinvasive squamous cell carcinoma. It is a difficult diagnosis; the subjectivity of histologic assessment and relative infrequency of in situ adenocarcinoma have presented challenges in the elucidation of the natural behavior of microinvasive adenocarcinoma. What is known is that it carries a good prognosis. When invasion is ≤2 mm, lymph node metastases essentially do not occur (*Obstet Gynecol.* 1985;65:46; *Obstet Gynecol.* 1997;89:88; *Int J Gynecol Pathol.* 2000;19:29).

3. **Invasive adenocarcinoma.** Infiltrating glands with cribriform and papillary structures are the architectural characteristics of invasive adenocarcinoma. A desmoplastic stromal reaction—a feature that helps to distinguish adenocarcinoma from both AIS and the hyperplastic entities described earlier—is present (e-**Fig. 34.16**).

   a. **Mucinous adenocarcinoma.** Most primary mucinous adenocarcinomas have cytologic features resembling endocervical glands. The cells are cuboidal to columnar and show nuclear pleomorphism, nuclear atypia, and many mitoses. The relatively abundant cytoplasm stains positively for mucin. Mucinous adenocarcinomas with goblet cells that have an overall morphology more similar to intestinal epithelium are termed intestinal variants.

   b. **Minimal deviation adenocarcinoma (adenoma malignum).** This rare entity comprises only 1% of primary adenocarcinomas of the cervix. The glandular epithelium is so bland in appearance that these lesions may not be recognized as malignant on biopsy or curettage specimens; increased mitotic activity and cytologic atypia may be present focally, but these findings are not prominent. The diagnosis rests on the presence of deep infiltration, aggregation of glands around vessels or nerves, and a stromal reaction—features that are easiest to assess on cone biopsy or hysterectomy. The incidence of this lesion is increased in Peutz–Jeghers syndrome.

   c. **Endometrioid adenocarcinoma.** Comprising 30% of cervical adenocarcinomas, endometrioid adenocarcinoma of the cervix is identical in appearance to its counterpart in the endometrium. When well differentiated, the lesion shows tall columnar cells without mucin. It may be very difficult to distinguish a cervical primary lesion from direct extension into the cervix of a tumor of the uterine corpus. Immunohistochemistry may be of some use in this situation, as endocervical adenocarcinomas are generally expected to express CEA and p16, while endometrial adenocarcinomas tend to be negative for these two markers and positive for vimentin and estrogen receptor. Care should be taken when using immunohistochemistry, because neither of these profiles has 100% specificity.

d. **Well-differentiated villoglandular adenocarcinoma** is considered to be a subtype of endometrioid adenocarcinoma. It shows an exophytic growth pattern with glandular and villous elements, little nuclear pleomorphism, and a low mitotic rate, quite similar to an intestinal villous adenoma (e-**Fig. 34.17**). There is value in the distinction, as this is a tumor of young women and has a favorable prognosis (*Gynecol Oncol.* 1997;64:147).

e. **Clear cell adenocarcinoma.** This tumor's association with in utero diethylstilbestrol (DES) exposure has made it widely recognized. Although rare, the tumor can occur in patients without a DES-exposure history as well. Clear cells with hobnail morphology are observed in solid, papillary, and tubular arrangements. The presence of this tumor in the cervix should prompt a search for a primary tumor of the ovary, endometrium, or vagina—sites where this entity is much more common.

f. **Serous adenocarcinoma** is another adenocarcinoma that only rarely occurs as a cervical primary tumor.

g. **Mesonephric adenocarcinoma.** This lesion differs from mesonephric remnants in its cytologic atypia, crowding, and increased mitotic activity. It arises in the deep lateral cervical walls and a variety of architectural patterns are characteristic, including tubular, papillary, solid, and retiform. The behavior of this very rare tumor is generally indolent, if the tumor is low stage.

D. **Other carcinomas**

1. **Adenosquamous carcinoma.** Both squamous and glandular differentiation are observed in this lesion. To be diagnostic, invasive glandular and squamous components must be present; that is, adenocarcinoma with adjacent squamous dysplasia is not adenosquamous carcinoma. The epidemiologic profile is similar to that of squamous cell carcinoma and adenocarcinoma.

2. **Glassy cell carcinoma** is considered a subtype of adenosquamous carcinoma that occurs in young women. It carries a poor prognosis because it is unresponsive to radiotherapy; progression is rapid, and distant metastases are common. Microscopically, the tumor consists of sheets of pleomorphic cells with granular eosinophilic cytoplasm, nucleoli, and brisk mitotic activity. The tumor is usually infiltrated by eosinophils and plasma cells. An in situ precursor lesion is not typically found in association with this tumor.

3. **Adenoid cystic carcinoma** is a rare cervical tumor found mostly in postmenopausal African American women who present with abnormal bleeding and a pelvic mass. This tumor shows cystic spaces filled with eosinophilic hyaline material or basophilic mucin surrounded by palisades of epithelial cells. The tumor architecture may be tubular, cribriform, or solid. Adenoid cystic carcinoma of the cervix typically shows more cytologic atypia than is present in its salivary gland counterpart but displays the same tendency for perineural invasion and local aggressiveness.

4. **Mucoepidermoid carcinoma (MEC)** is not currently recognized as a distinct entity in the WHO classification of cervical tumors. Tumors with striking similarity to the analogous tumor of the salivary gland do occur in the cervix, however, with epidermoid, intermediate, and mucin-producing cells. Interestingly, it has been shown that when strict histologic criteria are applied, cervical tumors with mucoepidermoid morphology harbor the same t(11;19)(q21;p13) as salivary gland MEC (*Am J Surg Pathol.* 2009;33:835).

This suggests that MEC may actually be an entity distinct from adenosquamous carcinoma in the cervix.

5. **Adenoid basal carcinoma.** This tumor occurs in a population similar to that of adenoid cystic carcinoma. It also shows a nested cribriform architecture. The epithelium, however, is composed of more uniform, round to oval, basophilic cells, often with squamous differentiation, without significant atypia or increased mitotic activity. There is often associated CIN. Correct identification of this lesion is important because it is low grade and does not have aggressive behavior; in fact, some have suggested that the tumor is more appropriately termed adenoid basal epithelioma (*Am J Surg Pathol.* 1998;22:965).

E. **Neuroendocrine neoplasms.** A variety of neuroendocrine neoplasms may occur in the cervix, although rarely. The classification of these tumors is similar to that of neuroendocrine tumors of the lung.

1. **Carcinoid.** These benign tumors are organoid in their architecture and are composed of small, oval to spindle cells with granular cytoplasm. Mitoses are rare in typical carcinoid tumors. Immunoreactivity with neuroendocrine markers synaptophysin, chromogranin A, and neuron-specific enolase is the rule.

2. **Atypical carcinoid.** Moderate cytologic atypia and the presence of 5 to 10 mitotic figures/10 high-power fields (HPFs) are sufficient to classify a carcinoid as atypical; at least small foci of necrosis are often present (*Arch Pathol Lab Med.* 1997;121:34). These tumors generally retain the organoid architecture of typical carcinoids. Their biologic behavior is difficult to assess systematically due to the subjectivity involved in separating atypical carcinoids from typical carcinoids and large cell neuroendocrine carcinomas.

3. **Large cell neuroendocrine carcinoma.** These tumors show frequent vascular invasion, have higher mitotic activity than atypical carcinoids (>10 mitotic figures/10 HPFs s), and show loss of the organoid architecture seen in less aggressive neuroendocrine tumors. There may be focal adenocarcinoma-like areas with abundant cytoplasm and large nucleoli. Necrosis is frequent. The prognosis is poor, similar to that of small cell carcinoma.

4. **Small cell carcinoma.** Histologically identical to its counterpart in the lung, small cell carcinoma (also known as high-grade neuroendocrine carcinoma) is a tumor of variably sized, round to oval to spindle cells with scanty cytoplasm, high mitotic activity, nuclear molding, and frequent crush artifact (e-**Fig. 34.18**). Necrosis may be extensive. Clinical series are small due to the rarity of the tumor, but the prognosis is uniformly poor.

F. **Mesenchymal neoplasms.** A wide variety of sarcomas may be primary to the cervix, including leiomyosarcoma, embryonal rhabdomyosarcoma, endometrioid stromal sarcoma, alveolar soft part sarcoma, and angiosarcoma (e-**Fig. 34.19**).

G. **Mixed epithelial and mesenchymal neoplasms**

1. **Adenosarcomas** are polypoid lesions that microscopically consist of large papillae of malignant stroma covered with benign endocervical epithelium. The stroma can have many different appearances; it can consist of plump, mitotically active spindle cells or more undifferentiated round cells similar to those of small cell carcinoma. Heterologous sarcomatous elements may be present, with skeletal muscle, cartilage, adipose, or osseous differentiation. Prognosis after excision is apparently good, although only small numbers of cases have been reported.

2. **Malignant mixed Müllerian tumor (MMMT),** or carcinosarcoma, also presents as a polypoid mass. In contrast to its more common counterpart in the uterine corpus, the malignant epithelial component is more often squamous or basaloid, as opposed to glandular. The sarcomatous component is usually

TABLE 34.2 TNM Staging and FIGO Classification of Carcinomas of the Uterine Cervix

TNM classification

Primary tumor (T)

TNM Categories	FIGO Stages	
TX		Primary tumor cannot be assessed
T0		No evidence of primary tumor
Tis	0	Carcinoma in situ (preinvasive carcinoma)
T1	I	Cervical carcinoma confined to uterus (extension to corpus should be disregarded)
T1a	IA	Invasive carcinoma diagnosed only by microscopy
T1a1	IA1	Stromal invasion no >3.0 mm in depth and 7.0 mm or less in horizontal spread
T1a2	IA2	Stromal invasion >3.0 mm and not >5.0 mm with a horizontal spread 7.0 mm or less
T1b	IB	Clinically visible lesion confined to the cervix or microscopic lesion greater than T1a2/1A2
T1b1	IB1	Clinically visible lesion 4.0 cm or less in greatest dimension
T1b2	IB2	Clinically visible lesion >4 cm in greatest dimension
T2	II	Tumor invades beyond uterus but not to pelvic wall or to lower third of the vagina
T2a	IIA	Without parametrial invasion
T2a1	IIA1	Clinically visible lesion 4.0 cm or less in greatest dimension
T2a2	IIA2	Clinically visible lesion >4.0 cm in greatest dimension
T2b	IIB	With parametrial invasion
T3	III	Tumor extends to pelvic wall, involves lower third of vagina, or causes hydronephrosis or nonfunctioning kidney
T3a	IIIA	Tumor involves lower third of vagina, no extension to pelvic wall
T3b	IIIB	Tumor extends to pelvic wall or causes hydronephrosis or nonfunctioning kidney
T4	IVA	Tumor invades mucosa of bladder or rectum or extends beyond true pelvis
M1	IVB	Distant metastasis

Regional lymph nodes (N)

NX	Regional lymph nodes cannot be assessed
N0	No regional lymph node metastasis
N1	Regional lymph node metastasis

Distant metastasis (M)

MX	Distant metastasis cannot be assessed
M0	No distant metastasis
M1	Distant metastasis

Stage grouping

Stage 0	Tis	N0	M0
Stage IA	T1a	N0	M0
Stage IA1	T1a1	N0	M0
Stage IA2	T1a2	N0	M0
Stage IB	T1b	N0	M0
Stage IB1	T1b1	N0	M0
Stage IB2	T1b2	N0	M0
Stage IIA	T2a	N0	M0
Stage IIB	T2b	N0	M0
Stage IIIA	T3a	N0	M0
Stage IIIB	T1,T2,T3a	N1	M0
	T3b	Any N	M0
Stage IVA	T4	Any N	M0
Stage IVB	Any T	Any N	M1

From: Edge SB, Byrd DR, Compton CC, et al., eds. *AJCC Cancer Staging Manual.* 7th ed. New York, NY: Springer; 2010. Used with permission.

homologous, with a spindle-cell morphology similar to that of fibrosarcoma. In limited series of MMMT of the cervix, it appears that the prognosis is better than that of MMMT of the uterine corpus.

H. **Hematolymphoid neoplasms.** Lymphoma of the cervix is usually a part of systemic disease.

I. **Melanoma.** Primary melanoma of the cervix is rare. Vaginal bleeding and a cervical mass is a common presentation. The tumor is usually low stage at presentation, but the prognosis is dismal. Morphologically, the tumor is similar to melanomas of other sites, although cervical melanomas have been noted for a tendency toward a spindle-cell morphology. Melanin pigment is variable from tumor to tumor. It is important to identify a junctional component in this lesion if it is to be classified as primary to the cervix; otherwise, a thorough search for another primary site is indicated.

J. **Secondary malignancies.** Most metastases to the cervix arise from tumors at other sites in the reproductive tract. Aside from the uterus and ovary, the gastrointestinal tract and breast are the most common origins of cervical metastases.

V. **PATHOLOGIC AND CLINICAL STAGING OF MALIGNANCIES**

A. **American Joint Committee on Cancer (AJCC) and International Federation of Gynecology and Obstetrics (FIGO) criteria.** The AJCC criteria for the staging of cervical cancer with the corresponding FIGO clinical staging categories are outlined in Table 34.2.

B. **Additional information.** The final report in any case of malignancy should explicitly include all of the information required for assigning a stage as well as other information of clinical interest not required for staging; Synoptic reports should be used to uniformly convey this information. For the cervix, the report should include: (1) the histologic type and grade; (2) the presence or absence of precursor lesions (either CIN or AIS); (3) tumor size, including depth and width; (4) whether the malignancy is unifocal or multifocal; (5) presence or absence of lymphovascular space invasion; (6) presence or absence of vaginal, paracervical/parametrial, or uterine extension; (7) margin status; and (8) presence or absence of lymph node or distant metastases.

Cytopathology of the Uterine Cervix

Michael E. Hull

I. **SPECIMEN TYPES**

A. **Liquid-based preparations** are the most widely used modality for cervical screening (Pap test). A brush is used to sample the cervix and the sample is placed in appropriate transport fluid for the proprietary system used in the laboratory, be it ThinPrep (Hologic, Inc., Marlborough, MA) or SurePath (BD Diagnostics-TriPath, Burlington, NC). Advantages of this modality include a cleaner background, a monolayer of cells, increased diagnostic sensitivity, and ease of performance of HPV assays.

B. **Conventional smears** are made by using a spatula and/or brush to sample the cervix, smearing the endo- and ectocervical samples on a glass slide, and then immediately fixing the sample. Papanicolaou staining is performed in the laboratory.

II. **EXFOLIATIVE CYTOLOGY OF THE CERVIX**

A. **Squamous cells.** A spectrum of squamous cells, ranging from small parabasal and metaplastic cells with dense cytoplasm and relatively high N/C ratios (e-Fig. 34.20), to intermediate cells with medium-sized round nuclei with open chromatin and polygonal cytoplasmic outlines (e-Fig. 34.21), to superficial cells with polygonal shapes and small pyknotic nuclei (e-Fig. 34.22) is seen in normal cervical smears and liquid-based preparations.

B. **Glandular cells.** The classic appearance of endocervical glandular cells is sheets of regularly spaced cells forming a so-called "honeycomb" pattern (e-Fig. 34.23); varying degrees of disruption of this architecture herald reactive and neoplastic changes. Endometrial cells are smaller and form more three-dimensional aggregates in cytology preparations; they are also typically more degenerated than endocervical cells. Careful attention to nuclear details such as the chromatin pattern and nuclear contours is required to separate glandular neoplasia from reactive atypia.

III. **THE BETHESDA SYSTEM** was developed in 1988 with the objective of standardizing terminology to promote better communication between the laboratory and clinicians. It is in its second edition (2001).

A. **Adequacy.** A statement of adequacy is required. Cellularity should be 5000 cells for a liquid-based preparation, and this can be reproducibly and quickly estimated with experience and with the use of reference images. Having 75% of squamous cells obscured by blood or inflammation renders a specimen unsatisfactory, as does improper labeling or slide breakage.

B. **Negative for intraepithelial lesion or malignancy**

1. **Microorganisms** should be reported. Various causes of vaginitis can be detected cytologically.

   Trichomonas vaginalis is seen as a pear-shaped structure, ~30 μm in diameter. It has a small pale nucleus and red cytoplasmic granules. The flagella are often difficult to appreciate (e-Fig. 34.24).

   Bacterial vaginosis is marked by the presence of "clue cells," which are coccobacilli-coated squamous cells (e-Fig. 34.25). This is reported as "shift in flora suggestive of bacterial vaginosis."

   Actinomyces infection shows filamentous organisms and the "sulfur granules" described above. This infection is associated with IUDs.

   Candida albicans is responsible for most cases of vulvovaginal candidiasis. Although the fungus can be a commensal microorganism, when it is accompanied by acute inflammation, the infection is usually symptomatic. Budding yeast and/or pseudohyphae are seen (e-Fig. 34.26).

   Herpes genitalis is usually caused by HSV type 2. Nuclear enlargement, chromatin margination, multinucleation, nuclear inclusions, and nuclear molding are evident (e-Fig. 34.27).

2. **Other nonneoplastic findings**

   a. **Reactive changes/repair in squamous cells** include nuclear enlargement (up to twice the size of an intermediate cell) with or without multinucleation, smooth nuclear contours, small nucleoli, and mild nuclear hyperchromasia. In reparative change, there is vacuolization of the cytoplasm and some of the cells may be elongated, clustering together in a streaming pattern. Repair implies disruption of the epithelium with subsequent increased proliferation. The relative abundance of cytoplasm and lack of true nuclear atypia differentiate this from neoplastic squamous proliferations (e-Fig. 34.28). Reactive endocervical cells may show even greater nuclear enlargement, multinucleation, mild hyperchromasia, and prominent nucleoli (e-Fig. 34.29).

   b. **IUD.** The recognition of IUD-related changes is particularly important in cervical smears, as the singly dispersed cells with vacuolated cytoplasm and large nuclei seen in this reactive condition can mimic adenocarcinoma. Despite nuclear enlargement, truly atypical nuclei are not seen. Correlation with the history is key when IUD-type changes appear.

    c. **Normal appearing glandular cells' status posthysterectomy** may represent metaplastic change, adenosis, or misplaced fallopian tube remnants. They are not considered an epithelial cell abnormality.

C. **Epithelial cell abnormality**

  1. **Squamous cell**

    a. **Atypical squamous cells of undetermined significance (ASCUS)** have nuclei 2.5 to 3 times the size of an intermediate cell nucleus. There is minimal nuclear hyperchromasia and a somewhat increased N/C ratio. Reflex HPV testing is recommended. While the predictive value of an ASCUS/HPV-positive sample varies with patient age, in general, the risk of the presence of CIN2 or greater on follow-up of an ASCUS/HPV-positive Pap test is similar to that of a low-grade squamous intraepithelial lesion (LSIL) Pap test, that is, 20% to 30% (*N Engl J Med.* 2007;357:1579).

    b. **Atypical squamous cells cannot exclude HSIL** are approximately the size of squamous metaplastic cells, with associated nuclear enlargement resulting in an appearance approaching that of a high-grade squamous intraepithelial lesion (HSIL). They usually lack the severe hyperchromasia and abnormal nuclear contours of HSIL, however. Colposcopy is indicated after this interpretation, since 30% of patients will have CIN2 or greater on follow-up (*Am J Obstet Gynecol.* 2003;183:1383).

    c. **Low-grade squamous intraepithelial lesion (LSIL)** is a cytologic lesion with nuclei greater than three times the size of an intermediate nucleus. Despite the increased nuclear size, N/C ratios are relatively preserved. Irregular nuclear contours and hyperchromasia are needed to make this interpretation. Multinucleation and koilocytic halos are common, but not required (e-**Fig. 34.30**).

    d. **High-grade squamous intraepithelial lesion (HSIL)** displays cells with severe nuclear hyperchromasia and contour irregularities, but the nuclei are generally smaller than those of LSIL. These severely dysplastic cells are singly dispersed and in syncytia (e-**Fig. 34.31**).

    e. **Squamous cell carcinoma** has nuclear abnormalities that are equal to or more severe than those of HSIL, with the addition of prominent nucleoli (e-**Fig. 34.32**). An inflammatory/proteinaceous background (the so-called "tumor diathesis") favors invasive squamous cell carcinoma, although the diathesis is seen less prominently in liquid-based preparations.

  2. **Glandular cell**

    a. **Atypical glandular cells** show nuclear enlargement, mild nuclear hyperchromasia, variable pleomorphism, and increased N/C ratios. Often in these cases, only incomplete features of adenocarcinoma are present. Although not always possible, every attempt should be made to state whether the abnormal cells are endometrial or endocervical in origin.

    b. **AIS of the endocervix** shows glandular groups with nuclear stratification, crowding, and sometimes a characteristic "feathering." The nuclei are generally elongated and lack nucleoli (e-**Fig. 34.33**).

      Adenocarcinoma of the endocervix can be detected by cervical cytology in ~80% of cases. However, only 22% of endometrial adenocarcinoma cases are evident in Pap tests (*Acta Cytol.* 2007;51:47). The cells of endocervical carcinoma can be arranged singly or in three-dimensional clusters, and they show clearly malignant nuclear features including pleomorphism, hyperchromasia, irregular nuclear contours, and occasional large nucleoli. Cytoplasmic vacuoles are often present (e-**Fig. 34.34**). Cytologically, it can be difficult to distinguish endometrial and endocervical origins.

D. **Other.** The Bethesda System calls for the use of this category in cases showing endometrial cells in patients ≥40 years of age. Clinical correlation is required to assess the significance of such cells. The absence of a squamous intraepithelial lesion must also be documented in the report when "other" is utilized.

IV. **ANCILLARY TESTING.** HPV testing is recommended in most cases of ASCUS. It is performed on the unused portion of a liquid-based sample. This testing can be done using the Digene Hybrid Capture 2 assay (QIAGEN, Inc., Valencia, CA), in situ hybridization (Ventana Medical Systems, Inc., Tucson, AZ), or polymerase chain reaction-based assays. These assays test for a number of high-risk HPV subtypes. Although new assays are available that provide the actual genotype of the infecting virus, the utility of this more specific information has yet to be determined.

A. **Markers of HPV integration** such as E6 and E7 mRNA assays and p16 immuno-histochemistry, among others, are under investigation. Their place in cervical cancer screening in not well defined, but the hope is that positivity for this type of marker will be more specific than high-risk HPV infection alone for the eventual development of a high-grade squamous intraepithelial lesion or invasive squamous cell carcinoma.

B. **Automated screening of cervical cytology specimens** is now in wide use, with FDA approval. The system used depends upon the proprietary liquid-based Pap test used in the laboratory.

SUGGESTED READINGS

ACOG Committee on Practice Bulletin. ACOG Practice Bulletin no. 109: Cervical cytology screening. *Obstet Gynecol.* 2009;114:1409.

Committee on Adolescent Health Care. ACOG Committee Opinion no. 436: Evaluation and management of abnormal cervical cytology and histology in the adolescent. *Obstet Gynecol.* 2009;113:1422.

Ganesan R, Ferryman SR, Meier L, et al. Vasculitis of the female genital tract with clinicopathologic correlation: A study of 46 cases with follow-up. *Int J Gynecol Pathol.* 2000;19:258.

Lennerz JK, Perry A, Mills JC, et al. Mucoepidermoid carcinoma of the cervix: another tumor with the t(11;19)-associated CRTC1-MAML2 gene fusion. *Am J Surg Pathol.* 2009;33:835.

Wright TC Jr, Massad LS, Dunton CJ, et al. 2006 American Society for Colposcopy and Cervical Pathology-sponsored Consensus Conference. 2006 consensus guidelines for the management of women with cervical intraepithelial neoplasia or adenocarcinoma in situ. *J Low Genit Tract Dis.* 2007;11:223.

Vagina

Rao Watson, John D. Pfeifer,
and Phyllis C. Huettner

I. **NORMAL STRUCTURE.** The vagina is derived from the müllerian ducts and is composed of three layers: mucosa, muscularis propria, and adventitia. The mucosa is composed of squamous epithelium overlying a lamina propria that contains a rich vascular and lymphatic network with scattered stromal cells that may show multinucleation.

II. **BENIGN CONDITIONS**

A. **Infectious diseases**

1. **Vulvovaginal candidiasis** is a common condition that predominantly affects adult women in their second and third decades. Up to 70% of women will experience at least one episode in their lifetime. Common predisposing factors include antibiotic use, steroid use, oral contraceptive use, immunosuppression, and uncontrolled diabetes. Pruritus, erythema, and thick white vaginal discharge are the most common symptoms. Histologically, squamous epithelial hyperplasia with hyperkeratosis and/or parakeratosis is seen. Foci of neutrophilic infiltration of the squamous epithelium are commonly present. *Candida* can be present in the form of budding yeasts as well as pseudohyphae, highlighted on GMS or other special stains.

2. **Bacterial vaginosis** is most commonly found among adult women. It is caused by *Gardnerella vaginalis,* a bacillus which usually grows when the vaginal flora shifts toward a more acidic environment. A watery, malodorous discharge without significant inflammation is a common symptom. Microscopically, the bacteria overgrow and cover the squamous cells, producing so-called clue cells.

3. **Trichomoniasis,** a sexually transmitted disease, is caused by *Trichomonas vaginalis,* an oval protozoon with flagella. Microscopically, the organisms are identified by their bluish-pink body, elongated nuclei, and flagella.

4. **Herpes simplex infection** is a sexually transmitted disease caused by herpes simplex virus (HSV). Grossly, the virus causes a mucosal ulceration within a few days to 2 weeks following the exposure. These lesions are highly infectious until crusting, with final scarring occurring within 2 to 3 weeks of initial symptoms. The majority of cases are caused by HSV-2, and recurrence is higher with infection by HSV-2 than by HSV-1.

   Microscopically, the ulcerated lesions are characterized by epithelial necrosis with associated degenerated cells containing viral inclusions, best identified at the periphery of the ulcer. The cells with viral inclusions have characteristic features including multinucleation and ground glass nuclei with a rim of chromatin condensation at the nuclear border surrounded by a cytoplasmic halo.

5. **Actinomyces-like organisms** are most commonly seen in women with noncopper intrauterine contraceptive devices.

B. **Inflammatory diseases**

1. **Atrophic vaginitis** occurs most commonly in postmenopausal women, but can also occur during the postpartum period. Grossly, the primary finding is punctate hemorrhage of the vaginal mucosa. Microscopically, the squamous cells show decreased glycogen due to lower estrogen levels. Atrophy can be distinguished from vaginal intraepithelial neoplasia (VAIN) by the monotony

of the cell population, uniform chromatin, the lack of cytologic atypia, and the low mitotic rate.

2. **Crohn disease** can result in rectovaginal fistula formation and is associated with fibrosis, chronic inflammation, and granulomas. The differential diagnosis includes vaginal fistulas of other etiologies including radiation therapy, perforated colonic diverticulum, or as a complication of hysterectomy.

3. **Stenosis,** ulceration, and necrosis are well-described sequelae of radiation therapy. Stenosis can also follow severe bullous erythema multiforme (Stevens–Johnson syndrome).

C. Cysts
1. **Müllerian cysts** are the most common type of vaginal cyst and can be lined by endocervical-, endometrial-, or endosalpingeal-type epithelium (e-**Fig. 35.1**).*

2. **Epithelial inclusion cysts** are lined by keratinizing squamous epithelium and filled with white sebaceous and keratinous debris. They most commonly arise in areas of previous trauma such as episiotomy sites.

3. **Mesonephric cyst.** Also known as Gartner duct cysts, they are usually located along the anterolateral wall of the vagina (along the path of the mesonephric duct). This type of cyst is lined by low cuboidal, nonmucinous epithelium.

4. **Bartholin gland cysts** are thought to develop from obstruction of the ducts of Bartholin glands, which normally open on to the vestibule. The cyst lining varies from squamous to transitional to mucin secreting (e-**Fig. 35.2**).

D. **Adenosis** occurs in about 30% of women who were exposed to diethylstilbestrol (DES) in utero and is associated with an increased risk of clear cell adenocarcinoma (see section on clear cell adenocarcinoma below). Adenosis usually involves the upper third of the vagina, but the middle third or lower third are affected in about 10% of cases. Grossly, adenosis presents as a red erythematous granular lesion. Microscopically, adenosis is defined by the presence of columnar epithelium of endometrial or endocervical type in the vaginal mucosa or underlying submucosa (e-**Fig. 35.3**).

E. **Endometriosis** of the vagina comprises <10% of cases of pelvic endometriosis. The diagnosis requires the presence of müllerian-type epithelium (most commonly endometrioid) and endometrial-type stroma. Hemosiderin-laden macrophages are often present as well. The presence of endometrial type stroma can be used to distinguish endometriosis from adenosis (e-**Fig. 35.4**).

III. **BENIGN NEOPLASMS.** The WHO classification of vaginal tumors is given in Table 35.1.
A. Epithelial
1. **Squamous papilloma** is usually asymptomatic and can occur at any age. Grossly, it usually presents as a cluster of papillary lesions. Microscopically, squamous papillomas have a fibrovascular core and are lined by benign squamous epithelium.

2. **Fibroepithelial polyps** most commonly occur in adult women during their reproductive years. They occur in the lower third of the vagina and grossly have a soft and papillary surface. Microscopically, they are composed of squamous epithelium with underlying hypocellular fibrovascular stroma. Atypical myofibroblasts are common in the stroma, and scattered multinucleated cells with bizarre atypical nuclei may also be seen (e-**Fig. 35.5**). However, rhabdomyoblasts and a cambium layer are not present and mitotic figures are rare; these features, together with patient age, distinguish fibroepithelial polyp from sarcoma botryoides.

---

*All e-figures are available online via the Solution Site Image Bank.

| TABLE 35.1 | WHO Histologic Classification of Tumors of the Vagina |

Epithelial tumors
Squamous tumors and precursors
  Squamous cell carcinoma, not otherwise specified
    Keratinizing
    Nonkeratinizing
    Basaloid
    Verrucous
    Warty
  Squamous intraepithelial neoplasia
  Benign squamous lesions
    Condyloma acuminatum
    Squamous papilloma (vaginal micropapillomatosis)
    Fibroepithelial polyp
Glandular tumors
  Clear cell adenocarcinoma
  Endometrioid adenocarcinoma
  Mucinous adenocarcinoma
  Müllerian papilloma
  Adenoma
Other epithelial tumors
  Adenosquamous carcinoma
  Adenoid cystic carcinoma
  Adenoid basal carcinoma
  Carcinoid
  Small cell carcinoma
  Undifferentiated carcinoma

Mesenchymal tumors and tumorlike conditions
Sarcoma botryoides
Leiomyosarcoma
Endometrioid stromal sarcoma, low grade
Undifferentiated vaginal sarcoma
Leiomyoma
Genital rhabdomyoma
Deep angiomyxoma
Postoperative spindle cell nodule

Mixed epithelial and mesenchymal tumors
Carcinosarcoma (malignant müllerian mixed tumor)
Adenosarcoma
Malignant mixed tumor resembling synovial sarcoma
Benign mixed tumor

Melanocytic tumors
Malignant melanoma
Blue nevus
Melanocytic nevus

Miscellaneous tumors
Tumors of germ cell type
  Yolk sac tumor
  Dermoid cyst
Others
  Peripheral primitive neuroectodermal tumor/Ewing tumor
  Adenomatoid tumor

Lymphoid and hematopoietic tumors
Malignant lymphoma
Leukemia

Secondary tumors

From: Tavassoli FA, Devilee P, eds. *World Health Organization Classification of Tumours. Pathology and Genetics. Tumours of the Breast and Female Genital Organs.* Lyon: IARC Press; 2003. Used with permission.

3. **Condyloma acuminatum** is caused by human papilloma virus (HPV) serotypes 6 and 11. Microscopically, it is composed of papillary fibrovascular cores lined by squamous epithelium with acanthosis, hyperkeratosis, and parakeratosis, with associated viral cytopathic effect or koilocytosis characterized by nuclear enlargement and irregularity, chromatin clumping and hyperchromasia, occasional bi- or multinucleation, and perinuclear clearing.

B. **Mesenchymal**

1. **Leiomyoma** is the most common benign mesenchymal tumor of the vagina in adults, with a mean age at presentation of 40 years. Leiomyomas rarely affect children. The tumor most commonly develops in the submucosa. Grossly, it consists of a well-circumscribed, firm mass with a white-tan cut surface. Microscopically, the tumor is composed of fascicles of spindle cells with elongated uniform nuclei, fine chromatin, smooth nuclear membranes, and a moderate amount of eosinophilic cytoplasm. Mitotic figures are rare.

2. **Genital rhabdomyoma** is a rare tumor of the vagina that shows skeletal muscle differentiation. It affects middle-aged women, and patients usually present with vaginal bleeding or dyspareunia. Grossly, it is a solid, polypoid to nodular lesion that creates a bulging mass under the mucosa. Microscopically, rhabdomyoma is composed of loosely interweaving bundles of spindle cells with oval nuclei, abundant eosinophilic cytoplasm, and occasional cross-striations. Nuclear pleomorphism and mitotic activity are absent. Immunohistochemical stains for skeletal muscle markers such as desmin, myogenin, and myo-D1 are positive. Rhabdomyoma can be distinguished from rhabdomyosarcoma on the basis of the absence of a dense layer of atypical neoplastic cells beneath the epithelium, cytologic atypia, and mitotic activity.

3. **Angiomyofibroblastoma** is a benign tumor that occurs in the vagina and vulva. Grossly, it has a well-circumscribed outline with a white-tan cut surface, and can range from 0.5 to 14 cm in maximal dimension. Microscopically, it is composed of fascicles of spindle cells that have abundant eosinophilic cytoplasm, elongated nuclei, and minimal to no atypia, although scattered multinucleated cells may be present. Architecturally, the cells form alternating hyper- and hypocellular areas, with accentuation of the hypercellular areas around vessels. The absence of red blood cell extravasation and stromal mucin distinguishes this entity from aggressive angiomyxoma. Surgical excision is the treatment of choice.

4. **Deep "aggressive" angiomyxoma** predominantly affects the sacroiliac soft tissue and perineum of women in their fifth decade. Grossly, it presents as a large mass with a gelatinous, soft cut surface. Microscopically, it is composed of bland spindle cells with delicate eosinophilic cytoplasmic processes scattered throughout a hypocellular myxoid stroma. Medium to large thick-walled hyalinized vessels are commonly present; loose fibrillar arrangements of collagen fibers (so-called myoid bundles) are typically found around the thick-walled vessels (e-Fig. 35.6). The stromal cells are usually immunopositive for smooth muscle actin (SMA) and desmin.

5. **Postoperative spindle cell nodule** is a pseudosarcomatous lesion that most commonly appears at the site of an excision, a few weeks to months after the surgery. Grossly, it presents as a small friable reddish mass in the vaginal vault. Microscopically, it is composed of fascicles of spindle cells with stromal granulation tissue and extravasated red blood cells. Although atypical mitotic figures can be seen, atypical nuclear cytology is not present.

   The differential diagnosis of postoperative spindle cell nodule includes vaginal leiomyosarcoma. A clinical history of a recent surgery can aid diagnosis.

6. **Müllerian papilloma** is a benign papillary tumor of childhood. It typically occurs in the upper vaginal wall of children with a mean age of 5 years.

TABLE 35.2 TNM Staging Scheme and American Joint Committee on Cancer Staging Guidelines for Carcinomas of the Vagina

Primary tumor (T)

TNM Categories	FIGO[a] Stages	
TX		Primary tumor cannot be assessed
T0		No evidence of primary tumor
Tis		Carcinoma in situ (preinvasive carcinoma)
T1	I	Tumor confined to vagina
T2	II	Tumor invades paravaginal tissues but does not extend to pelvic wall
T3	III	Tumor invades to pelvic wall
T4	IVA	Tumor invades mucosa of bladder or rectum, and/or extends beyond the true pelvis; note that the presence of bullous edema is not sufficient evidence to classify a tumor as T4
M1	IVB	Distant metastasis

Regional lymph nodes (N)

NX	Regional lymph nodes cannot be assessed
N0	No regional lymph node metastasis
N1	Regional lymph node metastasis

Distant metastasis (M)

MX	Distant metastasis cannot be assessed
M0	No distant metastasis
M1	Distant metastasis

Stage grouping

Stage 0[b]	Tis	N0	M0
Stage I	T1	N0	M0
Stage II	T2	N0	M0
Stage III	T3	N0	M0
	T1,T2,T3	N1	M0
Stage IVA	T4	Any N	M0
Stage IVB	Any T	Any N	M1

[a]International Federation of Gynecology and Obstetrics Classification.
[b]FIGO staging no longer includes Stage 0 (Tis).
From: Edge SB, Byrd DR, Compton CC, et al., eds. *AJCC Cancer Staging Manual.* 7th ed. New York, NY: Springer; 2010. Used with permission.

Microscopically, it is composed of a complex branching fibrovascular core, surrounded by hypocellular stroma and covered by bland cuboidal to columnar epithelial cells that show no atypia. Mitotic figures are not seen.

IV. MALIGNANT NEOPLASMS

A. **Epithelial.** The AJCC staging guidelines for vaginal carcinomas are given in Table 35.2.

1. **Vaginal intraepithelial neoplasia (VAIN)** is a premalignant, HPV-associated lesion that primarily affects women 20 to 40 years old. The risk factors for VAIN are the same as for cervical intraepithelial neoplasia and include a low age at first intercourse and an increased number of sexual partners. HPV serotypes 6 and 11 are associated with low-grade VAIN (VAIN 1), and HPV serotypes 16, 31, 33, 35, and 39 are associated with most cases of high-grade VAIN (VAIN 2 and 3). The majority of low-grade lesions regress spontaneously, although about 5% of cases of low-grade VAIN progress to higher

grades of dysplasia and invasive carcinoma. Progression into higher grades may take several years to a decade.

Grossly, VAIN appears as an exophytic to verrucopapillary lesion. Microscopically, the squamous epithelium shows nuclear atypia (nuclear enlargement, hyperchromasia, and irregular nuclear membranes) with koilocytosis and an increased number of mitotic figures. Grading is based on the extent to which the thickness of the squamous epithelium shows atypia; VAIN 1, 2, and 3 are defined as the loss of maturation of the lower third (e-Fig. 35.7), lower two-thirds (e-Fig. 35.8), and full thickness (e-Fig. 35.9) of the squamous epithelium, respectively. Clinical management of VAIN 1 is simple observation of the patient; the preferred treatment of VAIN 2 or 3 is local excision or laser ablation.

2. **Squamous cell carcinoma** of the vagina accounts for 85% of vaginal carcinomas and occurs most commonly in women between the ages of 60 and 80 years. In younger women, squamous cell carcinoma is usually associated with HPV infection. Squamous cell carcinoma often metastasizes to the regional lymph nodes and has a predilection for distant metastasis to lung and bone.

3. **Verrucous carcinoma** is a variant of squamous cell carcinoma. It is a slowly growing, well-differentiated tumor with a warty gross appearance. Microscopically, it demonstrates verruciform architecture with minimal nuclear epithelial atypia, and a pushing rather than infiltrative margin. Local excision is the treatment of choice. Local or distant metastasis is extremely rare.

4. **Clear cell adenocarcinoma** rarely occurs in women who do not have a history of DES exposure. The lifetime risk of developing clear cell adenocarcinoma in women exposed to DES is about 0.1%, with a mean age of 20 years. In women who have not been exposed to DES, clear cell adenocarcinoma develops in the postmenopausal years around the age of 60. Patients typically present with bleeding or a grossly visible mass of the cervix or the vagina.

   Histologically, clear cell carcinoma is composed of cells with pleomorphic and hyperchromatic nuclei with abundant clear cytoplasm; hobnailing is often a prominent feature. The malignant cells may form papillary or tubulocystic structures. The most common metastatic sites are the regional lymph nodes and lung.

5. **Other epithelial malignancies.** Primary adenocarcinoma of the vagina of non–clear-cell type is rare; most non–clear-cell adenocarcinomas represent metastasis from the endocervix or endometrium, or other sites such as the ovary, colon, or breast. The non–clear-cell types of adenocarcinoma that most frequently involve the vagina include mucinous, papillary serous, endometrioid, and adenosquamous (e-Fig. 35.10).

B. **Mesenchymal**

1. **Sarcoma botryoides** (a subtype of embryonal rhabdomyosarcoma) is the most common malignant vaginal tumor in children, usually affecting girls <5 years. It is commonly located submucosally and grossly appears as grape-like clusters of tumor that fill (and in some cases protrude from) the vagina. Microscopically, the tumor is composed of cells with elongated small nuclei and a moderate amount of bright eosinophilic cytoplasm. For diagnosis, at least one microscopic field must show the malignant cells forming a condensed layer (a so-called cambium layer) beneath an intact squamous epithelium (*Pediatr Dev Pathol.* 1998;1:550). The tumor cells are immunopositive for skeletal muscle markers such as actin, desmin, myo-D1, and myogenin. Surgical excision with radiation and chemotherapy is the treatment of choice, and the prognosis is usually excellent.

2. **Leiomyosarcoma** is the most common malignant vaginal sarcoma of adults. Grossly, the tumor is typically a mass of 3 to 5 cm in maximal dimension.

Microscopically, the tumor is identical to its counterparts at other sites in the female reproductive tract (e-**Fig. 35.11**).

The criteria for distinguishing leiomyosarcoma from smooth muscle tumors of uncertain biologic potential are not as well defined for vaginal tumors as for tumors of the myometrium. Current recommendations are that tumors >3 cm in maximal dimension with an infiltrating margin, moderate to marked cytologic atypia, and ≥5 mitoses per 10 high-power fields be diagnosed as leiomyosarcoma (*Obstet Gynecol.* 1979;53:689).

C. Other tumors

1. **Malignant melanoma** of the vagina is a rare tumor. It most commonly occurs in postmenopausal women in the lower third of the vagina. Grossly, it can present as a bulky palpable mass with or without pigmentation. Microscopically, the cells have the same cytomorphology as the cells of cutaneous malignant melanoma. Immunohistochemical stains for S-100, HMB45, MelanA, and vimentin are positive in the malignant cells; immunostains for cytokeratin are negative. Vaginal melanomas are treated surgically; radiation and chemotherapy have not proven effective. The prognosis is very poor and the recurrence rate is high.

2. **Metastasis** to the vagina from primary tumors of other sites is uncommon. As noted above, metastasis usually originates from malignancies of the cervix, endometrium, ovary, colon, and breast.

36 Vulva

Danielle H. Carpenter, John D. Pfeifer,
and Phyllis C. Huettner

I. **NORMAL ANATOMY.** The vulva or external female genital region encompasses the mons pubis, labia majora, labia minora, clitoris, and vestibule. The entire vulva except for the vestibule is covered by keratinized, stratified squamous epithelium. The epithelium of the vestibule is glycogenated squamous epithelium. The lateral aspects of the labia majora and the mons pubis contain hair follicles. Sebaceous glands are present in the labia majora and the perineum. The clitoris is lined by keratinizing stratified squamous epithelium overlying paired corpora cavernosa that contain vascular spaces surrounded by nerves.

The urethral meatus, major vestibular glands (Bartholin glands; e-Fig. 36.1),* minor vestibular glands, paraurethral glands (Skene glands), and vagina all open onto the vulva. The Bartholin glands are paired glands that open posterolaterally on the hymenal ring; they are composed of acini lined by cuboidal mucus-secreting epithelium that drain into a duct that may be lined by mucus-secreting, transitional, or squamous epithelium, depending on the location from deep to surface. Skene glands open on either side of the urethral meatus and are composed of acini lined by mucus-secreting epithelium that open into ducts lined by transitional epithelium.

II. **GROSS EXAMINATION, TISSUE SAMPLING, AND HISTOLOGIC SLIDE PREPARATION**

A. **Vulvar biopsies.** Vulvar biopsies should be oriented as for skin biopsies (see Chap. 38) and three H&E stained levels examined.

B. **Vulvar resections** It is helpful to ask the surgeon to orient the specimen with a diagram or labeled sutures so that orientation can be maintained during processing. The margins of resection should be inked and, depending on the location of the resection, the periurethral, vaginal, and perianal margins need to be noted. In cases with an obvious malignant neoplasm, one section per centimeter of tumor, including the areas closest to the deep margin; lateral margin; and/or other margins are recommended. In cases where no tumor is observed grossly, the entire specimen should be submitted. Because many gynecologic oncologists consider resection for squamous cancer in this area to be adequate only if tumor is >8 mm from the margin (*Cancer.* 2002;95:2331), radial rather than shave margins should be taken of all but the most obviously negative margins so that the distance from tumor to margin can be measured.

III. **DIAGNOSTIC FEATURES OF COMMON DISEASES OF THE VULVA.** Many inflammatory and neoplastic conditions that affect the skin will also affect the vulva. These are discussed in the skin chapters (see Chaps. 38 and 39). This section only covers those conditions for which the vulva is a common site of disease.

A. **Inflammation**

1. **Bartholin abscess** presents as a painful swelling in the area of the Bartholin gland. Microscopically, there is acute inflammation of the Bartholin duct, glands, and connective tissue, with purulent luminal contents. The etiology includes *Neisseria gonorrhea, Staphylococcus,* or other aerobic or anaerobic organisms. Treatment includes excision, drainage, and appropriate antibiotics.

2. **Hidradenitis suppurativa** presents as painful subcutaneous nodules in areas containing apocrine glands, particularly the vulva and axilla. Initial changes

---

*All e-figures are available online via the Solution Site Image Bank.

include acute and chronic inflammation around hair follicles, which progress to abscess formation, sinus tract formation, and dermal scarring (e-**Fig. 36.2**). Treatment may include laser ablation or total excision of the involved area.

3. **Crohn's disease** may present as vulvar or perianal erythema, ulceration, abscesses, or fistulas between bowel and vulva or between two different areas of vulva. Microscopically, there is acute and chronic inflammation of the deep dermis, often with associated noncaseating granulomas, fistulas, or sinus tracts (e-**Figs. 36.3** and **36.4**).

B. **Infection**

1. ***Candida* infection** is often a chronic inflammatory condition of the vulva that may be associated with diabetes. It often presents as pruritis and clinically shows areas of redness with thickened, edematous skin. Microscopically, there is acanthosis with acute and chronic inflammatory cells in the epithelium, and parakeratosis with neutrophils. Often fungal organisms are visible on H&E stain in the keratin layer; they are easily identified by silver stains.

2. **Syphilis** is a sexually transmitted disease caused by the spirochete *Treponema pallidum*. The primary lesion of syphilis, the chancre, develops in about half of the women within 3 weeks of infection and is characterized by one to sometimes multiple painless, clean-based ulcers. The ulcer heals in 2 to 6 weeks without a scar. Secondary syphilis develops within 6 weeks to 6 months and is characterized by the development of a rash on the palms, soles, and mucosal surfaces, as well as elevated plaques and papules (termed condyloma lata) on the vulva and mucosal surfaces. On microscopic sections, the chancre shows epidermal ulceration, dermal acute and chronic inflammation with numerous plasma cells, and severe arteritis. Condyloma lata are characterized by marked epidermal acanthosis and hyperkeratosis, dermal inflammation with numerous plasma cells, and arteritis. The organisms may be detected on Warthin–Starry, Steiner, or Dieterle stains; no organisms are seen in some cases of active infection.

3. **Human papilloma virus (HPV) infection.** Condyloma acuminatum, also referred to as genital warts, is the result of sexually transmitted infection caused by HPV types 11 (75% of cases) or 6 (25% of cases). They present as asymptomatic, usually multiple or confluent, papillary or papular lesions, and may occur anywhere on the vulva or perianal region.

   Microscopically, condylomata of the vulva typically have a fibrovascular stalk. The epithelium exhibits acanthosis, papillomatosis, hyperkeratosis, dyskeratosis, and an accentuated granular cell layer (e-**Fig. 36.5**). Viral cytopathic effect, termed koilocytosis, takes the form of cytoplasmic clearing around enlarged nuclei with irregular nuclear outlines and clumped chromatin (e-**Fig. 36.6**). Vulvar condylomata usually follow a protracted course. They may grow rapidly during pregnancy and then regress after delivery. Small condylomas may be treated with topical agents while large ones are excised, or treated with laser ablation or cryotherapy.

4. **Herpes simplex virus (HSV).** Infection with HSV type 2, or less commonly type 1, is typically heralded by fever, dysuria, and severe pain. Painless vesicles then appear which progress to an intensely painful ulcer. The ulcer typically heals in about 2 weeks. Microscopically, epithelial ulceration is surrounded by virally infected keratinocytes that exhibit multinucleation, "ground glass" nuclear chromatin, or eosinophilic nuclear inclusions (e-**Fig. 36.7**).

5. **Molluscum contagiosum** is a sexually transmitted disease in adults caused by infection with the *Molluscum contagiosum* poxvirus. The lesions are small, 3 to 6 mm diameter papules with a characteristic central depression or umbilication, and are usually asymptomatic although perianal lesions may be pruritic. Microscopic features (e-**Fig. 36.8**) include formation of a cup-shaped papule with marked epidermal acanthosis, and intracytoplasmic inclusions

that are initially eosinophilic but become more basophilic as the lesion ages. Most lesions regress spontaneously.

C. Noninfectious squamous lesions

1. **Lichen sclerosus** presents as symmetric plaque-like areas of white, thinned epithelium that may be superficially ulcerated. In advanced cases, there may be scarring of involved areas and stenosis of the introitus.

    Microscopically, there is typically a band-like lymphocytic infiltrate in the upper dermis with spongiotic changes to the basal layer of the epidermis and loss of melanocytes from the overlying epidermis. Thinning of the epidermis with flattening of the rete and a zone of collagenous connective tissue immediately beneath the epidermis is frequently present (e-Fig. 36.9) and was the basis for the previous nomenclature "lichen sclerosis et atrophicus." However, it is now recognized that a spectrum of histologic changes can be seen in the disease, ranging from a predominantly lichenoid infiltrate without dermal collagenization to prominent dermal scarring with minimal chronic inflammation. Treatment involves high-dose corticosteroids. Postmenopausal women with lichen sclerosus have a small risk of developing differentiated VIN (see below) and squamous cell carcinoma.

2. **Lichen simplex chronicus** (formerly "squamous cell hyperplasia") typically occurs in adults and presents as a localized area of pruritus (*J Reprod Med.* 2007;52:3). It is thought to be a nonspecific response triggered by a variety of irritants. Clinically, the area is white or red, with accentuated skin markings and sometimes areas of excoriation. The characteristic feature on microscopy is marked acanthosis without atypia, increased mitotic activity, inflammation, often with features that overlap other specific dermatoses (e-Fig. 36.10). Hyperkeratosis may be present. The dermis is normal. Treatment includes limiting exposure to irritants, topical corticosteroids, and antipruritic agents.

D. Cystic lesions

1. **Bartholin cyst.** Obstruction of the Bartholin duct leads to the accumulation of secretions and the formation of a cystic dilatation of the duct. The epithelium lining these cysts may be squamous, transitional, or mucinous. Cysts can be treated by drainage, marsupialization, or excision of the gland.

2. **Keratinous cysts** occur at any age and typically affect the labia majora. They are small, measuring just a few millimeters in maximal dimension, and are filled with white cheesy material without hair. Microscopically, they are lined by stratified squamous or flattened epithelium. They can be excised if symptomatic.

3. **Mucus cysts** occur in the vestibule and are lined by mucinous epithelium with or without squamous metaplasia. They are probably the result of occlusion of minor vestibular glands.

IV. TUMORS. The WHO classification of tumors of the vulva is presented in Table 36.1.

A. Benign tumors and tumor-like lesions

1. **Fibroepithelial polyps** are also known as acrochordons or skin tags. They may be hyperpigmented, hypopigmented, or flesh-colored, and typically occur on hair-bearing skin. They usually have a papillomatous or pedunculated growth pattern and a soft cut surface. Microscopically, the epithelium may be thickened with hyperkeratosis, or may be flattened. The stroma contains loose bundles of collagen and may be edematous. Fibroepithelial polyps are clinically insignificant but can be excised if they are cosmetically unacceptable.

2. **Papillary hidradenoma** is a benign tumor that originates from apocrine sweat glands. It presents as a dome-shaped mass, usually <2 cm in diameter, arising between the labium majus and labium minus. The mass may ulcerate and bleed but is usually asymptomatic. Microscopically, papillary hidradenoma forms tubules and acini lined by a luminal layer of epithelial cells and an outer

TABLE 36.1   WHO Histologic Classification of Tumors of the Vulva

Epithelial tumors
Squamous and related tumors and precursors
  Squamous cell carcinoma, not otherwise specified
    Keratinizing
    Nonkeratinizing
    Basaloid
    Warty
    Verrucous
    Keratoacanthoma-like
Variant with tumor giant cells
Others
  Basal cell carcinoma
  Squamous intraepithelial neoplasia
    VIN 3/squamous cell carcinoma in situ
Benign squamous cell lesions
  Condyloma acuminatum
  Vestibular papilloma (micropapillomatosis)
  Fibroepithelial polyp
  Seborrheic and inverted follicular keratosis
  Keratoacanthoma
Glandular tumors
  Paget's disease
  Bartholin gland tumors
    Adenocarcinoma
    Squamous cell carcinoma
    Adenoid cystic carcinoma
    Adenosquamous carcinoma
    Transitional cell carcinoma
    Small cell carcinoma
    Adenoma
    Adenomyoma
    Others
Tumors arising from specialized anogenital mammary-like glands
  Adenocarcinoma of mammary gland type
  Papillary hidradenoma
  Others
Adenocarcinoma of Skene gland origin
Adenocarcinoma of other types
Adenoma of minor vestibular glands
Mixed tumor of the vulva
Tumors of skin appendage origin
  Malignant sweat gland tumors
  Sebaceous carcinoma
  Syringoma
  Nodular hidradenoma
  Trichoepithelioma
  Trichilemmoma

Soft tissue tumors
  Sarcoma botryoides
  Leiomyosarcoma
  Proximal epithelioid sarcoma

(continued)

TABLE 36.1	WHO Histologic Classification of Tumors of the Vulva (*Continued*)

Alveolar soft part sarcoma
Liposarcoma
Dermatofibrosarcoma protuberans
Deep angiomyxoma
Superficial angiomyxoma
Angiomyofibroblastoma
Cellular angiofibroma
Leiomyoma
Granular cell tumor
Others

Melanocytic tumors
Malignant melanoma
Congenital melanocytic nevus
Acquired melanocytic nevus
Blue nevus
Atypical melanocytic nevus of the genital type
Dysplastic melanocytic nevus

Miscellaneous tumors
Yolk sac tumor
Merkel cell tumor
Ewing tumor/peripheral primitive neuroectodermal tumor

Hematopoietic and lymphoid tumors
Malignant lymphoma (specify type)
Leukemia (specify type)

Secondary tumors

From: Tavassoli FA, Devilee P, eds. *World Health Organization Classification of Tumours. Pathology and Genetics. Tumours of the Breast and Female Genital Organs.* Lyon: IARC Press; 2003. Used with permission.

layer of myoepithelial cells (e-**Figs. 36.11** and **36.12**). Cytologic atypia and mitotic activity are rare. These lesions exhibit a pseudocapsule, and caution should be exercised before interpreting compression of glandular epithelium at the periphery as invasion. Local excision is curative.

3. **Granular cell tumors** may be seen in many sites but about 7% involve the vulva. They usually present as a painless, slowly growing subcutaneous mass involving the labia majora, clitoris, or mons pubis. On gross examination, they are not encapsulated. Microscopically, they are composed of sheets of large cells with abundant, eosinophilic, granular cytoplasm, and relatively small, uniform nuclei separated by hyalinized stroma. The epithelium overlying a granular cell tumor often exhibits pseudoepitheliomatous hyperplasia (e-**Figs. 36.13** and **36.14**). It is important not to interpret this finding as squamous cell carcinoma on a superficial biopsy. The cytoplasm of the neoplastic cells is PAS positive and diastase resistant; immunohistochemically, the cytoplasm is positive for S-100 and myelin basic protein.

Granular cell tumor is treated with wide local excision; margins should be assessed carefully as the tumor may recur if not completely excised. Malignant granular cell tumors of the vulva are very rare and are best diagnosed in the presence of distant metastases.

4. **Leiomyomas** are the most common soft-tissue tumor of the vulva. They present as painless masses. Like leiomyomata elsewhere, they are grossly well circumscribed with a firm, whorled cut surface. Microscopically, they

TABLE 36.2	Comparison of VIN Types	
	VIN of the usual type (u-VIN)	**Differentiated VIN (d-VIN)**
Age	• Younger, reproductive age	• Postmenopausal
Etiology	• HPV related	• Not HPV related
		• Associated with lichen sclerosis
Histology	• Easily identifiable nuclear atypia and abnormal mitoses	• More subtle nuclear atypia; abundant eosinophilic cytoplasm
	• Viral cytopathic effect	• No viral cytopathic effect
	• Warty, basaloid, mixed subtypes	
Grading	• VIN 1, VIN 2, or VIN 3	• Considered VIN 3
Progression	• Lower	• Higher (keratinizing SCC)

are identical to leiomyomata in the uterus, composed of interlacing fascicles of smooth muscle cells with no atypia, necrosis, and only occasional mitotic figures. The criteria for distinguishing benign from malignant smooth muscle tumors in the vulva are not as well established as they are in the uterus. Excision is the treatment of choice.

B. Malignant neoplasms and their precursors

1. **Vulvar intraepithelial neoplasia (VIN).** Although most cases of VIN are associated with HPV infection, the correlation is not as strong as with cervical intraepithelial neoplasia (CIN). It is generally agreed that there are two broad types of VIN: VIN of the usual type (u-VIN) and differentiated VIN (d-VIN). The salient features of u-VIN and d-VIN are presented in Table 36.2 (*Crit Rev Oncol Hematol.* 2008; 68:131).

   a. **u-VIN** is analogous to CIN. It is almost always caused by high risk HPV infection (HPV16 most frequently). The gross appearance is variable; it usually forms discrete plaques which may be flat, hyperkeratotic, or pigmented.

      Microscopically, u-VIN shows nuclear enlargement, irregularity, and hyperchromasia. Mitotic figures are common and are frequently atypical. Warty-type u-VIN has a growth pattern similar to a condyloma and microscopically exhibits acanthosis, hyperkeratosis, and parakeratosis; koilocytotic atypia and multinucleation are common. Basaloid-type u-VIN is usually flat without hyperkeratosis or parakeratosis; the cells are small and resemble the cells of the basal epithelium, and features of viral cytopathic effect are not prominent. Mixed types with both warty and basaloid features also occur. VIN 1 is diagnosed when the dysplastic cells involve the lower third of the epithelium; in VIN 2, the dysplastic cells involve the lower two-thirds of the epithelium, and in VIN 3, the dysplastic cells involve the full thickness of the epithelium (e-**Figs. 36.15** and **36.16**). The treatment for u-VIN is excision.

   b. **d-VIN** is much less commonly associated with high-risk HPV and is often seen in the setting of lichen sclerosis or lichen simplex chronicus.

      Microscopically, d-VIN has more subtle dysplastic changes than u-VIN. Characteristic findings include acanthosis, parakeratosis, and elongation of the rete ridges often with keratinization at the tips of the rete. The cells do not show viral cytopathic effect, but rather have enlarged nuclei with prominent nucleoli and abundant eosinophilic cytoplasm (e-**Fig. 36.17**). Frequently, there is edema between keratinocytes with prominence of the intercellular bridges. Though the atypia is frequently confined to the basal layers, d-VIN is considered VIN 3 and because of the high risk of squamous cell carcinoma. Excision is the treatment of choice.

2. **Squamous cell carcinoma** may be an incidental finding in a resection for VIN, may develop in the background of lichen sclerosus or an inflammatory dermatosis, or may develop in women with no history of VIN. Tumors may be exophytic, endophytic, or plaque-like and may be located anywhere on the vulva.

On microscopic examination, nests of invasive carcinoma will exhibit nuclear atypia, increased mitotic activity, and will be associated with a reactive and desmoplastic stroma. A characteristic feature is keratinization in nests deep in the stroma (e-**Fig. 36.18**). Tumors may show warty, keratinizing, verrucous, basaloid, or mixed features.

In addition to the size of the tumor, the thickness of invasive tumor (as measured from the top of the granular cell layer to the point of deepest invasion) as well as the depth of invasion (as measured from the dermal–epidermal junction at the tip of the nearest normal dermal papilla to the point of deepest invasion) should be recorded. Lymphovascular space invasion is also an important prognostic feature and should be noted if found. The staging scheme for vulvar carcinomas is presented in Table 36.3.

The role of sentinel lymph node biopsy in the management of patients with vulvar squamous cell carcinoma continues to be evaluated (*Curr Opin Obstet Gynecol.* 2004;16:65). The intensity of the histopathologic evaluation (including immunohistochemistry) determines the frequency at which metastases are identified, which is important since even small metastases/isolated tumor cells are associated with a small but increased risk for the presence of more extensive metastatic disease (*Curr Opin Oncol.* 2010;22:481). The prognostic importance of different sizes and numbers of nodal metastases is reflected in the current FIGO staging system (see Table 36.3).

3. **Melanoma,** though rare, is the second most common malignancy of the vulva after squamous cell carcinoma. Common presenting symptoms include bleeding, a mass, and pain. Vulvar melanomas may be flat or polypoid and are usually pigmented, often with satellite lesions. Vulvar melanomas very uncommonly arise from a nevus.

The clinical and microscopic features of vulvar melanoma are the same as those of melanomas arising elsewhere (e-**Figs. 36.19** and **36.20**) and are covered in detail in Chapter 40. Important features to note are the thickness, presence or absence of ulceration, histologic pattern, degree of inflammation, presence of vascular or perineural invasion, and the presence of satellitosis. Most vulvar melanoma exhibit an acral-lentiginous pattern; however, those arising on vulvar skin are more likely to be superficial spreading. Treatment is wide local excision aiming for 1 to 2 cm margins, which can be difficult to obtain in the vulva without compromising vital structures. The prognosis for vulvar melanoma is poorer than for melanoma of other skin sites.

4. **Paget's disease** tends to affect elderly women and presents with patchy, erythematous, excoriated areas of vulvar skin and epithelium. Microscopically, the squamous epithelium is infiltrated by enlarged cells, either individually or in clusters, that hug the epidermal–dermal junction (e-**Fig. 36.21**). These cells have abundant mucinous cytoplasm, large nuclei with small nucleoli, and often form small glands within the epithelium. These Paget cells may also involve the adnexal structures.

Immunohistochemistry is very helpful in distinguishing Paget's disease from melanoma, which may appear morphologically similar. The neoplastic cells of Paget's disease will be positive for cytokeratin and CEA (e-**Fig. 36.22**), but negative for HMB 45; melanoma has the opposite staining pattern.

Cases of Paget's disease associated with underlying carcinoma (usually vulvar adnexal adenocarcinoma, rectal adenocarcinoma, or bladder carcinoma) have a significantly worse prognosis, so careful gross and microscopic

TABLE 36.3	TNM Classification of Carcinomas of the Vulva

TNM categories	FIGO stages	
TX		Primary tumor cannot be assessed
T0		No evidence of primary tumor
Tis		Carcinoma in situ (preinvasive carcinoma)
T1a	IA	Lesions 2 cm or less in size, confined to the vulva or perineum and with stromal invasion 1.0 mm or less
T1b	IB	Lesions >2 cm in size or any size with stromal invasion >1.0 mm, confined to the vulva or perineum
T2	II	Tumor of any size with extension to adjacent perineal structures (lower/distal 1/3 urethra, lower/distal 1/3 vagina, anal involvement)
T3	IVA	Tumor of any size with extension to any of the following: upper/proximal 2/3 of urethra, upper/proximal 2/3 vagina, bladder mucosa, rectal mucosa, or fixed to pelvic bone
TX		Regional lymph nodes cannot be assessed
N0		No regional lymph node metastasis
N1		One or two lymph nodes with the following features:
N1a	IIIA	1 lymph node metastasis each 5 mm or less
N1b	IIIA	1 lymph node metastasis 5 mm or greater
N2	IIIB	Regional lymph node metastasis with the following features:
N2a	IIIB	Three or more lymph node metastases each <5 mm
N2b	IIIB	Two or more lymph node metastases 5 mm or greater
N2c	IIIC	Lymph node metastasis with extracapsular spread
N3	IVA	Fixed or ulcerated regional lymph node metastasis
M0		No distant metastasis
M1	IVB	Distant metastasis (including pelvic lymph node metastasis)

Anatomic stage prognostic groups (TNM and FIGO)

Stage 0	Tis	N0	M0
Stage I	T1	N0	M0
Stage IA	T1a	N0	M0
Stage IB	T1b	N0	M0
Stage II	T2	N0	M0
Stage IIIA	T1, T2	N1a, N1b	M0
Stage IIIB	T1, T2	N2a, N2b	M0
Stage IIIC	T1, T2	N2c	M0
Stage IVA	T1, T2	N3	M0
	T3	Any N	M0
Stage IVB	Any T	Any N	M1

From: Edge SB, Byrd DR, Compton CC, et al., eds. *AJCC Cancer Staging Manual.* 7th ed. New York, NY: Springer, 2010. Used with permission.

examination of excision specimens is warranted. In cases that lack an associated invasive malignancy, radical surgical excision does not seem to provide any benefit compared with wide local excision (*Gyn Oncol.* 2000;77:183).

SUGGESTED READINGS

de Hullu JA, van der Zee AG. Surgery and radiotherapy in vulvar cancer. *Crit Rev Oncol Hematol.* 2006;60:38.

Tavassoli FA, Devilee P, eds. *Tumours of the Breast and Female Genital Organs.* 1st ed. Lyon, France: International Agency for Research on Cancer; 2003.

37 Placenta

Phyllis C. Huettner

I. **NORMAL ANATOMY.** The normal, unfixed term placenta weighs 350 to 550 g, trimmed of membranes and cord. The placenta consists of three parts: fetal membranes, umbilical cord, and placental disk.

The fetal membranes insert at the edge of the disk and envelop the fetus and amniotic fluid. Microscopically, they are composed of a cuboidal amniotic epithelium with underlying connective tissue, a chorionic layer (composed of connective tissue, intermediate trophoblast, and degenerated villi), and sometimes a layer of decidua (gestational endometrium) (e-Fig. 37.1).*

The umbilical cord is composed of two umbilical arteries (e-Fig. 37.2) and one umbilical vein (e-Fig. 37.3) surrounded by Wharton's jelly, a paucicellular connective tissue matrix. Its outer surface is lined by a layer of cuboidal amniotic epithelium.

The placental disk is typically oval and microscopically composed of chorionic villi surrounded by maternal blood in the intervillous space. The chorionic villi contain vessels of the fetal circulatory tree embedded in mesenchymal stroma (e-Fig. 37.4). A layer of cytotrophoblast encompasses the villous stroma, and this is surrounded by a layer of syncytiotrophoblast that is in contact with the intervillous space. The maternal surface of the placental disk, which is adjacent to the uterine wall, contains variable amounts of fibrin, intermediate trophoblast, and decidua. The umbilical cord inserts near the center of the placental disk, and branches of the umbilical cord vessels arborize over the shiny fetal surface of the disk. Microscopically, the fetal surface of the disk is lined by amnion and chorion.

II. **GROSS EXAMINATION, TISSUE SAMPLING, AND HISTOLOGIC SLIDE PREPARATION**

A. **Fetal membranes.** The fetal membranes should be assessed for completeness. The presence of green, blue, or brown staining, indicating meconium or hemosiderin staining, should be noted. The membranes should be inspected for amniotic bands, nodules of amnion nodosum or squamous metaplasia, and hemorrhage. The distance from the insertion to the disk edge should be measured as this gives a rough estimate of where the placenta was implanted in the uterus. A strip of membranes should be cut from the rupture site to the disk insertion site, one end grasped by a forceps, and the strip rolled around the forceps; this membrane roll should be eased off the forceps into formalin. At least one cross-section of this membrane roll should be examined.

B. **Umbilical cord.** The length of the cord is measured, including any detached segments. Note should be made of marginal insertion (at the disk edge), or velamentous/membranous insertion (into the membranes). Abnormalities of cord color (meconium staining) should be noted. Focal abnormalities such as stricture, hematoma, knots, nodules, plaques, or amniotic bands should be noted and measured. Cross-sections should be made at regular intervals throughout the cord length, and the number of vessels and the presence of thrombi should be noted. At least two cross-sections of cord should be examined microscopically, avoiding the area just above the insertion site where the two umbilical arteries fuse.

---

*All e-figures are available on line via the Solution Site Image Bank.

C. **Disk.** The disk should be assessed for completeness and measured in three dimensions. After examining and removing the membranes and cord, the unfixed disk should be weighed. The fetal surface of the disk, which is covered by amnion and chorion, is examined for the same abnormalities as the membranes. The branches of the umbilical cord vessels are examined for lacerations, calcifications, and thrombi. The maternal surface of the disk is examined for retroplacental hematomas, indentations, or other focal abnormalities. The disk is then sliced at 1-cm intervals, and each slice is examined and palpated. The color, location (central vs. peripheral), size, texture (firm vs. spongy), demarcation (whether well circumscribed or ill defined), and number of all focal lesions are recorded. An estimate of the percentage of the placental parenchyma involved by each type of process is noted. Any organized blood clot in the container is measured. At least two sections of central placenta that include fetal and maternal surfaces as well as sections of focal lesions should be submitted.

D. **Multiple gestation.** Placentas from twin gestations may have completely separate disks, a fused disk with two gestational sacs, or a fused disk and just one gestational sac (monoamniotic). If present, the dividing membranes should be inspected. The percentage of placental parenchyma associated with each twin should be determined. A roll of the dividing membranes should be made as for the fetal membranes, and at least one cross-section of the roll should be examined microscopically to confirm the gross and ultrasound impression of chorionicity. The chorionic plate vessels should be inspected for anastomoses. In monochorionic or monoamniotic placentas, the type of anastomoses (artery to artery, artery to vein, vein to vein) should be investigated by air injection and recorded, keeping in mind that arteries cross over veins. Note should be made of unpaired large vessels as these likely represent areas of physiologically important deep artery-to-vein anastomoses.

III. **DIAGNOSTIC FEATURES OF COMMON DISORDERS OF THE PLACENTA**

A. **Fetal membranes**

1. **Meconium.** With recent meconium passage the fetal plate and membranes will be yellowish-green and slimy. With longstanding meconium passage, the membranes, fetal plate, and even the umbilical cord will be dull brown. Microscopically, the amniotic epithelium is stratified and tufted with pyknotic nuclei. There is marked edema between the amnion and chorion. Macrophages in this area are filled with yellowish-brown, waxy, meconium pigment (e-Fig. 37.5). Pigmented macrophages may also be seen in the chorion and decidua.

   Meconium passage may be the result of neurologic maturity in the fetal intestines, but may also be associated with chronic in utero hypoxia, or stressors closer to delivery. Rarely, meconium induces vascular necrosis in umbilical vessels.

2. **Hemosiderin deposition** may stain the fetal plate and membranes brown or green. Often there is old blood clot where the disk meets the fetal membranes. Circumvallation (see Section III.D) may also be present. Microscopically, the membranes do not show the epithelial stratification, tufting, and edema seen with meconium. Membrane macrophages contain refractile pigment that is positive with an iron stain. Sometimes a layer of hemosiderin is deposited in the basement membrane beneath the amniotic epithelium (e-Fig. 37.6). Diffuse chorioamniotic hemosiderosis is an indication of chronic peripheral separation and is associated with oligohydramnios in the absence of membrane rupture, preterm delivery, and chronic lung disease.

3. **Amnion nodosum** forms small, grayish-white, discrete nodules or plaques that may occur anywhere on the cord or fetal membranes but are most common on the fetal plate near the cord insertion. These nodules, which represent vernix caseosa, are easy to remove with a cotton swab. Microscopically, they consist

of fetal squamous cells, amniotic epithelial cells, and sometimes fetal hair (e-**Fig. 37.7**). Sometimes nodules of amnion nodosum become re-epithelialized by contiguous amniotic epithelium.

Amnion nodosum is the result of oligohydramnios. It therefore serves as a marker of conditions such as renal agenesis that may cause decreased fluid production, and can also alert to possible complications of oligohydramnios such as pulmonary hypoplasia and limb positioning abnormalities.

4. **Squamous metaplasia.** Plaques or nodules of squamous metaplasia are present in nearly every placenta. They are tan-white and may be seen anywhere on the cord, membranes, or fetal plate of the disk but are most common on the fetal plate near the cord insertion. Squamous metaplasia is difficult to remove with a cotton swab. Microscopically, squamous metaplasia in the placenta is identical to that present elsewhere in the body. Squamous metaplasia is not clinically significant.

5. **Amniotic bands** may appear as shredded amnion on the fetal surface of the placenta or as thin adhesion-like threads connecting one part of the fetal plate to another, connecting the fetal plate to the umbilical cord, or attached to the fetal digits or other fetal parts. Microscopically, they are composed of fibrous tissue often with no attached amnion. Amniotic bands are associated with a wide variety of abnormalities in the fetus including digital amputations (e-**Fig. 37.8**), cleft lip and palate, and body-wall defects. Characteristically, the defects are asymmetric, no two cases are identical, and the spectrum of defects in any given case does not fit into a recognizable genetic syndrome. Amniotic band syndrome only extremely rarely recurs in a subsequent gestation.

6. **Fetus papyraceous.** Occasionally, a mummified remnant of an embryo from much earlier in gestation will be compressed on the fetal membranes (e-**Fig. 37.9**), referred to as fetus papyraceous. It may represent an unrecognized twin gestation or may be the result of selective termination of a higher order gestation.

B. **Umbilical cord**

1. **Length abnormalities.** The normal umbilical cord is 55 to 60 cm long. Short cords (<35 to 40 cm) occur in about 5% of cords; they are usually associated with conditions of decreased fetal movement such as amniotic bands, oligohydramnios, body-wall defects, fetal neuromuscular disorders, and arthrogryposis. Long cords (>80 cm) occur in about 5% of cords; long cords are associated with an increased likelihood for encirclement around the fetal neck or other body part, knots, cord prolapse, and marked cord twisting.

2. **Single umbilical artery (SUA).** The incidence of SUA (e-**Fig. 37.10**) is about 1%, and SUA is about 4 times more common in twins. There is a strong association between SUA and congenital malformations, mortality, and low birth weight. SUA is likely an acquired defect as the incidence is lower earlier in gestation; in fact, the absence of the artery may be the cause of associated malformations. In some cases of SUA, a small, atrophic remnant of the second artery can be seen (e-**Fig. 37.11**). SUA is also strongly associated with other cord and placental abnormalities such as velamentous insertion, marginal insertion, extrachorialis, and shape abnormalities.

3. **Abnormal cord insertion**

   a. **Marginal insertion.** In marginal insertion, the umbilical cord inserts at the edge of the disk (e-**Fig. 37.12**). This occurs in 6% to 18% of placentas and is not clinically significant.

   b. **Velamentous insertion.** In velamentous insertion, the umbilical cord inserts into the fetal membranes (e-**Fig. 37.13**). This insertion abnormality is seen in about 1% of placentas. In about 75% of these cases, the vessels branch within the membranes before the branches insert into the placental disk;

in 25% of cases, the cord vessels run through the membranes without branching. Because the branches of the umbilical cord are not protected by Wharton's jelly, they are at risk for compression, thrombosis, and laceration.

4. **Umbilical cord knots.** About 1% of umbilical cords have a true knot (e-**Fig. 37.14**), which may be loose or tight. Differences in the diameter and color of the cord on either side of the knot should be noted. Cords with size differences, particularly with a dusky appearance between the knot and the fetus, are likely to be associated with an adverse outcome. The cord on either side of the knot should be examined microscopically for thrombi, a feature that suggests a clinically important knot. The knot should be untied in the fresh state to look for persistent grooving of Wharton's jelly, a feature that suggests chronic tightening. The fetal mortality rate for umbilical cord knots is reported to be between 5% and 11%.

5. **Umbilical cord coiling.** The normal cord has a left-handed twist, a feature that is thought to increase turgor, preventing compression of cord vessels. A coiling index can be determined by counting the number of complete turns divided by the length of the cord (which can be compared to a standard reference). About 5% of cords will have no twist, a finding that has been correlated with increased fetal mortality, operative delivery for fetal distress, abnormal karyotype, preterm delivery, and fetal heart rate abnormalities. Hypocoiled cords, with a coiling index below the 10th percentile, and hypercoiled cords, with a coiling index above than 90th percentile, have also been associated with a variety of adverse outcomes.

6. **Umbilical cord stricture** is a focal area of cord that is markedly narrowed with a depletion of Wharton's jelly, fibrosis, and often thrombosis of the umbilical cord vessels. The most common location for a stricture is the area adjacent to the umbilicus. There is a high association between cord stricture and stillbirth, especially early in gestation. Most cases also show excess twisting.

7. **Umbilical cord hematomas** occur once in every 5500 deliveries, although small hematomas have been documented in 1.5% of cases following ultrasound-guided cord blood sampling. Hematomas nearly always occur in the portion of cord closest to the fetus and present as a fusiform swelling with a dark, hemorrhagic color. It is important not to confuse a true hematoma, which will be obvious at the time of delivery, with blood accumulation in the cord as a result of clamping, blood drawing, or other manipulation during or after delivery. Large hematomas have a perinatal mortality rate of 50%, whereas small ones have very low fetal morbidity or mortality.

C. **Circulatory disorders**

1. **Infarcts** are firm and well circumscribed, with one edge usually abutting the maternal surface of the disk (e-**Fig. 37.15**). Early infarcts are red whereas older infarcts are white. Sometimes there is central hemorrhage. Microscopically, there is collapse of the intervillous space, which crowds the villi together (e-**Fig. 37.16**). Depending on the age, the trophoblast may be pale and degenerative (recent) or show little staining with only ghost outlines of villi (longstanding).

Infarcts are common, occurring in 10% to 25% of term placentas from normal pregnancies, typically at the periphery. Extensive infarction, infarcts >3 cm, infarcts that occur in the central placenta, and infarcts in the first or second trimester of pregnancy are clinically significant and often indicate significant underlying maternal disease such as pre-eclampsia, collagen vascular disease, or a hereditary thrombophilic condition. Infarcts are caused by an interruption in the maternal blood supplied by a given spiral artery to an area of placental tissue.

The normal placenta can lose 15% to 20% of the parenchyma without adversely affecting the fetus. However, in placentas that are chronically underperfused, such as in pre-eclampsia, a lesser degree of infarction may be clinically significant. Extensive infarction may cause fetal hypoxia, intrauterine growth restriction, periventricular leukomalacia in preterm infants, or fetal death.

2. **Massive perivillous fibrin deposition.** When large amounts of fibrin are deposited in the placenta, a firm, white or yellow, slightly gritty, ill-defined mass is formed (e-**Fig. 37.17**). Often small pockets of red, villous tissue are interspersed within strands of white fibrin. Microscopically, there is expansion of the intervillous space by eosinophilic fibrinoid material pushing the villi away from each other (e-**Fig. 37.18**); clusters of cytotrophoblast proliferate in the fibrinoid material, and the villi entrapped in this fibrinoid material become ischemic. The amount of fibrin deposition needed for diagnosis of massive perivillous fibrin deposition or to be associated with an adverse outcome for the fetus is not well established. Some studies have found that entrapment of 20% of the central-basal terminal villi is associated with adverse outcomes (*Arch Pathol Lab Med.* 1994;18:698); others have defined clinically significant fibrin deposition as fibrin extending from the fetal to maternal surface and entrapping 50% of villi on at least one slide (*Pediatr Dev Pathol.* 2002;5:159). Massive perivillous fibrin is associated with intrauterine growth restriction, periventricular leukomalacia in preterm infants, and fetal death, and may recur in subsequent pregnancies.

3. **Maternal floor infarct.** The term maternal floor infarct is a misnomer in that it is a form of fibrin deposition, not infarction. It is defined as perivillous fibrin deposition surrounding at least one-third of the villi adjacent to the basal plate, often with extension of fibrin into the underlying decidua. An alternative definition is that basal villi of the entire maternal floor be encased in fibrin at least 3 mm thick on at least one slide. As in massive perivillous fibrin deposition, the villi in maternal floor infarct that are surrounded by fibrin undergo ischemic changes.

   Maternal floor infarct is quite uncommon, seen in far <1% of placentas. It is associated with stillbirth, intrauterine growth retardation, preterm delivery, and neurodevelopmental impairment. It may recur in subsequent pregnancies.

4. **Subchorionic fibrin deposition** is common and appears as firm, oval, tan-white, slightly raised plaques of the fetal surface of the placenta, beneath the amnion and chorion. On cut section, it is laminated and clearly beneath the membranes but above the villous tissue (e-**Fig. 37.19**). Microscopically, sections show layers of blood and fibrin beneath the chorion. Subchorionic fibrin plaques are not clinically significant.

5. **Retroplacental thrombohematomas** occur in about 4.5% of placentas. They are organized blood clots beneath the maternal surface of the placenta that indent the placental surface. Recent retroplacental hematomas are soft, red, easily dislodged, and are often seen in the specimen container rather than adherent to the placenta by the time the placenta arrives in the laboratory. Older hematomas are firm, brown, and densely adherent with definite placental indentation (e-**Fig. 37.20**). Microscopically, retroplacental hematomas consist of organized blood clot and fibrin, and the underlying placental parenchyma may be infarcted depending on how long the hematoma has been present (e-**Fig. 37.21**). Sometimes the villi immediately beneath the thrombohematoma exhibit villous stromal hemorrhage in which the vessels are disrupted and the stroma contains extensive red cells (e-**Fig. 37.22**).

Retroplacental hematoma is an important cause of stillbirth. Although retroplacental hematoma and the clinical syndrome of placental abruption share many of the same risk factors, in only a third of cases with clinically identified abruption will a retroplacental hematoma be found on placental examination (likely associated with rapid delivery before clot can form), and in only a third of cases in which retroplacental hematoma is identified will there be a history of placental abruption (likely small and clinically insignificant).

6. **Intervillous thrombohematomas** are very common lesions, seen in up to 50% of normal placentas and 78% of placentas from complicated pregnancies. They are well-circumscribed, round to oval, very firm lesions with a laminated cut surface (e-**Fig. 37.23**). Recent intervillous thrombohematomas are red, whereas older ones are white. They are usually located midway between the fetal and maternal surfaces. Microscopically, they are composed of layers of red cells and fibrin devoid of villi. A thin rim of infarcted villous tissue may be present at their periphery.

   The blood in intervillous thrombohematomas is of both maternal and fetal origin, and so they serve as markers of fetomaternal hemorrhage. There is a very good correlation between the number of intervillous thrombohematomas in the placenta and the degree of fetomaternal hemorrhage as measured by the Kleihauer–Betke test on maternal blood. Fetomaternal hemorrhage may be associated with fetal anemia, fetal thrombocytopenia, fetal death, and maternal sensitization to fetal antigens that are not shared.

7. **Subamniotic hematomas** are liquid collections of blood that pool between the amnion and chorion of the fetal plate (e-**Fig. 37.24**). Microscopically, they may be difficult to demonstrate as the blood drains out once a cut is made. Subamniotic hematomas are thought to result from trauma to chorionic plate vessels when traction is placed on the cord during delivery of the placenta. It is not usually clinically significant because this occurs after delivery of the infant. Occasionally, subamniotic hematomas are the result of injury to vessels during amniocentesis to assess lung maturity or other procedures.

8. **Marginal hematomas** occur in about 2% of placentas. They are wedge-shaped collections of blood at the margin of the placenta where the fetal membranes meet the placental disk (e-**Fig. 37.25**). Often there is blood clot beneath the free membranes in this area. Sometimes a thin layer of blood forms on the adjacent maternal surface of the placenta, but it does not indent or infarct the placenta and therefore is not clinically significant.

9. **Massive subchorial thrombosis** (Breus mole) is a very rare condition, occurring in <1 in 1000 placentas. It is defined as a red thrombus measuring at least 1 cm in thickness immediately beneath the chorionic plate (e-**Fig. 37.26**). Microscopically, sections show an organizing blood clot. The pathogenesis of this rare condition is uncertain.

10. **Fetal thrombotic vasculopathy.** Occlusion of vessels in the fetal circulatory system can involve the large umbilical cord vessels, the chorionic plate vessels, or the smaller fetal vessels within the chorionic villi. Because there is one continuous circulation between the fetus and the placenta during gestation, thrombotic lesions in the placenta, particularly when extensive, may serve as a marker for thrombotic or embolic lesions in the circulation of the fetus itself. The prevalence of fetal thrombotic vasculopathy is not known.

    On gross examination, collections of avascular terminal villi appear as well-circumscribed pale areas of parenchyma of varying sizes that retain the same spongy consistency as the surrounding placental tissue (e-**Fig. 37.27**). Microscopically, these areas appear as villi with dense, eosinophilic, nearly acellular stroma with an absence of vessels (e-**Fig. 37.28**). The villi are normally spaced without collapse of the intervillous space as is seen in infarcts, a lesion with which avascular terminal villi may be confused grossly. A second pattern, formerly termed as hemorrhagic endovasculitis but now referred to as villous stromal-vascular karyorrhexis, is characterized by karyorrhexis of fetal cells such as endothelium, stroma, or blood cell elements (e-**Fig. 37.29**). In this pattern, the villi are more cellular than in avascular terminal villi, with degenerating fetal capillaries and fragmented red cells. Fetal vascular obstruction in the placenta is usually related to stasis, hypercoagulability, or vascular damage.

11. **Chorangiomas** are placental hemangiomas. They are found in about 1% of placentas and are usually small. Typical chorangiomas are well circumscribed, red or gray, and have a firmer consistency than the surrounding parenchyma (e-**Fig. 37.30**). Sometimes fibrous septae form lobules within the chorangioma. Microscopically, chorangiomas are composed of small capillary-type vessels with a few intermixed larger vessels (e-**Fig. 37.31**). Occasional cases may be more cellular, show calcification or degeneration, or exhibit some cytologic atypia. Chorangiomas do not undergo malignant transformation, and most are incidental findings with no clinical consequences. Large or multiple chorangiomas may cause polyhydramnios, preterm delivery, antepartum bleeding, hydrops fetalis, fetal anemia or thrombocytopenia, fetal growth restriction, and cardiomegaly. Infants with placentas containing chorangiomas have a higher than expected incidence of hemangiomas elsewhere.

12. **Chorangiosis** is defined as the presence of ≥ 10 capillaries per terminal villus in 10 terminal villi in at least three different regions of the placenta (e-**Fig. 37.32**). Care should be taken to distinguish chorangiosis from congestion that makes the vessels appear more prominent. Chorangiosis is found in about 5% of placentas, typically at term. It is associated with congenital anomalies, maternal diabetes, maternal anemia, smoking, twin gestation, and delivery at high altitude.

D. **Implantation disorders**

1. In **placenta accreta**, the placenta is abnormally adherent. On gross examination, the placenta is often severely disrupted or fragmented due to attempts to remove it manually. Sometimes thick areas of gray myometrial tissue will be visible on the maternal surface. Microscopically, the key feature is an absence of decidua between villi and myometrium (e-**Fig. 37.33**). The presence of fibrin and trophoblast between villi and myometrium is typical of accreta. Trophoblast is cytokeratin immunopositive, which is a feature that can be used to distinguish it from decidual cells.

2. **Placenta extrachorialis.** Usually the fetal membranes insert at the edge of the disk. In placenta extrachorialis, the membranes insert away from the disk edge, leaving a portion of the disk uncovered by fetal membranes. There are two types of extrachorialis, and they are best distinguished on gross examination. In circummarginate placentation, the junction between the membranes and the disk is relatively smooth and flat. In circumvallate placentation, this junction forms a thick, rolled ridge (e-**Fig. 37.34**). A given placenta may exhibit partial or complete extrachorial placentation and may exhibit a combination of circummarginate and circumvallate placentation. The percentage of the disk circumference involved by each type should be recorded.

   Circummarginate placentation is not clinically significant. Complete circumvallate placentation is thought to be caused by chronic abruption or peripheral separation at the disk edge and is often associated with diffuse chorioamniotic hemosiderosis.

3. **Shape abnormalities.** The placental disk is usually oval or round, but a variety of shape abnormalities may be seen, the most common or important of which follow.

a. **Succenturiate (accessory) lobe.** In about 3% to 5% of placentas, a small portion of placenta (the succenturiate lobe) is completely separated from the main disk by membranes devoid of underlying villi. The umbilical cord almost always inserts into the main disk; the branches of the main vessels that supply the succenturiate lobe are at an increased risk of thrombotic events.

b. **Bilobed placenta.** Occasionally, the placenta will form two distinct lobes of approximately equal size, usually connected at one edge by villous tissue. The umbilical cord usually inserts between the lobes. The clinical significance of bilobed placenta, if any, has not been established.

E. **Maternal disease.** Many of the most common and clinically important maternal diseases affecting women during pregnancy have the shared feature of low uteroplacental blood flow, which results in a characteristic set of changes in the placenta and a growth-retarded fetus.

1. **Pre-eclampsia** is the most common maternal disease to occur during pregnancy, complicating from 2% to 7% of all pregnancies. It is defined as the development of hypertension with proteinuria or generalized edema after 20 weeks gestation. Eclampsia is diagnosed when seizures occur in the setting of pre-eclampsia. Pre-eclampsia is a leading cause of maternal and fetal morbidity and mortality.

On gross examination, the placentas of pre-eclamptic women are often small. Decidual vasculopathy may be present (in the placentas of normal women, intermediate trophoblast remodels the intramyometrial segments of the spiral arteries late in the first trimester or early in the second trimester by replacing smooth muscle and elastic tissue with fibrinoid material, converting these vessels into flaccid tubes and thereby dramatically increasing the blood flow to the placenta; in pre-eclampsia, the remodeling of these intramyometrial segments of spiral arteries does not occur). One form of decidual vasculopathy is absence of this physiologic transformation; this condition can only be diagnosed in the decidual tissue adherent to the maternal surface of the placenta. A second form of decidual vasculopathy is acute atherosis; in this condition the spiral arteries exhibit fibrinoid necrosis, infiltration by lipid-laden macrophages, and often a chronic inflammatory infiltrate (e-**Fig. 37.35**). Vessels with acute atherosis, while already narrow, often have superimposed thrombi further reducing the blood flow through them. Acute atherosis can be diagnosed in the decidual tissue adherent to the maternal surface of the placenta but is most frequently seen in decidual spiral arteries in the membrane roll.

The villi exhibit changes related to low uteroplacental blood flow. They are small with an increased number of syncytial knots (e-**Fig. 37.36**) and exhibit a prominent cytotrophoblast layer, increased villous stroma, and a thickened trophoblastic membrane (**n**). Placentas from pre-eclamptic women are more likely to have infarcts, and the infarcts are more likely to be larger and/or more numerous. There is also an increased incidence of retroplacental hematomas in the placentas of pre-eclamptic women.

The *h*emolysis, *e*levated *l*iver enzyme levels, *l*ow *p*latelet count syndrome (HELLP) and acute fatty liver of pregnancy complicate a subset of pregnancies with pre-eclampsia. Although there is a much higher rate of preterm delivery, fetal mortality, maternal complications, and maternal mortality with these two syndromes compared with pre-eclampsia, the placental findings are not significantly different from those of women with pre-eclampsia alone.

2. **Diabetes.** The placental findings in diabetes are variable because the duration and severity of the disease are highly variable. Women with longstanding diabetes and significant vascular disease may show placental changes similar to those seen in pre-eclampsia. The placentas in the majority of cases,

however, are larger and heavier than normal. The microscopic findings are not specific but are nonetheless characteristic. The villi are often edematous and immature for gestational age. The cytotrophoblast is prominent. There is irregular thickening of the trophoblastic basement membrane. Chorangiosis, avascular terminal villi, and SUA are increased in frequency.

Women with diabetes are more likely to deliver stillborn infants or infants with malformations and/or macrosomia. There is no relationship between these adverse outcomes and the severity of the placental findings.

3. **Maternal thrombophilic disorders.** There is increased interest in the relationship between hereditary thrombophilic disorders (such as protein C and S deficiency, factor V Leiden, and hyperhomocysteinemia) and pregnancy complications. Although controversial, it appears that various hereditary thrombophilic conditions, alone and in combination, are associated with an increased number and larger infarcts, acute atherosis, spiral artery thrombi, retroplacental hematomas, and fetal thrombotic vasculopathy.

4. **Sickle cell disease.** The placentas from women with sickle cell disease may be small and may have an increased number of infarcts. A characteristic finding is the presence of sickled maternal erythrocytes in the intervillous space (e-**Fig. 37.37**). Sickled maternal red cells may also be seen in the placentas of women with sickle cell trait.

F. **Multiple gestations**
   1. **Types of placentation**
      a. **Diamniotic dichorionic.** In this type of placentation, the placental disks may be completely separate or fused. Each fetus is enveloped by its own gestational sac composed of amnion and chorion. The dividing membranes are thick. Sections show amniotic epithelium from each twin with fused chorion from both twins (e-**Fig. 37.38**).

      Dizygous (fraternal) twins exhibit diamniotic dichorionic placentation, but about 25% of monozygous (identical) twins also exhibit this type of placentation if the blastocyst splits within the first 3 days postfertilization. Because diamniotic dichorionic twins do not share vascular anastomoses, these twins are the least likely to have complications such as fetal loss, preterm delivery, and twin–twin transfusion syndrome (TTTS).

      b. **Diamniotic monochorionic placentation.** In this type of placentation, the placental disks are typically fused. Each fetus is enveloped by its own gestational sac lined by amnion. A single chorionic layer surrounds both sacs so that the dividing membranes are composed of only fused amnion from each sac with no intervening chorion (e-**Fig. 37.39**).

      Twins with monochorionic placentation are monozygous. This type of placentation is seen in about 75% of monozygous twins and results when the blastocyst splits between 4 and 7 days after fertilization. Twins with monochorionic placentation usually share vascular anastomoses and are therefore at risk for complications such as fetal loss, preterm delivery, and TTTS.

      c. **Monoamniotic placentation.** In monoamniotic placentation, the twins share a gestational sac, and therefore there are no dividing membranes (e-**Fig. 37.40**). Twins with monoamniotic placentation are monozygous, but only 1% of twins are monoamniotic. This type of placentation results when the blastocyst splits between 8 and 13 days after fertilization. Monoamniotic twins have a very high rate of complications, with only 50% surviving to term. They share vascular anastomoses, so are at risk for the associated complications noted above for monochorionic twins. In addition, because they share the same gestational sac, these twins have a high rate of umbilical cord accidents.

2. **TTTS** complicates about 15% of monochorionic twin gestations. It is the result of a chronic imbalance of blood flow across the two placental circulations. The vascular anastomoses normally seen in monochorionic placentas may be artery-to-artery, vein-to-vein, or artery-to-vein. The artery-to-vein anastomoses are usually at the capillary level and are not visible on gross examination, but are the most important physiologically as they allow blood to flow in only one direction and therefore can result in a chronic blood flow imbalance. Twins with artery-to-artery anastomoses are much less likely to develop TTTS because these anastomoses tend to cancel any circulatory imbalances that occur. Hemodynamic imbalance may also be affected by the type of cord insertion (especially a velamentous cord in the donor twin) and extensive infarction or other abnormalities of the placenta in one twin (with resultant increased placental resistance).

Often the twins are discrepant in size. The donor twin supplies blood for both twins and is hypovolemic, oliguric, and oligohydramnic. The donor twin may be anemic and hypoglycemic, with small and pale organs. The placental territory of this twin is usually large, bulky, and pale with edematous villi and increased nucleated red cells in fetal vessels. The recipient twin experiences circulatory overload resulting in polyuria, polyhydramnios, and eventually hydrops fetalis; this twin develops heart failure, hemolytic jaundice, and kernicterus, with heavy and congested organs. The placental territory of this twin is small, firm, and congested.

G. **Infection.** Intrauterine infections can have important consequences for the fetus including abortion, stillbirth, active infection after birth, and long-term sequelae such as cerebral palsy, blindness, deafness, and learning disabilities. There are two patterns of placental infection: ascending and transplacental. Ascending infections are the most common and are typically caused by bacteria. They result in inflammation of the fetal membranes (chorioamnionitis) and inflammation of the umbilical cord (funisitis). Transplacental infections are much less common and may be caused by viruses, protozoa, and some bacteria. The placenta usually shows chronic and sometimes acute inflammation within the villi (villitis). Most cases of villitis, however, do not have an infectious etiology but instead represent villitis of unknown etiology (VUE).

1. **Ascending infections** are caused by aerobic or anaerobic organisms that travel through the cervix or uterine soft tissues to the amniotic cavity. Ascending infections complicate about 4% of term deliveries but a much higher percentage of preterm deliveries. Both the mother and the fetus (after about 20 weeks) respond to the infection. Maternal neutrophils emigrate from vessels in the decidua through the chorion and eventually into the amnion (e-**Fig. 37.41**). They also marginate from the intervillous space to the subchorionic fibrin under the fetal plate of the placenta, and eventually emigrate through the chorion and amnion of the fetal plate. Fetal neutrophils emigrate from chorionic plate vessels toward the amnion. They also emigrate from the umbilical cord vessels, a process termed funisitis (e-**Fig. 37.42**). A staging and grading system has been developed to assess the extent and severity of both the maternal and fetal inflammatory response (*Pediatr Dev Pathol*. 2003;6:435).

In term gestations there is a relationship between the time elapsed since membrane rupture and the likelihood of developing chorioamnionitis; in preterm gestations it is thought that the chorioamnionitis precedes and contributes to the development of membrane rupture. There is also a relationship between acute chorioamnionitis, funisitis, and adverse fetal outcome such as neonatal sepsis, neonatal pneumonia, cerebral palsy, chronic lung disease, and necrotizing enterocolitis. Some of these complications may be directly related to infection and others to the effect of prematurity, but the fetal response to infection that includes release of cytokines and other molecules (termed the fetal inflammatory response syndrome) also likely plays a role in pathogenesis. Adverse outcomes are more tightly linked to funisitis, and are greater for arteritis than phlebitis; funisitis associated with vascular thrombi has the highest complication rate of all. These associations have provided the rationale for staging and grading the inflammatory response in the fetal membranes and umbilical cord as referenced above.

2. **Transplacental infections** reach the placenta by hematogenous spread from the mother. They are usually caused by viruses or protozoa such as those of *Toxoplasma gondii*, rubella, cytomegalovirus (CMV), and herpes simplex virus (HSV) (TORCH) infections, but some bacteria, most notably *Treponema pallidum* and *Listeria monocytogenes,* may also be spread transplacentally.

The tissue response pattern to infections spread transplacentally is villitis. In cases of villitis, there are usually no findings on gross examination, although occasionally small yellow nodules may be seen. Microscopically, the villi contain an inflammatory infiltrate, usually composed of only lymphocytes and histiocytes but occasionally containing plasma cells and neutrophils (e-**Fig. 37.43**). Sometimes multinucleated giant cells are seen. Villitis may be necrotizing or nonnecrotizing; necrotizing villitis, in which there is destruction of the trophoblastic membranes with fibrin deposition causing affected villi to agglutinate, is most common. This abnormal agglutination, rather than the inflammation, is the feature that is most easily recognized on low-power examination. Usually, villitis is randomly distributed throughout the placenta, but sometimes villitis only involves the basal villi. There are subtle features that suggest a specific etiology in some cases; some of the most common of these are detailed below.

a. **CMV.** On gross examination, the placenta may be small, normal, or enlarged and pale. The characteristic microscopic features are necrotizing lymphoplasmacytic villitis, stromal hemosiderin, necrotizing vasculitis, and areas of villous vessel sclerosis. Cases often show areas of active villitis as well as areas of scarred villi. In about 20% of cases, viral inclusions are seen involving the fetal capillaries, villous stromal cells, or trophoblast (e-**Fig. 37.44**). Immunohistochemistry, in situ hybridization, and polymerase chain reaction (PCR) may all be used to confirm a diagnosis of CMV in cases with a clinical suspicion or suggestive microscopic features.

CMV infections are usually acquired in utero and are more commonly the result of a primary infection rather than reactivation of latent viral infection. Infected women are usually asymptomatic.

b. **HSV** infections are typically acquired during delivery through an infected birth canal and therefore usually do not cause abnormalities in the placenta. Occasionally, however, the virus may be transmitted as an ascending infection, causing acute necrotizing lymphoplasmacytic chorioamnionitis with viral inclusions in the amniotic epithelium, or acute funisitis. The virus may also be transmitted hematogenously, giving rise to necrotizing or nonnecrotizing villitis. Immunohistochemistry and in situ hybridization may be helpful in confirming infection. Disseminated HSV infection may cause severe disease or death of a newborn.

c. **Parvovirus B19.** On gross examination, the placenta is often large for gestational age and pale, as would be expected in any condition causing fetal anemia. Microscopically, the villi are edematous and there are numerous nucleated fetal red cells in the villous vessels. Many of the red cell precursors contain eosinophilic intranuclear glassy inclusions with peripheral margination of the chromatin (e-**Fig. 37.45**). Immunohistochemistry or in situ hybridization may be useful in confirming the diagnosis.

Parvovirus causes a mild disease with a rash in children and is usually asymptomatic in adults. Pregnant women are more severely affected with a flu-like syndrome and polyarthralgia; most fetuses are unaffected by maternal infection. Because red cell precursors, endothelial cells, and cardiac myocytes are specific targets for parvovirus, fetal anemia and eventual hydrops fetalis can cause fetal death.

d. **Human immunodeficiency virus (HIV)** is usually transmitted from mother to child at delivery or through breastfeeding in the postnatal period. Transplacental transmission is the least common method of spread. The role of the placenta in promoting or preventing the spread of HIV is unclear. There are typically no gross abnormalities. The microscopic features are not specific and are controversial.

e. **Syphilis** is caused by the spirochete *T. pallidum*. Placentas from cases of syphilis may be normal but are often markedly enlarged, bulky, and edematous. Microscopically, many cases show a classic triad of large, hypercellular, immature villi; villous vascular proliferation with perivascular fibroblastic proliferation and medial hypertrophy; and villitis that is usually chronic but may be acute, plasmacytic, or granulomatous. However, this triad is seen in only 43% of cases, although two of the three features are seen in another 47% of cases. In addition to the triad, some cases show necrotizing funisitis or lymphoplasmacytic deciduitis. Special stains for spirochetes may identify organisms, although often the number of organisms is very low (e.g., one per slide). PCR identifies cases even when staining is negative.

f. **Toxoplasmosis** is caused by the protozoal organism *T. gondii,* and the placental findings in congenital toxoplasmosis are highly variable. The placenta may be normal but is often very large and edematous. Microscopically, the villitis is subtle and nonnecrotizing or results in fibrotic villi. The inflammatory infiltrate is lymphohistiocytic. Occasionally, true granulomas are present in the inflammatory infiltrate. In addition to villitis, some cases show a plasmacytic infiltrate in the decidua, chronic chorioamnionitis and funisitis, and thrombosis and calcification of the large vessels of the chorionic plate. The encysted organisms may be present in the cord, membranes, decidua, or villi but it are not associated with inflammation and are very difficult to identify. Tachyzoites released from the cysts cause marked inflammation and necrosis. Immunohistochemistry, immunofluorescence, and PCR may all aid in the diagnosis.

g. *Listeria monocytogenes.* The pathologic features of listerial infections differ in several respects from those of other transplacental infections. The placenta is typically normal on gross examination but occasionally small, yellowish-white microabscesses can be seen. Microabscesses, which feature an abundance of neutrophils between the villous stroma and the trophoblast as well as extensive necrosis, are present microscopically. Occasionally, palisaded histiocytes and multinucleated giant cells will be seen. Usually, acute chorioamnionitis is also present. The organism is a small rod-shaped or curved gram-positive coccus that can be found in amniotic epithelial cells, and immunohistochemistry may be more sensitive than routine special stains for its identification.

Listeriosis can have devastating consequences for the fetus. It may cause spontaneous abortion, prematurity, neonatal sepsis, meningitis, and death. Infections at birth are typically associated with sepsis and death.

3. **VUE.** In most cases of villitis, an infectious etiology is not identified; these cases are referred to as VUE. Serologic studies of both the infant and mother can be used to exclude many infectious causes if clinically indicated. Most cases of VUE are seen in the third trimester, and the placenta is normal on

gross examination. Microscopically, about 85% of cases are very mild or mild; most are necrotizing and have a lymphohistiocytic inflammatory infiltrate. Sometimes there is vasculitis of the stem villus vessels with associated downstream avascular terminal villi. The inflammatory cells in VUE are of maternal origin.

There are two theories about the pathogenesis of VUE. One theory proposes that VUE is a response to an unrecognized infectious agent, although many cases have been studied with increasingly sophisticated techniques and no agent has been identified. The other theory proposes that VUE is an immunologic phenomenon, specifically a host-versus-graft reaction; the maternal origin of the inflammatory cells, the tendency of VUE to recur, and the increased incidence of autoimmune diseases in the mother all support this theory.

In most cases of VUE, the fetus is unaffected. Adverse fetal outcomes in the form of intrauterine growth restriction, long-term neurologic deficits, oligohydramnios, abnormal nonstress tests, abnormal pulsed flow Doppler studies, abnormal biophysical profiles, and perinatal mortality are related to the severity of the villitis.

Skin: Nonneoplastic Dermatopathology

Samuel J. Pruden II, Kimberley G. Crone, and Anne C. Lind

I. **NORMAL MICROANATOMY.** Microscopically, the skin is composed of three compartments: the epidermis (a keratinizing epithelium), the dermis (a connective tissue matrix), and the subcutis (a layer of adipose tissue). Specific features and the relative size of each of these compartments vary with body site and age and reflect the many functions of the skin. Familiarity with regional anatomical differences helps recognition of subtle abnormalities, provides a clue to the site of a biopsy if that information is not provided, and aids in the formulation of a differential diagnosis that is appropriate to specific anatomic locations.

The epidermis, a stratified squamous epithelium, rests on a normally invisible basement membrane. The keratinocytes of the basal layer (stratum basale) have a generative function and are anchored to the basement membrane by hemidesmosomes. Immediately above the basal layer is the variably thick "prickle" or "spinous" cell layer (stratum spinosum). This name refers to the slender eosinophilic processes that extend between adjacent keratinocytes as seen by light microscopy. These processes correspond to the desmosomes or cytoplasmic attachment plaques. Above the spinous layer is the granular layer (stratum granulosum), which features fine intracytoplasmic basophilic keratohyaline granules. The granular cell layer is 1 to 3 cells thick and forms a water-tight barrier. The most mature and outermost cell layer of the epidermis, the cornified layer (stratum corneum), is composed of flat keratinocytes without nuclei. Keratinocytes are derived from ectoderm and produce type I small acidic (K9–20) and type II large neutral-to-basic (K1–8) keratins. Transit time through all layers of the epidermis is ~28 days.

Cells other than keratinocytes are also present in the epidermis. Melanocytes originate in the neural crest and are normally located in the basal layer slightly beneath the basal keratinocytes. They are histologically distinct, having a rounded, hyperchromatic nucleus as compared with the more elongated nucleus of the basal keratinocyte. They sometimes show a pericytoplasmic clearing/vacuole. This is an artifact of fixation and is attributable to their lack of desmosomes. The melanocyte to basal keratinocyte ratio varies from 1:10 on truncal skin to 1:3 on facial skin, and the ratio is affected by solar damage/sun exposure as well as anatomic site. Melanocytes produce melanin, which has an ultraviolet light-protective function. Melanin is packaged in melanosomes that are exported via slender, elongated, dendritic processes that extend between keratinocytes.

Langerhans cells are usually histologically invisible and function as antigen-presenting cells. They are suprabasal dendritic cells that, when seen in aggregates, have a coffee-bean shaped nucleus. Langerhans cells are visible only via special stains or in aggregates in chronic inflammatory disorders and in Langerhans cell histiocytosis. Merkel cells are located along the stratum basale and are also histologically invisible. They have recently been determined to be derived from progenitor keratinocytes and are presumed to serve in tactile perception.

Small, slender, regularly spaced downward extensions of the epidermis (rete) divide the superficial dermis into papillae. The papillary dermis, located immediately beneath the basement membrane, is composed of fine collagen and elastic tissue fibers and contains the capillary loops of the vascular plexus. The reticular dermis, with its haphazardly arranged thick collagen bundles and elastic tissue fibers, is separated from the papillary dermis by the superficial vascular plexus. Elastic fibers, a component of both the papillary and the reticular dermis, are usually visible only with the aid of special stains. The dermis provides structural support and flexibility to the skin.

The dermis also contains adnexal structures, arrector pili muscles, nerves, and blood vessels. Adnexal structures in the skin include hair follicles and the eccrine, apocrine, and sebaceous glands. Eccrine glands develop as downgrowths of the epidermis. They are present as secretory coils in the deep dermis and have a vertically oriented duct that communicates directly through the epidermis by way of a pore called the acrosyringium. Alternatively, apocrine glands develop from the follicular unit and communicate to the surface via a connection through the follicular infundibulum. Like the eccrine gland they have a deep coil and a vertically oriented duct, although the apocrine coil has a larger central space than the eccrine coil and has the classic eosinophilic cytoplasmic apical bleb. Like the apocrine gland, sebaceous glands are outgrowths of the follicular infundibula. They form lobules that connect to the follicle via a small duct and are composed of peripheral basaloid cells and central mature sebocytes with vacuolated cytoplasm.

Hair follicles have varied features depending on the type of hair they produce and, if they are a terminal hair, whether they are actively growing (anagen), resting (telogen) or involuting (catagen). The infundibular portion of the follicle is histologically identical to the epidermis. This portion extends from the epidermal surface to the sebaceous duct. The isthmus has trichilemmal keratinization and extends from the sebaceous duct to the insertion point of the arrector pili muscle (the bulge). The lower segment of the follicle extends from the bulge to the bulb, the classic ball-and-claw that is seen at the base of every hair follicle.

The subcutis is composed of mature adipose tissue separated into lobules by fibrous septae. Fully lipidized adipocytes have a slender, crescentic, barely visible nucleus that has been displaced to the periphery of the cell by the accumulated lipid. The deep vascular plexus separates the subcutis from the reticular dermis.

II. COMMON DESCRIPTIVE TERMS

A. Acantholysis: Loss of attachment(s) between keratinocytes (e-**Fig. 38.1**).*

B. Acanthosis: Thickening of the epidermis (e-**Fig. 38.2**).

C. Bulla: Fluid containing space in the epidermis, >1cm in size.

D. Dyskeratosis: Abnormal keratinization that results in altered eosinophilic cytoplasm; individual dyskeratotic cells may be referred to as Civatte or colloid bodies (e-**Fig. 38.3**).

E. Epidermotropism: Migration of malignant cells into the epidermis (e-**Fig. 38.4**).

F. Exocytosis: Migration of benign, nonepithelial cells into the epidermis, commonly seen in association with spongiosis (e-**Fig. 38.5**).

G. Hypergranulosis: Thickening (increased number of layers) of the granular layer (e-**Fig. 38.6**).

H. Hyperkeratosis: Thickening of the stratum corneum.

---

*All e-figures are available online via the Solution Site Image Bank.

I. Orthokeratosis: Appropriately mature stratum corneum composed of superficial keratinocytes without nuclei. Seen in a characteristic loose "woven" (basketweave) pattern on nonacral skin, and densely compact on the acral skin of the palms and soles (e-**Fig. 38.7**).

J. Parakeratosis: Abnormally retained keratinocyte nuclei in the stratum corneum (e-**Fig. 38.8**).

K. Spongiosis: Fluid/edema creating a space between adjacent cells in the stratum spinosum, which makes the desmosomes appear prominent (e-**Fig. 38.9**).

L. Vacuolar change: Clearing of basal keratinocyte cytoplasm secondary to inflammation at the epidermal–dermal junction (e-**Fig. 38.10**).

III. GROSS EXAMINATION AND TISSUE SAMPLING. The skin biopsy/excision is generally received in the laboratory in a fixative such as 10% formalin. If special studies are required, a nonfixative preservative (e.g., Michel's medium) is required. The gross description should include all pertinent information, including tissue size in centimeters (length × width × thickness), presence or absence of epidermis, color, presence or absence of hair (especially if from the scalp), and alterations to the epidermal surface (including documentation of the dimensions, color, and distance to the nearest margin of discrete lesions). All surfaces, except the epidermis, must be inked before sectioning. Avoiding the use of black ink facilitates interpretation of commonly used special stains, immunostains, natural pigments, and some exogenous pigments. If the clinician has provided orientation for specific margin identification, inking with two or more colors is required.

Shave or punch biopsies with a greatest epidermal dimension of <0.3 cm are submitted for processing without sectioning. Specimens with a greatest epidermal measurement of at least 0.4 cm are sectioned vertically through the epidermis resulting in pieces of relatively uniform thickness (∼0.2 to 0.3 cm thick) (Figs. 38.1 and 38.2). As seen in Fig. 38.1, if an epidermal lesion is present, sectioning that will best represent the lesion and its relationship to the nearest margin is optimal. Biopsy tissue is otherwise sectioned along the longest epidermal axis,

Punch Biopsy

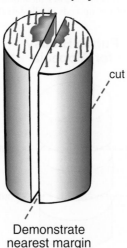

cut

Demonstrate
nearest margin

Figure 38.1 Gross processing of a punch biopsy.

Shave Biopsy

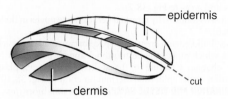

Figure 38.2 Gross processing of a shave biopsy.

thus maximizing microscopic visualization (which is particularly important when incisional/wedge biopsies are performed).

Punch biopsies of the scalp for evaluation of alopecia are sectioned horizontally (every 0.2 to 0.3 cm) to permit evaluation of follicular density and architecture at various tissue levels (Fig. 38.3). One plane of section should separate the tissue at the level of the deep reticular dermis. The two pieces of tissue are placed with each superficial surface down in the tissue cassette and are subsequently embedded with this same orientation. This allows sections that include complete sequential discs that include en face sections of all of the follicles in the specimen. If embedded and sectioned appropriately, the superficial sections will also include a peripheral rim of epidermis and basement membrane zone. The deeper levels will highlight the infundibulum and isthmus; the lower segment will highlight the hair bulb.

Elliptical biopsies and excisions are approached, in general, in a similar fashion. If an ellipse is oriented by a suture or any other means, inks of different colors are applied to the two long margins to allow specific margin identification under the microscope. Sections of an ellipse should be taken at regular intervals of 2 to 3 mm to allow a reasonable assessment of the true margin. Laboratories vary in their handling of the tip ends of ellipses; the recommended method is

Punch Biopsy
for Alopecia

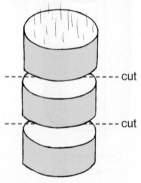

Figure 38.3 Gross processing of an alopecia biopsy.

Unoriented Ellipse   **Oriented Ellipse**

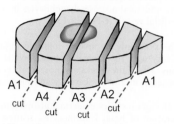 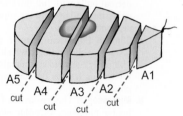

Figure 38.4 Gross processing of an elliptical excision specimen.

illustrated in Figure 38.4. To prevent embedding errors, cassettes should never be overcrowded. Sponges can help prevent distortion of the tissue during processing; for example, submit punch biopsies on one sponge, and lay the pieces of a shave biopsy flat between two sponges. If alternative embedding is required, as for alopecia biopsies, clear instructions to the histology technicians are helpful in ensuring appropriate sections.

Frozen sections may be helpful in evaluating margins of cutaneous carcinomas and may (rarely) be requested if a life-threatening condition (such as toxic epidermal necrolysis [TEN]) requires tissue diagnosis prior to treatment. Frozen sections for diagnosis or margin examination of melanocytic neoplasms are never indicated and may compromise diagnosis on the basis of subsequent permanent sections. The majority of dermatopathology diagnoses are best made on adequately processed, fixed tissue.

IV. INFLAMMATORY DERMATOSES

A. Lichenoid/interface: Characterized by basal keratinocyte damage; may have a band of lymphocytes in the upper dermis (lichenoid) or show only vacuolar alteration of basal keratinocytes and dyskeratosis (interface).

1. Lichen planus

a. Clinical: Multiple, flat topped papules and plaques, pruritic, sometimes featuring superficial white lines (Wickham's striae), most common in adults, can involve skin, hair, nails, and mucous membranes.

b. Microscopic: Compact hyperkeratosis, acanthosis, band of lymphocytes at the epidermal–dermal junction, dyskeratotic keratinocytes in (Civatte bodies) and under (colloid bodies) the epidermis, rete with a "saw-tooth" pattern, melanophages (e-**Fig. 38.11**).

2. Lichen planus-like keratosis

a. Clinical: A single red, scaly plaque on sun-damaged skin (arms and chest/shoulders); the clinical impression is frequently that of a basal cell carcinoma or other nonmelanoma skin cancer.

b. Microscopic: Basketweave orthokeratosis with patchy parakeratosis, obscuring band of lymphocytes at the epidermal–dermal junction, flattened/atrophic epidermis sometimes, vacuolar alteration, dyskeratosis, melanophages (e-**Fig. 38.12A** and **B**).

3. Erythema multiforme (EM)/Stevens–Johnson syndrome (SJS)/TEN

a. Clinical: EM is a clinical reaction pattern characterized by symmetric, targetoid lesions seen best on the palms and soles; it may involve the mucosa, and it is associated with multiple "triggers" (most commonly HSV). SJS and TEN always have mucosal ulcerations with cutaneous sloughing. SJS involves <10% of body surface area (BSA) whereas TEN >30% BSA.

b. **Microscopic:** Vacuolar alteration of basal keratinocytes, aggregates of dyskeratotic keratinocytes throughout the epidermis, possible subepidermal bulla with full-thickness epidermal necrosis, lymphocytes in the epidermis and around the superficial vessels (e-**Fig. 38.13**).

4. **Lupus erythematosus**
   a. **Clinical:** Lupus can involve the skin only or involve multiple organ systems. Skin findings, which vary with the clinical disease, include a "butterfly"-shaped erythematous rash on the cheeks and nose, scaly erythematous lesions on sun-exposed skin and/or scarring, and alopecic plaques.
   b. **Microscopic:** The spectrum of changes includes epidermal atrophy, follicular plugging, vacuolar alteration of basal keratinocytes, scattered dyskeratotic keratinocytes, thickened basement membrane, superficial and deep perivascular and periadnexal infiltrate of lymphocytes, some extravasated erythrocytes, and interstitial dermal mucin (e-**Fig. 38.14**). Direct immunofluorescence of a well-established lesion usually shows linear–granular immunoglobulin G (IgG), IgM, and/or complement deposition at the basement membrane.

5. **Graft versus host disease (GVHD)**
   a. **Clinical:** GVHD may be hyperacute (rarely, <14 days from transplant), acute, or chronic. Acute cutaneous GVHD is often a morbilliform eruption with sudden onset that favors acral sites (palms, soles, head, and neck) and may occur before gastrointestinal or hepatic manifestations. Chronic GVHD may clinically resemble lichen planus (lichenoid GVHD) or morphea (sclerodermoid GVHD).
   b. **Microscopic:** Acute GVHD shows epidermal atrophy with a spectrum of changes at the basement membrane zone (see the section on grading). Because the process is mediated by lymphocytes, lymphocytes in the epidermis and superficial dermis are required for the diagnosis. The histologic changes of acute GVHD are indistinguishable from those seen in response to marrow engraftment (cutaneous eruption of lymphocyte recovery). Grading of acute GVHD:

   Grade 0: No histologic alteration by skin biopsy.

   Grade 1: Vacuolar alteration.

   Grade 2: Dyskeratotic keratinocytes in the epidermis and/or adnexal epithelium (e-**Fig. 38.15**).

   Grade 3: Clefting of the epidermis from the dermis.

   Grade 4: Complete separation of the epidermis from the dermis.

   Grades 1 to 4 require the presence of lymphocytes in the dermis and epidermis (the number of lymphocytes may vary); eosinophils may also be present and do not necessarily support the diagnosis of a reaction to a medication.

B. **Psoriasiform:** Characterized by regular elongation of the rete.
   1. **Psoriasis**
      a. **Clinical:** It has diverse clinical forms (vulgaris, pustular, erythrodermic, guttate), the most common being psoriasis vulgaris, which presents as erythematous plaques with a thick scale on the extensor surfaces (knees, elbows). Guttate psoriasis is often more acute and has many raindrop-like, mildly scaly papules.
      b. **Microscopic:** Confluent parakeratosis, absent granular cell layer, regular elongation of the rete, neutrophils in the stratum corneum (Munro's microabscess) and stratum spinosum (spongiform pustule of Kogoj), widely dilated papillary dermal vessels, increased mitoses, and a

lymphocytic infiltrate in the dermis characterize psoriasis vulgaris (e-**Fig. 38.16**). Guttate psoriasis has mounds of parakeratosis, but lacks the regular acanthosis of psoriasis vulgaris.

2. **Lichen simplex chronicus**
    a. **Clinical:** Thick, hyperkeratotic (and sometimes hyperpigmented) plaques, commonly on the back of the neck, extensor forearms, and legs, or genital region, caused by chronic rubbing or scratching.
    b. **Microscopic:** Compact orthokeratosis, a thickened stratum granulosum, thick and elongated rete. The papillary dermis characteristically has collagen fibers that run toward the skin surface (so-called vertical streaks). The low-power impression may be that of acral-type skin. Acral-type epidermis when paired with dermal hair follicles points to a diagnosis of lichen simplex chronicus (e-**Fig. 38.17**).

3. **Other.** Other entities with a psoriasiform pattern include dermatophytosis, pityriasis rubra pilaris, mycosis fungoides, and chronic spongiotic dermatitis.

C. **Spongiotic:** Characterized by expanded space between adjacent keratinocytes of the spinous layer. Acute spongiosis has spongiosis and vase-shaped vesicles but no or minimal parakeratosis; subacute spongiosis has definitive parakeratosis; chronic spongiosis has psoriasiform hyperplasia and areas of compact orthokeratosis mixed with parakeratosis.

1. **Eczema/atopic dermatitis/allergic or irritant contact dermatitis**
    a. **Clinical:** Erythematous scaly patches or plaques, variable distribution, any age/gender; age/gender and distribution vary with the inciting agent; atopic dermatitis in children is classically periflexural.
    b. **Microscopic:** Parakeratosis, spongiosis, variable acanthosis, and a superficial perivascular inflammatory infiltrate that may be purely lymphocytic or may have lymphocytes mixed with other inflammatory cells such as eosinophils; the degree of change depends on the chronicity of the lesion.

2. **Pityriasis rosea**
    a. **Clinical:** Scaly erythematous patches/plaques; classically distributed in a "Christmas tree-like" pattern on the back; less common patterns exist, including lesions on the extremities (inverse pityriasis rosea).
    b. **Microscopic:** Mounds of parakeratosis, irregular acanthosis, patchy spongiosis, and a mild superficial perivascular lymphocytic infiltrate with extravasated erythrocytes. Prominent exocytosis of lymphocytes is occasionally present and erythrocytes may extend into the epidermis. (e-**Fig. 38.18**).

3. **Eosinophilic spongiosis**
    a. **Clinical:** Varied, depending on etiology. Etiologies include allergic contact dermatitis, arthropod bite reactions, drug eruptions, the urticarial phase of pemphigus or pemphigoid, and the first stage of incontinentia pigmenti.
    b. **Microscopic:** Spongiosis with exocytosis of eosinophils; the degree of either may vary, and the epidermis may be acanthotic (e-**Fig. 38.19**).

4. **Other.** Other entities that have a spongiotic tissue pattern include early and partially treated psoriasis and mycosis fungoides.

D. **Vesiculobullous:** Characterized by a vesicle or bullae.
1. **Bullous pemphigoid**
    a. **Clinical:** Tense blisters on an erythematous base, may be pruritic, may be generalized, usually in the elderly. Variants include pemphigoid gestationis, which occurs in pregnancy, and cicatricial pemphigoid, which has mucosal involvement and resolves with mucosal scarring.
    b. **Microscopic:** Subepidermal vesicle/bulla with a dermal infiltrate of eosinophils. A variant without significant inflammation also occurs

(e-**Fig. 38.20**). Direct immunofluorescence shows linear deposition of IgG and C3 at the basement membrane zone. Collagen IV can be demonstrated at the floor of the blister by immunoperoxidase or immunofluorescence stains.

2. **Pemphigus vulgaris**
   a. **Clinical:** Painful oral erosions and flaccid cutaneous blisters that extend easily with lateral pressure (Nikolsky's sign).
   b. **Microscopic:** Suprabasilar acantholysis without dyskeratosis (e-**Fig. 38.21A** and **B**). Direct immunofluorescence shows intercellular IgG and complement. Indirect immunofluorescence may also be useful for diagnosis and to follow response to therapy.

3. **Porphyria cutanea tarda**
   a. **Clinical:** Blistering of sun-exposed skin, especially hands and face; milia (small subepidermal cysts) may develop. Patients may have hypertrichosis.
   b. **Microscopic:** Subepidermal blisters with minimal inflammation. The dermal papillae extend into the blister floor (festooning) (e-**Fig. 38.22**). The thickened vascular basement membrane(s) can be highlighted by periodic acid-Schiff (PAS) stain.

4. **Epidermolysis bullosa acquisita**
   a. **Clinical:** Blister formation at sites of trauma, generally in adults.
   b. **Microscopic:** Subepidermal bulla with a sparse inflammatory infiltrate. Direct immunofluorescence shows basement membrane linear deposition of IgG and complement as in bullous pemphigoid; however, collagen IV will be seen at the roof of the blister by immunoperoxidase or immunofluorescence stains.

5. **Dermatitis herpetiformis**
   a. **Clinical:** Highly pruritic, small vesicles and/or excoriations on the extensor surfaces (elbows, knees, and buttocks/sacrum) associated with gluten sensitivity.
   b. **Microscopic:** Neutrophils in the dermal papillae with a small subepidermal cleft (e-**Fig. 38.23**). Direct immunofluorescence shows granular IgA at the dermal papillae.

E. **Granulomatous:** Characterized by a variable number and arrangement of epithelioid histiocytes.
   1. **Necrobiotic granuloma**
      a. **Granuloma annulare**
         i. **Clinical:** Clinically variable; lesions may be localized or generalized, annular and erythematous, papules, plaques or patches, subcutaneous nodules or perforating.
         ii. **Microscopic:** Epithelioid histiocytes palisade around dermal collagen with nuclear dropout; there may be an associated lymphocytic infiltrate, and interstitial mucin may be increased in the center. The interstitial variant has less definitive architectural features and may appear at scanning power as a vaguely patterned, hypercellular dermis. Subcutaneous granuloma annulare has a tumor-like presentation with central necrosis with mucin, palisaded histiocytes, and a hypervascular rim containing chronic inflammatory cells (e-**Fig. 38.24**).
      b. **Necrobiosis lipoidica**
         i. **Clinical:** A chronic plaque with a depressed yellow center and an erythematous, raised rim/border, usually pretibial; female predilection; may be associated with diabetes.
         ii. **Microscopic:** Dermal collagen is fibrotic; layers of fibrosis alternate with zones of histiocytes and plasma cells. The abnormalities fill the dermis and may extend into the septae of the subcutis (e-**Fig. 38.25**).

2. **Sarcoidal granuloma (sarcoidosis)**
   a. **Clinical:** Highly variable, but with a predilection to areas of cutaneous injury/scars; up to one-third of patients with sarcoidosis will have skin lesions. Presentations include annular lesions, areas of hypopigmentation, ichthyosis-like changes, alopecia, subcutaneous nodules, and erythema nodosum.
   b. **Microscopic:** Naked, noncaseating granulomata are classic. The type of dermal granulomatous inflammation is highly variable in patients with documented systemic sarcoidosis (e-**Fig. 38.26**).

F. **Vasculopathic:** Characterized by damaged/incompetent endothelial cells. This broad category includes vascular damage mediated by neutrophils, lymphocytes, eosinophils, or histiocytes; vascular occlusive disease related to thrombi, emboli, or vascular deposits of calcium; noninflammatory vascular damage; urticaria; and neutrophilic dermatoses.

1. **Acute vasculitis** (leukocytoclastic vasculitis)
   a. **Clinical:** Palpable purpura, generally on the extremities. Clinical variants include Henoch–Schönlein purpura, hemorrhagic edema of childhood, urticarial vasculitis, and mixed cryoglobulinemia.
   b. **Microscopic:** Involves the vessels at the interface of the papillary and reticular dermis (the superficial vascular plexus) with perivascular neutrophils, nuclear debris, fibrinoid necrosis of the vessel walls, and extravasation of erythrocytes. Direct immunofluorescence may be positive (e.g., Henoch–Schönlein purpura) for IgA and complement (e-**Fig. 38.27**).

2. **Granuloma faciale**
   a. **Clinical:** Reddish brown plaque(s) on the face.
   b. **Microscopic:** A dense, mixed inflammatory infiltrate separated from the epidermis by a grenz (uninvolved) zone; eosinophils, neutrophils, lymphocytes, mast cells, and plasma cells fill the superficial to mid papillary dermis; there are associated classic dilated, thin-walled blood vessels (e-**Fig. 38.28**).

3. **Lymphocytic vasculitis**
   a. **Clinical:** Highly varied; diverse clinical conditions ranging from primary dermatoses, morbilliform viral exanthema, to connective tissue diseases; all have a lymphocytic vasculitis as all or part of their histology.
   b. **Microscopic:** Superficial perivascular lymphocytes arranged tightly around the vessels with plump endothelial cells and with variable numbers of extravasated erythrocytes; there is no fibrinoid necrosis or leukocytoclasis.

4. **Vaso-occlusive vasculopathies**
   a. **Clinical:** Varied presentations include purpura, livedo reticularis and ulcer/infarct.
   b. **Microscopic:** Occlusion of any of the vessels in the cutaneous vasculature with cellular thrombi (in Coumadin necrosis, heparin necrosis, disseminated intravascular coagulation, TTP, heritable disorders of coagulation) or acellular/hyaline thrombi (essential cryoglobulinemia). Cholesterol emboli may be seen after instrumentation; marrow emboli may be seen after trauma; vascular calcification can lead to vascular occlusion if extreme (calciphylaxis).

5. **Neutrophilic dermatosis (Sweet's syndrome)**
   a. **Clinical:** Erythematous plaques, abrupt onset, tender and nonpruritic; most common on the head, neck and upper extremities; accompanied by fever/constitutional symptoms and leukocytosis; up to 20% associated with malignancy.

b. **Microscopic:** Diffuse superficial dermal infiltrate of neutrophils; presence or absence of vasculitis and/or folliculitis is controversial. There may be associated marked papillary dermal edema leading to pseudobullae.

6. **Urticaria**
   a. **Clinical:** Wheals that are pruritic and generally last <24 hours, at any body site. Persistence for >24 hours, burning rather than itching, and resolution of a lesion with a purpuric macule suggest a diagnosis of urticarial vasculitis.
   b. **Microscopic:** At low power may appear histologically normal; sparse perivascular and interstitial infiltrate of neutrophils, eosinophils, lymphocytes, mast cells, and plasma cells without extravasation of erythrocytes or necrosis. Dermal edema may be noted, and there may be neutrophils in the vascular lumina (e-**Fig. 38.29**).

7. **Pigmented purpuric dermatosis/capillaritis**
   a. **Clinical:** Multiple clinical variants.
      i. Schamberg disease – multiple, small, "cayenne-pepper"-like macules sprinkled on the lower extremities, usually transient and self-limited. Most common in young adults.
      ii. Lichen aureus – solitary or multiple, golden-brown plaques on trunk or extremities; most common in young adults; may persist for years.
   b. **Microscopic:** Lymphocytes surround the capillaries of the papillary dermis, with scattered extravasated erythrocytes; an iron stain will highlight siderophages. Some vacuolar alteration, as seen in lichenoid dermatitis, may be present. All variants have similar histology and are best distinguished by their clinical presentation (e-**Fig. 38.30**).

8. **Noninflammatory purpura**
   a. **Clinical:** Purplish/erythematous discoloration of a small (petechia) or large (purpura/ecchymosis) area of skin at any body site. No age/gender predilection.
   b. **Microscopic:** Erythrocytes in the dermis without associated inflammation; amount/degree varies. In senile purpura, there are telangiectatic blood vessels and there is usually severe solar elastosis (e-**Fig. 38.31**).

G. **Panniculitis:** Characterized by inflammatory changes to the septa or lobules of the subcutaneous adipose tissue.

1. **Erythema nodosum (Septal)**
   a. **Clinical:** Single or multiple, painful, erythematous nodules on the anterior lower leg/shin, although other sites can be involved; predilection for young adults. This is a cutaneous reaction that is associated with multiple systemic diseases and medications, including inflammatory bowel disease, sarcoidosis, infections (viral, bacterial, and rickettsial), leukemia/lymphoma, antibiotics, salicylates, and oral contraceptives.
   b. **Microscopic:** Adipose tissue septa are affected, and the lobules are relatively spared. Early lesions have neutrophils in the septa, and late lesions have variable numbers of lymphocytes, multinucleate giant cells, histiocytes, and eosinophils; septa become fibrotic over time (e-**Fig. 38.32**).

2. **Erythema induratum/nodular vasculitis (Lobular)**
   a. **Clinical:** Single or multiple erythematous nodules on the posterior lower leg/calf; any age/gender may be affected.
   b. **Microscopic:** Adipose tissue lobules are infiltrated by histiocytes in well-to poorly formed granulomata; lymphocytes, neutrophils, and plasma cells may be present. A mixed cellularity vasculitis is usually seen, and some vessels of the subcutis can have the classic alterations of an acute/necrotizing vasculitis (e-**Fig. 38.33A and B**).

3. Subcutaneous fat necrosis of the newborn (Lobular)

   a. Clinical: Firm, sometimes nodular areas in body sites associated with increased adipose tissue (shoulders/buttocks/cheeks) of an otherwise healthy newborn infant. Some infants develop acute or delayed hypercalcemia.

   b. Microscopic: Adipose tissue lobules with numerous multinucleate histiocytes that contain classic, radiating, needle-like inclusions; lymphocytes and histiocytes may also be present (e-**Fig. 38.34**).

4. Calcifying panniculitis (Lobular)

   a. Clinical: Highly varied depending on the underlying systemic pathology including disorders of coagulation, peripheral vascular disease, localized trauma/inflammation, and calciphylaxis of renal failure.

   b. Microscopic: Stippled basophilic calcium deposits in and around vessels that range in size from capillaries to arterioles, with lipophages, variable inflammation, and variable erythrocyte extravasation.

5. Membranous lipodystrophy (Lobular)

   a. Clinical: Varied disease processes are associated with this histologic alteration. It is most commonly seen in lipodermatosclerosis (sclerosing panniculitis) which manifests as indurated plaques of the inferior lower extremities resulting in an "inverted champagne bottle" clinical appearance.

   b. Microscopic: Small cysts in the lobules of the subcutis that have a complex eosinophilic cuticle with frond-like excrescences (arabesque); minimal/no inflammatory response (e-**Fig. 38.35**).

6. Other. Inflammatory and/or structural alterations with varied clinical and histologic presentations can also be seen in the subcutaneous adipose tissue as a result of primary inflammatory dermatoses such as lupus (profundus), human immunodeficiency virus (HIV) infection, pancreatitis, alpha 1-antitrypsin deficiency, or in response to venous insufficiency, trauma, or infection.

V. COMMON CUTANEOUS INFECTIONS

A. Viral

1. Molluscum contagiosum

   a. Clinical: Single to multiple, small (1 to 2 mm), umbilicated papules, most common in children and young adults, no site or gender predilection. In immunosuppressed persons, lesions may be numerous and large (>1 cm).

   b. Microscopic: Exo-/endophytic, acanthotic, and papillomatous epidermis, with classic homogeneous eosinophilic cytoplasmic inclusions (Henderson–Patterson bodies) that displace and compress keratinocyte nuclei into small peripheral crescents; keratinocyte cytoplasm has a violaceous hue (e-**Fig. 38.36**).

2. Verruca vulgaris

   a. Clinical: Single to multiple, hyperkeratotic (verrucous) lesions, no age or gender predilection, occur(s) most commonly on exposed skin.

   b. Microscopic: Compact orthokeratosis with parakeratosis at the peaks of a papillomatous epidermis, hypergranulosis due to increased number and size of irregular keratohyaline granules (viral keratohyaline), keratinocytes with large irregular hyperchromatic nuclei with a conspicuous perinuclear halo (koilocytes), and elongated rete that bow inward toward the center of the lesion. Any of these alterations can be lost over time (e-**Fig. 38.37**).

3. Verruca plana

   a. Clinical: Usually multiple, small, flat-topped, flesh-colored to pink papules; most common on the face and hands; occur at any age in both genders; may spread to adjacent skin by trauma such as scratching or shaving.

   b. **Microscopic:** Hyperorthokeratosis (basketweave), hypergranulosis/viral keratohyaline, some scattered koilocytes, epidermal acanthosis with a relatively flat surface and base (e-**Fig. 38.38**).

4. **Condyloma acuminatum**

   a. **Clinical:** Single or multiple, flesh-colored, papillomatous papules/plaques; external genitalia, perineum, and anus.

   b. **Microscopic:** Variable parakeratosis with compact orthokeratosis, acanthosis with mild papillomatosus, viral keratohyaline, and koilocytes in varying amounts. If dysplasia/dysmaturation of the keratinocytes is noted, testing for high-risk human papilloma virus (HPV) serotypes (e.g., serotypes 16 and 18) can be performed. Striking cytologic atypia can also be incited by topical treatment with agents such as podophyllin (e-**Fig. 38.39**).

5. **Myrmecia/deep palmoplantar wart**

   a. **Clinical:** Single to multiple, small, hyperkeratotic, variably papillomatous; restricted to acral or periungual skin (hands/feet).

   b. **Microscopic:** Exo-/endophytic, compact hyperortho- and parakeratosis, viral keratohyaline, prominent basophilic nuclei, koilocytes, multiple large irregular eosinophilic cytoplasmic inclusions. Nuclear size is not affected by the viral inclusions, and the nucleus is not displaced by the inclusions (e-**Fig. 38.40**).

6. **Herpes (HSV/varicella zoster virus)**

   a. Clinical: Variable.

      i. Primary herpes simplex – Painful grouped vesicles which ulcerate; ulcer frequently has a scalloped border.

      ii. Primary varicella – Vesicles on an erythematous base following a one to two day prodrome; vesicles are highly pruritic and accompanied by fever; trunk is a favored site; lesions appear in crops, crust in <24 hours; most commonly seen in children.

      iii. Recurrent varicella (zoster) – Commonly restricted to a dermatome (an area innervated by one nerve); may otherwise appear similar to HSV infection.

      iv. Herpes folliculitis – Painful, erythematous nodules.

   b. **Microscopic:** Acantholysis, dyskeratosis, multinucleate keratinocytes with irregularly shaped nuclei, chromatin displaced to the nuclear membrane by central homogeneous basophilic material that corresponds to the viral protein. Neutrophils, hemorrhage, and necrosis are invariably present, but variable in amount. Herpetic lesions commonly display perilesional interface dermatitis and sebocytis. In herpes folliculitis, similar changes are restricted to some portion of the hair follicle epithelium and the epidermis is usually spared (e-**Fig. 38.41**).

B. **Fungal.** The most common fungi present on the surface of the skin is the yeast form of *Malassezia* sp. (*Pityrosporum*). These small, ovoid forms in the stratum corneum are incidental findings and, unless seen deep to the infundibulum of the hair follicle and associated with inflammation, are usually not reported.

1. **Dermatophytosis**

   a. **Clinical:** Variable; pustules at the advancing border suggest tinea.

      i. Tinea corporis – Annular, erythematous plaques with scale; any site/age/gender.

      ii. Tinea capitis/tinea barbae – Folliculitis of scalp or face.

      iii. Tinea faciei – Facial erythema and scaling.

      iv. Tinea pedis/athlete's foot – Itchy, scaly rash on feet.

      v. Onychomycosis – Thickened and/or discolored nails.

b. **Microscopic:** Fungal hyphae are present in the stratum corneum, usually/ often visible without the use of special stains such as Gomori methenamine silver (GMS)/PAS. All other changes are highly variable, including parakeratosis, intracorneal neutrophils, and dermal inflammation. Clippings of nails for the evaluation of fungal nail infections/ onychomycosis are processed after softening in a phenol solution (such as a depilatory) and should always be stained for organisms because the hyphae are usually invisible without special stains (e-**Fig. 38.42**).

2. **Angioinvasive fungus**

a. **Clinical:** Necrotic papules/plaques in severely immunosuppressed persons; frequent, but not invariable, systemic symptoms.

b. **Microscopic:** Ischemic necrosis of the epidermis and superficial dermis; extravasation of erythrocytes; fungal hyphae present in mid to deep dermal blood vessels of all sizes with extension through the vascular wall; inflammation type and amount highly variable and may be absent (e-**Fig. 38.43**).

3. **Traumatically implanted fungus/dematiaceous fungus**

a. **Clinical:** Variable from scaly and erythematous to nodular and verrucous; often at sites of trauma or implantation of vegetable matter; clinician may see foreign material such as a wood splinter. Verrucous lesions are common in chromomycosis; draining sinuses in mycetoma.

b. **Microscopic:** Pseudocarcinomatous epidermal hyperplasia and/or ulceration; mixed acute, chronic, and granulomatous inflammation; brown/ golden hyphae and spore forms (Medlar bodies/"copper pennies") can be seen depending on the organism (e-**Fig. 38.44**).

VI. DERMAL DEPOSITS

A. Myxoid

1. Myxoma

a. **Clinical:** Usually solitary, flesh-colored, papule or nodule; most common in adults, with no site predilection.

b. **Microscopic:** Pools of acellular, hypovascular, wispy blue material in the papillary and/or reticular dermis; usually moderately well circumscribed but not encapsulated. Stains such as colloidal iron or Alcian blue at low pH can be used to confirm the presence of interstitial mucin (e-**Fig. 38.45**).

2. Digital mucous cyst

a. **Clinical:** Solitary dome-shaped papule or nodule that may appear cystic, on the distal finger/toe in proximity to joint or nail; middle-aged to elderly adults, slightly more common in women.

b. **Microscopic:** Compact hyperorthokeratosis with variable other epidermal change(s); acellular, wispy blue material in the papillary dermis; there may be cystic degeneration.

3. Calcinosis cutis

a. **Clinical:** Varied, ranging from small firm papules, to plaques, to tumor nodules.

b. **Microscopic:** Basophilic deposits usually in the dermis, varying from small areas with a cracked geographic appearance, to large well-circumscribed pools with less intense basophilia and a homogeneous appearance (e-**Fig. 38.46**).

4. Osteoma cutis

a. **Clinical:** Highly varied. One common variant presents as multiple firm papules, most common on the face at the sites of acne scars; may be seen as a secondary change in cysts, benign cutaneous neoplasms, or malignant cutaneous neoplasms.

      b. Microscopic: Trabecular bone with fatty replacement of the marrow cavity and/or hematopoiesis; osteoblasts in Haversian canals; sometimes osteoclasts (e-**Fig. 38.47**).

5. Gout

    a. Clinical: Nodules/dermal deposits; ear or periarticular sites.

    b. Microscopic: Dermal/subcutaneous nodular amorphous pink deposits with variable surrounding foreign body giant cell reaction. After processing, birefringent needles are not detectable (e-**Fig. 38.48**).

6. Amyloid

    a. Systemic

      i. Clinical: Papular or nodular lesions; purpura.

      ii. Microscopic: Hyaline deposits in the dermis or amyloid rings around blood vessels and adipocytes.

    b. Primary cutaneous

      i. Clinical: Macular and lichen amyloidosis are seen as pebbled/pigmented areas on the upper back and shins, respectively; nodular amyloid presents as solitary or multiple nodules in varied locations.

      ii. Microscopic: Macular amyloidosis appears histologically normal at scanning power; classic amyloid deposits are seen in the dermal papillae; lichen amyloidosis is similar to macular with the added abnormality of lichen simplex chronicus; nodular amyloidosis has large dermal aggregates of amyloid and plasma cells.

VII. KERATINOUS CYSTS. These are epithelial-lined cystic structures in the dermis and/or subcutis. They vary in manner of keratinization and/or cyst contents.

A. Infundibular type

    1. Clinical: Solitary, slow growing, dome-shaped, mobile nodule with a small opening to the skin (punctum); most common on the face, neck, and trunk.

    2. Microscopic: Lined by stratified squamous epithelium with orthokeratotic (basketweave) keratin and an intact granular layer, but devoid of rete. The cyst contains laminated loose keratin (e-**Fig. 38.49**).

B. Trichilemmal type (pilar, or isthmus/catagen)

    1. Clinical: Solitary or multiple, smooth, mobile, firm nodule(s); most common on the scalp of females.

    2. Microscopic: Lined by stratified squamous epithelium with an abrupt transition to compact orthokeratotic keratin; granular layer is absent or minimally present; keratinocytes grow larger toward the lumen. The cyst contains compact eosinophilic keratin, which may be focally calcified (e-**Fig. 38.50**).

C. Steatocystoma

    1. Clinical: Uncommon, solitary (simplex) or multiple (multiplex), smooth, firm, yellow or skin-colored cystic papules and nodules; most common on the trunk and proximal extremities.

    2. Microscopic: An undulating cyst lined by a thin, stratified squamous epithelium that is covered by a homogeneous eosinophilic cuticle; sebaceous glands may communicate with the cyst cavity, which is usually devoid of contents (e-**Fig. 38.51**).

D. Vellus hair cyst

    1. Clinical: Multiple, small, asymptomatic skin-colored papules; most common on the chest and axillae of children or young adults.

    2. Microscopic: Small cyst lined by stratified squamous epithelium showing either epidermal or trichilemmal keratinization; contains multiple small vellus hairs intermixed with keratin (e-**Fig. 38.52**).

VIII. DISORDERS OF COLLAGEN AND ELASTIN

A. Morphea/localized scleroderma

1. **Clinical:** One or more depressed, firm, bound-down plaques; they are slightly erythematous to violaceous during the inflammatory stage; they develop an ivory white appearance with chronicity; most common on the trunk or extremities in children or young adults, with a slight female predominance.

2. **Microscopic:** Thick hypocellular collagen bundles replace the usual haphazardly arranged reticular dermal collagen; adipose tissue around eccrine coils may be absent; arrector pili muscles may show hypertrophy; dermal–subcutaneous interface is flattened; plasma cells may be present and, in early-stage/inflammatory-stage morphea, deep interstitial plasma cells may be the only alteration (e-**Fig. 38.53**).

B. Lichen sclerosus et atrophicus

1. **Clinical:** Slightly depressed, pale patches/plaques with a tissue paper-like surface; preferentially involves the female genitalia; more common past middle age; extragenital lesions most common on hair-bearing skin; called *balanitis xerotica obliterans* when the glans penis/prepuce is affected. Genital lesions give rise to squamous cell carcinoma in a minority of cases.

2. **Microscopic:** The unusual combination of compact hyperkeratosis and epidermal atrophy is a clue to the diagnosis at scanning magnification. Early lesions are lichenoid, mimicking lichen planus; lesions eventually develop homogenization/pallor of the papillary dermal collagen, which is acellular but contains prominent dilated vessels. Evidence of a preexisting lichenoid infiltrate may be seen as a band of lymphocytes with melanophages beneath the altered collagen (e-**Fig. 38.54**).

C. Pseudoxanthoma elasticum

1. **Clinical:** Small, flesh-colored papules with the appearance of plucked chicken skin, most common on the neck/axillae; may be associated with retinal changes (angioid streaks) and incompetence of blood vessels manifested by hypertension, cerebrovascular accidents, and sudden cardiac death. Involvement of the vessels of the gastrointestinal system may result in bleeding/hemorrhage. Hereditary, with both autosomal dominant and recessive forms that map to chromosome 16. A nonhereditary, acquired variant affects only the skin and is most common in the periumbilical region of obese multigravid women.

2. **Microscopic:** Short, coiled, beaded basophilic/amphophilic elastic tissue fibers are present in the superficial reticular dermis (e-**Fig. 38.55**). Calcium is deposited on these abnormal elastic fibers and can be demonstrated by a calcium stain such as von Kossa.

D. Solar elastosis

1. **Clinical:** Wrinkled skin at sites of extensive sun exposure, usually seen in the elderly or in persons with excess exposure to ultraviolet light.

2. **Microscopic:** Amorphous, acellular basophilic material replaces the papillary and superficial reticular dermis (e-**Fig. 38.56**).

IX. DISORDERS OF EPIDERMAL MATURATION AND KERATINIZATION

A. Acantholytic dyskeratosis

1. **Clinical:** Varied, including malodorous, erythematous lesions in seborrheic areas; solitary pruritic lesions on the trunk; solitary warty lesions most commonly on the head and neck.

2. **Microscopic:** Suprabasilar cleft, acantholysis, dyskeratosis, elongated rete (villi), and distinctive granular keratinocytes that are perfectly round (corps ronds), or parakeratotic and acantholytic (corps grains) (e-**Fig. 38.57**).

B. Granular parakeratosis
1. **Clinical:** Brownish keratotic plaques at sites where skin rubs against skin; most common in the axillae; may be pruritic.
2. **Microscopic:** Keratohyaline granules are present in a confluent, thick layer of parakeratotic keratin (e-**Fig. 38.58**).

C. Porokeratosis
1. **Clinical:** Multiple clinical types; most commonly multiple erythematous macules with a thread-like palpable scale at their border on sun-damaged skin (disseminated superficial actinic porokeratosis [DSAP]).
2. **Microscopic:** All lesions of porokeratosis have one or more cornoid lamellae consisting of a thin spire of parakeratotic keratin arising from an area of the epidermis without a granular layer and usually associated with isolated, scattered, dyskeratotic keratinocytes. If the entire lesion is sampled, a cornoid lamella can be seen at both edges/sides of the lesion. DSAP has an atrophic epidermis between the cornoid lamella and a patchy/discontinuous band of lymphocytes in the superficial dermis (e-**Fig. 38.59**).

39 Nonmelanocytic Tumors of the Skin

Nathan C. Walk, Yumei Chen, Anne C. Lind, Friederike Kreisel, and Dongsi Lu

I. BENIGN TUMORS OF THE EPIDERMIS

A. Seborrheic keratosis

1. **Clinical:** Single or multiple discrete papules or plaques, typically measuring 0.5 to 1.0 cm, variably pigmented and with a "stuck-on" appearance, only on hair-bearing skin; most commonly found in people >30 years of age.

2. **Microscopic:** Exophytic or endophytic lesion sharply demarcated from adjacent epidermis, composed of basaloid and often homogeneous cells mixed with squamoid cells. Intraepidermal pseudocysts filled with loose orthokeratotic keratin are usually present. There are many microscopic patterns of seborrheic keratoses, the most common being hyperkeratotic, acanthotic, reticulated, and clonal. Features of irritation are commonly seen (e-Fig. 39.1).

B. Clear cell acanthoma

1. **Clinical:** Uncommon, slow growing, pink to brown, dome-shaped nodule or small plaque, most frequently on the leg of middle-aged and elderly individuals.

2. **Microscopic:** Acanthotic epidermis with a sharply demarcated proliferation of keratinocytes with pale/clear cytoplasm with associated parakeratosis, agranulosis, and neutrophils in the stratum corneum and spinosum. Periodic acid–Schiff (PAS) stain highlights cytoplasmic glycogen (e-Fig. 39.2).*

C. Large cell acanthoma

1. **Clinical:** A sharply demarcated, scaly patch on the sun-exposed skin of middle-aged and elderly individuals.

2. **Microscopic:** Sharply demarcated acanthosis, keratinocyte nuclear and cytoplasmic enlargement (about 2× normal), hypergranulosis and hyperorthokeratosis (e-Fig. 39.3).

II. PREMALIGNANT AND MALIGNANT TUMORS OF THE EPIDERMIS

A. Actinic keratosis

1. **Clinical:** Scaly, erythematous papules or nodules on sun-exposed skin of the head and neck, upper and lower extremities; more common in fair-skinned individuals.

2. **Microscopic:** Patchy parakeratosis and agranulosis that often spare adnexal ostia, irregular downward buds of atypical (dysplastic) basal keratinocytes. Dyskeratotic cells are sometimes present. Dysplasia does not involve the full thickness of the epidermis, and solar elastosis is frequently seen (e-Fig. 39.4).

3. **Genetics:** Approximately 50% of actinic keratoses show *TP53* mutations and overexpression of cyclin D1, whereas 16% have independent activation of *Ras*. Loss of heterozygosity is commonly seen on chromosome 3p (31%), 9p (39%), 9q (22%), 13q (52%), 17p (64%), and 17q (46%); human papilloma virus (HPV) is detected in 41% of cases.

---

*All e-figures are available online via the Solution Site Image Bank.

B. **Squamous cell carcinoma in situ (Bowen disease)**

1. **Clinical:** Sharply demarcated, scaly, often hyperkeratotic macule, papule, or plaque; most common in sun-exposed areas (particularly the face and legs); more common in fair-skinned, older individuals.

2. **Microscopic:** Keratinocytes with enlarged, hyperchromatic nuclei and minimal cytoplasm occupy the full thickness of the epidermis; variable acanthosis, hyperparakeratosis, agranulosis, dyskeratosis, mitoses above the basal layer and loss of maturation; the neoplastic cells populate adnexal structures (e-**Fig. 39.5**).

3. **Genetics:** Increased expression and mutation of *TP53* have been observed. Allelic deletion of one or more chromosome 9q markers has also been detected in occasional lesions.

C. **Invasive squamous cell carcinoma** (The American Joint Committee on Cancer [AJCC] Tumor, Node, Metastasis [TNM] staging scheme for cutaneous squamous cell carcinoma and other cutaneous carcinomas is given in Table 39.1.)

1. **Clinical:** Early lesions are firm, skin-colored, or erythematous nodules; later lesions are shallow ulcers with firm, elevated, or indurated surroundings, sometimes with crust or scale; most common in fair-skinned, older individuals on sun-exposed areas and in immunocompromised patients. Metastatic potential depends on location, histology, and precursor lesions/etiology.

2. **Microscopic:** Acanthosis, invasion of the dermis by individual or nested keratinocytes with variable amounts of cytoplasm and nuclear pleomorphism, dyskeratosis, and swirls of parakeratotic keratin (keratin pearls); there may be dermal desmoplasia and variable inflammation. Acantholysis, perineural invasion, and sarcomatoid change predict more aggressive behavior (e-**Fig. 39.6**).

D. **Basal cell carcinoma**

1. **Clinical:** Variable presentation; most commonly a dome-shaped, firm papule with a pearly, telangiectatic surface; slowly growing; primarily on the head, neck, and trunk. The most common skin cancer in Caucasians; rarely metastasizes unless neglected.

2. **Microscopic:** Variable histology; Common features include basaloid cells with hyperchromatic nuclei and scant cytoplasm, usually connected to an unremarkable or ulcerated epidermis. Basaloid islands show peripheral palisading, mitoses, and apoptosis; a retraction artifact separates the basaloid cells from the surrounding basophilic, variably mucinous stroma (e-**Fig. 39.7**).

3. **Genetics:** Mutations of genes *PTCH1* on chromosome 9q22.3 and *SMD* on chromosome 7q31–32 involved in activating hedgehog signaling pathway have been identified in both sporadic basal cell carcinomas and basal cell nevus syndrome, a rare autosomal dominant (AD) disorder.

III. **TUMORS OF THE CUTANEOUS APPENDAGES.** Tumors of the cutaneous appendages have a somewhat nebulous nomenclature. A traditional system organizes the tumors on the basis of their origin from one of the normal cutaneous appendages: hair follicle, sebaceous gland, eccrine gland, or apocrine gland. However, complex adnexal tumors also occur that have abnormalities of two or more of the normal skin constituents, including the epidermis itself, and there is sometimes controversy as to a tumor's precise histogenesis (i.e., eccrine vs. apocrine, and so on). The following is a succinct review of the major tumors derived from the skin appendages.

A. **Benign appendage tumors.** Benign adnexal tumors have architectural symmetry when viewed at low power and, usually, a distinctive cleft between the stroma of the tumor and the native dermal collagen.

1. **Hair follicle tumors**

a. **Trichofolliculoma**

i. **Clinical:** Rare, solitary, small (<1 cm), skin-colored papule on the face. A tuft of fine hairs protrudes from the center.

TABLE 39.1	Tumor, Node, Metastasis (TNM) Staging Scheme for Cutaneous Squamous Cell Carcinoma and Other Cutaneous Carcinomas

Primary tumor (T)[a]

TX	Primary tumor cannot be assessed
T0	No evidence of primary tumor
Tis	Carcinoma in situ
T1	Tumor 2 cm or less in greatest dimension with less than two high-risk features[b]
T2	Tumor >2 cm in greatest dimension or tumor any size with two or more high-risk features[a]
T3	Tumor with invasion of maxilla, mandible, orbit, or temporal bone
T4	Tumor with invasion of skeleton (axial or appendicular) or perineural invasion of skull base

Regional lymph nodes (N)

NX	Regional lymph nodes cannot be assessed
N0	No regional lymph node metastases
N1	Metastasis in a single ipsilaterial lymph node, 3 cm or less in greatest dimension
N2	Metastasis in a single ipsilateral lymph node, >3 cm but not >6 cm in greatest dimension; or in multiple ipsilateral lymph nodes, none >6 cm in greatest dimension; or in bilateral or contralateral lymph nodes, none >6 cm in greatest dimension
N2a	Metastasis in a single ipsalateral lymph node, >3 cm but not >6 cm in greatest dimension
N2b	Metastasis in multiple ipsilaterial lymph nodes, none >6 cm in greatest dimension
N2c	Metastasis in bilateral or contralateral lymph nodes, none >6 cm in greatest dimension
N3	Metastasis in a lymph node, >6 cm in greatest dimension

Distant metastasis (M)

M0	No distant metastases
M1	Distant metastases

Anatomic stage/prognostic groups

Stage	T	N	M
Stage 0	Tis	N0	M0
Stage I	T1	N0	M0
Stage II	T2	N0	M0
Stage III	T3	N0	M0
	T1	N1	M0
	T2	N1	M0
	T3	N1	M0
Stage IV	T1	N2	M0
	T2	N2	M0
	T3	N2	M0
	T Any	N3	M0
	T4	N Any	M0
	T4	N Any	M0
	T any	N Any	M1

[a]Excludes cSCC of the eyelid.
[b]High-risk features for the primary tumor (T) staging.
From: Edge SB, Byrd DR, Compton CC, et al., eds. *AJCC Cancer Staging Manual.* 7th ed. New York, NY: Springer; 2010. Used with permission.

    ii. **Microscopic:** One or more cystically dilated hair follicles with radiating follicles that project into a relatively cellular stroma. The secondary hair follicles are of variable maturity and may give rise to more hair follicles (e-**Fig. 39.8**).

b. Trichoepithelioma

    i. **Clinical:** Usually solitary, skin-colored papule, most common on the central face; if multiple, associated with AD inheritance. The desmoplastic variant is a solitary, firm annular lesion with a raised border and central depression that occurs exclusively on the face.

    ii. **Microscopic:** A relatively well-circumscribed dermal tumor composed of islands of basaloid cells with pilar differentiation in a cellular stroma; papillary mesenchymal bodies are characteristic. Small keratinous cysts and foci of calcification are often present. The tumor epithelium may mimic basal cell carcinoma, but there is no retraction artifact or mucinous stroma (e-**Fig. 39.9**). The desmoplastic variant shows a well-circumscribed lesion in the upper and mid-dermis composed of cords or small nests of basaloid cells in a sclerotic stroma (e-**Fig. 39.10**). It may be confused with a syringoma or a morphea-form basal cell carcinoma.

c. Trichoadenoma (of Nikolowski)

    i. **Clinical:** Rare nodule on the face or buttocks.

    ii. **Microscopic:** A well-demarcated dermal tumor composed of multiple cyst-like structures lined by multilayered keratinizing pilar-type squamous epithelium. The cysts contain keratinous debris and no hair shafts (e-**Fig. 39.11**).

d. Dilated pore of Winer

    i. **Clinical:** Common, usually solitary, comedo-like lesion on the head and neck, or trunk.

    ii. **Microscopic:** A cystically dilated hair follicle, filled with loose keratin and lined by acanthotic stratified squamous epithelium with irregular budding (e-**Fig. 39.12**).

e. Trichilemmoma

    i. **Clinical:** A solitary, small, skin-colored/pink or brown papule on the face and neck; multiple lesions are associated with Cowden syndrome.

    ii. **Microscopic:** A well-circumscribed, endo-exophytic tumor composed of clear squamoid cells with glycogenated cytoplasm. The tumor extends from the epidermis with a lobular configuration. There is a thin peripheral rim of palisading columnar cells and variable, thick, eosinophilic basement membrane (e-**Fig. 39.13**).

f. Pilomatrixoma (Calcifying epithelioma of Malherbe)

    i. **Clinical:** Firm, deeply located nodule, most common on the face and upper extremities; onset frequently in childhood.

    ii. **Microscopic:** A sharply demarcated tumor in the lower dermis and, often, the subcutis. The tumor is composed of large, irregularly shaped tumor islands and intervening stroma. Two basic cell types are present: basaloid cells and "shadow" or "ghost" cells. The basaloid cells resemble the cells in basal cell carcinoma and are present at the periphery of the tumor islands. The shadow cells, which have eosinophilic cytoplasm, distinct cell borders, and no nuclear staining, occupy the center of tumor islands. Several layers of transitional cells with intermediate features may be present. In addition, dystrophic calcification, a mixed inflammatory infiltrate, hemosiderin, melanin, bone, and foreign body giant cells can be seen (e-**Fig. 39.14**).

g. Fibrofolliculoma/trichodiscoma

    i. **Clinical:** Skin-colored papules, most common on the face; may be solitary or multiple. Multiple lesions are seen in Birt–Hogg–Dubé syndrome, which has an AD inheritance and carries a high risk for developing renal tumors, pulmonary cysts, and pneumothorax.

    ii. **Microscopic:** Spectrum of changes with fibrofolliculoma at one end and trichodiscoma at the other. Fibrofolliculoma is composed of thin strands of follicular epithelium extending from a hair follicle structure into a stroma that is well defined and composed of loose connective tissue with fine fibrosis. A trichodiscoma has a dominant stromal component that is characterized by strands of loose connective tissue with intermixed fibroblasts resembling an angiofibroma (e-**Fig. 39.15**).

2. **Eccrine tumors**

  a. **Syringoma**

    i. **Clinical:** Usually multiple, skin-colored, small, firm papules on the lower eyelids and cheeks, more common in women; onset is often at puberty.

    ii. **Microscopic:** Multiple small ducts in a dense fibrous stroma in the dermis. The ducts are lined by two layers of cuboidal epithelium, and sometimes are "tadpole" or "comma-like." Solid nests and strands of tumor cells can be present (e-**Fig. 39.16**).

  b. **Eccrine (or apocrine) mixed tumor (chondroid syringoma)**

    i. **Clinical:** Solitary, firm, dermal or subcutaneous nodule on the head and neck.

    ii. **Microscopic:** Well-circumscribed dermal tumor of small epithelial cells in solid nests, small clusters, and ducts in a prominent myxoid, cartilaginous, and/or fibrous stroma (e-**Fig. 39.17**).

  c. **Cylindroma**

    i. **Clinical:** Solitary nodule on the head and neck; predominantly in middle-aged to elderly women; rarely undergoes malignant transformation; if multiple, associated with AD inheritance and an occurrence as "turban tumors"

    ii. **Microscopic:** A poorly circumscribed dermal tumor composed of irregularly shaped nests of basaloid cells, surrounded by a thick eosinophilic basement membrane. The cellular nests fit together in a "jigsaw" pattern (e-**Fig. 39.18**).

  d. **Spiradenoma**

    i. **Clinical:** Usually solitary, firm, tender or painful dermal nodule. There is no characteristic distribution. They occur primarily in young adults.

    ii. **Microscopic:** One or more sharply demarcated dermal nodule(s) of basaloid cells. Two types of cells are present: small lymphocyte-like cells with hyperchromatic nuclei and larger epitheliod cells with more open chromatin. There may be a thin pseudocapsule; a few duct-like structures are present (e-**Fig. 39.19**).

  e. **Poroma group (including eccrine poroma, dermal duct tumor, and hidroacanthoma simplex)**

    i. **Clinical:**

      (a) **Eccrine poroma**—solitary, sessile or slightly pedunculated, pink nodule often on the plantar or palmar skin, or other locations with sweat glands.

      (b) **Dermal duct tumor**—a solitary, firm nodule on the head, neck, and extremities.

      (c) **Hidroacanthoma simplex**—a solitary plaque or nodule on the extremities and trunk; clinically resembles seborrheic keratosis or basal cell carcinoma.

    ii. **Microscopic:**

      (a) **Eccrine poroma**—a circumscribed tumor composed of columns of basaloid cells extending from the lower epidermis into the dermis within a loose, vascular stroma. Ducts and, rarely, small cysts may be seen in the tumor columns. There is a sharp demarcation from the epidermis (e-**Fig. 39.20**).

(b) Dermal duct tumor—islands of basaloid cells similar to those of eccrine poroma, located entirely in the dermis. An epidermal connection may be found if multiple sections are examined.

(c) Hidroacanthoma simplex—islands of basaloid cells similar to those of poroma, confined to the epidermis.

f. Acrospiroma (nodular hidradenoma; solid-cystic hidradenoma; apocrine/eccrine hidradenoma; clear cell hidradenoma)

  i. Clinical: Solitary nodule, 0.5 to 2.0 cm or more, no site predilection, disputed histogenesis. Nomenclature for this entity is confusing.

  ii. Microscopic: Variable histologic appearance, as reflected by the nosology; usually a circumscribed, nonencapsulated, multilobular, central dermal tumor with variable proportions of cystic and solid areas; tumor cells have variable clear or eosinophilic cytoplasm and are round, fusiform, or polygonal. Duct-like structures are typically present and may have a squamous appearance. The stroma varies from rather fine fibrous tissue to dense hyalinized collagen (e-**Fig. 39.21**).

3. Sebaceous hyperplasia and tumors

a. Sebaceous hyperplasia

  i. Clinical: Yellow to whitish papules with central umbilication, typically on the face of older individuals. It may mimic a basal cell carcinoma.

  ii. Microscopic: Multiple large, but otherwise normal, sebaceous lobules centered on a large central orifice; solar elastosis is frequently present (e-**Fig. 39.22**).

b. Sebaceous adenoma

  i. Clinical: Rare, solitary or multiple, pink or flesh-colored, usually <1 cm nodule(s) on the face or scalp of adults; may be associated with Muir–Torre syndrome (visceral carcinoma).

  ii. Microscopic: Multiple circumscribed sebaceous lobules usually centered in the superficial to mid-dermis; composed of peripheral basaloid germinative cells, central mature sebaceous cells, and a variable zone of transitional forms. Mature cells usually outnumber the basaloid cells (e-**Fig. 39.23**).

  iii. Genetics: Loss of protein expression of DNA mismatch repair genes (*MSH-2*, *MSH-6*, *MLH-1*, and *PMS-2*) has been found in a number of patients with sebaceous adenoma. There is a high correlation between lost expression of mismatch repair (MMR) proteins and microsatellite instability (MSI).

4. Apocrine tumors

a. Apocrine hidrocystoma (apocrine cystadenoma)

  i. Clinical: Solitary, translucent to bluish nodule, predominantly occurring on the face.

  ii. Microscopic: Several large cysts in the dermis; the cyst wall is composed of an outer myoepithelial layer and an inner layer of cuboidal to columnar cells with apocrine decapitation secretion; pseudopapillary projections may be present (e-**Fig. 39.24**).

b. Syringocystadenoma papilliferum

  i. Clinical: Varied; most commonly a raised, warty plaque on the scalp; associated with nevus sebaceous in approximately one-third of the cases.

  ii. Microscopic: Deep invaginations of duct-like structures extend from an acanthotic, variably papillomatous epidermis into the dermis; they are lined by squamous epithelium in the upper portion and by two-layer, sweat duct-like epithelium in the lower portion; numerous plasma cells are present in the connective tissue stroma of the papillae (e-Fig. 39.25).

   iii. **Genetics:** Allelic deletions of the *patched* gene on chromosome 9q22 and loss of heterozygosity of chromosome 9p21 have been reported in syringocystadenoma papilliferum.

5. **Complex adnexal tumors: Nevus sebaceous of Jadassohn (organoid nevus)**
   a. **Clinical:** Solitary, yellow or waxy, patch or plaque with alopecia on the scalp (most common), face, neck, or trunk; present at birth or first noticed in early childhood.
   b. **Microscopic:** A complex hamartoma involving the epidermis, pilosebaceous unit, and ducts/glands. There is variable epidermal acanthosis, papillomatosis, and abnormally formed/abortive hair follicles with bulbs that do not extend into the subcutis; increased numbers of large sebaceous glands are present around and after puberty; dilated apocrine glands are found in up to 50% of cases (e-Fig. 39.26). Secondary tumors may develop, such as syringocystadenoma papilliferum.

B. **Malignant tumors of the cutaneous appendages** are rare and far less common than their benign counterparts. As with the benign tumors discussed earlier, a malignant neoplasm can arise from any of the normal skin appendages, and there may be more than one component to a particular tumor. Only extramammary Paget disease will be discussed.
   1. **Clinical:** A red, scaly plaque, typically in areas rich in apocrine glands such as the anogenital region and, less commonly, the axilla; usually pruritic and slowly spreading. An underlying adnexal carcinoma is present in approximately 20% to 25% of cases; visceral carcinoma (rectal, prostate, bladder, cervix, or urethra) is present in 10% to 15% of cases.
   2. **Microscopic:** Similar to mammary Paget disease, there are large, predominantly intraepidermal, epithelioid tumor cells with large, pleomorphic nuclei and abundant pale cytoplasm that may or may not contain mucin. The tumor cells are concentrated in the lower epidermis and randomly dispersed throughout the epidermis; they may also be seen in the superficial dermis. Special stains may be needed to distinguish extramammary Paget disease from melanoma in situ and squamous cell carcinoma in situ with pagetoid features. The tumor cells are positive by mucicarmine and PAS stain; carcinoembryonic antigen (CEA), epithelial membrane antigen (EMA), and low-molecular-weight keratin immunostains are positive; Melan-A/Mart-1 and S-100 immunostains are negative (e-Fig. 39.27).

IV. **BENIGN AND MALIGNANT TUMORS OF MESENCHYMAL ORIGIN.** Classification of mesenchymal neoplasms is based on the mature, nonneoplastic tissue from which they are believed to be derived: blood vessel, nerve, smooth muscle, skeletal muscle, bone, cartilage, fibrous tissue, neuroendocrine tissue, or hematopoietic elements. Many of these tumors are discussed elsewhere in this text (see Chaps. 43 to 44 and 46 covering hematolymphoid and soft tissue malignancies, respectively); only the most common entities will be discussed here.
   A. **Vascular tumors**
      1. **Lobular capillary hemangioma (pyogenic granuloma)**
         a. **Clinical:** Common, rapidly developing polypoid or pedunculated, red, eroded papules or nodules that bleed easily; seen on mucous membranes and skin.
         b. **Microscopic:** An exophytic, frequently ulcerated, proliferation of capillaries divided into lobules by fibrous tissue septae; variably cellular, often surrounded by a collarette of epidermis (e-Fig. 39.28).

2. **Arteriovenous hemangioma (acral arteriovenous tumor)**
    a. **Clinical:** A solitary, usually asymptomatic, red or purple, enlarging or bleeding papule, averaging 4 mm in diameter; most common on the lips, perioral skin, nose, and eyelids of middle-aged to elderly men.
    b. **Microscopic:** Well-circumscribed, nonencapsulated vascular tumor in the upper to mid-dermis, composed of closely packed, large caliber, thick-walled and thin-walled vessels (e-Fig. 39.29).
3. **"Cherry" angioma (senile angioma, Campbell de Morgan spot)**
    a. **Clinical:** Solitary or multiple tiny, bright red papules, predominantly on the trunk and proximal extremities; common in adults, almost universal in the elderly.
    b. **Microscopic:** Early lesions with one or more dilated interconnecting thin-walled vessels in the papillary dermis. Established lesions are polypoid with an epidermal collarette and are composed of dilated and congested vascular channels in the papillary dermis (e-Fig. 39.30).
4. **Angiokeratoma**
    a. **Clinical:** Single to multiple red to black papule(s) or plaque(s) that may be warty or hyperkeratotic; multiple variants exist with characteristic clinical presentations and carrying various eponyms.
    b. **Microscopic:** Markedly dilated and congested papillary dermal vessels form cavernous channels that have an intimate association with the epidermis; irregular acanthosis and variable hyperkeratosis (e-Fig. 39.31).
5. **Lymphangioma (cystic lymphatic malformation)**
    a. **Superficial lymphangioma (lymphangioma circumscriptum)**
        i. **Clinical:** Multiple, localized, scattered, or grouped translucent vesicles or papulovesicles; may be red or purple due to intralesional hemorrhage and thrombus formation; usually congenital, sometimes presents later in childhood and is rare in adults. There may be a deeper component.
        ii. **Microscopic:** Multiple dilated, thin-walled lymphatic channels in the papillary and upper reticular dermis; epidermis is sometimes acanthotic and forms a collarette (e-Fig. 39.32).
    b. **Deep lymphangioma (including cavernous lymphangioma and cystic hygroma)**
        i. **Clinical:** Usually solitary, rubbery, skin-colored nodules that may result in swelling of the soft tissue; most common on the face, trunk, and extremities; varies from spongy to a large cystic tumor. Most are present at birth or the first few years of life.
        ii. **Microscopic:** Variable; in general, there are irregularly dilated vascular channels of variable size in the dermis, the subcutis, and deeper tissue. The vessels are thin- or thick-walled, and contain luminal proteinaceous fluid or lymphocytes. There is no endothelial atypia or mitotic activity. The intervening stroma is unremarkable or fibrotic (e-Fig. 39.33).
6. **Glomus tumor and glomangioma**
    a. **Clinical:** Painful, solitary or multiple, red to purple subungual macule(s); may be a nodule at other sites. Glomangioma is less painful.
    b. **Microscopic:** Well-circumscribed or encapsulated dermal tumor composed of sheets of glomus cells surrounding blood vessels. The glomus cells are homogeneous with eosinophilic cytoplasm and dense, round nuclei. The tumor stroma is fibrous and often pale-staining (e-Fig. 39.34). A glomangioma is predominantly vascular and has fewer glomus cells (e-Fig. 39.35). The glomus cells are positive for smooth muscle actin and negative for endothelial markers such as CD31.
7. **Kaposi sarcoma**
    a. **Clinical:** Early lesions are ecchymotic macules or patches; later lesions are bluish or purple papules, nodules, plaques, and tumors; all are palpable. There are four clinical subtypes with similar cutaneous findings:

Classic, African (endemic), Epidemic (human immunodeficiency virus [HIV]-associated), and Iatrogenic (immunosuppressive therapy related). Regardless of type, it is a low-grade malignancy that is slowly progressive but may involve internal organs. The etiologic agent is human herpes virus type 8 (HHV-8) in all types.

   b. **Microscopic:** Early lesions show a dermal proliferation of irregular slit-like vascular channels with extravasated erythrocytes, hemosiderin, and plasma cells. The endothelial cells are plump or inconspicuous; there is no significant cytologic atypia. The vascular channels infiltrate between collagen bundles and surround existing blood vessels (promontory sign) and appendages (e-**Fig. 39.36**). As the lesions evolve into papules, plaques, and nodules, there are increased spindle cells between the poorly defined slit-like vessels. Intracytoplasmic eosinophilic hyaline globules (PAS positive) can be identified within the tumor cells (e-**Fig. 39.37**).

8. **Epithelioid hemangioendothelioma**
   a. **Clinical:** Firm, tan-pink subcutaneous nodules and plaques, uncommonly involving the dermis, measuring several centimeters in maximal diameter; common sites are the trunk and extremities. The lesion is seen primarily in adults and has a slight female predilection; 40% of tumors recur, and ~15% develop distant metastasis.

   b. **Microscopic:** Sheets and cords of large polyhedral tumor cells in the subcutis/dermis. The tumor cells have amphophilic cytoplasm, prominent cytoplasmic vacuoles, and round nuclei often with small nucleoli; the cells have a tendency to grow around preexisting large vessels. The stroma is variably fibrous or myxoid. Mitotic figures and necrosis may be seen and may indicate worse clinical behavior. The tumor cells are immunoreactive for endothelial cell markers CD31, CD34, von Willebrand factor, and thrombomodulin (e-**Fig. 39.38**).

9. **Angiosarcoma**
   a. **Clinical:** Single or multifocal, purpuric or black plaque(s) on the head and neck of elderly patients, or purplish-red papules or polypoid tumors in the chronically edematous skin associated with lymphedema and/or prior radiation.

   b. **Microscopic:** Poorly circumscribed and often multifocal proliferation of anastomosing, infiltrative vascular channels in the dermis and subcutis with prominent extravasation of erythrocytes and hemosiderin. The vascular channels are lined by crowded, variably plump, and atypical endothelial cells; papillary processes sometimes extend into the lumens of the vessels. Poorly differentiated tumors with an epithelioid cellular morphology may resemble carcinoma or melanoma. The tumor cells are immunopositive for endothelial cell markers such as CD31, CD34, factor VIII-related antigen, and *Ulex europaeus* (e-**Fig. 39.39**).

B. **Neural and neuroendocrine tumors**
   1. **Traumatic neuroma**
      a. **Clinical:** Usually firm, pea-sized nodule in the subcutis and deep soft tissue at sites of previous injury; may be painful.

      b. **Microscopic:** Irregularly arranged nerve fascicles embedded in fibrous scar tissue. Each fascicle is surrounded by fibrous tissue and perineural cells. There are scattered mast cells (e-**Fig. 39.40**).

   2. **Solitary circumscribed neuroma (palisaded and encapsulated neuroma)**
      a. **Clinical:** Uncommon, usually solitary, skin-colored or pink papule, most common on the face of middle-aged adults; slow-growing, painless, and <6 mm in diameter.

      b. **Microscopic:** Well-circumscribed and partially encapsulated dermal nodule composed of fascicles of bland spindle cells with amphophilic cytoplasm and serpiginous nuclei that appear parallel to each other within a single fascicle. No intervening fibrous tissue is present (e-Fig. 39.41).

3. Neurofibroma

   a. **Clinical:** Soft, skin-colored, pedunculated papules or nodules. Multiple lesions in a segmental or widespread distribution are related to neurofibromatosis.

   b. **Microscopic:** A nonencapsulated dermal or subcutaneous tumor characterized by loosely arranged, wavy spindle cells in a pale-staining stroma. There are increased small caliber vessels and mast cells in the stroma. The spindle cells tend to surround adnexal structures rather than displace them (e-Fig. 39.42).

4. Cutaneous schwannoma (neurilemmoma)

   a. **Clinical:** Uncommon, slowly growing, usually solitary tumor/nodule with a predilection for the limbs of adults. The neoplasm can be either sporadic or associated with neurofibromatosis 2 (NF-2). Schwannomas are more commonly seen in the deep soft tissue, intracranially, or intraspinally.

   b. **Microscopic:** Similar to their soft tissue counterpart; form a circumscribed and encapsulated subcutaneous/dermal nodule. The tumor cells are spindled Schwann cells with indistinct cytoplasmic borders arranged in interlacing fascicles. There are hypercellular areas (Antoni A) containing rows or palisades of nuclei aligned around eosinophilic cellular processes (Verocay bodies) and hypocellular (Antoni B) areas. No axons are present (e-Fig. 39.43).

5. Merkel cell carcinoma

   a. **Clinical:** A rapidly growing, often ulcerated, red nodule or plaque usually arising on the sun-exposed skin of the elderly, particularly on the head, neck, and extremities. An association with polyoma virus infection (specifically, Merkel cell polyoma virus [MCPyV]) has been demonstrated in the majority of cases. AJCC TNM staging scheme for Merkel cell carcinoma is given in Table 39.2.

   b. **Microscopic:** Trabeculae, nests, and sheets of small cells with scant cytoplasm, indistinct cytoplasmic borders, vesicular nuclei with nuclear molding, and multiple small nucleoli that infiltrate the entire dermis and sometimes the subcutis. There are numerous apoptotic forms and mitoses. Local intralymphatic spread is commonly seen. The tumor cells are positive for neuron-specific enolase, chromogranin, and synaptophysin and have a characteristic "paranuclear dot-like" staining pattern for low-molecular-weight keratin such as CK20. The tumor cells are negative for CD45, S-100, and TTF-1, allowing distinction from hematopoietic and melanocytic neoplasms, as well as metastatic small cell carcinoma of the lung (e-Fig. 39.44).

   c. **Genetics:** Deletion of chromosome 1p36 is commonly seen; numerous other chromosomal abnormalities have been described, of which trisomy 6 is the most common.

6. Granular cell tumor

   a. **Clinical:** Asymptomatic, solitary, skin-colored nodule <3 cm in diameter; multiple lesions in ~10% of cases; most common in African American adults and women. Malignant counterpart is exceedingly rare.

   b. **Microscopic:** A nonencapsulated dermal-based tumor composed exclusively of large polyhedral cells with abundant fine to coarsely granular eosinophilic cytoplasm, and small oval centrally located nuclei. The granular cells infiltrate between collagen bundles and surround adnexa. The epidermis may be markedly acanthotic as in pseudocarcinomatous hyperplasia (e-Fig. 39.45). Tumor cells are usually positive for S-100, except in a subset of congenital lesions reported as CD34-positive granular cell dendrocytosis.

TABLE 39.2	Tumor, Node, Metastasis (TNM) Staging Scheme for Merkel Cell Carcinoma

Primary tumor (T)

TX	Primary tumor cannot be assessed
T0	No evidence of primary tumor (e.g., nodal/metastatic presentation without associated primary)
Tis	In situ primary tumor
T1	≤2 cm maximum tumor dimension
T2	>2 cm but not >5 cm maximum tumor dimension
T3	Over 5 cm maximum tumor dimension
T4	Primary tumor invades bone, muscle, fascia, or cartilage

Regional lymph nodes (N)

NX	Regional lymph nodes cannot be assessed
N0	No regional lymph node metastasis
cN0	Nodes negative by clinical exam[a] (no pathologic node exam performed)
pN0	Nodes negative by pathologic exam
N1	Metastasis in regional lymph node(s)
N1a	Micrometatasis[b]
N1b	Macrometastasis[c]
N2	In transit metastasis[d]

Distant metastasis (M)

M0	No distant metastasis
M1	Metastasis beyond regional lymph nodes
M1a	Metastasis to skin, subcutaneous tissues or distant lymph nodes
M1b	Metastasis to lung
M1c	Metastasis to all other visceral sites

Anatomic stage/prognostic groups

Stage	T	N	M
Stage 0	M0	Tis	N0
Stage IA	M0	T1	pN0
Stage IB	M0	T1	cN0
Stage IIA	M0	T2/T3	pN0
Stage IIB	T2/T3	cN0	M0
Stage IIC	T4	N0	M0
Stage IIIA	Any T	N1a	M0
Stage IIIB	Any T	N1b/N2	M0
Stage IV	Any T	Any N	M1

[a]Clinical detection of nodal disease may be via inspection, palpation, and/or imaging.
[b]Micrometastases are diagnosed after sentinel or elective lymphadenectomy.
[c]Macrometastases are defined as clinically detectable nodal metastases confirmed by therapeutic lymphadenectomy or needle biopsy.
[d]In transit metastasis: a tumor distinct from the primary lesion and located either (1) between the primary lesion and the draining regional lymph nodes or (2) distal to the primary lesion.
From: Edge SB, Byrd DR, Compton CC, et al., eds. *AJCC Cancer Staging Manual.* 7th ed. New York, NY: Springer; 2010. Used with permission.

C. **Fibrous and fibrohistiocytic tumors**
   1. **Keloid**
      a. **Clinical:** Firm, pink to purple, mildly tender, bosselated tumors that usually develop at sites of previous injury; most common on the upper back, shoulders, presternal area, and ear lobes of dark-skinned individuals.
      b. **Microscopic:** A nodule of haphazardly arranged, broad, homogeneous, brightly eosinophilic collagen bundles outlined by large, pale-staining fibroblasts in the superficial dermis (e-**Fig. 39.46**).

2. **Dermatofibroma**
   a. **Clinical:** Brownish, round, firm dermal nodules, usually <1 cm in diameter; most common on the legs of young adults.
   b. **Microscopic:** Poorly circumscribed dermal proliferation of spindled fibroblasts, histiocytes, and blood vessels. Fibroblasts at the periphery surround the collagen bundles ("collagen-trapping"). Dermatofibromas are histologically varied, and there are many corresponding named variants such as cellular, aneurysmal, "Monster" cell, and so on. The epidermis typically shows acanthosis, basal keratinocyte hyperpigmentation, and a broad flattened rete or a basaloid proliferation which can be mistaken for basal cell carcinoma in a superficial shave biopsy (**e-Fig. 39.47**).

3. **Dermatofibrosarcoma protuberans**
   a. **Clinical:** Solitary or multiple polypoid nodules arising in an indurated plaque on the trunk or extremities of adults; slowly growing locally aggressive tumor; rarely metastasizes.
   b. **Microscopic:** A cellular dermal tumor composed of homogeneous spindle cells arranged in a storiform or cartwheel pattern. The tumor cells infiltrate between adnexa, and there is characteristically extension into the subcutis with fat trapping. Occasional mitotic figures can be found, and atypia is mild. The epidermis is normal, atrophic, or ulcerated (**e-Fig. 39.48**).
   c. **Genetics:** The tumor characteristically exhibits the translocation t(17;22)(q22;q13), which results in production of a COLIA1–PDGFB fusion protein.

4. **Giant cell fibroblastoma:** A histologic variant of dermatofibrosarcoma protuberans, primarily affecting children; it has a strong male predominance and a similar anatomic distribution; harbors the same translocation as dermatofibrosarcoma protuberans.
   a. **Clinical:** Grossly, it is a firm yellow or gray tumor with a gelatinous or rubbery consistency without hemorrhage or necrosis.
   b. **Microscopic:** The tumor is usually hypocellular and composed of wavy spindle cells and scattered giant cells with hyperchromatic and angulated nuclei. The stroma is variable from myxoid, to collagenous, to sclerotic. Scattered mast cells are seen within the stroma. Irregular branching "angiectoid" spaces resembling dilated lymphatics may be seen, lined by spindled or multinucleated cells morphologically identical to those of the surrounding stroma (**e-Fig. 39.49**). The lining and stromal cells are immunopositive for CD34 and immunonegative for CD31, S-100, actin, desmin, and EMA.

5. **Angiofibroma**
   a. **Clinical (major types)**
      i. **Fibrous papule of the face:** A solitary, firm, dome-shaped, often flesh-colored lesion on the nose or central face.
      ii. **Pearly penile papules:** Tiny white papules, 1 to 3 mm in diameter, arranged in groups or rows on the coronal margin of the penis.
      iii. **Adenoma sebaceum (tuberous sclerosis):** Multiple papules or nodules with a predilection for the butterfly area of the face.
      iv. **Digital fibrokeratoma:** A solitary, thin, tall horn on a digit.
   b. **Microscopic:** Dermal fibrosis; dilated small vessels; and variably enlarged, angulated, or stellate fibroblasts. Concentric fibrosis around the blood vessels is more prominent in adenoma sebaceum than in fibrous papule of the face (**e-Fig. 39.50**). The epidermis of digital fibrokeratomas shows hyperkeratosis and acanthosis of acral skin (**e-Fig. 39.51**).
   c. **Genetics:** Mutations of two genes, *TSC1* on chromosome 9 and *TSC2* on chromosome 16, are identified in patients with tuberous sclerosis.

6. **Acrochordon (skin tag, soft fibroma, fibroepithelial polyp, and so on)**
   a. **Clinical:** Flesh-colored, pedunculated papules or nodules with irregular or smooth surfaces. Most common on the axilla, neck, groin, and eyelids; incidence increases with age; more common in obese women.
   b. **Microscopic:** Polypoid, variable epidermal change, well vascularized, loose dermal connective tissue. A variable amount of fat can be seen in the dermis of larger lesions (soft fibroma). No appendages are present (e-Fig. 39.52).

7. **Epithelioid sarcoma**
   a. **Clinical:** Epithelioid sarcoma has recently been divided into two distinct subtypes.

   The distal type presents as one or more slowly growing, firm, painless, tan-white subcutaneous nodules with an indistinct infiltrating margin. The tumor occurs most commonly on the distal extremities, particularly the hand and wrists. Ulceration and sinus formation may be present weeks or months after the lesion is first noted. The local recurrence rate is near 80%; distant metastasis occurs in 30% to 45% of cases, most commonly to the lymph nodes and lung.

   The proximal type is not characteristically a tumor of the skin or subcutaneous tissue, but instead involves the pelvis, perineum, and/or genital tract. It is discussed in more detail in Chapter 47.
   b. **Microscopic:** The proximal type arises in the subcutaneous or soft tissue (it is rarely dermal) and has a nodular arrangement of tumor cells that tend to palisade around geographic central degeneration/necrosis. A lymphohistiocytic infiltrate often surrounds the tumor nodules. The tumor cells are large and polygonal with abundant deeply eosinophilic cytoplasm, round to oval nuclei, and prominent nucleoli. Plump spindled tumor cells are sometimes present. Mitoses are frequent. The tumor cells are positive by immunohistochemistry for low- and high-molecular-weight keratins, EMA, and vimentin and are also positive for CD34 in 60% to 70% of cases. The architectural features are similar to those seen in deep granulomatous processes such as deep granuloma annulare.

D. **Fatty and muscular tumors**
   1. **Lipoma**
      a. **Clinical:** Common, asymptomatic, soft, subcutaneous nodule.
      b. **Microscopic:** Unremarkable mature adipocytes are surrounded by a thin fibrous capsule; there is a paucity of fibrous septae.
   2. **Angiolipoma**
      a. **Clinical:** Often multiple, painful, subcutaneous nodules of the extremities or trunk; usually appears after puberty.
      b. **Microscopic:** Varying proportions of mature adipose tissue and small-caliber blood vessels with fibrin thrombi, surrounded by a thin fibrous capsule, and arranged vaguely into lobules by fine incomplete fibrous septae (e-Fig. 39.53).
   3. **Leiomyoma**
      a. **Clinical:** Solitary or multiple red nodules, often painful.
      b. **Microscopic: Pilar leiomyoma** is a circumscribed, nonencapsulated tumor composed of interlacing smooth muscle bundles (e-Fig. 39.54). **Scrotal leiomyomas** are similar but often have ill-defined or focally infiltrative margins. **Angioleiomyoma** is a deep dermal/subcutaneous, well-circumscribed nodule of interlacing smooth muscle bundles between multiple thick walled vessels (e-Fig. 39.55).
   4. **Leiomyosarcoma**
      a. **Clinical:** Rare, dermal or subcutaneous nodule or plaque, most common on the extremities. Dermal leiomyosarcomas frequently extend into the

subcutaneous tissue; there are no confirmed cases of metastases from dermal tumors. Subcutaneous leiomyosarcomas have greater tendency for local recurrence and metastasis.

   b. Microscopic: Interlacing, hypercellular smooth muscle bundles with pleomorphic and hyperchromatic nuclei, and occasional mitoses (at least one per 10 high-power fields).

V. CUTANEOUS LYMPHOID INFILTRATES.

These infiltrates are highly varied and encompass reactive lymphoid infiltrates, primary cutaneous lymphoma, and cutaneous involvement by systemic disease/nodal lymphoma. With the exception of mycosis fungoides (MF), determination of whether the skin is the primary or a secondary site of a lymphoma requires a complete clinical examination for appearance and distribution of cutaneous lesions, presence or absence of lymphadenopathy and/or organomegaly, systemic symptoms, and peripheral blood smear abnormalities. In contrast to nodal lymphomas, of which B-cell lymphomas comprise the vast majority, ~70% of cutaneous lymphomas are of T-cell origin, of which MF is the most common (accounting for about 50% of all cutaneous lymphomas overall). The World Health Organization/European Organization for Research and Treatment of Cancer (WHO/EORTC) classification and the current WHO classification are the most current classifications on cutaneous lymphomas and are uniformly accepted by pathologists, dermatopathologists, dermatologists, and oncologists worldwide. Table 39.3 summarizes the WHO/EORTC classification of cutaneous lymphomas. Since MF and primary cutaneous CD30+ lymphoproliferative disorders are the most common cutaneous lymphomas, only these will be discussed in more detail below.

A. Mycosis fungoides

   1. Clinical: Patches, plaques, and/or tumors with a wide anatomic distribution; most common in middle-aged to elderly persons, but documented in children. Usually pruritic, may present with or develop erythroderma; clinical course is usually indolent. MF is, as a rule, limited to the skin, with widespread distribution and a protracted disease course. Extracutaneous spread may occur in advanced stages, mainly to lymph nodes, liver, spleen, lungs, and blood. Malignant cells of MF involving the blood in advanced stages are cerebriform in appearance and called Sézary cells. Disease progression involving peripheral blood must be distinguished from primary Sézary syndrome, a rare T-cell lymphoma that presents as a triad of erythroderma, generalized lymphadenopathy, and malignant T-cells (Sézary cells) in the peripheral blood. The staging scheme for MF and Sézary syndrome is outlined in Table 39.4, and the histopathologic staging of lymph nodes in MF and Sézary syndrome are outlined in Table 39.5.

   2. Microscopic: Histologic features vary with clinical presentation. Epidermal changes range from atrophic to psoriasiform. Spongiosis may be disproportionate to the intraepidermal lymphocytes.

   a. Patch stage/early MF is histologically subtle. A patchy, paucicellular band of lymphocytes is present in a fibrotic papillary dermis; lymphocytes extend into the epidermis (epidermotropism); intraepidermal lymphocytes are larger than the dermal lymphocytes and have hyperchromatic, cerebriform nuclei; lymphocytes are separated from keratinocytes by a halo and file along the basal layer of the epidermis (so-called "string of beads" pattern). Aggregates of atypical intraepidermal lymphocytes (Pautrier microabscesses) are rare. Dermal lymphocytes align along collagen bundles (e-Fig. 39.56).

   b. Plaque stage has easily identifiable Pautrier microabscesses in the epidermis and a more prominent band of lymphocytes in the upper dermis (e-Fig. 39.57).

   c. Tumor stage shows a dense nodular or diffuse infiltrate filling the dermis and extending into the subcutis. Epidermotropism may be lost. There may be transformation to a large cell phenotype. The infiltrate is

TABLE 39.3 A WHO/EORTC Classification of Cutaneous Lymphomas

Cutaneous T-cell and NK-cell lymphomas
Mycosis fungoides (MF)
MF variants and subtypes
    Folliculotropic MF
    Pagetoid reticulosis
    Granulomatous slack skin
Sézary syndrome
Adult T-cell lymphoma
Primary cutaneous CD30+ lymphoproliferative disorders
    Primary cutaneous anaplastic large cell lymphoma (cALCL)
    Lymphomatoid papulosis
Subcutaneous panniculitis-like T-cell lymphoma
Extranodal NK/T-cell lymphoma, nasal type
Primary cutaneous peripheral T-cell lymphoma, unspecified
    Primary cutaneous aggressive epidermotropic CD8+ T-cell lymphoma (provisional)
    Cutaneous $\gamma/\delta+$ T-cell lymphoma (provisional)
    Primary cutaneous CD4+ small/medium-sized pleomorphic T-cell lymphoma (provisional)

Cutaneous B-cell lymphomas
Primary cutaneous marginal zone B-cell lymphoma
    Primary cutaneous immunocytoma
    Primary cutaneous plasmacytoma
    Follicular hyperplasia with monotypic plasma cells
Primary cutaneous follicle centre lymphoma
    Growth patterns: follicular, follicular and diffuse, diffuse
Primary cutaneous diffuse large B-cell lymphoma, leg type
Primary cutaneous diffuse large B-cell lymphoma, other
Primary cutaneous intravascular large B-cell lymphoma
Precursor hematologic neoplasm
CD4+/CD56+ hematodermic neoplasm (formerly blastic NK cell lymphoma)

From Willemze R, Jaffe ES, Burg G, et al. WHO-EORTC classification for cutaneous lymphomas. *Blood* 2005;105:3768–3785.

characteristically CD3+, CD5+, CD4+, and CD8−; a minority of cases are CD3+, CD5+, CD4−, and CD8+; CD2 and CD7 may be lost in the neoplastic lymphocytes.

3. **Genetics:** Some human leukocyte antigen (HLA) class II alleles (specifically HLA-B8, Aw31, and Aw32) are more prevalent among patients with MF. Clonal T-cell receptor (TCR) gene rearrangements have been detected (mostly alpha/beta, rarely gamma/delta receptors). There is also an increased rate of aberrations involving multiple chromosomes, including chromosomes 1, 6, 11, 8, 17, 13, 15, and 9, in advanced stage disease.

B. **Primary cutaneous CD30 + lymphoproliferative disorders** are the second most common form of cutaneous T-cell lymphomas and represent a spectrum of diseases including primary cutaneous anaplastic large cell lymphoma (cALCL), lymphomatoid papulosis (LyP), and borderline cases. Primary cALCL and LyP show considerable histologic overlap and are best distinguished on the basis of clinical presentation and course.

1. **Primary cALCL**

    a. **Clinical:** Solitary or localized, large (>2 cm), often ulcerated, red/brown tumors; mostly in adults. Partial regression is common; complete spontaneous regression is rare; extracutaneous involvement is possible.

    b. **Microscopic:** Nodular or diffuse dermal infiltrate composed of sheets of cohesive CD30+ atypical cells, frequently involving the superficial

TABLE 39.4	Tumor, Node, Metastasis (TNM) Staging Scheme for Mycosis Fungoides and Sézary Syndrome

ISCL/EORTC revision to the classification of mycosis fungoides and Sézary syndrome

Skin

T1	Limited patches,[a] papules, and/or plaques[b] covering <10% of the skin surface. May further stratify into T1a (patch only) vs. T1b (plaque ± patch)
T2	Patches, papules, or plaques covering 10% or more of the skin surface. May further stratify into T2a (patch only) vs. T2b (plaque ± patch)
T3	One or more tumors[c] (≥1 cm diameter)
T4	Confluence of erythema covering 80% or more of the body surface area

Node

N0	No clinically abnormal peripheral lymph nodes[d]; biopsy not required
N1	Clinically abnormal peripheral lymph nodes; histopathologically Dutch grade 1 or NC1 LN0–2
N1a	Clone negative[e]
N1b	Clone positive[e]
N2	Clinically abnormal peripheral lymph nodes; histopathologically Dutch grade 2 or NC1 LN3
N2a	Clone negative[e]
N2b	Clone positive[e]
N3	Clinically abnormal peripheral lymph nodes; histopathology Dutch grades 3–4 or NC1 LN4; clone positive or negative
Nx	Clinically abnormal peripheral lymph nodes; no histologic confirmation

Visceral

M0	No visceral organ involvement
M1	Visceral involvement (must have pathology confirmation[f] and organ involved should be specified)

Peripheral blood involvement

B0	Absence of significant blood involvement: 5% or less of peripheral blood Lymphocytes are atypical (Sézary) cells[g]
B0a	Clone negative[e]
B0b	Clone positive[e]
B1	Low blood tumor burden: >5% of peripheral blood lymphocytes are atypical (Sézary) cells but does not meet the criteria of B2
B1a	Clone negative[e]
B1b	Clone positive[e]
B2	High blood tumor burden: 1000/μL. Sézary cells[g] or more with positive clone[e]

[a]For skin, patch indicates any size lesion without significant elevation or duration. Presence/absence of hypo- or hyperpigmentation, scale, crusting, and/or poikiloderma should be noted.

[b]For skin, plaque indicates any size skin lesion that is elevated or indurated. Presence or absence of scale, crusting, and/or poikiloderma should be noted. Histologic features such as folliculotropism or large-cell transformation (>25% large cells), CD30+ or CD30−, and clinical features such as ulceration are important to document.

[c]For skin, tumor indicates at least one 1 cm diameter solid or nodular lesion with evidence of depth and/or vertical growth. Note total number of lesions, total volume of lesions, largest size lesion, and region of body involved. Also noted if histologic evidence of large-cell transformation has occurred. Phenotyping for CD30 is encouraged.

[d]For node, abnormal peripheral lymph node(s) indicates any palpable peripheral node that on physical examination is firm, irregular, clustered, fixed or 1.5 cm or larger in diameter. Node groups examined on physical examination include cervical, supraclavicular, epitrochlear, axillary, and inguinal. Central nodes, which are not generally amenable to pathologic assessment, are not currently considered in the nodal classification unless used to establish N3 histopathologically.

[e]A T-cell clone is defined by PCR or Southern blot analysis of the T-cell receptor gene.

[f]For viscera, spleen and liver may be diagnosed by imaging criteria.

[g]For blood, Sézary cells are defined as lymphocytes with hyperconvoluted cerebriform nuclei. If Sézary cells are not able to be used to determine tumor burden for B2, then one of the following modified ISCL criteria along with a positive clonal rearrangement of the TCR may be used: (1) expanded CD4+ or CD3+ cells with CD4/CD8 ratio of 10 or more, (2) expanded CD4+ cells with abnormal immunophenotype including loss of CD7 or CD26.

From Olsen E, Vonderheid E, Pimpinelli N, et al. Revisions to the staging and classification of mycosis fungoides and Sézary syndrome: a proposal of the International Society for Cutaneous Lymphomas (ISCL) and the cutaneous lymphoma task force of the European Organization of Research and Treatment of Cancer (EORTC). *Blood*. 2007;11:1713 with permission of the American Society of Hematology.

TABLE 39.5	Histopathologic Staging of Lymph Nodes in *Mycosis fungoides* and Sézary Syndrome

Updated ISCL/EORTC Classification **Dutch system NC1–VA classification**

N1	Grade 1: dermatopathic lymphadenopathy (DL)	LN0: no atypical lymphocytes
		LN1: occasional and isolated atypical lymphocytes (not arranged in clusters)
		LN2: many atypical lymphocytes or in 3–6 cell clusters
N2	Grade 2: DL; early involvement by MF (presence of cerebriform nuclei >7.5 μm	LN3: aggregates of atypical lymphocytes; nodal architecture preserved
N3	Grade 3: partial effacement of LN architecture; many atypical cerebriform mononuclear cells (CMCs)	LN4: partial/complete effacement of nodal architecture by atypical lymphocytes or frankly neoplastic cells
	Grade 4: complete effacement	

From Olsen E, Vonderheid E, Pimpinelli N, et al. Revisions to the staging and classification of mycosis fungoides and Sézary syndrome: a proposal of the International Society for Cutaneous Lymphoma (ISCL) and the cutaneous lymphoma task force of the European Organization of Research and Treatment of Cancer (EORTC). *Blood*. 2007;11:1713 with permission of the American Society of Hematology.

subcutis. The atypical cells have large rounded or irregular vesicular nuclei; prominent, centrally placed nucleoli; and ample clear to amphophilic cytoplasm. A nonneoplastic mixed inflammatory infiltrate is present (e-**Fig. 39.58**). The large lymphocytes in cALCL are negative for anaplastic lymphoma kinase-1 (ALK-1), which is frequently positive in systemic anaplastic large cell lymphoma (ALCL).

    c. Genetics: Clonal rearrangement of TCR genes is detected in >90% of cases of primary cALCL. However, the translocation t(2;5)(p23;q35) characteristic of systemic ALCL is rarely, if ever, found in primary cALCL.

  2. Lymphomatoid papulosis (LyP)

    a. Clinical: Recurrent crops of papules, nodules, and plaques at different stages of evolution, mainly on the trunk and extremities of young adults. Spontaneous regression occurs within a few weeks or months; the course may last for decades. Correlation with clinical lesion size, behavior, and distribution is required for diagnosis. Patients with LyP should be monitored lifelong since 5% to 25% of patients develop a second lymphoma, such as Hodgkin lymphoma or anaplastic large cell lymphoma.

    b. Microscopic: Three histologic subtypes exist:

      i. Type A: Wedge-shaped, mixed cellular infiltrate of small lymphocytes, eosinophils, neutrophils, and histiocytes, mixed with variable numbers of large atypical lymphocytes that may have hyperchromatic nuclei or resemble the neoplastic cells of ALCL (e-**Fig. 39.59**).

      ii. Type B: Histology similar to plaque stage MF.

      iii. Type C: Histology similar to ALCL. The characteristic immunophenotype of the tumor cells is CD30+/CD3+/CD4+ and CD8/EMA negative.

    c. Genetics: Clonal rearrangement of TCR gene can be found in at least 40% of LyP lesions. Chromosome deletions and rearrangements of chromosomes 1, 7, 9, and 10 have also been demonstrated.

VI. CUTANEOUS METASTASIS (FROM VISCERAL CARCINOMA). The skin is an uncommon site for metastasis from visceral malignancies. Carcinoma may reach the skin by direct extension from an underlying tumor, by lymphatic and/or hematogenous spread as part of systemic involvement, or by accidental implantation during a diagnostic or surgical procedure. Metastases tend to occur on the skin near the primary malignancy; metastasis to sites distant from the primary tumor is more common in tumors that demonstrate angioinvasion (e.g., primary tumors of the kidney or lung).

Rarely, a cutaneous metastasis is the first indication of a visceral malignancy; the umbilicus, and less frequently the scalp, is a particularly common site of involvement in this setting. Adenocarcinoma is more frequently observed as a cutaneous metastasis than is squamous cell carcinoma or urothelial carcinoma. Cutaneous metastases are variable in clinical appearance and can occur either as solitary or multiple papules/nodules, or as mimics of inflammatory/infectious conditions.

A. Sister Mary Joseph nodule

1. **Clinical:** This condition was named after Sister Mary Joseph (1856–1939), a surgical assistant for Dr. William Mayo, who noted the association between paraumbilical nodules observed during skin preparation for surgery and metastatic intra-abdominal cancer confirmed at surgery. It is usually a solitary, firm, indurated nodule, sometimes with surface fissuring or ulceration; it is variable in size and can be painful. Common underlying tumors include gastrointestinal malignancy (>55%, male predominance) and ovarian malignancies (34%).

   Sister Mary Joseph nodules account for 60% of all malignant umbilical tumors (primary or secondary). Most patients die within months after the appearance of the umbilical tumor.

2. **Microscopic:** Most commonly, a dermal-based adenocarcinoma with histology resembling the primary malignancy. Signet-ring cell morphology may be present, especially from a gastric primary (e-**Fig. 39.60**).

B. Metastatic breast carcinoma

1. **Clinical:** Typically small papules, ranging from 1 to 2 mm in diameter to large tumor masses, on the anterior chest wall. Intralymphatic spread of tumor cells (inflammatory carcinoma) can manifest as a diffuse, warm, indurated plaque (carcinoma erysipeloides). Scalp metastasis can present as alopecia (alopecia neoplastica), which is also seen in metastases from other visceral sites, especially from a lung primary.

2. **Microscopic:** Usually a poorly differentiated adenocarcinoma. Ductal and sometimes lobular arrangements are present. The proportion of intravascular tumor varies (e-**Fig. 39.61**).

C. Metastatic renal cell carcinoma

1. **Clinical:** Typically erythematous, vascular papule or nodule, may be misdiagnosed as lobular capillary hemangioma or Kaposi sarcoma; solitary in 15% to 20% of cases. The scalp is a common site of involvement.

2. **Microscopic:** Usually well-circumscribed, dermal nodule(s) composed of sheets and nests of polygonal tumor cells with clear cytoplasm, distinct cytoplasmic borders, and enlarged hyperchromatic nuclei; associated with a delicate rich vascular stroma, red blood cell extravasation, and hemosiderin deposition. The histologic features can be bland, and the differential diagnosis includes other primary and metastatic tumors with clear cell morphology (e-**Fig. 39.62**).

40 Skin: Melanocytic Lesions

Anne C. Lind, Nils Becker, Emily A. Bantle, and Louis P. Dehner

I. **BACKGROUND.** Melanocytes are melanin-synthesizing cells derived from the neural crest. During the first 3 months of gestation, they migrate into the ectoderm where they normally occupy a space slightly beneath the basal keratinocytes. They can be differentiated from adjacent keratinocytes by their rounded and slightly hyperchromatic nucleus as compared with the more elongated or ovoid nucleus with evenly dispersed chromatin of the basal keratinocyte. In addition, melanocytes usually exhibit a pale often eccentric rim of eosinophilic cytoplasm and are separated from the neighboring basal keratinocytes and/or basement membrane by a clear space or halo (**e-Fig. 40.1**).* Occasionally, dendritic processes can be seen as they extend between the keratinocytes. The ratio of melanocytes to basal keratinocytes depends on the body site. On the trunk and extremities it is approximately 1:7 to 10, while the ratio on the face and external genitalia is about 1:3.

The main function of melanocytes is the production of melanin, a tyrosine-derived photoprotectant which converts UV radiation into heat, thus preventing UV-related DNA damage. Melanin is exported via melanosomes, which are membrane-bound and have an internal lattice-like structure. Melanin granules are deposited on the lattice, eventually obscuring this architectural feature. Melanin pigment found in the skin is classified as eumelanin (brown or black pigment) or pheomelanin (yellow-red pigment), the latter of which is rich in sulfur.

In addition to the general considerations for gross examination of skin specimens (Chap. 38), a complete description of the background skin color and the clinical "ABCDs" (see section on melanoma) is required for biopsies or excisions of a pigmented lesion. Therefore, the size of the surface lesion, distance to or presence at the margin, color regularity or irregularity, and border, should all be included in the gross description.

Diagnosis of a melanocytic lesion is based on multiple architectural and cytologic criteria. In most cases, these microscopic features result in a specific diagnosis that reliably correlates with the anticipated biologic behavior of the melanocytic proliferation. Features associated with benignancy include symmetry, circumscription, maturation, predominance of nested melanocytes, cohesive nests of melanocytes, and melanocytes with regular nuclear borders and without nucleoli or atypical mitoses. A comparison of the histologic criteria for benign and malignant melanocytic proliferations can be found in Table 40.1. The status of the margins should be included routinely on all pathology reports of melanocytic proliferations, even in punch biopsy specimens. Although there admittedly is no consensus on this point, the margin status provides additional information that is often clinically useful.

Immunohistochemical stains can be helpful in distinguishing melanocytic from nonmelanocytic lesions, confirming nodal micrometastases, or demonstrating confluence or nonconfluence of melanocytes. Although several stains are available, including S100, Melan-A (MART-1), HMB-45, MITF, and NKI-C3, no immunostain is capable of reliably differentiating malignant from benign melanocytic lesions.

---

*All e-figures are available online via the Solution Site Image Bank.

TABLE 40.1	Histopathologic Features in the Differential Diagnosis of Benign and Malignant Melanocytic Proliferations	
Microscopic feature	**Nevus**	**Melanoma**
Symmetry	+	− or ±
Circumscription	+	− or ±
Nested melanocytes	+	±
Cohesive nests	+	±
Regular nuclear border	+	−
Absence of nucleoli	+	−
Atypical mitoses	−	±
"Deep" mitoses	−	+

Because of the histologic diversity of melanocytic lesions, there are instances in which the morphologic features that support a benign diagnosis (nevus) and those that support a malignant diagnosis (melanoma) seem to be equally represented. Occasionally, even among experts, there is no consensus regarding the benign or malignant nature of a melanocytic lesion based on the histomorphology. In these cases, as in definitive melanomas, a complete excision is necessary, and consultation with a pathologist or dermatopathologist either within the department or from an outside institution should be sought.

When a melanocytic lesion exhibits borderline features, chromosomal studies are sometimes helpful to determine a definitive diagnosis. Two main methods are utilized for this purpose: comparative genomic hybridization (CGH) and fluorescence in situ hybridization (FISH). It has been shown that most nevi maintain chromosomal stability and therefore do not exhibit DNA gains and/or losses. Melanomas, by comparison, have variable gains and losses across multiple genes, while Spitz nevi have either a normal genotype or an isolated amplification of chromosome 11p.

II. **BENIGN MELANOCYTIC PROLIFERATIONS.** Any nevus, by definition, is benign. A melanocytic nevus, when the histologic diagnosis is given without modifiers such as "with severe atypia," is a benign proliferation/hamartoma of melanocytes in the epidermis, epidermis and dermis, or dermis alone. In general, a melanocytic nevus is a small (<6 mm), symmetric, well-circumscribed proliferation of nested melanocytes, and the melanocytes that are deepest in the dermis are smaller than superficial melanocytes, a process known as maturation. The basic histologic criteria, as shown in Table 40.1, apply to most nevi. However, there are multiple histologic subtypes of nevi, some with exceptions to these criteria. Therefore, knowledge of the histologic subtypes, and the exceptions they present, is helpful. A summary of these variants and their malignant counterparts is provided in Table 40.2 and The World Health Organization (WHO) classification of melanocytic tumors is given in Table 40.3.

A. **Lentigo simplex**
   1. **Clinical:** It is an acquired pigmented lesion that is small in size and has a flat appearance. It is evenly colored and can usually be found on sun-exposed skin in persons <40 years of age.
   2. **Microscopic:** Rete are long and slender and have increased numbers of cytologically unremarkable melanocytes, without aggregates (nests) of melanocytes. Melanin pigment is increased in the basal keratinocytes (e-Fig. 40.2).

B. **Junctional melanocytic nevus**
   1. **Clinical:** It is an acquired pigmented lesion that is small in size and has a flat appearance. Like lentigo simplex, it is evenly colored and can usually be found on sun-exposed sites.

TABLE 40.2	Histologic Types of Melanocytic Nevus and Their Borderline or Malignant Counterpart

Benign	Borderline or malignant
Junctional melanocytic nevus with or without AD	Melanoma in situ, lentiginous or superficial spreading type
Compound melanocytic nevus with or without AD	Melanoma of nevoid type, melanoma arising in nevus or malignant melanoma
Dermal melanocytic nevus	Metastatic or recurrent melanoma
Spitz nevus	"Spitzoid" melanoma or "borderline" atypical Spitz tumor
Pigmented spindle cell nevus of Reed	Spindle cell melanoma
Deep penetrating nevus	Spindle cell melanoma
Halo nevus	Melanoma with intense host reaction
Balloon cell nevus	Melanoma with balloon cell features
Congenital nevus with proliferative nodule(s)	Melanoma arising in congenital nevus
Blue nevus	Melanoma with regression
Cellular blue nevus	Spindle cell melanoma or malignant cellular blue nevus

AD, architectural disorder.

2. **Microscopic:** Nests/aggregates of melanocytes are present at the tips of the rete. There may be increased numbers of cytologically unremarkable melanocytes along the sides of the rete, but there is no confluent growth of melanocytes (e-**Fig. 40.3**).

3. **Note:** The presence of a purely junctional nevus should be viewed with some concern in an individual >50 years. In these cases, it is helpful to take into consideration the size of the lesion and also to determine whether the junctional population of melanocytes has a confluent or nonconfluent pattern of proliferation. The diagnosis of junctional nevus should be made hesitantly on skin with significant solar elastosis.

C. **Compound melanocytic nevus**
   1. **Clinical:** It is an acquired pigmented lesion that is small in size. It is usually slightly raised, evenly colored, and is normally found on sun-exposed skin. However, like intradermal nevi, it may have a variety of configurations from polypoid to papillomatous.
   2. **Microscopic:** This nevus has features of both a junctional and an intradermal nevus. There are nests/aggregates of melanocytes at the tips of the rete and nests/aggregates of melanocytes in the dermis. The proportion of epidermal melanocytes to dermal melanocytes is variable (e-**Fig. 40.4**).
   3. **Note:** Care should always be taken to make certain that the deep dermal melanocytes are smaller, do not have nucleoli, and lack mitotic figures. A second population or clone of nevoid cells should be viewed with concern. There is no more diagnostically treacherous lesion than the nevoid or nevus-like melanoma.

D. **Intradermal melanocytic nevus**
   1. **Clinical:** An intradermal melanocytic nevus is a raised (papular), nonpigmented lesion that may have a variety of configurations from polypoid to papillomatous, reflecting in part the appearance of the epidermis. It can be mistaken clinically for a skin tag (fibroepithelial polyp) or a basal cell carcinoma.
   2. **Microscopic:** Nested and individual melanocytes are found only in the dermis (e-**Fig. 40.5**). The dermal component of compound or intradermal nevi can show so-called neurotization with a resemblance to a neurofibroma, contain

| **TABLE 40.3** | WHO Histologic Classification of Melanocytic Tumors |

Malignant melanoma
Superficial spreading melanoma
Nodular melanoma
Lentigo maligna
Acral–lentiginous melanoma
Desmoplastic melanoma
Melanoma arising from blue nevus
Melanoma arising in a giant congenital nevus
Melanoma of childhood
Nevoid melanoma
Persistent melanoma

Benign melanocytic tumors
Congenital melanocytic nevi
  Superficial type
  Proliferative nodules in congenital melanocytic nevi
Dermal melanocytic lesions
  Mongolian spot
  Nevus of Ito and Ota
Blue nevus
  Cellular blue nevus
Combined nevus
Melanotic macules, simple lentigo, and lentiginous nevus
Dysplastic nevus
Site-specific nevi
Acral
Genital
Myerson nevus
Persistent (recurrent) melanocytic nevus
Spitz nevus
Pigmented spindle cell nevus (Reed)
Halo nevus

From: Weedon D, LeBoit P, Burg G, et al., eds. *World Health Organization Classification of Tumours. Pathology and Genetics. Skin Tumours.* Lyon, France: IARC Press; 2005. Used with permission.

spaces with a pseudovascular appearance, and have scattered multinucleated cells as a feature of presumed senescence.

E. **Spitz nevus (spindle and/or epithelioid cell nevus)**

1. **Clinical:** It is commonly found on the head and neck or extremities of children and adolescents, with decreasing incidence with increasing age. It may arise suddenly and can rarely be multiple. Frequently, Spitz nevi are not pigmented; consequently, the clinical differential diagnosis might include a vascular lesion (angioma) or juvenile xanthogranuloma.

2. **Microscopic:** Common features include compact hyperorthokeratosis, hypergranulosis, and acanthosis. The melanocytes can be spindled, epithelioid, or mixed and are arranged in vertically oriented nests (mimicking clusters of bananas) at the epidermal–dermal junction; often a cleft/space between the epidermis and nested melanocytes is present (e-**Fig. 40.6**). Epithelioid melanocytes have large nuclei and abundant eosinophilic cytoplasm. Numerous ectatic, thin-walled vascular spaces may be seen in the papillary dermis (which accounts for the clinical impression of a vascular lesion). Superficial mitoses may be seen; however, atypical mitoses, clustered mitoses, or deep mitoses should raise the possibility of a Spitz-like or spitzoid melanoma,

regardless of age or site. Pagetoid spread may be seen in an otherwise typical Spitz nevus. Caution is required when considering the diagnosis of an epithelioid Spitz nevus in a person past middle age and/or on sun-damaged skin. The designation of "Spitz tumor" has been suggested for the Spitz nevus with atypical features (e-**Fig. 40.7**), if not all Spitz nevi. Although the diagnostic challenge presented by a melanocytic lesion with Spitz features is admittedly difficult, the overwhelming majority of Spitz nevi occurring in children and adolescents have benign behavior.

F. Pigmented spindle cell nevus of Reed
  1. **Clinical:** A pigmented spindle-cell nevus of Reed is a heavily but evenly pigmented, small, acquired lesion in the shoulder/pelvic girdle region. It is most common in women in their second and third decades.
  2. **Microscopic:** It is a symmetric and well-circumscribed proliferation of spindled melanocytes in the epidermis and superficial dermis with a pattern reminiscent of a woven basket. Fascicles of spindled cells are oriented vertically, horizontally, and tangentially. A broad zone of melanophages in the superficial dermis is invariably present beneath the melanocytes (e-**Fig. 40.8**). The relationship of the Reed nevus to the Spitz nevus is uncertain.

G. Blue nevus
  1. **Clinical:** It is a congenital or acquired, small lesion that is flat to slightly raised. Unlike most other melanocytic lesions, it is blue rather than black or brown. They occur most commonly on the head, neck, and extremities.
  2. **Microscopic:** A common blue nevus is a superficial, dermal, lentil-shaped, variably cellular proliferation of spindled and dendritic melanocytes that interdigitate between collagen bundles. Melanophages are frequently admixed. The epithelioid variant has, as the name implies, melanocytes with a more epithelioid appearance (e-**Fig. 40.9**). The differential diagnosis of a common blue nevus includes dermal melanocytosis.

H. Cellular blue nevus
  1. **Clinical:** It is a large (1 to 2 cm) heavily pigmented, blue to blue-black, raised lesion that is most common on the scalp or buttocks.
  2. **Microscopic:** This lesion is characterized as a mid- to deep-dermal multinodular biphasic proliferation. The nodular centers are composed of small epithelioid melanocytes, with pale to amphophilic cytoplasm. The nodules are surrounded by a rim of pigmented spindled melanocytes and melanophages. There may be extension of the nodules into the contiguous subcutis in some cases. Despite the striking tumor-like appearance, a consideration of malignancy should not be entertained in the absence of necrosis, atypical mitosis, and prominent nucleoli (e-**Fig. 40.10**).

I. Dermal melanocytosis (Nevus of Ota, Nevus of Ito, Mongolian spot, Hori nevus)
  1. **Clinical:** These nevi are characteristically flat, slate-gray to blue to dark brown patches on the face, shoulder, sacrum, or bilateral temples. They predominantly occur in people of Asian descent and are more common in females.
  2. **Microscopic:** These lesions have identical features and some overlap with those of a blue nevus. Instead of a superficial lentil-shaped lesion they are present in the mid- to deep-dermis as ill-defined, paucicellular infiltrates of pigmented, spindled, and/or dendritic melanocytes (e-**Fig. 40.11**).

J. Congenital and congenital-pattern nevi
  1. **Clinical:** Congenital or congenital-pattern nevi are pigmented lesions that are usually present at birth or that appear during infancy. They are classified as small (<2 cm), intermediate (2 to 20 cm), or large (>20 cm). They are frequently varied in pigmentation and have irregular borders. These nevi may be hairy and/or become progressively more hairy. Involvement of the leptomeninges by benign or malignant melanocytes in a child with a large or giant congenital nevus is known as neurocutaneous melanosis.

2. **Microscopic:** A junctional component exists in these lesions in early infancy, but the melanocytes are predominantly dermal with time. Individual nevoid to small epithelioid melanocytes in the dermis extend along or into dermal structures (such as the adnexa, arrector pili muscles, and small peripheral nerves) and into lymphovascular spaces. The subcutis and deeper structures may also be infiltrated by nevus cells. The epidermal melanocytic pattern is highly variable, ranging from no significant melanocytic proliferation, to nested melanocytes, to confluent lentiginous hyperplasia. Mitotic figures, but not atypical forms, may be present at any level. Proliferative nodules composed of monomorphous melanocytes and with brisk mitotic activity may be present and might lead to an erroneous interpretation of melanoma.

An apparent congenital nevus, especially from the scalp, with a more complex pattern of spindle cells, perivascular pseudorosettes, and tactoid bodies likely represents a so-called neurocristic hamartoma.

A congenital-pattern nevus is regarded as an acquired lesion that has a dermal growth pattern similar to that of a congenital nevus, including a predominance of individual cells rather than nests, and preferential growth in or along adnexal structures (e-**Fig. 40.12**).

K. **Deep penetrating nevus**
1. **Clinical:** It is a pigmented lesion that is usually acquired during early adulthood. It is of small size and found most commonly on the upper half of the body. Occasionally, it may resemble a blue nevus.
2. **Microscopic:** Deep penetrating nevi show dermal fascicles and nodules of epithelioid to spindled melanocytes with conspicuous granular, gray-brown cytoplasm admixed with melanophages and some nevoid melanocytes. They may extend to the subcutis in a mixed pushing and infiltrative pattern. Nuclear pleomorphism, mitotic figures, and nucleoli may be noted. This lesion may be seen as one component of a combined nevus. The combination of the cytologic and architectural features may lead to a concern for melanoma (e-**Fig. 40.13**).

L. **Halo nevus**
1. **Clinical:** A halo nevus shows a characteristic central zone of pigment with a circumferential rim of hypo-/depigmentation. It may be raised or flat and sometimes is noted as a recent change in a preexisting pigmented lesion.
2. **Microscopic:** Sections show a junctional, compound, or intradermal melanocytic nevus which has been obscured or nearly obscured by a dense band of lymphocytes. Regressive changes (immature fibroplasia, neovascularization, paucicellular lymphocytic infiltrate, melanophages) may be seen at the perimeter. The lymphocytic infiltrate should not impart a sense of asymmetry, and the epidermal melanocytes, if present, should be predominantly nested (e-**Fig. 40.14**).

M. **Nevus with architectural disorder/Clark nevus/dysplastic nevus**
1. **Clinical:** Nevi with architectural disorder are highly variable in appearance, ranging from small, symmetric, and evenly pigmented to large (>6 mm), irregularly shaped, and irregularly pigmented. Nevi with architectural disorder are a cutaneous marker for the dysplastic nevus syndrome where multiple atypical nevi (>100) can be present. Nevi with architectural disorder are a controversial entity of uncertain significance outside of this syndrome. The lack of uniformity in diagnostic terms is one sign of this controversy.
2. **Microscopic:** This junctional or compound melanocytic proliferation has its diagnostic features centered on the epidermal–dermal junction. The nested melanocytes bridge between adjacent rete, nested melanocytes arise between or from the sides of rete (rather than the tips), eosinophilic collagenous tissue drapes beneath the epidermis in a festoon-like pattern (lamellar fibroplasia), and there is nonconfluent lentiginous melanocytic hyperplasia. The

melanocytes may have a bland, nevoid appearance; have a size greater than that of the basal keratinocytes (mild cytologic atypia); have increased size and variable chromatin patterns (moderate cytologic atypia); or have increased size, variable chromatin patterns, pleomorphism, and nucleoli (severe cytologic atypia). A nevus with architectural disorder and severe cytologic atypia should be considered a borderline melanocytic proliferation; a conservative but complete excision should be encouraged (e-**Fig. 40.15**).

N. Nevi on special sites
  1. **Clinical:** The clinical appearance varies with site. Special sites include umbilicus, acral skin (palms/soles), areola, and mucocutaneous sites such as the conjunctiva, anus, and external genitalia.
  2. **Microscopic:** In addition to the features associated with junctional and/or compound nevi, the junctional melanocytic proliferations at these sites may have an increase in the number of individual melanocytes with either a lentiginous or pagetoid pattern, loss of cohesion, and asymmetry.

O. Combined melanocytic nevus
  1. **Clinical:** They vary in appearance. They may be flat, raised, or both and may be variably pigmented. Although they can present at any age, they are most common in the first three decades. The combination of features in these lesions (asymmetry, color variations, and possible border irregularities) often raises concern for melanoma.
  2. **Microscopic:** Combined melanocytic nevi may have any of the features of the previously described nevi in a side-by-side arrangement or top-to-bottom arrangement. One of the more common combinations is a compound melanocytic nevus and a blue nevus; the most worrisome combinations include a compound melanocytic nevus with a deep penetrating nevus, or a side-by-side Spitz nevus and compound nevus.

P. Recurrent melanocytic proliferations
  1. **Clinical:** These are characterized by a sudden appearance or reappearance of pigment in a scar from a previously biopsied or excised nevus and/or melanoma. In some instances, the patient may not be able to provide reliable information regarding the biologic nature and/or diagnosis of the previous lesion.
  2. **Microscopic:** Lentiginous melanocytic hyperplasia and randomly scattered, irregular nests of melanocytes are present above an immature or mature dermal scar. The features of a recurrent nevus may be indistinguishable from a recurrent melanoma and have been referred to as "pseudomelanoma." Adjacent lesional tissue outside of the scar and/or knowledge of the initial biopsy or excision findings is imperative for arriving at the correct diagnosis (e-**Fig. 40.16**).

Q. Nevus ambiguous. This category could include any/all melanocytic lesions that have some of the classic features of a distinctive subtype (such as a Spitz nevus) but are variant in others.

III. **MELANOMA** is a malignant melanocytic neoplasm that can occur in any tissue on any body site. Ninety percent of all melanomas arise in the skin, and only cutaneous melanoma will be considered in this section.

Melanoma accounts for only a small percentage (3% to 5%) of primary cutaneous malignancies; basal cell carcinoma and squamous cell carcinoma are far more prevalent (95% to 97%). However, melanoma accounts for >50% of cancer deaths from a primary cutaneous malignancy. The incidence of melanoma has increased over the past 25 years, but the recognition and diagnosis of lower stage lesions account for a substantial proportion of this increased incidence. As expected, the overall survival has shown improvement as pathologically lower stage lesions are diagnosed. Melanoma is most common in individuals >50 years of age but affects persons of all ages, including infants. It is slightly more common in males, in whom the pattern of distribution is slightly different. In males, melanoma is more common on the trunk/head and neck; in females, melanomas on the lower extremities are more common. There are numerous histologic types (see Table 40.3), and early study results suggest that the genetic signature of melanoma is different depending on its association with sun exposure (chronic, intermittent, or none; *N Engl J Med.* 2005;353:2135). While the majority of melanomas have easily recognized histologic patterns, some subtypes, such as nevoid and spitzoid, are unsettlingly similar to benign melanocytic lesions. In addition, amelanotic melanomas have a clinically more challenging appearance due to their lack of pigmentation. They are considered to be poorly differentiated melanomas.

Clinical features may vary slightly with anatomic site and/or histologic subtype; however, in general, a melanoma is Asymmetric, has an irregular Border, its Color is uneven, and it has a Diameter that is >6 mm. These clinical features have been described as the ABCDs of pigmented lesions. The patient may report a change in a preexisting pigmented lesion and/or complain of pruritus. A clinical description of a worrisome pigmented lesion can be helpful, especially in the case of a biopsy with borderline atypical histologic features. It should always be considered that a partial biopsy may not be representative of the overall pathology.

A. Melanoma in situ
  1. **Microscopic:** There is an increase in the number of atypical, enlarged melanocytes found only in the epidermis. These cells show a spectrum of nuclear enlargement and hyperchromatism. There may be prominent pagetoid spread (i.e., melanocytes are present above the suprapapillary plate) in a superficial spreading pattern, or confluent spread of melanocytes at the level of the basal keratinocytes in a lentiginous pattern. Nests may or may not be present, but if present are randomly distributed and vary in size and shape. Melanocytes are not seen in the dermis, although features of regression may be seen and warrant a comment because invasion may have been present earlier (e-**Fig. 40.17**).
  2. **Differential diagnosis:** Sun-induced melanocytic hyperplasia, recurrent melanocytic proliferations, lentiginous dysplastic melanocytic nevus, pagetoid Spitz nevus, and psoralen and ultraviolet A light (PUVA) lentigo.

B. Malignant melanoma—superficial spreading type
  1. **Clinical:** Superficial spreading melanoma often occurs on the trunk of men and lower extremities of women; however, it can be found on any body site.
  2. **Microscopic:** Increased numbers of melanocytes with enlarged nuclei and increased amounts of cytoplasm are present at all levels of the epidermis, pagetoid spread is easily identified, and melanocytes with similar cytologic features are present in the dermis. In the dermis, melanocytes may be seen as individual cells, in small clusters, and/or in sheets (e-**Fig. 40.18**).
  3. **Differential diagnosis:** Compound melanocytic nevus.

C. Malignant melanoma—lentiginous type (lentigo maligna melanoma)
  1. **Clinical:** This type usually develops on the face or sun-exposed areas of the upper extremities of elderly patients.
  2. **Microscopic:** Increased numbers of melanocytes with enlarged nuclei and a mild increase in cytoplasm are present in a confluent pattern at the level of the basal keratinocytes without sparing of the suprapapillary plates. Poorly formed and randomly scattered nests of melanocytes may be present; pagetoid cells are not seen. An artifactual subepidermal cleft might be noted, and melanocytes might extend along the adnexal epithelium. In this variant, cytologic atypia might not be prominent. Melanocytes are present in the dermis (e-**Fig. 40.19**).
  3. **Differential diagnosis:** Sun-induced melanocytic hyperplasia, recurrent melanocytic proliferations (benign or malignant), and lentiginous dysplastic melanocytic nevus.

D. Malignant melanoma—nodular type

1. **Clinical:** These can be found on any body site. Characteristically, they lack an initial radial growth phase, leading to a nodular or polypoid appearance.

2. **Microscopic:** Melanocytes with atypical, but often monotonous, nuclear and cytoplasmic features including enlarged nuclei, irregular nuclear borders, increased amounts of cytoplasm, and abundant mitotic activity (including atypical forms) are present in the dermis in a large nodule or sheet. There may be no apparent intraepidermal melanocytic proliferation, and if malignant melanocytes are present in the epidermis, they do not span the entire dermal tumor. Ulceration is frequently noted (e-Fig. 40.20).

E. Malignant melanoma—desmoplastic-neurotropic type

1. **Clinical:** It has a predilection for the head and neck region and is often non-pigmented.

2. **Microscopic:** There is a predominantly dermal proliferation of individual, large, spindled melanocytes with prominent nuclear pleomorphism. Melanocytes are noted between collagen bundles and along nerves. The lesion may be poorly defined and variably cellular. Unlike most types of cutaneous melanoma, the desmoplastic melanoma may be S-100 negative and generally is nonreactive with other markers of melanocytic differentiation such as Melan-A/MART-1 and/or HMB-45. Apparent expression of smooth muscle actin (SMA) has been noted (e-Fig. 40.21).

3. **Differential diagnosis:** Malignant fibrous histiocytoma, scar, dermatofibroma, sclerotic dermatofibrosarcoma protuberans, and leiomyosarcoma.

F. Malignant melanoma—nevoid type

1. **Microscopic:** Sections show a symmetric, well-circumscribed, nested proliferation of small, nevoid melanocytes with dermal maturation. At low power, it may be indistinguishable from a compound melanocytic nevus. At higher power, deep dermal melanocytes have prominent nucleoli and mitoses (e-Fig. 40.22).

2. **Differential diagnosis:** Melanocytic nevus.

G. Malignant melanoma—spitzoid type

1. **Microscopic:** Epithelioid and spindled melanocytes in a predominantly nested pattern are seen in an acanthotic and hyperkeratotic epidermis. The epidermal architectural features are strikingly similar to a Spitz nevus. Dermal melanocytes may be preferentially present in sheets or in large confluent nests, and lack maturation. There is a degree of nuclear pleomorphism that exceeds the atypia seen in the usual Spitz nevus. Mitotic figures, including atypical forms, may be present at all levels of the dermis and may be asymmetrically distributed. A lymphocytic response, if present, may abut the deep aspect of the lesion and provide a suggestion of asymmetry. Frequently the nuclear to cytoplasmic ratio is greater than that of a Spitz nevus, and there is no apparent decrease in nuclear size between the superficial and deep dermal melanocytes (e-Fig. 40.23).

2. **Differential diagnosis:** Spitz nevus.

IV. MICROSCOPIC STAGING OF MELANOMA. The Tumor, Node, Metastasis (TNM) classification of malignant melanoma as published in the American Joint Committee on Cancer (AJCC) guidelines from 2010 is provided in Table 40.4. The following changes have been made from the 2002 guidelines: The use of the mitotic rate per mm^2 instead of Clark level for categorizing T1 melanomas, the inclusion of at least one melanoma-associated immunohistochemical marker in the detection of nodal metastases (unless a diagnosis can be made by cellular morphology), and the removal of the prior existing 0.2 mm threshold for positive lymph nodes.

A. Breslow thickness is the single most important prognostic parameter associated with an invasive melanoma. An optical micrometer, calibrated to the microscope, is aligned perpendicularly to the epidermis, and the melanoma is

TABLE 40.4	Pathologic Tumor, Node, Metastasis (TNM) Classification of Malignant Melanoma (AJCC, 2010)

Primary tumor (T)

TX	Primary tumor cannot be assessed (includes shave biopsies and regressed melanoma); pTX includes shave biopsies and regressed melanomas
T0	No evidence of primary tumor
Tis	Melanoma in situ (atypical melanocytic hyperplasia, melanocytic dysplasia, not an invasive malignant lesion)
T1	Tumor ≤ 1 mm in thickness
	T1a: Without ulceration and mitosis $<1/mm^2$
	T1b: With ulceration or mitosis $\geq 1/mm^2$
T2	Tumor 1.01–2.00 mm in thickness
	T2a: Without ulceration
	T2b: With ulceration
T3	Tumor 2.01–4.00 mm in thickness
	T3a: Without ulceration
	T3b: With ulceration
T4	Tumor >4.00 mm in thickness
	T4a: Without ulceration
	T4b: With ulceration

Regional lymph nodes (N)

NX	Regional lymph nodes cannot be assessed
N0	No regional lymph node metastasis
N1	Metastasis in one regional lymph node
	N1a: Micrometastasis (diagnosed after sentinel lymph node biopsy)
	N1b: Macrometastasis (clinically detectable and pathologically confirmed)
N2	Metastasis in two or three regional lymph nodes
	N2a: Micrometastasis
	N2b: Macrometastasis
	N2c: Satellite or in-transit metastasis without regional nodal metastasis
N3	Metastasis in four or more regional lymph nodes, or matted metastatic regional lymph nodes, or satellite or in-transit metastasis with metastasis in regional lymph node(s)

Distant metastasis (M)

MX	Distant metastasis cannot be assessed
M0	No distant metastasis
M1	Distant metastasis
	M1a: Skin, subcutaneous tissue, or lymph nodes beyond the regional lymph nodes
	M1b: Lung metastasis
	M1c: All other visceral sites, or any site with elevated serum lactate dehydrogenase (LDH)

Pathologic staging

Stage 0	Tis	N0	M0
Stage IA	T1a	N0	M0
Stage IB	T1b	N0	M0
	T2a	N0	M0
Stage IIA	T2b	N0	M0
	T3a	N0	M0

(continued)

TABLE 40.4	Pathologic Tumor, Node, Metastasis (TNM) Classification of Malignant Melanoma (AJCC, 2010) (*Continued*)		
Stage IIB	T3b	N0	M0
	T4a	N0	M0
Stage IIC	T4b	N0	M0
Stage IIIA	T1–4a	N1a, 2a	M0
Stage IIIB	T1–4a	N1b, 2b, 2c	M0
	T1–4b	N1a, 2a	M0
Stage IIIC	T1–4b	N1b, 2b, 2c	M0
	Any T	N3	M0
Stage IV	Any T	Any N	M1

From Balch CM, Gershenwald JE, Soong S-J, et al. *Final Version of 2009 AJCC Melanoma Staging and Classification.* JCO December 20, 2009;27:36:6199–6206.

measured from the top of the granular cell layer through the dermal melanocytes at the thickest portion of the melanoma, avoiding the adventitial dermis along adnexal structures. Measurements of the clinical lesion (width and breadth) together with the measured Breslow thickness provide an estimate of tumor volume.

B. **Ulceration.** The presence or absence of ulceration is documented on all gross and microscopic examinations. Ulceration may correlate with proliferative activity and predicts more aggressive clinical behavior. The presence of ulceration modifies the T stage of a melanoma. Ta melanomas are not ulcerated; Tb indicates ulceration and predicts a biologic behavior closer to the next T category.

C. **Mitotic rate per mm^2.** The mitotic rate now replaces the Clark level in subclassifying T1 melanomas. It is evaluated in the most mitotically active areas of the tumor and reported as the number of mitoses per mm^2.

D. **Satellite and/or in-transit metastasis.** This is characterized by the presence of a focus of melanoma within 2 cm of the primary melanoma, but separated from the main tumor nodule by uninvolved dermis and/or subcutis. An in-transit metastasis is a focus of metastatic melanoma in the skin in a distance >2 cm from the primary melanoma but not beyond the first draining lymph node basin. Either of these events affects staging adversely and has a biologic impact that is comparable to that of nodal metastases.

E. **Sentinel lymph node examination.** Varying protocols and varying attitudes regarding this procedure exist. A common approach involves the following steps.
   1. Nodes are grossly identified, and each is submitted in a separate cassette.
   2. All nodes are bivalved through the hilum.
   3. The cut faces of the bivalved node are placed face down in the tissue cassette.
   4. Histotechnicians waste as little tissue as possible when cutting from the face of the paraffin block.
   5. Slides are cut at 4 to 5 μm thickness. Slides representing levels 1, 10, and 20 are stained with hematoxylin and eosin (H&E). Slides representing levels 2, 11, and 21 are saved on charged slides for potential immunoperoxidase studies. Slides representing levels 3, 12, 22 are retained for additional studies if needed.
   6. The H&E-stained slides are examined; if there is diagnostic melanoma present, a diagnosis is rendered and stains are not performed.
   7. If there is no obvious melanoma, or if there are suspicious areas that could represent melanoma, melanocyte-specific immunostains (such as Melan-A) are performed on the reserved slides. Final diagnosis is given only after these studies are completed.

V. NONMELANOCYTIC PIGMENTED LESIONS. The pathologist is sometimes presented with a biopsy or excision of skin for a clinically pigmented lesion, often with the clinical description of "atypical pigmented lesion; rule out melanoma." Lesions that are not composed of melanocytes microscopically, but can mimic a nevus or melanoma clinically, include: pigmented seborrheic keratosis (e-**Fig. 40.24**), pigmented basal cell carcinoma (e-**Fig. 40.25**), pigmented actinic keratosis, solar lentigo (e-**Fig. 40.26**), dermatofibroma (e-**Fig. 40.27**), postinflammatory pigmentary alteration (e-**Fig. 40.28**), intracorneal hemorrhage (calcaneal petechiae) (e-**Fig. 40.29**), tinea nigra (e-**Fig. 40.30**) and Monsel's solution in a biopsy site (e-**Fig. 40.31**).

SUGGESTED READINGS

Banerjee SS, Harris M. Morphological and immunophenotypic variations in malignant melanoma. *Histopathology.* 2000;36:387–402.

Barnhill RL, Piepkorn M, Busam KJ. *Pathology of Melanocytic Nevi and Malignant Melanoma.* 2nd ed. New York, NY: Springer; 2004.

Crowson AN, Magro CM, Mihm MC. *The Melanocytic Proliferations. A Comprehensive Textbook of Pigmented Lesions.* New York, NY: Wiley-Liss; 2001.

Culpepper KS, Granter SR, McKee PH. My approach to atypical melanocytic lesions. *J Clin Pathol.* 2004;57:1121–1131.

Elder D, van den Oord J. Pathology and pathophysiology of melanocytic disorder. *Histopathology.* 2002;41(Suppl. 2):120–146.

Massi G, Leboit PE. *Histological Diagnosis of Nevi and Melanoma.* Berlin, MA: Steinkopff Darmstadt/Springer; 2004.

Thompson JF, Morton DL, Kroon BBR. *Textbook of Melanoma.* New York, NY: Martin Dunitz; 2004.

Nervous System

<table>
<tr><td>

41

</td><td>

Central Nervous System: Brain, Spinal Cord, and Meninges

Richard J. Perrin, Sushama Patil, and Arie Perry

</td></tr>
</table>

I. **INTRODUCTION.** The task of evaluating a neuropathologic specimen often seems daunting, given the complexity of this organ system and its ever-enlarging list of diseases. However, when a methodical approach is applied using clinical, radiologic, histological and, increasingly, molecular information, the chances of error can be significantly reduced.

II. **ANATOMY AND HISTOLOGY.** The central nervous system (CNS) consists of cerebrum, cerebellum, brain stem, spinal cord, meninges, 12 paired cranial nerves, and the blood vessels supplying these structures. The brain and spinal cord are enclosed within the skeletal confines of the cranium and vertebral canal. The mature (adult) brain weighs around 1200 to 1400 g. The meninges covering the brain and spinal cord are of two principal types: (1) the dense fibrous dura mater and (2) the more delicate leptomeninges (pia and arachnoid mater). The cerebrum is divided into right and left hemispheres by a thick dural fold, the falx cerebri. A second dural fold between the cerebrum and the cerebellum (tentorium cerebelli) divides the brain into infra- and supratentorial compartments. Infratentorially, the midbrain, pons, and medulla oblongata (cranial to caudal) form the brain stem, which is connected to the cerebellum by means of three (superior, middle, and inferior) cerebellar peduncles. The supratentorial compartment contains cerebral cortex (frontal, temporal, parietal, and occipital lobes), white matter, and deep gray nuclei, such as basal ganglia, thalamus, and hypothalamus. The term "neuraxis" is sometimes used to refer to brain and spinal cord; thus, lesions that involve brain parenchyma are said to be "intra-axial" (e.g., astrocytoma, central neurocytoma, ependymoma), and those located outside of the parenchyma are referred to as "extra-axial" (e.g., meningioma, hemangiopericytoma [HPC], solitary fibrous tumor [SFT], and schwannoma of cranial nerve VIII). Similarly, in the spine, the terms "intramedullary" and "extramedullary" are used to denote lesions within or adjacent to the spinal cord parenchyma, respectively.

The CNS is composed of two tissue types, namely gray and white matter, that differ qualitatively on gross and microscopic examination. Neuronal cell bodies and dendrites reside mostly in the gray matter (cortex and deep gray nuclei), and axons create the framework of the white matter. Glial cells (astrocytes, oligodendroglial cells, and microglia) are present in different proportions in these tissues. Oligodendrocytes are more populous in the white matter; their processes form the sheaths of myelin that insulate CNS axons. The eosinophilic, finely granular to fibrillary material between cell bodies is often referred to as "neuropil" and is formed by the processes of neurons (axons and dendrites) and glial cells. Neuronal morphology varies significantly, with cell body size ranging from <15 μm (e.g., small neocortical granular stellate neurons) to 100 μm (Betz cells of the primary motor cortex). For descriptive purposes, neocortical pyramidal neurons are often considered the morphologic prototype. These cells contain abundant amphophilic cytoplasm, clumpy basophilic Nissl substance, a large round central nucleus, a prominent nucleolus, coarse proximal cytoplasmic processes, and a prominent apical dendrite oriented perpendicular to the cortical surface. Ependymal glial cells form a ciliated cuboidal epithelium that lines the ventricles and central canal and focally transitions with epithelium of the choroid plexus. The choroid plexus, which produces cerebrospinal fluid (CSF) within the ventricles, is papillary; its branching fibrovascular cores are lined by a specialized epithelium with a hobnailed apical surface.

III. INTRAOPERATIVE EVALUATION, GROSS EXAMINATION, AND TISSUE SAMPLING. Evaluation of a surgical neuropathology specimen often begins with an intraoperative consultation, which may be requested by the surgeon (1) to confirm the presence of lesional tissue, (2) to provide a preliminary diagnosis that will guide surgical management (e.g., aggressive surgery for ependymoma, limited biopsy for lymphoma, culture sample to microbiology for abscess), and (3) to sample fresh or frozen tissue for ancillary studies (e.g., Western blot for Creutzfeldt–Jakob disease [CJD], molecular pathology, tumor banking, karyotyping). For optimal evaluation, specimens should ideally be submitted on Telfa nonstick gauze pads saturated with normal saline. Tissue that has been soaked in saline is certainly acceptable, but is more likely to fragment during transport and may demonstrate more severe freezing artifacts. Fresh brain tissue, especially small biopsy specimens, should never be placed on dry gauze or tissue paper, because subsequent tissue retrieval from these materials is almost impossible. Water content may be reduced through very gentle blotting on a clean dry plastic surface, but fresh brain tissue is very fragile, and improper handling can introduce cellular "touch" and "crush" artifacts.

For intraoperative diagnosis, small portions of the fresh specimen should be chosen for freezing, for cytologic "smear" or "touch" preparations, and for possible ultrastructural examination. Freezing or otherwise exhausting the entire specimen for intraoperative diagnosis should be avoided, for several reasons. First, the techniques available during intraoperative examination seldom yield sufficient information for a definitive final diagnosis; most diagnoses require the fine histologic detail afforded by paraffin sections and information from immunohistochemical stains and other ancillary molecular tests. Second, freezing introduces artifacts (e.g., ice crystals, clumping of nuclear chromatin). Third, on some occasions, surgical attempts to obtain additional diagnostic material from the patient cause bleeding or other complications that prevent further tissue acquisition.

The manner in which intraoperative specimens are processed for diagnosis is important. Before any tissue is frozen, a block of embedding compound (commonly referred to as "OCT"), formed within an empty tissue well within the cryostat, should be frozen fast to a cryostat "chuck." After freezing, the chuck and OCT block are removed sharply and inverted; the tissue should be placed centrally on the flat surface of the frozen OCT block, immediately covered with a minimal amount of liquid OCT, and frozen from above by a flat, prechilled metallic weight (**e-Fig. 41.1**).* This process maximizes rate of freezing and minimizes (but does not eliminate) ice crystal formation. Cytologic evaluation by smear preparation is extremely helpful because it lacks freezing artifacts and preserves nuclear details. Smears can be prepared by gently compressing a very small amount of representative tissue between two glass slides, gently sliding them apart, and immediately fixing both smeared slides in 95% alcohol (**e-Fig. 41.2**). Lastly, a small tissue fragment (1 mm^3) should also be fixed in glutaraldehyde and

---

*All e-figures are available online via the Solution Site Image Bank.

processed for potential electron microscopic studies, particularly if the intraoperative diagnosis is unclear.

Gross examination and tissue sampling for permanent sections is less complicated. Most neuropathologic specimens are small and/or fragmented, limiting full appreciation of meaningful gross features. Even when large resection specimens are submitted intact, gross abnormalities are often absent or subtle. In fact, radiographs are commonly considered the "gross pathology" for CNS biopsies. In either case, specimens are usually entirely submitted for histologic analysis after adequate formalin fixation (a few hours for smaller specimens and overnight fixation for large specimens). Because most neuropathologic processes are heterogeneous, even when the diagnosis seems clear, if a resection specimen is too large for complete processing, it should still be extensively sampled. For similar reasons, Cavitronic UltraSound Aspirator (CUSA) material should not be dismissed as worthless; such material may be somewhat less preserved than resected tissue due to partial autolysis and other artifacts, but occasionally it provides essential clues to the final diagnosis.

A. **CNS biopsy for special circumstances.** Brain and sometimes meningeal biopsies for nonneoplastic indications are occasionally performed (e.g., nonresolving chronic meningitis, neurosarcoidosis). Similarly, a "blind" frontal lobe biopsy is sometimes obtained for neurodegenerative disorders that do not have a clearly defined etiology, particularly in younger patients. When a prion protein disease like CJD is suspected, the neuropathologist should be given advance notice and should be involved from the outset. One piece of cortex from the biopsy should be snap frozen for Western blot analysis by a reference laboratory such as the National Prion Disease Pathology Surveillance Center (NPDPSC) (special shipping containers must be used, and specific procedures must be followed; see http://www.cjdsurveillance.com/). The remaining tissue should be fixed in 10% neutral buffered formalin for 24 hours, followed by immersion in 88% to 98% formic acid (undiluted stock solution) for 1 hour, prior to routine processing. If initial histologic examination reveals pathologic features consistent with CJD or fails to suggest an alternative diagnosis to explain the clinical findings, paraffin-embedded material (blocks or unstained slides) must accompany the frozen specimen to the reference laboratory to allow immunohistochemistry to be performed. CJD pathology can be patchy within the brain (even when the abnormal protein is widespread), and rare cases of CJD are caused by a protease-sensitive prion requiring immunohistochemical rather than immunoblot analysis for definitive diagnosis (*Ann Neurol.* 2010;68:162). Lab equipment (gloves, instruments, etc.) are decontaminated with 1N sodium hydroxide solution for a minimum of 1 hour or, alternatively, in 10% or 20% bleach solution for 1 hour, followed by autoclaving. Many disinfection protocols that may be more or less appropriate for particular circumstances have been reported (*Infect Control Hosp Epidemiol.* 2010;31:107). Frozen tissue diagnosis should not be attempted on tissues suspected of prion protein diseases.

B. **Ancillary studies**
   1. **Electron microscopy (EM).** The utilization of EM for diagnosis of CNS lesions is labor intensive, time-consuming, and expensive, and it is mainly used to evaluate nerve and muscle biopsies. However, ultrastructural evaluation remains invaluable for many other neuropathologic diagnoses, including CADASIL (see Section VIII.D), neuronal ceroid lipofuscinoses, and for distinguishing ambiguous brain tumor cases, particularly meningioma and ependymoma.
   2. **Immunohistochemistry** is now routinely used in evaluation of complex surgical neuropathology cases, especially in the area of tumor neuropathology. Frequently utilized antibodies and their immunoreactivity for common tumor types are summarized in Table 41.1.

TABLE 41.1 Typical Immunoprofiles of Common CNS Neoplasms

Tumor	Positive (+)	Positive or negative (±)	Negative (−)
PA	GFAP	NF (few entrapped axons)	IDH-1, YKL-40
GBM (primary)	GFAP, YKL-40, NF (axons), S-100, CK		IDH-1, CAM 5.2
DA	S-100, GFAP, IDH-1[a]		CK[b], LCA, SYN, HMB-45
Oligodendroglioma	S-100, GFAP[c], IDH-1		CK[b], LCA
Ependymoma	S-100, GFAP, D2-40, and CD99 (lumens)	SYN (dot-like)	LCA, SYN, IDH-1-
Choroid plexus tumors	S-100, CK, VIM, transthyretin[d]	EMA (luminal), CK	EMA, CEA
Metastatic carcinoma	EMA and CK, CK7 (lung), CK20 (colon), TTF1 (lung), CAM 5.2	GFAP	GFAP, LCA, HMB-45, IDH-1
Melanoma	S-100, HMB-45, Melan-A (MART-1)	CEA, S-100, SYN	GFAP, CK, LCA, IDH-1
Lymphoma	LCA, CD20 (L26), CD79a		CK, GFAP, HMB-45, SYN, CD3
Meningioma	EMA, VIM, PR[f], BAF47	EMA[e]	GFAP, HMB-45
HPC	VIM, CD99, bcl-2, Factor XIIIa[h]	S-100, CD34, CK[g]	EMA, CK, GFAP, S-100
Medulloblastoma	SYN, BAF47	CD34	CK, LCA, EMA
AT/RT	VIM, EMA, CK, actin	S-100, GFAP	PLAP, β-hCG, LCA, **BAF47**[i]
GG	SYN, NF, CG, GFAP	SYN, GFAP, desmin, AFP	CK, EMA, PLAP
Central neurocytoma	SYN, Neu-N	Neu-N	NF, CG, CK, LCA
Schwannoma	S-100[j], CD34, Coll IV[j]	GFAP, S-100	EMA, NF, CK
Paraganglioma	SYN, CG, S-100[l]	GFAP, HMB-45[k]	GFAP, CK, HMB-45
HB	S-100, NSE, inhibin	NF	CK, EMA
Germinoma	OCT4, D2-40[m], c-kit (CD117)[m], PLAP	GFAP	AFP, EMA, HMB-45, LCA
Yolk sac tumor	AFP, CK	β-hCG[n], CK	β-hCG, GFAP, OCT4, EMA
Choriocarcinoma	β-hCG, CK, EMA	PLAP, c-kit[m]	AFP, OCT4, GFAP, HMB-45
Embryonal carcinoma	CK, OCT4, PLAP, CD30	PLAP	β-hCG, LCA, HMB-45
Teratoma	CK, EMA	c-kit[m], AFP, EMA, D2-40[m]	β-hCG, c-kit

[a]IDH-1 stains the majority of diffuse gliomas including secondary GBM, but not primary GBM.
[b]CAM 5.2 recommended, because CK (AE1/AE3) AE1/AE3 stains reactive astrocytes and frequently stains gliomas.
[c]Strongly positive in minigemistocytes and gliofibrillary oligodendrocytes.
[d]Not specific for choroid plexus.
[e]Positive in myeloma.
[f]Nuclear PR reactivity is strong in most WHO I meningiomas, weaker or absent in WHO grade II and III.
[g]Positive in secretory variant.
[h]Characteristic pattern of scattered, individual immunoreactive cells.
[i]Loss of BAF-47 immunoreactivity is observed in the vast majority of ATRT; reactivity is retained in most other pathologies.
[j]Diffuse, strong expression.
[k]Positive in melanotic schwannomas.
[l]Positive in sustentacular cells.
[m]Membranous pattern in germinoma, cytoplasmic in embryonal carcinoma/yolk sac tumor.
[n]Positive in syncytiotrophoblasts, present in a minority of the cases.

GFAP, glial fibrillary acid protein; NF, neurofilament; IDH-1, isocitrate dehydrogenase 1; YKL-40, chitinase-3-like 1; CK, cytokeratin; CAM5.2, cytokeratin negative in glial cells; TTF1, thyroid transcription factor 1; LCA, leukocyte common antigen; SYN, synaptophysin; D2-40, podoplanin; EMA, epithelial membrane antigen; VIM, vimentin; PR, progesterone receptor; CEA, carcinoembryonic antigen; PLAP, placental alkaline phosphatase; AFP, α-fetoprotein; β-hCG, β-human chorionic gonadotrophin; BAF47, also called SNF5 and INI1; CG, chromogranin; Coll IV, collagen type IV; NSE, neuron-specific enolase.

a. **Glial markers.** The most commonly used glial marker in neuropathology practice is glial fibrillary acid protein (GFAP). This intermediate filament protein is fairly (but not completely) specific for glial lineage. However, it does not reliably distinguish astrocytic, oligodendroglial, and ependymal tumors from one another, and may also be encountered in other tumors with glial differentiation such as choroid plexus tumors, medulloblastomas and/or primitive neuroectodermal tumors (PNETs), gangliogliomas (GGs). GFAP can even be detected to some extent in nonglial neoplasms, such as nerve sheath and cartilaginous tumors.

b. **Neuronal markers.** The most commonly used neuronal markers include neurofilament (NF) protein, synaptophysin (SYN), chromogranin, and Neu-N.

SYN is one of the more sensitive markers of neuronal differentiation. It is typically found even in the most primitive neuronal tumors (medulloblastomas and PNETs) and is very useful for highlighting neoplastic ganglion cells, pituitary adenomas and carcinomas, carcinoid tumors, neurocytomas, and paragangliomas. One major disadvantage of SYN is that it fails to differentiate native (entrapped) neuropil from tumor neuropil. Additionally SYN stains a proportion of tumors (e.g., pilocytic astrocytomas [PAs]) that are generally not considered to have neuronal differentiation. In some cases, however, this feature is actually somewhat useful; classic oligodendrogliomas show dot-like paranuclear reactivity for SYN.

NF is a heteropolymer unique to neurons and axons. Mature neuronal tumors, such as GGs, often stain for NF; however, more primitive neuronal tumors such as medulloblastomas are often negative. Additionally, NF also stains normal axons, a property that is of great utility for demonstrating an infiltrative growth pattern by highlighting entrapped axons (e-**Fig. 41.3**).

Neu-N is a marker of advanced neuronal differentiation; it has the advantage of clearly marking neuronal nuclei and cell bodies rather than surrounding neuropil. As a result, it is particularly useful for identifying architectural abnormalities in cortical dysplasia, and for highlighting neuronal loss (e.g., in mesial temporal sclerosis) and neurons entrapped within invasive tumors. Surprisingly, most neoplastic ganglion cells in GGs are negative for Neu-N; this feature can be useful because entrapped cortical neurons are virtually always strongly positive.

c. **Epithelial markers.** The commonly used epithelial markers include cytokeratin (CK; AE1/AE3), epithelial membrane antigen (EMA), and CAM 5.2. CKs are used predominantly in the diagnosis of metastatic carcinomas, but are also used to identify craniopharyngiomas, chordomas, and choroid plexus tumors. Due to cross-reactivity with GFAP, gliomas (and reactive astrocytes) may show CK reactivity, a major pitfall in the differential between glioblastoma (GBM) and metastatic carcinoma. In such instances, CAM 5.2 is recommended, because gliomas (and reactive astrocytes) are virtually always negative. EMA is frequently used in the identification of meningiomas, which, unlike true epithelial tumors, usually display minimal to no CK expression (secretory meningioma is an exception). EMA is also useful in the diagnosis of ependymomas, along with CD99 and D2–40 antibody (podoplanin).

d. **S-100 protein** is a marker of neuroectodermal cells, including melanocytes, glia, Schwann cells, chondrocytes, and the sustentacular cells in tumors such as paraganglioma, pheochromocytoma, and olfactory neuroblastoma. In conjunction with collagen IV, which stains basement membranes, S-100 is particularly helpful for demonstrating

Schwann cell differentiation in benign and malignant peripheral nerve sheath tumors (MPNSTs).

e. **Proliferation markers** are used in conjunction with mitotic counts in brain tumors to guide determination of tumor grade and prognosis. The most widely used marker is Ki-67, which labels nuclei that are not in the G_0 phase of the cell cycle.

f. **"Molecular test" markers.** Recently, several antibodies have been developed that can be used in lieu of more complicated molecular tests for diagnosis and prognosis of various neoplasms.

  i. **INI1/BAF47 deletions** are detected in ~70% of the atypical teratoid/rhabdoid tumors (AT/RTs); however, loss of the corresponding INI1 protein is even more common than the genetic alteration. Loss of INI1 nuclear immunoreactivity in tumor cells is used as a surrogate for genetic testing to demonstrate biallelic inactivation of the gene.

  ii. **Isocitrate dehydrogenase (IDH1/IDH2) mutations** have been detected in the majority of diffuse gliomas, with the notable exception of primary (de novo) GBM, and appear to play a fundamental and early role in oncogenesis (*N Eng J Med.* 2009;360:765). The most common mutation is in the IDH1 gene (R132H), and is recognized by monoclonal antibody IDH-1. Diagnostically, this immunohistochemical stain shows greatest promise for its potential to distinguish low-grade diffuse glioma from gliosis (*Am J Surg Pathol.* 2010;34:1199; *Acta Neuropathol.* 2010;119:509). Prognostically, the presence of this mutation is favorable, as such tumors appear to show greater response to therapy.

3. **Molecular diagnostics** involves the measurement of diagnostically or prognostically relevant pathologic features at the DNA (epigenetic, genomic [nuclear or mitochondrial], mRNA, or protein levels.

The most common and practical approaches to detect changes in DNA (deletions of chromosomal regions, amplifications of oncogenes, or loss of specific tumor suppressor genes) include fluorescence in situ hybridization (FISH) and quantitative polymerase chain reaction (PCR) techniques. FISH has the advantages of simplicity, morphologic preservation, and minimal tissue and purity requirements. However, FISH is insensitive to very small deletions/amplifications, substitution mutations, or epigenetic modification (e.g., methylation).

The most notable use of FISH in surgical neuropathology is to detect losses of chromosomal arms 1p and 19q testing as a prognostic and/or management tool for adult patients with oligodendroglial tumors (*Adv Anat Pathol.* 2005;12:180). Other clinical applications of FISH include detection of EGFR amplification and/or 10q deletions to distinguish the small cell variant of GBM from anaplastic oligodendroglioma; 22q11.2 deletion (INI1 locus) to distinguish AT/RT from variants of medulloblastoma (*Hum Pathol.* 2001;32:156); isochromosome 17q (i17q) and *NMYC* or *CMYC* amplifications to diagnose and predict outcome for medulloblastomas, large cell/anaplastic medulloblastomas and other aggressive forms of CNS-PNET; meningioma-associated deletions (*NF2, DAL1,* 1p, 14q) to distinguish anaplastic meningiomas from other malignancies or benign meningiomas from foci of meningothelial hyperplasia; and (9p21) to provide prognostic information about higher-grade meningiomas.

A common use of PCR-based techniques is to detect O6-methylguanine-DNA methyltransferase (MGMT) gene methylation, which blocks MGMT transcription. As the MGMT gene product plays an important role in DNA repair, GBMs with this epigenetic modification show greater sensitivity to alkylating agents (like temozolomide) and radiation therapy (*N Eng J Med.* 2005;352:987).

IV. **BASIC ELEMENTS OF CNS PATHOLOGY.** The cells and tissues of the CNS are capable of displaying diverse histologic abnormalities. A few of these are pathognomonic for a given disease, but most diseases require a constellation of findings to suggest a diagnosis.

A. **Neurons.**

1. **Axonal injury.** When an axon is damaged and the associated neuron survives, the axon itself may form a swelling, or axonal spheroid, at the site of injury. If the axon is severed, in most cases the distal portion will disintegrate in an active cellular process called Wallerian degeneration. In some cases, the axotomized neuron will undergo "chromatolysis," in which the cell body appears mildly swollen and achromatic; this change reflects a loss of Nissl substance that occurs as the cell alters its metabolism to allow repair of its damaged axon.

2. **Apoptosis.** If neuronal injury is severe enough to cause cell death, neurons may undergo apoptosis (as occurs in the basis pontis and subiculum from hypoxic ischemic injury late in gestation, a pattern labeled with the misnomer pontosubicular necrosis). Alternatively, neurons may undergo necrosis.

3. **Necrosis.** The classic histologic appearance of acute neuronal necrosis includes (1) variably intense cytoplasmic eosinophilia (accounting for the name "red neurons") and (2) shrunken pyknotic nuclei (e-**Fig. 41.4**). Red neurons require 12 to 24 hours to develop within a living brain; individuals who die within minutes or a few hours of an ischemic stroke do not show red neurons in affected region(s). Although red neurons are commonly caused by ischemia, many insults (e.g., hypoxia, hypoglycemia, epilepsy, herpes simplex virus [HSV] infection) can also cause neuronal necrosis. It is important to note that a common artifact caused by overmanipulation of fresh brain tissue can cause normal healthy neurons to (superficially) resemble red neurons. Neurons affected by this "dark cell change" usually show more basophilia than red neurons, a nucleus that is less distinct within the cell body, and an apical dendrite that resembles a spiral or corkscrew (e-**Fig. 41.5**).

4. **Ferrugination.** Occasionally, damaged neurons around the edge of a remote infarct or traumatic injury become encrusted with basophilic iron and calcium salts. This condition is often referred to as mineralization or ferrugination.

5. **Binucleation** of neurons, rare in normal brains, is infrequently noted in dysplastic/malformative processes (e.g., tuberous sclerosis, TS), in certain neoplasms (e.g., GG), and in Alzheimer disease (AD) (*Neuropathol Appl Neurobiol.* 2008;34:457) (e-**Fig. 41.6**).

6. **Intraneuronal inclusion bodies** form within neurons under many different circumstances. Some are pathognomonic, some are associated with one or more diseases, and others appear to have no pathologic significance.

   a. **Pick bodies** are round, tau-positive intracytoplasmic neuronal inclusions. In Pick disease (a form of frontotemporal dementia), these are argyrophilic by Bielschowsky and Bodian (but not Gallyas) silver stains and are abundant in neurons of the cortex, hippocampus, and dentate gyrus. A similar (but less abundant, Gallyas positive) inclusion is seen in corticobasal degeneration.

   b. **Lewy bodies** (LBs). Classic LBs, which occur within pigmented neurons of the brainstem, are spherical cytoplasmic inclusions with an eosinophilic core and a pale halo (e-**Fig. 41.7**). By contrast, cortical LBs appear as subtle spheres of homogeneous eosinophilia. Making detection even more difficult, cortical LBs are not argyrophilic. Fortunately, LBs all show immunoreactivity for ubiquitin and α-synuclein (e-Fig. 41.8). These lesions (along with similar inclusions [Lewy neurites] that appear within cell processes) are seen in Lewy body disorders (e.g., Parkinson disease [PD], and dementia with Lewy bodies [DLBs]).

c. **Marinesco bodies** are small, eosinophilic, strongly ubiquitin-positive intranuclear inclusions located chiefly in pigmented brain stem neurons (e-Fig. 41.9). These have no known pathologic significance.

d. **Neurofibrillary tangles (NFTs)** (e-Fig. 41.10) are argyrophilic intracytoplasmic filamentous aggregates of hyperphosphorylated tau protein. Although characteristic of AD, they also appear in many other neurodegenerative disorders, and in rare GGs.

e. **Hirano bodies** are brightly eosinophilic rod-shaped or elliptical cytoplasmic inclusions that occur within the proximal dendrites of neurons, particularly in the hippocampus. Although not specific, they are particularly numerous in brains with AD pathology (e-Fig. 41.11).

f. **Granulovacuolar degeneration (GVD)** is common in hippocampal pyramidal neurons in AD, and less common in older brains without AD. GVD resembles many small bubbles, each with a small basophilic granule.

g. **TDP-43 neuronal cytoplasmic inclusions (NCIs),** as the name suggests, are immunoreactive for TDP-43. Although NCIs are characteristic of a subset of frontotemporal dementias, they are not specific, and may be seen in the temporal lobe in other neurodegenerative diseases (e.g., AD).

h. **Bunina bodies** are eosinophilic ubiquitin and TDP-43 immunoreactive intracytoplasmic inclusions that form in motor neurons in cases of familial and sporadic amyotrophic lateral sclerosis (ALS).

B. **Astrocytes**

1. **Reactive astrocytosis.** Normally, astrocytes are evenly dispersed (albeit with regional variation), mitotically silent, and GFAP positive. In most forms of brain injury, astrocytes become hypertrophic, increase their GFAP content, and may proliferate. Reactive astrocytes have prominent stellate processes and, often, abundant eccentrically distributed glassy cytoplasm that inspires the moniker "gemistocyte." Nevertheless, reactive astrocytes generally maintain an even distribution, and do not exhibit nuclear atypia (radiation exposure is an exception). Grossly, tissues affected by chronic astrocytosis are usually firm; thus, the term "gliotic" is used to describe brain tissues that appear unusually firm or rubbery.

2. **Bergmann gliosis** refers to an accumulation of astrocytic nuclei (usually in association with neuron loss) within the Purkinje cell layer of the cerebellum.

3. **Alzheimer type II astrocytes,** with swollen pale nuclei and minimal visible cytoplasm, appear in hyperammonemic states (e.g., liver failure, Wilson disease). In the cortex and striatum, these nuclei are round with a prominent nucleolus (e-Fig. 41.12); in the pallidum, dentate nucleus, and brainstem, they are irregular and lobated.

4. **Corpora amylacea** are basophilic, round, concentrically lamellated aggregates of polyglucosan (polyglucosan bodies) that develop within astrocytic processes. Common in normal brains, particularly near ventricular and pial surfaces, these become more numerous with age. Similar structures (Lafora bodies) form in far greater numbers in astrocytes and neurons (and in eccrine sweat glands) in Lafora body disease.

5. **Rosenthal fibers (RFs)** are brightly eosinophilic, somewhat refractile, irregular/beaded structures that range from ~10 to 40 μm in diameter. EM reveals them as swollen astrocytic processes filled with electron-dense amorphous granular material and glial filaments. RFs are commonly observed in PA, but

are also commonly seen in nonneoplastic tissues adjacent to slowly growing neoplasms (e.g., craniopharyngioma, ependymoma), cysts, and syrinx; such RF-abundant tissue reaction is called piloid gliosis (e-**Fig. 41.13**).

   6. **Eosinophilic granular bodies (EGBs),** although not present in nonneoplastic astrocytes, are found in slowly growing astrocytic and glioneuronal tumors (PA, GG, and pleomorphic xanthoastrocytoma [PXA]). EGBs appear on H&E sections (or cytologic smear preparations) as refractile clusters of small, round hyaline droplets, and are PAS-positive (e-**Fig. 41.14**).

C. **Microglia.** Normal residents of the brain, microglial cells are of monocytic lineage (and are consequently immunoreactive for leukocyte common antigen [LCA/CD45] as well as CD68 and CD163). In response to various signals, these cells undergo activation, whereupon they change their morphology (appearing as irregular elongated "rod cells"), become motile, and intensify their communication with other cells via secreted factors (e.g., cytokines and interleukins). They may also participate in limited phagocytosis. Small clusters of activated microglial cells (microglial nodules) are characteristic of viral encephalitis and may be seen decorating dying neurons, in a process called neuronophagia. Capacity for phagocytosis increases in the setting of injury, infection, or demyelinating disease when microglia differentiates into macrophages. Monocytes and macrophages may also be recruited into the CNS from the systemic circulation. Occasionally, brisk mitotic activity among macrophages in these settings (particularly in tumefactive multiple sclerosis (MS), which radiographically resembles GBM) can cause diagnostic confusion with gliomas. Gliomas themselves often contain a large number of microglial cells, which appear to play a role in tumorigenesis (*Cancer Res.* 2008;68:10358).

D. **Cerebral edema** is an increase in brain volume due to increased water content. Depending on its pathogenesis, cerebral edema can be classified as vasogenic, cytotoxic, osmotic, or interstitial (resulting from obstructive hydrocephalus). However, combinations of different edema types often coexist. In vasogenic edema, the fluid collection is predominantly extracellular and results from breakdown of the blood–brain barrier. In cytotoxic edema, the fluid accumulation is intracellular, the result of impaired Na/K-ATPase function in glial cells caused by toxins, ischemia, or various other conditions. Osmotic edema results when osmolality of the brain interstitial fluid exceeds that of the plasma. Interstitial edema results from transependymal flow from the ventricles in the setting of obstructive hydrocephalus.

E. **Hydrocephalus,** an abnormal increase in the intracranial volume of CSF associated with dilatation of all or part of the ventricular system, may be classified as communicating, noncommunicating (obstructive), normal pressure, or *ex vacuo.*

   1. **Noncommunicating** hydrocephalus results from physical blockage of CSF flow, usually by tumor compressing a narrow channel, such as the foramen of Monro or the cerebral aqueduct.

   2. **Communicating** hydrocephalus results from impaired resorption of CSF at the arachnoid granulations, as may occur in the setting of subarachnoid hemorrhage or meningitis; less commonly, it may result from increased CSF production, for example, by a choroid plexus papilloma.

   3. **Normal pressure hydrocephalus (NPH),** characterized classically by the clinical triad of dementia, ataxia, and incontinence, is poorly understood. NPH may represent a circumstance in which production and resorption of CSF reach a new equilibrium after a prolonged period of impaired resorption.

   4. **Hydrocephalus *ex vacuo*** describes a state of ventricle expansion due to loss of adjacent parenchyma or generalized cerebral atrophy (as occurs in AD).

F. **Intracranial pressure** (ICP) and **brain herniation.** Normally, the cranial cavity contents (blood, brain, and CSF) are maintained in volumetric balance within the rigid skull and dura. ICP increases when this balance is strained, as may result from diffuse brain edema, increased cerebral blood flow and blood volume, or development of space-occupying lesions (e.g., tumor, abscess, hematoma, or large edematous infarct). Elevated ICP, if not treated, can cause herniation; herniation syndromes include subfalcine (cingulate gyrus), transtentorial (uncal), and cerebellar tonsillar/brainstem herniations.

G. **Duret (secondary brain stem) hemorrhage** occurs when penetrating pontine arteries (which arise perpendicularly from the basilar artery) become kinked in association with brainstem herniation; the resulting acute hemorrhagic infarction of the pons is often fatal.

V. **NEOPLASMS OF THE CNS.** For most CNS tumors, incidence varies greatly with age and gender. Among adults, metastases, GBM, and meningioma are the most common CNS neoplasms; among children, PA, medulloblastoma, and ependymoma are far more common. Likewise, tumors often differ in their radiographic features and propensity for certain anatomic sites. For this reason, microscopic evaluation of a CNS biopsy specimen is incomplete without considering the neuroradiologic findings that describe the targeted lesion in situ. Indeed, neuroradiologic assessment can be considered to be the neuropathology surrogate for gross examination. Imaging studies are particularly helpful when evaluating small biopsy samples. The World Health Organization (WHO) currently lists more than 100 types of CNS tumors and their variants (Table 41.2). Table 41.3 organizes common CNS tumor diagnoses on the basis of location, patient age, and imaging characteristics.

Histologic features are also critical for diagnosis. Because a final diagnosis may not be obvious from an initial histomorphologic examination, it is worthwhile to begin with a broad differential based on a specimen's general histopathologic pattern. Table 41.4 lists eight major histopathologic patterns that may be encountered, along with their most commonly associated diagnostic entities. Once a differential diagnosis has been formulated on the basis of these data, closer examination of microscopic details can refine the differential further and suggest what ancillary tests (if any) are required to arrive at a final diagnosis.

A. Gliomas

1. **Diffuse (infiltrating) astrocytomas (DAs), WHO grade II.** Diffuse gliomas are the most frequent primary CNS neoplasms. Because they are diffusely infiltrative, complete resection is nearly impossible. On MRI, DAs are nonenhancing, T1 hypointense, T2/FLAIR hyperintense, ill-defined intra-axial masses that can occur throughout the neuraxis, but commonly involve the cerebral hemispheres. Clinically, they present with new-onset seizures (the most common symptom), headaches, or functional neurologic deficits. Grossly, these lesions may appear gray-tan to gelatinous and obscure the native gray-white junction. Microscopically, tumor cells invade adjacent cortex along white matter tracts. They aggregate around neurons and blood vessels and beneath pial and ependymal surfaces to produce the so-called secondary structures of Scherer. The cytologic features of astrocytic tumor cells can vary widely from uniform and minimally atypical, to highly pleomorphic both in cytoplasmic and nuclear features (e-Fig. 41.15). Cells with elongate, irregular, hyperchromatic nuclei with minimal cytoplasm are seen in fibrillary astrocytomas, whereas cells with eccentrically located nuclei and abundant eosinophilic cytoplasm characterize the gemistocytic variant. Tumor cells are often, but not invariably, immunoreactive to GFAP. A recently identified immunohistochemical marker, antibody IDH-1, is proving invaluable for distinguishing the majority of DAs (but not primary GBMs) from gliosis. Mitotic activity is very low or nonexistent.

2. **Anaplastic astrocytoma (AA), WHO grade III,** is a diffusely infiltrating glioma with a mean age of presentation in the fifth decade. AA may appear

TABLE 41.2	WHO Classification and Grading of CNS Tumors			
	I	II	III	IV
Tumors of neuroepithelial tissue				
Astrocytic tumors				
PA	*			
PMA		*		
SEGA	*			
PXA		*		
DA		*		
Fibrillary astrocytoma				
Gemistocytic astrocytoma				
Protoplasmic astrocytoma				
AA			*	
GBM				*
Giant cell GBM				*
GS				*
Gliomatosis cerebri			*	
Oligodendroglial tumors				
Oligodendroglioma		*		
Anaplastic oligodendroglioma			*	
Oligoastrocytic tumors				
Oligoastrocytoma		*		
Anaplastic oligoastrocytoma			*	
Ependymal tumors				
Subependymoma	*			
Myxopapillary ependymoma	*			
Ependymoma		*		
Cellular		*		
Papillary		*		
Clear cell		*		
Tanycytic		*		
Anaplastic ependymoma			*	
Choroid plexus tumors				
Choroid plexus papilloma	*			
Atypical choroid plexus papilloma		*		
Choroid plexus carcinoma			*	
Other neuroepithelial tumors				
AB				
CGs of the third ventricle		*		
AGs	*			
Neuronal and mixed neuronal-glial tumors				
Dysplastic gangliocytoma of cerebellum (Lhermitte–Duclos)	*			
Desmoplastic infantile astrocytoma/GG	*			
DNT	*			
Gangliocytoma	*			
GG	*			
Anaplastic GG			*	
Central neurocytoma		*		
Extraventricular neurocytoma		*		
Cerebellar liponeurocytoma		*		

(continued)

TABLE 41.2 WHO Classification and Grading of CNS Tumors (*Continued*)

	I	II	III	IV
PGNT	*			
RGNT of the fourth ventricle	*			
Paraganglioma	*			
Tumors of the pineal region				
Pineocytoma	*			
PPTID		*	*	
Pineoblastoma				*
PTPR		*	*	
Embryonal tumors				
Medulloblastoma				*
Desmoplastic/nodular medulloblastoma				*
Medulloblastoma with extensive nodularity				*
Anaplastic medulloblastoma				*
Large cell medulloblastoma				*
CNS PNET				*
CNS neuroblastoma				*
CNS ganglioneuroblastoma				*
Medulloepithelioma				*
Ependymoblastoma				*
AT/RT				*
Tumors of cranial and paraspinal nerves				
Schwannoma (neurilemoma, neurinomas)	*			
Cellular	*			
Plexiform	*			
Melanotic	*			
Neurofibroma	*			
Plexiform				
Perineurioma, NOS	*	*	*	
Perineurioma (intraneural)	*			
Malignant perineurioma			*	
MPNSTs		*	*	
Epithelioid MPNST		*	*	
MPNST with mesenchymal differentiation		*	*	
Melanotic MPNST		*	*	
MPNST with glandular differentiation		*	*	
Tumors of the meninges				
Meningioma				
Meningothelial	*			
Fibrous (fibroblastic)	*			
Transitional (mixed)	*			
Psammomatous	*			
Angiomatous	*			
Microcystic	*			
Secretory	*			
Lymphoplasmacyte-rich	*			
Metaplastic	*			
Chordoid		*		
Clear cell		*		
Atypical		*		

(*continued*)

TABLE 41.2	WHO Classification and Grading of CNS Tumors (*Continued*)			
		I	II	III	IV

	I	II	III	IV
Papillary			*	
Rhabdoid			*	
Anaplastic (malignant)			*	
Mesenchymal, nonmeningothelial tumors				
Lipoma				
Angiolipoma				
Hibernoma				
Liposarcoma				
Fibromatosis				
SFT				
Inflammatory myofibroblastic tumor				
Fibrosarcoma				
Malignant fibrous histiocytoma				
Leiomyoma				
Leiomyosarcoma				
Rhabdomyoma				
Rhabdomyosarcoma				
Chondroma				
Chondrosarcoma				
Osteoma				
Osteosarcoma				
Osteochondroma				
Hemangioma				
Epithelioid hemangioendothelioma				
HPC		*		
Anaplastic HPC			*	
Angiosarcoma				
Kaposi sarcoma				
Ewing sarcoma–PNET				
Primary melanocytic lesions				
Diffuse melanocytosis				
Melanocytoma				
Malignant melanoma				
Melanomatosis				
Other neoplasms related to the meninges				
HB	*			
Tumors of the hematopoietic system				
Malignant lymphomas/primary CNSLs				
B-cell lymphoma				
DLBCL				
Low-grade B-cell lymphoma				
Marginal zone B-cell lymphoma				
Plasmacytoma				
Intravascular B-cell lymphoma				
T-cell lymphoma				
Anaplastic large-cell lymphoma				
NK/T-cell lymphoma				
Hodgkin's disease				

(continued)

| **TABLE 41.2** | WHO Classification and Grading of CNS Tumors (*Continued*) |

	I	II	III	IV
Histiocytic tumors				
LCH				
Rosai–Dorfman disease				
Erdheim–Chester disease				
Haemophagocytic lymphohistiocytosis				
JXG				
Malignant histiocytic disorders (histiocytic sarcoma)				
GCTs				
Germinoma				
Embryonal carcinoma				
Yolk sac tumor				
Choriocarcinoma				
Teratoma				
Mature				
Immature				
Teratoma with malignant transformation				
Mixed GCT				
Tumors of the sellar region				
Craniopharyngioma		*		
Adamantinomatous		*		
Papillary		*		
Granular cell tumor of the neurohypophysis		*		
Pituicytoma		*		
Spindle cell oncocytoma of the adenohypophysis		*		

Modified from: Louis DN, Ohgaki H, Wiestler OD, Cavenee WK, eds. *WHO Classification of Tumours of the Central Nervous System.* Lyon: IARC Press; 2007. Used with permission.

de novo, or through progression of a preexisting DA. Like DA, AA preferentially involves the cerebral hemispheres. On MRI, AA is similar to DA, but may show faint focal enhancement. Histologically, AA is distinguished by increased cellularity, pleomorphism, and increased proliferative index. The defining feature that distinguishes AA from DA is mitotic activity, which should be evaluated in the context of sample size. In a limited (needle/core) biopsy, a single mitosis is sufficient to designate a glioma as anaplastic. However, in large resections there should be at least a few mitoses before the tumor is considered anaplastic. By definition, AAs do not have microvascular proliferation or necrosis.

3. **Glioblastoma (multiforme; GBM), WHO grade IV,** is the most malignant form of astrocytoma and also the most common glioma subtype. GBMs occur mostly in adults with a peak age of onset in the sixth to seventh decades. On imaging, GBMs show heterogeneous or ring enhancement, and are differentiated from AA histologically by endothelial hyperplasia (EH) and/or necrosis; the latter is often characterized as pseudopalisading (hypercellular tumor cells arranged radially around a zone of central necrosis). EH, also referred to as microvascular proliferation or endothelial proliferation, is defined by the presence of multilayered vessel walls with enlarged, often cytologically atypical and mitotically active endothelial (and smooth muscle/pericytic) cells, sometimes forming glomeruloid structures with multiple lumina (**e-Fig. 41.16**). Recently, it has been demonstrated that some of the cells in these abnormal vessels are created through metaplasia of

TABLE 41.3 Common CNS Tumor Diagnosis by Location, Age, and Imaging Characteristics

Location	Child/young adult	Older adult
Cerebral/supratentorial	GG (TL, cyst-MEN) DNT (TL, intracortical nodules) PNET (solid, E) AT/RT (infant) PXA (cyst-MEN)	Grade II–III glioma (NE) GBM (ring E, butterfly) Mets (gray-white junctions, E) Lymphoma (periventricular, E)
Cerebellar/infratentorial	PA (cyst-MEN) Medulloblastoma (vermis, E) Ependymoma (4th v., E) Choroid plexus papilloma (4th v.) AT/RT (infant)	Mets (multiple, E) HB (cyst-MEN) Choroid plexus papilloma (4th v.)
Brain stem	"brain stem glioma" (pons) PA (dorsal brain stem)	Gliomatosis cerebri (multifocal)
Spinal cord (intra-axial)	Ependymoma PA (cystic)	Ependymoma DA (ill-defined) Paraganglioma (filum terminale) Myxopapillary ependymoma (filum terminale)
Extra-axial/dural	Secondary lymphoma/leukemia	Meningioma Metastases HPC/SFT Secondary lymphoma/leukemia
Intrasellar	Pituitary adenoma Craniopharyngioma Rathke's cleft cyst	Pituitary adenoma Rathke's cleft cyst
Suprasellar/hypothalamic/ optic pathway/3rd v.	Germinoma/GCT Craniopharyngioma PA PMA (E)	Colloid cyst (3rd v.)
Pineal	Germinoma/GCT Pineocytoma Pineoblastoma Pineal cyst	Pineocytoma Pineal cyst
Thalamus	PA AA/GBM	AA/GBM Lymphoma
Cerebellopontine angle	Vestibular schwannoma (NF2)	Vestibular schwannoma Meningioma
Lateral ventricle	Central neurocytoma SEGA (TS) Choroid plexus papilloma Choroid plexus carcinoma (infant)	Central neurocytoma SEGA (TS) Choroid plexus papilloma Subependymoma
Nerve root/paraspinal	Neurofibroma (NF1) MPNST (NF1)	Schwannoma Meningioma Secondary lymphoma Neurofibroma (NF1) MPNST

CNS, central nervous system; MEN, mural enhancing nodule; NE, nonenhancing; E, enhancing; DNT, dysembryoplastic neuroepithelial tumor; MPNST, malignant peripheral nerve sheath tumor; SEGA, subependymal giant cell astrocytoma; TL, temporal lobe; PNET, primitive neuroectodermal tumor; AT/RT, atypical teratoid rhabdoid tumor; GBM, glioblastoma; v., ventricle; AA, anaplastic astrocytoma; NF, neurofilament.

TABLE 41.4 Major Histopathologic Patterns in Surgical Neuropathology

I. Parenchymal infiltrate with hypercellularity
- Diffuse glioma
- CNS lymphoma
- Infections
- Inflammatory demyelinating disease
- Organizing infarct
- Reactive gliosis

II. Discrete mass (pure)
- Metastasis
- Ependymoma
- Subependymoma
- SEGA
- Central neurocytoma
- Pineocytoma
- Primitive/embryonal tumor (e.g., AT/RT)
- Choroid plexus papilloma
- CCM/cavernous angioma/cavernoma
- HB

III. Solid and infiltrative process
- PA
- PXA
- GBM/GS
- GG
- DNT
- Primitive/embryonal tumor (e.g., medulloblastoma/PNETs)
- Choroid plexus carcinoma
- GCTs
- Craniopharyngioma
- CNS lymphoma
- Sarcoma
- Abscess and other forms of infection

IV. Vasculocentric process
- CNS lymphoma
- Lymphomatoid granulomatosis
- Intravascular lymphoma
- Vasculitis
- Meningioangiomatosis
- Acute demyelinating encephalomyelitis (ADEM)
- Amyloid angiopathy and lobar hemorrhage
- ABRA
- Arteriolosclerosis
- CADASIL
- Vascular malformation
- Infection (e.g., *Aspergillus*)
- Neurosarcoidosis
- Thromboembolic disease

(continued)

TABLE 41.4	Major Histopathologic Patterns in Surgical Neuropathology (*Continued*)

V. Extra-axial mass
- Meningioma
- HPC
- SFT
- Sarcomas
- Schwannoma
- Metastasis
- Melanoma/melanocytoma
- Secondary lymphoma/leukemia/plasmacytoma
- Paraganglioma
- Sarcoidosis/granulomatous diseases
- Inflammatory pseudotumors
- Calcifying pseudotumor of neuraxis
- Histiocytosis (e.g., Rosai–Dorfman disease)

VI. Meningeal infiltrate
- Meningeal carcinomatosis (or lymphomatosis, gliomatosis, melanomatosis, meningiomatosis, etc.)
- Meningitis
- Sarcoidosis/granulomatous diseases
- Collagen vascular disease
- Inflammatory disorder (e.g., Castleman disease)

VII. Destructive/necrotic process
- Cerebral infarct
- Tumor with treatment effect
- Infection
- Vasculitis
- Severe demyelinating disease

VIII. Subtle pathology or near normal biopsy
- Hypothalamic hamartoma
- Low-grade glioma
- Cortical dysplasia/tuber
- Mesial temporal sclerosis
- Heterotopia
- Ischemic disease
- Neurodegenerative disease
- Benign cysts
- Reactive gliosis
- Hepatic encephalopathy
- Cerebral edema
- Viral encephalitis

Modified from Short Course Syllabus #37, USCAP, 2006.

neoplastic glioma cells (*Nature* 2010;468:824). There are several morphologic variants of GBM.

a. **Small cell GBM (scGBM)** usually presents *de novo* rather than progressing from a lower-grade astrocytoma. The term "small cell" is not intended to draw a morphologic comparison to the neuroendocrine carcinoma of the lung with the same name; instead, it may be considered a foil of the previously named giant cell GBM. scGBM has some features that resemble high-grade oligodendroglioma, and other features that provide genuine diagnostic clues. At low magnification, the hypercellular sheets of scGBM appear bland. At higher power, scGBM shows slightly oval or elongate nuclei with mild hyperchromasia and delicate chromatin, perinuclear halos, microcalcifications, and "chicken-wire"-like branching capillaries. However, unlike most oligodendrogliomas, its mitotic rate is remarkably high (e-**Fig. 41.17**). This dissonance (bland histology and abundant mitotic figures) is often the first clue to the diagnosis (*Adv Anat Pathol.* 2005;12:180). Other helpful clues include radiographic ring-enhancement and, when present, focal EH and pseudopalisading necrosis. However, a subset of anaplastic oligodendrogliomas can show these features, and one-third of scGBMs do not.

Immunohistochemical and molecular characteristics can be used to distinguish scGBM and oligodendrogliomas. The tumor cells in scGBM often contain thin, GFAP-positive cytoplasmic processes; GFAP reactivity in oligodendrogliomas is usually restricted to minigemistocytes, gliofibrillary oligodendrocytes, and entrapped reactive astrocytes. The MIB-1 (Ki-67) labeling index is typically much higher in scGBM than in most anaplastic oligodendrogliomas, although the ranges of these indices overlap. More importantly, reactivity with antibody IDH-1 is uniformly absent in scGBM (a primary GBM) and present in the majority of oligodendrogliomas. Additionally, FISH studies have shown EGFR amplifications in ~70% and deletions of chromosome 10q in >90% of the scGBMs (e-**Fig. 41.18**); these are rare in oligodendroglioma. In contrast, codeletion of chromosomal arms 1p and 19q, common in oligodendrogliomas, is not observed in scGBM.

b. **Gliosarcoma (GS) WHO grade IV,** a variant of GBM, is often superficially located and, radiographically, deceptively circumscribed. GS exhibits astrocytic and sarcomatous elements, the latter usually resembling fibrosarcoma or malignant fibrous histiocytoma. However, GS may also exhibit bone, cartilage, muscle, and even epithelial lines of differentiation; when the latter is present, the tumor may be called adenoid GBM. Molecular studies have demonstrated similar genetic abnormalities within all histologic elements of the tumor, suggesting a clonal origin. The sarcomatous elements in GS are reticulin rich, typically negative for GFAP, and positive for vimentin, smooth muscle actin, muscle-specific action (MSA), etc., based on the sarcomatous differentiation pattern. In contrast, the glial regions are reticulin poor and GFAP positive.

4. **Gliomatosis cerebri** is an extensively infiltrative glioma, often of astrocytic type, that involves three or more lobes of the cerebrum and often extends into brain stem, cerebellum, and/or spinal cord as well. Microscopically, gliomatosis most often has features of AA but is associated with a poor prognosis regardless of the grade. Foci of progression to GBM are not uncommon.

5. **Circumscribed astrocytomas**

a. **Pilocytic astrocytoma (PA), WHO grade I** (e-**Fig. 41.19**), is a slowly growing, rather circumscribed neoplasm frequently occurring in children and young adults, with a predilection for cerebellum. It also occurs in the optic pathway, hypothalamus, dorsal brain stem, spinal cord, and rarely, cerebral hemispheres. Classically, these tumors appear in imaging studies as cystic lesions with an enhancing mural nodule. In the brain stem, they may occur as exophytic lesions. Histologically, these tumors have a biphasic pattern in which compact pilocytic areas are interspersed with microcystic loose and/or spongy areas. PA is variably cellular and populated by bipolar cells with long hair-like (piloid) processes. RFs and EGBs commonly occur within the compact (dense) regions and, although not specific for PA, provide very helpful diagnostic clues. Mitotic activity is low. The blood vessels within PAs are commonly hyalinized, and often exhibit linear glomeruloid tufts of EH. This feature, particularly when coupled with the marked nuclear atypia that commonly occurs in PA, can lead to confusion with high-grade glioma. However, the EH and nuclear atypia of PA have no prognostic significance. PAs usually follow a benign clinical course.

b. **Pilomyxoid astrocytoma (PMA), WHO grade II,** is a piloid neoplasm closely related to PA that presents in infants at a median age of 10 months, and favors the hypothalamus and optic chiasm. On MRI, PMA appears circumscribed and solid, hypointense on T1 and hyperintense on T2, and shows homogenous contrast enhancement. The histologic hallmark of PMA is the presence of monomorphous bipolar cells in a markedly mucoid matrix, with a prominent angiocentric arrangement that resembles the perivascular pseudorosettes of ependymoma (e-Fig. 41.20). As defined, PMA does not show RFs or EGBs. Nuclear atypia is uncommon. Mitoses can be present. Vascular proliferation resembling that in PA is characteristic. Necrosis may be seen. The tumor cells show strong and diffuse immunoreactivity for GFAP, S-100, and vimentin. A subset of tumor cells is also positive for SYN. Clinically, PMAs behave more aggressively than PAs, with frequent local recurrences and, often, CSF seeding at the time of diagnosis.

6. **Pleomorphic xanthoastrocytoma (PXA), WHO grade II,** is an epileptogenic neoplasm commonly located in the superficial cortical regions of the temporal lobe, often with meningeal attachment. Histologically, this tumor is composed of large pleomorphic, variably GFAP-positive astrocytes intermingled with less conspicuous spindled cells (e-Fig. 41.21). Some of the tumor cells have bizarre nuclei and nuclear pseudoinclusions, and multinucleated giant cells are common. EGBs are almost always evident. Xanthomatous tumor cells, although diagnostically helpful, only occur in 25% of the cases. Other features include perivascular plasmalymphocytic cuffing and scant mitoses. Reticulin silver stain highlights a network of basal laminae that surrounds individual tumor cells. Neuronal differentiation is often evidenced by reactivity for SYN and NF protein; reactivity for CD34 is frequently observed. Grade II PXAs have a relatively favorable prognosis (81% 5-year survival). Anaplastic (WHO grade III) transformation, characterized by less pleomorphism, increased proliferative activity, necrosis, and/or microvascular proliferation, occurs in 15% of the PXAs; reticulin staining is often diminished in these cases.

7. **Subependymal giant cell astrocytoma (SEGA), WHO grade I,** is almost exclusively found in children and young adults with tuberous sclerosis (TS). These well-circumscribed, intraventricular tumors usually occur near the foramen of Monro and cause symptoms associated with obstructive hydrocephalus. Imaging studies reveal contrast enhancement and calcification. Histologically, the tumor cells may be spindled, epithelioid, or gemistocyte-like, and may appear in sweeping fascicles, large clusters, or perivascular pseudorosettes. The gemistocyte-like cells have abundant glassy eosinophilic cytoplasm and nuclei resembling those of ganglion cells, with fine granular chromatin and prominent nucleoli (e-Fig. 41.22). The hybrid astrocytic and neuronal features of SEGAs are also reflected in their immunohistochemical profile, with focal reactivity for both GFAP and one or more neuronal markers (e.g., SYN). Mitoses are rare. Microvascular proliferation and necrosis are typically absent.

8. **Oligodendrogliomas, WHO grade II,** comprise 10% to 25% of all the adult gliomas, behave less aggressively than astrocytomas, and show slower progression and longer patient survival. The most useful histologic feature for distinguishing oligodendroglial neoplasms from astrocytic tumors is nuclear morphology; oligodendroglioma nuclei are nearly spherical, with delicate chromatin, crisp envelopes, and inconspicuous nucleoli (e-**Fig. 41.23**). Other helpful features include clear perinuclear haloes that often result as an artifact of routine histologic processing; a delicate hexagonal array of capillaries that resembles chicken wire; and mucin-rich microcystic spaces, microcalcifications, predominantly cortical involvement, and perineuronal satellitosis. Immunohistochemically, classic oligodendroglioma cells show no reactivity for GFAP. However, oligodendrogliomas often contain three cell types that do show such reactivity, specifically mini-gemistocytes, gliofibrillary oligodendrocytes, and reactive astrocytes. The mini-gemistocyte, named for its superficial resemblance to the larger astrocytic gemistocyte, has a belly of glassy, eosinophilic cytoplasm and an eccentrically placed oligodendroglial nucleus. Gliofibrillary oligodendrocytes are indistinguishable from classic oligodendroglial tumor cells on H&E stained sections, but show a GFAP-positive rim of cytoplasm and a tadpole-like tail. Entrapped, nonneoplastic astrocytes generally retain their characteristic stellate morphology.

In addition to oligodendrogliomas, several other tumors exhibit the so-called fried egg appearance with rounded nuclei and clear perinuclear haloes; most notably dysembryoplastic neuroepithelial tumor (DNT), PA, central neurocytoma, clear cell ependymoma, and mixed oligoastrocytoma (MOA). Nevertheless, this differential diagnosis can usually be resolved using clinical information, other histologic clues (e.g., RFs, EGBs, atypical astrocytic nuclei), immunohistochemical stains (e.g., GFAP, Neu-N, SYN, NF, IDH-1, EMA, CD99, D2-40, MIB-1), and FISH studies.

Ancillary genetic testing of oligodendrogliomas (*Adv Anat Pathol.* 2005;12:180) is now routinely performed. Several studies utilizing FISH techniques have established the presence of 1p and 19q codeletions in 60% to 90% of the oligodendrogliomas (e-**Fig. 41.24**); these tumors behave less aggressively, are more sensitive to chemotherapy and radiation, and are thus considered genetically favorable. Apart from the obvious prognostic implications, identification of 1p and 19q codeletions also helps to differentiate oligodendroglioma-like mimics from true oligodendrogliomas. Unfortunately, pediatric oligodendrogliomas generally do not show codeletion; those that do harbor the codeletion frequently occur in teenagers and older children and likely represent the adult type oligodendroglioma (*J Neuropathol Exp Neurol.* 2003;62:53).

9. **Anaplastic oligodendroglioma, WHO grade III.** On the basis of WHO criteria, anaplastic oligodendroglioma must have "significant mitotic activity, EH, or necrosis" along with increased cellularity and marked atypia (*WHO Classification of Tumors of the Central Nervous System.* Lyon, France: IARC Press; 2007). High-grade oligodendrogliomas additionally often show greater cytologic pleomorphism, epithelioid morphology, prominent nucleoli, and sharper cell borders. Necrosis is more often infarct-like rather than pseudopalisading. The exact number of mitoses required for diagnosis has not been established, but a mitotic index of six or more per ten high-power fields (40×) is often used to assign anaplastic grade III (based on *J Neuropathol Exp Neurol.* 2001;60:248) in the absence of EH or necrosis. Anaplastic transformation can be focal or widespread. Some oligodendrogliomas appear otherwise low grade, but contain hypercellular nodules with increased mitotic activity; such cases may be designated

oligodendroglioma with focal anaplasia, WHO grade III. Neuroimaging studies of anaplastic oligodendroglioma often, but not invariably, show patchy or homogeneous contrast enhancement. Ring enhancement is uncommon and predicts poor prognosis. scGBM is usually considered in the differential diagnosis.

10. **Mixed oligoastrocytoma (MOA).** Although the majority of gliomas, when adequately sampled and well fixed, show classical features of either oligodendroglioma or astrocytoma, many cases show ambiguous or intermixed features and are therefore included in the category of MOA. MOAs exhibit low diagnostic concordance rates even among expert neuropathologists (*J Neuropathol Exp Neurol.* 2003;62:1118), largely due to the absence of specific markers for either astrocytic or oligodendroglial differentiation. Histologically, the oligodendroglial and astrocytic components manifest either as geographically separate or, more often, as intermingled forms. Unlike the classical oligodendroglioma, only a small subset of MOAs exhibits 1p and 19q codeletions. When MOAs exhibit an increased mitotic index, EH, or palisading necrosis, they are designated as anaplastic (WHO grade III); in the absence of EH or necrosis, the threshold for mitotic index is not well established, but the threshold of six or more mitotic figures per ten high-power fields (40×) is often applied (*J Neuropathol Exp Neurol.* 2001;60:248). MOAs with necrosis are sometimes referred to as GBM with oligodendroglial component, WHO grade IV (*J Clin Oncol.* 2006;24:5419); they have a prognosis better than that of classic GBMs, but worse than that of anaplastic MOAs lacking necrosis.

B. **Ependymal neoplasms**

1. **Ependymoma, WHO grade II** (e-Fig. 41.25). Ependymomas occur as discrete enhancing masses. In children, they favor a fourth ventricular location; in young adults, the spinal cord. However, these associations are not absolute, and supratentorial tumors, often unassociated with the ventricles, can present in either age group. CSF dissemination occurs in <5% of the cases. Calcification in ependymoma is common when the lesion is located intracranially, whereas cyst formation is common in supratentorial cases. Smear preparations of ependymoma show uniform round to oval nuclei, distinct nucleoli, and spindled to epithelioid morphology; histologically, the tumor cells form perivascular pseudorosettes and, in 5% to 10% of the cases, true ependymal rosettes. True rosettes (or ependymal canals) have central lumens reminiscent of the young central canal of the spinal cord, whereas perivascular pseudorosettes have vessels at the center, surrounded by a nucleus-free zone of radially oriented tumor cell processes. Ependymal canals, elongate versions of true rosettes, are typically seen in only the most differentiated examples. Immunohistochemically, most ependymomas exhibit reactivity for GFAP. Many cases also show reactivity for EMA, CD99, and/or podoplanin (antibody D2-40) along the luminal surface of true rosettes/ependymal canals or within paranuclear intracytoplasmic dot-like structures, thought to represent intracytoplasmic lumina. In difficult cases, EM studies can confirm ependymal differentiation by demonstrating long zipper-like intercellular junctions, microvilli, cilia, and/or intracytoplasmic lumina. Variants of ependymoma include the clear cell (mimics oligodendroglioma), cellular (mimics medulloblastoma or PNET), tanycytic (mimics schwannoma or PA), and papillary (mimics choroid plexus tumors) subtypes. Rarely, ependymomas may contain cells with melanin pigment, or xanthomatous, signet ring, giant cell, or neuronal features. Poor prognostic indicators include age <3 years, posterior fossa location, and anaplastic tumor grade. Grade II ependymomas have a 5-year progression-free survival rate of 60% to 80% as compared with 25% to 50% in anaplastic ependymomas.

2. **Anaplastic ependymoma, WHO grade III.** Several grading systems have been proposed for ependymomas, but no consensus has been achieved. According to the WHO 2007 criteria, anaplastic ependymomas are characterized by increased cellularity, brisk mitotic activity, pseudopalisading necrosis, and microvascular proliferation. Necrosis by itself in the absence of pseudopalisading does not warrant the diagnosis of anaplasia, because lower-grade ependymomas also can show degenerative changes.

3. **Myxopapillary ependymoma, WHO grade I,** is a slowly growing tumor of young adults that occurs almost exclusively in the cauda equina region, where it arises from the filum terminale. Grossly, these tumors are encapsulated, intradural, sausage-shaped masses with a gelatinous interior. Histologically, the tumors show variable proportions of ependymal and papillary patterns. In papillary areas, the tumor cells form irregularly ovoid rings of cuboidal-to-columnar epithelium, each ring formed around a hyalinized central vessel, some fibrous stroma, and a rim of pale basophilic mucin. Pale basophilic often bubbly mucinous (myxoid) material also separates the papillae. In ependymal areas, the tumor cells are spindled and slender, and are arranged in loose fascicles and rather extravagant perivascular pseudorosettes (e-Fig. 41.26). The tumor cells are immunoreactive for GFAP, S-100 protein, and vimentin, with variable staining for EMA, CD99, and podoplanin (antibody D2–40). These tumors have a favorable prognosis following complete resection. If untreated or incompletely resected, rare cases can progress and invade perispinal tissues. Occasional ependymal tumors in this location show a mixture of myxopapillary and typical ependymoma features; the clinical behavior of such tumors is incompletely understood.

4. **Subependymoma, WHO grade I,** is a benign, slowly growing, solid tumor related to ependymoma. They are often asymptomatic, discovered incidentally on CT and MRI studies performed for other reasons. Occasionally, they undergo intratumoral hemorrhage and become life threatening by exerting mass effect. Prognosis is excellent following resection. Grossly, they are sessile or pedunculated masses within the ventricles (lateral > fourth > third). Histologically, they are lobulated and well demarcated. The tumor nuclei resemble those of ependymoma and appear in irregular clusters within a dense fibrillar background formed by tumor cell processes (e-Fig. 41.27). Mitotic figures are rare. Occasional pseudorosettes are not unusual. Secondary degenerative changes include microcyst formation, hemosiderin deposition, vascular hyalinization, myxoid change, and calcification. Nuclear pleomorphism and microvascular proliferation are occasionally seen; these do not warrant a higher-grade diagnosis. It is worth noting that subependymoma may appear as part of a compound ependymal tumor; in such cases, tumor grading should be assigned according to the ependymal component.

C. **Choroid plexus tumors**

1. **Choroid plexus papilloma, WHO grade I** (e-Fig. 41.28), is a benign lesion commonly located in the lateral ventricles in children, and in the fourth ventricle in adults. It typically presents with symptoms associated with obstructive hydrocephalus. Histologically, choroid plexus papilloma resembles normal choroid plexus. However, its fibrovascular cores are lined by a cuboidal-to-columnar epithelium that lacks the superficial intercellular spaces that impart a cobblestone appearance to normal choroid plexus. Mitotic activity is low. Clear cytoplasmic vacuoles are noted in some cases. Occasionally, infarct-like necrosis may be present, but has no prognostic significance. Focal ependymal differentiation is common. Tumor cells show immunoreactivity for S-100, CAM 5.2, transthyretin, and GFAP (focally) but not for EMA and carcinoembryonic antigen (CEA).

2. **Choroid plexus carcinoma, WHO grade III** (e-Fig. 41.29), usually presents in children <3 years of age as an enhancing, intraventricular mass. These tumors are highly aggressive, often metastasize via the CSF, and are nearly uniformly fatal. Histologically, the tumors are more solid and complex than papillomas. High-grade cytology and frequent mitoses are the rule. Foci of necrosis are characteristic, and microvascular proliferation may be seen. Focal small cell features may mimic embryonal tumors (e.g., PNET). Immunoreactivity for S-100, CAM 5.2, and transthyretin is characteristic; is variable for GFAP; and is not typically observed for EMA and CEA. The differential diagnosis includes anaplastic ependymoma (GFAP+, CAM 5.2−, EMA+/−), GBM (GFAP+, CAM 5.2−), medulloblastoma/PNET (SYN+, CAM 5.2−), and metastatic carcinoma (in older patients, EMA+, CEA+/−, S-100 +/−, CAM 5.2+).

D. **Other glial neoplasms.**

1. **Angiocentric glioma (AG), WHO grade I** (e-Fig. 41.30). First reported in 2005, AG is a rare supratentorial tumor associated with epilepsy in children and young adults. Radiographically, AG appears as a T2/FLAIR hyperintense, nonenhancing mass that expands the cortex with minimal mass effect. In some cases, a projection of the tumor extends to the ventricle. Histologically, AG shows uniform, slender spindled glial cells, often arranged either radially from or parallel to vessels, and, occasionally, perpendicular to the pia. AG shows some ependymal features, including dot-like immunoreactivity for EMA, and microvilli and zipper-like junctions by EM. The proliferation index is low.

2. **Astroblastoma (AB), not yet graded** (e-Fig. 41.31). As with AG, AB is associated with epilepsy in children and young adults, but AB is also associated with headaches and vomiting, and shows a female predominance. On MRI, AB is usually large, lobulated, well demarcated, solid with an occasional cystic component, T2-isointense with gray matter, and enhancing. Histologically, AB bears some resemblance to ependymoma, but has stout (rather than fibrillar) cell processes that form the defining astroblastic pseudorosettes. Vascular hyalinization is usually robust; in some tumors, this architectural pattern assumes a papillary appearance. Like ependymoma and AG, AB shows dot-like immunoreactivity for EMA; reactivity for GFAP highlights the abbreviated cell processes within pseudorosettes. ABs showing >5 mitoses per ten 40× fields, anaplastic nuclear features, increased cellularity, microvascular proliferation, and pseudopalisading necrosis are considered anaplastic/malignant, but may still be resectable due to this tumor's noninfiltrating growth pattern.

3. **Chordoid glioma of the third ventricle (CG), WHO grade II,** is a rare tumor of adults that occurs almost exclusively in the vicinity of the anterior third ventricle and hypothalamus. Radiographically, CG is solid, well demarcated, T2 intense, and strongly contrast enhancing. Histologically, as its name suggests, CG focally resembles chordoma, showing cords and clusters of eosinophilic epithelioid cells within a bubbly basophilic mucinous matrix; where mucin is lacking, the cells (strongly GFAP positive, modestly reactive for EMA) appear in sheets. Lymphoplasmacytic infiltrates are typically seen. Immunoreactivity for GFAP (and absence of whorls, psammoma bodies, and physaliferous cells) distinguishes CG from chordoid meningioma and chordoma.

E. **Neuronal and glioneuronal neoplasms**

1. **Ganglion cell tumor (GG and gangliocytoma), WHO grade I.** Ganglion cell tumors are epileptogenic and appear most often in the temporal lobes. On imaging, they commonly enhance and appear solid, cystic, or both. A cyst with an enhancing mural nodule is a common (but not specific) pattern. Microscopically, they are usually cortically based, microcystic, variably

fibrotic, and calcified, and they often show perivascular lymphocytic cuffing (e-Fig. 41.32). Dysmorphic neurons (that may exhibit cytomegaly, vacuolated cytoplasm, coarse Nissl substance, irregular multipolar processes, and/or nuclear abnormalities including binucleation) are the defining feature. Architecturally, the ganglion cells are clumped or haphazardly arranged in comparison with the laminar well-ordered arrangement of the normal cortex. GGs have a variable glial component, typically astrocytic; glial predominant GG may resemble DA or PA. Other features commonly noted include EGBs and RFs (although the latter is more common at the tumor periphery, and may result from piloid gliosis). Cortical dysplasia may be seen adjacent to GG. High-grade glial transformation is exceedingly rare and difficult to define. The glial component is immunoreactive for GFAP; the neuronal component is variably immunoreactive for SYN, NF, and chromogranin, but is usually immunonegative or minimally positive for Neu-N. A subset of cells both within and adjacent to the tumor often shows immunoreactivity for CD34; these CD34+ cells are "spider-like," characterized by long, stellate, ramified processes, and are thought to represent progenitor cells. GGs have a favorable prognosis after surgical resection.

2. **Desmoplastic infantile astrocytoma and desmoplastic infantile ganglioglioma** (DIA/DIG), **WHO grade I** (e-Fig. 41.33), typically occur in children younger than 2 years, and are located superficially within the frontoparietal region. Radiologically, they are very large, attached to the dura, brightly enhancing, and are associated with a very large, occasionally multiloculated cyst. Histologically, the tumors are biphasic. In the collagen IV- and reticulin-rich phase, the tumor cells are arranged in a storiform or fascicular pattern. The astrocytic cells, spindled and gemistocytic, are often inconspicuous within the desmoplastic background, but can be identified by GFAP immunostaining. The neuronal component (present in DIG, absent in DIA) is also subtle because the polygonal neuronal tumor cells are often considerably smaller than those of conventional GG. The other component of the tumor resembles PNET, with abundant small cells and many mitotic figures, and lacks reticulin and collagen. EH and necrosis may be observed but are not associated with an unfavorable prognosis.

3. **Dysplastic cerebellar gangliocytoma (DCG) (Lhermitte–Duclos disease), WHO grade I.** This unique cerebellar neoplasm is often associated with Cowden syndrome (autosomal dominant PTEN/MMAC-1 mutation). Patients with DCG often present with cerebellar dysfunction and/or obstructive hydrocephalus. DCG, which is T1 hypointense and T2 hyperintense, has a characteristic striped appearance with both modalities. Microscopically, DCG presents as a unilateral expansion of cerebellar folia wherein the internal granular layer is replaced by dysmorphic ganglion cells; there is no glial component. Abnormal vascular proliferation is sometimes noted, and white matter is occasionally vacuolated. Evaluation for other features of Cowden syndrome (breast and gastrointestinal lesions) is warranted in patients with DCG.

4. **Central neurocytoma, WHO grade II** (e-Fig. 41.34), occurs in the lateral ventricles near the foramen of Monro in young or middle-aged patients with obstructive hydrocephalus. On imaging studies, these masses are large, globular, enhancing, and often calcified. Histologically, the tumor cells have a uniform appearance with round nuclei, finely granular chromatin, inconspicuous nucleoli, sparse eosinophilic or clear cytoplasm, and delicate fibrillar cell processes (in contrast to the coarse processes of glial tumors). The cells often appear in solid monotonous sheets that may also exhibit prominent chicken-wire vasculature, and/or neurocytic (Homer-Wright) rosettes, and/or perivascular pseudorosettes, and/or calcifications. Thus, the

differential diagnosis often includes oligodendroglioma and ependymoma. In most cases, the brain/tumor interface of central neurocytoma is solid/pushing rather than infiltrative. Immunohistochemistry shows diffuse and strong immunoreactivity with SYN, variable reactivity for Neu-N and NF, and focal reactivity for GFAP. Occasionally, neurocytomas occur within the parenchyma of the cerebral hemispheres, cerebellum, or spinal cord; these extraventricular neurocytomas often exhibit more pronounced ganglion cell and astrocytic differentiation. A small subset of neurocytomas (central and extraventricular) with microvascular proliferation, necrosis, and elevated mitotic/proliferative index (MIB-1 labeling index of 2% or more) show more rapid recurrence, and are identified as atypical, although they are still considered WHO grade II.

5. **Dysembryoplastic neuroepithelial tumor (DNT), WHO grade I,** is a benign, slowly growing tumor of adolescents and young adults who have a history of longstanding, drug-resistant partial seizures. On imaging, DNT appears in an area of expanded cerebral cortex, with a predilection for the medial temporal lobe. DNT is T1 hypointense, T2/FLAIR hyperintense, and nodular; some complex varieties show enhancement (see below). Microscopically, simple DNT demonstrates only the specific glioneuronal element; patterned intracortical mucin-rich nodules each exhibit a network of bundled axons and delicate capillaries that divide the mucin into microcystic pools. This network is decorated by oligodendroglioma-like cells and occasional stellate astrocytes, and some of the microcytic pools show morphologically normal "floating" neurons (**e-Fig. 41.35**). Mitotic figures are rare to absent. Complex DNT consists of the specific glioneuronal element with an additional component referred to as glial nodules which are histologically identical to PA, GG, diffuse glioma, or another glial neoplasm. Cortical dysplasia may be seen adjacent to DNTs. Simple DNTs are commonly misdiagnosed as oligodendrogliomas and, if sampling is incomplete, complex DNTs may be misdiagnosed according to the glial nodule subtype that is present. Therefore, review of clinical history and radiographic imaging is essential in evaluating specimens from temporal lobe epilepsy surgical resections. DNT has a benign course and postsurgical seizure resolution is common.

6. **Papillary glioneuronal tumor (PGNT), WHO grade I,** is a contrast-enhancing, well-circumscribed, solid or cystic lesion that arises most commonly in the periventricular white matter, usually in the temporal lobe (*Am J Surg Pathol.* 1998;22:1171). Patients, most commonly young adults, present with seizures, headaches, and vision disturbance. Histologically, as the name suggests, these tumors have glial and neuronal elements, and a papillary appearance. The glial element (GFAP-positive) forms a loose layer of spindled-to-cuboidal cells closely apposed to the surfaces of hyalinized fibrovascular cores; between these pseudopapillary structures are the neuronal tumor cells (SYN positive), which can range morphologically from neurocytic to ganglion cell-like. Mitotic activity, atypia, vascular proliferation, and necrosis are rare to absent (**e-Fig. 41.36**).

7. **Rosette-forming Glioneuronal Tumor of the Fourth Ventricle (RGNT), WHO grade I.** This tumor, most common in young adults, always involves the ventricular system of the posterior fossa, and in unusual cases may extend upwards into the proximal supratentorial ventricles (*Am J Surg Pathol.* 2002;26:582). Consequently, RGNT usually presents with sequelae of obstructive hydrocephalus. MRI shows RGNT to be circumscribed and solid, T2 hyperintense, T1 hypointense and, in some cases, heterogeneously enhancing. Histologically (**e-Fig. 41.37**), RGNT is biphasic, characterized by a uniform population of small neurocytic cells and a second glial element that resembles PA. The neurocytic cells have hyperchromatic round

nuclei and a small amount of cleared cytoplasm; classically, they form single or clustered rosettes and pseudorosettes within a relatively hypocellular eosinophilic matrix of astrocytic tumor cell processes. The centers of these rosettes and pseudorosettes are more intensely eosinophilic and contain fine, SYN-immunoreactive cell processes. The surrounding matrix shows immunoreactivity for GFAP, and may exhibit EGBs and RFs. Surgical resection is curative.

F. Pineal parenchymal tumors

1. **Pineocytoma, WHO grade I,** is more common in adults. On MRI, pineocytoma appears as a T1 hypo- or isointense, T2 hyperintense, uniformly enhancing, often calcified, discrete mass in the region of the pineal gland. Through mass effect, pineocytoma often causes increased ICP and upward gaze palsy (Parinaud syndrome). Histologically, pineocytoma tumor cells (SYN+, Neu-N+) have round-to-oval nuclei, salt and pepper chromatin, inconspicuous nucleoli, and poorly demarcated cell borders, and often form pineocytic rosettes (large, exaggerated Homer-Wright rosettes) (e-Fig. 41.38). Mitotic activity is very low. Pineocytomas may be difficult to distinguish from normal pineal tissue in a small biopsy, although a lobular pattern with gliovascular septae favors the latter.

2. **Pineoblastoma, WHO grade IV,** is a rapidly growing malignant tumor that predominantly occurs in children and very young adults. Occasionally, pineoblastomas occur in association with bilateral retinoblastoma (trilateral retinoblastoma). On MRI, pineoblastomas are inconsistent: hypo- to isointense on T1, hypo- to hyperintense on T2, with homogeneous or heterogeneous enhancement. Their borders appear more infiltrative than those of pineocytoma, and leptomeningeal metastasis (through CSF dissemination) is common at presentation. Grossly, they are soft, friable, and poorly demarcated. Hemorrhage and necrosis may be present. Calcification is rare. Histologically, they resemble other small blue cell tumors (e.g., medulloblastoma, PNET). The primitive-appearing cells have little cytoplasm, hyperchromatic molded nuclei, and are densely packed in sheets occasionally interrupted by Homer-Wright rosettes, Flexner–Wintersteiner rosettes (which have a central lumen), and zones of necrosis. Mitotic activity is generally high. Invasion of the adjacent pineal gland and leptomeninges is common. Immunoreactivity for neuronal markers (e.g., NF, SYN, chromogranin, and neuron-specific enolase) is weak and focal relative to that seen in pineocytoma. Occasionally, these tumor cells may additionally express antigens related to photoreceptor or pineal differentiation, including retinal S-antigen, rhodopsin, and melatonin.

3. **Pineal parenchymal tumor of intermediate differentiation (PPTID), WHO grade II–III,** is a recently recognized entity that occurs more commonly in adults. Histologically, PPTID is rather cellular, lacks pineocytic rosettes, and has slightly more pronounced cytologic atypia and a higher mitotic/proliferative rate than pineocytoma (MIB-1 indices from 10% to 16% for PPTID vs. 1% to 2% for pineocytoma). PPTID appears in two main patterns: diffuse, with mildly irregular round-to-oval nuclei arranged in a sheet-like pattern, and pseudolobulated, wherein tumor cells are divided into lobules delineated by vessels. A higher grade (III) is assigned to PPTID when the mitotic index exceeds six mitoses per ten 40× fields or when immunoreactivity for NF protein is nearly absent; for this reason, definitive grading is best reserved for resection rather than limited biopsy specimens. Recurrence and survival rates are intermediate between those of pineoblastoma and pineocytoma.

4. **Papillary tumor of the pineal region (PTPR), WHO grade II or III,** has been reported in children and adults, with a peak in the third decade. MRI shows a large, well-circumscribed, T2-intense, enhancing (occasionally cystic)

mass in the vicinity of the pineal gland. Histologically, PTPR exhibits papillary features; large, pale-to-eosinophilic tumor cells form columnar epithelia around hyalinized vessels (e-**Fig. 41.39**). In other, more solid areas, tumor cells with round-to-oval nuclei and clear or vacuolated cytoplasm may form true ependymal rosettes. Mitotic activity is variable (0 to 10 per 10 high-power fields), and necrosis may be seen; EH is usually not observed. PTPR does not infiltrate the pineal gland.

This histologic appearance resembles that of ependymoma. Further, both tumors can show focal membranous and dot-like reactivity for EMA (consistent with the fact that PTPR is thought to arise from the specialized ependymal cells of the subcommissural organ). The key features that distinguish PTPR are minimal reactivity for GFAP and strong reactivity for CK18. Because PTPR has only recently been described, official grading criteria have not yet been defined; however, a mitotic index of five or more per ten 40× fields has been associated with poorer prognosis.

G. **Embryonal tumors**, most common in children, are so-named because their "small blue cell" histology is reminiscent of elements of the embryonic nervous system. These tumors are bulky, grow rapidly, and seed the CSF pathways. All embryonal tumors are inherently malignant (WHO grade IV); however, the prognoses for these tumors vary widely, as some respond very well to current treatments.

1. **Medulloblastoma, WHO grade IV,** the most common embryonal CNS tumor, is thought to originate from remnants of the external granular layer or from the fourth ventricular germinal matrix. On imaging, they are often T1 hypointense, T2 hyperintense, noncalcified, homogeneously contrast-enhancing cerebellar masses with restricted diffusion. In approximately one-third of the classic cases, the tumor has already seeded the CSF pathways focally (with so-called drop metastases in the lumbosacral spinal cord) or diffusely (with so-called icing of the subarachnoid space) at the time of presentation. Distant metastases, most often involving bone and lymph nodes, are rare. Several histologic subtypes of medulloblastoma have been described including classic/undifferentiated, desmoplastic/nodular, "with extensive nodularity," large cell, and anaplastic.

Classic/undifferentiated medulloblastoma (e-**Fig. 41.40**), the most common subtype, appears as a patternless sheet of abundant small tumor cells with hyperchromatic nuclei and minimal apparent cytoplasm. The nuclei show a degree of molding and are often described as round-to-oval or carrot-shaped. Nucleoli are inconspicuous. Mitotic figures and apoptotic bodies are often abundant. Microvascular proliferation and necrosis may be present, but are not prominent. About 40% of the cases exhibit Homer-Wright rosettes. In addition to seeding the CSF, this tumor often reinvades the cerebellar parenchyma from the subarachnoid space via Virchow–Robin spaces.

The *desmoplastic/nodular variant* (e-**Fig. 41.41**) has a characteristic low-power appearance of rounded, pale islands separated by dark internodular tissue. The pale islands (reticulin free) contain cells with a relatively neurocytic phenotype that features round to oval nuclei, open chromatin, moderate cytoplasm, cell processes that form a neuropil-like stroma, and little mitotic activity. The internodular tissue (reticulin rich) is formed by densely packed, primitive-appearing cells with hyperchromatic malleable nuclei, smudged chromatin, little cytoplasm, and high proliferative activity. This variant is genetically distinct and has a slightly more favorable prognosis than other subtypes (*Acta Neuropathol.* 2006;112:5).

Another prognostically favorable variant is *medulloblastoma with extensive nodularity.* This rare tumor, found almost exclusively in infants, radiographically may resemble a cluster of grapes (T1 imaging, postcontrast). Histologically, it resembles the desmoplastic variant, but is dominated by pale, reticulin-free nodules with neuronal differentiation; primitive areas are diminished. After treatment, this tumor has been reported to undergo complete gangliocytic differentiation.

In contrast, the rare *large cell variant* of medulloblastoma behaves relatively aggressively and is less responsive to therapy. The cells of large cell medulloblastoma have relatively more cytoplasm than those of classic medulloblastoma, as well as larger nuclei, vesicular chromatin, and prominent nucleoli. It is worth noting, however, that this large cell histologic pattern may not be uniform within a tumor, and intermixed anaplastic tissue is often associated.

Anaplastic medulloblastomas feature cellular pleomorphism, cytomegaly, hyperchromasia, a markedly elevated mitotic index, atypical mitoses, abundant apoptotic bodies, apoptotic lakes, and cell wrapping (e-Fig. 41.42). Although the common cooccurrence of large-cell and anaplastic features has led some to advocate a combined large-cell/ anaplastic medulloblastoma category, anaplasia can be observed in classic medulloblastomas that lack large-cell features.

Medulloblastomas are generally immunopositive for SYN and variably positive for GFAP, and have high MIB-1 (Ki-67) labeling indices. Cytogenetic and FISH studies of medulloblastomas often show loss of chromosome 17p and, when coupled with duplication of its long arm, formation of isochromosome 17q (i17q). i17q is encountered in about 30% of medulloblastomas and is considered a relatively specific diagnostic marker; whether it is associated with poorer prognosis is less clear. Other genetic aberrations that clearly are associated with aggressive behavior and shortened survival times are amplification of C-MYC, and less commonly MYCN, oncogenes. These amplifications are observed in 4% to 17% of medulloblastomas and are observed in a greater percentage of anaplastic/large cell medulloblastomas. In contrast, immunoreactivity for nuclear beta-catenin, which is observed in 15% to 20% of sporadic cases, is associated with favorable prognosis.

The 5-year survival rate for medulloblastoma overall is 60%, following current treatment protocols (gross total resection, craniospinal radiation therapy, and adjuvant chemotherapy). Patients with the extensively nodular variant fare relatively better; other patients, particularly when younger than 3 years and/or with limited surgical resections and/or with CSF dissemination, have relatively unfavorable prognoses.

2. **CNS-PNET, WHO grade IV,** is often histomorphologically identical to classic medulloblastoma but occurs outside the cerebellum. On imaging, CNS-PNET is contrast enhancing and may exhibit calcification, hemorrhage, and/or necrosis. Some features of neuronal differentiation (e.g., diffuse and widespread immunoreactivity for SYN, NF proteins, NSE) are common; reactivity for GFAP is usually strong within only a subset of cells. As with medulloblastoma, several variants of CNS-PNET have been described. Tumors with extensive neuronal differentiation have been alternatively termed "cerebral neuroblastomas" or, when ganglion cells are observed, ganglioneuroblastoma. Other rare cases showing multilayered true rosettes (with central lumens) that blend into a surrounding sheet of dense tumor cells are called ependymoblastoma (e-Fig. 41.43). A newly recognized tumor has several of these features (*Pediatr Develop Pathol.* 2000;3:346) and is aptly named "ETANTR" (embryonal tumor with abundant neuropil and true rosettes) (e-Fig. 41.44); whether this aggressive tumor is distinct or represents a variant of CNS/PNET is not yet clear. A final variant of CNS/PNET

is medulloepithelioma, defined by arrangements of neoplastic neuroepithelium reminiscent of the developing neural tube that appear among other areas with PNET-like histology.

3. **AT/RT, WHO grade IV** (e-Fig. 41.45), is a densely cellular tumor of infants and young children (most are <3 years old, with a male predominance) that can occur anywhere in the neuraxis. Radiographically, AT/RT is usually large, cystic, hemorrhagic, focally necrotic, and heterogeneously enhancing; not uncommonly, nodular leptomeningeal spread is found at presentation. Histologically, AT/RT is defined by rhabdoid cells with eccentrically placed vesicular nuclei, prominent nucleoli, and large eosinophilic paranuclear whorls of intermediate filaments. The rhabdoid cells may appear only focally, or not at all, in a biopsy specimen; tissue heterogeneity is common in AT/RT. A small blue cell component is seen in 65% of the cases and may predominate. For this reason, AT/RT can easily be confused with medulloblastoma (particularly the large cell/anaplastic variant) or CNS-PNET. Other areas of AT/RT may show glial, mesenchymal, epithelial, or papillary features, potentially conjuring an even broader differential diagnosis. AT/RT typically shows immunoreactivity for vimentin, EMA, CK, and smooth muscle actin, and often, for SYN and GFAP as well. Because AT/RT can mimic other entities and is relatively common among infantile CNS tumors, a very low threshold should be maintained to rule out this diagnosis when confronted with a tumor in a child under 3 years of age. A highly sensitive and specific immunohistochemical stain that differentiates AT/RT from other embryonal tumors targets the BAF47/INI1 protein, the product of the INI1/BAF47/hSNF5 tumor suppressor gene on chromosome 22q11. AT/RT results from biallelic inactivation of this gene, and hence virtually all AT/RTs show loss of intranuclear reactivity for BAF47/INI1. These are highly aggressive tumors; mean survival is 17 months.

H. **Tumors of the meninges**

1. **Meningiomas,** which bear resemblance to the arachnoidal cells that normally inhabit the inner surface of the dura, are most often intracranial and extra-axial, appearing over the cerebral convexities, parasagittally along the falx cerebri, along the skull base or tentorium, or in the optic nerve sheath. Less commonly, meningiomas appear within the spine, where thoracic segments are favored. Rarely, meningiomas occur within a ventricle, presumably arising from the tela choroidea, a leptomeningeal invagination at the base of the choroid plexus. Most meningiomas occur in adults between 20 and 60 years of age, with a peak incidence around 45 years and a slight female preponderance (female to male ratio of 3:2). Spinal meningiomas are particularly more common in women (female to male ratio of 9:1). Radiation-induced meningiomas (which can appear two or more decades after radiotherapy for other brain tumors or for *Tinea capitis*) are well recognized but rare. Many benign meningiomas (WHO grade I) grow slowly and come to clinical attention incidentally or only after they have grown to very large size and have begun to cause headaches, seizures, or focal neurologic deficits by compressing adjacent structures. In contrast, atypical (WHO grade II) and anaplastic (WHO grade III) forms can be aggressive, show more rapid growth, a greater propensity to recur following resection, and, in some cases, invasion of the CNS. It is important to note, however, that even a benign meningioma can show invasion of soft tissue and bone, and may come to clinical attention after invading the orbits or sinuses; invasion of soft tissue and bone is not considered a criterion for WHO grading. On imaging, meningiomas are extra-axial, homogeneously enhancing lesions. Trailing of the enhancement into adjacent dura is a useful radiologic sign (the so-called dural tail) but can also be observed in other

dura-based tumors. Hyperostosis of the adjacent skull is a suggestive radiographic finding that is somewhat more specific, and is often associated with bone invasion.

Grossly, meningiomas are spherical to lobulated, firm or rubbery, usually well circumscribed, and firmly attached to the inner surface of the dura. Meningiomas that occur along the sphenoid wing may grow "en plaque" as flat, carpet-like masses. Most invade the underlying dura or dural sinuses but do not involve the pia or the underlying CNS.

The microscopic features of meningioma are highly variable, and 13 histologic variants are recognized by the WHO classification system (e-**Fig. 41.46**). However, the patterns that characterize these variants often appear together within a single tumor. Although cytologic smear preparations of meningioma are occasionally nondiagnostic, they usually show three-dimensional clusters (sometimes exhibiting whorls) of epithelioid to spindled cells, reflecting the cells' rather cohesive nature. Tumor cell nuclei are generally round to oval and often contain intranuclear pseudoinclusions (cytoplasmic invaginations) and nuclear clearings; these latter features are characteristic, but not specific. Likewise, concentric microcalcifications (psammoma bodies) provide some diagnostic reassurance. Histologically, the most common cytoarchitectural patterns in meningioma are fibrous (fascicles of spindled cells) and meningothelial (dominated by whorls and fascicles); identification of these patterns—even focally—may provide the strongest initial clue to diagnosis, particularly when an uncommon histologic pattern dominates the specimen. Nevertheless, familiarity with the variants of meningioma is critically important to avoid misdiagnosis, particularly when specimens are small. In such cases, immunohistochemistry is indispensible for confirming the diagnosis. Some of the common differential diagnoses for meningioma subtypes are provided in Table 41.5. Most meningiomas display patchy or weak membranous reactivity for EMA and reactivity within nuclei for progesterone receptor (PR) (although reactivity for PR is less common among atypical and anaplastic tumors). Relevant for the often-encountered differential diagnosis of schwannoma versus meningioma for a spindled CNS neoplasm, collagen IV reactivity is not observed in meningioma, and S100 reactivity is typically patchy rather than diffuse. In unusual circumstances, when immunohistochemistry fails to provide diagnostic clarity, EM may be helpful; meningioma cells have interdigitating cell processes with scattered desmosomes, and do not secrete a basement membrane. FISH for common genetic changes may also be useful for guiding diagnosis (see below).

a. **Histologic variants, grading, and prognosis.** Roughly 80% of meningiomas are considered histologically benign (WHO grade I) and have a low risk of recurrence after gross total resection (~5% at 5 years, ~20% at 20 years). Atypical (WHO grade II) meningiomas constitute 15% to 20% of cases and have a higher risk of recurrence (~30% or more at 5 years). Anaplastic (WHO grade III) meningiomas account for 1% to 2% of cases, are associated with even higher recurrence rates, and often prove fatal (median survival <2 years). After histologic grade, the most influential prognostic factor for recurrence is extent of surgical resection; subtotally resected benign meningiomas have a recurrence rate of ~30% to 40% at 5 years. Other prognostic factors include male gender and young age; each is unfavorable. Genetic characteristics of a meningioma also influence prognosis, as discussed below.

One determinant of WHO grade is the histologic pattern. Meningothelial, fibrous, transitional, psammomatous, angiomatous, microcystic, secretory, lymphoplasmacyte-rich, and metaplastic variants are considered WHO grade I unless they have additional superimposed

TABLE 41.5	Common Differential Diagnosis for Meningioma Subtypes[a]
Variant	**Differential diagnoses**
Meningothelial/transitional	Metastatic carcinoma Meningothelial hyperplasia
Fibrous/fibroblastic	Schwannoma
Psammomatous	Reactive process
Angiomatous (vascular)	HB Atypical meningioma (degenerative atypia)
Microcystic	Diffuse or PA Clear-cell meningioma
Secretory	Metastatic adenocarcinoma (e.g., thyroid)
Lymphoplasmacyte-rich	Inflammatory process
Metaplastic (bone, cartilage, xanthomatous, myxoid, fat, etc.)	Soft tissue tumors
Clear cell (WHO grade II)	Metastatic RCC Microcystic meningioma HB
Chordoid (WHO grade II)	Chordoma CG of the third ventricle Epithelioid hemangioendothelioma
Papillary (WHO grade III)	Papillary ependymoma AB HPC Metastatic malignancy
Rhabdoid (WHO grade III)	Metastatic malignancy AT/RT GBM/GS

[a]Modified from Short Course Syllabus #37, USCAP, 2006.
WHO, World Health Organization; GBM, glioblastoma.
Modified from: Louis DN, Ohgaki H, Wiestler OD, Cavenee WK, eds. *WHO Classification of Tumours of the Central Nervous System*. Lyon: IARC Press; 2007. Used with permission.

features that independently reach criterion for assignment of a higher grade. Tumors dominated by chordoid or clear cell histology, on the other hand, show greater propensity to recur and are classified as WHO grade II. Tumors with abundant papillary and rhabdoid histology show an aggressive clinical course and warrant a diagnosis of WHO grade III. When a tumor exhibits more than one pattern, the dominant histologic subtype dictates which grade is assigned. Nevertheless, when a histologic pattern characteristic of a higher grade is observed even focally, mention should be made in the resulting pathology report.

b. **Atypical meningioma, WHO grade II** (e-Fig. 41.47). In addition to meningiomas with a dominant clear cell or chordoid pattern, meningiomas in this category include those with increased mitotic activity (four or more mitotic figures per ten high-power fields) or three or more of the following histologic features: (1) generally increased cellularity; (2) small cell change, in which focal areas show small dense nuclei and diminished cytoplasm, reminiscent of clusters of lymphocytes; (3) prominent (macro) nucleoli; (4) uninterrupted patternless or sheet-like growth (loss of architecture); and (5) foci of spontaneous or geographic necrosis not induced by embolization or radiation (*Am J Surg Pathol*. 1997;21:1455).

Consistent with increased mitotic activity, atypical meningiomas also generally exhibit moderately elevated Ki-67 (MIB-1 antibody) labeling indices. Because measurements of Ki-67 labeling index can show interinstitutional variability, this feature is not officially considered in the WHO grading system. However, it does represent a reasonable surrogate for mitotic activity when cytologic preservation is poor or when a specimen is particularly small.

c. **Brain invasion.** Brain invasion by meningioma is characterized by entrapped islands of brain parenchyma at the periphery of the tumor and/or irregular tongue-like protrusions of tumor tissue in attached brain parenchyma. On H&E sections, this phenomenon can be quite subtle, so immunohistochemistry for GFAP is often warranted for confirmation (e-**Fig. 41.48**). Brain invasion may occur in tumors that are otherwise histologically benign, atypical, or anaplastic. Although brain invasion has historically been assumed to be a malignant feature, clinicopathologic correlation studies have revealed statistical outcomes more consistent with atypical meningiomas. Therefore, brain-invasive meningiomas are considered WHO grade II even when their histologic patterns are otherwise benign.

d. **Anaplastic (malignant) meningioma, WHO grade III.** Anaplastic meningiomas that are not overtly papillary or rhabdoid must exhibit a markedly elevated density of 20 or more mitotic figures per ten $40\times$ fields or show histologic features of frank malignancy reminiscent of carcinoma, melanoma, or high-grade sarcoma (*Cancer* 1999;85:2046) (e-**Fig. 41.49**). Consequently, the differential diagnosis for these anaplastic meningiomas often includes one or more of these malignant tumors. Complicating this situation somewhat is the tendency for meningioma to harbor metastatic carcinoma from outside the CNS (most commonly breast and lung). In such cases, when immunohistochemical data are insufficient to support a diagnosis with confidence, ultrastructural and FISH studies probing for genetic changes common to meningioma may be useful.

e. **Genetic changes in meningioma.** Most meningiomas of all grades show loss of chromosome 22q, site of the NF2 gene, thought to be important for tumor development. A genetic alteration with prognostic implications is loss of the CDKN2A/p16 region on 9p21. Characteristic of the majority of anaplastic meningiomas, loss of 9p21 is associated with decreased survival; tumors that lack this alteration show survival patterns more consistent with atypical rather than anaplastic grade.

2. **Hemangiopericytoma (HPC), WHO grade II–III,** and **Solitary Fibrous Tumor (SFT), ungraded, but benign** (e-Fig. 41.50). Historically, these two uncommon tumors have been regarded as distinct entities, but their overlapping clinical and histologic features suggest that they may represent ends of a continuum. Radiologically, they resemble meningioma; they are dura-associated, solid, uniformly enhancing, and appear in a similar anatomical distribution. However, unlike meningioma, HPC does not show intratumoral calcification and can be associated with bone lysis rather than hyperostosis. Additionally, HPC appears hypervascular by angiography, and may receive a dual blood supply from the meninges and brain. Microscopically, this hypervascularity is contributed by slit-like vascular channels lined by flattened endothelial cells and frequent ectatic, thin-walled and branching "staghorn vessels." Although such vessels are not specific, they provide a very helpful diagnostic clue.

The parenchyma of these tumors is usually biphasic. Hypocellular areas of SFT are strongly collagenous and hyalinized; cellular areas of SFT are composed of a patternless or mildly fascicular arrangement of elongated spindled-to-oval cells that are intermixed with brightly eosinophilic, interlaced collagen bundles. Mitotic figures are sparse, and other classically anaplastic features are not observed. When the cellular areas of SFT become particularly dense, they may resemble HPC. Cellular areas of HPC contain oval-to-epithelioid cells with round nuclei and scant cytoplasm that are densely arranged in a random or vaguely nested pattern with little intervening stroma; collagen is not prominent. Within this dense background, paucicellular areas of HPC appear as pale islands. A diagnosis of anaplasia for HPC requires either >5 mitotic figures per ten 40× fields or the presence of necrosis, plus two or more of the following: hypercellularity, moderate or severe nuclear atypia, and hemorrhage. In ambiguous cases, special stains can guide diagnosis; HPC shows at best only focal immunoreactivity for CD34 but has abundant stromal reticulin fibers that surround cells individually and in small groups; SFT stains strongly for CD34 and is reticulin-poor. Both neoplasms show immunoreactivity for vimentin, bcl-2, and CD99, and no reactivity for S-100, CD31, EMA, and PR. FISH studies can also be helpful, as loss of chromosome 22q has not been reported in HPC. It is worth noting, however, that loss of 9p21, a poor prognostic marker in high-grade meningiomas, has been reported in about 25% of HPCs.

I. **Hemangioblastoma (HB), WHO grade I.** Sporadic cases of this benign, slowly growing, highly vascular neoplasm occur most often in the posterior fossa of adults, favoring the cerebellum. HBs located elsewhere (e.g., brain stem, spinal cord, retina, cerebrum), particularly when multiple and/or occurring in younger patients, are more commonly associated with von Hippel–Lindau disease (VHL); therefore, discovery of an HB with any of these unusual characteristics warrants thorough screening for other manifestations of VHL (e.g., endolymphatic sac tumor, pheochromocytoma, pancreatic cyst or islet tumor, renal cyst or clear cell carcinoma, and papillary cystadenoma of the epididymis). On imaging studies, the classic HB is well-circumscribed, intra-axial, and cystic, with an enhancing mural nodule that is hypervascular on angiography. Microscopically, hemangioblastomas have two main components: stromal and vascular. Stromal cells show variable morphology, but typically are large and polygonal with vacuolated lipid-laden cytoplasm (e-**Fig. 41.51**). Karyomegaly and nuclear degenerative atypia among these stromal cells are common and without significance. The vascular component is characterized by thin-walled channels lined by flattened endothelial cells. On the basis of the relative prominence of these two components, two histologic variants have been described: cellular and reticular. The less common stroma-rich cellular variant may show greater Ki-67 labeling index and propensity to recur than the more common reticular variant. Mast cells are common within HBs and foci of extramedullary erythropoiesis are present in a minority of cases. Occasionally, these tumors produce brisk piloid gliosis in the adjacent brain parenchyma. On the basis of radiographic and histologic patterns, the differential diagnosis often includes PA and metastatic renal cell carcinoma (RCC), requiring immunohistochemical stains such as D2–40/podoplanin or inhibin (positive in stromal cells), as well as EMA, CD10, and RCC (all variably positive in RCC) and GFAP (positive in PA and most often negative in stromal cells).

J. **Tumors of the sella and/or suprasellar region (other than pituitary adenomas).**

1. **Craniopharyngiomas, WHO grade I,** due to their location, may present clinically with hormonal abnormalities, vision disturbance, and obstructive hydrocephalus. These partly cystic, histologically benign epithelial tumors are thought to originate from Rathke's pouch epithelium. On MRI, these tumors often show T1 bright cyst contents and postcontrast enhancement of solid areas and any cyst capsule(s). Two morphologically distinct

subtypes have been described, adamantinomatous and papillary; the former shows heterogeneous calcifications on CT, whereas the less common papillary variant does not.

a. **Adamantinomatous craniopharyngiomas** occur more commonly in children aged 5 to 15 years, but show a second peak in the fifth and sixth decades. Grossly, cyst contents have the appearance of dark green-brown machine oil. Calcifications are frequently noted. Microscopically, this variant resembles adamantinoma of the bone (tibia) and ameloblastoma of the jaw. The adamantinomatous variant is formed by a complex squamous epithelium that shows: basal palisading (a columnar orientation of the most peripheral layer of nuclei); an overlying zone of moderate cellularity in which focal areas resemble a network of processes over a cleared background (stellate reticulum); and central keratinization, which produces nodules of pale, anucleate, cohesive cell remnants (wet keratin) (e-Fig. 41.52). Areas of xanthogranulomatous inflammation and abundant cholesterol clefts are common. The border of this tumor is usually irregular and adherent to surrounding structures, and the adjacent parenchyma typically shows robust piloid gliosis. Although histologically benign, its adherent somewhat invasive nature leads to frequent recurrence even after gross total resection. Consequently, adamantinomatous craniopharyngioma can cause considerable morbidity, particularly given its close association with the optic chiasm and pituitary.

b. **The papillary variant** (e-Fig. 41.53) is less common, is not typically seen in children, and most commonly occurs in the third ventricle or suprasellar region rather than in the sella itself. Grossly, it is seldom cystic; any cysts observed contain clear fluid rather than "machine oil." Calcifications are absent, and the interface with the brain is smoother and less adherent. Histologically, the papillary variant is formed by a well-differentiated, nonkeratinizing squamous epithelium that overlies broad, loose fibrovascular cores. The basal layer shows increased density, but without strong palisading. Beyond the apical surface, the tissue degrades (undergoes dehiscence), effectively leaving crude pseudopapillae of viable tissue around stromal cores. Occasionally, the epithelium may show focal cilia or goblet cells. In spite of clearer demarcation from the adjacent brain tissue in the papillary variant, the tumor has a similarly high rate of recurrence as the adamantinomatous variant.

K. **Germ cell tumors (GCTs).** Included in this category are germinoma, teratoma, yolk sac tumor, embryonal carcinoma, and choriocarcinoma. Typically, these brain tumors occur in children or young adults. A pineal location, classically associated with increased intracranial pressure and Parinaud syndrome, is more common in males; a suprasellar location, classically associated with diabetes insipidus, vision changes and hypopituitarism, is slightly more common in females. In some cases, both areas are involved. Less common sites include the basal ganglia and thalamus. On MRI, most GCTs are heterogeneously T2 hyperintense and show heterogeneous enhancement. Calcification and complexity are common in teratomas, and hemorrhage is strongly associated with choriocarcinoma. Histologically, these tumors are homologous to their gonadal and mediastinal counterparts. Occasionally, the marked lymphocytic infiltrate and/or granulomatous response seen in germinomas can mask the underlying large, clear cells with central round nuclei and large nucleoli that define the neoplasm. In such cases, immunostaining for c-kit (membranous pattern), OCT4 (nuclear pattern), and placental alkaline phosphatase (PLAP) (cytoplasmic and membranous pattern) may be applied to aid diagnosis (Table 41.1, e-Fig. 41.54). Rare germinomas contain syncytiotrophoblastic elements and should not be confused with choriocarcinoma. Pure germinomas are exquisitely radiosensitive and have an excellent prognosis; those with syncytiotrophoblastic cells show a greater tendency to recur, and modestly less favorable survival. Mature teratomas follow a benign clinical course and may be cured by gross total resection. Yolk sac tumors, embryonal carcinoma, and choriocarcinoma (and mixed tumors composed of more than one of these elements) confer less favorable prognoses.

L. **Lymphomas and histiocytic tumors.**

1. **Primary CNS lymphomas (PCNSLs)** are malignant lymphomas that occur in the absence of systemic lymphoma. PCNSL is more common among but not exclusive to elderly or immunosuppressed patients. On imaging, PCNSLs occur as single or multiple homogeneously enhancing lesions; some appear well circumscribed (resembling, e.g., a metastasis or tumefactive MS) and others appear somewhat diffuse (resembling a diffuse glioma). A periventricular location is common. These lesions often respond dramatically to steroid therapy, at least initially; although this radiographic response may provide a diagnostic clue, steroid treatment is usually withheld when possible until a tissue diagnosis is secured.

   Microscopically, PCNSLs appear as parenchymal and angiocentric infiltrates of highly atypical lymphocytes (e-**Fig. 41.55**) accompanied by nonneoplastic CD3+ T cells. The neoplastic cells usually have centroblast-like or immunoblast-like morphology and are immunoreactive for B-lymphocyte markers (e.g., CD20, CD79a); most PCNSLs are considered diffuse large B-cell lymphomas (DLBCLs). Affected vessels show mural expansion by this mixed population, a feature that can be highlighted by reticulin stain. In some cases, nonneoplastic foamy histiocytes and reactive astrocytes may also be abundant in the parenchyma. Necrosis and evidence of Epstein–Barr virus (EBV) (by immunostain or in situ hybridization for EBV-encoded RNA [EBER]) are features associated with acquired immunodeficiency syndrome (AIDS) or immunosuppression-associated PCNSL.

   Uncommon variants of lymphoma that affect the CNS include: *lymphomatoid granulomatosis,* an angiodestructive EBV-driven high-grade B-cell lymphoma that affects the brain in 25% of cases (more commonly, the lung and skin) and features fibrinoid angionecrosis and poorly formed granulomas (lymphohistiocytic nodules); and *intravascular B-cell lymphoma,* a high-grade extranodal B-cell lymphoma characterized by its restriction to vessel lumina. Both of these variants lead to vascular occlusion and infarcts. *T-cell lymphomas* are encountered only rarely as PCNSLs. When lymphoma metastasizes to the CNS (secondary CNS lymphoma) it typically appears in epidural, dural, or leptomeningeal locations and is accompanied by systemic disease.

2. **Histiocytic Disorders**

   a. **Langerhans cell histiocytosis (LCH)** is the term officially endorsed by the Histiocyte Society to replace previous terms (e.g., Hand–Schüller–Christian disease [HSCD], eosinophilic granuloma, histiocytosis X, etc.) LCH primarily affects children, with a median age of 12 years. The most common manifestation involves an isolated osteolytic lesion of the skull (eosinophilic granuloma) that may also involve the underlying meninges and cortex. When multiple, such lesions may be accompanied by hypothalamic involvement (consistent with HSCD). Although it is rare to encounter isolated involvement of the hypothalamus, pituitary, and optic chiasm (e-**Fig. 41.56**), this region shows radiographic changes in ~50% of cases with disseminated LCH, and 25% of children with multifocal disease present with diabetes insipidus. Histologically (e-**Fig. 41.57**), LCH is characterized by Langerhans cells accompanied by variable amounts of nonneoplastic reactive elements that may include eosinophils, neutrophils, macrophages, lymphocytes, plasma cells, and multinucleated giant cells. Langerhans cells are recognizable morphologically by their grooved "coffee bean" nuclei; immunohistochemically by reactivity for S100, CD1a, and langerin (CD207); and ultrastructurally by the presence of Birbeck granules.

b. **Non-LC Histiocytic disorders** are far less common in the CNS. Intracranial *Rosai–Dorfman disease* (e-**Fig. 41.58**) affects children and adults and can mimic meningioma; it most often affects the meninges as a contrast-enhancing mass, and may induce a nonneoplastic hyperplastic response in the associated arachnoidal cells. However, the other constituents of the tumor include plasma cells, lymphocytes, and, most importantly, scattered large pale histiocytes (S-100+, CD68+, CD1a–) with prominent nucleoli. In a majority of cases, these large histiocytes exhibit the diagnostic feature of emperipolesis (engulfment of lymphocytes or plasma cells). *Erdheim–Chester disease* affects adults and may involve any part of the CNS or its coverings. Meningeal and perivascular lesions feature foamy histiocytes (S100 variable, CD68+, CD1a–, factor XIIIa+) but cells in the parenchyma may resemble activated microglia or neoplastic astrocytes; sparse lymphocytes, plasma cells, eosinophils, and multinucleated histiocytes may also be seen. Definitive diagnosis usually requires correlation with clinical and radiologic evidence of systemic involvement, particularly bone pain and sclerosis of the long bones. *Juvenile xanthogranuloma* (JXG) (e-**Fig. 41.59**) usually appears as an isolated cutaneous nodule in children, but can also occur as an isolated lesion in the brain or meninges. The histiocytes of this lesion are S-100-, CD68+, CD1a–, Factor X111a+, CD11c+, and lysozyme negative, an immunophenotype similar to that of plasmacytoid monocytes. Scattered Touton giant cells, lymphocytes, and eosinophils are commonly seen. JXG is benign, but may cause seizures. *Histiocytic sarcoma* is a very rare tumor that shows cytologic atypia, necrosis, and a high proliferative index; stains only with macrophage markers CD68 and CD163; and is associated with poor prognosis.

M. **Metastatic tumors to the CNS** are the most common CNS neoplasms, and occur in up to 30% of adult and 6% to 10% of pediatric cancer patients. Common sources in adults include carcinomas of lung, breast, kidney, and colon, as well as melanomas. In children, leukemia, lymphoma, osteogenic sarcoma, rhabdomyosarcoma, and Ewing sarcoma are the most common primaries. Radiologically, the majority of CNS metastases implant in the cerebral hemispheres at the junction of cortex and white matter, appear well circumscribed, and show ring-like or diffuse contrast enhancement. Histologically and immunophenotypically, metastases usually resemble their primary tumors at least focally; it is therefore always worthwhile to review slides from a putative primary tumor whenever possible.

VI. INFLAMMATORY AND INFECTIOUS DISORDERS

A. **Inflammatory demyelinating disorders** are characterized by myelin loss with relative preservation of axons; this finding is often accompanied by abundant foamy macrophages and perivascular lymphocytes. Classic radiographic examples of myelin disorders are not generally biopsied, but when clinical and/or radiologic data are unusual or ambiguous, neurosurgery may be recommended to obtain a tissue sample.

1. **Multiple sclerosis (MS)** is an idiopathic demyelinating disorder with genetic, environmental, and infectious influences. Historically, several subtypes have been described, including relapsing-remitting, secondary progressive, primary progressive, acute monophasic (Marburg disease), and acute tumefactive. The relapsing–remitting form (RRMS), characterized by intermittent attacks and partial recovery from neurologic deficits during periods of

remission, is more common in young adults (women > men with a ratio of 2:1) and is the most common form in the United States (~80% of cases). Less common forms involve rapid, unremitting clinical deterioration—either *de novo* (primary progressive MS [PPMS]) or in the setting of RRMS (secondary progressive MS [SPMS]). Demyelinative MS plaques in these subtypes most often involve white matter periventricularly, and in the optic pathway, brain stem, and/or spinal cord. Radiographically, chronic inactive plaques are hypointense on T1 and diffusion-weighted images; plaques with active inflammation are hyperintense on T2 and show postcontrast enhancement. This latter feature can be responsible for some radiological diagnostic uncertainty in cases of Marburg disease or acute tumefactive MS. In acute tumefactive MS, a large isolated plaque appears as a T2-hyperintense, peripherally enhancing lesion that resembles a high-grade glioma or lymphoma. Although the rim of enhancement around the demyelinative lesion may be incomplete at the cortical side (forming a horseshoe-shaped profile that would be highly unusual in a neoplasm), this feature is not robust enough for conclusive diagnosis; consequently, such lesions, although uncommon, are often biopsied. At frozen section, tumefactive MS can represent a great diagnostic challenge; in such cases, examination of a cytologic smear preparation is often very helpful as it preserves important cellular details that can be obscured by freezing artifact. Microscopically, an active demyelinative MS plaque shows (1) loss of myelin, (2) relative preservation of axons, (3) perivascular nonneoplastic lymphocytic infiltrates, (4) numerous foamy macrophages, (5) reactive astrocytosis, and (6) cerebral edema. Mitotic activity among astrocytes and macrophages may be brisk, but nuclear atypia should be minimal. Granular mitoses and Creutzfeldt cells (which contain multiple micronuclei), although not specific for MS lesions, are characteristic. Myelin loss with axonal sparing (which distinguishes this lesion from an axon-destroying infarct) is best visualized by comparing Luxol fast blue–PAS (LFB–PAS) stained sections to others stained with Bielschowsky silver or NF protein immunohistochemistry (e-Fig. 41.60). On LFB–PAS sections, the border of demyelination is usually abrupt, and blue-green debris (representing partially metabolized myelin) is visible within macrophages. In rare cases that cannot be satisfactorily diagnosed with special stains, FISH studies can be applied to evaluate for glioma-associated chromosomal changes.

2. **Acute disseminated encephalomyelitis (ADEM)/perivenous encephalomyelitis** represents an unusual autoimmune response among children and young adults that is induced by recent infection by measles (most commonly, but also), mumps, varicella, influenza, rubella, *Campylobacter jejuni*, or *Mycoplasma pneumoniae* or vaccination (smallpox or rabies). Symptoms include headache, fever and vomiting, followed by weakness, ataxia, and visual and sensory loss with progression to stupor and seizures. Radiologically, ADEM usually appears as many small T2-weighted and FLAIR hyperintensities in subcortical and periventricular white matter and the spinal cord; the deep gray matter and cortex may also be affected. This clinicoradiographic pattern is characteristic enough that biopsy is not always performed. Nevertheless, when obtained, biopsy material shows perivenous demyelination with axonal sparing, mononuclear infiltrates, macrophages, activated microglia, and occasional petechial hemorrhages. ADEM is thought to result from a myelin-directed, cross-reactive immune response to a foreign antigen.

3. **Demyelinating viral infections.** Viral infections that commonly cause CNS demyelination include human immunodeficiency virus (HIV leukoencephalopathy and vacuolar myelopathy [HIVL, HIVVM]), human T-cell lymphotropic virus-1 (HTLV-associated myelopathy/tropical spastic

paraparesis [HAM/TSP]), JC virus (progressive multifocal leukoencephalopathy [PML]), and measles virus (subacute sclerosing panencephalitis [SSPE]).

a. **HIVL/HIVVM.** White matter damage by HIV is thought to be mediated by virally infected macrophages and giant cells; oligodendrocytes are not directly infected. HIVL is often associated with HIV-associated encephalitis (HAVE) but begins earlier, often introducing cognitive impairment (up to 50% of AIDS patients develop dementia ascribed to HIVL and HIVE). Histologically, HIVL may show subtle white matter pallor, with variable numbers of microglial nodules, macrophages, and multinucleated giant cells. HIVVM targets the spinal cord in ~25% of AIDS cases, producing vacuolar myelopathy in the dorsal and lateral columns that resembles subacute combined degeneration.

b. **HAM/TSP,** characterized by paraparesis, spasticity, and hyperreflexia of the lower extremities and positive Babinski sign, affects 1% to 5% of individuals who are seropositive for HTLV-1. As the clinical presentation suggests, HAM/TSP preferentially affects the lateral columns (corticospinal tracts), most severely in the thoracic spinal cord; corresponding changes (T2 hyperintensity, thoracic spinal cord atrophy) are visible radiologically. Although biopsy is uncommonly undertaken, histology of the cord shows leptomeningeal and perivascular lymphocytic infiltrates, foamy macrophages, widespread myelin loss, and axonal dystrophy of the lateral columns.

c. **PML** is caused by reactivation of a latent JC papovavirus (much of the general population is seropositive) in the setting of immunosuppression (e.g., lymphoproliferative disorders, AIDS, monoclonal antibody treatments for autoimmune diseases). Patients experience 3 to 6 months of progressive neurologic symptoms that reflect the anatomic distribution of the lesions, which favor the subcortical and deep cerebral white matter, cerebellum, brainstem and, rarely, the spinal cord. Personality changes are often prominent, followed by dementia and death. In some cases, restoration of immunocompetency may halt the disease; in other cases, the restored inflammatory response hastens clinical decline (the so-called immune reconstitution inflammatory syndrome [IRIS]). On MRI, the lesions of PML are T2-hyperintense, T1-hypointense, and nonenhancing; however, enhancement is common in the setting of IRIS. Histologically, PML shows foci with myelin loss, a variably modest lymphocytic infiltrate (more pronounced in IRIS), and, within the center of larger lesions, few oligodendrocytes. Some oligodendrocytes show the hallmark lesion of PML, a large nucleus with marginated chromatin and a glassy inclusion that appears plum colored on H&E sections (e-Fig. 41.61). Ultrastructurally, the papovavirus particles exhibit a "stick and ball" or "spaghetti and meatballs" pattern. Also noted within and around these lesions are pseudoneoplastic astrocytes with atypical nuclei; these cells do not appear to produce or contain virus particles, and should not be mistaken for astrocytoma. Immunohistochemistry for JC virus proteins, EM, and in situ hybridization studies may be used to confirm the presence of the virus.

d. **SSPE** (e-Fig. 41.62) is a rare sequela of measles in which a defective measles paramyxovirus targets oligodendrocytes and neurons resulting in a slowly progressive encephalitis that results in coma and death. SSPE may present as many as 3 to 10 years after initial infection. Early in the course, radiographic findings are minimal; periventricular T2- and FLAIR hyperintensities appear late. Antimeasles IgG titers in CSF may be elevated. Histologically, SSPE shows large areas of myelin loss and neuron loss, leptomeningeal and perivascular lymphocytic infiltrates, and, most importantly, eosinophilic viral inclusions in the nuclei of oligodendrocytes and neurons. Diagnosis may be confirmed through immunohistochemistry for measles virus associated proteins.

B. CNS Infections may be broadly classified into meningitides, encephalitides, and abscesses.

1. **Meningitis** may be caused by bacteria, mycobacteria, viruses, fungi, and parasites. Although CSF analysis is often sufficient for diagnosis, biopsy is occasionally necessary.

    a. **Bacterial meningitis** is characterized in its acute stage by abundant neutrophils within the subarachnoid space, and subpial reactive gliosis. Organisms are usually difficult to identify. In the chronic stage, neutrophils are supplanted by mononuclear cells, and granulation tissue and fibrosis may appear.

    b. **Tuberculous meningitis** can mimic bacterial meningitis, but more commonly exhibits a patchy granulomatous infiltrate of epithelioid histiocytes, multinucleated giant cells, and mononuclear cells. As with bacterial meningitis, organisms are difficult to identify, even with acid-fast stains; ancillary testing (PCR, culture) may aid diagnosis.

    c. **Viral meningitis** often shows meningeal and perivascular lymphocytic infiltrates that may extend into Virchow–Robin spaces. Because these infiltrates can be minimal and patchy, absence of inflammation on biopsy does not rule out the diagnosis. Identification of microglial nodules in the parenchyma supports an additional diagnosis of viral encephalitis.

    d. **Fungal meningitis** provokes a mononuclear/granulomatous inflammatory response similar to that of tuberculous meningitis, but the organisms are usually easily identified by histochemical stains. Nevertheless, culture is required for definitive speciation. In contrast to yeast forms (*Histoplasma, Blastomyces, Cryptococcus*), pseudohyphal and hyphal organisms (*Candida, Aspergillus, Zygomycetes, Fusarium, Coccidioides*) can be angioinvasive and compromise blood supply leading to infarction.

2. **Encephalitis** is most often caused by viruses, and less commonly by parasites.

    a. **Viral encephalitis** is recognized histologically by the presence of meningeal and perivascular lymphocytes accompanied by parenchymal microglial nodules. Occasionally, a microglial nodule may be observed around a dying neuron (termed neuronophagia). Hundreds of viruses can cause encephalitis, and most do so without forming distinctive inclusions, so serologic/laboratory tests and clinical observations are usually required for diagnosis. Nevertheless, a small subset of pathogens is responsible for most clinically significant cases.

        i. **West Nile Virus (WNV)** has become the leading cause of epidemic viral encephalitis in the United States within the last decade, and now spans the continent. This arbovirus (arthropod-borne) infection has a peak incidence in the summer or early autumn. In the acute phase, WNV can induce a neutrophil response that is visible in the meninges and CSF. In the chronic phase, microglial nodules are most abundant in the spinal cord, thalamus, and substantia nigra pars compacta. WNV encephalitis is best diagnosed by detection of specific IgM in the CSF rather than by PCR.

        ii. **Herpes encephalitis** is the most common cause of sporadic viral encephalitis is the United States. Asymmetric, bilateral involvement of the temporal lobes is characteristic, and when severe involves hemorrhage and necrosis. Clinically, involvement of the temporal lobes may cause hallucinations, agitation, personality changes, and psychosis. PCR testing of CSF for HSV shows high sensitivity and specificity, but sensitivity might be lower early in the course of infection. Histologically, in addition to perivascular lymphocytes and microglial nodules, biopsy material may show areas of necrosis with foamy macrophages and hemorrhage. Intranuclear Cowdry A ("owl's eye") and Cowdry B (eosinophilic translucent) inclusions may also be visible in some cases. Immunohistochemistry or in situ hybridization for HSV-1 and HSV-2 may be applied to confirm the diagnosis.

iii. **Varicella zoster virus (VZV) encephalitis** is more common with immunosuppression, and targets several structures leading to different injuries. By infecting and damaging large- and medium-sized vessels, VZV causes bland and hemorrhagic infarcts. By damaging small vessels, VZV causes small, deep, ovoid ischemic lesions, and then infects the newly exposed oligodendrocytes, creating areas of demyelination; intranuclear Cowdry A inclusions (e-**Fig. 41.63**) are often visible within glial cells at the lesion's edges. Less commonly, VZV infects ependymal cells causing ventriculitis.

iv. **HIV encephalitis** (microglial nodule encephalitis), in conjunction with HIV leukoencephalopathy, is associated with the dementia that complicates AIDS. The histopathology features widespread, robust microglial nodules with associated lymphocytes, reactive astrocytes, and occasional multinucleated giant cells that harbor the virus. Neurotoxic cytokines and other damaging chemical agents (e.g., reactive oxygen species) may also play a role in this poorly understood dementia, which is also associated with cortical and subcortical atrophy.

v. **Rocky Mountain spotted fever** is caused by rickettsia, but can mimic viral encephalitis and is therefore mentioned here. The organism targets vascular endothelium and smooth muscle cells, and thus produces vasculitis, thrombosis, microinfarcts, and petechial hemorrhage without fibrinoid necrosis. Microglial nodules and mononuclear infiltrates with a leptomeningeal and perivascular distribution are commonly seen.

b. **Parasitic encephalitis**

i. **Neurocysticercosis** (e-**Fig. 41.64**), caused by the pork tapeworm, *Taenia solium,* is the most common CNS parasitic infection worldwide and a common cause of seizures. The larvae form thin-walled cysts in muscle, brain, eyes, liver, and lung. Each cyst contains a scolex that can be detected radiographically or histologically and serves as the pathognomonic feature of the lesion. Death of the organism triggers a brisk mixed and granulomatous inflammatory response. Over months to years, inflammation subsides; the cyst becomes fibrotic and, eventually, a small calcified nodule.

ii. **Cerebral malaria** affects fewer than 10% of infected individuals, favoring those without immunity (<4 years of age, foreign visitors). Presenting symptoms include fever, headache, backache, photophobia, vomiting, variable neurologic deficits, and seizures. The disorder is caused by the deposition/lodging of parasitized erythrocytes within the microvasculature of the brain, which is accompanied by petechial hemorrhages in the white matter around necrotic vessels. Over time, the ring hemorrhages are resorbed by microglia, macrophages, and astrocytes, forming Dürck granulomas. Prompt treatment with corticosteroids and antimalarial drugs reduces mortality.

iii. **Amebic encephalitis (AE)** is caused by several organisms, including *Naegleria fowleri, Balamuthia mandrillaris,* and *Acanthamoeba* species; *Entamoeba histolytica* tends to form abscesses. *N. fowleri*—usually encountered during fresh water swimming—enters the CNS through the cribriform plate; the other parasites enter hematogenously from other infected organs. Clinically, AE with *N. fowleri* presents in previously healthy children and young adults as acute meningitis and progresses to coma and death in 2 to 3 days. Histologically, mononuclear inflammation of the meninges is scanty, but the adjacent brain shows extensive hemorrhagic necrosis. Organisms are visible in the subarachnoid space and around vessels. These trophozoites bear a striking resemblance to foamy macrophages but have a prominent central nucleolus. AE with *B. mandrillaris* and *Acanthamoeba* has a similar dismal prognosis, but a more chronic course.

iv. **Toxoplasmosis** is seen in neonates as a congenital infection (one of the TORCH infections) that leads to microcephaly with dystrophic calcifications. Later in life, infection may cause fever, a maculopapular rash, and malaise or may be asymptomatic. In the setting of subsequent immunosuppression (particularly AIDS) a dormant infection can undergo reactivation and present with multiple deep-seated and/or cortical enhancing lesions. Grossly, the focal lesions of cerebral toxoplasmosis are multiple, discrete, and necrotic; less commonly, toxoplasmosis may appear as a more diffuse encephalitis. Histologically (e-**Fig. 41.65**), the necrotic lesions show peripheral mixed inflammatory infiltrates, neovascularization, and gliosis. Perivascular inflammation and fibrinoid necrosis of vessels may also be seen. Although H&E stains are usually adequate for identifying *Toxoplasma gondii,* immunostains for the protozoan offer greater sensitivity and specificity. In unusual cases when cerebral toxoplasmosis manifests diffusely without necrotic foci, histologic changes include microglial nodules and reactive astrocytosis.

3. **Brain abscess** may be caused by bacteria, protozoa, or fungi. Most cases result from direct spread from the paranasal sinuses, middle ear, or dental root; in other cases, the organism travels hematogenously from another site. In children, congenital heart defects may allow septic emboli to bypass the pulmonary circulation; in adults, lung infections and endocarditis are the most common sources of hematogenous inoculation. Damaged brain tissue and immunosuppression contribute in some cases. Abscesses mature over a 2-week period. Days 1 to 2 involve endothelial swelling and neutrophil invasion; over days 3 to 4, necrosis and macrophages are prominent, and lymphocytes and plasma cells join the infiltrate; over days 5 to 7, granulation tissue forms around the necrotic center; and over days 8 to 14, the capsule becomes strengthened by collagen and fibrosis, traversed by radially oriented capillaries and surrounded by gliosis.

C. **Granulomatous inflammation**
1. **Sarcoidosis** affects the CNS in 5% of the cases, most often involving the basal meninges, cranial nerves, optic tracts, and/or hypothalamus. Facial nerve palsy is the most common presenting symptom, but other focal deficits also occur, reflecting loss of function of involved structures. CNS-only sarcoidosis is quite rare, but cases of systemic sarcoidosis that also affect the CNS often receive neurosurgical/neuropathologic attention because the neurologic symptoms are so worrisome. Radiographically, the involved structures show postcontrast enhancement. Grossly, the meninges and cranial nerves may appear nodular and thickened. Microscopically, affected structures show epithelioid granulomas with giant cells (e-**Fig. 41.66**). Necrosis, although it may be seen focally, is not a usual feature of neurosarcoidosis, and should encourage consideration of other diagnoses. Because sarcoidosis is a diagnosis of exclusion, reasonable efforts to exclude other etiologies for granulomatous inflammation (e.g., fungal, tuberculous, and

rheumatologic) must be made. Ultimately, a pathologic diagnosis no more specific than granulomatous inflammation (accompanied by an appropriate written comment) is usually warranted.

VII. SEIZURE DISORDERS. Surgically curable seizure disorders are broadly classified into neoplastic and nonneoplastic lesions. Distinct neoplastic entities that generate chronic seizures include DNT, GGs, and PXAs, and are discussed above. Common nonneoplastic entities are discussed below.

A. Hippocampal (mesial temporal) sclerosis (HS) is a disorder characterized by neuronal loss and gliosis of the hippocampus and, in some cases, adjacent mesial temporal structures such as the amygdala and entorhinal cortex. Clinically, HS is associated with longstanding complex partial seizures, most often beginning near the turn of the first decade of life. Radiographically, the hippocampus is small, and affected structures show T2 and FLAIR hyperintensity and evidence of hypometabolism. Surgical treatment often involves amygdalo-hippocampectomy. Histologically, the hippocampus shows variable neuronal loss and gliosis, most pronounced in areas CA1 (Sommer's sector) and CA4 (the endfolium of Ammon's horn) (e-**Fig. 41.67**). In more advanced cases, area CA3 and the subiculum may be similarly affected. Neurons within the dentate gyrus are often reduced in number and, in some cases, may appear dispersed or split into two layers. Because this diagnosis requires accurate identification of neuronal populations defined only by anatomic landmarks, the hippocampal specimen must be carefully oriented when it is sectioned for histology; ideally, it is resected in one piece that can be sectioned perpendicular to its long axis to reveal the desired classic "seahorse" architecture. Not uncommonly, HS resection specimens demonstrate a second pathology (a minute tumor or a malformation of cortical development [MCD]) that could otherwise independently account for seizures; such findings mirror the clinicopathologic experience that seizure activity can both engender and arise from HS. After resection, the vast majority of patients experience a significant reduction in seizure frequency or are cured altogether.

B. Malformation of cortical development (MCD/cortical dysplasia) is a general term applied to a wide range of developmental abnormalities that affect the cortex. These abnormalities come to attention most often as epileptogenic foci, and are thought to account for up to 25% of cases of intractable epilepsy.

Grossly and radiographically, MCD may appear as (1) ectopic bands or nodules of cortical tissue in the white matter (heterotopias); (2) a firm, focal cortical expansion (cortical tuber); (3) an area of smooth, unfolded cortical ribbon (agyria/lissencephaly); (4) an area of cortical ribbon with few, broad gyri (pachygyria); (5) an area of cortex with many small irregular gyri and fused sulci (polymicrogyria); (6) an area with a blurred gray-white junction (some focal cortical dysplasias, FCDs); or (7) ostensibly normal tissue (other FCDs).

Histologically, MCD shows similar variability. Heterotopias contain gray matter neuropil and abnormally arranged neuronal elements. Cortical tubers are formed by aggregates of large "balloon cells" with abundant glassy eosinophilic cytoplasm and an eccentrically placed neuron-like nucleus (e-**Fig. 41.68**). Tubers may occur sporadically in isolation or in greater numbers in the setting of TS; the lesion itself is histologically identical in the two settings. Agyria and pachygyria appear most commonly as a four-layered (rather than six-layered) cortical ribbon. Polymicrogyria has been described as having two-layered and/or four-layered areas within the cortex, but the most consistent feature is a fusion of two adjacent molecular layers through what would otherwise be a sulcus.

FCD, like MCD, represents a collection of entities; these have been conveniently organized within the classification of Palmini et al. (*Neurology*

2004;62[Suppl 3]:S2). Particularly in subtle cases, immunohistochemistry for NeuN (to accentuate neuronal cytoarchitecture), NF protein (to stain the somata of enlarged, atypical neurons), GFAP and CD34 (to reveal poorly defined, highly branched cells associated with MCDs) may facilitate diagnosis (*Acta Neuropathol.* 1999;97:481).

C. **Other seizure-associated disorders** encountered less often are hemimegalencephaly, Rasmussen encephalitis, hypothalamic hamartoma, and Sturge–Weber angiomatosis.

VIII. VASCULAR DISORDERS

A. **Vascular malformations** are classified into four groups: arteriovenous malformation (AVM), cerebral cavernous malformation/cavernoma (CCM), capillary telangiectasia (CT), and venous angioma (VA). CT and VA are asymptomatic and virtually never encountered in surgical pathology, so will not be discussed further.

1. **Arteriovenous malformations (AVMs)** are usually supratentorial and are thought to be congenital. About 50% come to clinical attention in the third, fourth, or fifth decades due to hemorrhage. Other AVMs induce seizures or, less often, slowly grow and cause a constellation of progressively worsening headaches and focal neurologic deficits. Angiography and MRI provide a diagnosis, reveal abnormal flow characteristics, and identify the supplying and draining vessels of these lesions to facilitate intervention strategy. Grossly, superficially located AVMs typically show dilated, thick-walled draining veins on the cortical surface; cut sections show a disorganized mass of blood vessels of varying mural thickness and diameter, with associated atrophic, relatively firm (gliotic) brain parenchyma. Histologically, AVMs are characterized by an array of abnormal blood vessels that show evidence of remodeling and degenerative changes (arteries with medial hyperplasia, collagen deposition, and complex restructuring of the internal elastic lamina; veins with thick collagenous walls). In some vessels, mixed arterial and venous features can be identified. Amongst the abnormal blood vessels, the intervening parenchyma shows atrophy, astrocytosis and, often, hemosiderin deposits. Masson trichrome stain and an elastin stain Verhoeff-Van Gieson (VVG) can be used to reveal features of the vascular pathology that are subtle on routine sections. If embolization has been performed prior to resection, intravascular foreign material may be identified; if sufficient time has elapsed, a foreign body giant cell reaction may be visible.

2. **CCM** (also called cavernous angioma, cavernous hemangioma, and cavernoma) is a vascular malformation characterized by large, thin-walled ectatic vessels or sinusoids that are closely packed with minimal intervening brain parenchyma (**e-Fig. 41.69**). CCMs are usually supratentorial, but may occur anywhere in the CNS or leptomeninges. Autopsy studies have estimated the prevalence of sporadic CCMs to be approximately 1 in 200 individuals. As many as 50% of the patients with these lesions develop seizures and/or recurrent headaches. Additionally, these lesions exhibit an annual 1% chance of hemorrhage. Because such hemorrhages are not at high pressure, they are usually not fatal; however, they may cause focal neurologic deficits and do increase the risk of seizures and subsequent hemorrhage severalfold. Brainstem lesions are associated with worse prognosis. Radiographically, T2-weighted images show a heterogeneous center with a surrounding rim of hypodensity that corresponds to deposits of hemosiderin; gradient-echo MRI shows greater sensitivity for this ferruginous penumbra and therefore can detect smaller lesions. Grossly, CCMs appear spongy and dark red with golden brown hues due to hemosiderin deposition and, occasionally, calcifications. Microscopically, the vascular component shows only a single layer of endothelium and lacks a muscular layer and an internal

elastic lamina. The peripheral rim of resected tissue contains hemosiderin-laden macrophages and gliotic parenchyma with axonal spheroids. Areas of fibrosis, xanthomatous degeneration, and calcification are common. Although most cases are sporadic, some are familial with an autosomal dominant inheritance, and affected individuals often have multiple CCMs.

B. **Primary angiitis of the CNS (PACNS).** Inflammation of the CNS vasculature may occur as part of a systemic vasculitis (e.g., Giant cell arteritis, polyarteritis nodosa) or may be CNS specific (PACNS). PACNS more commonly afflicts males in late middle age. Symptoms are highly variable, but are generally multi-focal, intermittent, progressive and, by definition, strictly neurologic. On MRI, PACNS may show nothing more than multiple ischemic microinfarcts; the angiographic finding of alternating luminal stenosis and dilatation (beads on a string), while characteristic, is neither sensitive nor specific for the disorder. CSF cytology may show mild lymphocytic pleocytosis, another nonspecific finding. To establish the diagnosis, meningeal/brain biopsy is performed. Histologically, the key feature of PACNS is segmental granulomatous inflammation of small- and medium-sized arteries featuring transmural lymphocytic infiltrates and expansion of the intima by histiocytes and multinucleated giant cells. Fibrinoid necrosis is characteristic but not required for diagnosis. The associated parenchyma often shows changes associated with ischemic injury. As is the case for sarcoidosis, other potential causes of granulomatous vasculitis (including acid-fast bacilli, fungus, and intravascular amyloid) must be excluded, and the most appropriate pathologic diagnosis is often simply "granulomatous vasculitis." Although prognosis is poor without treatment, immunosuppression (prednisone, with or without cyclophosphamide) has been effective in some cases.

C. **Congophilic (or cerebral) amyloid angiopathy (CAA)** is characterized by deposits of amyloid in leptomeningeal and superficial cortical vessels. By far, the most common substrate of this disease is amyloid-beta 1 to 40; ~80% of the neuropathologically confirmed AD cases show CAA at least focally. Not surprisingly, therefore, CAA commonly affects the elderly. These deposits can disrupt physiological autoregulation of blood flow and may contribute to cognitive dysfunction. Most often CAA comes to clinical attention only when it becomes severe enough to compromise vessel integrity. The superficial lobar hemorrhage that can result from CAA can cause mass effect and may resemble intratumoral hemorrhage; consequently, surgical evacuation is often performed for decompression, occasionally with some degree of parenchymal resection to determine the cause. Parenthetically, this circumstance illustrates why CNS hematoma evacuation specimens must be examined very thoroughly for even the smallest fragments of brain tissue. Microscopically, involved vessels show amyloid deposits that can be appreciated on routine and special stains (Congo red and thioflavin S) (e-Fig. 41.70). Immunohistochemistry can be used to identify the amyloidogenic peptide involved; cases that do not show reactivity for amyloid-beta may be tested for rarer forms that are caused by cystatin C (Icelandic type), integral membrane protein 2B (ITM2B, British type or Danish type), gelsolin (Finnish type), or transthyretin (meningo-vascular amyloidosis). Although inflammation is usually absent, specimens must be evaluated for amyloid-beta related angiitis (ABRA), a form of granulomatous vasculitis (e-Fig. 41.71) that may respond to immunosuppressive therapy.

D. **Cerebral Autosomal Dominant Arteriopathy with Subcortical Infarcts and Leukoencephalopathy (CADASIL)** (e-Fig. 41.72) is caused by missense mutations of the *Notch3* gene. The abnormal protein accumulates in granules (PAS-positive, osmiophilic) within the walls of small arteries, the smooth muscle layer degenerates, and the vessel walls become thickened and fibrotic; this process gradually diminishes capacity for and regulation of perfusion. CADASIL usually presents in the fifth or sixth decade of life with classic migraine, multiple sub-cortical ischemic strokes, psychiatric disturbance, and later, dementia. In this context, T2 hyperintensities in anterior temporal lobes and external capsules on MRI are strongly suggestive. Although the symptoms of CADASIL arise from the brain, the disease also affects peripheral tissues including the skin. His-tologic and ultrastructural examination of arterioles in the skin or brain pro-vides the diagnosis. Notably, a rare, otherwise identical clinical/radiologic syn-drome with an autosomal recessive inheritance pattern (appropriately named CARASIL, linked to the *HTRA1* gene) lacks granular osmiophilic inclusions.

E. **Cerebral infarcts.** Most often, biopsies of infarcts are performed when "glioma" is in the differential diagnosis, particularly in young patients. Gross and micro-scopic features of a cerebral infarct change over time. In the acute stage (1 to 3 days), red necrotic neurons, vacuolated neuropil, and variable neu-trophilic infiltrates are present. Subacute infarcts (days to weeks) demon-strate capillary proliferation with prominent endothelial cells, numerous foamy macrophages, and reactive astrocytes that are typically more common at the periphery. Because such reparative lesions may exhibit mitotic figures, necro-sis, and microvascular proliferation consistent with GBM, care must be taken to recognize the reactive and histiocytic components, particularly during an intraoperative microscopic evaluation. Large infarcts eventually evolve into cystic lesions with a weblike network of delicate blood vessels, sparse gliotic parenchymal remnants, and a few residual macrophages. Infarcts disrupt and destroy axons, a feature often helpful in distinguishing infarcts from demyeli-native processes such as MS in which the axons are relatively spared. Once an infarct is diagnosed, identifying its cause is the next step; if the specimen at hand provides no insight, clinical correlation is required.

IX. **NEURODEGENERATIVE DISORDERS.** Although some of these affect children and ado-lescents, most come to clinical attention after the fifth or sixth decades. An increas-ing number of neurodegenerative diseases can be diagnosed by identifying changes in DNA, biologic fluids, peripheral biopsy material, or radiographic images. Nev-ertheless, few treatments are currently available in clinic for neurodegenerative disorders, and most of them remain idiopathic, progressive, and fatal. Conse-quently, CNS biopsy performed explicitly to diagnose a neurodegenerative disease is rare. These disorders usually appear in a surgical pathology specimen inciden-tally (e.g., when some brain is removed to evacuate a life-threatening hematoma) or when unusual clinical/radiologic data suggest that securing a definitive tissue diagnosis warrants the risk of brain biopsy. Recognizing these disorders in surgical specimens may become more critical as treatments become available.

A. **Alzheimer disease (AD),** the most common neurodegenerative disorder, is char-acterized histologically by neuron loss, gliosis, and the presence of extracellular beta-amyloid peptide deposits (diffuse, cored, and neuritic plaques) and NFTs (NFT, intraneuronal aggregates of hyperphosphorylated tau protein) in the neocortex and hippocampus (e-**Fig. 41.73**). Plaque deposition begins 10 to 15 years before the onset of very mild dementia of the Alzheimer type (DAT, the appropriate term for the clinical manifestations of AD). The degree of cognitive impairment appears to correlate with the severity and extent of NFT pathology, which begins in the mesial temporal lobes and subsequently spreads outward to involve the parietal and frontal lobes; the occipital lobe is relatively spared. Neuroimaging techniques (to assess atrophy, metabolism, and amyloid burden within the brain) and CSF biomarker measurements (e.g., of amyloid-beta peptide and tau protein) are likely to allow reasonable antemortem con-firmation of AD pathology in the near future (*Nature* 2009;461:916–922), but recognition of the histologic changes will remain important.

Currently, there are three leading sets of criteria for the neuropatho-logic diagnosis of AD: Khachaturian, Consortium to Establish a Registry for

Alzheimer's Disease (CERAD), and National Institute on Aging (NIA/Reagan). Technically, the Khachaturian system, which evaluates only the presence of amyloid plaques within any portion of neocortex, is the only one that can be applied faithfully to a limited brain biopsy; officially, CERAD requires sampling of numerous cortical areas (possible only at autopsy) for a semiquantitative assessment of neuritic plaques, and NIA/Reagan additionally requires assessment of the anatomical distribution of NFT pathology within the brain. Nevertheless, since NFT pathology correlates most reliably with the degree of cognitive impairment and the frontal lobe is generally affected later in the disease process, the presence of plaques and NFTs in a biopsy specimen from the frontal lobe should suggest that AD pathology may be responsible for/contributing to a patient's cognitive symptoms. The deposits of AD are best visualized by modified Bielschowsky silver staining, thioflavin S or T staining (using fluorescence microscopy), or by immunohistochemistry for amyloid-beta peptide and for phosphorylated tau protein. As discussed above, CAA often accompanies AD pathology.

B. **Lewy body disease (LBD).** This generic term is intended to unify several clinico-pathologic diagnoses that feature this intraneuronal inclusion and the related Lewy neurite (e-Fig. 41.8). Lewy body pathology, either alone or in conjunction with AD, is associated with about 10% to 15% of dementia cases. LB pathology has been proposed (in the setting of clinical PD) to begin within a few selectively vulnerable brainstem nuclei and to spread rostrally, reaching the prefrontal neocortex in later stages (*Neurobiol Aging* 2003;24:197). In parallel, many patients with PD develop dementia about 10 years after motor symptoms. Therefore, identification of these lesions in a frontal lobe biopsy specimen at sufficient density provides reasonable evidence that a patient may be suffering from dementia related to LBD (*Neurology* 2005;65:1863). Because these lesions are very subtle on H&E sections of the neocortex, and because they are not argyrophilic on Bielschowsky-stained sections, immunohistochemistry for (ideally, phosphorylated) alpha-synuclein is required for definitive identification; this stain should therefore be applied routinely, particularly when symptomatology is suggestive of PD or dementia with LBs, or when other relevant pathologies are not detected.

C. **Creutzfeldt–Jakob Disease (CJD)** (e-Fig. 41.74). The need to diagnose or rule out CJD as a cause of rapidly progressive dementia (developing in ~2 years or less) is one of the leading clinical scenarios prompting brain biopsy. CJD is a transmissible spongiform encephalopathy (TSE; other types include Gerstmann–Strauss–Scheinker [GSS] syndrome, fatal insomnia, and kuru) that is classically characterized by a clinical triad of myoclonus, periodic shortwave EEG activity, and rapidly progressive dementia. Diffusion weighted (DWI) and FLAIR MRI commonly show restricted diffusion within the striatum and cerebral cortex. Although the condition is transmissible, most cases are sporadic, affecting one person per million individuals per year with a peak age of onset at age 60; 10% of the cases are familial and are attributable to mutations in the prion protein. Only rare examples are iatrogenic, resulting from inoculation with tissues or instruments inadvertently contaminated by protease-resistant prion protein from another individual with CJD. Microscopically, CJD cases show neuronal loss, gliosis, and spongiform change consisting of small, sharply defined, punched out vacuoles. These histologic changes appear in an anatomic pattern suggested by radiographic changes, but evaluation is typically limited to a right frontal cortex biopsy specimen. Within the cortex, the spongiform change of CJD should span the entire thickness of the cortical ribbon; other dementing conditions may show vacuolation that appears similar and is limited to superficial layers. It is worth noting, however, that the histologic changes in CJD may be anatomically patchy, and therefore very subtle or invisible in a limited biopsy specimen. It is also worth noting that biopsies of individuals with CJD may also show preexisting histologic changes associated with other dementing illnesses, therefore, identification of abundant amyloid plaques, NFTs, or LBs does not rule out the possibility of CJD. For this reason, immunoblotting and immunohistochemical analysis for the abnormal protease-resistant protein are essential for definitive diagnosis.

D. **New variant CJD (nvCJD)** is a rare form of TSE linked to bovine spongiform encephalopathy (BSE). Unlike CJD, nvCJD affects a younger demographic (adults younger than 40 years), typically has a longer clinical course characterized by behavioral changes more often than dementia, and shows an additional thalamic abnormality on DWI, T2, and FLAIR MRI. Microscopically, the most characteristic feature is the presence of numerous amyloid plaques (the so-called florid plaques that are PRP-positive, amyloid-beta negative) in the cerebral and cerebellar cortices. The few hundred cases reported since 1996 have been clustered in the UK and France and are thought to stem from an outbreak of BSE that affected the UK cattle industry in 1986. Perhaps reflecting the incubation period and changes in cattle industry practices, the incidence of nvCJD in the UK has dwindled over the last decade, so the diagnosis is now quite rare.

Cytopathology of the Central Nervous System

Souzan Sanati and Lourdes R. Ylagan

I. **SPECIMEN TYPES.** The most common specimen type obtained for cytologic evaluation of pathologic conditions of the central nervous system (CNS) is cerebrospinal fluid. Rarely, stereotactic fine needle aspiration (FNA) of cysts or masses of the CNS is used to provide specimens for cytologic diagnosis.

A. **Cerebrospinal fluid (CSF).** Several methods have been developed in the last decade for concentration of samples obtained via lumbar puncture, including cytocentrifugation and membrane filtration. Slides prepared via the cytocentrifugation technique using a cytofunnel (http://www.shandon.com) are usually Diff-Quik stained since leukemic involvement of the CSF is the most common malignant diagnosis; the limited amount of material obtained (0.5 to 1.0 ml) usually precludes allocating material for Papanicolaou and other stains. Although the precise proportions vary by practice setting, most CSF specimens obtained for headaches and mental status changes show reactive (e-**Fig. 41.75**) or nonspecific features, and usually contain benign lymphocytes and monocytes (e-**Fig. 41.76**). Other normal cells which can be found in CSF specimens include ependymal and choroidal cells (e-**Fig. 41.77**).

1. **Traumatic tap.** CSF samples that consist predominantly of peripheral blood are diagnosed as "negative for malignant cells" with the caveat that the sample may represent a traumatic tap (which occurs in about one-quarter of the cases). When a CSF sample shows leukemic involvement in the presence of peripheral blood, the possibility of CSF sample contamination by peripheral blood blasts should be raised and a repeat sample should be obtained.

2. **Infectious processes.** Peripheral blood contamination can result in the presence of variable numbers of polymorphonuclear neutrophils in a CSF sample; however, abundant neutrophils in the absence of blood contamination should raise the possibility of acute meningitis. Prompt diagnosis is crucial, since it can be fatal if not treated promptly (e-**Fig. 41.78**). Aseptic meningitis gives a picture

of an increased number of mature appearing lymphocytes and monocytes (e-Fig. 41.79). Suspicion of an infectious process should prompt additional work up including microbiologic cultures and molecular methods to identify the source of infection. With the advent of highly active antiretroviral therapy (HAART), AIDS related CSF lesions have become rare in recent years (*J Neurovirol.* 2005;11(Suppl 3):72).

3. **Lymphoma and leukemia.** A primary diagnosis of lymphoma or leukemia should not be made in the absence of flow cytometric analysis of the cells to demonstrate a clonal process. A diagnosis of involvement by lymphoma or leukemia may be rendered if malignant appearing lymphoid cells or cells consistent with blasts are present (e-Figs. 41.80 to 41.85) in a patient with a previously proven history of lymphoma or leukemia.

4. **Metastasis.** Cytologic examination of CSF can be used to document CNS involvement in patients who have a known history of metastatic carcinoma (e-Fig. 41.86) or melanoma (e-Fig. 41.87), as well as leukemia or lymphoma (e-Fig. 41.88) as noted above. In cases of metastasis, the diagnosis should be confirmed by immunocytochemical stains or by comparison of the cytologic material with the patient's primary malignancy. The diagnostic approach to the rare metastatic tumors of unknown origin that present in the CSF is the same as for tumors of unknown origin presenting at other sites (*Semin Oncol.* 1993;20:206).

B. **Stereotactic brain FNA** is an uncommon procedure, and the choice of the preparatory method is dependent upon the type of tissue aspirated. Involvement by a known primary lesion should be confirmed by comparison of the cytologic specimen with the prior diagnostic material. Fluid or purulent fine needle aspirates should be cultured as well as submitted for cytologic evaluation.

C. **Diagnostic categories**

1. **Negative for malignancy.** This diagnosis is rendered for CSF specimens in which only benign cellular elements, and primarily mature appearing lymphocytes and/or monocytes are present.

2. **Atypical cytology.** This diagnosis is rendered when there are rare atypical cells but for which there is inadequate material for ancillary studies. This diagnosis should prompt the collection of additional material for either flow cytometric or immunocytochemical evaluation.

3. **Suspicious for malignancy.** This diagnosis is rendered when there are rare cells highly concerning for involvement by a malignant process, but when the findings are nonetheless insufficient for definitive diagnosis.

4. **Positive for malignancy.** This diagnosis is rendered when there is both quantitative and qualitative evidence of a malignant neoplasm. Ancillary tests can be used to provide a definitive diagnosis as to the type of neoplasm.

D. **Special techniques.** Special techniques, such as confirmatory FISH, can be performed on CSF samples (e-Fig. 41.89).

42

Nerve Biopsies

Robert E. Schmidt

Successful use of nerve biopsy requires a discussion between the clinician and neuropathologist since the clinical differential diagnosis may dictate an unusual sampling scheme, for example, vasculitis in which multiple cross-sections may be required for diagnosis.

I. **NORMAL PERIPHERAL NERVE AND METHODS OF ANALYSIS.** The sural nerve, a cutaneous sensory nerve to the lateral foot, is typically biopsied without stretching or use of intraneural anesthetic. The nerve is divided into a portion for fixation in formalin for paraffin embedding, and a portion for fixation in glutaraldehyde for plastic sections and possible electron microscopy. The entire nerve is typically used rather than dissected into individual fascicles. The portion (~1 cm) of the nerve fixed in formalin should be cut into 3 mm segments and examined in cross-section with paraffin-embedded H&E sections, thioflavin-S histochemistry, and possible immunohistochemistry.

An **H&E-stained cross section** of the sural nerve (e-Fig. 42.1)* contains 6 to 12 fascicles, each surrounded by flattened perineurial cells. Outside the perineurium is the epineurium, containing connective tissue and an anastomotic vascular network. Often individual myelinated axons can be seen in H&E-stained material (e-Fig. 42.2). The endoneurium (the space inside of the perineurial cell layer and outside the axon/Schwann cell units) contains fluid, collagen, capillaries, venules, fibroblasts, macrophages/monocytes, and scattered mast cells. Immunohistologic localization is useful for the demonstration of neurofilaments (a rough measure of axon number, e-Fig. 42.3), amyloid, immunoglobulins, subtypes of inflammatory cells, and growth factors and their receptors.

Plastic-embedded sections of 1 μm thickness (e-Fig. 42.4) provide a wealth of information. Myelinated axons range in diameter from 2 to 18 μm and are coarsely separated into small (mean of 4 μm) and large (~12 μm) myelinated axon populations (e-Figs. 42.5 and 42.6) with myelin thickness related directly to axonal diameter. The patterns of nerve damage visible in plastic sections may be characteristic (although rarely pathognomonic) of certain disease entities or pathogenetic processes. Qualitative information is provided on the degree of myelinated axon loss, distribution of axon loss, presence of active axonal degeneration (AD) or demyelination, identification of regenerative clusters of axons, swollen axons, onion-bulb formation, the nature of cellular infiltrates, or amyloid deposition. Groups of unmyelinated axon populations are detectable in plastic sections (e-Fig. 42.6).

Ultrastructure provides additional detail and is the only definitive method to evaluate unmyelinated axons (e-Fig. 42.7), which are three- to fourfold more numerous than myelinated axons in the sural nerve and typically are <2 μm in diameter.

If necessary, lengths of individual lightly fixed, osmicated myelinated axons can be dissected or "teased" out of a fascicle with pins. Each myelin internode, maintained by a single Schwann cell, ranges from 0.2 to 1.8 mm in length, increasing

---

*All e-figures are available online via the Solution Site Image Bank.

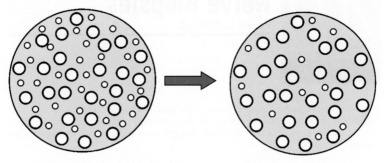

Figure 42.1 Selective loss of small myelinated axons. Normal fascicle is on the left.

linearly with axon diameter. Ongoing activity or residua of past episodes of demyelination or AD are readily identified.

Morphometry provides quantitative data concerning axon number and axon size-frequency distribution. Large axons are lost in uremia, abetalipoproteinemia, thallium, arsenic, acute intermittent porphyria, cisplatin, vincristine, and Friedreich ataxia. Small axons are selectively damaged (Fig. 42.1) in amyloidosis, some forms of diabetic neuropathy, acute pandysautonomia, Fabry disease, and hereditary sensory and autonomic neuropathies (HSANs).

II. THREE BASIC PATHOLOGIC MECHANISMS CHARACTERIZE NEUROPATHIES

A. **Axonal degeneration** is the most common pattern in biopsies, resulting in degeneration of the axon and its myelin sheath (**e-Figs. 42.8** and **42.9**). Often the distal portions of the longest axons are preferentially involved (i.e., distal axonopathy or dying-back neuropathy). Myelin destruction and its early catabolism occurs in the Schwann cell, producing the myelin "ovoid" of teased fibers and is subsequently continued in hematogenously and endogenously derived macrophages which engulf the debris. Early regenerative events begin immediately with the proliferation of Schwann cells and their processes which accumulate within the original basal lamina of the axon/Schwann cell unit as "bands of Büngner" which are conduits for regenerating axonal sprouts. Schwann cells increase their synthesis of growth factors as trophic and tropic stimuli. Maturing axons form regenerative clusters (**e-Fig. 42.10**) of thinly myelinated axons within the original Schwann cell's basal lamina and, with time, one axon emerges and begins to function and the others regress. Such a regenerated axon characteristically has a myelin sheath relatively thin for its axon's caliber. Teased fiber preparations show a distinctive and uniform internodal length regardless of axon diameter. The end-stage of a chronic neuropathy may consist of rare preserved axons, scattered fibroblasts, and Schwann cells and may provide little information concerning the process which preceded it.

AD shares mechanisms with Wallerian degeneration (WD) which is the reaction of axons and myelin distal to a crush injury. In WD, many axons show simultaneous involvement and are often at the same histologic stage; in AD, it is typical to find degenerating, regenerating, and normal axons together, some of which may have a distinctive pathologic signature (Fig. 42.2).

B. **Segmental demyelination** represents preferential damage to one or several internodes of the myelin sheath, directly to myelin or to its Schwann cell, with relative axonal sparing as seen in this teased fiber preparation (**e-Fig. 42.11**). Schwann cell proliferation results in the replacement of each lost myelin internode by several shorter internodes resulting in variation in internodal length along individual teased fibers.

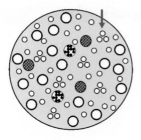 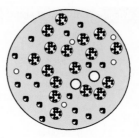

**Axonal
Degeneration**

**Wallerian
Degeneration**

Figure 42.2 AD vs. WD. AD is typically characterized by simultaneous AD, regenerative clusters (*arrow*), and axons with pathologic signatures (*crosshatched*) compared with synchronous and uniform degeneration of most axons in a fascicle in WD.

C. Secondary demyelination preferentially, nonrandomly involves selected axons, which may be atrophic or damaged, while entirely sparing others. It may reflect an abnormal axon-Schwann cell interaction resulting in secondary myelin loss. Uremic neuropathy is the prototype.

III. TOXIN-INDUCED NEUROPATHIES. A huge number of toxins and drugs (Table 42.1), including many whose neuropathic toxicity limits their clinical usefulness, produce neuropathy, likely with different mechanisms. One group of ADs targets axonal transport, and others selectively affect neurofilaments or microtubules. Acrylamide can result in distinctive neurofilament and tubulovesicular aggregates involving distal portions of axons. Zinc pyridinethionine and bromophenylacety-lurea preferentially target reversal of the polarity of axonal transport resulting in terminal swellings. Lead, diphtheria toxin, perhexiline, lysolecithin, and hexachlorophene are prominent toxins preferentially directed at the Schwann cell/myelin sheath, resulting in demyelination. Many therapeutic agents may induce peripheral nerve disease. Heavy metals (e.g., arsenic, mercury, thallium, gold) are well known for their toxic effects on peripheral nerves. Neuropathic industrial and environmental agents have resulted in epidemics of toxic neuropathy.

IV. ISCHEMIC NEUROPATHIES. The nerve vascular supply (i.e., vasa nervorum) is rich and anastomotic, requiring a substantial decrease in nerve blood flow to interrupt function. Vasculitis (i.e., vasculopathy with angionecrosis) is frequently patchy, resulting in asymmetric nerve involvement (mononeuritis multiplex), emphasizing the need for thorough sampling of the nerve biopsy. Polyarteritis nodosa, the vasculitic prototype, is characterized by epineurial arteries damaged by polymorphonuclear leukocytes, macrophages, monocytes, fibrin (e-Figs. 42.12 and 42.13), and a range of axonopathy rarely culminating in infarction. There may be inter- or intrafascicular variability in axon loss (Fig. 42.3, and e-Figs. 42.14 and 42.15). Fibrotic recanalized vessels mark previous sites of vasculitic damage.

Patients with collagen vascular diseases may clinically present with mononeuritis multiplex, histologically comparable to that of polyarteritis nodosa or a minimal epineurial perivascular mononuclear cell infiltrate (i.e., microvasculitis) lacking angionecrosis. Epineurial perivascular collections of a few mononuclear cells are common, and some authors consider them, in isolation, to be of little pathologic importance in the absence of loss of vascular continuity or vasculopathy. Alternatively, they may represent an early or mild vascular injury, or represent

TABLE 42.1	Partial List of Agents Causing Toxic Neuropathies	
Metals	**Toxins**	**Drugs**
Aluminum	Acrylamide	Almitrine
Arsenic	Allyl chloride	Amiodarone
Cadmium	Buckthorn	Bortezomib
Gold	Carbon disulfide	Chloroquine
Lead	Dimethylaminopropionitrile	Cisplatin
Lithium	Dioxin	Clioquinol
Mercury	Ethanol	Colchicine
Tellurium	Ethylene oxide	Cyanide
Thallium	Hexacarbons and solvents	Dapsone
	Latrotoxin	Dichloroacetate
	Organophosphorus esters	Disulfiram
	Perchloroethylene	Doxorubicin
	Styrene	Ethambutol
	Toluene	Etoposide
	Toxic oil syndrome	Glutethimide
	Trichloroethylene	Hydralazine
	Vacor	Isoniazid
	Vinyl chloride	Metronidazole
	Xylene	Misonidazole
		Nitrofurantoin
		Nitrous Oxide
		Nucleosides
		Perhexiline
		Phenytoin
		Podophyllin
		Polychlorinated biphenyls
		Procainamide
		Pyridoxine (Vitamin B_6)
		Sodium cyanate
		Statins
		Suramin
		Tacrolimus (FK506)
		Taxanes [Paclitaxel (Taxol), docetaxel]
		Thalidomide
		Vinca alkaloids (Vincristine, Vinblastine)
		Zinc pyridinethionine

an area adjacent to more substantial vasculopathy. Immunoglobulin and complement deposition within the vascular wall in collagen vascular diseases may reflect the deposition of circulating immune complexes not specific for nerve.

V. METABOLIC NEUROPATHIES constitute a pathogenetically heterogeneous group.

    A. Diabetes. There is a complex spectrum of neuropathies in diabetes which may have different pathogenetic mechanisms:

        1. Symmetrical sensori (motor) polyneuropathy is the most well known variety of diabetic neuropathy, presenting with distal, largely sensory problems which may culminate in stocking-glove anesthesia. Patients may develop neuropathy after years of recognized diabetes or present de novo with neuropathic symptoms. Typically, distal axon loss is accompanied by vasculopathy (e-Fig. 42.16). Schwann cells, perineurial cells, and endothelial cells are enveloped by thickened basement membranes, thought to reflect

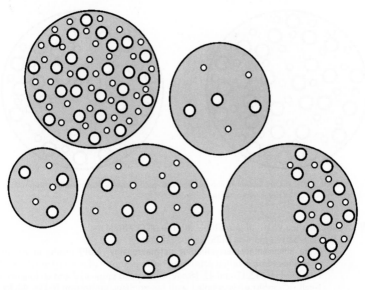

Figure 42.3 Ischemic pattern of axon loss. Intra- and interfascicular variability of axon loss is typical but not pathognomonic of a vasculitic/ischemic pathogenesis.

resistance to degradation because of the formation of advanced glycation end products. Some patients with painful dysesthesias and a normal electrophysiologic exam show loss of intraepidermal axons in skin biopsies, a procedure becoming routine practice in some institutions. Multiple ischemic insults may summate to produce a symmetrical and uniform axon loss distally, but this mechanism has not been universally accepted. Diabetes-induced oxidative stress may reflect deranged metabolism and/or mitochondriopathy.

2. **Asymmetric neuropathies** include radiculoplexus neuropathy (diabetic amyotrophy), truncal radiculopathy, upper limb mononeuropathy, and cranial nerve (chiefly III) palsies characterized by an inflammatory microvasculitis and/or perineuritis, possible immune complex and complement deposition, and a mild to marked axonopathy.

3. **Diabetic autonomic neuropathy** produces a large range of symptoms contributed by the sympathetic and parasympathetic nervous systems (also enteric and visceral sensory). Autonomic axons may be involved in symmetrical sensorimotor polyneuropathy or as more restricted involvement of autonomic fibers in the gut, bladder, penis, and other organs. Studies of human diabetics and rodents show markedly swollen dystrophic axons and synapses in prevertebral sympathetic ganglia.

B. **Uremia** results in demyelination of relatively atrophic axons (i.e., secondary demyelination).

C. **Others.** Deficiencies of pyridoxine, thiamine, vitamin E (found in abetalipoproteinemia, cystic fibrosis, and biliary atresia), niacin, cobalamin, and multiple nutritional deficiencies (apparently resulting in an epidemic in Cuba) are associated with several forms of neuropathy. Hypothyroidism, acute intermittent porphyria, galactosemia, hepatic failure, acromegaly, chronic respiratory insufficiency, and critical illness may also be associated with neuropathy.

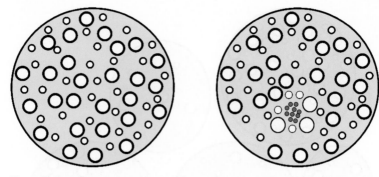

Figure 42.4 AIDP. Patchy loss of myelin in large and small axons is accompanied by an inflammatory infiltrate (*solid dots*). Normal fascicle is on the left.

VI. NEUROPATHIES WITH AN IMMUNE-MEDIATED MECHANISM

A. Guillain–Barré syndrome (GBS)

1. **Acute inflammatory demyelinating polyneuropathy (AIDP)** results in patchy myelin loss with residual debris and the appearance of naked demyelinated axons (**e-Figs. 42.17** and **42.18**). A perivascular epineurial and endoneurial T-cell rich infiltrate is coupled with macrophage infiltration (**e-Fig. 42.19**) and results in distinctive macrophage-mediated stripping of layers of otherwise normal appearing myelin (Fig. 42.4, **e-Figs. 42.20 to 42.22**). Circulating antibodies against endoneurial targets may secondarily gain access through a damaged blood nerve barrier or be locally synthesized. Plasmapheresis and intravenous immunoglobulins may be useful treatment modalities. Eventually, Schwann cells proliferate and remyelinate the denuded internode (**e-Fig. 42.23**). Axonopathy and axon loss is seen, probably because of a noxious endoneurial environment containing cytokines and oxidative mediators.

2. **Acute motor axonal neuropathy (AMAN) and acute motor and sensory axonal neuropathy (AMSAN).** In these axonal forms of GBS, the axon rather than myelin is the primary target and may produce AMAN or AMSAN dysfunction. Macrophages may be found adjacent to nodes of Ranvier or entering the periaxonal space, possibly targeting axons with a variable degree of AD. Antibody may target a constituent of the node of Ranvier to which it binds, fixes complement forming a membrane attack complex, recruits macrophages, and results eventually in AD. Axonal GBS may be associated with a more aggressive course with poorer outcome, electrophysiologic and pathologic evidence of prominent axonopathy, relatively increased incidence of enteric *Campylobacter jejuni* infection, and a role for antibody directed against GM1 ganglioside. Different patterns of nerve injury seen in GBS may reflect the strain of infecting organism or host-HLA alleles.

3. **Miller Fisher variant of GBS** is distinguished from AIDP/AMAN by a distinctive presentation of ataxia, areflexia, and ophthalmoplegia, and antibodies against the ganglioside GQ_{1b} which is concentrated at the nodes of Ranvier, particularly those of the oculomotor nerves.

B. Chronic inflammatory demyelinating polyradiculoneuropathy (CIDP) is characterized by a symmetric progressive or relapsing/remitting, sensory and motor polyradiculoneuropathy, particularly involving proximal nerves. Perineurial inflammation and onion-bulbs reflect its chronicity, but do not occur in all

cases. CIDP may be a chronic form of GBS in which there is failure of regulatory T-cells to suppress the typically monophasic attack of GBS. Its autoimmune pathogenesis involves CD4+ and CD8+ T-cells, and possibly also antimyelin antibodies. HLA subtype frequencies (e.g., HLA-DR2) differ between GBS and CIDP.

C. **Antimyelin associated glycoprotein (MAG) neuropathy** is a slowly progressive demyelinating neuropathy with an associated IgM monoclonal gammopathy (monoclonal gammopathy of unknown significance, MGUS) in which the antibody is directed against MAG, a molecule which supports myelin integrity. Anti-MAG antibodies deposited on portions of the myelin sheaths of peripheral nerve axons result in altered myelin periodicity, demyelination, and AD. Immunosuppression and plasmapheresis have resulted in transient improvement. Rituximab, a mouse–human chimeric antibody against the B cell surface marker CD20, is reported to have clinical benefit.

D. **Antiglycolipid, antisulfatide, and antiganglioside neuropathies** have been associated with a wide range of clinically identifiable acute and chronic neuropathy syndromes.

E. **Anti-Hu antibody neuropathy** is associated with paraneoplastic sensory neuropathy and likely reflects development of antibodies against shared antigens of small cell lung carcinoma and dorsal root ganglion neurons. Infiltration of CD8+ T cells is also present.

F. **Autoimmune autonomic neuropathy** resulting in autonomic failure following a viral illness may be mediated by circulating antibodies against ganglionic nicotine acetylcholine receptor.

VII. **GENETIC NEUROPATHIES**

A. **Hypertrophic (onion-bulb) neuropathies**

The concentric proliferation of Schwann cells in response to multiple episodes of demyelination and subsequent remyelination results in onion-bulbs, the defining pathologic hallmark of a group of neuropathies. Onion-bulbs are visible in H&E-stained nerves (e-Fig. 42.24), a pattern accentuated with immunolabeling for Collagen type IV (e-Fig. 42.25). Onion bulbs are best illustrated in plastic embedded nerve (e-Fig. 42.26) and with electron microscopy (e-Fig. 42.27). Nerves may be palpably enlarged and conduction velocities markedly decreased. Genetic analysis has identified mutations in myelin constituents (Po, PMP22, myelin basic protein), including those localized to noncompact myelin near the paranode (MAG, connexin 32, neurofascin 155) and axonal proteins (Caspr, contactin, kinesin). A more complete catalogue can be found at several websites (e.g., http://www.molgen.ua.ac.be/CMTMutations/).

1. **Hypertrophic Charcot–Marie–Tooth disease (CMT1)** is inherited as an autosomal dominant condition resulting from a duplication or point mutation in the *PMP-22* gene or a point mutation in Po myelin protein (both needed for myelin compaction), a defect in the early growth response 2 gene (*EGR2*), or mutations of periaxin (a Schwann cell protein regulating its shape and axonal communication). Animal models have established a role for macrophage and lymphocytic infiltration in disease pathogenesis. X-linked CMT demonstrates a defect in the gene for connexin-32.

2. **Other types (Table 42.2).** Dejerine–Sottas disease (DSS, includes HMSN-III+) begins in early life, some cases of which have a demonstrable genetic defect in *PMP-22*, periaxin, *GDAP1*, *EGR2*, or myelin protein Po. Refsum's disease, caused by phytanic acid oxidase deficiency, also results in an onion-bulb neuropathy.

B. **Hereditary neuropathy with pressure palsies (HNPP).** Teased fiber preparations of this dominantly inherited neuropathy demonstrate marked focal hyper-myelination (called tomaculi or sausages) characterized by redundant myelin

TABLE 42.2 Forms of Hereditary Neuropathy with Onion-Bulbs and Tomaculi

Designation	Inheritance	Gene defect	Pathology
CMT1A	AD	PMP22	Onion bulbs (OB)
CMT1B	AD	Po	OB
CMT1C	AD	EGR2	OB
		LITAF/SIMPLE	OB
CMT1X	XD	Connexin 32	Axonal/OB
CMT2A	AD	Kinesin Family Member IB (Kif1b)	Axonal/±OB
CMT2B	AD	RAB-7	Axonal/±OB
CMT2D	AD	Glycyl tRNA synthetase	Axonal
CMT2E	AD	Neurofilament-L	Axonal
		PMP22, Po, Connexin 32	Axonal
CMT3 (DSS)	AD or AR (or de novo)	PMP22, Po, EGR2 Periaxin, GDAP1	OB
CMT4A	AR	GDAP1	OB
CMT4B.1	AR	Myotubularin Related protein 2	Demyel + folds
CMT4B.2	AR	Set binding factor-2	OB + focal thickening
CMT4C	AR	SH3 & tetratricopeptide repeat domain 2	OB + focal thickening
CMT4D (HMSN-LOM)	AR	N-myc downstream Regulated gene 1 (*NDRG1*)	OB
CMT4E	AR/AD	EGR-2, Po	Severe myelin loss
CMT4F	AR/AD	Periaxin, PMP22, Po, EGR2	OB (+tomaculi)
HNPP	AD	PMP22	Demyel + tomaculi

folds, demyelination, and remyelination. Evidence suggests monosomy of the *PMP-22* gene due to loss of a portion of chromosome 17.

C. **Hereditary giant axonal neuropathy** results in axons distended by aggregates of neurofilaments and thinned myelin sheaths, a variety of CNS symptoms, and so-called kinky hair. Schwann cells and endothelial cells may also have aggregates of intermediate filaments. This neuropathy results from the disruption of the gene coding for the synthesis of gigaxonin which interferes with the microtubule network and its dynein motor.

D. **Hereditary sensory and autonomic neuropathies (HSANs).** Included in this group are neuropathies with autonomic and sensory dysfunction, dominant and recessive forms of acral sensory neuropathy, familial dysautonomia, and congenital sensory neuropathy with anhidrosis, all of which are characterized by neuron loss in sensory and various sympathetic and parasympathetic ganglia.

VIII. **AMYLOID AND RELATED NEUROPATHIES.** Amyloid represents an extracellular deposit of proteins arranged in a β-pleated sheet conformation forming 10 to 20 nm unbranched filaments which stain with Thioflavin-S fluorescence and Congo Red (the latter polarizes light resulting in an apple green color). Amyloid neuropathy occurs in (i) primary (nonhereditary) amyloidosis (also composed of immunoglobulin-derived amyloid); (ii) amyloidosis associated with dysglobulinemia, and (iii) hereditary amyloidoses (e.g., Andrade's disease) in which the deposited amyloid is derived from transthyretin or other materials. Amyloid may be deposited within the endoneurium, in the endoneurial and epineurial vasculature (e-**Figs.** 42.28 and 42.29), or within epineurial connective tissue. Axon loss, particularly small axons, is typical. Immunostains may identify the amyloid source (e.g., kappa light chains in a myeloma patient).

TABLE 42.3	Subtypes of HIV-Associated Neuropathy	
Subtype of neuropathy (NP)	**Clinical stage**	**Mechanism**
1. Distal sensory NP	Advanced HIV	Macrophage-mediated axonopathy
2. Toxic antiretroviral drug NP	Advanced HIV	Mitochondrial DNA synthesis
3. Mononeuritis multiplex		
Vasculitic form	Moderately advanced	Immune complex deposition
CMV multiple monoNP	Advanced HIV	CMV infection Schwann cells, vessels
4. Inflammatory demyelinating NP		
GBS (demyelinating or axonal)	Early HIV	Immune dysfunction
CIDP	Early HIV	Immune dysfunction
5. Opportunistic infectious NP		
CMV polyradiculopathy	Advanced HIV	CMV necrotizing NP
Herpes Zoster radiculopathy	Advanced HIV	VZV: Schwann cells and endothelium
6. Neoplastic (lymphoma)	Advanced HIV	Endoneurial infiltration
7. Autonomic neuropathy	Advanced HIV	
8. Diffuse infiltrative lymphocytosis	Moderately advanced	CD8 lymphocytosis/ vasculopathy

IX. INFECTIOUS NEUROPATHIES

A. Herpes Zoster (shingles) presents as a painful cutaneous vesicular rash corresponding to a dermatome in which DRG varicella virus has emerged from latency, initially established at the time of childhood chickenpox infection. In response to immunologic cues or other stimuli, virus activates, travels distally within axons forming a cutaneous eruption (rarely myelitis), and produces hemorrhagic ganglioradiculitis (e-**Fig. 42.30**), infecting satellite and Schwann cells and neurons in trigeminal ganglia and DRG.

B. Leprosy. This is caused by *Mycobacterium lepra* infection and results in loss of cutaneous sensation and motor function as the result of direct infection (lepromatous form) or as a result of a granulomatous response to the organism (tuberculoid form). The tuberculoid form involves the skin and adjacent nerves, in which few organisms are found (complicating distinction from sarcoid neuropathy). In patients with a compromised immune response to the organism, endoneurial fibrosis is accompanied by numerous organisms which can be demonstrated within Schwann cells (particularly those of unmyelinated axons) and endoneurial macrophages (lepra cells). The organism is particularly fond of Schwann cells, binding to laminin-α_2 (*Science.* 2002;296:927).

C. AIDS. Several different types of neuropathy may develop in patients infected with HIV (Table 42.3) including GBS, CIDP, and necrotizing vasculitis (*Muscle Nerve.* 2003;28:542). Distal sensory polyneuropathy (DSP) shows prominent HIV-infected macrophage activation and lymphocytic (CD8+ > CD4+) infiltration with local release of proinflammatory cytokines (IFN-γ, TNF-α, and IL-6) in the vicinity of degenerating axons and DRG neurons. The viral product gp120 results in neuronal apoptosis and direct local toxicity to axons and may increase vulnerability to dideoxynucleoside-induced neurotoxicity. Antiretroviral treatment may produce a clinical picture closely resembling DSP, possibly due to direct mitochondrial toxicity. Skin biopsy is a sensitive and early monitor of the development of DSP, demonstrating loss of epidermal axons and axonal swellings, often in the absence of neuropathic changes in the sural nerve.

   D. Lyme disease. Cranial and peripheral nerves show an epineurial or perineurial perivascular lymphocytic/plasmacytic infiltrate (perivasculitis) and AD. Organisms are not typically seen in involved nerves.

X. TRAUMATIC NEUROPATHY exists in many forms. Chronic nerve compression and entrapment is characterized by focal loss of myelin. More severe trauma with loss of nerve continuity may produce a traumatic neuroma, that is, a combination of degenerative and regenerative responses resulting in a disorganized aggregate of collagen and axonal "minifascicles" (e-**Figs. 42.31** and **42.32**). The distinctive appearance of minifascicles can be seen with immunohistochemistry for neurofilaments (which stains axons, e-**Fig. 42.33**) or epithelial membrane antigen (EMA, which stains the perineurium, e-**Fig. 42.34**), and in plastic sections (e-**Fig. 42.35**).

SUGGESTED READINGS

Kennedy WR. Opportunities afforded by the study of unmyelinated nerves in skin and other organs. *Muscle Nerve.* 2004;29:756–767.

Midroni G, Bilbao JM. *Biopsy Diagnosis of Peripheral Neuropathy.* Boston, MA: Butterworth-Heinemann; 1995.

Pestronk A. Neuromuscular Division Website, Washington University School of Medicine, http://www.neuro.wustl.edu/neuromuscular/

Spencer PS, Schaumburg HH, Ludolph AC. *Experimental and Clinical Neurotoxicology.* New York, NY: Oxford University Press; 2000.

Zochodne DW. Diabetes mellitus and the peripheral nervous system: Manifestations and mechanisms. *Muscle Nerve.* 2007;36:144–166.

Hematopoietic System

43

Lymph Nodes
Anjum Hassan and Friederike Kreisel

I. **NORMAL ANATOMY.** Lymph nodes are the most widely distributed collections of lymphoid tissue within the lymphoreticular system, which also includes the thymus, tonsils, adenoids, spleen, and Peyer patches. Due to their easy accessibility, lymph nodes are the most frequently examined lymphoid tissue for a lymphoreticular disorder. Microscopically, the lymph node shows four compartments: The most obvious are the primary and secondary follicles, which are usually found near the capsule, surrounding the follicles and extending deeper into the node is the paracortex. The third and fourth compartments represent the medullary region and the sinuses, respectively (**e-Fig. 43.1**).*

II. **GROSS EXAMINATION, TISSUE SAMPLING, AND HISTOLOGIC SLIDE PREPARATION.** Fresh lymphoid tissue should be examined by gross inspection, touch preparation, or frozen section examination to assess whether the:

A. Tissue represents adequate sampling, and

B. Tissue needs to be allocated for various ancillary studies essential to a correct diagnosis. The fresh lymph node should be cut perpendicularly along the long axis, and material for ancillary studies procured as follows:

1. Wet touch preparations fixed in 95% alcohol or formalin, for H&E or Papanicolaou staining

2. Air-dried touch preparations for Giemsa or Wright–Giemsa staining, cytochemistry (myeloperoxidase, nonspecific esterase, etc.), or cytogenetics [i.e., fluorescence in situ hybridization (FISH)]

3. Rapidly frozen tissue for immunohistochemistry, cytochemistry, or genetic analysis

4. Fresh tissue (in RPMI 1640 medium or saline) for flow cytometry

5. Sterile fresh tissue for microbial cultures or cytogenetic analysis (karyotyping or FISH)

6. Thin-shaved tissue rapidly fixed in glutaraldehyde for electron microscopy

7. Paraffin-embedded tissue after fixation for routine H&E-staining, immunohistochemistry, and special stains [e.g., Giemsa, periodic acid-Schiff (PAS), elastin, trichrome, Leder, etc.]

Procuring tissue for histology takes priority over other studies. The most commonly used fixative for permanent sections is 10% neutral buffered formalin. B5 fixative is commonly used in addition to 10% neutral buffered

---

*All e-figures are available online via the Solution Site Image Bank.

formalin because of the sharp nuclear detail it produces. However, this mercuric chloride-based fixative is very expensive and poses an environmental hazard. Furthermore, molecular studies cannot be carried out on B5-fixed paraffin-embedded tissue, because it will generally yield poor polymerase chain reaction (PCR) amplification results.

III. DIAGNOSTIC FEATURES OF COMMON BENIGN DISEASES OF LYMPH NODES. In reactive lymphadenopathy, there are five different architectural patterns to be recognized, with many showing a mixed pattern of response.

A. Follicular hyperplasia (e-Fig. 43.2) is characterized by an increase in number and size of B-cell germinal centers and is common in lymph node–draining sites of chronic inflammation. This pattern is also present in syphilitic lymphadenitis where, in addition to the marked lymphoid hyperplasia, thickening of the capsule by chronic inflammation, fibrosis, and neovascularization with arteritis and phlebitis, and a marked plasma cell infiltrate in the medullary region predominate. Rheumatoid lymphadenopathy and acute human immunodeficiency virus (HIV) lymphadenitis are other examples of marked follicular hyperplasia.

B. Diffuse (paracortical) hyperplasia shows expansion of the T-cell paracortical areas. This pattern is commonly seen in viral lymphadenitis [Epstein–Barr virus (EBV), cytomegalovirus (CMV), herpes] and vaccinia lymphadenitis revealing an expansion of the paracortex with increased immunoblasts, imparting a mottled appearance. Follicular hyperplasia and sinus dilation are often concurrent findings in this entity, resulting in a mixed pattern of lymphoid hyperplasia. Phenytoin lymphadenopathy represents a relatively pure diffuse hyperplasia showing an expanded paracortical T-zone with numerous large immunoblasts, eosinophils, plasma cells, and neutrophils.

C. Sinus hyperplasia describes increased cellularity within the medullary sinuses of lymph nodes. Sinus histiocytosis is seen in numerous nonspecific responses to chronic inflammation, as well as in lymph nodes draining solid tumors. Sinus histiocytosis with massive lymphadenopathy (Rosai–Dorfman) disease is characterized by markedly dilated sinuses filled with CD68+, S100+ histiocytes showing emperipolesis. Lipophagic reactions causing sinus histiocytosis with accumulation of phagocytosed fat include mineral oil ingestion, Whipple disease, and lymphangiography procedures. Prominent vacuoles in the histiocytes can generate a signet-ring cell histiocytosis, a pattern that should not be confused with signet-ring-cell carcinoma. Finally, vascular transformation of lymph node sinuses (e-Fig. 43.3) shows a sinus pattern, and it is important to distinguish this entity from Kaposi sarcoma (e-Fig. 43.4). The latter can be distinguished from the former by the proliferation of spindle-shaped Kaposi sarcoma cells forming cleft-like vascular spaces that contain erythrocytes, many of which are extravasated.

D. Granulomatous lymphadenopathy describes formation of epithelioid granulomas in lymph nodes. Caseating granulomas are epithelioid granulomas that form central necrosis and caseation and are typically seen in *Mycobacterium tuberculosis* lymphadenitis. Special stains for mycobacteria in paraffin-embedded tissue (Ziehl–Neelson, Fite–Faraco) will detect the bacilli as bright red, slender, beaded microorganisms (e-Figs. 43.5 and 43.6). *Mycobacterium leprae* lymphadenitis and histoplasma lymphadenitis are other examples of caseating granulomatous inflammation. Necrotizing, noncaseating granulomas are present in cat-scratch disease (e-Fig. 43.7) caused by *Bartonella henselae,* in which suppurative granulomas with stellate microabscesses surrounded by palisading histiocytes predominate. Kikuchi-Fujimoto lymphadenopathy is characterized by necrotizing granulomas containing karyorrhectic debris, but lacking neutrophils; this form of necrotizing lymphadenitis characteristically occurs in young Asian women. Nonnecrotizing, noncaseating granulomas are characteristic of sarcoidosis lymphadenopathy (e-Fig. 43.8), composed primarily of epithelioid histiocytes with scattered multinucleated giant cells, lymphocytes, and plasma cells. This type of epithelioid granuloma can also be seen in draining lymph nodes of Crohn's disease.

E. **Acute lymphadenitis** is an acute inflammation in lymph nodes draining an infected focus. Acute lymphadenitis is almost exclusively bacterial in nature, and morphologic features range from focal infiltration by neutrophils to necrosis and suppuration with abscess formation.

It should be mentioned that in most cases of benign reactive lymphadenopathy, a combination of more than one architectural pattern is present in the same lymph node.

IV. INCIDENCE AND EPIDEMIOLOGY OF NON-HODGKIN LYMPHOMAS

A. **B-cell lymphomas.** B-cell lymphomas constitute the vast majority of lymphomas in North America and Europe, accounting for nearly 90% of all lymphomas. Diffuse large B-cell lymphoma (DLBCL) (~31%) (e-**Fig. 43.9**) and follicular lymphoma (~22%) (e-**Fig. 43.10**) are the most common types. Immunosuppression, specifically due to HIV infection and immunosuppressive therapy to prevent graft versus host disease, is associated with a markedly increased incidence of mature B-cell lymphomas, particularly DLBCL and Burkitt lymphoma (e-**Fig. 43.11**).

Some of the low-grade B-cell lymphoproliferative disorders include follicular lymphoma grades 1 and 2, chronic lymphocytic leukemia/small lymphocytic lymphoma (CLL/SLL) (e-**Fig. 43.12**), nodal and extranodal marginal zone B-cell lymphoma (e-**Fig. 43.13**), and lymphoplasmacytic lymphoma, which are generally indolent, but incurable and usually present in a disseminated stage with bone marrow involvement. Mantle cell lymphoma (e-**Figs. 43.14** and **43.15**) and DLBCL represent "intermediate-grade" B-cell lymphomas that generally show a more aggressive clinical behavior, but are potentially curable. The same applies to high-grade B-cell lymphomas, which include Burkitt lymphoma and precursor B-lymphoblastic leukemia/lymphoma.

B. **T-cell lymphomas.** Mature T-cell and natural killer (NK)-cell malignancies are rare, accounting for only 10% to 12% of all non-Hodgkin lymphoma (NHL), and usually are more aggressive than B-cell lymphomas. The most common subtypes are peripheral T-cell lymphoma, unspecified (~4% of all adult NHLs and ~30% of peripheral T-cell lymphomas) (e-**Fig. 43.16**) and anaplastic large cell lymphoma (~3% of all adult NHLs) (e-**Fig. 43.17**). In general, T-cell and NK-cell malignancies are much more common in Asia and are linked to viral infection with EBV (NK-cell lymphomas) (e-**Fig. 43.18**) and human T-cell leukemia virus (HTLV-1) (adult T-cell leukemia/lymphoma) (e-**Fig. 43.19**). The current 2008 World Health Organization classification of lymphoid malignancies is summarized in Table 43.1.

V. PATHOPHYSIOLOGY OF NON-HODGKIN LYMPHOMAS

A. **B-cell lymphomas.** Mature B-cell malignancies mimic stages of normal B-cell differentiation; therefore, classification is generally based on their morphologic and immunophenotypic resemblance to the normal B-cell counterpart (Fig. 43.1) (*Best Pract Res Clin Haematol.* 2005;18:11). Normal B-cell development begins in the bone marrow where precursor B-lymphoblasts undergo immunoglobulin VDJ gene rearrangement and develop into IgM+, IgD+ naïve B-cells with surface immunoglobulin light chain and CD5 expression. These resting B-cells circulate in the blood and occupy primary follicles and mantle zones of secondary follicles. Malignant counterparts of CD5+ naïve B-cells are believed to be CLL and mantle cell lymphoma. Upon antigen stimulation, naïve B-cells undergo blastic transformation, migrate into the center of the primary follicle, and form the germinal center. These centroblasts are large lymphoid cells with vesicular chromatin and several eccentrically located nucleoli. They express BCL-6 and CD10 but switch off BCL-2 protein expression, therefore becoming susceptible to death through apoptosis. Centroblasts undergo intense proliferation that is accompanied by somatic

TABLE 43.1 2008 WHO Classification of Lymphoid Neoplasms

Mature B-cell neoplasms
Chronic lymphocytic leukemia/small lymphocytic lymphoma
B-cell prolymphocytic leukemia
Splenic B-cell marginal zone lymphoma
Hairy cell leukemia
Splenic B-cell lymphoma/leukemia, unclassifiable
Splenic diffuse red pulp small B-cell lymphoma
Hairy cell leukemia-variant
Lymphoplasmacytic lymphoma
Heavy chain diseases (gamma heavy chain/mu heavy chain/alpha heavy chain diseases)
Plasma cell neoplasms
MGUS
Plasma cell myeloma
Solitary PC of bone
Extraosseous PC
Monoclonal immunoglobulin deposition diseases
Extranodal marginal zone B-cell lymphoma of MALT lymphoma
Nodal marginal zone B-cell lymphoma
Follicular lymphoma
Primary cutaneous follicle center lymphoma
Mantle cell lymphoma
DLBCL, NOS
T-cell/histiocyte-rich large B-cell lymphoma
Primary DLBCL of the CNS
Primary cutaneous DLBCL, leg type
EBV positive DLBCL of the elderly
DLBCL associated with chronic inflammation
Lymphomatoid granulomatosis
Primary mediastinal (thymic) large B-cell lymphoma
Intravascular large B-cell lymphoma
ALK positive large B-cell lymphoma
Plasmablastic lymphoma
Large B-cell lymphoma arising in HHV8-associated multicentric Castleman disease
Primary effusion lymphoma
Burkitt lymphoma
B-cell lymphoma, unclassifiable, with features intermediate between DLBCL and Burkitt lymphoma
B-cell lymphoma, unclassifiable, with features intermediate between DLBCL and CHL

Mature T-cell and NK-cell neoplasms
T-cell prolymphocytic leukemia
T-cell large granular lymphocytic leukemia
Aggressive NK-cell leukemia
EBV positive T-cell lymphoproliferative diseases of childhood
Systemic EBV+ T-cell lymphoproliferative disease of childhood
Hydroa vacciniforme-like lymphoma
Adult T-cell leukemia/lymphoma
Extranodal NK-/T-cell lymphoma, nasal type
Enteropathy-associated T-cell lymphoma
Hepatosplenic T-cell lymphoma
Subcutaneous panniculitis-like T-cell lymphoma
Mycosis fungoides

(continued)

TABLE 43.1 2008 WHO Classification of Lymphoid Neoplasms (*Continued*)

Sézary syndrome
Primary cutaneous CD30+ T-cell lymphoproliferative disorders
Primary cutaneous peripheral T-cell lymphomas, rare subtypes
Primary cutaneous gamma–delta T-cell lymphoma
Primary cutaneous CD8 positive aggressive epidermotropic cytotoxic T-cell lymphoma
Primary cutaneous CD4 positive small/medium T-cell lymphoma
Peripheral T-cell lymphoma, NOS
Angioimmunoblastic T-cell lymphoma
Anaplastic large cell lymphoma, ALK positive
Anaplastic large cell lymphoma, ALK negative

From: Swerdlow SH, Campo E, Harris NL, et al., eds. *WHO Classification of Tumours of Haematopoietic and Lymphoid Tissues.* Lyon: IARC Press; 2008. Used with permission.

hypermutation of their rearranged variable-region genes, giving rise to cells carrying receptors with high affinity for the stimulating antigen. This leads to a large pool of B-lymphoid cells with intraclonal diversity. Centroblasts then mature into centrocytes, representing intermediate-sized lymphoid cells with irregular, cleaved nuclei and inconspicuous nucleoli. Centrocytes with mutations resulting in decreased affinity for antigen die by apoptosis, whereas centrocytes with high affinity for antigen are rescued from apoptosis by re-expressing BCL-2. Malignant counterparts of germinal center-derived B-cells are follicular lymphoma, a subset of DLBCL, and Burkitt lymphoma. Via interactions with follicular dendritic cells through CD23 and with T lymphocytes through CD40 ligand (CD40L), centrocytes switch off BCL-6 expression and differentiate into either memory cells or plasma cells. Memory cells are found in the marginal zone of follicles; they typically express immunoglobulin M (IgM) and lack expression of IgD, CD5, CD10, or CD23. Plasma cells home to the bone marrow; they lack surface immunoglobulin and pan-B-cell expression, but express CD79a, CD138, and cytoplasmic IgG or IgA. Neither memory cells nor plasma cells undergo further somatic hypermutations. Marginal zone B-cell lymphoma corresponds to postgerminal center cells, possibly memory cells of marginal zone type. Plasma cell myeloma is the malignant counterpart of bone marrow-homing IgG- or IgA-producing plasma cells.

B. **T lymphocytes.** Two major classes of T lymphocytes exist on the basis of the structure of the T-cell receptor (TCR). Approximately 95% of all T-cells are $\alpha\beta$ T-lymphocytes that can be subdivided into CD4+ helper T-cells or CD8+ cytotoxic T-cells. Only 5% of T-cells are $\gamma\delta$ cells, which are primarily found in the splenic pulp and intestinal epithelium and are not MHC restricted in their function, because they do not express CD4 or CD8. The TCR is composed of either the $\alpha\beta$ or $\gamma\delta$ chains, each consisting of an external variable (V) and constant (C) domain. The TCR is complexed with CD3 that contains γ, δ, and ε chains. NK cells do not have a complete TCR, but usually express the ε chain of the CD3 in the cytoplasm; therefore, NK cells will stain positively with a polyclonal antibody to CD3. The malignant counterparts of $\gamma\delta$ T-cells are believed to be hepatosplenic T-cell lymphoma (e-**Fig. 43.20**) and enteropathy-type T-cell lymphoma (e-**Fig. 43.21**). NK cells share some immunophenotypic markers and functions with cytotoxic CD8+ T-cells; these include expression of CD2, CD7, CD8, CD56, CD57, granzyme B, perforin, and T-cell intracellular antigen (TIA-1).

Due to their broad cytologic spectrum, absence of immunophenotypic markers of monoclonality, and general lack of specific genetic abnormalities, clinical presentation plays a major role in the subclassification of T-cell and

Normal and Abnormal Counterparts of B-Cell Progeny†

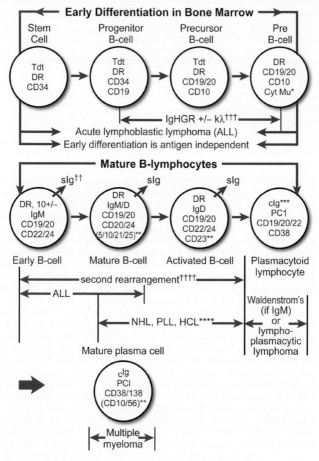

Figure 43.1 Brief overview of normal B-cell progeny and malignant counterparts.

NK-cell malignancies (Fig. 43.2). For example, hypercalcemia is associated with adult T-cell leukemia; hemophagocytic syndrome occurs more frequently in cytotoxic T-cell or NK-cell malignancies; persistent severe neutropenia is a relatively common clinical feature in T-cell granular lymphocyte leukemia (e-**Fig. 43.22**); and systemic symptoms of edema, pleural effusion, ascites, arthritis combined with anemia, and polyclonal hypergammaglobulinemia are relatively specific for angioimmunoblastic T-cell lymphoma (e-**Fig. 43.23**).

Normal T-Cell Progeny ††

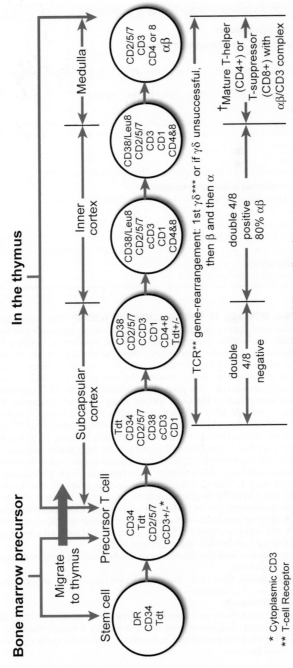

* Cytoplasmic CD3
** T-cell Receptor
*** Gamma-Delta chains expressed on immature thymocytes and Natural Killers cells only
† Mature T-cells can circulate in peripheral blood and tissues
†† Only positive markers are noted. Markers partially expressed or about to lose expression are noted by a "+/-".

Figure 43.2 Brief overview of normal T-cell progeny.

689

TABLE 43.2	An Algorithm for the Workup of Lymphomas

Cell type: Are the cells lymphoid?

In a tissue section, what is the low-power architecture?

Cell size

Are the majority of cells small (same size as a lymphocyte)? Or large (~3 times as big as a lymphocyte, or even bigger)?

Is there an even mixture of small and large cells? Are they anaplastic?

Nuclear shape

Do the cells have round nuclei with a smooth contour (noncleaved)? Or a round shape with a bumpy or notched contour (irregular)? Or a variable shape with deeply folded or grooved nuclei (cleaved)?

Histologic grade

Is necrosis present? Is there a "starry sky" appearance? Are mitoses easy to find?

Lineage (by flow cytometry or immunohistochemistry)

Are the cells of B lineage (generally CD20+) or T lineage (generally CD3+)?

Maturation

Are the cells at a precursor (TdT+) or a mature (TdT−) stage of maturation?

If mature and of B lineage, are they prefollicular, follicular, postfollicular, or effector cell stage?

If mature and of T lineage, are they at a thymic or postthymic/effector cell stage?

Disease specific markers

Do the cells express cyclin D1, bcl6, ALK-1, and so on?

VI. **A RATIONAL APPROACH TO GENERAL LYMPHOMA WORKUP.** The classification of lymphomas may appear difficult; however, a systematic approach can be used to efficiently narrow the differential diagnosis for most cases. Needless to say, knowledge of clinical history and a basic complete blood count are required to guide the initial steps of the evaluation (e.g., to direct the immunophenotypic workup of the sample by flow cytometry), because tissue sections are often not available until the next day. The general algorithm (see Table 43.2) starts with the low-power appearance of the tissue section. Is the architecture nodular, follicular, diffuse, or mixed? What is the cell size; small (close to a normal lymphocyte), medium, or large (about three times the size of a normal lymphocyte)? What is the nuclear shape (cleaved nuclei of follicular lymphoma or round nuclear contours of chronic lymphocytic lymphoma)? Is the process high grade (necrosis, starry sky appearance, high mitotic rate)? The workup continues with a determination of the lineage and stage of maturation. As mentioned above, flow cytometry is usually extremely helpful in delineating the lineage, provided care is taken to save fresh tissue in RPMI medium and order appropriate markers; alternatively, immunohistochemistry can be performed on formalin-fixed, paraffin-embedded tissue. The workup concludes with evaluation of disease-specific markers such as cyclin D1 and anaplastic large cell lymphoma kinase (ALK-1), which can only be evaluated by immunohistochemistry in tissue sections.

Antigen markers useful in delineating and subclassifying lymphoid malignancies are the following:

A. **Leukocyte marker.** CD45 [also known as leukocyte common antigen (LCA)] is expressed on all leukocytes.

B. **Markers of immaturity**
   1. TdT (terminal deoxynucleotidyl transferase, a specialized DNA polymerase; nuclear expression present only in pre-B and pre-T lymphoblasts)
   2. CD34 (present on pluripotent hematopoietic stem cells and progenitor cells of many lineages)

3. CD10 (CALLA, common acute lymphoblastic leukemia antigen); expressed on marrow pre-B-cells and mature follicular center B-cells)
4. CD22 (present on pre-B-cells)
5. cμ (cytoplasmic μ heavy chain)

C. **Primarily B-cell associated markers**
1. CD19 (present on marrow pre-B-cells, mature B-cells, but not on plasma cells; no paraffin-reactive antibody available)
2. CD20 (present on marrow pre-B-cells, mature B-cells, but not on normal plasma cells)
3. CD79a (present on mature and pre-B-cells, as well as on plasma cells)
4. CD22 [transmembrane molecule, present on mature B-cells (cCD22) and pre-B-cells (cCD22)]

D. **Markers helpful in subclassifying mature B-cell lymphomas**
1. CD5 (expressed on all T-cells and small subset of B-cells, expressed on neoplastic CLL and mantle cell lymphoma cells)
2. CD10
3. CD11c (expressed in high levels on monocytes, macrophages, and NK cells, as well in moderate levels on granulocytes; expressed on subsets of T and B-cells)
4. CD23 (present on activated mature B-cells)
5. CD38 (primarily expressed on mature B-cells and plasma cells)
6. CD43 (leukosialin, expressed on the surface of all leukocytes except resting B-cells; CD43 expression in B-cell lymphomas is highly correlated with CD5 and is therefore an indicator of aberrant B-cell populations)
7. BCL-6 (expressed normally in germinal center lymphocytes in the normal lymph node; it is distributed in a pattern reciprocal to that of BCL-2)
8. BCL-2 (present on T-cells and normal mantle B lymphocytes; aberrantly expressed in majority of B-cell lymphomas)
9. Cyclin D1 (cell cycle regulatory protein rearranged through the t(11;14) of mantle cell lymphoma; also expressed weakly in hairy cell leukemia and plasma cell dyscrasias; nuclear protein detectable in paraffin-embedded sections)
10. CD138 (Syndecan-1, expressed on most cases of myeloma, but also present in carcinomas)

E. **Markers of clonality:** κ and λ immunoglobulin light chains

F. **Primarily T cell- and NK cell-associated markers:**
1. CD1 (expressed on cortical thymocytes and Langerhans cell histiocytes)
2. CD2 [present on all T-cells (thymic and peripheral T-cells) and NK cells]
3. CD3 (lineage-specific marker for T-cells; cytoplasmic form also expressed in NK cells)
4. CD5 (expressed on all T-cells and a small subset of B-cells)
5. CD7 (expressed on all T-cells and a small subset of myeloid precursor cells)
6. CD8 (present on cytotoxic subset of peripheral T-cells and on a subset of thymocytes and NK cells)
7. CD16 (present on NK cells and granulocytes)
8. CD56 (present on NK cells and subset of T lymphocytes; also present on myeloma cells)
9. TIA-1 (cytotoxic granule-associated RNA binding protein), granzyme B, and perforin (proteins released by cytotoxic T-cells, inducing apoptosis) are expressed in cytotoxic T-cells and NK cells

G. **Flow cytometry** can easily detect clonality in B-cell malignancies (normal κ to λ light chain ratio ranges between 1:1 and 4:1). Clonality for T-cell malignancies can only be detected by molecular or cytogenetic studies.

H. **Southern blot analysis** is considered the gold standard for identifying clonal immunoglobulin heavy chain (*IgH*) gene or *TCR* gene rearrangements.

T lymphocytes normally rearrange four different *TCR* genes (*TCRα, β, γ,* and *δ*) to encode a unique antigen receptor expressed on their surface, and Southern blot analysis targets the *TCRβ* gene. In contrast to normal tissue, where only one band corresponding to the germline configuration is visible with this technique, both B-cell and T-cell malignancies will yield an additional band corresponding to the clonal population.

I. **PCR.** Because Southern blot analysis is labor intensive and expensive to perform, many laboratories have turned to PCR amplification methods to detect clonal *IgH* and *TCR* gene rearrangements.

The 200 variable segments of the *IgH* gene contain three highly variable and mutation-prone regions called complementary determining regions (CDR1, 2, and 3) that are interspersed between four conserved framework regions (FR1, 2, 3, and 4) that provide reliable targets for consensus primers. About 70% of B-cell malignancies harbor clonal rearrangements that are detectable with framework 3 primers, and about 15% to 20% of additional clonal rearrangements can be detected when framework 2 primers are used. Therefore, most laboratories use primers targeting frameworks 2 and 3 to detect at least 80% of all B-cell lymphomas.

The rearranged *TCRγ* gene is most suitable for clonal detection by PCR amplification in T-cell malignancies, because most T lymphocytes harbor rearrangements in 1 of the 11γ segments. Because many of these segments are homologous to one another, they can be targeted by a single consensus primer set. *TCRδ* and *TCRα* cannot be targeted because *TCRδ* is deleted during *TCRα* gene rearrangement and *TCRα* has such a diversity of possible rearrangements that these cannot be covered by current probe technology.

J. **Cytogenetic analysis** is a morphologic study of chromosomes to assess changes in their number and structure.

1. **Conventional karyotyping** requires viable cells, and analysis of chromosomes is performed according to their size and banding pattern after chromosome staining. Although this study has become critical in the diagnosis and classification of acute leukemias, it is not frequently used as part of a routine diagnostic workup for lymph node biopsies.

2. **FISH** uses one or more labeled probes directed toward specific portions of chromosomes. It is helpful in locating specific translocations, deletions, and amplifications of chromosomal regions. The advantage of FISH (see Chap. 59) is that it can be performed on nondividing nuclei (interphase nuclei), eliminating the need for cell culture. Furthermore, interphase FISH can be performed on a wide range of specimen types, such as peripheral blood smears, cytospin preparations, or paraffin-embedded tissue. Many of the classic chromosomal translocations that characterize specific lymphomas can be identified with interphase FISH techniques. Tables 43.3 and 43.4 summarize the characteristic morphologic, immunophenotypic, and genetic features of B-cell and T/NK-cell malignancies, respectively.

VII. **PLASMA CELL NEOPLASMS.** Plasma cells represent terminally differentiated B-cells. Their neoplasms are characterized by secretion of a single homogenous immunoglobulin product known as the monoclonal or "M" component, which can be detected by serum and urine protein electrophoresis. The World Health Organization categorizes plasma cell neoplasms into monoclonal gammopathy of undetermined significance (MGUS), plasma cell myeloma, plasmacytomas (PCs), immunoglobulin deposition diseases, and osteosclerotic myeloma (POEMS syndrome).

A. **Patients with MGUS** are asymptomatic with no evidence of lytic bone lesions, but reveal a clonal plasma cell population in the bone marrow of <10% and an associated small M component of <30 g/L. No lytic lesions or myeloma-related organ damage is present and a B-cell lymphoma with plasmacytic differentiation should be excluded.

TABLE 43.3 **Characteristic Features of Different B-Cell Malignancies**

Disease	Clinical presentation	Morphology	Immunophenotype	Genetics
CLL/SLL	Mostly asymptomatic, may present with fatigue, autoimmune hemolytic anemia, hepatosplenomegaly, lymphadenopathy; peripheral absolute lymphocytosis	PB: Small cells with coarsely clumped chromatin and inconspicuous nucleoli LN: Proliferation centers composed of "paraimmunoblasts" and prolymphocytes	CD20 (weak), CD19, IgM, IgD, CD22 (weak), CD5, CD23, CD79a, CD43	Trisomy 12, deletions at 13q14, deletions at 11q22–23 50%–60% have somatic hypermutations, IgH clonally rearranged
Prolymphocytic leukemia	Marked splenomegaly without lymphadenopathy, rapidly rising lymphocyte count (>100 × 10^9/L)	PB: Medium-sized cells with round nucleus, moderately condensed chromatin, and prominent central nucleolus	CD20 (bright), CD19, IgM, CD22, CD79a, FMC7, CD23 typically absent, CD5 present in 1/3 of cases	Complex karyotypes are common, abnormalities of TP53 in ~50%, IgH clonally rearranged
Hairy cell leukemia	Predominantly middle-aged men, splenomegaly, pancytopenia with monocytopenia	PB: Small- to medium-sized cells with circumferential hairy projections Spleen: Red pulp infiltration (macroscopy: "bloody lakes")	CD19, CD20, CD22 (bright), CD79a, CD11c (bright), CD25 (bright) CD103, TRAP, DBA.44 in tissue sections	No specific cytogenetic abnormality, IgH clonally rearranged
Lymphoplasmacytic lymphoma/ Waldenström macroglobulinemia	Monoclonal IgM serum paraprotein with associated hyperviscosity symptoms	Mixture of small lymphocytes, plasmacytoid lymphocytes, and plasma cells, Dutcher bodies	CD19, CD20, CD22, CD79a, CD38, surface and cytoplasmic IgM, no expression of CD5, CD23, or CD10	No specific cytogenetic abnormality, IgH clonally rearranged
Splenic marginal zone B-cell lymphoma	Splenomegaly, sometimes associated with autoimmune thrombocytopenia or anemia, peripheral lymphadenopathy uncommon	PB: Small- to medium-sized cells with polar villi (villous lymphocytes) Spleen: Both white pulp and red pulp infiltration	CD19, CD20, CD79a, IgM and IgD, no expression of CD5, CD23, CD10, or CD43	Allelic loss of chromosome 7q21–32 in 40% of cases, trisomy 3 in rare cases, IgH clonally rearranged

(continued)

TABLE 43.3 Characteristic Features of Different B-Cell Malignancies *(Continued)*

Disease	Clinical presentation	Morphology	Immunophenotype	Genetics
Extranodal marginal zone B-cell lymphoma (MALT lymphoma)	History of chronic inflammatory or autoimmune disorders (*Helicobacter pylori* gastritis, Hashimoto thyroiditis, Sjögren syndrome), GI tract most common site of involvement	Polymorphous infiltrate of centrocyte-like cells, monocytoid cells, small lymphocytes, scattered immunoblasts and lymphoid cells with plasmacytic differentiation, "overrun follicles," lymphoepithelial lesions	CD19, CD20, CD79a, IgM, no expression of CD5, CD23, CD10	t(11;18)(q21;q21) in ~25% to 50% of cases, t(14;18)(q32;q21) (IgH/MALT1), IgH clonally rearranged
Nodal marginal zone B-cell lymphoma	Localized or generalized lymphadenopathy	Marginal zone and interfollicular areas infiltrated by centrocyte-like B-cells, monocytoid B-cells, or small lymphocytes; plasma cell differentiation may be present	CD19, CD20, CD79a, IgM, no expression of CD5, CD23, CD10	The translocations associated with extranodal MZL are not detected; IgH clonally rearranged
Follicular lymphoma	Widespread peripheral and central lymphadenopathy, bone marrow involved in 40% of cases	Follicular pattern of closely packed neoplastic follicles composed of either small cleaved centrocytes or large centroblasts Grade 1: 0–5 centroblasts/hpf Grade 2: 6–15 centroblasts/hpf Grade 3: >15 centroblasts/hpf	CD19, CD20, CD22, CD79a, BCL-6, BCL-2, CD10	t(14;18)(q32;q21) → rearrangement of the BCL-2 gene leading to overexpression of the BCL-2 protein and survival advantage of malignant cells; IgH clonally rearranged
Mantle cell lymphoma	Lymphadenopathy, most common extranodal site is the GI tract (multiple lymphomatous polyposis)	May show vaguely nodular, diffuse or mantle zone pattern, medium-sized lymphoid cells with irregular nuclear contours, may be blastoid in appearance	CD19, CD20, CD5, FMC-7, CD43, cyclin-D1, lack of expression of CD23, CD10, BCL-6	t(11;14)(q13;q32), translocation between IgH and BCL-1 genes; IgH clonally rearranged

Entity	Clinical Features	Morphology	Immunophenotype	Genetics
Diffuse large B-cell lymphoma (DLBCL)	Rapidly enlarging, often symptomatic mass, often disseminated disease	Sheets of large cells with nuclear size equal or exceeding normal macrophage nucleus Morphologic variants: Centroblastic, immunoblastic, T cell/histiocyte rich, anaplastic	CD19, CD20, CD22, CD79a, CD10, and BCL-6 co-expression: germinal center B-like (better overall survival than activated B-type)	IgH clonally rearranged, ~30% with abnormalities of 3q27 region involving BCL6
Mediastinal (thymic) large B-cell lymphoma	Mostly women in their third to fifth decade, large anterior mediastinal mass, sometimes with impending superior vena cava syndrome	Large cells with associated delicate interstitial fibrosis causing compartmentalization, possible thymic remnants, biopsy samples often small and obscured by profuse sclerosis and crush artifact	CD19, CD20, CD30 (weak), Ig and HLA class I and II expression is often absent	IgH clonally rearranged; hyperdiploid karyotype, gains in chromosome 9p
Burkitt lymphoma	Highly aggressive lymphoma often presenting at extranodal sites or as acute leukemia, risk for central nervous system involvement, "endemic" Burkitt lymphoma with involvement of jaws and other facial structures, "sporadic" Burkitt lymphoma with abdominal masses	Medium-sized cells with basophilic vacuolated cytoplasm and regular nuclei with several small nucleoli, tingible-body macrophages imparting "starry-sky" appearance	CD19, CD20, CD22, CD10, CD79a, BCL-6, no expression of TdT, BCL-2, Ki-67 index of 100%	IgH clonally rearranged; t(8;14) in most cases, t(2;8) and t(8;22) rare

CLL, chronic lymphocytic leukemia; SLL, small lymphocytic lymphoma; MALT, mucosa-associated lymphoid tissue; Ig, immunoglobulin; GI, gastrointestinal; PB, peripheral blood; LN; hpf, high-powered field; TRAP, tartrate-resistant acid phosphatase; HLA, human leukocyte antigen; TdT, terminal deoxynucleotidyl transferase.

TABLE 43.4 Characteristic Features of Different T-Cell and NK-Cell Malignancies

Disease	Clinical presentation	Morphology	Immunophenotype	Genetics
T-cell prolymphocytic leukemia	Aggressive disease with hepatosplenomegaly and generalized lymphadenopathy, marked lymphocytosis, usually >100 × 10⁹/L, anemia and thrombocytopenia	PB: Medium-sized cells with nongranular cytoplasm, visible nucleolus, and cytoplasmic protrusions or blebs	CD3, CD2, CD7, CD4+/CD8− in 60%, CD4+/CD8+ in 25%, CD4−/CD8+ in 15%	inv(14)(q11;q32) in 80%, t(14;14) (q11;q32) in 10% involving TCR-α/β and TCL-1, clonally rearranged TCR
T-cell large granular lymphocyte leukemia	Indolent clinical course, severe neutropenia with/without anemia, mild to moderate lymphocytosis, moderate splenomegaly, rheumatoid arthritis, circulating immune complexes, hypergamma-globulinemia	PB: Large granular lymphocytes with abundant cytoplasm and fine or coarse azurophilic granules; BM: Interstitial infiltrate	CD3, TCR-α/β, CD8 in 80%, co-expression of TIA-1, CD57, perforin, granzyme B, Fas (CD95) and FasL	Clonally rearranged TCR, no unique cytogenetic abnormality
Aggressive NK-cell leukemia	More prevalent among Asians; fever, leukemic blood picture, constitutional symptoms, cytopenias, hepatosple-nomegaly, multiorgan failure due to ↑ serum soluble Fas ligand level	PB: Lymphoid cells larger than normal LGL with slightly basophilic cytoplasm containing granules, hyperchromatic nucleus	CD2, cCD3 ε, CD56, TIA-1, granzyme B, perforin, EBV, no expression of surface CD3 or CD57	TCR not clonally rearranged, EBV present in clonal episomal form
Adult T-cell leukemia	Endemic in Japan, the Caribbean basin, parts of Central Africa, linked to HTLV-1, hypercalcemia, hepatosplenomegaly, ↑LDH, associated T-cell immunodeficiency with opportunistic infections	PB: Medium- to large-sized cells with polylobated nucleus ("flower cells")	CD2, CD3, CD5, CD4, CD25, lack CD7 expression	Clonally integrated HTLV-1, clonally rearranged TCR

Extranodal NK-/T-cell lymphoma, nasal type	More prevalent in Asia, Mexico, Central, and South America, extensive midfacial destructive lesions, other extranodal sites include skin, soft tissue, testis, GI tract	Extensive ulceration and necrosis, angiocentric and angiodestructive growth pattern, hyperchromatic nucleus, intermixed inflammatory cells	CD2, CD56, cCD3 ε, granzyme B, TIA-1, perforin, surface CD3 not expressed	TCR not clonally rearranged, EBV present in clonal episomal form
Enteropathy-type T-cell lymphoma	Associated with celiac disease and ulcerative jejunitis	Ulcerating mucosal mass in jejunum or ileum, broad cytologic spectrum, intermixed inflammatory cells	CD3, CD8+/−, CD103, TIA-1, granzyme, perforin	Clonally rearranged TCR, HLA DQA1*0501, DQB1*0201 genotype of celiac disease
Hepatosplenic T-cell lymphoma	Peak incidence in adolescents and young adults, marked hepatosplenomegaly with lymphadenopathy, more common in patients with immunosuppression	Sinusoidal infiltration of liver, spleen, and bone marrow by monotonous small- to medium-sized cells	CD3, TCR-γ/δ, TIA-1, negative for CD4, CD8, TCR-α/β, and perforin	Clonally rearranged TCR, isochromosome 7q, trisomy 8
Subcutaneous panniculitis-like T-cell lymphoma	Multiple subcutaneous nodules, may be associated with hemophagocytic syndrome with pancytopenia, fever, and hepatosplenomegaly	Diffuse, lacelike infiltrate in subcutis without sparing septae; epidermis uninvolved; necrosis, karyorrhexis, rimming of fat cells	CD3, CD8, granzyme B, perforin, TIA-1	Clonally rearranged TCR
Mycosis fungoides	Long natural history, multiple skin lesions, patch → plaque → tumor, frequently on trunk	Epidermotropic infiltrate of tumor cells with "cerebriform" nuclei, Pautrier's microabscesses	CD2, CD3, CD5, CD4, TCR-α/β, no expression of CD7	Clonally rearranged TCR
Sézary syndrome	Aggressive variant of mycosis fungoides; erythroderma, lymphadenopathy, and circulating Sézary cells	PB: Minimum of 1000 Sézary cells per mm^3, "cerebriform" nuclei	Increased CD4/CD8 ratio lacking expression of CD7	Clonally rearranged TCR

(continued)

TABLE 43.4 Characteristic Features of Different T-Cell and NK-Cell Malignancies (*Continued*)

Disease	Clinical presentation	Morphology	Immunophenotype	Genetics
Angioimmunoblastic T-cell lymphoma	Immunodeficiency secondary to lymphoma, skin rash, edema, pleural effusion, ascites, cytopenia, polyclonal hypergammaglobulinemia, + rheumatoid factor	Mixture of polymorphous lymphocytes some with clear cytoplasm, plasma cells, eosinophils, and immunoblasts; arborizing HEV; prominence of FDC meshwork outside follicles	CD2, CD3, CD4 with co-expression of CD10, follicular dendritic cells are highlighted by CD21, CD23, CD35, immunoblasts are CD20+ and EBV+	Clonally rearranged TCR, trisomy 3, trisomy 5, additional X chromosome
Peripheral T-cell lymphoma, unspecified	Predominantly nodal-based lymphomas that cannot be better classified, generalized disease	Broad cytologic spectrum, T-zone variant with preservation of follicles, Lennert variant with many epithelioid clusters	CD2, CD3, mostly CD4, may express CD30	Rearranged TCR
Anaplastic large cell lymphoma	10%–30% of childhood lymphomas advanced stage (III or IV) with frequent extranodal involvement	Hallmark cells = large cells with abundant cytoplasm and horseshoe-shaped nuclei	CD30 (membrane and Golgi), ALK-1 (60%–85%), EMA+, CD43, CD2, CD4	Rearranged TCR t(2;5) involving NPM and ALK

NK, natural killer; HTLV, human T-cell leukemia virus; LDH, ; GI, gastrointestinal; PB, peripheral blood; BM, bone marrow; LGL, large granular lymphocytes; HEV, high endothelial vessels; FDC, follicular dendritic cells; TCR, T-cell receptor; TIA, T-cell restricted intracellular antigen; FasL, Fas ligand; EBV, Epstein–Barr virus; ALK-1, anaplastic large cell-1; EMA, epithelial membrane antigen; TCL-1, T-cell leukemia/lymphoma 1; HLA, human leukocyte antigen.

TABLE 43.5 Criteria for the Diagnosis of Plasma Cell Myeloma

Symptomatic plasma cell myeloma
PC on tissue biopsy or
  clonal bone marrow plasmacytosis (usually >10% plasma cells)
M-protein in serum or urine: usually (but not always) serum IgG >30 g/dL or IgA >25 g/dL;
  κ or λ light chain excretion >1.0 g/d on 24-h urine electrophoresis
Related organ or tissue impairment (anemia, hypercalcemia, lytic lesions, renal insufficiency,
  recurrent infections, etc.)
Asymptomatic (smoldering) plasma cell myeloma
M-protein in serum at myeloma levels (>30 g/L)
  and/or
Clonal bone marrow plasmacytosis (10% or more)
No related organ or tissue impairment

B. **Plasma cell myeloma** usually is characterized by multifocal bone marrow plasmacytosis causing osteolytic lesions, pathologic fractures, bone pain, hypercalcemia, and anemia (e-Figs. 43.24 and 43.25). The diagnostic criteria for plasma cell myeloma are outlined in Table 43.5. These criteria must be manifest in a symptomatic patient with progressive disease to diagnose symptomatic plasma cell myeloma. Clinical variants include asymptomatic (smoldering) myeloma when patients are asymptomatic and have no lytic bone lesions (Table 43.5); nonsecretory myeloma where serum M-protein may be absent but cytoplasmic M-protein can be demonstrated by immunohistochemistry (in the majority of patients) and abnormalities in serum light chains are demonstrable by serologic testing (*Br J Hematol.* 2003;121:749); and plasma cell leukemia (PCL) when clonal plasma cells equal or exceed 20% of the leukocyte differential count. Up to 5% of patients with plasma cell neoplasia may present with PCL. Morphologically, the circulating plasma cells may resemble plasmacytoid lymphocytes; therefore, immunophenotypic studies are extremely helpful in this setting. Unlike other myelomas, PCL usually lacks aberrant expression of CD56 and is more likely to be associated with abnormal or unfavorable cytogenetics (Table 43.6).

C. **Plasmacytomas** manifest as a localized osseous or extraosseous lesion with no radiographic or morphologic evidence of bone marrow involvement (e-Figs. 43.26 to 43.29). The most common osseous location is the vertebral body, and the most common extraosseous location is the upper respiratory tract.

D. **Monoclonal immunoglobulin deposition diseases** present with visceral and soft tissue deposits of immunoglobulin light chains, heavy chains, or both. An example of monoclonal light chain deposition is primary amyloidosis, a rare disease characterized by deposition of an abnormal immunoglobulin. These immunoglobulin light chains are predominantly λ, secreted by monoclonal plasma cells, ingested and processed by macrophages, and discharged into

TABLE 43.6 Diagnostic Criteria of Monoclonal MGUS and PC

Type	Marrow plasmacytosis	Serum M component	Lytic lesions	Organ or tissue impairment
MGUS	<10%	Less than myeloma levels (IgG <35 g/dL; IgA <25 g/dL)	None	None
PC	None	Absent or low	Present	None

Ig, immunoglobulin.

extracellular matrix as β-pleated sheets containing amyloid P component. The deposits are visible as homogenous, pink material in tissue sections that are green birefringent by Congo red staining. The clinical consequences are related to deposition of amyloid in organs, resulting in organomegaly and organ malfunction. Rarely, plasma cell or lymphoplasmacytic neoplasms secrete abnormal light or, less often, heavy chains or sometimes both, which may cause similar but nonamyloid deposits in organs, most commonly in kidneys (*Hematol Oncol Clin North Am.* 1992;6:323; *N Eng J Med.* 1993;329: 1389).

E. **POEMS** syndrome represents an osteosclerotic myeloma with associated clinical features including polyneuropathy, organomegaly, endocrinology, monoclonal gammopathy, and skin changes. Lymph-node biopsies in these patients may demonstrate Castleman-like features, specifically its plasma cell variant (*Blood.* 2003;101:2496–2506). The bone marrow shows plasmacytosis only in the vicinity of sclerotic lesions with <5% plasma cells elsewhere (*Blood Rev.* 1996;10:75–80).

F. **Immunophenotype.** Neoplastic plasma cells typically express monotypic cytoplasmic immunoglobulin and lack surface immunoglobulin expression. Most cases lack CD19 and CD20 expression, whereas CD79a, CD38, and CD138 (syndecan-1) are found in the majority of cases. CD56 is aberrantly expressed in up to 70% of myelomas. Expression of cyclin D1 is also a feature of plasma cells, specifically in multiple myeloma (see Section VII.G), and diagnosis of mantle cell lymphoma must be avoided on the basis of an isolated finding of cyclin D1 positivity. Other antigens that are aberrantly expressed and could be helpful in detection of minimal residual disease or targeted therapy include CD20, CD117, CD52, or CD10 (*Am J Clin Pathol.* 2004;121:482–488; *Blood.* 2008;12:4017–4023). CD56 negative myelomas show more extensive marrow infiltration, lower osteolytic potential, frequent plasmablastic morphology, and a tendency toward leukemic transformation (*Br J Haematol.* 2002;117:882–885).

G. **Myeloma genetics.** Plasma cell neoplasms demonstrate clonally rearranged immunoglobulin heavy and light chains by molecular studies; cytogenetic methods to detect chromosomal abnormalities include cytokine-stimulated bone marrow biopsy for conventional karyotyping and FISH. Combined, these modalities increase the frequency of detectable genetic aberrations in myeloma to over 90% (*Cancer Res.* 2004;64:1546–1558). Complex karyotypes with multiple chromosomal gains and losses are the most frequent abnormalities, the most common being gains in chromosomes 3, 5, 7, 9, 11, 15, and 19 and losses in chromosomes 8, 13, 14, and X (*Blood.* 1995;85:2490). Monosomy or partial deletion of 13 (13q14) is the most common structural chromosomal abnormality. In about 40% of cases, translocations involving one of five recurrent oncogenes are seen. The most common translocation is t(11;14)(q13;q32), involving the *BCL1* locus on chromosome 11q13 (*CYCLIN D1*) and the immunoglobulin heavy (*IgH*) chain locus on 14q23, which leads to over expression of cyclin-D1 (*Brit J Hematol.* 1998;101:189; *Blood.* 2002;99:2185; *J Clin Oncol.* 2005;23:6333). Other translocation partners for the *IgH* locus are 4p16.3 (*FGFR-3* and *MMSET*), 6p21 (*CCND3*), 16q23 (*C-MAF*), and 20q11 (*MAFB*) (Table 43.7).

VIII. **CASTLEMAN DISEASE.** Castleman disease is an important consideration in the differential diagnosis of lymphomas due to its clinical presentation. It can occur at any age but has a predilection for young adults, often presenting as a mass, most often in the mediastinum, although cervical, abdominal, and axillary nodes may all be the sites of origin (*Cancer.* 1972;29:670; *Semin Diag Pathol.* 1988;5:346; *Mod Pathol.* 1992;5:525). In some cases, generalized lymphadenopathy with B-symptoms, anemia, thrombocytopenia, and pemphigus mimic the clinical

TABLE 43.7	Commonly Occurring Cytogenetic Abnormalities in Multiple Myeloma[a]	
Abnormality	**% Occurrence**	**Prognostic implications**
I. Numerical[b]		Favorable
a. Hyperdiploidy	61%–68%	Unfavorable
b. Hypodiploidy	10%–30%	
II. Complex		
Partial or complete deletion of 13 and 11q, del 17q13	Ranging from 1%–25%	Unfavorable
t(11;14), t(6;14)[c]	cyclinD1 15%–18%, D3 3%	Favorable
t(4;14), t(14;16), t(14;20)[c]	FGFR 15%, MAFB 2%	Unfavorable

[a]Up to 90% of cases show abnormalities using FISH techniques. By conventional cytogenetics, 30%–50% of patients show an abnormal karyotype.
[b]Most common abnormalities are trisomy 3, 7, 9, and 11; monosomy 13; and, in females, monosomy X.
[c]t(4;14) and t(11;14) are the most common translocations. See text for the oncogenes.

presentation of lymphoma. Classically, Castleman disease is divided into two clinical entities.

Hyaline-vascular Castleman disease shows capsular thickening and overt nodularity of lymph node architecture. The diagnostic features are generally seen in lymphoid follicles, namely hyperplasia and expanded mantle zones with lymphocytes arranged in concentric layers. The germinal centers appear regressed and vascularized, with some blood vessels that traverse tangentially to impart a lollipop appearance. Multiple germinal centers can be seen per follicle (e-**Figs. 43.30** to **43.32**). The paracortical areas are also highly vascularized, containing a mix of cells with an increased number of plasmacytoid/monocytoid lymphocytes accompanied in some cases by a variable increase in plasma cells. While immunophenotypic findings do not differentiate lymph node involvement by hyaline-vascular Castleman disease from reactive follicles, a CD21 stain is especially helpful for demonstrating expanded concentric meshworks of follicular dendritic cells. However, ancillary studies (including flow cytometry and immunohistochemistry) must be performed to exclude Hodgkin lymphoma, NHLs, and plasma cell neoplasms. Surgical resection of the involved node is usually curative (*Virchows Arch A Pathol Anat Histopathol.* 1993;423:369).

Plasma cell type Castleman disease is less common than the hyaline-vascular type. It can be unicentric (localized to one site of presentation), although it more commonly presents as multicentric disease (systemic illness with malaise, fevers, night sweats, and cytopenias). Polyclonal plasmacytosis in the bone marrow, hypergammaglobulinemia, and elevated IL-6 levels are important clues to diagnosis; elevated IL-6 levels are more common in the unicentric plasma cell type. Histologically, the paracortical regions show marked polyclonal plasmacytosis (monoclonal lambda–light chains can be seen in up to 30% of cases); the nodal architecture is otherwise well preserved with follicles varying from reactive to regressed. A variety of other disease entities need to be excluded using appropriate ancillary studies including HIV lymphadenopathy, autoimmune/chronic inflammatory conditions, other lymphomas (most importantly HHV-8 associated plasmablastic lymphoma), and even metastatic carcinoma. An association with POEMS syndrome has been noted (see Section VII.E); human herpes virus (HHV)-8 plays a pathogenic role in HIV and non-HIV associated settings and can often be documented in lesional tissue by immunohistochemical stains (ORF73/latency-associated nuclear antigen-1), although an HHV-8 association is more commonly seen in cases with monoclonal plasmacytosis (*Human Pathol.* 1985;16:162; *Histopathology.* 1989;14:11; *AIDS.* 1996;10:61). While unicentric plasma cell type Castleman disease can be cured with surgical excision, systemic therapy may be required in multicentric forms.

IX. **HODGKIN LYMPHOMA.** Hodgkin lymphoma typically presents as a primarily nodal disease characterized by a predominance of reactive cells with a paucity of neoplastic Reed–Sternberg (RS) cells or variants. Hodgkin lymphoma comprises two distinct entities: classical Hodgkin lymphoma (CHL) and nodular lymphocyte–predominant Hodgkin lymphoma (NLPHL). These two entities differ in their clinical appearance, morphology, immunoglobulin transcription of the neoplastic cells, and immunophenotype.

A. **CHL** accounts for ~95% of Hodgkin lymphoma and is subdivided into four categories: nodular sclerosis (~70%), mixed cellularity (~20% to 25%), lymphocyte rich (~5%), and lymphocyte depleted (<5%). The neoplastic cell is the classical RS cell or its variants (mononuclear forms, mummified forms, or lacunar cells).

1. Nodular sclerosis CHL commonly presents with a mediastinal mass. Histology reveals scattered RS cells embedded in a mixed inflammatory background of mostly T lymphocytes, plasma cells, eosinophils, neutrophils, and histiocytes, compartmentalized into nodules by thick strands of collagen fibrosis (e-**Figs. 43.33** to **43.35**).

2. Mixed cellularity CHL presents with scattered RS cells in a diffuse or vaguely nodular mixed inflammatory background without nodular sclerosing fibrosis.

3. In lymphocyte-rich CHL, the nonneoplastic cellular background is composed of predominantly T lymphocytes. Other inflammatory cells are rare.

4. Lymphocyte-depleted CHL is rare and occurs most commonly in association with HIV infection. Histologically, sheets of RS cells predominate without a significant lymphocytic or mixed inflammatory infiltrate.

   The main clinical findings of CHL at diagnosis are painless peripheral lymphadenopathy, most commonly involving the cervical region, and constitutional symptoms such as fever, night sweats, weight loss, and infections due to immunosuppression. Many of the pathologic and clinical features reflect an abnormal immune response due to the wide variety of cytokines and chemokines (Table 43.8), produced by the RS cells (*Blood.* 2002;99:4283). The etiology of CHL is largely unknown. Studies based on the month of diagnosis have revealed peaks in February and March, and the lymphoma appears to be more prevalent in adolescents and young adults with higher socioeconomic status (*Hematol Oncol.* 2004;22:11). The association between EBV and CHL has been demonstrated in numerous seroepidemiologic studies in which antibody titers to EBV and viral capsid antigens have been consistently found to be higher in the lymphoma cases compared with controls. There also have been reports of clustering of CHL within the same family, especially among siblings of same sex and close age. Certain human leukocyte antigen (HLA) types, such as A1, B5, and B18, appear also to be clearly associated with this lymphoma (*Hematol Oncol.* 2004;22:11).

B. **Nodular lymphocyte predominant Hodgkin lymphoma (NLPHL)** is characterized by scattered large neoplastic L&H cells (lymphocytic and/or histiocytic cells, popcorn cells) residing in nodular meshworks of follicular dendritic processes, filled with nonneoplastic lymphocytes mostly of B-cell lineage (e-**Figs. 43.36** and **43.37**). Clinically, patients present with localized peripheral lymphadenopathy. The disease develops slowly, with fairly frequent relapses, but remains responsive to chemotherapy and usually is not fatal. About 3% to 5% of cases evolve into DLBCL.

C. **Pathophysiology.** The cellular origin of neoplastic cells in both CHL and NLPHL was finally determined when clonally rearranged immunoglobulin

TABLE 43.8	Role of Cytokines in CHL	
Cytokine	**Biologic activity**	**Comments**
IL-1	Potent proinflammatory cytokine, induction of fever and acute phase proteins	Associated with B-symptoms
IL-5	Eosinophil differentiation, proliferation, and activation	Associated with blood and tissue eosinophilia
IL-6	Plasma cell differentiation, stimulation of IL-1, and TNF-α production	Associated with thrombocytosis and tissue plasmacytosis
IL-8	Neutrophil recruitment factor	Associated with tissue neutrophilia
IL-9	T-cell and mast cell growth factor	May be acting as a growth factor for RS cells
IL-10	Impaired immune response	Associated with EBV+ cases
IL-13	B-cell proliferation and survival; Ig class switching to IgG4 and IgE	Autocrine growth factor for RS cells
TGF-β	Inhibition of IL-2R upregulation and IL-2–dependent T- and B-cell proliferation, potent stimulator of fibroblast proliferation and collagen synthesis	Associated with tissue fibrosis

IL, interleukin; IL-2R, interleukin 2 receptor; TGF, transforming growth factor; Ig, immunoglobulin; TNF-α, tumor necrosis factor-α; EBV, Epstein–Barr virus.

genes were amplified from purified Hodgkin cells obtained by microdissection (*Proc Natl Acad Sci USA.* 1994;91:10962). Additionally, the detection of somatic mutations within the rearranged immunoglobulin genes suggests a germinal center or postgerminal center B-cell to be the precursor of Hodgkin cells. Although tumor cells of both CHL and NLPHL harbor rearranged immunoglobulin genes, these are not expressed in CHL due to lack of immunoglobulin messenger RNA (mRNA). Further studies have shown that the absence of immunoglobulin transcription is caused by inactivation of the immunoglobulin promoter through impaired or absent activation of the octamer-dependent transcription factor Oct2 and/or its coactivator BOB.1. Immunohistochemistry for Oct2 and BOB.1 usually is negative in classical RS cells, unlike L&H cells in NLPHL that express these two markers (*Blood.* 2001; 91:496).

Normally, when B-cells are no longer capable of expressing immunoglobulin, they rapidly undergo apoptosis. However, although classical RS cells do not express immunoglobulin chains due to the absence of immunoglobulin mRNA, they are resistant to apoptosis. One mechanism preventing apoptosis is believed to be persistent activation of the nuclear transcription factor, nuclear factor kappa B (NFκB), in classical RS cells caused by mutations within members of the IκB family, which are natural inhibitors of NFκB, or by aberrant activation of IκB kinase (*Lancet Oncol.* 2004;5:11).

D. **Immunophenotype studies.** Immunohistochemistry markers important in the diagnosis of Hodgkin lymphoma are:
   1. CD30 (expressed on classical RS cells in ~98% of cases)
   2. CD15 (expressed on classical RS cells in ~80% of cases; also expressed in neutrophils)
   3. CD20 (may be expressed in a small subset of classical RS cells; strongly positive in L&H cells, positive in intermixed nonneoplastic small B lymphocytes)

4. CD45 (LCA) (negative in classical RS cells, strongly positive in L&H cells, positive in accompanying nonneoplastic inflammatory cells)

5. CD79a (negative in classical RS cells, strongly positive in L&H cells, positive in intermixed nonneoplastic small B lymphocytes)

6. Epithelial membrane antigen (EMA) negative in classical RS cells, positive in L&H cells in ~50% of cases)

7. BCL-6 (positive in L&H cells in nearly all cases)

8. CD3 (positive in intermixed T lymphocytes, L&H cells are ringed by CD3+ T-cells)

9. CD57 (positive in intermixed cytotoxic T-cells, L&H cells are ringed by CD57+ T-cells)

10. BSAP (B cell–specific activator protein and product of the *PAX 5* gene; positive in both classical RS cells and L&H cells)

11. EBV (positive in classical RS cells in ~40% of cases)

X. STAGING OF LYMPHOMAS AND PLASMA CELL MYELOMA

A. **Hodgkin and non-Hodgkin lymphomas.** Formal documentation of anatomic extent of disease is required in all patients newly diagnosed with lymphoma prior to therapeutic intervention. Clinical staging takes into account variables such as history and physical examination, imaging studies, blood chemistry determination, complete blood count, and bone marrow biopsy. If a patient presents with relapsed disease, determination of anatomic extent of the disease is recommended but a new clinical stage is usually not assigned. The most widely used anatomic staging classification for Hodgkin and non-Hodgkin lymphomas is the Ann Arbor classification, which has been adopted by the American Joint Committee on Cancer (AJCC) as the official system for lymphoma staging (see Table 43.9).

1. Definition of lymph node regions is based on the definitions proposed by the Rye Symposium in 1965 and adopted by both the Ann Arbor and AJCC systems. The currently accepted classification groups of lymph nodes are right cervical (includes cervical, supraclavicular, occipital, and preauricular nodes); left cervical; right axillary; left axillary; right infraclavicular; left

TABLE 43.9	Ann Arbor Staging for Hodgkin and Non-Hodgkin Lymphoma
Stage I	Involvement of single lymphatic site (i.e., nodal region, Waldeyer's ring, thymus, or spleen) (I); or localized involvement of a single extralymphatic organ or site in the absence of any lymph node involvement (IE) (rare in Hodgkin lymphoma).
Stage II	Involvement of two or more lymph node regions on the same side of the diaphragm (II); or localized involvement of a single extralymphatic organ or site in association with regional lymph node involvement with or without involvement of other lymph node regions on the same side of the diaphragm (IIE). The number of regions involved may be indicated by a subscript, as in, for example, II3.
Stage III	Involvement of lymph node regions on both sides of the diaphragm (II), which also may be accompanied by extralymphatic extension in association with adjacent lymph node involvement (IIIE) or by involvement of the spleen (IIIS) or both (IIISE). Splenic involvement is designated by the letter S.
Stage IV	Diffuse or disseminated involvement of one of more extralymphatic organs, with or without associated lymph node involvement; or isolated extralymphatic organ involvement in the absence of adjacent regional lymph node involvement, but in conjunction with disease in distant site(s). Stage IV includes any involvement of the liver or bone marrow, lungs (other than by direct extension from another site), or cerebrospinal fluid.

TABLE 43.10 Staging Systems for Multiple Myeloma

| | Durie–Salmon staging system | | | | | | ISS criteria | |
| | | | Serum urine M-immunoglobulins protein | | | Serum Cr | | | |
Stage	Hb	Serum calcium	Osteolytic lesion	IgG	IgA		A	B	β_2M	Albumin
I	>10 g/dL	≤12 mg/dL	Normal or single lesion	<50 g/dL	<30 g/dL	<4 g/24 h	<2.0 mg/dL	>2.0 mg/dL	<3.5 mg/dL	>3.5 g/dL
II	Not stage I or III						<2.0 mg/dL	>2.0 mg/dL		
III	<8.5 g/dL	>12 mg/dL	Advanced multiple lytic lesions	>70 g/dL	>50 g/dL	>12 g/24 h	<2.0 mg/dL	>2.0 mg/dL	>5.5 mg/dL	—

Hb, hemoglobulin; Cr, creatinine; β_2M, β_2 microglobulin; Ig, immunoglobulin; —, not required for staging.

infraclavicular; mediastinal; hilar; para-aortic; mesenteric; right pelvic; left pelvic; right inguinofemoral; and left inguinofemoral.

2. Definition of extranodal involvement (such as by direct extension into lung, thyroid, liver, etc.) is designated by an "E" alongside the anatomic stage. Involvement of bone marrow, cerebrospinal fluid, liver, or pleura equates to stage IV by convention.

B. **Staging of multiple myeloma.** The AJCC recommends the Durie-Salmon staging system for multiple myeloma. This system takes into account various complete blood count variables, blood chemistries, M-protein levels, and imaging studies.

A newer, simpler, and more cost-effective alternative is the International Staging System (ISS), previously the International Prognostic Index. This system uses two simple blood parameters, specifically β_2 microglobulin (β_2-M) and albumin. The ISS has been proven to be useful for staging myeloma (*J Clin Oncol.* 2005;23:3412) and is currently recommended for widespread use. A comparison of these myeloma staging systems is depicted in Table 43.10.

Lymph Node Cytopathology

Julie Elizabeth Kunkel

I. **INTRODUCTION.** Diagnosis of NHL by FNA requires a multiparametric approach that couples cytomorphology with ancillary studies, including flow cytometry, immunohistochemistry, FISH, cytogenetics, and molecular studies. Using a combined approach, diagnosis of NHL based on FNA and core needle biopsy specimens has >96% sensitivity and specificity when compared with excisional biopsy (*Am J of Clin Pathol.* 2011;135:4). Proper triage of a lymph node FNA at the time of immediate evaluation depends on the distinction between reactive lymphadenopathy, a lymphomatous process, or a metastasis from a known or unknown primary to direct subsequent distribution of tissue for appropriate studies (cell block, flow cytometry, FISH, etc.).

The lymphoid cells from FNA specimens characteristically are dyshesive, and the background frequently shows lymphoglandular bodies (cytoplasmic fragments of disrupted lymphocytes). In general, NHL exhibits a monotonous population of atypical lymphoid cells in contrast to the polymorphous appearance of normal and reactive lymph nodes. Cytologically, NHL is classified as small cell lymphoma, intermediate cell lymphoma, and large cell lymphoma on the basis of the cell size in comparison with histiocytes. Small cell lymphoma includes small lymphocytic lymphoma, lymphoplasmacytic lymphoma, follicular lymphoma (grade 1), mantle cell lymphoma, and marginal zone lymphoma. Intermediate cell lymphoma is further divided into lymphoblastic lymphoma and Burkitt lymphoma. Large cell lymphoma usually refers to DLBCL, but also includes T-cell and NK-cell lymphoma.

II. **REACTIVE LYMPHADENOPATHY.** The aspirate is characterized by a polymorphous population of lymphoid cells with variable size and shape that predominantly contains small lymphoid cells with smooth nuclear contours and coarse chromatin, intermixed with scattered intermediate cells and large immunoblast-like cells. Scattered plasma cells, histiocytes, and tingible body macrophages are present. Lymphohistiocytic aggregates are also seen, consisting of collections of lymphoid cells and histiocytes held together by dendritic reticular cells (**e-Fig. 43.38**) (*Acta Cytol.* 1987;31:8).

Clusters of neutrophils are indicative of suppurative lymphadenopathy. Collections of epithelioid histiocytes are consistent with granulomatous lymphadenitis (**e-Fig. 43.39**) (*Sarcoidosis.* 1987;4:38) and may be seen in infectious and noninfectious processes; special stains and culture are required for identification of fungi and mycobacteria. Fungal hyphae and yeast forms can occasionally be identified as negative images on Diff-Quik–stained smears (e-Fig. 43.40).

III. SMALL-CELL LYMPHOMA

A. **Small lymphocytic lymphoma.** The aspirate contains a monotonous population of small lymphoid cells with round nuclear contours, characteristic checkerboard-like clumpy chromatin, and indistinct nucleoli (e-Fig. 43.41). Scattered large prolymphocytes/paraimmunoblasts with vesicular chromatin, prominent central nucleoli, and pale cytoplasm are present.

B. **Lymphoplasmacytic lymphoma.** The smear contains a mixed population of small lymphoid cells, plasmacytoid cells, and plasma cells.

C. **Follicular lymphoma.** The aspirate is composed predominantly of small centrocytes (that have irregular and grooved nuclear membranes) that are intermixed with scattered centroblasts (that have a large noncleaved nuclei with multiple small peripheral nucleoli) and immunoblasts (that have single prominent central nucleolus) (e-Fig. 43.42). Lymphoid aggregates without abundant histiocytes are not infrequently found (*Cancer.* 1999;87:216; *Cancer.* 2006;108:1). Although the cytologic criteria for grading follicular lymphoma are not well established, the percentage of centroblasts on smears has been proposed as a basis for grading by several groups (*Am J Clin Pathol.* 1997;108:143; *Clin Pathol.* 2002;117:880).

D. **Mantle cell lymphoma.** The aspirate is composed of a monotonous population of small to intermediate-sized lymphoid cells with variable nuclear membrane contour irregularity, dispersed chromatin, and inconspicuous nucleoli (e-Fig. 43.43) (*Cancer.* 1999;87:216).

E. **Nodal marginal zone B-cell lymphoma.** The aspirate contains a rather polymorphous lymphoid population composed predominately of small lymphoid cells with round nuclei and clumpy chromatin, with scattered plasmacytoid cells and immunoblast-like large cells (*Diagn Cytopathol.* 1999;20:190). Some intermediate-sized lymphoid cells that have a monocytoid appearance and exhibit a moderate amount of pale cytoplasm are also present (e-Fig. 43.44). Lymphoepithelial lesions are not identified on smears. Due to its polymorphous appearance, diagnosis based on the cytopathologic findings alone is challenging without ancillary studies.

IV. INTERMEDIATE CELL LYMPHOMA

A. **Lymphoblastic lymphoma.** The aspirate is composed of a monotonous population of intermediate-sized lymphoid cells with fine granular chromatin, irregular nuclear membrane contours, inconspicuous nucleoli, and scant basophilic cytoplasm (e-Fig. 43.45). Mitoses are frequently identified (*Acta Cytol.* 1992;36:887).

B. **Burkitt lymphoma.** The aspirate contains a monotonous population of intermediate-sized lymphoid cells with round nuclei, finely dispersed chromatin, and multiple distinct nucleoli. The cytoplasm is scant, deep blue, and contains small lipid-filled vacuoles (e-Fig. 43.46). Tingible body macrophages and mitosis are prominent (*Cytopathol.* 1995;12:201) and are indicative of brisk cell turnover.

V. LARGE CELL LYMPHOMA

A. **DLBCL.** The aspirate shows a monotonous population of large atypical lymphoid cells. The centroblastic variant contains centroblasts with irregular nuclear membrane contours, coarse chromatin, and multiple small nucleoli (e-Fig. 43.47). The immunoblastic variant shows immunoblasts with irregular nuclear membrane contours, open chromatin, and single prominent nucleoli. The T-cell rich B-cell lymphoma variant is composed predominantly of small mature lymphocytes and scattered large immature lymphoid cells with polymorphic nuclei and prominent nucleoli. The cytological diagnosis of this variant is challenging (*Diagn Cytopathol.* 1998;18:1).

B. Peripheral T-cell lymphoma, unspecified type. The aspirate is polymorphic and contains scattered large atypical lymphocytes with convoluted nuclear membranes. The background shows a reactive pattern and is composed of small mature lymphocytes, plasma cells, neutrophils, eosinophils, and macrophages. Ancillary studies are necessary for diagnosis (*Diagn Cytopathol.* 2000;23:375).

C. Anaplastic large cell lymphoma. The aspirate shows both singly dispersed and poorly cohesive groups of malignant cells with large and pleomorphic nuclei, prominent nucleoli, and a moderate amount cytoplasm. Horseshoe- and "donut"-shaped nuclei, as well as binucleated and multinucleated RS-like tumor cells, are also present. Immunostains are necessary for diagnosis (*Acta Cytol.* 1996;40:779). Mistaking this entity for carcinoma may be a diagnostic pitfall due to the cellular cohesion and pleomorphism.

D. Myeloid sarcoma is an extramedullary solid collection of myeloid cells. The disease may be present in a lymph node and may be a harbinger of leukemia or evidence of relapsed disease. Aspirates show tumor cells in any stage of myeloid differentiation ranging from blasts to more mature myeloid forms; however, in some cases, myeloid differentiation may be entirely absent. The differential diagnosis often includes large cell lymphoma; correct characterization rests on histochemical and flow-cytometric analyses (*Ann Diagn Pathol.* 2000;4:1).

VI. HODGKIN LYMPHOMA. The aspirate of classic Hodgkin lymphoma contains rare to scattered RS cells. The classic binucleated RS cells have markedly enlarged nuclei, macronucleoli, and a moderate amount of basophilic cytoplasm (e-Fig. 43.48). The mononuclear variant has cells with markedly enlarged, irregular, and multilobated nuclei with macronucleoli (e-Fig. 43.49). The characteristic reactive lymphoid background includes mainly mature lymphocytes, scattered eosinophils, neutrophils, plasma cells, and occasional epithelioid histiocytes (e-Fig. 43.49) (*J Clin Pathol.* 1986;86:286). Diagnosis is challenging due to the scarcity of the RS cells, and the cytopathologic diagnosis of NLPHL from FNA specimens is very difficult if not impossible. Nonetheless, when FNA biopsy is used in conjunction with immunohistochemistry as a screening test for Hodgkin lymphoma, the approach has a positive predictive value that has been reported to be >90% in some studies (*Cytopathology.* 1994;5:226; *Acta Cytol.* 2001;45:300).

VII. METASTATIC MALIGNANCY. The most common indication for lymph node FNA biopsy is metastatic malignancy. The reported sensitivity of diagnosis based on FNA specimens in this clinical setting is >90%, with a specificity of >98% (*Cytopathology.* 1996;15:382; *Diagn Cytopathol.* 2003;28:175). The aspirate shows a nonlymphoid population of cells with malignant cytological features. An absence of a background of lymphocytes and nodal elements is important to report if it is uncertain whether the epithelial malignancy represents a nodal metastasis; examples include breast cancers present in the axillary tail which may be mistaken clinically for axillary nodal metastases, and hilar lung masses which may represent central tumors versus metastatic involvement of hilar nodes. In the case of nodal effacement by tumor, this distinction may not be possible.

In the case of a known primary, comparison with the primary malignancy usually will confirm the diagnosis. For patients with a history of multiple malignancies, or cytomorphology that is not congruous with the reported history, immunostains must be employed to confirm the site of origin. If clinical uncertainty is present at the time of immediate evaluation, directing additional passes for cell block preparation will increase the diagnostic yield of material available for immunohistochemical profiling.

SUGGESTED READINGS

Immunobiology, (6th ed.) New York and London: Garland Publishing; 2005:149–153.
Swerdlow SH, Campo E, Harris NL, et al., *WHO Classification of Tumors; Pathology and Genetics; Tumors of Hematopoietic and Lymphoid Tissues,* 4th ed. Lyon, France: IARC Press; 2008.

44 Bone Marrow Pathology

Jeffery M. Klco and John L. Frater

I. **NORMAL GROSS AND MICROSCOPIC ANATOMY.** The bone marrow is generally considered the fourth largest organ in the human body and is composed of cells derived from a variety of lineages including stromal cells, adipocytes, lymphocytes, and hematopoietic precursors. The most frequently sampled areas are the posterior superior iliac crest and, much less frequently, the sternum and long bones. The bone marrow has an orderly microscopic anatomy. The most superficial part consists of a layer of dense cortical bone with an adjacent cover of dense fibrous periosteum. Deep into the cortex are the bony trabeculae, which consist of thin trabecular bone and the marrow cavity itself. The marrow cavity contains islands of maturing hematopoietic cells with intervening areas of fat, the latter of which increase with age.

The cellularity of the bone marrow is defined as the percentage of the marrow cavity composed of hematopoietic cells. In biopsies from the posterior iliac crest, marrow cellularity decreases with age, and is expressed by the formula: Marrow cellularity $= (100 - \text{patient age})\% \pm 20\%$. Thus, a 50-year-old individual would be expected to have a marrow cellularity of approximately $(100 - 50)\% \pm 20\%$, or 30% to 70%.

Under normal circumstances, maturing myeloid and erythroid elements occupy different regions of the marrow cavity. Myeloid precursors lie adjacent to the trabecular bone, and erythroid elements form "islands" of cells between trabeculae. The ratio of myeloid to erythroid elements is roughly 2:1. Megakaryocytes are irregularly distributed throughout the bone marrow. Under normal circumstances they are not present in clusters.

It is important to be cognizant of the multidisciplinary nature of hematopathology. Diagnoses in bone marrow pathology are not generally the product of morphologic analysis of the bone marrow core biopsy or peripheral blood and bone marrow aspirate smears alone. Clinical history is extremely important in separating morphologically similar diseases and should be provided by the patient's physicians. Also, the pertinent features of the physical examination, such as lymphadenopathy, splenomegaly, and hepatomegaly, are of importance. Other clinical laboratory information, such as complete blood counts and serum and/or urine protein electrophoresis, are often of interest. Radiographic data are of importance, particularly in the evaluation of a monoclonal protein.

II. **GROSS EXAMINATION AND TISSUE SAMPLING.** The same pathologist should review both the bone marrow aspirate smears and the core biopsies whenever possible to avoid ambiguities or outright contradictions. The bone marrow aspirate is generally performed before the biopsy. There are two kinds of aspirate smears: smears prepared directly from the specimen without pretreatment and smears prepared from concentrated aspirate fluid. Concentrated bone marrow aspirate smears and touch preparations prepared from the bone marrow core biopsy are particularly useful in the evaluation of specimens diluted with peripheral blood. Three to five smears are stained using the Wright–Giemsa or similar technique, one is stained for iron using the Prussian blue technique, and additional unstained smears are reserved for ancillary techniques such as fluorescence in situ hybridization (FISH), if necessary. Although examination of bone marrow cells with enzyme cytochemistry is likely to be rendered obsolete in the coming years, its use is still highly recommended by the World Health Organization (WHO) committee for the diagnosis of acute myeloid leukemia, and high-quality aspirate smears should be reserved for this purpose when an acute myelogenous leukemia is suspected. Additional bone marrow aspirates are obtained for flow cytometric, cytogenetic, and/or molecular genetic studies. Aspirate smears are generally reviewed using high power (600× to 1000×) and are important for evaluating individual cell detail. However, because the process of aspiration disrupts cell cohesion, the relationship of the various cell types and the marrow cellularity cannot be reliably assessed. An adequate bone marrow core biopsy adds this important information.

III. **DIAGNOSTIC FEATURES OF COMMON BENIGN DISEASES.** The number and scope of nonneoplastic bone marrow disorders are vast. Emphasis is given to commonly encountered bone marrow diseases and conditions that may simulate neoplasia.

   A. **Megaloblastic anemia.** It is often not necessary to perform a bone marrow biopsy in patients who present with anemia, because the most common forms of anemia (iron deficiency, megaloblastic, and anemia of chronic disease) may be diagnosed by laboratory analysis of the peripheral blood, clinical history, and response to iron, vitamin B_{12}, and/or folate replacement. Bone marrow biopsy is performed for patients with anemia that is unexplained or therapeutically resistant.

   It is important to note that megaloblastic anemia may simulate a neoplastic condition, particularly a myelodysplastic syndrome. Patients with megaloblastic anemia may present with marked cytopenias and pronounced dyspoiesis (e-Figs. 44.1 and 44.2).* Clues to discriminate this benign condition from a myelodysplastic syndrome include normal blast percentage, absence of karyotypic abnormalities, and improvement of cytopenias following administration of vitamin B_{12}/folate in megaloblastic anemia. Also, the degree of dyspoiesis in megaloblastic anemia often exceeds that encountered in most cases of neoplastic myelodysplasia.

   B. **Benign causes of lymphocytosis.** Numerous benign conditions may cause a transient increase in benign lymphocytes in the peripheral blood and can simulate chronic lymphocytic leukemia/small lymphocytic lymphoma (CLL/SLL), T-cell large granular lymphocytic leukemia, or other lymphoid leukemias. Stress lymphocytosis is a transient increase in morphologically normal peripheral blood lymphocytes encountered in individuals subjected to physiologic stresses, including individuals presenting to hospital emergency departments. An absolute increase in lymphocytes accompanied by "reactive" forms with increased basophilic cytoplasm and inconspicuous nucleoli may be seen in patients infected with Epstein–Barr virus (EBV, e.g., infectious mononucleosis) or, less commonly, cytomegalovirus or other viral pathogens. Interestingly, in cases of EBV infection the virus particles are present in morphologically normal lymphocytes, and the reactive lymphocytes represent cytotoxic T cells directed at the infected cells. Correlation with serum viral antibody titers is useful for arriving at the correct diagnosis and for avoiding unnecessary procedures such as bone marrow and lymph node biopsies. Many other infections are associated with lymphocytosis, including pertussis, in which the lymphocytes have characteristic clefted nuclei and thus may simulate peripheral blood involvement by a non-Hodgkin lymphoma. Persistent polyclonal B-cell hyperplasia, as its name implies, is often of longer duration than other benign forms of lymphocytes. It frequently affects women who smoke, and is associated with the human leukocyte antigen (HLA)-DR7 phenotype.

   C. **The granulocytic "left shift."** Other cases of leukocytosis represent a granulocytic shift to immaturity (colloquially known by the archaic term "left shift" that refers to the traditional placement of immature myeloid cell percentages to the left of neutrophils in classical peripheral blood smear reports). Because many

---

*All e-figures are available online via the Solution Site Image Bank.

of these cases also demonstrate eosinophilia and/or basophilia, it is important to distinguish them from neoplastic conditions, in particular chronic myelogenous leukemia or other myeloproliferative neoplasms. Most commonly, especially in hospitalized populations, a granulocytic shift to immaturity represents an acute response to bacterial or other infections. Transient increases in mature demarginated neutrophils may also follow surgery or other physical trauma. Unusual causes of increased peripheral blood neutrophils with or without immature granulocytes include chronic idiopathic neutrophilia, hereditary neutrophilia, and leukocyte adhesion factor deficiency.

D. **Benign causes of erythrocytosis.** Under normal conditions, the circulating red blood cell mass is maintained at a constant level by the actions of the cytokine erythropoietin, which is produced by renal peritubular cells. An absolute increase in circulating red blood cells (polycythemia) may be primary (most commonly due to the myeloproliferative neoplasm polycythemia vera) or secondary (due to increased production of erythropoietin). Thus, in establishing a diagnosis of polycythemia vera, a number of conditions must be excluded that may cause secondary erythrocytosis, including smoking, living in a high-altitude environment, and high oxygen-affinity hemoglobins.

E. **Benign causes of thrombocytosis.** There are numerous benign causes of thrombocytosis (defined as a peripheral blood platelet count in excess of 450×10^9/L). Common reactive causes of peripheral thrombocytosis include childbirth, major hemorrhage, iron deficiency anemia, chronic inflammatory conditions, infection, and acute stress events.

F. **Aplastic anemia.** Bone marrow aplasia is usually associated with bi- or pancytopenia rather than isolated anemia, and may be identified in a variety of clinical settings. It may occur secondary to a variety of drugs, most commonly chemotherapeutic agents, benzene, alcohol, and arsenic. It may also occur secondary to exposure to radiation, viral infection (e.g., viral hepatitis, EBV), or tuberculosis. An important cause of infection-mediated isolated anemia is infection with parvovirus B19. Other causes of bone marrow hypocellularity include paroxysmal nocturnal hemoglobinuria, Fanconi anemia, dyskeratosis congenital, and other very rare inherited bone marrow failure syndromes (*Int J Hematol.* 2002;76, Suppl 1:207).

The common morphologic finding in bone marrow biopsies from patients with aplastic anemia is marked panhypoplasia; a notable exception is parvovirus infection in which there is selective suppression of erythroid precursors. These specimens should be carefully scrutinized for evidence of significant dyspoiesis or increased blasts because a minority of myelodysplastic syndromes and acute myeloid leukemias present with markedly hypocellular bone marrow biopsies. These specimens should also be examined for evidence of infection as evidenced by granuloma formation in the case of tuberculosis, or intranuclear inclusions in the case of viral infection. The inclusions of parvovirus are ill defined and are localized to the nuclei of proerythroblasts and can be illuminated by immunohistochemistry against viral capsid proteins.

G. **Serous degeneration** (serous atrophy) is a pattern of bone marrow injury most often associated with acquired immunodeficiency syndrome (AIDS) and states of chronic nutritional deficiency such as starvation, chronic alcoholism, and anorexia nervosa (*Arch Pathol Lab Med.* 1992;116:504). The primary morphologic finding in the bone marrow is stromal edema with associated microvesicular change. The bone marrow is hypocellular in these regions due to loss of normal hematopoietic elements. The findings may be focal, alternating with regions of relatively preserved normal hematopoiesis. It is important to recognize that the subcortical bone marrow is normally hypocellular and occasionally demonstrates edema, possibly related to trauma associated with the biopsy procedure, and thus may mimic serous degeneration.

H. Granulomas may be encountered in bone marrow core biopsies and are occasionally noted in aspirate smears. Granulomas may be quite subtle and are usually composed of admixed histiocytes, lymphocytes, and plasma cells. Some granulomas contain foci of necrosis and infiltrating neutrophils. The causes of granuloma formation in the bone marrow are similar to those in other sites; the most common etiologies are infectious, autoimmune, or idiopathic. In addition, granulomas are occasionally encountered in the bone marrow of patients with Hodgkin lymphoma, although their presence is not indicative of marrow involvement by disease. Because it is impossible to predict with certainty the etiology of bone marrow granulomas, their presence usually warrants the use of stains to aid in the identification of acid-fast bacilli or fungi. However, it should be noted that special stains are far less sensitive than microbiologic culture in the detection of most infectious agents in the bone marrow, so microbiologic analysis of fresh bone marrow tissue is recommended when an infectious etiology is considered. An important item in the morphologic differential diagnosis of granulomas is the lipogranuloma, which is generally considered to be nonpathologic and consists of a collection of histiocytes and lymphocytes surrounding an area of fat demonstrating microvesicular change.

I. Benign lymphoid aggregates are present in the bone marrow of healthy individuals and at increased incidence in elderly individuals. Because they are common, it is important to recognize the attributes of benign aggregates and distinguish them from their malignant counterparts. Benign aggregates are often well circumscribed and are small to medium sized. They are composed of an admixture of cell types including small and mature-appearing lymphocytes (typically CD3+ T cells), histiocytes, and granulocytes. They frequently contain a central small-caliber vessel. Although they occasionally abut bony trabeculae, they do not demonstrate the paratrabecular pattern of growth seen in follicular lymphoma and other non-Hodgkin lymphomas involving the marrow. In some cases, immunohistochemistry or in situ hybridization for κ and λ immunoglobulin light chains can be used to further evaluate aggregates.

J. AIDS. Since the first cases of AIDS were reported in 1981, a number of associated diseases have been identified in the bone marrow. Commonly encountered morphologic changes in the bone marrow of human immunodeficiency virus (HIV)-infected individuals include granulomas, lymphoid aggregates, plasma cell aggregates, and dysplasia in one or more hematopoietic lineages (*Haemophilia*. 2001;7:47). Since the development of combined drug therapy, the incidence of secondary infections has decreased. However, infectious agents are still encountered in the bone marrow of individuals infected with HIV and, because impaired inflammatory responses are a hallmark of HIV infection, it is recommended that all bone marrow biopsies from patients with HIV be examined with special stains for fungi and mycobacteria.

Lymphoid aggregates occur with increased frequency in the bone marrow of HIV-infected individuals, are sometimes large with ill-defined borders, and grow along bony trabeculae; these are all features suggestive of malignancy. They may be extremely difficult to evaluate, especially in view of the increased incidence of non-Hodgkin lymphomas in this population. Ancillary studies may be useful in the evaluation of monoclonal B-cell or phenotypically abnormal/monoclonal T-cell populations.

Dyspoiesis is a common finding in the bone marrow of patients with HIV infection and can be seen in other viral infections such as hepatitis C. The significance of this finding may be difficult if not impossible to interpret because of the increased incidence of neoplastic myelodysplasia and acute leukemias in the HIV+ population. Blasts are not typically increased in HIV-associated dysplasia, and clonal cytogenetic abnormalities are not present.

K. **Hemophagocytic syndrome** is a potentially deadly condition in which cytokine-stimulated benign histiocytes phagocytose other hematopoietic cells in an uncontrolled fashion. The most common causes of hemophagocytic syndrome are related to activation of benign macrophages by cytokines produced by malignant cells, and unregulated phagocytosis by macrophages following infection. Malignancy-related hemophagocytic syndrome is most commonly associated with peripheral T-cell lymphoma, although other hematopoietic and lymphoid malignancies are also rarely associated with this complication, including acute myeloid leukemias with the translocation t(16;21)(p11;q22). The most common infectious cause of hemophagocytic syndrome is EBV. Regardless of the underlying cause, hemophagocytic syndrome presents with splenomegaly, fever, and wasting. Pancytopenia, elevated liver function tests, and coagulopathy are variably present. Evaluation of the bone marrow aspirate and core biopsy reveals variable numbers of macrophages containing phagocytosed hematopoietic cells (*Am J Surg Pathol.* 2001;25:865).

L. **Chédiak–Higashi syndrome** is an autosomal recessive inherited disorder that is caused by a mutation in the *CHS1-LYST* gene located at chromosome 1q42. The clinical features of this syndrome are related to abnormal lysosomal trafficking and include recurrent infection, oculocutaneous albinism, neurologic disorders, and a bleeding diathesis. Granulocytes, monocytes, and lymphocytes contain abnormal large granules derived from secondary or cytotoxic granules (**e-Fig. 44.3**) (*Platelets.* 1998;9:21).

M. **Mucopolysaccharidoses.** Alder–Reilly anomaly is identified in the granulocytes of patients with a group of uncommon diseases characterized by X-linked or autosomal recessive transmitted defects in the enzymes involved in mucopolysaccharide metabolism (Table 44.1A) (*Clin Lab Haematol.* 1996;18:39). Granulocytes in the peripheral blood and bone marrow have coarse azurophilic granules superficially resembling normal primary granules. Classification of cases of mucopolysaccharidosis requires chemical and/or molecular analysis.

N. **Lipid storage disorders.** There are numerous genetically mediated conditions related to defects in enzymes comprising the pathway of lipid metabolism (Table 44.1B). The most commonly encountered are Gaucher disease and Niemann–Pick disease. **Gaucher disease** demonstrates an autosomal recessive pattern of inheritance and is caused by a defect in the enzyme β-glucocerebrosidase. Clinically, patients present with bone pain and splenomegaly related to the proliferation of morphologically abnormal histiocytes at these sites. The cytoplasm of the macrophages has a "wrinkled tissue paper" appearance which represents the accumulation of glucocerebroside in these cells (**e-Fig. 44.4**). Occasional cases are associated with B-lineage malignancies (including plasma cell dyscrasias) and light chain amyloidosis (*J Intern Med.* 1999;246:587).

Patients with **Niemann–Pick** disease typically present with organomegaly, neuropathy, and abnormal laboratory findings similar to those identified in Gaucher disease. The pathophysiology of Niemann–Pick disease is related to autosomal recessively inherited defects in the enzyme sphingomyelinase, with the presence of sphingomyelin in affected cells. Macrophages in this disorder have been described as "sea-blue" due to the cytoplasmic accumulation of PAS-positive material representing sphingomyelin (*Ann Hematol.* 2001;80:620).

The remaining lipid storage diseases, which are somewhat less common, have clinical presentations similar to those of Gaucher and Niemann–Pick diseases. Some are associated with additional findings. For example, **Hermansky–Pudlak** syndrome is associated with platelet storage pool deficiencies and oculocutaneous albinism (*Platelets.* 1998;9:21).

IV. **DIAGNOSTIC FEATURES OF MALIGNANCIES**

A. **Myelodysplastic syndromes** are clonal hematopoietic disorders characterized in most cases by peripheral cytopenias (hemoglobin <10 g/dL, absolute neutrophil

TABLE 44.1	Storage Diseases

A. Mucopolysaccharidoses

Disease	Enzyme deficiency
Hurler syndrome (mucopolysaccharidosis type I H)	α-L-iduronidase
Scheie syndrome (mucopolysaccharidosis type I S)	α-L-iduronidase
Hurler–Scheie syndrome (mucopolysaccharidosis type I H-S)	α-L-iduronidase
Hunter syndrome (mucopolysaccharidosis type II)	Iduronidate α-sulfatase
Sanfilippo syndrome type A (mucopolysaccharidosis type III A)	Heparin N-sulfatase
Sanfilippo syndrome type B (mucopolysaccharidosis type III B)	α-N-Acetylglucosaminidase
Sanfilippo syndrome type C (mucopolysaccharidosis type III C)	α-Glucosaminide transferase
Sanfilippo syndrome type D (mucopolysaccharidosis type III D)	N-Acetylglucosamine-6-sulfatase
Morquio syndrome type A (mucopolysaccharidosis type IV A)	N-Acetylgalactosamine, 6-sulfate sulfatase
Morquio syndrome type B (mucopolysaccharidosis type IV B)	β-Galactosidase
Maroteaux–Lamy syndrome (mucopolysaccharidosis type VI)	N-Acetylgalactosamine-4-sulfatase
Sly syndrome (mucopolysaccharidosis type VII)	β-Glucuronidase

B. Lipid storage disorders

Disease	Enzyme deficiency	Substance stored
Gaucher disease	β-Glucocerebrosidase	Glucocerebroside
Niemann–Pick disease	Sphingomyelinase	Sphingomyelin
Gangliosidosis	β-galactosidase	GM$_1$ ganglioside
Tay–Sachs disease	Hexosaminidase A	GM$_2$ ganglioside
Sandhoff disease	Hexosaminidase A	GM$_2$ ganglioside
Fabry disease	α-Galactosidase	Ceramide trihexalose

count [ANC] $<1.8 \times 10^9$/L, and/or platelets $<100 \times 10^9$/L) and increased bone marrow cellularity (*Hematology Am Soc Hematol Educ Program.* 2006;199). The entities comprising this family of diseases are summarized in Table 44.2. Diagnosis is made by assessment of the bone marrow aspirate smear for significant dyspoiesis and correlation with the clinical history, including a failure to respond to iron, vitamin B$_{12}$, and folate replacement. Dyspoiesis is identified in one or more of the hematopoietic lineages. In the myeloid series, this most commonly manifests as abnormal nuclear lobation, including cells with pseudo-Pelger–Huët (hypolobate) nuclei, and cells with decreased cytoplasmic granules. Erythroid precursors demonstrate nuclear irregularities including budding, with occasional ringed sideroblasts (erythroid precursors with multiple punctate iron granules surrounding the nuclei that reflect iron abnormally trapped in mitochondria). Megakaryocytes contain multiple separate nuclei or are small with decreased nuclear lobation (e-**Figs. 44.5 to 44.8**). Importantly, these changes must be present in at least 10% of the cells in a given lineage to morphologically establish this diagnosis.

TABLE 44.2 Myelodysplastic Syndromes

Disease	Blood	Bone marrow	Cytogenetics (percentage of cytogenetically abnormal cases)	Outcome (median survival)
Refractory cytopenia with unilineage dysplasia	Uni- or bicytopenia No/rare blasts	Unilineage dysplasia <5% blasts <15% ringed sideroblasts	<50%	~2% progress to acute leukemia at 5 y
Refractory anemia with ringed sideroblasts	Anemia No blasts	≥15% ringed sideroblasts Erythroid dysplasia <5% blasts	<10%	1–2% progress to acute leukemia (6 y)
Refractory cytopenia with multilineage dysplasia	Bi/pancytopenia No/rare blasts No Auer rods <1 × 10⁹/L monocytes	Dysplasia in ≥10% of cells in 2 or more myeloid cell lines ≥5% blasts <15% ringed sideroblasts No Auer rods	~50%	~11% progress to acute leukemia at 2 y
Refractory cytopenia with multilineage dysplasia and ringed sideroblasts	Bi/pancytopenia No/rare blasts No Auer rods <1 × 10⁹/L monocytes	Dysplasia in ≥10% of cells in 2 or more myeloid cell lines ≥ringed sideroblasts <5% blasts No Auer rods	Unknown; probably similar to refractory cytopenia with multilineage dysplasia	Unknown; probably similar to refractory cytopenia with multilineage dysplasia
Refractory anemia with excess blasts-1 (RAEB-1)	Cytopenias <5% blasts[a] No Auer rods <1 × 10⁹/L monocytes	Uni/multilineage dysplasia 5–9% blasts No Auer rods[b]	~30–50%	~25%
Refractory anemia with excess blasts-2 (RAEB-2)	Cytopenias 5–19% blasts ± Auer rods <1 × 10⁹/L monocytes	Uni/multilineage dysplasia 10–19% blasts ± Auer rods	~30–50%	~33%
Myelodysplastic syndrome – unclassifiable	Cytopenias No/rare blasts No Auer rods	Unilineage dysplasia <5% blasts No Auer rods	Unknown	Unknown
Myelodysplastic syndrome associated with isolated del(5q)	Anemia Normal/increased platelet count <5% blasts	Normal/increased megakaryocytes with hypolobate nuclei <5% blasts Isolated del(5q) cytogenetic abnormality No Auer rods	100% (isolated del(5q) cytogenetic abnormality; cases with additional abnormalities should not be classified under this diagnosis)	Unknown median survival—probably many years

Notable exceptions:

[a] A diagnosis of RAEB-1 can be established if there are 2% to 4% myeloblasts in the peripheral blood with less than 5% blasts in the bone marrow.

[b] Cases with Auer rods and less than 10% bone marrow myeloblasts are designated as RAEB-2.

From: Swerdlow S, Campo E, Harris NL, et al., eds. *WHO Classification of Tumours of Haematopoietic and Lymphoid Tissues.* Lyon: IARC Press; 2008. Used with permission.

Detection of a cytogenetic abnormality is helpful, although the majority of cases of "low-grade" myelodysplasia (refractory cytopenia with unilineage dysplasia [i.e., refractory anemia], refractory anemia with ringed sideroblasts, and refractory cytopenia with multilineage dysplasia) have normal karyotypes. Common cytogenetic abnormalities include partial or complete deletions of chromosomes 5 and 7, del(20q), and/or trisomy of chromosome 8. Abnormalities of chromosome 7 or complex karyotypes (>3 cytogenetic abnormalities) carry a poor prognosis. 5q-syndrome is a special type of myelodysplastic syndrome in which dyspoiesis is most prominent in the megakaryocytic series, accompanied by thrombocytosis; this form of myelodysplasia is associated with long survival.

"High-grade" myelodysplasia (refractory anemia with excess blasts types 1 and 2) presents with a greater percentage of peripheral blood/bone marrow blasts compared to low-grade cases. In general, refractory anemia with excess blasts is more clinically aggressive than that with or without ringed sideroblasts, and has a variable propensity for progression to acute leukemia or bone marrow failure, both of which are essentially untreatable by any means short of a bone marrow transplant. Outcome in the myelodysplastic syndromes may be predicted using the International Prognostic Scoring System (IPSS), which takes into account blast percentage, karyotype, and the presence of cytopenias (*Leukemia.* 2005;19:2223).

B. Myeloproliferative neoplasms. The myeloproliferative neoplasms (formerly chronic myeloproliferative disorders) are characterized by an expansion of one or more of the hematopoietic lineages as evidenced by increased bone marrow cellularity and increased circulating white blood cells (usually granulocytes), erythrocytes, and/or platelets. Initially, blasts are present in normal to slightly increased numbers in the marrow. Although these are malignant disorders, the affected cell line(s) are usually morphologically normal, and pronounced dyspoiesis is not a characteristic feature of the chronic myeloproliferative disorders. In contrast to myelodysplasia, organomegaly (splenomegaly and/or hepatomegaly) is a common feature of this disease, and becomes more pronounced with disease progression as the bone marrow becomes dysfunctional and/or fibrotic.

Particularly in their early stages, it may be difficult to distinguish these diseases from reactive conditions affecting the marrow. Also, because the various myeloproliferative neoplasms have overlapping morphologic features, distinguishing between them may be very difficult. However, it is important to recognize and distinguish between the various members of this family of disorders because the different malignancies have variable propensities for high-grade (i.e., acute leukemic) transformation and bone marrow failure. Accordingly, the identification of disease-specific molecular markers in this family of diseases is the subject of intense scrutiny, and important molecular lesions have been identified. The first, *BCR-ABL,* has been known for many years, and is largely limited to chronic myelogenous leukemia and occasional cases of acute myeloid leukemia, precursor B-lymphoblastic leukemia/lymphoma, and biphenotypic acute leukemia, at least some cases of which likely represent blast phases of clinically silent chronic myelogenous leukemia.

BCR-ABL is most frequently encountered as the classic Philadelphia chromosome, t(9;22)(q34;q11), which juxtaposes the break cluster region gene (*BCR*) at chromosome 22q11 with the Abelson tyrosine kinase gene (*ABL*) at chromosome 9q34. The resultant BCR-ABL fusion protein is a constitutively activated tyrosine kinase directly responsible for the manifestations of disease in chronic myelogenous leukemia. In chronic myelogenous leukemia, BCR-ABL is typically of the 210 kd (p210) form, compared with BCR-ABL in precursor B-lymphoblastic leukemia/lymphoma which is generally 190 kd (p190). The p230 (230 kd) form of BCR-ABL is identified in cases of chronic myelogenous leukemia with a predominance of mature neutrophils rather than immature granulocytes. Previously, cases of chronic myeloproliferative disorders with the p230 form of BCR-ABL and neutrophilia were classified as chronic neutrophilic leukemia, but the WHO classification now recommends that such cases be classified as chronic myelogenous leukemia.

More recently, point mutations have been identified in Philadelphia chromosome–negative myeloproliferative neoplasms, the most prominent of which is the *JAK2* V617F point mutation involving the Janus tyrosine kinase 2 (*Am Soc Hematol Educ Program*. 2006;240). Other mutations have recently been identified in several genes, including myeloproliferative leukemia virus (*MPL*), TET oncogene family member 2 (*TET2*), additional sex combs-like 1 (*ASXL1*), casitas B-lineage lymphoma proto-oncogene (*CBL*), and the lymphocyte adaptor protein *LNK*, although none of these mutations appear to be specific for myeloproliferative neoplasms.

1. **Chronic myelogenous leukemia** is a well-characterized clinicopathologic entity because essentially all cases have the characteristic Philadelphia chromosome t(9;22)(q34;q11) and corresponding rearrangement of *BCR-ABL* (*Br J Haematol*. 1991;79, Suppl 1:34). This is a disorder derived from clonal expansion of an abnormal pluripotential hematopoietic stem cell. Affected individuals typically present with nonspecific constitutional symptoms and on physical examination are frequently found to have an enlarged spleen. Patients most often present in the chronic phase characterized by a peripheral leukocytosis composed of granulocytes (in various stages of maturation) with peripheral and bone marrow basophilia and eosinophilia (e-**Fig. 44.9**). The blast percentage in chronic phase is usually <2% of white blood cells in the peripheral blood and <5% in the bone marrow. Untreated, cases of chronic myelogenous leukemia invariably acquire additional genetic lesions (i.e., additional Ph chromosome, isochromosome 17q, or trisomy 8) resulting in a maturation arrest in the malignant population and terminate in an acute leukemic (blast) phase. The blast phenotype is myeloid in ~80% of cases and lymphoid in most of the remaining cases, and has a biphenotypic or ambiguous phenotype in rare individuals. Chronic myelogenous leukemia in blast phase is essentially untreatable by any means short of a bone marrow transplant. Increasingly, patients presenting with chronic myelogenous leukemia in chronic phase are treated with small molecular inhibitors such as imatinib mesylate, a tyrosine kinase inhibitor with a high degree of specificity for the BCR-ABL–encoded tyrosine kinase. However, an increasing problem is the development of resistance to imatinib mesylate, for which second- and third-generation tyrosine kinase inhibitors have been developed.

2. **Polycythemia vera** is a clonal stem cell disorder in which the majority of disease manifestations are related to expansion of the cells of the erythroid lineage as evidenced by increased hematocrit, blood volume, and blood viscosity (*Blood*. 2002;100:4272). The clinical features of this disease are related to this phenomenon. The skin has a plethoric appearance and there is an increased propensity for vascular thromboses, hemorrhage, and central nervous system phenomena including stroke, tinnitus, headache, and vertigo. The peripheral blood manifestations of disease are related to expansion of red blood cell mass. There is an increased red blood cell count (approximately 7,000,000 to 10,000,000/mm^3) and hemoglobin (usually >18.5 g/dL in men and >16.5 g/dL in women) without a corresponding increased reticulocyte count. Because polycythemia vera is related to expansion of a pluripotential hematopoietic stem cell, other cell lines are variably affected. Thus, some patients have an associated neutrophilic leukocytosis and/or thrombocytosis. Other clinical laboratory features of disease include an increased leukocyte alkaline phosphatase (LAP) score and increased serum vitamin B$_{12}$ levels, the

latter due to an increase in transcobalamin 1. Bone marrow analysis is performed to exclude other forms of myeloproliferative disorder and to assess baseline fibrosis. Usually, initial bone marrow analysis reveals increased bone marrow cellularity with multilineage expansion of hematopoiesis and minimal fibrosis.

In establishing a diagnosis of polycythemia vera, nonneoplastic erythrocytosis and erythrocytosis due to cytokine production by nonhematopoietic malignancies must be excluded. Common causes of secondary erythrocytosis include pathologic conditions (such as chronic pulmonary disease and smoking) and physiologic conditions (such as living in high-altitude locations). A *JAK2* mutation (most commonly V617F but mutations in exon 12 have also been identified) is found in the vast majority of cases and thus is now a major criterion for diagnosis.

In most cases, polycythemia vera is a clinically indolent condition. The treatment of choice for most patients is periodic phlebotomy to minimize the risks associated with increased blood viscosity. Less than 10% of patients develop bone marrow failure or acute leukemia.

3. **Essential thrombocythemia** is a clonal neoplasm derived from a pluripotential hematopoietic stem cell in which the majority of clinical and pathologic features are related to morphologically and physiologically abnormal megakaryocytes and platelets (*Haematologica.* 1999;84:17). There is usually a marked peripheral thrombocytosis, generally in excess of $1,000 \times 10^9$/L, although a sustained count of $>450 \times 10^9$/L is sufficient for diagnosis. The platelets are frequently morphologically abnormal, including forms with decreased granularity. The most prominent characteristic of the bone marrow is marked megakaryocytic hyperplasia. The megakaryocytes are frequently morphologically abnormal, with large overall size and hyperlobate (staghorn) nuclei. A definite diagnosis can be established after other myeloproliferative neoplasms are eliminated from consideration with ancillary studies. *JAK2* V617F mutations are found in ∼50% of cases (both of essential thrombocythemia and primary myelofibrosis). The major pathophysiologic consequences of the thrombocytosis and proliferation of megakaryocytes are episodic bleeding and thrombosis, which are major causes of morbidity and mortality. Less than 1% of cases progress to acute leukemia.

4. **Primary myelofibrosis** (chronic idiopathic myelofibrosis, agnogenic myeloid metaplasia, myelofibrosis with myeloid metaplasia) is another myeloproliferative neoplasm attributed to transformation of a pluripotential hematopoietic stem cell. Classically, there are two phases in the natural history of disease (*Hematol Oncol Clin North Am.* 2003;17:1211). The first phase, referred to as the cellular phase, is characterized by a marked expansion of all hematopoietic lineages; it is followed by the spent phase, characterized by progressive bone marrow failure and fibrosis. Because the cellular phase is often clinically silent, the majority of clinical findings are related to increasing bone marrow fibrosis, and include fatigue (due to anemia), bleeding (due to thrombocytopenia), and infection (due to granulocytopenia). Hepatosplenomegaly due to extramedullary hematopoiesis is a common physical finding.

The cellular phase is often characterized by peripheral granulocytic leukocytosis and/or thrombocytosis. The former is sometimes accompanied by eosinophilia or basophilia clinically mimicking chronic myelogenous leukemia. In the cellular phase, the bone marrow is hypercellular due to a panhyperplasia of all hematopoietic lineages. Megakaryocytes cluster in the bone marrow and are characteristically highly atypical including large forms with bulbous/hyperchromatic nuclei. Fibrosis is minimal at this stage of disease. With time, the bone marrow becomes increasingly fibrotic (which is

TABLE 44.3 WHO Criteria for Systemic Mastocytosis

Major criteria are as follows:

Multifocal infiltrates of mast cells ($\geq$15 mast cells constitute an aggregate) detected in sections of bone marrow and/or other extracutaneous organ(s), and confirmed by tryptase immunohistochemistry or other special stains.

Minor criteria are as follows:

a. In biopsy sections of bone marrow or other extracutaneous organs, >25% of the mast cells in the infiltrate are spindle-shaped or have atypical morphology, or, of all mast cells in the bone marrow aspirate smears, >25% are immature or atypical mast cells.

b. *Kit* point mutation at codon 816 in bone marrow, blood, or other extracutaneous organ(s)

c. Mast cells in bone marrow, blood, or other extracutaneous organs coexpress CD117 with CD2 and/or CD25.

d. Serum total tryptase persistently >20 ng/mL (unless there is an associated clonal myeloid disorder, in which case this parameter is not valid)

Note: The diagnosis of systemic mastocytosis may be made if one major and one minor criterion are present, or if three minor criteria are fulfilled.
From: Swerdlow S, Campo E, Harris NL, et al., eds. *WHO Classification of Tumours of Haematopoietic and Lymphoid Tissues.* Lyon: IARC Press; 2008. Used with permission.

best illustrated by a reticulin stain) and the patient becomes increasingly susceptible to the consequences of decreased peripheral white blood cells, red blood cells, and platelets. Death is most commonly due to infection or hemorrhage. Acute leukemia is an uncommon late sequela, occurring in <10% of individuals.

5. **Systemic mastocytosis.** Mastocytosis, the abnormal accumulation of mast cells in the skin and other tissues, has a wide range of clinical behavior. A benign form of disease is localized to the skin, occurs predominantly in younger individuals, and is characterized by spontaneous regression. In the systemic form of mastocytosis, mast cells are increased in many organs including the bone marrow (e-Figs. 44.10 to 44.12). The WHO criteria for systemic mastocytosis are summarized in Table 44.3. Systemic mastocytosis represents a clonal disorder in most cases: Mutations in the *kit* proto-oncogene (most commonly D816V) have been identified in many individuals, and presumably play a role in the pathophysiology of disease. In cases with associated eosinophilia, the *FIP1L1-PDGFRA* fusion gene has been identified. The same fusion gene has been identified in chronic eosinophilic leukemia/hypereosinophilic syndrome.

The clinical course of systemic mastocytosis is highly variable. Cases with cutaneous involvement (urticaria pigmentosa) are more likely to have a benign disease course, whereas individuals with peripheral blood involvement (mast cell leukemia) frequently die within weeks of diagnosis.

C. **Neoplasms characterized by eosinophilia and abnormalities of the platelet-derived growth factor receptors and fibroblast growth factor 1 receptor.** The WHO 2008 added an additional category of myeloid and lymphoid neoplasms (see Table 44.4) characterized by fusion genes resulting in aberrant signaling of platelet-derived growth factor receptor A (*PDGFRA*), platelet-derived growth factor receptor B (*PDGFRB*), and fibroblast growth factor receptor 1 (*FGFR1*). These cases all present with eosinophilia and thus other causes of eosinophilia should be ruled out, including T-cell non-Hodgkin lymphomas, infection, and drug therapy.

D. **Acute leukemia.** Compared with myelodysplastic and myeloproliferative neoplasms, acute leukemias frequently present with a greater tumor burden

TABLE 44.4 Summary of the WHO Classification of Lymphoid and Myeloid Disorders Associated with Eosinophilia

Disease	Common rearrangement	Clinical	Morphology	Progression to acute leukemia	Prognosis (sensitivity to imatinib)
Myeloid and lymphoid neoplasms with PDGFRA rearrangement	FIP1L1-PDGFRA (due to cryptic deletion at 4q12 which may require RT-PCR or FISH for detection)	M > F; wide age range; fatigue, splenomegaly and sequelae of high peripheral eosinophil count (>1.5 × 10⁹/L) including pruritus and cardiac failure	Eosinophilia with orderly maturation; mast cells are increased in bone marrow; typically mimics chronic eosinophilic leukemia	Uncommon, may be AML or T-LBL	Likely good if there is no organ damage from high eosinophil count (yes)
Myeloid and lymphoid neoplasms with PDGFRB rearrangement	ETV6-PDGFRB [t(5;12)(q31; p12)]; can be detected by conventional cytogenetics; Numerous variants have been reported	M > F, wide age range; splenomegaly and leukocytosis, including monocytes and eosinophils; mimics CMML	Hypercellular bone marrow with granulocytic predominance, including eosinophils, neutrophilic precursors and monocytes	Rare, typically myeloid	Likely good if there is no organ damage from high eosinophil count (yes)
Myeloid and lymphoid neoplasms with FGFR1 abnormalities (also known as 8p11 syndrome)	ZNF198-FGFR1 [t(8;13)(p11:q12) most common; numerous variants identified	M > F, median age ~30; variable clinical presentation; extensive extramedullary disease may be present	Varied, ranging from eosinophilia to T-lymphoblastic lymphoma	AML, T-LBL, B-ALL, mixed phenotype acute leukemia have all been reported	Poor (no)

Modified from: Swerdlow S, Campo E, Harris NL, et al., eds. *WHO Classification of Tumours of Haematopoietic and Lymphoid Tissues.* Lyon: IARC Press; 2008. Used with permission.

(i.e., with blast percentages of at least 20%) and are broadly categorized as myeloid or lymphoid according to their immunologic and enzyme cytochemical properties, the characteristic features of which are summarized in Tables 44.5 and 44.6. There are two important exceptions to the requirement of at least 20% blasts in acute myeloid leukemia. In the WHO classification, the presence of t(8;21)(q22;q22) [*AML1-ETO*], inv(16)(p13;q22)/t(16;16)(p13;q22) [*CBFβ-MYH11*], and t(15;17)(q22;q12) [*PML-RARα*] is classified as acute myeloid leukemia regardless of the percentage of blasts (e-**Figs. 44.13 to 44.17**). The second exception involves acute erythroid leukemia, for which blasts comprise at least 20% of the nonerythroid cell population, rather than at least 20% of all cells; because another requirement for acute erythroid leukemia is that at least 50% of all cells are erythroid precursors, cases with very high erythroid percentages may qualify as acute leukemia even in the presence of a very modest blast percentage. Immunophenotypic analysis of acute leukemia is discussed in Chapter 43.

Acute leukemias, particularly in children and the elderly, may present with isolated anemia and a lack of circulating blasts. Diagnosis requires detection of at least 20% blasts in the bone marrow and/or the presence of an acute myeloid leukemia–specific cytogenetic abnormality. Although replacement of the bone marrow by fibrosis, carcinoma, sarcoma, or other nonhematopoietic cell may result in anemia, it is generally accompanied by leukopenia and/or thrombocytopenia reflecting indiscriminate displacement of normal marrow constituents.

1. **B-lymphoblastic leukemia** is arbitrarily separated from its tissue analogue, lymphoblastic lymphoma, by the presence of a tissue mass and ≤20% bone marrow blasts in the latter (e-**Fig. 44.18**) and is no longer subdivided on the basis of immunophenotype since genetic features are more predictive of outcome. B-lymphoblastic leukemia is most common in children <6 years old; patients with purely lymphomatous disease are somewhat younger on average. Most cases express HLA-DR, terminal deoxynucleotidyl transferase (TdT), CD10, CD19, CD24, and cytoplasmic CD79a. CD10-negative cases often demonstrate rearrangements of the mixed-lineage leukemia (*MLL*) gene and coexpress one or more myeloid-associated antigens. In the pediatric population, cytogenetic and molecular genetic findings are highly predictive of disease outcome. Predictors of good outcome include the following: age 4 to 10 years at diagnosis, hyperdiploidy (51 to 65 chromosomes) in the blast population, and presence of translocation t(12;21)(p13;q22) [*TEL-AML1*]. Predictors of poor outcome include the following: age <4 years or >10 years, hypodiploidy, t(9;22)(q34;q11.2) [*BCR-ABL*], t(4;11)(q21;q23) [*AF4-MLL*], and t(1;19)(q23;q13.3) [*PBX-E2A*]. The prognostic significance of t(1;19) is controversial. Recently, mutations/deletions in the lymphoid transcription factor gene *IKZF1* (IKAROS) have been shown to be associated with a high rate of leukemic relapse and a poor outcome. Mutations in *PAX5* are also common.

   A special category of lymphoblastic leukemia is the **leukemic analogue of Burkitt lymphoma.** Patients with this disease commonly present with an abdominal mass (Western Europe and North America) or a jaw lesion (Africa). The bone marrow is commonly involved, and the blasts have deeply basophilic cytoplasm with many lipid vacuoles, express CD10 and monoclonal surface immunoglobulin light chain, and are generally CD34 and TdT negative (e-**Fig. 44.19**). Diagnosis requires demonstration of the translocation t(8;14)(q24;q32) [*MYC-IGH*] or, less commonly, the variant translocations t(2;8)(q11;q24) or t(8;22)(q24;q11) involving *MYC* and the κ and λ light chain genes, respectively.

TABLE 44.5   WHO Classification of Acute Myeloid Leukemias

Disease	Clinical	Morphology	Immunophenotype	Prognosis
A. Acute myeloid leukemia with recurrent genetic abnormalities				
Acute myeloid leukemia with t(8;21)(q22;q22); (RUNX1-RUNX1T1)	Often presents with extramedullary disease	Blasts with long slender Auer rods, abnormal granulation	CD13+, CD33+, MPO+, CD19+, CD34+, CD56+	Favorable
Acute myeloid leukemia with abnormal bone marrow eosinophils inv(16)(p13q22) or t(16;16)(p13;q22) (CBFβ/MYH11)	Occasionally presents with extramedullary disease	Abnormal eosinophils with large basophilic granules, decreased lobation	CD13+, CD33+, MPO+; frequently CD4+, CD14+, CD11b+, CD11c+, CD64+, CD36+, lysozyme+	Favorable
Acute promyelocytic leukemia (AML with t(15;17)(q22;q12); (PML/RARα and variants)	Coagulopathy, normal/low WBC (hypergranular variant); high WBC (hypogranular variant)	Abnormal promyelocytes with multiple Auer rods predominate	CD13+ (heterogeneous), CD33+ (bright), HLA-DR–, CD34–	Favorable
Acute myeloid leukemia with t(9;11)	Frequently occurs in children	Monocytic blasts predominate	Variable CD13 and CD33+, CD4+, CD14+, CD11b+, CD11c+, CD64+, CD36+, lysozyme+	Intermediate survival
Acute myeloid leukemia with t(6;9)(p23;q34); DEK-NUP214	Pancytopenia	Basophilia with multilineage dysplasia	CD13+, CD33+, myeloperoxidase+, HLA-DR+, CD34+, CD117+, TdT±	Poor
Acute myeloid leukemia with inv(3)(q21;q26.2) or t(3;3) (q21; q26.2); RPN1-EVI1	Normal/elevated platelet count	Multilineage dysplasia including marked dysmegakaryopoiesis	CD13+, CD33+, HLA-DR+, CD34+, CD117+, CD41/ CD61 ±	Poor
Acute myeloid leukemia with t(1;22)(p13;q13); RBM15-MLK1	Infants and young children; hepatosplenomegaly is common	Megakaryoblastic	CD41/CD61+, CD13+, CD33+. CD34–, HLA-DR–	Typically poor

B. Acute myeloid leukemia with multilineage dysplasia

1. Following myelodysplastic syndrome (MDS) or myelodysplastic/myeloproliferative disorder
2. MDS-related cytogenetic abnormality
3. Multilineage dysplasia (dysplasia in at least 50% of the cells in two cell lineages)

C. Acute myeloid leukemia and myelodysplastic syndromes, therapy-related

- Alkylating agent–related; typically has a 5–10-year latency with t-MDS stage
- Topoisomerase type II inhibitor–related (some may be lymphoid); 1–5-year latency with no t-MDS phase, commonly has balanced translocations including 11q23 abnormalities
- Other types

D. Acute myeloid leukemia not otherwise categorized

Acute myeloid leukemia minimally differentiated	Usually presents in adulthood, cytopenias	<3% of blasts MPO+, <3% of blasts NBE+	Often CD13+, CD33+, CD117+, CD34+, CD38+, HLA-DR+	Unfavorable
Acute myeloid leukemia without maturation	Usually presents in adulthood, cytopenias, occasionally with markedly increased WBC	Blasts comprise ≥90% of nonerythroid cells; ≥3% of blasts MPO+, <3% of blasts NBE+	Often CD13+, CD33+, CD34+, CD117+, MPO+	Unfavorable
Acute myeloid leukemia with maturation	Variable age range and symptomatology	≥3% of blasts MPO+, ≤3% of blasts NBE+; > 10% maturing granulocytic cells	Usually CD13+, CD33+, CD15+; variable CD117+, CD34+, HLA-DR+	Variable
Acute myelomonocytic leukemia	Anemia, fever, fatigue; WBC usually elevated	>20% blasts (including promonocytes); ≥20% monocytes and precursors; and ≥20% neutrophils and precursors; ≥3% of blasts MPO+, ≥3% of blasts usually NBE+[a]	Usually CD13+, CD33+; Often CD4+, CD14+, CD11b+, CD11c+, CD64+, CD36+, lysozyme+	Variable
Acute monoblastic leukemia	Most common in children, often presents with extramedullary disease, bleeding disorders	≥80% monocytic cells, of which ≥80% are monoblasts; <20% neutrophils and precursors; <3% of blasts MPO+, ≥3% of blasts NBE+	Variable CD13+, CD33+, CD117+; Often CD14+, CD4+, CD11b+, CD11c+, CD64+, CD68+, CD36+, lysozyme+	Unfavorable
Acute monocytic leukemia	Most common in adults, often presents with extramedullary disease, bleeding disorders	≥80% monocytic cells, of which the majority are promonocytes; <20% neutrophils and precursors; <3% of blasts MPO+, ≥3% of blasts NBE+	Variable CD13+, CD33+, CD117+; Often CD14+, CD4+, CD11b+, CD11c+, CD64+, CD68+, CD36+, lysozyme+	Unfavorable

(continued)

TABLE 44.5 WHO Classification of Acute Myeloid Leukemias (*Continued*)

Acute erythroid leukemia (erythroid/myeloid)	Adults; anemia	≥50% of entire nucleated population is erythroid and ≥20% myeloblasts in nonerythroid population; >3% of blasts may be MPO+	Erythroblasts are glycophorin A+ and hemoglobin A+; myeloblasts are CD13+, CD33+, CD117+, and MPO+	Unfavorable
Pure erythroid leukemia	Extremely rare	>80% of cells are immature erythroid cells; no significant myeloblast component; <3% of blasts MPO+, ≥3% of blasts NBE+	Blasts are sometimes glycophorin A+ and hemoglobin A+;	Unfavorable
Acute megakaryoblastic leukemia	Cytopenias	Dysplastic megakaryocytes, Blasts often have cytoplasmic pseudopods. Abnormal platelets and megakaryocyte fragments in peripheral blood; usually <3% of blasts MPO+ and >3% of blasts NBE+	Usually CD41+, CD61+; occasionally CD13+, CD33+; CD34–, CD45–, HLA-DR–	Poor
Acute basophilic leukemia	Very rare	Blasts are toluidine blue+; usually <3% of blasts MPO+, <3% of blasts NBE+	Usually CD13+, CD33+, CD34+, HLA-DR+, CD9+	Difficult to predict due to low number of reported cases, probably poor
Acute panmyelosis with myelofibrosis	Very rare, adults, pancytopenia with no/minimal splenomegaly	Panhyperplasia, dysplastic megakaryocytes; increased reticulin fibrosis	CD13+, CD33+, CD117+, MPO+; some cases express erythroid or megakaryocytic antigens	Poor

MPO, myeloperoxidase; WBC, white blood count; NBE, naphthyl butyrate esterase; HLA, human leukocyte antigen.
[a]The World Health Organization allows the diagnosis of acute myelomonocytic leukemia in the absence of NBE reactivity if the "cells meet morphologic criteria for monocytes."
From: Swerdlow S, Campo E, Harris NL, et al., eds. *WHO Classification of Tumours of Haematopoietic and Lymphoid Tissues*. Lyon: IARC Press; 2008. Used with permission.

TABLE 44.6 Common Mutations in Acute Myeloid Leukemia[a]

Mutation	Frequency	Clinical	Cytogenetics	Outcome
NPM1 (Nucleophosmin)[b]	25–35%	Typically de novo disease; high WBC and myelomonocytic morphology common; blasts typically CD34−	Frequently normal	Favorable
CEBPA (CCAAT/enhancer binding protein-alpha)[b]	5–10%	High PB blast count; typically AML with/without maturation	Frequently normal	Favorable
FLT3-ITD (FMS-like tyrosine kinase-internal tandem duplication	20–30%	High WBC; varied morphology (including acute promyelocytic leukemia)	Varied	Poor
IDH1/IDH2 (isocitrate dehydrogenase 1 and 2)[c]	IDH1: ~7%; IDH2: ~8%	Typically AML with/without maturation; uncommon in monocytic leukemias	Typically normal (frequently occurs with other mutations with exception TET2)	TBD
DNMT3a (DNA methyltransferase 3a)	20–25%	Common in myelomonocytic/monocytic leukemias	Normal cytogenetics (exclusive of good risk recurrent genetic abnormality AMLs)	Poor
TET2 (TET oncogene family member 2)	~7%	No distinct clinical presentation	Typically normal (frequently occurs with other mutations with exception IDH mutations)	TBD

[a]Other mutations identified in AML include c-KIT, N-RAS, K-RAS, WT1, RUNX1 and partial tandem duplication of MLL; these mutations are not specific for AML and their prognostic significance has yet to be determined in a large cohort of AML patients.
[b]Acute myeloid leukemia with mutated NPM1 and CEBPA are provisional entities in WHO (2008).
[c]IDH1, IDH2, DNMT3a and TET2 mutations have also been identified in other myeloid malignancies.
Adapted from JCO. 2011;29:475–486; Blood. 2011;118:5593–5603.

2. **T-lymphoblastic leukemia/lymphoma** is less common and involves an older demographic than its B-cell counterpart. Patients typically present with abundant blasts in the peripheral blood and a mediastinal mass. The blasts are generally TdT positive and demonstrate variable expression of other T-lineage antigens, most commonly CD3 and CD7. Genetic aberrations identified in this entity include translocations between $TCR\beta$ and $TCR\delta$ genes and a variety of partners; microdeletions of $TAL1$; activating mutations in $NOTCH$; and del(9q), which results in deletion of the tumor suppressor gene $CDKN2A$. Although T-lymphoblastic malignancies have historically had a poor prognosis, recent innovations in treatment have improved outcome.

E. **CLL/SLL and related disorders.** In patients (particularly elderly individuals) with unexplained lymphocytosis, an absolute increase in lymphocytes may represent peripheral blood involvement by low-grade non-Hodgkin lymphoma or leukemia such as CLL/SLL (Table 44.7). For most non-Hodgkin lymphomas, diagnosis is made following biopsy of an involved lymph node or extramedullary focus of disease, and bone marrow biopsy is performed for staging rather than precise classification. An exception to this is CLL/SLL, in which primary diagnosis is often made following flow cytometric analysis of the peripheral blood and demonstration of the characteristic immunophenotype (CD5+, CD10−, CD19 bright+, CD20 heterogeneously+, CD23+, FMC7−, and CD79b−).

Various non-Hodgkin lymphomas have different patterns of marrow involvement. Because B-cell lymphomas are more common than T-cell tumors, the former are better characterized. For example, follicular lymphoma and mantle cell lymphoma have a paratrabecular pattern of marrow involvement, whereas CLL/SLL is never paratrabecular (e-**Fig. 44.20**). In the case of CLL/SLL, the pattern of involvement of the marrow may be predictive of prognosis: cases with predominantly focal lesions are more indolent, whereas examples with a diffuse pattern of involvement are more aggressive. As in lymph nodes, the bone marrow infiltrate of CLL/SLL may contain proliferation (or growth) centers that represent aggregates of prolymphocytes (paraimmunoblasts) and presumably represent the proliferative component of the tumor mass (e-**Figs. 44.21 and 44.22**). Marginal zone lymphomas may demonstrate follicular colonization when they occur in bone marrows with lymphoid aggregates. Overall, the likelihood of marrow involvement by non-Hodgkin lymphoma is highly variable depending on type, ranging from very common (e.g., CLL/SLL) to rare (e.g., extranodal marginal zone lymphoma). Immunohistochemistry is typically not required in non-Hodgkin lymphoma staging biopsies, although it is occasionally helpful in delineating benign from malignant lymphoid aggregates.

F. **Hairy cell leukemia** is a rare form of chronic leukemia. Most commonly, the affected individual is a middle-aged man presenting with pancytopenia, including lymphopenia and monocytopenia, and an enlarged spleen. Occasionally, patients present with a leukemic blood picture mimicking CLL. The bone marrow is virtually always involved. Although identified in bone marrow aspirate preparations, hairy cells are more easily identified in the peripheral blood by the presence of cytoplasmic projections (hence the name "hairy cell leukemia," e-**Fig. 44.23**). The malignant cells frequently have an interstitial pattern of involvement of the bone marrow and for this reason are occasionally overlooked. Sometimes the pattern of marrow involvement recapitulates the pattern of splenic involvement by this malignancy with collections of extravasated red blood cells surrounded by ill-defined collections of hairy cells (e-**Figs. 44.24 and 44.25**). The malignant cells are positive with tartrate-resistant acid phosphatase (TRAP) enzyme cytochemistry. Flow cytometry identifies a characteristic pattern of reactivity: the hairy cells are CD5, CD10, and CD23 negative, but positive for the pan B-cell antigens CD19 and CD20. In addition, they typically demonstrate bright coexpression of CD11c and CD25, and are also positive for

TABLE 44.7 B-Lineage Lymphoid Leukemias and Lymphomas Involving the Bone Marrow

Disease	Phenotype	Morphology	Cytogenetics (significance)	Molecular genetics (impact on outcome)
Chronic lymphocytic leukemia/small lymphocytic lymphoma	CD5+, CD10−, CD19+ (bright), CD20+ (dim), CD23+, FMC7−, CD79b−, sIg light chain+ (dim) CD38± (unfavorable if +), Zap70± (unfavorable if +)	Usually small mature-appearing lymphocytes; diffuse, interstitial, or nodular patterns of marrow involvement (never paratrabecular)	13q14 deletions (favorable outcome), +12 (morphologically atypical, unfavorable outcome), 17p (*TP53*) deletions (unfavorable)	Presence of Ig heavy chain variable region mutation (favorable)
Mantle cell lymphoma	CD5+, CD10−, CD19+, CD20+ (bright), CD23−, FMC7+, CD79b+, sIg light chain+ (usually bright), cyclin D1+	Usually small lymphocytes with clefted/folded nuclei; diffuse, nodular, interstitial, or paratrabecular patterns of marrow involvement	t(11;14) [*BCL1-IGH*]	—
Follicular lymphoma	CD5−, CD10+, CD19+, CD20+, CD23−, sIg light chain+	Variable cytomorphology; diffuse, nodular, interstitial, or paratrabecular patterns of marrow involvement	t(14;18) [*BCL2-IGH*]	—
Marginal zone B-cell lymphoma	CD5−, CD10−, CD19+, CD20+, CD23−, sIg light chain+	Small lymphocytes, some with ample cytoplasm	t(11;18)(q21;q21) [*API2-MALT1*] identified in a subset of extranodal marginal zone lymphoma	—
Lymphoplasmacytic lymphoma/Waldenström macroglobulinemia	CD5−, CD10−, CD19+, CD20+, CD23−, sIg light chain+	Small lymphocytes, some with plasmacytoid features	t(9;14)(q13;q32) [*PAX5-IGH*] identified in ~50% of cases but is not limited to this type of lymphoma	—

sIg, surface immunoglobulin; Ig, immunoglobulin.
From: Swerdlow S, Campo E, Harris NL, et al., eds. *WHO Classification of Tumours of Haematopoietic and Lymphoid Tissues.* Lyon: IARC Press; 2008. Used with permission.

CD103 and FMC7 (*Semin Oncol*. 1998;25:6). Identification of this pattern of reactivity in the presence of appropriate cytomorphology essentially excludes other types of B-cell neoplasia, such as splenic marginal zone lymphoma and prolymphocytic lymphoma. Although hairy cell leukemia is largely resistant to conventional chemotherapies, it is sensitive to purine analogs (i.e., cladribine) and is associated with a prolonged median survival.

SUGGESTED READINGS

Foucar K. *Bone Marrow Pathology*. Chicago, IL: ASCP Press; 2001.

Jaffee ES, Harris NL, Stein H, et al. *World Health Organization Classification of Tumors. Pathology and Genetics of Tumors of Haematopoietic and Lymphoid Tissues*. Lyon, France: IARC Press; 2008.

Knowles DM, ed. *Neoplastic Hematopathology*, 2nd ed. Philadelphia, PA: Lippincott Williams & Wilkins; 2001.

45 Spleen

Mohammad O. Hussaini and Anjum Hassan

I. **NORMAL GROSS AND MICROSCOPIC ANATOMY.** The spleen is the largest lymphatic organ. In a normal adult, it weighs 50 to 250 g. Anatomically, the spleen is divided into white and red pulp, separated by an ill-defined interface known as the marginal zone (e-**Fig. 45.1A**).* For a schematic of splenic architecture, see Figure 45.1.

A. **White pulp.** The white pulp consists of periarteriolar lymphoid sheets (PALS), which contains lymphoid follicles. T lymphocytes are predominately located in periarteriolar lymphoid nodules and B lymphocytes are predominately located in the lymphoid follicles. The latter may contain germinal centers that become visible to the naked eye when enlarged, forming splenic nodules (malpighian corpuscles). In routine hematoxylin and eosin (H&E)-stained sections, the white pulp appears basophilic due to the dense heterochromatin in lymphocyte nuclei (e-**Fig. 45.1B**).

B. **Red pulp.** The red pulp has a red appearance in fresh specimens and in histologic sections because it contains a large number of red blood cells (e-**Fig. 45.1B**). It consists of splenic sinuses separated by splenic cords (the cords of Billroth), which are composed of a loose network of reticular cells and fibers with a large number of erythrocytes, macrophages, lymphocytes, plasma cells, and granulocytes. Special endothelial cells that express both endothelial and histiocytic markers (known as Littoral cells) line the sinuses. The sinusoidal lining epithelium is discontinuous, allowing for transport of blood cells between the splenic cords and sinuses.

II. **GROSS EXAMINATION AND TISSUE SAMPLING**

A. **Biopsy and fine needle aspiration cytology.** These procedures are rarely attempted because of the risk of hemorrhage and the likelihood of undersampling. However, some studies suggest increased chances of a definitive diagnosis when fine needle biopsy is combined with flow cytometry, with an overall accuracy of 91% and a major complication rate of <1% (*Am J Hematol.* 2001;67:93).

B. **Splenectomy.** Trauma, staging procedures, and surgical convenience account for >50% of all splenectomies. Therapeutic splenectomy for known diagnoses (idiopathic thrombocytopenic purpura [ITP], chronic myeloproliferative disorders, lymphomas, etc.) accounts for most of the remaining cases (*Cancer.* 2001;91:2001). Unexpected pathology is rarely found in splenectomy specimens, but significant splenomegaly (weight >300 g) or localizing lesions warrant careful prosection and ancillary studies.

C. **Processing.** The spleen is weighed, and its outer dimensions are recorded. Hilar fatty tissue is removed and processed for lymph nodes. The capsule should be described, noting texture and intactness. The spleen should be thinly sliced (every 2 to 3 mm); lesional distribution should be noted, followed by a description of the uninvolved spleen. Sections of any lesions (preferably following overnight formalin fixation of thin slices) and two representative sections of uninvolved spleen should be submitted for microscopic examination.

If clinically indicated, fresh lesional tissue in 1 mm pieces should be placed in RPMI medium and directed immediately to the flow cytometry lab with instructions regarding the appropriate protocol. Cytogenetic studies may be

---

*All e-figures are available online via the Solution Site Image Bank.

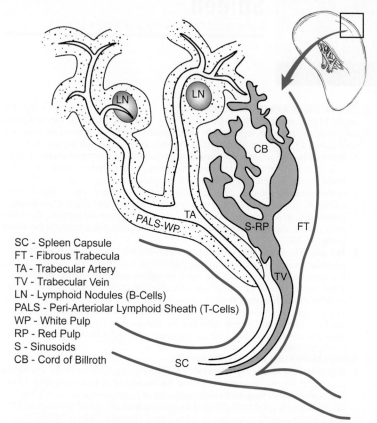

SC - Spleen Capsule
FT - Fibrous Trabecula
TA - Trabecular Artery
TV - Trabecular Vein
LN - Lymphoid Nodules (B-Cells)
PALS - Peri-Arteriolar Lymphoid Sheath (T-Cells)
WP - White Pulp
RP - Red Pulp
S - Sinusoids
CB - Cord of Billroth

Figure 45.1 Diagram of the spleen showing important anatomic landmarks and B- and T-cell distribution.

useful, especially for diagnosis of hematologic malignancies; using sterile technique, lesional material should be procured immediately after removal of the spleen in the operating room and directed to the cytogenetics lab. Samples can also be frozen, or fixed for electron microscopy. Freezing preserves many of the antigens for immunohistochemical evaluation in hematopoietic malignancies and enhances nucleic acid recovery for DNA- and RNA-based molecular diagnostic techniques (although most diagnostic molecular tests can be reliably performed on formalin fixed, paraffin embedded material).

III. GENERAL CONSIDERATIONS

A. Splenomegaly. Often the spleen becomes enlarged due to infectious causes or congestive states. Red pulp congestion is frequently observed and is the most common finding in such cases (Table 45.1).

B. Hypersplenism. Hypersplenism refers to destruction of one or more blood cell lines by the spleen (*Eur J Gastroenterol Hepatol.* 2001;13:317). It is the most important indication for elective splenectomy. Diagnostic criteria for hypersplenism include cytopenia of one or more blood cell lines, bone marrow

TABLE 45.1	Conditions Associated with Splenomegaly

I. Infection
  A. Infectious endocarditis
  B. Infectious mononucleosis
  C. Tuberculosis
  D. Histoplasmosis
  E. Syphilis
  F. Parasitic infections (e.g., malaria)
  G. Cytomegalovirus
II. Congestive states
  A. Cirrhosis
  B. Splenic vein thrombosis
  C. Heart failure
III. Hematologic malignancy
  A. Non-Hodgkin lymphoma
  B. Hodgkin lymphoma
  C. Myeloproliferative disorders
  D. Multiple myeloma
IV. Immune-related conditions
  A. Rheumatoid arthritis
  B. Systemic lupus erythematous
  C. Storage disorders (e.g., Gaucher disease)

Adapted from *Pathologic Basis of Disease,* 8th ed. Philadelphia, PA: W.B. Saunders; 2009.

hyperplasia, splenomegaly, and correction of cytopenia(s) following splenectomy. Of the many possible etiologies (see Table 45.2), congenital disorders such as hereditary spherocytosis (**e-Fig. 45.2**), infiltrative disorders such as leukemias and lymphomas (**e-Fig. 45.3**), and autoimmune disorders are the most common.

C. Hyposplenism. Hyposplenism refers to any deficiency or absence of a functioning spleen and is usually due to splenectomy. Splenic function is usually assessed by radiologic imaging or morphologic techniques. Peripheral blood smear examination may also be informative; findings suggesting hyposplenism can

TABLE 45.2	Disorders Associated with Hypersplenism

I. Abnormal sequestration of intrinsically defective blood cells in a normal spleen
  A. Congenital disorders of erythrocytes (hereditary spherocytosis, elliptocytosis; hemoglobinopathies, e.g., sickle cell disease, unstable hemoglobins)
  B. Acquired disorders of erythrocytes (autoimmune hemolytic anemias, malaria, babesiosis)
  C. Autoimmune thrombocytopenia and/or neutropenia
II. Abnormal spleen causing sequestration of normal blood cells
  A. Disorders of the monocyte/macrophage system (chronic congestion, storage diseases, parasitic infections, LCH, etc.)
  B. Malignant Infiltrative disorders (leukemias, lymphomas, plasma cell dyscrasias, metastatic carcinoma)
  C. Extramedullary hematopoiesis (severe hemolytic states, chronic idiopathic myelofibrosis)
  D. Chronic infections, for example, tuberculosis, brucellosis
  E. Vascular/stromal abnormalities (vascular tumors, peliosis, splenic cysts, hamartomas)
III. Miscellaneous conditions
  A. Hyperthyroidism
  B. Hypogammaglobulinemia
  C. Progressive multifocal leukoencephalopathy

TABLE 45.3	Disorders Associated with Hyposplenism

I. Congenital
  A. Asplenia
  B. Hypoplasia
  C. Immunodeficiency disorders
II. Acquired
  A. Splenectomy
  B. Acquired atrophy and/or infarction
    1. Sickle cell disease
    2. Vascular disorders (vasculitides, thromboembolic conditions)
    3. Essential thrombocythemia
    4. Malabsorption syndromes
    5. Autoimmune diseases
    6. Irradiation
    7. Cytotoxic chemotherapy
    8. Chronic alcoholism
    9. Hypopituitarism
  C. Functional asplenia with normal-sized or enlarged spleen
    1. Infiltration by leukemia, lymphoma, multiple myeloma, mastocytosis
    2. Early (splenomegalic) sickle cell disease
    3. Amyloidosis
    4. Sarcoidosis
    5. Benign and malignant vascular tumors
    6. Malabsorption syndromes
  D. Depressed immune function
    1. AIDS
    2. Status post
      a. Irradiation
      b. Cytotoxic chemotherapy
      c. Immunosuppressive agents, including corticosteroids
    3. Endocrine disorders
      a. Hypothyroidism
      b. Hypopituitarism
      c. Diabetes mellitus
    4. Chronic alcoholism

occur in any blood cell line, including erythrocytes (Howell–Jolly bodies [e-Fig. 45.4], poikilocytosis with target cells, acanthocytes, and nucleated red blood cells), platelets (thrombocytosis), and white blood cells (e.g., lymphocytosis, monocytosis, and eosinophilia). Other causes of hyposplenism include congenital hypoplasia (e.g., Fanconi anemia and sickle cell disease; e-Fig. 45.5), infiltrative disorders, old age, and many others (see Table 45.3).

  D. Accessory spleen. Alternatively termed "spleniculi," these are most commonly located in the splenic hilum, tail of the pancreas, and the gastrohepatic ligament (*N Engl J Med.* 1981;304:11). They are found in up to one-third of autopsy cases and share the same histologic and pathologic features as native spleen (see e-Fig. 45.6). Accessory spleens are clinically significant in patients requiring splenectomy for hypersplenism.

  E. Splenosis. Splenosis refers to splenic implants or regrowth of splenic tissue after trauma or surgical splenectomy. When associated with trauma, the most common location is in the abdominal cavity, but splenosis has been reported at virtually all anatomic sites, including the brain (*Am J Surg Pathol.* 1998;22:894).

Usually benign incidental findings, their clinical importance lies in their potential to mimic neoplastic and nonneoplastic splenic lesions.

IV. **REACTIVE SPLENIC DISORDERS.** These can be divided into diffuse and localized processes. Diffuse disease entities include reactive lymphoid hyperplasia (e-**Fig. 45.7A**), follicular hyperplasia, and disorders such as Castleman disease (see Chap. 43). Localized disease includes granulomatous disorders and infectious processes similar to those in other locations (see Chap. 43).

A. **Diffuse reactive processes.** Reactive lymphoid hyperplasia in the spleen may occur with or without germinal center formation. Because of the reactive nature of the latter, and its histologic lack of maturing germinal centers, this entity is variably referred to as "activated A," "early activated immune reaction," "reactive nonfollicular hyperplasia," and even "immunoblastic hyperplasia" (*Am J Surg Pathol.* 1981;5:551). Nongerminal center hyperplasia is often associated with viral infections, especially herpes simplex virus and Epstein–Barr virus (e-**Fig. 45.7B**), which explains the common occurrence of splenomegaly in patients with infectious mononucleosis.

Reactive lymphoid hyperplasia with germinal center formation (e-**Fig. 45.7C**) is commonly referred to as "follicular" hyperplasia. It is the most common pattern of lymphoid hyperplasia in the spleen and is seen in both acute and chronic immune reactions. Follicular hyperplasia is frequently observed in bacterial infection, often as an incidental finding. In fact, splenomegaly is characteristic in subacute bacterial endocarditis, alerting the clinician to this process in the appropriate clinical context.

B. **Focal reactive processes.** Localized reactive splenic processes can also present with splenomegaly.

1. **Granulomas.** The most common form of a focal benign process is granulomatous inflammation, ranging from lipogranulomatous inflammation (of unknown etiology) to caseating or noncaseating granulomatous inflammation. Caseating granulomas are primarily due to infectious disease, including tuberculosis and fungal infection; however, they are also seen in X-linked chronic granulomatous disease. Noncaseating granulomatous disease is most frequently associated with sarcoidosis (e-**Fig. 45.8**). For most granulomas in the spleen, no known etiology can be found (*Arch Pathol Lab Med.* 1974;98:261).

2. **Infarcts.** The spleen is a frequent site of systemic emboli, which commonly arise from cardiac valve lesions or mural thrombi. Infarcts are usually wedge-shaped with a hemorrhagic to pale-tan to fibrotic appearance depending on the age of lesion (see e-**Fig. 45.9**). Non-wedge-shaped infarcts arise in a variety of intrinsic hematopoietic and nonhematopoietic processes. Essential thrombocythemia and chronic idiopathic myelofibrosis are the hematopoietic disorders most frequently associated with infarcts; less common causes include paroxysmal nocturnal hemoglobinuria, sickle cell disease, and aplastic anemia. Among nonhematopoietic etiologies, vasculitides (e.g., polyarteritis nodosa, infections, and TTP/ITP associated) and splenic artery aneurysms are common culprits.

V. **NEOPLASTIC DISORDERS OF THE SPLEEN**

A. **Lymphoid neoplasms.** Lymphoid neoplasms can involve the spleen as primary disease or as a part of a generalized lymphomatous process. Splenomegaly is a nonspecific but classic component of many hematolymphoid disorders. A brief approach to the evaluation of the normal and neoplastic components of the spleen is presented in Table 45.4.

1. **Primary splenic lymphomas.** These account for <1% of all lymphomas and can of B- or T-cell origin (see Chap. 43). Not unexpectedly, B-cell lymphomas are more common, and diffuse large B-cell lymphoma (which usually presents as single or multiple circumscribed nodules of varying sizes) accounts for the

General Guidelines to Evaluate the Stromal Compartment	Generally speaking, the stromal compartment consists of blood vessels, monocytes/macrophages, and dendritic cells. Together these comprise the "filtration unit" of spleen and are components of "cords of Billroth."
A) Vascular endothelial cells	CD34, CD31, Factor VIII related antigen are useful in highlighting both normal and neoplastic lesions.
Littoral cells	Share features of both endothelial cells and monocyte/macrophages. Express CD8 uniformly
B) Monocyte/macrophage	CD68, lysozyme, and anti-chymotrypsin are useful stains. When evaluation of intracellular material or infectious organisms is desired, PAS, Gram stain, AFB, and GMS stains can be used.
C) Dendritic cells	Two major types: Interdigitating (IDC) and follicular (FDC). CD68, S100, CD1a, lysozyme, α_1-antitrypsin may show variable positivity in dendritic cells.
	FDCs are CD21+ CD35+; IDCs are S100+.
General Guidelines to Evaluate the B- and T-cell Lymphoid Compartments	In general, most lymphomas involve the white pulp (nodular/follicular low power appearance), but extensive disease may present as diffuse white pulp expansion.
a) Could this be a metastasis?	a) CD45, if lesion is not obviously lymphoid.
b) Is it a B- or T-cell process?	b) B-(CD20, CD79a) and T-(CD3,CD45RO) cell markers are always used in concert to assess number and distribution of cells.
c) Are these malignant B-cells?	c) Aberrant T-cell markers, CD43, and/or CD5 are often co-expressed in malignant B-cells. By immunohisto-chemistry (IHC), these must be evaluated with extreme care in B-cell distribution areas (normal T-cells, most marrow-derived (myeloid) cells, and macrophages can all express CD43 by IHC).
d) Are these follicles benign or reactive?	d) Bcl-2 is particularly helpful in differential diagnosis of follicular lymphoma and reactive follicular hyperplasia. Benign germinal centers retain the capacity to undergo apoptosis and do not express the antiapoptosis protein, Bcl-2. About 80% of follicular lymphomas express Bcl-2 in the follicles.
e) How should the lymphoid malignancy be subtyped?	e) Additional B- and T-cell markers must be used to further characterize phenotype of various lymphomas (see also Chap. 43, Tables 43.3 and 43.4)
Some Examples of Disorders with Predominantly Red Pulp Involvement	In general, disorders with large components of circulating cells have more extensive red pulp involvement.
a) Hairy cell leukemia	TRAP and DBA-44
b) Hepatosplenic T-cell lymphoma	CD3+, CD4−, CD8−, often CD56+, Markers of cytotoxic molecules (TIA, perforin, granzyme B) +, $\gamma\delta$ rearrangement
c) T-LGL	CD3+, CD8+
d) T-PLL	CD3+, usually CD4+
e) Acute leukemias and myeloproliferative disorders	For granulocytic or monocytic cells: MPO, CD34, CD117, CD68
	For erythroid cells: Glycophorin and hemoglobin
	For megakaryocytes: CD41, CD42b, CD61, Factor VIII
	For precursor lymphoid leukemias: Tdt, CD79a, CD3, CD10

Abbreviations: T-LGL, T-large granular lymphocyte lymphoma; PAS, periodic acid-Schiff; AFB, acid-fast bacilli; GMS, Gomori methanamine silver; IDC, interdigitating dendritic cells; FDC, follicular dendritic cells; IHC, immunohistochemistry; TRAP, tartrate-resistant acid phosphatase; MPO, myeloperoxidase; TdT, terminal deoxynucleotidyl transferase.

vast majority of cases (e-**Fig. 45.10**). The diagnostic approach to primary splenic lymphomas is identical to lymphomas presenting elsewhere (see Chap. 43).

2. **Secondary splenic lymphomas**
   a. **Hodgkin lymphoma (HL).** The spleen is the most common extranodal site of HL, both classic (e-**Fig. 45.11A**) and lymphocyte-predominant Hodgkin disease (LPHD), although the latter is extremely rare (*Cancer.* 1971;27:1277; *Cancer.* 1987;59:99). Diagnostic Reed–Sternberg cells or variants (e-**Fig. 45.11B and C**) are a requirement for the diagnosis of classic HL, especially in cases without previously documented history. Immuno-histochemical evaluation is often very helpful in the differential diagnosis of classic HL versus LPHD.
   b. **Non-Hodgkin lymphomas.** More than 50% of cases of low-grade lymphomas show splenic involvement either in the form of splenomegaly or splenic hilar lymph node involvement. Splenic involvement can be categorized as focal or diffuse, the latter mode being more common. Usually there is initial expansion of white pulp in a nodular pattern in cases of low grade B-cell lymphomas (e.g., small lymphocytic, mantle cell, follicular, or marginal zone) eventually evolving into a diffuse pattern. Both patterns are often observed in appropriately sampled splenectomy specimens. Intermediate and high-grade lymphomas (large cell, Burkitt, lymphoblastic) tend to form single or multiple tumor masses. General histopathologic considerations for the diagnosis of these lymphomas are similar to those occurring in lymph nodes (see Chap. 43).

3. **Lymphomas presenting with prominent splenomegaly**
   a. **Splenic marginal zone B-cell lymphoma (SMZL).** SMZL is an indolent disease, and splenectomy results in long-term remission (*Semin Diagn Pathol.* 2003;20:83). SMZL is sometimes accompanied by autoimmune thrombocytopenia or anemia, and circulating villous lymphocytes (with polar projections) are sometimes seen in peripheral blood. Cytogenetically, allelic loss of chromosome 7q31–32 has been described in up to 40% of cases, and complex karyotypic abnormalities appear to carry a worse prognosis (*Discov Med.* 2010;10:79; *Blood.* 2010;116:9).

      Histologically, expanded periarteriolar lymphoid sheets are seen, composed of small lymphocytes and monocytoid lymphocytes (e-**Fig. 45.12**). Immunophenotypic studies by flow cytometry should demonstrate a clonal B-cell process (surface light chain restriction), usually lacking coexpression of CD5, CD10, and CD23. Alternatively, immunohistochemistry can be performed (to document a B-cell phenotype and coexpression of CD43) coupled with in situ hybridization studies (for kappa and lambda light chains); the latter is usually helpful in highlighting the clonal plasma cell population, which forms part of the spectrum of B-cell differentiation in marginal zone B-cell lymphomas.
   b. **Hepatosplenic T-cell lymphoma (HSTL).** This rare lymphoma has a clinically aggressive course and usually afflicts young males. It is characterized by a triad of peripheral cytopenias (anemia and thrombocytopenia), sinusoidal tropism, and hepatosplenomegaly. The disease is somewhat more common in immunosuppressed settings, such as post solid organ transplantation, and splenomegaly may exceed 3000 g. The neoplastic process is based on the red pulp, with conspicuous infiltration of sinuses (e-**Fig. 45.13**). The differential diagnosis includes other red pulp-based diseases such as hairy-cell leukemia. Immunophenotypic and genetic studies demonstrate a clonal population of T cells, often double negative for CD4 and CD8, with the majority showing T-cell receptor $\gamma\delta$ gene rearrangements. Isochromosome 7q10 and trisomy 8 are the strongest genetic associations (*Nat Rev Gastroenterol Hepatol.* 2009;6:433).

c. **Mantle cell lymphoma (MCL).** In mantle cell lymphoma, prominent splenomegaly usually represents the leukemic phase or stage III or IV disease. Consequently, the morphologic pattern of involvement can be diffuse, nodular, or both (e-**Fig. 45.14**). Splenic involvement may occur in the absence of significant lymphadenopathy (*Virchows Arch.* 2000;437:591). The usual constellation of morphologic, immunophenotypic, and cytogenetic findings is required for diagnosis (see Chap. 43).

d. **Hairy cell leukemia (HCL).** HCL classically presents with peripheral cytopenias, particularly monocytopenia (*Leuk Lymphoma.* 1994;13:307), and splenomegaly in a young male with recurrent opportunistic infections (*Am J Clin Pathol.* 1977;67:415). In the spleen, HCL involves and expands the red pulp; the white pulp is usually inconspicuous (e-**Fig. 45.15**). The classic immunophenotype by flow cytometry (CD103+, CD11c+, CD25+) can be easily demonstrated utilizing peripheral blood in the presence of circulating "hairy cells" and is required for diagnosis. This immunophenotype is also helpful in distinguishing hairy cell leukemia from HSTL, T-large granular lymphocyte lymphoma (T-LGL), other T-cell neoplasms, and mast cell disease, all of which can morphologically mimic hairy cell leukemia in spleen. By immunohistochemistry, DBA 44, Annexin A1, and cyclin D1 stains are helpful (*Lancet.* 2004;363:1869; *Hematol Oncol Clin North Am.* 2006;20:1051). No common recurrent cytogenetic abnormality is specific, however, numerical abnormalities of chromosomes 5 and 7 have been reported (*Hematol Oncol Clin North Am.* 2006;20:1011).

4. **Other B- and T-cell lymphomas.** T-prolymphocytic leukemia and T-LGL commonly involve the spleen (see Chap. 43) as they are usually leukemic at presentation. Likewise B- cell lymphomas, presenting at stage III or IV (see Chap. 43) can also involve spleen. An example of stage IIIES follicular lymphoma involving spleen is shown in e-**Figure 45.16**.

B. Myeloid neoplasms

1. **Chronic myelogenous leukemia (CML).** CML is classically associated with splenomegaly. The spleen is also the most common extranodal site of involvement in the blast phase of CML (see e-**Fig. 45.17**). Morphologic findings leading to the diagnosis of CML are best evaluated in touch preparations, although histologic sections are also easy to interpret. Touch preparations are required for optimal enumeration of blasts. Immunohistochemical stains (CD34, c-kit) and cytochemical stains (Leder, myeloperoxidase) can also be useful in highlighting the blast population. Disease progression (accelerated phase) and transformation in CML is usually obvious both clinically and morphologically.

2. **Acute leukemias.** Acute leukemias present as diffuse involvement of the red pulp (e-**Fig. 45.18**). The spleen is rarely a primary site of myeloid disease, and involvement reflects systemic disease. Histopathologic and immunophenotypic considerations are similar to acute leukemias presenting with peripheral blood and bone marrow involvement (see Chap. 44). Evaluation of spleen specimens for commonly occurring cytogenetic abnormalities, by conventional cytogenetics or fluorescence in situ hybridization (FISH), is a standard part of the work up unless there is already a prior history of leukemia. Care must be taken to appropriately evaluate for therapy-related morphologic and phenotypic changes and clonal evolution that may alter treatment course or effectiveness for targeted therapies.

3. **Mast cell disease (MSD) and/or systemic mastocytosis (SM).** These myeloproliferative neoplasms frequently involve the spleen. The morphologic patterns of involvement vary from isolated white pulp accentuation with fibrosis, to red pulp involvement with diffuse infiltration, fibrosis, and/or

nodular perivascular infiltrates. The presence of eosinophils, plasma cells, and fibrosis are all clues that point to the presence of mast cells. Flow cytometry is often not helpful for mast cell disease primarily because of technical difficulties in gating the desired population, although expression of CD2 and CD25 by flow cytometry is a feature specific to neoplastic mast cells (both benign and neoplastic mast cells are CD45+, CD33+, CD68+, and CD117+). In tissue sections, Leder stain (naphthol ASD chloroacetate esterase), CD117, and tryptase are helpful in highlighting mast cells.

C. **Nonhematopoietic neoplasms and pseudoneoplasms.** A wide variety of mesenchymal cell types form the complex reticular support network of splenic pulp and consequently a wide variety of mesenchymal tumors can occur as primary splenic neoplasms. These can generally be divided into stromal lesions, vascular lesions, and tumor-like lesions.

1. **Stromal lesions**
   a. **Dendritic cell tumors.** Two different kinds of dendritic cells exist in the normal lymphoid support network: interdigitating dendritic cells (IDCs) which are normally S-100 protein and MHC II positive, and follicular dendritic cells (FDCs) which express CD35 and CD21. Splenic involvement can be seen in neoplastic disorders of either IDC and FDC (*Cancer.* 1997;79:294; *Am J Surg Pathol.* 2002;26:530). Grossly, involvement is usually nodular, although disseminated systemic disease may present with diffuse splenic involvement. Dendritic cell tumors tend to behave in an aggressive manner despite their bland histologic appearance. In the absence of a preceding history, dendritic cell tumors are diagnoses of exclusion, mandating a thorough immunophenotypic workup to exclude myeloid malignancies, lymphoid B- and T-cell malignancies, and nonhematopoietic malignancies. It is important to note that FDC neoplasia may be associated with the hyaline vascular type of Castleman disease (*Adv Anat Pathol.* 2009;16:236).

   b. **Histiocytic lesions.** These lesions range from Langerhans cell histiocytosis (LCH) to histiocytic sarcomas including Langerhans-cell sarcoma. Splenic involvement is rare, usually occurring in the setting of disseminated disease and grossly presenting as single or multiple solid nodules.

   Expression of S-100 and CD1a by the neoplastic cells is consistent with a diagnosis of LCH. The sarcomatous forms can be less differentiated and may variably show expression of HLA-DR, CD45, CD68, PLAP, and vimentin (*Am J Surg Pathol.* 2004;8:1133).

2. **Vascular lesions.** Vascular tumors are common in the spleen given its rich vascular framework. Both benign and malignant vascular lesions may present in the spleen. (*Am J Surg Pathol.* 1997;21:827).
   a. **Benign lesions**
      i. **Littoral cell angioma** is unique in its presentation in the spleen and grossly is characterized by multiple spongy, cystic nodules. The cystic spaces are lined by cuboidal epithelium with intracytoplasmic eosinophilic globules. The lumina often contain abundant desquamated cells. Vascular markers (CD31, Factor VIII related antigen) are characteristically expressed; expression of CD68 and CD21 is more variable. CD34, commonly expressed in normal sinusoids, is uniformly negative.
      ii. **Peliosis,** characterized by ectatic sinusoids and blood-filled cysts, can involve the spleen. The location of the cysts (adjacent to PALS and follicles) is helpful in establishing the diagnosis. The clinical importance of this lesion lies in its propensity to undergo spontaneous rupture.
      iii. **Hemangiomas** are a frequent incidental finding at splenectomy (e-Fig. 45.19).

iv. **Sclerosing angiomatoid nodular transformation (SANT)** is a rare nonneoplastic lesion characterized by angiomatoid nodules surrounded by sclerotic stroma and a lymphoplasmacytic infiltrate (e-**Fig. 45.20**). It should be differentiated from vascular neoplasms of the spleen and lymphomas showing lymphoplasmacytic differentiation (*Am J Surg Pathol.* 2004;28:1268).

b. **Malignant lesions**

i. **Littoral cell hemangioendothelioma and angiosarcomas** rarely present in spleen (*Am J Surg Pathol.* 2006;30:1036). They are usually solid, often prompting a differential diagnosis that includes other spindle cell sarcomas. CD31 and Factor VIII related antigen immunostains establish the vascular nature of these otherwise undifferentiated malignancies; some cases may also show CD34 expression. A translocation involving chromosomes 1 and 3 has been reported in a few cytogenetically analyzed hemangioendotheliomas (*Am J Surg Pathol.* 2001;25:684). Complex cytogenetic abnormalities, none consistent from case to case, have been reported in angiosarcomas (*Cancer Genet Cytogenet.* 1993;63:171; *Cancer Genet Cytogenet.* 1998;100:52; *Cancer Genet Cytogenet.* 2001;129:64).

ii. **Kaposi sarcoma,** in the setting of HIV/AIDS, must be considered in the differential diagnosis of any splenic vascular lesion. Kaposi sarcoma usually shows positive immunohistochemistry for HHV-8 and a variety of vascular markers.

3. **Pseudoneoplastic lesions.** Examples include splenic hamartoma (well-circumscribed lesions with an angiomatoid lobular-nodular configuration, resembling red pulp; usually CD8+ and CD68+), splenic cysts (with or without an epithelial cell lining; when an epithelial lining is present it is usually cytokeratin positive; e-**Fig. 45.21**), angiomyolipoma (focally HMB-45 positive), and lymphangioma.

Inflammatory pseudotumor is a reactive nodular process that shows a predominance of benign inflammatory cells and stromal cells with sclerosis (e-**Fig. 45.22**). Inflammatory pseudotumor must be distinguished from inflammatory pseudotumor-like FDC tumor (which is usually EBV-associated and shows immunohistochemical expression of CD21 and CD35) and lymphomas with lymphoplasmacytic differentiation (MZL and LPL, see Chap. 43).

4. **Metastatic tumors.** A variety of carcinomas and sarcomas can metastasize to the spleen, although the lack of afferent lymphatics renders the spleen generally less amenable to metastatic disease. Metastases therefore commonly arise in the setting of disseminated disease. The most common epithelial metastatic tumors are carcinomas of breast or lung origin. Sarcomas involving the spleen tend to be of dendritic/histiocytic or vascular lineage.

5. **Other neoplasms.** Benign fibromas, osteomas, and chondromas can also occur in the spleen.

SUGGESTED READINGS

Bowdler AJ. *The Complete Spleen.* 2nd ed. Towota, NJ: Humana Press; 2001.

Neiman RS, Orazi A, eds. *Disorders of Spleen.* 2nd ed. Philadelphia: W.B. Saunders; 1999.

Rosati S, Frizzera G. Pseudoneoplastic lesions of hematolymphoid system. In: Wick MR, Humphrey PA, Ritter JH, eds. *Pathology of Pseudoneoplastic Lesions.* New York: Lippincott-Raven; 1997:449.

Swerdlow SH, Campo E, Harris NL, et al. *WHO Classification of Tumors and Haematopoietic and Lymphoid Tissues.* Lyon: IARC; 2008.

Soft Tissue and Bone

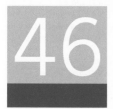

Soft Tissue

John D. Pfeifer and Louis P. Dehner

If the term "soft tissue" were restricted to only mesodermally derived structures, then nerves and neural tumors would not be considered in the discussion. Similarly, there are other examples of "soft tissue tumors (STTs)" which are present in organs but may not be derived from mesoderm. By convention, however, neural tumors, gastrointestinal stromal tumor, melanoma of soft parts, perivascular epithelioid cell tumor, and so on are regarded as "soft tissue neoplasms" despite the absence of any evidence of a well-characterized progenitor cell or mesenchymal stem cell (MSC, characterized immunophenotypically by reactivity for CD73, CD90, and CD105) with the multipotentiality to differentiate into a variety of tissues such as muscle, blood vessels, and fat (*Stem Cells.* 2011;29:397; *J Pediatr Hematol Oncol.* 2008;30:301).

I. **TISSUE PROCESSING**
   A. **Biopsy specimens.** Incisional or core biopsy of a suspected soft tissue neoplasm is performed to determine the appropriate management based on the pathologic type. The biopsy tissue should be placed immediately into 10% formalin or other appropriate fixative. The number of biopsy fragments should be recorded, as well as their aggregate dimension, and all the submitted tissue should be processed. Three H&E levels should initially be prepared for microscopic examination. For very small specimens, in order to avoid wasting tissue when refacing the block, it is strongly recommended that additional unstained slides be cut from the block during initial sectioning in the event additional studies such as immunohistochemistry are needed.
   B. **Resection specimens.** Excisional specimens are often complex and varied, and the macroscopic examination should be guided by tumor location, extent, and type. The margin of all intact specimens should be inked, and the gross distance from the tumor to the closest margin documented. The maximum dimension of the tumor should be recorded, as well as the color and consistency of the cut surface, and presence of hemorrhage and necrosis. In general, it is recommended that one section per centimeter of tumor should be submitted for microscopic examination (scout sections can be used to evaluate whether such thorough sampling is required for definitive diagnosis). The closest surgical margin should be evaluated by either shave or radial sections depending on the nature of the specimen.

   For those tumors in which a biopsy did not permit definitive diagnosis, tissue should be collected and processed for electron microscopy. Consideration should always be given to the need to send a sample of viable tumor for

TABLE 46.1 Recurring Cytogenetic Abnormalities Characteristic of Various Soft Tissue Neoplasms[a]

Tumor type	Cytogenetic aberration	Loci involved
Alveolar rhabdomyosarcoma	t(2;13)(q35;q14)	*PAX 3-FOXO1* fusion
	t(1;13)(p36;q14)	*PAX 7-FOXO1* fusion
Alveolar soft part sarcoma	der(17)t(X;17)(p11.2;q25)	*ASPL-TFE3* fusion
Angiomatoid fibrous histiocytoma	t(12;22)(q13;q12)	*EWSR1-ATF1* fusion
	t(2;22)(q33;q12)	*EWRS1-CREB1*
	t(12;16)(q13;q11)	*FUS-ATF1* fusion
Atypical lipomatous tumor/well-differentiated liposarcoma (ALT/WDLPS)	Supernumerary ring and/or marker chromosomes with amplification of 12q14-q15	Amplification of *MDM2, CDK4, HMGA2* genes
Clear cell sarcoma (melanoma of soft parts)	t(12;22)(q13;q12)	*EWSR1-ATF1* fusion
	t(2;22)(q32;q12)	*EWSR1-CREB1* fusion
Congenital infantile fibrosarcoma	t(12;15)(p13;q25)	*ETV6-NTRK3* fusion
Dedifferentiated liposarcoma	Supernumerary ring and/or marker chromosomes with amplification of 12q14-q15	Amplification of *MDM2, CDK4, HMGA2* genes
Dermatofibrosarcoma protuberans/giant cell fibroblastoma	t(17;22)(q22;q13) and derivative ring chromosomes	*COL1A1-PDGFB* fusion
Desmoid fibromatosis	Trisomy 8 or 20; loss of 5q	Somatic *CTNNB1* or *APC* mutations (only in deep tumors)
Desmoplastic small round cell tumor	t(11;22)(p13;q12)	*EWSR1-WT1* fusion
Elastofibroma	1q abnormalities	Unknown
Embryonal rhabdomyosarcoma	Loss of heterozygosity at 11p15; gains of 2, 7, 8, 11, 12, 20, 21, 13q21, 20; losses of 1p35–36.3, 7, 6, 9q22, 14q21–32, 17	Unknown
Epithelioid hemangioendothelioma	t(1;3)(p36;3q25)	*WWTR1-CAMTA1* fusion
Epithelioid sarcoma, proximal type	Alterations of 22q11.2	Biallelic inactivation of *hSNF5/INI1*
Ewing sarcoma/primitive neuroectodermal tumor	t(11;22)(q24;q12)	*EWSR1-FLI1* fusion
	t(21;22)(q22;q12)	*EWSR1-ERG* fusion
Extrarenal malignant rhabdoid tumor	Alterations of 22q11.2	Biallelic inactivation of *hSNF5/INI1*
Extraskeletal myxoid chondrosarcoma	t(9;22)(q22;q12)	*EWSR1-NR4A3* fusion
	t(9;17)(q22;q11.2)	*TAF2N-NR4A3* fusion
	t(9;15)(q22;q21)	*TCF12-NR4A3* fusion
Giant cell tumor of tendon sheath/diffuse-type giant cell tumors	Translocations involving 1p13, including t(1;2)(p13;q135)	*CSF1* fusions, including *CSF1-COL6A3*
Inflammatory myofibroblastic tumor	Translocations involving 2p23	*ALK* fusions with a variety of other genes

(continued)

TABLE 46.1	Recurring Cytogenetic Abnormalities Characteristic of Various Soft Tissue Neoplasms[a] (Continued)	
Tumor type	**Cytogenetic aberration**	**Loci involved**
Leiomyosarcoma	Structural alterations of 1, 7, 10, 13, 14	Unknown
Lipoblastoma	Rearrangements of 8q12	Rearrangement of *PLAG1* gene
Lipoma	Rearrangements 12q14-q15 and 6p21–22; deletions of 13q12–14	*HMGA2* and *HMGA1* fusions; unknown
Low-grade fibromyxoid sarcoma	t(7;16)(q33;p11) t(11;16)(p11;p11)	*FUS-CREB3L2* fusion *FUS-CREB3L1* fusion
Malignant peripheral nerve sheath tumor		Unknown
Myxoid/round cell liposarcoma	t(12;16)(q13;p11) t(12;22)(q13;q12)	*FUS-DD1T3* fusion *EWSR1-DD1T3* fusion
Nasopharyngeal angiofibroma	Gains of 1p, 7q, 10q, 12q, 16p, 16q, 17q, 19p, 20q, 22q	Activating mutations in *CTNNB1*
Soft tissue myoepithelial tumor	Translocations involving 22q12	*EWSR1* fusions with a variety of other genes
Synovial sarcoma	t(X;18)(p11;q11)	*SSX18-SSX1*, *SSX18-SSX2*, *SSX18-SSX4* fusions

[a]Only the most common abnormalities are indicated. For more details see Pfeifer JD. *Molecular Genetic Testing in Surgical Pathology*. Philadelphia, PA: Lippincott, Williams & Wilkins; 2006.

cytogenetic analysis. A sample of viable tumor should also be snap frozen and stored in the event it is needed for subsequent molecular evaluation, which plays an ever-increasing role in diagnosis as more and more types of STTs are shown to harbor characteristic genetic aberrations (Table 46.1).

II. **TERMINOLOGY REGARDING THE BIOLOGIC POTENTIAL OF SOFT TISSUE NEOPLASMS.**

A. The current WHO classification of STTs (Table 46.2) assigns each neoplasm to one of four categories, benign, intermediate (locally aggressive), intermediate (rarely metastasizing), and malignant. The four categories provide a standard nomenclature to indicate the biologic potential of the various STTs. It is important to emphasize that the intermediate categories are not defined on the basis of histologic grade, but rather biologic potential. Some of the latter tumors may have rather bland microscopic features as in the case of a desmoid fibromatosis, or hypercellular and mitotically active as in the case of some fibrohistiocytic tumors.

1. **Benign.** Most tumors in this category do not locally recur. If recurrence does occur, it is typically nondestructive. Complete local excision is curative. The common lipoma is an example of this category.

2. **Intermediate (locally aggressive).** Tumors in this category have a locally destructive and infiltrative growth pattern, and often locally recur. Wide excision is required for local control, but that is not necessarily an indemnification against a local recurrence. These tumors do not metastasize. An example of this tumor type is desmoid fibromatosis.

3. **Intermediate (rarely metastasizing).** Tumors in this category also have a locally destructive and infiltrative growth pattern. However, they also can give rise to distant metastases in a small subset of cases (typically <2%),

TABLE 46.2	WHO Classification of Soft Tissue Tumors

Adipocytic Tumors
Benign
Lipoma
Lipomatosis
Lipomatosis of nerve
Lipoblastoma/lipoblastomatosis
Angiolipoma
Myolipoma
Chondroid lipoma
Extra-renal angiomyolipoma
Extra-adrenal myelolipoma
Spindle cell/pleomorphic lipoma
Hibernoma

Intermediate (locally aggressive)
Atypical lipomatous tumor/well-differentiated liposarcoma

Malignant
Dedifferentiated liposarcoma
Myxoid liposarcoma/round cell liposarcoma
Pleomorphic liposarcoma
Mixed-type liposarcoma
Liposarcoma, not otherwise specified

Fibroblastic/myofibroblastic tumors
Benign
Nodular fasciitis
Proliferative fasciitis
Proliferative myositis
Myositis ossificans
Fibro-osseous pseudotumor of digits
Ischemic fasciitis
Elastofibroma
Fibrous hamartoma of infancy
Myofibroma/myofibromatosis
Fibromatosis colli
Juvenile hyaline fibromatosis
Inclusion body fibromatosis
Fibroma of tendon sheath
Desmoplastic fibroblastoma
Mammary-type myofibroblastoma
Calcifying aponeurotic fibroma
Angiomyofibroblastoma
Cellular angiofibroma
Nuchal-type fibroma
Gardner fibroma
Calcifying fibrous tumor
Giant cell angiofibroma

Intermediate (locally aggressive)
Superficial fibromatosis (palmar/plantar)
Desmoid-type fibromatoses
Lipofibromatosis

(continued)

TABLE 46.2 WHO Classification of Soft Tissue Tumors (*Continued*)

Intermediate (rarely metastasizing)
Solitary fibrous tumor and hemangiopericytoma
Inflammatory myofibroblastic tumor
Low-grade myofibroblastic sarcoma
Myxoinflammatory fibroblastic sarcoma
Infantile fibrosarcoma

Malignant
Adult fibrosarcoma
Myxofibrosarcoma
Low-grade fibromyxoid sarcoma/hyalinizing spindle cell tumor
Sclerosing epithelioid fibrosarcoma

So-called fibrohistiocytic tumors
Benign
Giant cell tumor of tendon sheath
Diffuse-type giant cell tumor
Deep benign fibrous histiocytoma

Intermediate (rarely metastasizing)
Plexiform fibrohistiocytic tumor
Giant cell tumor of soft tissues

Malignant
Pleomorphic MFH/undifferentiated pleomorphic sarcoma
Giant cell MFH/undifferentiated pleomorphic sarcoma with giant cells
Inflammatory MFH/undifferentiated pleomorphic sarcoma with prominent inflammation

Smooth muscle tumors
Angioleiomyoma
Deep leiomyoma
Genital leiomyoma
Leiomyosarcoma

Pericytic (perivascular tumors)
Glomus tumor
Malignant glomus tumor
Myopericytoma

Skeletal muscle tumors
Benign
Rhabdomyoma (adult type, fetal type, genital type)

Malignant
Embryonal rhabdomyosarcoma (including spindle cell, botryoid, anaplastic)
Alveolar rhabdomyosarcoma
Pleomorphic rhabdomyosarcoma

Vascular tumors
Benign
Hemangiomas of subcutaneous/deep soft tissue
Capillary
Cavernous
Arteriovenous
Venous
Intramuscular
Synovial
Epithelioid hemangioma
Angiomatosis
Lymphangioma

(continued)

TABLE 46.2   WHO Classification of Soft Tissue Tumors (*Continued*)

Intermediate (locally aggressive)
Kaposiform hemangioendothelioma

Intermediate (rarely metastasizing)
Retiform hemangioendothelioma
Papillary intralymphatic angioendothelioma
Composite hemangioendothelioma
Kaposi sarcoma

Malignant
Epithelioid hemangioendothelioma
Angiosarcoma of soft tissue

Chondro-osseous tumors
Soft tissue chondroma
Mesenchymal chondrosarcoma

Tumors of uncertain differentiation
Benign
Intramuscular myxoma
Juxtaarticular myxoma
Deep (aggressive) angiomyxoma
Pleomorphic hyalinizing angiectatic tumor
Ectopic hamartomatous thymoma

Intermediate (rarely metastasizing)
Angiomatoid fibrous histiocytoma
Ossifying fibromyxoid tumor
Mixed tumor/myoepithelioma/parachordoma

Malignant
Synovial sarcoma
Epithelioid sarcoma
Alveolar soft part sarcoma
Clear cell sarcoma of soft tissue
Extraskeletal myxoid chondrosarcoma
PNET/extraskeletal Ewing tumor
Desmoplastic small round cell tumor
Extra-renal rhabdoid tumor
Malignant mesenchymoma
Neoplasms with perivascular epithelioid cell differentiation (PEComa)
Clear cell myomelanocytic tumor
Intimal sarcoma

From: Fletcher CDM, Unni K, Mertens K, eds. *World Health Organization Classification of Tumours. Pathology and Genetics. Tumours of Soft Tissue and Bone.* Lyon: IARC Press; 2002. Used with permission.

     although the risk for metastasis of an individual tumor cannot be reliably predicted on the basis of morphologic features. Examples of this category include congenital infantile fibrosarcoma, dermatofibrosarcoma protuberans, and angiomatoid fibrous histiocytoma (AFH).

   4. Malignant. Tumors in this category also have a locally destructive and infiltrative growth pattern. However, they metastasize in high percentage of cases; low-grade sarcomas have a metastatic rate of 2% to 10%, and high-grade sarcomas metastasize in 20% to 100% of cases.

  B. Histologic grading of soft tissue sarcomas (STS). Although several grading systems of STSs have been proposed over the past 30 to 40 years, the two systems in widespread use are from the National Cancer Institute (NCI) and the French

TABLE 46.3	Grading of Soft Tissue Sarcoma[a]

FNCLCC Grading. The FNCLCC grade is determined by three parameters: differentiation (histology specific), mitotic activity, and extent of necrosis. Each parameter is scored: differentiation (1–3), mitotic activity (1–3), and necrosis (0–2). The scores are summed to designate grade.

Grade X Grade cannot be assessed
Grade 1 2 or 3
Grade 2 4 or 5
Grade 3 6—8

Differentiation. Tumor differentiation is histology specific and is generally scored as follows[b]:
Score 1 Sarcomas closely resembling normal, mature mesenchymal tissue
Score 2 Sarcoma of definite histologic type
Score 3 Synovial sarcomas, embryonal sarcomas, undifferentiated sarcomas, and sarcomas of unknown/doubtful type

Mitotic count. In the most mitotically active area of the sarcoma, ten successive high-power fields (HPFs) are assessed using a 40X objective.
Score 1 0–9 mitoses/10 HPFs
Score 2 10–19 mitoses/10 HPFs
Score 3 20 or more mitoses/10 HPFs

Tumor necrosis. Evaluated on gross examination and validated with histologic sections.
Score 0 No tumor necrosis
Score 1 ≤50% tumor necrosis
Score 2 >50% tumor necrosis

[a]Modified from *J Clin Oncol.* 1997;15:350; some soft tissue sarcomas in children have their own grading system as outlined in *Cancer.* 2010;116:2266.
[b]Many sarcomas have a histology-specific tumor differentiation score as outlined in *J Clin Oncol.* 1997;15:350.

Federation Nationale des Centres de Lutte Contre le Cancer (FNCLCC) (*Arch Pathol Lab Med.* 2006;130:2006; *Histopathology.* 2006;48:42) (Table 46.3). Three histologic features are the basis of the grading systems: tumor differentiation, necrosis, and mitotic count. However, many sarcomas have a specified histology-specific tumor differentiation score (*J Clin Oncol.* 1997;15:350), and some STSs in children have their own grading system (*Cancer.* 2010;116:2266). In general, the mitotic index and extent of necrosis are predictive of metastatic behavior and survival in adults whereas the mitotic index (less than or greater than 10 mitoses per 10 high-power fields (HPFs)) is the most significant prognostic variable in the case of non-rhabdomyosarcoma (RMS) STS in children.

It must be emphasized that it can be difficult to accurately assess a STS for grading purposes when it is resected after adjuvant chemotherapy.

III. **ADIPOCYTIC TUMORS.** This morphologic category of STTs includes some of the most commonly occurring neoplasms in adults which arise in the superficial and deep soft tissues. Generally, the deeper and larger the fatty tumor in adults, the greater the likelihood of a liposarcoma (LPS) (*ANZ J Surg.* 2007;77:524).

A. **Benign**

1. **Lipomas** are composed of mature adipocytes and are the most common soft tissue neoplasms in adults. Superficial lipomas arise in the subcutis; deep lipomas arise within the deep soft tissue; parosteal lipomas arise on the surface of bone; intramuscular and intermuscular lipomas arise within and between skeletal muscle; and lipoma arborescens arises in synovial membranes. Superficial tumors are generally <5 cm in maximum dimension, while deep tumors are often >5 cm. Lipomas are well circumscribed and have an oily light yellow cut surface, except in children whose tumors are pale white. Regardless of the anatomic site, the tumor is composed of mature

adipocytes separated into complete and incomplete lobules. Numerous histologic subtypes have been described but none has prognostic significance, including the following (*Adv Anat Pathol.* 2006;13:279).

a. **Angiolipoma** typically occurs in the subcutaneous tissue and consists of mature adipocytes with a variably prominent capillary network with scattered microthrombi. These vessels are typically found at the periphery of the lobules (**e-Fig. 46.1**).* These tumors may be multiple in the subcutis, and also occur in and around the spinal cord (*Childs Nerv Syst.* 2002;18:725).

b. **Myolipoma** (intramuscular lipoma) is found in the deep soft tissues of the abdominal cavity, inguinal region, and retroperitoneum. Mature adipose tissue is intermixed with mature smooth muscle or skeletal muscle.

c. **Chondroid lipoma** occurs in the limb girdle and proximal extremities. Cords and nests of lipoblasts as well as mature adipocytes are present in a myxoid to hyalinized chondroid matrix in the absence of true hyaline cartilage. Despite the presence of immature fat cells, surgical excision is curative. This tumor is distinct from chondrolipoma, which is characterized by hyaline cartilage within a lipoma.

d. **Spindle cell lipoma/pleomorphic lipoma** occurs predominantly on the posterior neck and shoulder area in middle aged and elderly men (only 10% of cases occur in women). The tumor presents as a mobile dermal or subcutaneous nodule that often has been present for many years. The microscopic features are variable: at one end of the spectrum are tumors composed of bland spindle cells with associated dense collagen bundles between mature adipocytes; at the other end are tumors with small hyperchromatic cells admixed with multinucleated giant cells between mature adipocytes. The spindle cells are immunopositive for CD34, and in some cases also for S-100 protein. This neoplasm is one of several cutaneous and STTs, which express CD34 (*J Cutan Pathol.* 2009;36:89). In the presence of atypical lipoblasts, spindle cell LPS must be considered since the latter tumor also rises in the subcutis (*Mod Pathol.* 2010;23:729).

2. **Lipomatosis** occurs in several different clinicopathologic settings, all of which are characterized by a diffuse overgrowth of mature adipose tissue. Regardless of the clinical subtype, the neoplastic cells are indistinguishable from those found in lipomas, which emphasizes the role of clinical history in arriving at the correct diagnosis.

a. **Diffuse lipomatosis** preferentially occurs in children <2 years old, and involves a substantial part of an extremity as well as the trunk, head and neck, pelvis, abdomen, or intestinal tract. In this setting, the phosphatase and tensin homolog (PTEN) hamartoma tumor syndrome as expressed in the Proteus syndrome, encephalocraniocutaneous lipomatosis, Bannayan–Ruvalcaba–Riley syndrome, and Cowden disease should be considered (*Genet Med.* 2009;11:687).

b. **Symmetric lipomatosis** occurs predominantly in middle aged men of Mediterranean ancestry, and is characterized by symmetric deposition of fat in the upper body.

c. **Pelvic lipomatosis,** which affects black males over a wide age range, usually manifests as an overgrowth of fat in perirectal and perivesical areas.

d. **Steroid lipomatosis** occurs in the setting of adrenocortical hormonal therapy or with endogenous endocrine abnormalities, and characteristically involves accumulation of fat in the face, sternal region, or middle of the upper back (the so-called buffalo hump).

---

*All e-figures are available online via the Solution Site Image Bank.

e. **HIV-lipodystrophy** in patients with AIDS occurs in those undergoing treatment with protease inhibitors or other forms of antiviral therapy, and is characterized by the accumulation of visceral fat with fat wasting in the face and limbs.

f. **Nevus lipomatosus** is a developmental anomaly presenting as a yellowish polypoid lesion of skin, typically in the lower abdominal-sacral-pelvic region (*J Dermatol.* 2000;27:16). It is characterized by mature adipose tissue in the papillary and reticular dermis. Soft fibroma and acrochordon have some overlapping features, but adipose tissue is not found in the papillary dermis in these latter two lesions.

3. **Lipomatosis** of nerve (neural fibrolipoma, fibrolipomatous hamartoma) is noted at birth or in early childhood, but is seen through the fourth decade. The median nerve and ulnar nerves are the usual sites of involvement, and a subset of cases is associated with macrodactyly. Perineurial and epineurial infiltration by a mixture of mature adipocytes and fibrous tissue typically separates individual nerve bundles. Another congenital fatty lesion related to peripheral nerves is *lumbosacral lipoma* in infants, which is characterized by a tethered filum terminale or conus medullaris (*Childs Nerv Syst.* 1997;13:298).

4. **Lipoblastoma** occurs in children (90% of cases occur in children under the age of 10 years) with a predilection for the lower extremity, but can also involve the trunk, mediastinum, abdomen-retroperitoneum, and head and neck (*Am J Surg Pathol.* 2009;33:1705). It is either a localized, well-circumscribed tumor (lipoblastoma) or has a diffuse infiltrating pattern (lipoblastomatosis). Like other fatty tumors, it has a lobulated architecture and is composed of a mixture of cell types including mature and immature adipocytes, a variable number of lipoblasts, multinucleated cells, signet-ring lipocytes, and stellate mesenchymal cells (e-**Fig. 46.2**). Grayish myxoid areas noted grossly have a resemblance to myxoid LPS, which can be problematic. Despite the presence of immature fat cells, this tumor is benign and does not metastasize, although approximately 20% to 25% of cases recur (most are examples of lipoblastomatosis). These tumors have the potential for maturation, and some cases have predominantly lipomatous features with residual immature myxoid areas at the periphery of the lobules. These tumors express for S-100 and CD34.

5. **Hibernoma** is a neoplasm composed of brown fat (adipocytes with multi-vacuolated granular cytoplasm) admixed with conventional adipose tissue. It occurs in young adults and is found in the neck, axilla, thigh, retroperitoneum, head and neck, trunk, and upper extremities (*Am J Dermatopathol.* 2009;31:685). The cut surface has a yellowish to brownish appearance, is usually oily and spongy; may be lobulated but is well demarcated; and can measure over 20 cm. Microscopically, lobules of brown fat are separated from conventional adipose tissue (e-**Fig. 46.3**).

B. **Intermediate (locally aggressive)**

1. **Atypical lipomatous tumor/well-differentiated LPS (ALT/WDLPS)** (50% to 55% of cases) occurs in adults in the fifth through eighth decade of life (*Cytogenet Genome Res.* 2007;118:138). The deep soft tissues of the lower extremity and retroperitoneum are usual primary sites; the paratesticular region and mediastinum are less common sites. Tumors arising in the retroperitoneum may attain sizes in excess of 20 cm and weigh 500 to 1000 g. The tumor has a lobulated, yellow to white, soft to firm cut surface that varies on the basis of lipomatous, fibrous, and myxoid components, and discrete margins are often difficult to discern from gross examination. Microscopically, the tumor is composed of cells with lipoma-like features except for the presence of scattered hyperchromatic, often

multinucleated and vacuolated cells with features of atypical lipoblasts. Four histologic subtypes are designated, namely adipocytic (lipoma-like), sclerosing, inflammatory, and spindle cell types, but more than one pattern may be present in the same neoplasm. Sclerosing foci are helpful in diagnosis because the areas of collagen contain atypical stromal cells (e-Fig. 46.4). Fluorescence in situ hybridization (FISH) for *MDM2* amplification characteristic of ALT/WDLPS is a sensitive and specific tool for distinguishing ALT/WDLPS from benign lipomatous neoplasms (*Mod Pathol.* 2008;21:943; *Adv Anat Pathol.* 2009;16:383).

Prognosis is largely determined by anatomic site and size. Smaller, more superficial tumors can be locally resected with negative margins, but those in the retroperitoneum are likely to recur because of positive surgical margins. Recurrent tumors may show evidence of so-called dedifferentiation (see below) which clearly demonstrates the overt malignant potential of ALT/WDLPS. Multifocal ALT/WDLPS is an uncommon but well-documented presentation.

C. Malignant

1. **Dedifferentiated LPS** shows a transition from ALT/WDLPS to a pleomorphic and/or high-grade spindle cell sarcoma (e-Fig. 46.5), either in the primary tumor (85% to 90% of cases) or in a recurrence (10% to 15% of cases) (*Virchows Arch.* 2010;456:167). The transition in pattern from ALT/WDLPS to high-grade sarcoma is usually abrupt. By convention, the focus of dedifferentiation should be at least several millimeters in greatest dimension. Because the area of dedifferentiation may be limited, thorough sampling and careful microscopic examination of all ALT/WDLPS is required in order to exclude the presence of dedifferentiation.

2. **Myxoid LPS/round cell LPS** peaks in incidence at the age of 30 to 40 years, occurs predominantly in the deep soft tissues of the extremities (more than two-thirds of cases arise in the musculature of the thigh), and is the most common type of LPS in the first two decades of life (*Ann Diagn Pathol.* 2000;4:252; *Am J Surg Pathol.* 2009;33:645). If this tumor is discovered in the retroperitoneum, it likely represents metastatic disease rather than a primary tumor (*Mod Pathol.* 2009;22:223).

   The cut surface of myxoid LPS is tan, glistening, and gelatinous; the round cell morphology is associated with a fleshy, white cut surface. Myxoid tumors are composed of uniform, round to oval, primitive nonlipogenic mesenchymal cells and small lipoblasts embedded in a myxoid stroma with a delicate arborizing capillary network (e-Fig. 46.6). In contrast, areas composed of sheets of high-grade primitive round cells are not accompanied by a myxoid stroma. It is not uncommon to identify a subset of round cells in myxoid LPS, usually in a perivascular distribution, but by convention round cell LPS has a composition of 80% or more of round cells. Immunohistochemically, the round cells are often S-100 protein positive. A poorer outcome is associated with round cell LPS, unlike the more favorable prognosis of pure myxoid LPS. Although the same two translocations are characteristic of both tumor types (Table 46.1), they do not correlate with prognosis (*Cytogenet Genome Res.* 2007;118:138).

3. **Pleomorphic LPS,** as the name implies, is by definition a high-grade sarcoma with a variable number of convincing pleomorphic lipoblasts. This tumor has a preference for the extremities, usually measures in excess of 10 cm, and primarily occurs in individuals over 40 years old. The tumor is either a well-circumscribed or an infiltrative mass with a variable appearance on cut surface ranging from solid to cystic, to necrotic, to hemorrhagic, to myxoid. Pleomorphic lipoblasts with enlarged hyperchromatic nuclei that are scalloped by cytoplasmic lipid vacuoles are not always numerous in the

background of highly atypical, even anaplastic round cells, spindle cells, and multinucleated tumor giant cells (e-Fig. 46.7). These tumors may have a prominent inflammatory infiltrate. Atypical, even bizarre mitotic figures are often present. Well-differentiated LPS can dedifferentiate to pleomorphic LPS (*Am J Surg Pathol.* 2010;34:1122; *Am J Surg Pathol.* 2010;34:837). In the absence of identifiable lipoblasts, these neoplasms are otherwise diagnosed as pleomorphic undifferentiated sarcomas but there is marked morphologic overlap between these tumors (*Am J Surg Pathol.* 2009;33:1594).

IV. FIBROBLASTIC/MYOFIBROBLASTIC TUMORS

A. Benign

1. **Nodular fasciitis** occurs in all age groups but has a predilection for young adults. It usually involves the subcutaneous tissue of the head and neck (especially in children), trunk, or upper extremities (e-Fig. 46.8). Dermal involvement is uncommon, but deeper fascial or intramuscular tumors are other presentations. Similar lesions may involve small to medium sized veins or the soft tissue of the outer table of the scalp (infantile cranial fasciitis), as intravascular and cranial fasciitis (e-Fig. 46.9), respectively. Uncommonly, the tumor develops at intraneural and intra-articular sites.

   These circumscribed, minimally infiltrative spindle cell proliferations have a fibrous to myxoid cut surface, and most are <2 cm in greatest dimension though some lesions can exceed 5 to 6 cm. Cystic degeneration is an uncommon gross feature, but one of the microscopic hallmarks is the presence of microcysts among the more cellular foci (*Arch Pathol Lab Med.* 2008;132:579). Collections of inflammatory cells, extravasated red cells, or osteoclast-like giant cells may be associated with the microcysts. Compactly cellular foci with storiform profiles or interlacing fascicles may reside adjacent to individual cells with a myxoid background in a tissue culture-like appearance (e-Fig. 46.8 and e-Fig. 46.9). More collagenized foci resemble a keloid. Mitotic figures, but not atypical ones, are expected in variable numbers. The spindle cells are strongly reactive for smooth muscle actin (SMA); unlike desmoid tumor, the cells are nonreactive for β-catenin (*Histopathology.* 2007;51:509).

2. **Proliferative fasciitis** and **proliferative myositis** primarily occur in middle aged and elderly patients. The subcutis in the upper extremity is the most common site of proliferative fasciitis, but some cases involve the trunk or lower extremity. Proliferative myositis is intramuscular, and primarily involves the trunk, shoulder girdle, and upper arm. Both lesions grow rapidly, measure between 3 and 5 cm, and are composed of plump fibroblastic and myofibroblastic spindled cells as in nodular fasciitis. However, the hallmark of proliferative fasciitis and proliferative myositis is the presence of large ganglion-like cells with an uneven distribution within the lesion. The ganglion-like cells may be mitotically active but atypical mitotic figures are not present. In addition to SMA, CD68 may be expressed in the ganglion-like cells.

3. **Ischemic fasciitis** occurs over bony prominences, usually due to impaired circulation and prolonged pressure in immobilized, often elderly individuals. A zonal architecture consists of central areas of coagulative necrosis and myxoid change, with fibroblastic and vascular proliferation at the periphery (*Am J Surg Pathol.* 2008;32:1546). There is some resemblance to deep granuloma annulare.

4. **Myositis ossificans** and **fibro-osseous pseudotumor of digits** are related lesions that occur in a broad age range of patients, though young adults are most frequently affected. Myositis ossificans has a propensity for the extremities, trunk, and head and neck, while fibro-osseous pseudotumor primarily occurs, as its name indicates, in the subcutis of the proximal

phalanx of the finger and toe. Both lesions are thought to be caused by soft tissue injury with resulting repair, which initially consists of a cellular fibroblastic focus resembling nodular fasciitis, followed by development of an equally cellular osteoblastic proliferation and a peripheral rind of osseous metaplasia (e-**Fig. 46.10**). A similar type of proliferative and metaplastic process arises in the periosteum. Biopsies from the fibroblastic and/or osteoblastic foci can be quite worrisome, but the mitotic activity is generally low and the mitotic figures are not atypical. The nuclei are not disproportionately large or hyperchromatic.

5. **Elastofibroma** is found predominantly in individuals over 50 years of age in the connective tissues between the chest wall and the inferior region of the scapula, deep to the rhomboid major and latissimus dorsi muscles, usually with attachment to the periosteum of the ribs. However, rare examples have been described in the axilla, ischial tuberosity, and greater trochanter (*Sarcoma* 2008;756565). The tumor can be unilateral or bilateral and has a gray-white, rubbery to fibrous cut surface with ill-defined margins. Microscopically, a paucicellular collagenized stroma (e-**Fig. 46.11**) contains elastic fibers with large, coarse, eosinophilic linear globules arranged in a so-called beads on a string pattern that is highlighted by a Weigert's elastic or pentachrome stain.

6. **Fibrous hamartoma of infancy (FHI)** is one of the "fibrous tumors of childhood" and is generally seen before 2 years of age (*J Am Acad Dermatol.* 2011;64:579). The anterior or posterior axillary fold, arm and shoulder, back, thigh, and groin are the preferred sites. The tumor forms an ill-defined mass in the subcutis and has a white fibrocollagenous gross appearance with interspersed fat. Microscopically, intersecting fibrous bands of variable thickness radiate through the subcutis and are associated with discrete nodules of immature mesenchyme or so-called neuroid nodules (e-**Fig. 46.12**). Without the latter nodules, there is a resemblance to another fibrous tumor of childhood, lipofibromatosis or infantile subcutaneous fibromatosis. When there is overgrowth of the subcutaneous fat by the fibrous component, the tumor acquires the features of fibromatosis or dermatofibrosarcoma protuberans. FHI has a low rate of recurrence (only 10% to 15%). Like most other fibrous tumors in infants and young children, FHI does not express β-catenin (*Pediatr Dev Pathol.* 2009;12:292).

7. **Myofibroma–myofibromatosis,** another fibrous tumor of childhood, though seen in adults on occasion, is composed of contractile myoid cells that seemingly originates within small vessels and extends into the surrounding dermis, soft tissues, various organs, and bone. A solitary mass in the head and neck in a young child (aged 0 to 3 years) is the most common of the three clinical presentations (Table 46.4), although there are no excluded sites for origin as the tumor can also involve skin, soft tissues,

TABLE 46.4	The Three Clinical Presentations of Myofibroma-Myofibromatosis in Children		
	Solitary	**Multicentric**	**Generalized**
Sites	Skin, soft tissue, bone	Skin and soft tissue, and/or bone	Skin, soft tissue, bone plus organs (lung, heart, liver, intestinal tract, brain)
Percentage of total cases	90	3–6	1–3
Prognosis	Excellent	Excellent	Poor

visceral organs, and the central nervous system. Individual tumors range from <1 to over 7 cm in greatest dimension and have a cut surface that ranges from firm and fibrous, to cystic and hemorrhagic. Immature plump to spindled cells are arranged in whorls and fascicles within a fibromyxoid stroma; smaller nodules at the periphery of the mass may be associated with a vessel(s) to suggest an angiocentric origin (e-**Fig. 46.13**). Hypercellular spindle cell foci are present in some cases with a resemblance to congenital infantile fibrosarcoma, but the tumor cells lack the t(12;15) translocation characteristic of the latter tumor. Other findings include a hemangiopericytoma-like pattern centrally, often with ischemic or hemorrhagic regions, dystrophic calcifications, and hyalinization. The spindle cells express vimentin and SMA, whereas the hemangiopericytoma-like foci are variably CD34 positive. The differential diagnosis of myofibroma includes nodular fasciitis; the distinction can be problematic since the two lesions have some overlapping morphologic and immunophenotypic features (*J Clin Pathol.* 2009;62:236).

8. **Angiomyofibroblastoma,** a rare tumor, occurs in women of reproductive age, where it arises in the rises in the pelviperineal region (vulva and vagina) as a painless, well-circumscribed, slowly enlarging mass (*Int J Gynecol Pathol.* 2005;24:26). In men, the neoplasm usually involves the paratesticular soft tissues or scrotum. Round to plump spindled myofibroblasts tend to cluster around blood vessels (e-**Fig. 46.14**); a subset of cases has a mature fatty component (*Int J Gynecol Pathol.* 2005;24:196). Binucleate and multinucleate cells are common in the absence of mitotic activity. These tumors are immunoreactive for desmin and estrogen and progesterone receptors. Some cases have an overlap with cellular angiofibroma and deep aggressive angiomyxoma (see below).

9. **Cellular angiofibroma** involves the superficial soft tissues of the vulva or inguinoscrotal region as well as the perineum, retroperitoneum, and subcutis of the chest (*J Cutan Pathol.* 2003;30:405). Grossly, the tumor is a well-circumscribed mass that usually measures <3 cm in diameter in women and <10 cm in men. The cut surface of the tumor has a yellow to tan-brown, soft to rubbery appearance. The tumor is composed of plump spindled cells with minimal eosinophilic cytoplasm, little cytologic atypia, and few mitotic figures; a background of delicate collagen fibers is present in tumors in females. The vascular component of the tumor is composed of small- to medium-sized vessels, with or without prominent hyaline walls, and is usually present throughout the entire lesion. Regressive/degenerative changes, including extravasated erythrocytes, hemosiderin deposition, cystic change, and intravascular thrombi are also present.

10. **Giant cell angiofibroma,** a slowly growing occasional painful tumor, has a predilection for the eyelids and orbital region of adults, although it has been identified in a number of other anatomic sites. The tumor is usually about 3 cm in greatest dimension, well-circumscribed, variably encapsulated, with cystic and/or hemorrhagic areas. Microscopically, cellular areas of round to spindled cytologically bland cells and multinucleated stromal cells (which often line pseudovascular spaces as is common in giant cell fibroblastoma) are set in a background of myxoid to collagenous stroma with small- to medium-sized blood vessels. Both the mononuclear and multinucleated cells are immunoreactive for CD34 and CD99, and occasionally also for BCL2.

11. **Nuchal-type fibroma** and **Gardner-associated fibroma** are virtually identical in terms of the microscopic features of dense, paucicellular collagenous bundles, which overgrow and occupy the dermis, subcutis, and deep soft tissues (*Cancer.* 1999;85:156). These tumors do not have the infiltrative

features of desmoid fibromatosis, however, a recurrence may be indistinguishable from a desmoid. As in desmoid tumors, there is nuclear immunopositivity for β-catenin. The possibility of Gardner syndrome should be raised in the presence of this tumor (*Am J Surg Pathol.* 2007;31:410). In the latter, multifocal lesions are seen.

B. Intermediate (locally aggressive)

1. **Superficial fibromatoses.** Palmar-plantar fibromatosis develops in males over 30 years of age (with a male to female ratio of 4:1) as an asymptomatic, isolated firm nodule, which evolves into cord-like bands between the nodules involving adjacent fingers. Plantar fibromatosis is seen more often in children and adolescents as painful subcutaneous nodules (*Am J Surg Pathol.* 2005;29:1095).

   The microscopic features evolve over time. Greater cellularity is present early on, consisting of bland plump to spindle cells that have a low mitotic rate and are set in a background of collagen and elongated vessels (**e-Fig. 46.15**). Older lesions are much less cellular and have a stroma that consists of dense, often hyalinized collagen. The extent of surgical excision is the primary determinant of the rate of recurrence. These tumors may demonstrate focal rather than diffuse nuclear positivity for β-catenin (*Mod Pathol.* 2001;14:895).

2. **Desmoid-type fibromatosis** (desmoid tumor, musculoaponeurotic fibromatosis) usually involves the head and neck region in children, and the proximal extremities and abdominal wall in adolescents and older females (*Hematol Oncol Clin North Am.* 2005;19:565). Both soft tissues and mesenteric desmoids may be associated with Gardner syndrome. A circumscribed mass measuring 5 to 10 cm with a firm white trabeculated surface is the typical gross appearance; the macroscopic circumscription may be deceptive since subtle and extensive infiltration into the interstitium between muscle bundles and along fascial planes is often present microscopically. Although desmoid tumor is classically a proliferation of fibroblasts, a number of patterns are seen, ranging from spindle cells forming bundles and fascicles in a dense collagenous background, to plump fibroblasts in a pale less fibrotic stroma (**e-Fig. 46.16**). Small blood vessels may be conspicuous, and when red blood cell extravasation is present, the lesion can resemble nodular fasciitis. Some mitotic figures may be present, and scattered small lymphoid nodules may be noted at the interface with surrounding normal tissues. If skeletal muscle is involved, it is usually infiltrated with remnants of muscle embedded in the fibrous proliferation (**e-Fig. 46.17**). SMA expression is common, and 46% to 50% of cases have nuclear reactivity for β-catenin (*Am J Surg Pathol.* 2007;31:1299).

3. **Lipofibromatosis (infantile subcutaneous fibromatosis),** another fibrous tumor of childhood, is a slowly growing, painless, ill-defined neoplasm occurring in a variety of sites including the distal extremities (*Am J Surg Pathol.* 2000;24:1491). Grossly, the tumor is an ill-defined white-tan to yellow mass that usually measures <5 cm in greatest dimension. Spindled fibroblastic cells form bands that surround and may separate lobules of fat; the growth pattern resembles fibrous hamartoma but without the nodules of immature mesenchyme. The tumor may express CD34, BCL2, S-100, actin, epithelial membrane antigen and CD99, an unusual phenotypic profile for a fibrous tumor.

4. **Infantile digital fibroma–fibromatosis** (inclusion body fibromatosis, recurring digital fibrous tumor of Reye) presents in the fingers and/or toes (10% to 30% of cases are multifocal), excluding the thumb and great toe, as a firm nodule or nodules. Rare examples of extradigital lesions have been reported (*Am J Surg Pathol.* 2009;33:1). The fibrous proliferation resembles

a desmoid tumor, with confluent infiltration and replacement of the dermis and deeper soft tissues including the skeletal muscle. Isolated adnexal structures are surrounded by the moderately cellular spindle cell proliferation. Paranuclear bodies consisting of actin microfilaments are one of the unique features of this tumor. These tumors are immunopositive for SMA, calponin, CD99, and CD117.

5. **Juvenile nasopharyngeal fibroma** occurs almost exclusively in adolescent males, often presenting with epistaxis. Extensive local growth occurs in the confined spaces of the nasopharynx and into the paranasal sinuses and pterygopalatine fossa (*Int J Pediatr Otorhinolaryngol.* 2011;75:1088). These tumors are firm and have a white-tan cut surface. A diffuse bland fibrous proliferation with a prominent component of small blood vessels is the typical microscopic appearance. This tumor is seen in the setting of familial adenomatous polyposis. The stromal cells express nuclear β-catenin.

C. Intermediate (rarely metastasizing)

1. **Solitary fibrous tumor (SFT)** and **hemangiopericytoma (HPC)** are grouped together as related (if not identical) neoplasms in the WHO classification (*Histopathology* 2006;48:36).

   a. **SFT** is classically found on the pleura (*Semin Diagn Pathol.* 2006;23:44), but has been reported in many different locations (including the dura, intestinal tract, mesentery, liver, skin, thyroid, lung, and orbit) in a broad age group. The tumor is a well-circumscribed, nonencapsulated, firm, white mass measuring 8 cm or less, and may show hemorrhage and focal myxoid change. Bland plump to spindle-shaped cells with a patternless architecture surround branching blood vessels of the type associated with HPC (**e-Fig. 46.18**). The cellularity often varies within individual tumors, and the hypocellular background stroma can have a myxoid fibrous appearance, and can resemble a nerve sheath tumor or low-grade fibromyxoid sarcoma (LGFMS). The tumor cells are immunoreactive for CD34 and CD99, but a subset of tumors also shows reactivity for SMA, BCL2, EMA, and even focal positivity for desmin, cytokeratin, and/or S-100. D2–40 may be positive in a small subset of SFTs, but immunoreactivity is more common in mesotheliomas (*Appl Immunohistochem Mol Morphol.* 2010;18:411).

   Malignant SFTs are usually 10 cm or greater in size and have increased mitotic activity (≥4 mitoses per 10 HPFs), focal necrosis, increased cellularity, marked cytologic atypia in a patchy distribution, infiltrative margins, and show p53 expression (*Arch Pathol Lab Med.* 2010;134:1645). However, the clinical behavior of an individual tumor is not always correlated with the histologic features. Some tumors have a solidly cellular fibrosarcoma-like pattern yet behave in a relatively innocuous fashion.

   b. By the current WHO classification scheme, the diagnosis of *HPC* is limited to STTs that morphologically resemble the cellular areas of SFT (**e-Fig. 46.19**), and that are composed of cells that have the immunoprofile of SFT. By this definition most cases of HPC occur in the deep soft tissues, primarily in the retroperitoneum of the pelvis, but also in the limb girdle and proximal upper or lower extremity. Most tumors are <15 cm in greatest dimension. Microscopically, the tumor cells have a uniform ovoid to spindled appearance in a background of small clefted to branching vascular spaces which are highlighted by CD34 immunoreactivity. Variable immunostaining for SMA is present. Mature adipose tissue is found in the lipomatous variant of HPC. Other settings for HPC include dural-intracranial, sinonasal, or infantile presentations; the latter is regarded as a pattern of infantile myofibroma–myofibromatosis

(*J Clin Neurosci.* 2010;17:469; *J Pediatr Hematol Oncol.* 2011;33:356; *Am J Surg Pathol.* 2003;27:737). As a final note, an HPC-like pattern of growth is seen in synovial sarcoma, malignant peripheral nerve sheath tumor (MPNSTs), mesenchymal chondrosarcoma, infantile fibrosarcoma, thymoma (spindle cell), and endometrial stromal sarcoma, emphasizing the need for careful microscopic examination, immunohistochemistry, and molecular studies for correct diagnosis.

2. **Inflammatory myofibroblastic tumor (IMT)** has a predilection for the mesentery, small intestine (ileocecal region), lung, and bladder, throughout childhood and into young adulthood. Approximately 5% to 10% of IMTs have systemic, constitutional manifestations (fever, anorexia, weight loss, hypochromic microcytic anemia, and/or hypergammaglobulinemia, thrombocytosis), likely due to IL-6 production by the tumor.

The tumor forms a white to tan, whorled, fleshy to myxoid, circumscribed mass measuring 1 to 25 cm in diameter that may also show areas of necrosis, hemorrhage, and calcification. Three basic histologic patterns can be found in any one tumor, although one or two may dominate (**e-Fig. 46.20**): dense fascicles of spindle cells with a mixed population of plasma cells, lymphocytes, and eosinophils in the background; loosely cellular foci with a myxoid and edematous background resembling nodular fasciitis; and hypocellular, collagenized foci with minimal inflammation and dystrophic calcifications. Mitotic figures are found among the spindle cells, but they are not atypical. Some tumors have a predominant round cell or epithelioid pattern, which should raise the possibility of an anaplastic lymphoma kinase (ALK)–positive inflammatory myofibroblastic sarcoma with only a minor spindle-cell component (*Am J Surg Pathol.* 2011;35:135). The differential diagnosis of IMT includes two unrelated lesions, calcifying fibrous pseudotumor with psammomatous calcifications and inflammatory fibroid tumor, the latter usually is present in the stomach or in the small intestine (*Int J Surg Pathol.* 2002;10:189; *Adv Anat Pathol.* 2007;14:178).

Immunohistochemically, a subset of tumors (approximately 50% to 60%, corresponding to those cases that harbor a rearranged *ALK* gene) shows cytoplasmic staining for the *ALK* gene product (*Am J Surg Pathol.* 2001;25:1364). However, virtually all cases are immunoreactive for vimentin; most show reactivity for SMA and variable reactivity for muscle-specific actin (MSA) and desmin; and 25% to 30% are reactive for cytokeratin. ALK-positive tumors may have a more favorable clinical outcome than the ALK-negative tumors (*Am J Surg Pathol.* 2007;31:509). Some IMTs may have a population of IgG4 plasma cells, but this finding does not imply a relationship to the IgG4-related sclerosing disorders (*Mod Pathol.* 2011;24:606).

3. **Congenital infantile fibrosarcoma (CIF)** occurs in children aged 2 years or younger (and can be present at birth) and usually presents in the superficial or deep soft tissues of the distal extremities, although cases also present in the trunk, head and neck, intestinal tract, deep pelvic tissues and heart (*J Clin Oncol.* 2010;28:318). This tumor can be mistaken clinically for a vascular tumor.

The cut surface of the tumor (which can measure up to 10 to 15 cm in diameter) ranges from white to tan, fleshy to firm, and may show areas of hemorrhage, necrosis, and/or myxoid and cystic degeneration; careful gross examination usually shows that the tumor has an infiltrative irregular margin. Several histologic patterns are seen. Interlacing, broad fascicles of spindle cells resembling the herringbone pattern of adult-type fibrosarcoma or monophasic synovial sarcoma are present in some tumors (**e-Fig. 46.21**). Alternatively, the tumor may be composed of more primitive appearing,

TABLE 46.5	Differential Immunohistochemical Profile of Adult-Type Fibrosarcoma and Other Spindle Cell Sarcomas					
	FS	SS	LMS	MPNST	SFT	DFSP
Vim	+	+	+	+	+	+
CK	−	±	−	±	−	−
EMA	−	±	−	±	−	−
SMA	±	−	+	−	−	−
S-100	−	±	±	±	−	−
CD34	−	−	−	−	+	+
CD99	−	+	−	−	−	−

FS, fibrosarcoma; SS, synovial sarcoma; LMS, leiomyosarcoma; MPNST, malignant peripheral nerve sheath tumor; SFT, solitary fibrous tumor; DFSP, dermatofibrosarcoma protuberans; VIM, vimentin; CK, cytokeratin; EMA, epithelial membrane antigen; SMA, smooth muscle actin; S-100, S-100 protein.

shorter spindle cells in a poorly organized pattern, which can raise concern for an embryonal rhabdomyosarcoma (ERMS) or an undifferentiated primitive sarcoma. Small foci of palisading necrosis or confluent areas of hemorrhage are helpful diagnostic features in CIF. Mitotic figures are readily identified. Nuclear pleomorphism, atypical mitoses, and a pale background stroma should raise the possibility of ERMS; immunohistochemistry is useful in the exclusion of the latter neoplasm (Table 46.5). Demonstration of the t(12;15)(p13;q25) translocation (the same translocation present in cellular mesoblastic nephroma) may be necessary in problematic cases. As noted earlier, foci resembling CIF may be present in myofibroma and myofibromatosis (*Pediatr Dev Pathol.* 2008;11:355).

D. **Malignant**
1. **Adult fibrosarcoma (AFS)** is a diagnosis of exclusion, rendered only after other types of spindle cell neoplasms (such as dermatofibrosarcoma, congenital-infantile fibrosarcoma, solitary fibrous tumor, monophasic synovial sarcoma, and MPNST) have been ruled out on the basis of immunohistochemistry and molecular genetic studies (Tables 46.1 and 46.5). Once these studies are performed, 60% to 80% of putative AFSs can be reclassified into another type of sarcoma (*Am J Surg Pathol.* 2010;34:1504). When strictly defined, AFS is primarily seen between the ages of 50 and 75 years, and has a predilection for the deep soft tissues of the head and neck, trunk, and extremities.

    Fibrosarcoma forms a well-circumscribed mass that has a white to tan appearance and a firm consistency on cut surface. Sweeping fascicles of compact spindle cells produce the quintessential herringbone pattern (e-**Fig. 46.22**). The background stroma shows a variable collagen content. Immunopositivity is limited to vimentin and, focally, SMA.

2. **Sclerosing epithelioid fibrosarcoma (SEF)**, a rare variant of fibrosarcoma, occurs over a wide age range, usually in the deep soft tissues of the lower extremities and limb girdles (*Clin Orthop Reh Res.* 2008;466:1485), but has been reported in bone (*Sarcoma.* 2010;431627). The tumor produces a well-circumscribed mass measuring up to 20 cm in greatest dimension, and has a firm white cut surface, although cystic and myxoid areas may be present. The rounded or epithelioid cells that compose the mass have minimal eosinophilic to clear cytoplasm, a low mitotic rate, and are arranged in acini, strands, and nests within a dense collagenous matrix. The tumor cells express vimentin but not CD34, HMB45, and CD45 (*Cancer Genet Cytogenet.* 2000;119:127). A small subset of cases shows focal weak expression of EMA and/or cytokeratin. Foci of SEF-like round cells in a collagenous

background have been reported in LGFMS (*Ann Diagn Pathol.* 2011; *Am J Surg Pathol.* 2007;31:1387).

3. **Low grade fibromyxoid sarcoma (LGFMS)**, another variant of fibrosarcoma, presents as a painless deep soft tissue mass (intra or extramuscular) that has, in some cases, been present for many years. Other sites of origin include the chest wall, thoracic cavity, head and neck, and retroperitoneum. Most tumors present in the fourth to fifth decades, but 5% of cases are diagnosed as early as the second decade; in younger patients, LGFMS is smaller and more superficial. Microscopically, a prominent capsule or pseudocapsule surrounds an 8 to 10 cm mass, which is composed of bland spindle cells with alternating and blending, fibrogenic and myxoid areas, with variable cellular density from one area to another (**e-Fig. 46.23**). Mitotic figures are sparse in number. A subset of tumors (~40%) contains poorly formed giant collagen rosettes consisting of a central hyalinized core surrounded by a rim of fibroblasts with epithelioid features. Another small subgroup has foci of increased cellularity and cytologic atypia of the type usually found in intermediate grade fibrosarcomas, but the prognostic significance of this finding has yet to be established. Both the t(7;16) and t(11;16) translocations are present in LGFMS with or without giant collagen rosettes (*Virchows Arch.* 2010;456:153). Fusion-gene positive tumors are EMA positive; are immunoreactive for CD99 and BCL2; but do not express SMA, S-100, and desmin (*Arch Pathol Lab Med.* 2006;130:1358).

4. **Myxofibrosarcoma (MYFS)** occurs over a wide age range, but has a predilection for individuals over 60 years of age; this tumor is also seen in young adults. Most cases present in the dermis and subcutis; only about one-third occur in the deep soft tissues of the lower (50% to 60% of cases) and upper extremities (25% to 30%). Rare cases occur in the breast, heart, retroperitoneum, paratesticular tissues, and orbit. Most tumors have a myxoid and infiltrative appearance, but more solid foci are present on gross examination. A multinodular growth pattern, variable cellularity within a myxoid stroma, and incomplete fibrous septa that course through the tumor are consistent microscopic features (*Hum Pathol.* 2004;35:612). Low-grade tumors, generally smaller and superficial, are hypocellular with a prominent myxoid matrix that contains only scattered plump or stellate tumor cells, with a relatively low number of mitotic figures. High-grade MYFS, generally larger and deeper, show marked cellular pleomorphism, multinucleated giant cells, a high mitotic rate (with easily identified atypical mitotic forms), and areas of solid growth (**e-Fig. 46.24**). The tumor cells express vimentin, but otherwise do not have a characteristic immunophenotype. Progression to a higher-grade sarcoma is seen in recurrent MYFS. Complex karyotypes have been identified and are similar to those seen in leiomyosarcoma (LMS) and undifferentiated pleomorphic sarcoma (*Virchows Arch.* 2010;456:201).

5. **Acral myxoinflammatory fibroblastic sarcoma** (inflammatory myxohyaline tumor) is a low-grade neoplasm in most cases arising in an articular–juxtaarticular location of the hands, feet, or digits of adult although examples in nonacral sites are seen (*Ann Diagn Pathol.* 2002;6:272; *J Cutan Pathol.* 2008;35:192). Clinically, the tumor is a dermal-subcutaneous nodule, measuring 2 to 3 cm, with a multinodular architecture. Microscopically, the tumor has a fibrous and myxoid stroma containing a mixed population of spindled to epithelioid cells, ganglion-like cells, Reed–Sternberg-like cells, bizarre multinucleated giant cells, and multivacuolated lipoblast-like cells. The tumor cells are immunopositive for CD34 and CD68.

V. **FIBROHISTIOCYTIC TUMORS.** As the name suggests, these neoplasms are composed of cells that have fibrohistiocytic morphology. However, electron microscopy and immunohistochemistry have firmly established that the cells comprising these tumors (other than the foamy macrophages) are, in fact, not histiocytes but rather primitive mesenchymal cells, fibroblasts, and myofibroblasts. The circulating or bone marrow fibrocyte is another potential candidate progenitor cell for this group of tumors (*Lab Invest.* 2007;87:858).

A. Benign

1. **Synovial tendon–based tumors.** It is uncertain whether synovial tumors are best classified as fibrohistiocytic tumors (as in the WHO classification) or as tumors differentiating toward synovial cells. In any event, this family of articular and extra-articular neoplasms includes giant cell tumor of tendon sheath (GCTTS) and diffuse-type giant cell tumor. Both tumors share translocations of chromosome 1p13 (Table 46.1), which often also involve 2q35 resulting in formation of a *COL6A3-CSF1* fusion gene (*Proc Natl Acad Sci USA.* 2006;103:690).

   a. **GCTTS** (also known as **giant cell tumor of tendon sheath, localized type; nodular tenosynovitis**) is a localized tumor that arises from the synovium of joints, bursae, and tendon sheath or adjacent tissues. The hand, and less often the wrist, ankle, foot, knee, elbow, and hip, are various sites of the tumor, which clinically presents as a painless mass, mainly in adults. GCTTS forms a firm lobulated yellowish-brown to tan circumscribed mass that measures 0.5 to 4 cm; erosion into adjacent bone is seen in larger lesions. Mononuclear cells with rounded to plumb-spindled features, foamy macrophages, siderophages, and multinucleate giant cells with a variably prominent hyalinized stroma (e-**Fig. 46.25**) are the microscopic elements of this multinodular neoplasm.

   b. **GCTTS, diffuse type (pigmented villonodular tenosynovitis)** presents as an intra-articular proliferation predominantly in the knee and hip joint, whereas the extra-articular tumor predominantly involves the periarticular soft tissues in the region of the knee and thigh (some extra-articular tumors have been localized to muscle and subcutis). This tumor has been reported in Noonan and NF1 syndromes. The tumor has a resemblance to GCTTS, although giant cells are less numerous or absent altogether. Pseudosynovial and blood-filled pseudoalveolar spaces are a common finding in the otherwise monotonous mononuclear proliferation (e-**Fig. 46.26**). Mitotic activity is usually present (in rare cases >5 mitoses per 10 HPFs), but atypical mitotic figures are absent. The immunoprofile of CD68, MSA, and desmin expression is the same as for GCTTS.

   Classification of this neoplasm as an intermediate (locally aggressive) tumor is based on the fact that over 45% of intra-articular and up to 50% of extra-articular tumors recur. Clearly malignant tumors are associated with the metastasis; this subgroup has a high mitotic rate (over 20 mitoses per 10 HPFs), necrosis, and cellular atypia (*Am J Surg Pathol.* 1997;21:153).

2. **Deep benign fibrous histiocytoma** is very likely the subcutaneous and deep soft tissue counterpart to cutaneous fibrous histiocytoma–dermatofibroma. There is a predilection for the extremities and head and neck region, although this tumor is also seen in the retroperitoneum and mediastinum (*Am J Surg Pathol.* 2008;32:354). The tumor is a circumscribed mass, commonly <4 cm in greatest dimension, that displays a similar range of histologic features as in the dermal-based lesions including a storiform architecture of spindle cells intermixed with mononuclear and multinucleated giant cells, hemosiderotic macrophages, xanthomatized histiocytes, and aneurysmal erythrocyte-filled spaces. Necrosis and frequent mitotic figures should be noted with concern.

3. **Fibrohistiocytic lesions** that typically occur in the skin (see Chap. 38) are dermal dendrocytic proliferations like the reticulohistiocytoma, Langerhans cell histiocytosis, and juvenile xanthogranuloma (*Am J Surg Pathol.* 2003;27:579; *Histopathology.* 2010;56:148).

B. **Intermediate (rarely metastasizing)**

1. **Plexiform fibrohistiocytic tumor (PFH)** primarily occurs in the first three decades of life with a preference for the extremities and head and neck (*Ann Diagn Pathol.* 2007;11:313). Grossly, it is a firm, multinodular and poorly circumscribed mass that usually measures <3 cm in greatest dimension in the dermis and subcutis. Microscopically, the architectural pattern is that of nodules or elongated groups of cells with a plexiform arrangement. Three cell types are present in the nodules: central multinucleated giant cells, mononuclear histiocyte-like cells, and spindled fibroblast-like cells (e-**Fig. 46.27**). Since one of the cell types may dominate, an appreciation of the overall architecture is important for diagnosis since the nodules can have few, if any, multinucleated cells and the spindle cell foci can resemble fibromatosis. The tumor cells express SMA and vimentin; CD68 reactivity is also present but is confined to the giant cells and mononuclear histiocyte-like cells. Approximately 30% to 35% of cases locally recur and <5% metastasize to regional lymph nodes and beyond (*Arch Pathol Lab Med.* 2007;131:1135; *Am J Dermatopathol.* 2004;26:141). A histogenetic relationship between PFH and cellular neurothekeoma has been proposed since there are overlapping microscopic and immunophenotypic features (*Am J Surg Pathol.* 2009;33:905; *Am J Surg Pathol.* 2007;31:329).

2. **Giant cell tumor of soft tissue** occurs in the superficial soft tissue of the lower and upper extremities, and occasionally at other sites. It is a circumscribed, nodular mass that has a soft, fleshy, gray to red-brown cut surface. Individual nodules of the mass measure up to 1.5 cm and are separated by fibrous septa that contain hemosiderin-laden macrophages. Microscopically, admixed mononuclear round to oval cells and multinucleated osteoclast-like giant cells are set in a richly vascular stroma. Mitotic activity can be brisk (up to 30 mitotic figures per 10 HPFs are often present), but cellular pleomorphism and atypia are absent. Metaplastic bone is noted in up to 50% of cases, and definitive foci of vascular invasion are identified in 30% of cases. The multinucleated giant cells are strongly CD68 immunopositive, whereas the mononuclear cells express SMA and vimentin but show only focal CD68 immunoreactivity.

C. **Malignant**

1. **Pleomorphic malignant fibrous histiocytoma (MFH)/undifferentiated high-grade pleomorphic sarcoma** is the diagnostic term reserved for those obvious high-grade sarcomas typically presenting in the deep soft tissues, which lack a lineage-specific immunophenotype. Considerable reassessment and revisionism have been directed toward the question of whether MFH represents a specific tumor type or a final common pathway of high-grade sarcomas (*Am J Surg Pathol.* 1992;16:213; *Am J Surg Pathol.* 1996;20:131; *Am J Surg Pathol.* 2001;25:1030). These neoplasms are characterized by complex cytogenetic rearrangements that can involve over 30% of the genome (*Virchows Arch.* 2010;456:201).

The tumor preferentially arises in the extremity and trunk, including the retroperitoneum. Individuals over 40 years of age present with a rapidly enlarging mass, and about 5% have metastatic disease at diagnosis, usually in the lung. The tumor measures 15 to 20 cm, if not greater, and has a white to tan-white, fleshy to fibrous cut surface, with areas of necrosis and hemorrhage. The microscopic pattern is often complex (e-**Fig. 46.28**), with field to field variation in terms of spindle cells, rounded to ovoid cells, and multinucleated cells. Myxoid foci can resemble areas of pleomorphic LPS but have an absence of convincing lipoblasts. One consistent microscopic feature of the tumor is high nuclear grade with numerous atypical mitotic figures; extensive necrosis with cystic degeneration and hemorrhage are other common features. Some of these tumors are immunoreactive for SMA and/or desmin, and so the differential diagnosis includes pleomorphic LMS or myofibrosarcoma (*Histopathology*. 2001;38:499). The CD68 positivity present in most cases is regarded by many as nonspecific. In the retroperitoneum, sarcomatoid carcinoma of the kidney, pancreas, and gallbladder should be excluded.

2. **Giant cell MFH/undifferentiated pleomorphic sarcoma with giant cells** is a rare neoplasm, which is composed of undifferentiated pleomorphic cells with associated stromal osteoclastic giant cells (in contrast to pleomorphic multinucleated tumor cells). Since it is now recognized that a prominent stromal osteoclastic giant cell reaction is a feature of many poorly differentiated carcinomas as well as sarcomas, putative cases of giant cell MFH should be carefully studied to exclude the presence of an even focal definable line of differentiation indicative of a specific carcinoma or sarcoma type. LMS and carcinoma of the breast, pancreas, biliary tract, and urinary tract are reported with similar osteoclast-like giant cells.

3. **Inflammatory MFH/undifferentiated pleomorphic sarcoma with prominent inflammation** is a diagnosis now reserved for an undifferentiated high-grade pleomorphic sarcoma with a prominent neutrophilic infiltrate, in addition to histiocytes, eosinophils, and xanthoma cells. Most cases arise in the retroperitoneum. Some of these tumors may be dedifferentiated LPS (*J Pathol*. 2004;203:822).

VI. **SMOOTH MUSCLE TUMORS.** Smooth muscle tumors are neoplasms in most cases, but a small subset of cases are hamartomas that usually present in children. Neoplasms in this category are ubiquitous in distribution from the skin and soft tissues, to visceral sites including the gastrointestinal and female reproductive tracts. In most cases, the pathologic distinction between the benign and malignant smooth muscle neoplasm is reasonably straightforward, with the exception of the leiomyoma of deep soft tissues and some tumors arising in the uterus (*Histopathology*. 2006;48:97). Many of the biologic features of this group of tumors are perplexing. For example, superficial, often small LMSs of skin may have the same microscopic features as their large deep counterparts even though the former often have a favorable prognosis (*J Am Acad Dermatol*. 2002;46:477). Similarly, an entirely benign appearing leiomyoma of the uterus can have an intravascular growth pattern with a capacity to "metastasize" to the heart and lungs (*Obstet Gynecol Surv*. 2010;65:189).

A. **Benign**

1. **Angioleiomyoma** (vascular leiomyoma) is a deep dermal or subcutaneous neoplasm often associated with pain that in women typically occurs in the lower extremities, but in men more often occurs in the head and upper extremities (*Skeletal Radiol*. 2008;37:339). These tumors, usually measuring 2 cm or less, consist of three subtypes: a solid subtype of mature smooth muscle cells with virtually no mitotic activity and small slit-like vascular channels; a venous subtype composed of less compact smooth muscle bundles, with venous-type vascular channels that blend with the intravascular smooth muscle; and a cavernous subtype with dilated vascular channels with indistinct smooth muscle walls. The differential diagnosis includes angiomyomatous hamartoma, which is an inguinal or popliteal lymph node–based lesion (*Ann Diagn Pathol*. 2008;12:372).

B. **Leiomyoma of deep soft tissue** is a rare neoplasm that, as its name suggests, usually develops in deep subcutis, skeletal muscle, the pelvic retroperitoneum, and the abdominal cavity (typically in the omentum and mesentery). This tumor can measure in excess of 30 cm. It is composed of bland appearing highly differentiated smooth muscle cells that have minimal atypia and a very low mitotic rate (for tumors in the extremities and intra-abdominal tumors in males, the mitotic rate is <1 mitosis per 50 HPFs; for peritoneal/retroperitoneal tumors in females, the mitotic rate is ≤5 per 50 HPFs). While degenerative changes such as fibrosis, myxoid change, hyalinization, and calcification may be present, necrosis is absent. The diagnosis of a deep leiomyoma should be approached with caution and should rely on the absence of virtually any mitotic activity and atypia (*Adv Anat Pathol.* 2002;9:351; *Ann Diagn Pathol.* 2003; 7:60).

Pilar leiomyoma and uterine smooth muscle tumors are discussed elsewhere (see Chaps. 39 and 33, respectively). There is a substantial literature on the cytogenetics of uterine leiomyomas, but considerably less on the extrauterine counterparts (*Cancer Genet Cytogenet.* 2005;158:1).

C. Malignant

1. **Leiomyosarcoma (LMS)** is typically a malignancy presenting in mid-life and beyond. There are four clinicopathologic settings: a retroperitoneal mass; a tumor arising from a large blood vessel with a preference for veins of the lower extremity and inferior vena cava; a subcutaneous or intramuscular tumor of the extremities; and a dermal-based neoplasm. Uterine and intestinal LMSs are not considered in this chapter, although the uterus is the most common primary site overall for LMS (*Adv Anat Pathol.* 2011;18:60).

   Except for cutaneous LMS, these tumors usually measure in excess of 6 cm and have a trabeculated or smooth, glistening, white-gray cut surface. High-grade tumors are accompanied by necrosis and hemorrhage. Architecturally, the tumors are composed of intersecting bundles of eosinophilic spindle cells with elongated nuclei with blunted ends (e-**Fig. 46.29**). Nuclear pleomorphism and an increased mitotic rate with atypical mitotic forms are characteristic. Poorly differentiated LMS is a pleomorphic high-grade sarcoma whose smooth muscle differentiation is highlighted by immunoreactivity for SMA, desmin, and h-caldesmon. Focal expression of keratin, EMA, CD34, and S100 may be present. These tumors typically have complex karyotypes with gains and losses across multiple chromosomes (*Virchows Arch.* 2010;456:201).

   A distinct clinicopathologic group of smooth muscle neoplasms are recognized in the immunocompromised setting; these tumors are associated with genomic integration of Epstein–Barr virus (EBV) (*J Clin Pathol.* 2007; 60:1358; *Am J Surg Pathol.* 2006;30:75; *J Cutan Pathol.* 2011;38:731) and have been described in both visceral, soft tissue and cutaneous sites. These tumors have low-grade spindle cell features to the extent that the traditional criteria for the diagnosis of LMS are not met in all cases, and are designated as EBV-associated smooth muscle tumors in some cases.

VII. PERICYTIC (PERIVASCULAR) TUMORS.
Tumors in this category show evidence of myoid/contractile perivascular cell differentiation. Morphologically, they have a tendency to grow in a circumferential perivascular pattern.

A. Benign

1. **Glomus tumor** usually occurs in the subungual region of the hand, wrist, and foot, but not to the exclusion of other sites including the bone, lung, and intestinal tract (*Arch Pathol Lab Med.* 2008;132:1448). Those tumors are <1 cm in greatest dimension in most cases, and are painful with minimal tactile stimulation or exposure to cold. Microscopically, these tumors consists of a mixture of glomus cells (characterized as uniform, small, rounded cells with eosinophilic to amphophilic cytoplasm and a central nucleus), smooth muscle cells, and central vascular space (e-**Fig. 46.30**). On the basis

of the relative proportion of these three elements, there are three subtypes of glomus tumor: solid, composed of nests of glomus cells surrounding capillary-sized vessels; glomangioma, composed of small clusters of glomus cells surrounding dilated vessels; and glomangiomyoma, in which there is a transition from typical round glomus cells to elongated cells that resemble mature smooth muscle. Glomangiomas may be multiple or familial, and are likely vascular malformations (*Arch Dermatol.* 2004;140:971).

2. **Myopericytoma,** previously interpreted as a hemangiopericytoma, usually arises in the subcutis of the distal extremities (*J Clin Pathol.* 2006;59:67). Less than 2 cm in greatest dimension, this tumor is unencapsulated but well circumscribed. Microscopically, the tumor is composed of a densely cellular population of oval to spindle-shaped cells with eosinophilic to amphophilic cytoplasm arranged in multilayered concentric profiles around compressed blood vessels. Mitotic figures are inconspicuous. There is diffuse immunopositivity for SMA and focal immunopositivity for CD34.

B. **Malignant.** Malignant glomus tumor (glomangiosarcoma) is rare and seemingly arises from a benign-appearing glomus tumor. The characteristic findings are a visceral or subfascial origin, a size >2 cm, marked nuclear atypia, and atypical mitotic figures. However, a subset of tumors does not have all of these findings; these cases are designated as tumors of uncertain malignant potential (*Am J Surg Pathol.* 2001;25:1). The round cell type is composed of poorly differentiated round cells, so SMA and pericellular type IV collagen are required for diagnosis. A spindle cell variant has features of LMS or fibrosarcoma.

VIII. SKELETAL MUSCLE

A. Nonneoplastic disorders

1. **Preparation of skeletal muscle biopsies.** Histopathologic examination of skeletal muscle biopsies, whether obtained through an open biopsy or through a needle biopsy, continues to have a critical role in the evaluation of patients with suspected myopathy (*Curr Neuro Neurosci Rep.* 2004;4:81). One portion of the biopsy should be formalin fixed and paraffin embedded according to standard laboratory protocols; another should be frozen for enzyme histochemistry studies; and the remainder should be fixed in glutaraldehyde for electron microscopic studies. While the histopathologic evaluation of skeletal muscle biopsies is a key component in the evaluation of neuromuscular disorders, and can be used to diagnose a variety of inherited, inflammatory, and toxic myopathies, it should only be performed in the context of a thorough history and clinical examination that has included appropriate laboratory studies (including measurement of serum creatine kinase) and electromyography. A number of inflammatory, toxic, and axial myopathies have characteristic histopathologic findings, and immunohistochemical studies can be utilized to characterize inflammatory infiltrates when present (*Autoimmunity.* 2006;39:161).

2. **Muscular dystrophies** and other *congenital myopathies* are diagnosed primarily on the basis of clinical and electromyographic features. Increasingly, the histopathologic evaluation of muscle biopsies in these settings has been supplanted by genetic testing as an increasing number of diseases has been characterized at a genetic level (*Pediatr Dev Pathol.* 2006;9:427; *Brain Pathol.* 2001;11:206).

3. **Mitochondrial myopathies,** which traditionally have been diagnosed on the basis of the demonstration of so-called ragged-red fibers by Gomori trichrome stain, are increasingly diagnosed on the basis of genetic testing since the genetic abnormalities in mitochondria that underlie these disease have recently been characterized (*Submicrosc Cytol Pathol.* 2006;38:201; *Biosci Rep.* 2007;27:23).

B. Benign

1. **Rhabdomyoma** by definition shows skeletal muscle differentiation, and includes cardiac rhabdomyoma and extra-cardiac rhabdomyoma (which has two subtypes: fetal and adult). Both cardiac and fetal rhabdomyomas may be hamartomas rather than true neoplasms; tuberous sclerosis and nevoid basal cell carcinoma syndrome accompany these tumors, respectively (*Ear Nose Throat J.* 2004;83:716; *Pediatrics.* 2006;118:e1146; *Congenital Heart Dis.* 2011;6:183).

   a. **Fetal rhabdomyoma** occurs almost exclusively in children under the age of 10 years, with a predilection for the postauricular region and chest wall (*Am J Surg Pathol.* 2008;32:485). The tumor forms a nodule in the subcutis or deeper soft tissues that has a circumscribed noninfiltrative pattern and is composed of bundles of fetal myotubes with interspersed small immature-appearing mesenchymal cells. The classic or myxoid pattern must be differentiated from ERMS, the latter of which has a less well-organized pattern, hyperchromatic nuclei, and mitotic figures. The so-called intermediate or cellular pattern (juvenile rhabdomyoma) is characterized by skeletal muscle differentiation beyond the fetal myotube stage.

   b. **Adult rhabdomyoma** is solitary in 75% to 80% of cases, but in about 25% of cases is multinodular, even multicentric. There is an overwhelming predilection for the head and neck region (especially the larynx and pharynx) (*Am J Otolaryngol.* 2011;32:240). Microscopically, lobules of large uniform polygonal cells with abundant granular, vacuolated, or eosinophilic cytoplasm; well-defined cell borders; and round nuclei with a prominent nucleolus are present. Cytoplasmic cross striations and rod-like inclusions are also present, in addition to abundant glycogen. Complete excision is recommended, since recurrence occurs in >40% of cases that have been incompletely excised.

   c. **Genital rhabdomyoma** presents almost exclusively in the vagina in women between the ages of 35 and 50 years as a solitary 1 to 3 cm polyp that may have been present for several years. Microscopically, bland, interlacing, haphazardly arranged rounded to strap-like cells that have abundant eosinophilic cytoplasm with cross striations, cytoplasmic glycogen, and a centrally located round nucleus with a prominent nucleolus are present. The tumor cells are embedded in a fibrous stroma with dilated vessels. Local excision is curative.

C. Malignant

1. **Embryonal rhabdomyosarcoma (ERMS)** is the most common soft tissue sarcoma of childhood (50% to 60% of cases), typically presents before 10 years of age, and accounts for 75% to 85% of all rhabdomyosarcomas in children. The other types of rhabdomyosarcomas, alveolar and pleomorphic types, comprise 20% to 30% and 5% or less, respectively. ERMS has a predilection for the head and neck (25% to 35% of cases) and pelvis-genitourinary tract (30% to 40% of cases). Unlike alveolar rhabdomyosarcoma (ARMS), a minority of ERMS presents in the peripheral soft tissues. The three basic microscopic patterns of ERMS are botryoid, spindle, and not otherwise specified (NOS), which proportionately account for 5%, 10%, and 85% of cases, respectively. The botryoid and spindle subtypes have a "superior" outcome, whereas the NOS subtype has an "intermediate" to "poor" prognosis (*Pediatr Dev Pathol.* 1998;1:550).

   The preoperative–pretreatment staging of childhood RMS is a multitier system, which includes the status of the tumor before treatment utilizing a TMN-based system (Table 46.6). The prognostically favorable sites of RMS in children include the orbit, nonparameningeal head and neck, common

TABLE 46.6	Pretreatment TNM Staging of Childhood Rhabdomyosarcoma[a]				
Stage	Sites	T invasiveness	T size	Regional nodes	Metastases
I	Orbit	T1 or T2	a or b	N0N1 or NX	M0
	Head and neck[b]	T1 or T2	a or b	N0N1 or NX	M0
	Genitourinary[c]	T1 or T2	a or b	N0N1 or NX	M0
II	Bladder/prostate	T1 or T2	a	N0 or NX	M0
	Extremity	T1 or T2	a	N0 or NX	M0
	Cranial	T1 or T2	a	N0 or NX	M0
	parameningeal	T1 or T2	a	N0 or NX	M0
	Others[d]				
III	Bladder/prostate	T1 or T2	a	N1	M0
	Extremity	T1 or T2	b	N0N1 or NX	M0
	Cranial	T1 or T2	b	N0N1 or NX	M0
	parameningeal	T1 or T2	b	N0N1 or NX	M0
	Others[d]				
IV	All	T1 or T2	a or b	N0 or N1	M1

[a]TNM pretreatment staging classification for the Intergroup Rhabdomyosarcoma Study-IV.
[b]Excluding parameningeal.
[c]Nonbladder/nonprostate.
[d]Includes trunk, retroperitoneum, and so on.
T, tumor; T1, confined to anatomic site of origin; T2, extension and/or fixation to surrounding tissue; a, <5 cm in diameter; b, ≥5 cm in diameter; N0, no clinically involved regional lymph nodes; N1, clinically involved: NX, clinical status unknown; M0, no distant metastasis; M1, distant metastasis present.
From *Pediatr Dev Pathol.* 1998;1:550.

bile duct, bladder, paratesticular soft tissues, and prostate; these are also sites of predilection for the favorable histology botryoid ERMS. All other sites are regarded as unfavorable where either the intermediate histology ERMS (NOS) or the unfavorable ARMS is the pathologic subtype. Tumor size (less than or greater than 5 cm) is another important variable in outcome with smaller RMSs having a better prognosis.

Because most ERMSs occur at sites which do not lend themselves to primary surgical resection with the prospect of negative tumor margins, biopsies and posttreatment excisions are the two specimen types seen most often for pathology examination. In general, ERMS is a soft, often gelatinous-myxoid mass whose shape and size accommodate its anatomic site. When the tumor arises in a hollow space or viscus like the nasopharynx, common bile duct, bladder, uterine cervix, or vagina, it has a polypoid configuration with the botryoid pattern of small primitive cells concentrated beneath the surface epithelium; interspersed among the small cells, differentiated rhabdomyoblasts may be identified. Otherwise, the tumor (which may measure up to 20 cm in diameter) has a rounded to ovoid configuration without a definite capsule or pseudocapsule; the cut surface has a faint multilobular appearance in which hemorrhage is more common than necrosis. The consistency of the tumor reflects the cellularity and the character of the stroma.

It is misleading to characterize ERMS as a uniform "round cell" neoplasm since the morphology of the tumor cells is often quite diverse, ranging from short spindle or round cells, to ovoid cells with or without a delicate cytoplasmic tail, to larger cells with pale vacuolated to eosinophilic cytoplasm (e-Fig. 46.31). The intercellular space often has a pale mucoid to myxoid appearance, which is seen on occasion in Ewing sarcoma/primitive neuroectodermal tumor (EWS/PNET) and malignant rhabdoid tumor. Where there is stroma, the tumor cells are larger, more compact, and more likely to have bright eosinophilic cytoplasm. In many tumors, the fact that no two high magnification microscopic fields have identical features reflects the polymorphous character of many ERMS. Diffuse and/or lobular growth patterns are seen either as a dominant or as a mixed feature. Those tumors composed predominately of spindle cells resemble a LMS or fibrosarcoma, but with immature rhabdomyoblasts present among the spindle cells.

A difficult assessment is the determination of "viable" tumor in a posttreatment biopsy. By convention, if the biopsy contains tumor cells with features seen in the pretreatment biopsy, residual viable tumor is the appropriate interpretation. Differentiated rhabdomyoblasts with negative Ki-67 (MIB-1) staining are considered nonproliferative and nonviable.

The immunophenotype correlates with the degree of skeletal muscle differentiation. Primitive ERMS may show only vimentin expression, although myoD1 and/or myogenin nuclear positivity is often present, but in a minority of the tumor cells. Most ERMSs are positive for desmin in 15% to 50% of tumor cells, whereas myogenin tends to display a bright nuclear signal in 15% to 30% of cells in contrast to ARMS in which myogenin shows near 100% nuclear positivity (*Am J Surg Pathol.* 2008;32:1513). Differentiating rhabdomyoblasts show desmin and/or MSA expression, while differentiated cells also are immunoreactive for myosin.

2. **Alveolar rhabdomyosarcoma (ARMS),** like EWS/PNET and hematolymphoid malignancies, is one of the quintessential malignant round cell neoplasms of childhood. Most cases are diagnosed in adolescents and young adults, although ARMS is seen infrequently in infants (*Cancer.* 2011;117:3493). Primary sites include the extremities, paraspinal and perineal regions, and the paranasal sinuses. Microscopically, the tumor has two general patterns: solid sheets of uniform high-grade round cells without extracellular mucin, and the classic alveolar pattern with tumor cells attached to incomplete fibrovascular septa dividing the loosely arranged cells into nests (e-**Fig. 46.32**). Both patterns can be seen in metastatic ARMS (the initial encounter with the tumor may be in a lymph node or bone metastasis since ARMS may present with disseminated metastatic disease). Most ARMSs are strongly and diffusely immunopositive for desmin and myogenin (*Pathol Oncol Res.* 2008;14:233). ALK protein overexpression is found in 40% to 50% of cases (*Pediatr Dev Pathol.* 2009;12:275).

The demonstration of the *FOX01 (FKHR)* breakapart by FISH is an important adjunct in the diagnosis of ARMS, with a positive result in approximately 75% to 80% of cases (*Am J Pathol.* 2009;174:550). The *PAX3-FOX01* fusion gene (resulting from t(2;13)) is more common (present in 70% to 80% of fusion positive cases) than the *PAX7-FOX01* fusion gene (resulting from t(1;13)). Fusion-negative ARMS has a gene profile and prognosis more like ERMS, but the significance of this observation remains unsettled (*J Clin Oncol.* 2010;28:2151) since specific fusion type and pattern of ARMS do not appear to correlate with outcome. Rarely RMS has a mixed pattern of ARMS and ERMS; these tumors represent a diagnostic dilemma, which may be resolved by FISH to determine the fusion status of the tumor.

3. **Pleomorphic rhabdomyosarcoma** is a high-grade sarcoma that presents in the deep soft tissues (*Am J Surg Pathol.* 2009;33:1850). These rare neoplasms occur overwhelmingly in adults. A poorly differentiated pleomorphic sarcoma resembling pleomorphic undifferentiated sarcoma and/or an equally high-grade spindle cell sarcoma are the histologic features. The eosinophilic cytoplasm may or may not have cross striations. Both desmin and

myogenin are positive; pancytokeratin and CD34 are reactive in a minority of cases.

4. **Sclerosing rhabdomyosarcoma,** a rare putative variant of rhabdomyosarcoma, may have a pattern of gene amplification of chromosome 12q more like LPS (*Hum Pathol.* 2009;40:1347).

5. **Ectomesenchymoma** is a rare neoplasm that occurs in children for the most part. It may have ERMS- or ARMS-like features, with populations of cells with a range of neural differentiation, from ganglion cells to more primitive neuroectodermal cells that express a variety of neural and myogenic markers. This tumor has a predilection for the head and neck including the CNS (*Pediatr Dev Pathol.* 2000;3:290; *J Neurosurg.* 2011;7:94). These tumors seem to bridge the molecular interface between RMS and MPNST (*Diagn Mol Pathol.* 2007;16:243; *Acta Neuropathol.* 2007;113:695).

IX. **VASCULAR TUMORS.** Vascular or vasoformative lesions constitute a pathogenetically heterogenous group of lesions composed of endothelial-lined vascular spaces with a circumscribed or more diffuse pattern of growth. These lesions are solitary or less often multifocal. They may be initially noted at or shortly after birth or become clinically evident in later childhood or adulthood. The skin and underlying soft tissues are the most common sites of presentation, but there are few anatomic sites or organs that are excluded from involvement (*Am J Surg Pathol.* 2010;34:942). In terms of pathogenesis, vascular lesions are reactive (etiology either known or unknown), malformative, or neoplastic.

A. **Inflammatory lesions.** Inflammatory disorders of the vessels, including the vasculitides, are covered in the chapter on the cardiovascular system (see Chap. 9).

B. **Reactive vascular proliferations.** This heading includes lesions that are generally thought to be reactive and nonneoplastic, although many mimic vascular tumors clinicopathologically.

1. **Papillary endothelial hyperplasia (PEH, Masson vegetant hemangioma)** is usually subdivided into a primary type (occurring in a vein in the head and neck or fingers) and a secondary type (arising in a preexisting hemangioma, hemorridal vein, or thrombohematoma) (*Auris Nasus Larynx.* 2009;36:363). Microscopically, numerous, small, delicate papillae with hyaline cores project into a vascular lumen (**e-Fig. 46.33**). Often there is a transition between an organizing fibrin clot and the PEH. A single layer of plump endothelial cells without appreciable cytologic atypia is characteristic, and helps differentiate it from angiosarcoma, which does not arise from a blood vessel or hematoma. With continued organization of the clot, the papillae fuse and form an anastomosing network of vessels with eventual recanalization.

2. **Glomeruloid hemangioma** is an uncommon, multifocal, primarily intravascular capillary proliferation that is associated with Castleman disease and the POEMS (*p*olyneuropathy, *o*rganomegaly, *e*ndocrinopathy, *M*-protein, and *s*kin changes) syndrome. Glomeruloid capillary proliferations within blood vessels of the dermis, deep soft tissue, or viscera are the microscopic features. Glomeruloid capillary tufts have an outer layer of pericytes but are lined by bland endothelial cells with or without cytoplasmic vacuolation.

3. **Lobular capillary hemangioma** (LCH) is one of the more common vascular lesions which is seen primarily in the skin where satellite lesions may occur, but the anatomic distribution is widespread in the head and neck (nasal and oral cavities), liver, and gastrointestinal tract. Microscopically, the lesion is pedunculated with a collarette of epidermis and is composed of lobular arrays of uniform capillary-sized vessels with a central thick-walled feeder vessel (**e-Fig. 46.34**). Ulceration of the epidermis with inflammation and

hemorrhage can obscure the underlying pathology, with superimposed granulation tissue (*J Eur Acad Dematol Venereol.* 2001;15:106). Extramedullary hematopoiesis may be seen. Other presentations include as a more dermal-based tumor producing a nodule rather than a polyp, and as an intravascular process. Lesions with more slit-like vascular spaces with a retained lobular architecture can resemble Kaposi sarcoma.

4. **Bacillary angiomatosis** has a close clinical and pathologic resemblance to LCH, but also features an interstitial neutrophilic infiltrate and amorphous deposits of Warthin–Starry positive aggregates of *Bartonella henselae* or *B. quintana*. Virtually all cases of bacillary angiomatosis occur in immunocompromised individuals (*Am J Dermatopathol.* 2011;33:513; *Clin Dermatol.* 2009;27:271).

5. **Vascular transformation of lymph nodes** (nodal angiomatosis) occurs as a secondary change in lymph nodes due to lymphatic and/or venous obstruction. Ectatic capillary-sized vessels within the subcapsular space and nodal sinuses are the microscopic features. The differential diagnosis is Kaposi sarcoma.

C. Benign

1. **Hemangioma** is the most common cutaneous and soft tissue tumor of infancy and childhood, and accounts for ~7% of benign STTs overall. Although most hemangiomas are superficially located, the liver and parotid gland may be involved in infants (*J Pediatr Surg.* 2007;42:62; *Ann Diagn Pathol.* 2002;6:339). There has been substantial revision in the classification of vasoformative lesions into vascular neoplasms or malformations based in part on glucose transporter 1 (GLUT-1) immunoreactivity in the majority of vascular neoplasms and its absence in malformations (*Hum Pathol.* 2000;31:11; *Clin Plast Surg.* 2005;32:99).

   a. **Capillary hemangioma** is the most common type of hemangioma and has a predilection for the head and neck. It is usually diagnosed in infants and young children, hence the designation infantile hemangioma. These lesions have rapid proliferative and prolonged involutional stages; the latter can continue into early to late childhood. The tumor is clinically a purple to reddish macule or nodule centered in the skin or subcutaneous tissue. Microscopically, cellular lobules during the proliferative phase may have few identifiable vascular lumina and readily identifiable mitotic figures. With involution, the vascular spaces are well defined, mitoses are absent, and a collagenous stroma becomes more prominent in the interstitium. The current classification of infantile hemangioma as a benign vasoformative lesion reflects the observation that GLUT-1 immunoreactivity is present in the majority of cases (*Clin Plast Surg.* 2011;38:31).

   b. **Congenital hemangioma** is present at birth and has two subtypes, involution congenital hemangioma and noninvoluting congenital hemangioma (*J Am Acad Dermatol.* 2004;50:875; *Cardiovasc Pathol.* 2006; 303:2006). The two subtypes have distinctive microscopic features and are GLUT-1 immunonegative unlike infantile hemangioma (*Arch Facial Plast Surg.* 2005;7:307).

   c. **Tufted angioma** typically presents in infancy and is characterized by scattered cellular vascular nodules associated with variably prominent dilated lymphatic spaces in the dermis and subcutis (*Arch Dermatol.* 2010;146:758). The endothelial cells may be spindled as in the related kaposiform hemangioendothelioma (KHE), or more epithelioid in appearance (e-**Fig. 46.35**). The tumors have in common expression for D2–40 and may be complicated by Kasabach–Merritt syndrome. Neither tufted angioma or KHE is GLUT-1 positive.

d. **Verrucous hemangioma** is composed of a mixture of cavernous and capillary vessels immediately beneath a hyperkeratotic, acanthotic epidermis.

e. **Cherry angioma** is suspected to represent an involuted LCH (*J Cutan Pathol.* 2011;38:740).

f. **Cavernous hemangioma** (likely a vascular malformation) occurs in the same age range and anatomic distribution as infantile hemangioma, but is less common; shows virtually no tendency to regress; and may be locally destructive due to extrinsic pressure on adjacent structures. A pattern of grouped, dilated, thin-walled blood vessels with an inconspicuous endothelial lining is the microscopic appearance. The blue-rubber-bleb nevus syndrome (characterized by cavernous hemangiomas of the skin and gastrointestinal tract) and Maffucci syndrome (cavernous hemangiomas and enchondromas) are two associated syndromes.

g. **Arteriovenous hemangioma,** also known as arteriovenous malformation, is associated with arteriovenous shunts. It is found more commonly in the skin than in the deep soft tissue where it is composed of a mixture of arterial vessels and thick-walled veins with variable circumscription. Focal vascular thrombosis, PEH, and dystrophic calcifications may be present.

h. **Venous hemangioma** (venous malformation) typically presents during adulthood in the deep soft tissue. Ectatic vessels often show thrombosis, PEH, and dystrophic calcification.

i. **Spindle cell hemangioma** occurs in young adults and is found in the skin and subcutis of the distal extremities, especially the hand. Thin-walled cavernous vessels lined by bland flattened endothelium are admixed with solid areas composed of plump spindle cells resembling Kaposi sarcoma. The tumor involves a large preexisting vessel in many cases. Recurrences are common (>50% of cases), often with a discontinuous growth pattern. This lesion should be distinguished from KHE, which has spindled endothelial cells.

j. **Synovial hemangioma,** as the name implies, arises in synovial-lined spaces, most commonly in the knee in the second decade of life. Microscopically, variably sized thin-walled vascular spaces occupy the stroma of hyperplastic synovium with associated marked hemosiderin deposition. The differential diagnosis includes pigmented villonodular synovitis and trauma-associated hemarthrosis as in hemophilia.

k. **Intramuscular angioma** (intramuscular hemangioma, skeletal muscle hemangioma) most frequently arises in the lower extremity, particularly the muscles of the thigh. It is a poorly circumscribed and diffusely infiltrating mass in the muscle composed of variably sized vessels ranging from large thick-walled veins to cavernous vascular spaces, small arteries, and capillaries, and thus has features more in keeping with an arterial-venous malformation than a true neoplasm. Despite the presence of mitotic activity and intraluminal capillary tufting, freely anastomosing vascular channels are not present. Mature adipose tissue may be a component of the intramuscular mass.

2. **Epithelioid hemangioma** occurs mainly in females between 20 and 40 years of age as a small, dull erythematous plaque of the head and neck. Microscopically it is a well-circumscribed nodule in the dermis or subcutis, or less frequently in the deep soft tissue, that has a vague lobular pattern of clustered small capillary-sized vessels around a feeder vessel. The endothelial cells are plump and have abundant cytoplasm with impingement upon the lumen of the vascular channel (so-called tombstone appearance). The neoplasm occurs rarely in the skeletal system and penis (*Am J Surg Pathol.* 2004;28:523; *Am J Surg Pathol.* 2009;33:270). When lymphocytes and

eosinophils are prominent, the lesion is an example of **angiomatoid hyperplasia with eosinophilia** (*J Cutan Pathol.* 2010;37:1045).

3. **Angiomatosis** is, by definition, a poorly circumscribed, diffuse network of vascular structures within a soft tissue site. In virtually all cases it presents during childhood or adolescence as diffuse soft tissue swelling. The demonstration that the vessels are GLUT-1 immunonegative is consistent with the interpretation that angiomatosis is a malformation. There are two histologic patterns: mixed-vessel-type lesions resembling intramuscular angiomas, and capillary-predominant type lesions with a lobular pattern. The various syndromic associations include Klippel–Trenaunay–Weber, Parkes-Weber, Bannayan–Riley–Ruvalcaba, Maffucci, and Proteus syndromes (*Semin Musculoskelet Radiol.* 2009;13:255).

4. **Lymphangioma** is a cavernous and/or cystic vascular lesion composed of dilated lymphatic channels that occurs most commonly in the head and neck of young children (e.g., a hygroma). Thin-walled dilated lymphatic vessels of varying size are lined by flattened endothelium that is strongly immunopositive with the D2–40 antibody (*Histopathology.* 2005;46:396). Scattered lymphoid aggregates may lie beneath the endothelium (**e-Fig. 46.36**). Lymphangioma is regarded as a lymphatic malformation.

5. **Atypical vascular lesion of the breast** presents as papules, nodules, or erythema several years (average 5 years, range 2 to 20 years) after external radiation for carcinoma of the breast. This lesion is composed of thin-walled vascular spaces resembling lymphatics and is confined to the superficial dermis. An infiltrating, more diffuse pattern into the deeper dermis and atypia of endothelial cells should be viewed with concern (*J Am Acad Dermatol.* 2007;57:126).

6. **Several other lesions** have been added to the seemingly ever expanding universe of vascular tumors. **Epithelioid angiomatous nodule** presents as one, or less often multiple, nodules with a wide distribution (*Pathol Res Pract.* 2009;205:753). The cellular nodules occupy the dermis and are composed of epithelioid endothelial cells. Some mitoses are present, and overall the lesion has features of an epithelioid hemangioma. **Pseudomyogenic hemangioendothelioma** arises in the extremities, for the most part as a dermal-subcutaneous or deep soft tissue mass. Plump spindle cells with prominent eosinophilic cytoplasm are arranged in loose or storiform fascicles (*Am J Surg Pathol.* 2011;35:190). Epithelioid cells are seen as a minor component, as are neutrophils. The tumor is immunopositive for AE1/AE3, FLI1, and CD31 expression. **Polymorphous hemangioendothelioma** is a lymph node–based vascular neoplasm (*Am J Surg Pathol.* 1997;21:1083). **Composite hemangioendothelioma** is, as its name implies, a vascular neoplasm with epithelioid, spindle cell, and angiosarcoma-like features (*Pathology.* 2011;43:176).

D. **Intermediate (locally aggressive)**

1. **Kaposiform hemangioendothelioma (KHE)**, a rare locally aggressive neoplasm, presents most commonly in the first year of life in the extremities or trunk (75% of cases) or retroperitoneum (20% of cases) (*Eur J Int Med.* 2009;20:106). One or multiple masses, or a more diffusely infiltrative process, are the various clinical manifestations. As the designation KHE implies, the individual lobules consist of a mixture of capillary-sized vessels that blend with more slit-like spindled vessels, with an absence of mitoses and an absence cytologic atypia (*Am J Surg Pathol.* 2004;28:559). KHE is immunoreactive for D2–40 (*Am J Surg Pathol.* 2010;34:1563). Approximately 20% of cases are complicated by the Kasabach–Merritt syndrome. A possibly related entity with a similar coagulopathy is multiple lymphangioendotheliomatosis (*Arch Dermatol.* 2004;140:599).

E. Intermediate (rarely metastasizing)

1. **Retiform hemangioendothelioma,** an uncommon neoplasm, arises in the skin of the distal extremity or trunk in young to middle-aged adults, and has a recurrence rate of 40% to 50% without wide excision. Grossly, the tumor is a reddish-purple slowly growing plaque centered in the reticular dermis, usually less than 2 to 3 cm in maximal dimension. Microscopically, the tumor is characterized by elongated, arborizing, narrow vessels that resemble the rete testis. The endothelial cells are monomorphic with a low mitotic rate, hyperchromatic nuclei, and hobnail morphology. The stroma between the vascular channels is prominent and often shows a pronounced lymphocytic infiltrate, but unlike angiosarcoma, the vascular spaces do not dissect through the dermal collagen. The tumor is immunopositive for CD31, but not for D2–40 or VEGFR-3 (*Am J Dermatopathol.* 2008;30:31).

2. **Papillary intralymphatic angioendothelioma** (Dabska tumor) occurs in infants and children in the skin (reticular dermis) as a slowly growing nodule or plaque without a site predilection (*Dermatology.* 2000;201:1). Thin-walled vascular spaces contain intraluminal papillary tufts of endothelial cells with a hobnail morphology as in retiform hemangioendothelioma. Papillary intralymphatic angioendothelioma (as well as retiform hemangioendothelioma) have been reported in bone (*Orthopedics.* 2004;27:327; *Pathol Int.* 2011;61:382).

3. **Kaposi sarcoma** is a low-grade clonal endothelial proliferation caused by human herpesvirus 8 (HHV8) infections. The clinicopathologic features of Kaposi sarcoma are discussed in more detail in the chapter on nonmelanocytic tumors of the skin (Chap. 39).

F. Malignant

1. **Epithelioid hemangioendothelioma** (intravascular bronchioloalveolar tumor) is a low-grade malignant endothelial neoplasm that occurs in patients of all ages, although it is rare in early childhood. The superficial and deep soft tissues, viscera (liver), and bone are various primary sites. About 10% of patients have multiorgan disease at the time of presentation. A t(1;13) translocation that produces a *WWTR1-CAMTA1* gene fusion has recently been shown to be a characteristic feature of the tumor, regardless of anatomic site (*Genes Chromosomes Cancer.* 2011;50:44).

   Grossly, the tumor presents as a poorly circumscribed multilobular infiltrative mass, measuring up to 10 cm in greatest dimension. Microscopically, the tumor consists of cords, short strands, solid nests, or individual cells that have rounded to slightly spindled features (e-**Fig. 46.37**). The cells are low grade with a low mitotic rate. Endothelial differentiation is evident by the formation of intracytoplasmic lumina (producing signet ring-like features) but distinct endothelial-lined vascular channels are not prominent. The neoplastic cells are embedded within a chondroid-like to hyalinized stroma. Atypical morphologic features, including an increased mitotic rate, increased nuclear pleomorphism, more spindled cytology, and necrosis correlate with more aggressive behavior. The tumor cells express CD31, CD34, and *Ulex europaeus* antigen, and variably express factor XIII-related antigen. Of note, 25% to 30% of tumors show focal cytokeratin expression which can lead to an incorrect diagnosis of metastatic signet ring cell carcinoma. The distinction from an epithelioid hemangioma is not obvious in all cases.

2. **Angiosarcoma,** a rare malignancy composed of endothelial cells, recapitulates the functional and morphologic features of normal endothelium to a variable degree (*Lancet Oncol.* 2010;11:983). The tumor is divided into several groups: cutaneous angiosarcoma (with or without an association with lymphedema—Stewart–Treves syndrome); angiosarcoma of the breast;

radiation-induced angiosarcoma; and angiosarcoma of the deep soft tissue. The malignancy is a poorly circumscribed hemorrhagic mass that measures from 1 to 2 cm to >10 cm, with histologic features that vary from hemangioma-like (but with scattered, enlarged, atypical endothelial cells with occasional mitotic figures and an infiltrating growth pattern) to a high-grade spindle cell sarcoma with a hemorrhagic background (e-**Fig. 46.38**). Intraluminal papillae lined by hyperchromatic cells are sometimes present. Vascular channels with a dissecting pattern of infiltration through the dermis or other surrounding tissues should be viewed with concern (see atypical vascular lesion of breast discussed above).

Epithelioid angiosarcoma, a well-recognized variant of angiosarcoma in the deep soft tissues, is composed of malignant epithelioid cells with abundant eosinophilic or amphophilic cytoplasm, large vesicular nuclei, and prominent nuclei (e-**Fig. 46.39**). In sites such as a pleura and peritoneum, the initial impression may be malignant mesothelioma or metastatic carcinoma (*Arch Pathol Lab Med.* 2011;135:268).

X. CHONDRO-OSSEOUS TUMORS

A. Benign

1. **Chondroma** occurs over a broad age range usually in the fingers and toes, with a juxtaarticular and tendinous predilection. Chondromas are typically composed of lobules of mature hyaline cartilage, but there are histologic variants: chondroblastic chondroma (when the lesion is cellular), fibrochondroma (when there is prominent fibrosis), and osteochondroma (when there is prominent ossification). Chondromyxoid fibroma and chondroblastoma typically arise in bone but have been reported in juxtacortical or soft tissue sites (*Am J Surg Pathol.* 2007;31:1662; *Diagn Cytopathol.* 2003;28:76). If the chondroid tumor is from the base of the skull, chondroid chordoma should be considered in the differential diagnosis.

B. Malignant

1. **Mesenchymal chondrosarcoma** is a neoplasm of the soft tissues or other extraosseous sites (25% to 30% of cases) or bone (70% to 75%), with some preference for the head and neck (meninges, orbit), spine, and lower extremities. Most cases are diagnosed between 15 and 40 years of age, but the tumor may be seen in the neonate (*Pediatr Dev Pathol.* 2008;11:309). Microscopically, nodules of neoplastic hyaline cartilage are separated by undifferentiated malignant small round cells, with or without a hemangiopericytoma-like appearance. The tumor cells are immunopositive for vimentin, desmin, EMA, and SOX9, and focally also express β-catenin (*Hum Pathol.* 2010;41:653; *Ann Diagn Pathol.* 2010;14:8). The tumor cells are nonreactive for FLI1 (*Appl Immunohistochem Mol Morphol.* 2011;19:233).

2. **Extraskeletal osteosarcoma** usually arises in the deep soft tissue, most commonly in the thigh, although the buttock, shoulder girdle, trunk, and retroperitoneum are other sites in individuals between 40 and 60 years of age (*J Thorac Oncol.* 2009;4:927). About 10% of patients have a history of prior radiation or trauma to the site. Malignant bone is usually most prominent in the center of the tumor, while more peripheral regions of the neoplasm tend to be more densely cellular (this zonation is the reverse of the pattern present in myositis ossificans and can be a useful feature for differential diagnosis).

XI. PERIPHERAL NERVE TUMORS.

The tumors of presumed peripheral nerve or nerve sheath derivation comprise some of the more common soft tissue neoplasms in routine practice.

A. Traumatic neuroma

is a nonneoplastic proliferation in response to nerve injury, often after a surgical procedure. It is a firm, tender nodule measuring <5 cm that consists of small crowded nerve fascicles arranged in a haphazard architectural pattern, that are composed of Schwann cells and fibroblasts in a fibromyxoid stroma (e-**Fig. 46.40**).

B. **Mucosal neuromas** on the lips, mouth, eyelids, and intestines are manifestations of multiple endocrine neoplasia IIB. The irregular nerve bundles in the submucosa have a prominent perineurium. The stroma often has a myxoid quality.

C. **Neurofibromas** are divided into three types on the basis of a growth pattern: localized, diffuse, and plexiform.

1. **Localized neurofibroma** is sporadic, usually superficial and solitary, and unassociated with a genetic syndrome. The dermis and subcutis are the sites of predilection. Microscopically, the circumscribed nodule is composed of spindle cells with wavy nuclei and strands of collagen in a neurofibrillary background with scattered mast cells. The differential diagnosis is a dermal melanocytic nevus with extensive neurotization.

2. **Plexiform neurofibromas** are manifestations of neurofibromatosis 1 (NF1), as are diffuse neurofibromas (*Lancet Neurol.* 2007;6:340). These tumors develop in early childhood as superficial soft tissue masses, and vary in size and extent of local involvement. An entire length of nerve can be transformed into the so-called bag-of-worms appearance in which multiple nerve bundles characteristically show expansion of the endoneurium by a myxoid stroma, with later extension beyond the perineurium into the adjacent soft tissue (e-**Fig. 46.41**). The interstitium is composed of thickened irregular fibrous bundles with interspersed short to fusiform spindle cells, and a diffuse pattern may accompany the plexiform component in the surrounding soft tissues. Foci of increased cellularity with associated enlarged, hyperchromatic nuclei should be viewed with concern for malignant transformation (e-**Fig. 46.42**). Nuclear reactivity for p53 is an additional finding of concern.

3. **Diffuse neurofibroma** has a predilection for the head and neck as a plaquelike elevation of the skin. The dermis and subcutis are effaced by a uniformly cellular proliferation within a fibrillary collagenous matrix containing Schwann cells with short uniform nuclei (e-**Fig. 46.43**) and occasional Meissner body-like formations. Some tumors are associated with other mesenchymal elements including ectatic vessels and mature entrapped adipose tissue. The overgrowth of subcutaneous fat is similar to that seen in dermatofibrosarcoma protuberans and infantile subcutaneous fibromatosis.

D. **Schwannoma** (neurilemoma) most often occurs in patients between 20 and 40 years old, but is also seen in children. Most schwannomas present as a solitary mass in the head and neck, on the flexor surfaces of the upper and lower extremities, or in association with spinal and paraspinal sensory nerves. Multiple or bilateral schwannomas are manifestations of NF2 and schwannomatosis (*Annu Rev Pathol.* 2007;2:191; *Rev Neurol Dis.* 2009;6:E81). Cellular and plexiform schwannomas may occur in children and in NF2; pigmented or melanotic schwannomas are one of the features of the Carney complex (*Ann Endocrinol.* (Paris) 2010;71:486).

The tumors vary in size, but virtually all are invested by a true capsule of the epineurium which can be difficult to demonstrate in some sites in the head and neck. A white to yellow-white mucoid cut surface with or without cystic degeneration and hemorrhage are the gross features. Most tumors are <5 cm in greatest dimension, although those that arise in the paraspinal retroperitoneum can be larger. The characteristic low-power microscopic pattern (e-**Fig. 46.44**) consists of alternating Antoni A areas (consisting of organized spindle cells with (e-**Fig. 46.45**) or without Verocay bodies) and Antoni B areas (consisting of less cellular regions in which the oval to spindled cells are arranged more haphazardly in a loose fibrous matrix). Thickened hyalinized vessels are prominent in many cases. There is considerable histologic variability in schwannomas; despite atypical findings, especially in so-called ancient-type schwannomas, these tumors rarely undergo malignant transformation (characterized by invasion through the capsule, epithelioid or small cell transformation, high-grade nuclear abnormalities, and atypical mitotic figures). It is noteworthy that epithelioid morphology alone is an insufficient criterion for malignancy because there is an epithelioid variant of schwannoma. The tumor cells are diffusely immunopositive for S-100 protein and collagen type IV, with delicate pericellular reactivity reflecting basement membrane-like deposition.

E. **Granular cell tumor** occurs in virtually all age ranges, although more frequently in adults than children. There is a predilection for the skin and sites in the head and neck, but this tumor occurs throughout the body. One unique type, the congenital epulis of the anterior gingival region in neonates, does not express S-100 protein (nonneural granular cell tumor). Several histologic patterns are seen, including closely apposed nests and ribbons, infiltrating cords, and confluent sheets of uniform polygonal to slightly spindled cells with a central nucleus that is surrounded by abundant uniform granular cytoplasm (**e-Fig. 46.46**). Pseudoepitheliomatous hyperplasia may be present in the overlying epidermis or squamous mucosa. Malignancy is rare, but is well documented (*Am J Surg Pathol.* 1998;22:779). Strong immunoreactivity for S-100, neuron specific enolase, and CD68 is the usual phenotype of the neural granular cell tumor.

F. **Neurothekeoma** (nerve sheath myxoma), a rare tumor in children and young adults, presents in the head, neck, and shoulders. Microscopically, nodules of bland, plump spindle cells are present in a myxoid matrix separated by fibrous connective tissue (**e-Fig. 46.47**). The cells show little pleomorphism and have a low mitotic rate. Increased cellularity, cytologic atypia, increased mitotic figures, extension into adjacent or deep soft tissues, and even vascular invasion are regarded as atypical variants (*Am J Surg Pathol.* 1998;22:1067).

G. **Perineurioma** is an uncommon neoplasm composed of perineural cells whose expression of epithelial membrane antigen is similar to meningothelial cells. The two types of perineurioma are those that arise within or external to a nerve (*Arch Pathol Lab Med.* 2007;131:625). The tumor has several histologic patterns including a lacy and reticulated network of delicate to somewhat plump fusiform spindle cells, and a more cellular pattern of storiform perivascular spindle cells. The background may be sclerotic or more typically myxoid. There are now several examples of peripheral nerve sheath neoplasms which have hybrid features of schwannoma and perineurioma (*Am J Surg Pathol.* 2009;33:1554); these tumors arise in the peripheral soft tissues and even within lymph nodes (*Pediatr Dev Pathol.* 2011).

H. **Malignant peripheral nerve sheath tumor (MPNST)** that arise from peripheral nerves are currently classified as MPNSTs. A sarcoma can be classified as an MPNST if it has arisen from a peripheral nerve, if it has arisen from a pre-existing benign nerve sheath tumor (in most cases, a neurofibroma), or if it demonstrates histologic and immunophenotype features that reflect Schwannian differentiation. Overall, 5% to 10% of STs are MPNSTs, especially in late adolescence and early adulthood.

These tumors are typically large (in excess of 5 cm) with a fleshy mucoid cut surface and large areas of hemorrhage and necrosis. Microscopically, they are composed of fascicles or broad sweeping profiles of malignant spindle cells that have wavy or comma-shaped nuclei. The cellular density often varies producing a "light-cell, dark-cell" appearance (**e-Fig. 46.48**). Nuclear palisading is present in some tumors, as are hyalinized cords and nodules that may resemble large rosettes. The immunophenotype tends toward Schwannian differentiation with

S-100 positivity (only in 50% of cases), but the tumors are more commonly positive for CD57 (Leu 7), collagen type IV, and myelin basic protein (*Arch Pathol Lab Med.* 2009;133:1370). Chromosomal losses are more common than amplifications (*Virchows Arch.* 2010;456:201).

Variant patterns of MPNST show rhabdomyoblastic differentiation (malignant triton tumor), glandular formation, and heterotopic bone and/or cartilage formation. These variants are encountered with some frequency in the setting of NF1 (the setting in which 40% to 50% of all MPNSTs are seen) (*Neurosurg Clin N Am.* 2008;19:533).

XII. TUMORS OF UNCERTAIN DIFFERENTIATION. For many of the tumors in this category, either the cell type that produces the tumor or the normal cell type that the tumor is recapitulating, or both, is unknown.

A. Benign

1. **Intramuscular myxoma** occurs primarily in adults between 40 and 60 years as a solitary, painless, slowly growing mass within the muscle of the thigh, buttocks, or limb girdle. Most tumors measure 5 cm in maximal dimension, and are well circumscribed with a pale gelatinous or myxoid cut surface. The tumor cells are small, bland, stellate to spindle in shape, have a very low mitotic rate, and are present in an abundant myxoid matrix that contains an inconspicuous vascular network (**e-Fig. 46.49**). Focal areas of increased cellularity and vascularity with collagenous background are present in some cases whose presence may cause concern (*Am J Surg Pathol.* 1998;22:1222). Simple excision is followed by a recurrence rate of <5% of cases (*Histopathology.* 2001;39:287). The differential diagnosis of myxoma includes many other myxoid tumors of the soft tissues (*Histopathology.* 1999;35:291; *Ann Diagn Pathol.* 2000;4:99). One or more myxomas of the soft tissues with fibrous dysplasia defines Mazabraud syndrome. Multiple cutaneous and mucosal myxomas are manifestations of Carney complex (*Lancet Oncol.* 2005;6:501; *Neuroendocrinology.* 2006;83:189).

2. **Juxtaarticular myxoma,** as the name suggests, usually arises in the vicinity of a large joint (primarily the knee). The lesion has a predilection for males between 20 and 40 years of age, and is usually <5 cm maximal dimension. This tumor is indistinguishable from an intramuscular myxoma, but is probably a different entity than the latter (*Virchows Arch.* 2002;440:12). Some cases may have hemorrhage and hemosiderin deposition, chronic inflammation, and fibrosis.

3. **Digital myxoma** (digital mucus cyst), usually occurs on a finger, and in adult women as a painful nodule <1 cm in diameter. Histologically, it resembles intramuscular myxoma. **Cutaneous myxoma** (also known as superficial angiomyxoma) is a cutaneous or subcutaneous lesion which occurs primarily in adults between 30 and 50 years of age; it must be differentiated from nerve sheath myxoma of peripheral nerve sheath origin and neurothekeoma (*Mod Pathol.* 2011;24:343).

4. **Deep aggressive angiomyxoma** is a slowly growing locally infiltrative tumor that usually occurs in the pelviperineal soft tissue of women, but is also seen as a scrotal mass (*Int J Gynecol Pathol.* 2005;24:26; *Int J Urol.* 2003;10:672; *Histopathology.* 2009;54:156). It forms a soft poorly circumscribed mass measuring 10 to 20 cm in greatest dimension that has a gelatinous cut surface. Small stellate to spindled cells with ill-defined cytoplasm and bland nuclei are set in a myxoid stroma rich in collagen fibers (**e-Fig. 46.50**). Numerous, variably sized, thick or thin walled vascular channels are present, from which smooth muscle seems to spin off and merge with the surrounding stroma. The tumor cells express vimentin and desmin, and also usually show nuclear expression of estrogen and progesterone receptors.

The tumor has a propensity to recur, which is not unexpected given its infiltrative and poorly defined margin. Local control is usually possible without radical surgery, and the tumor does not metastasize.

5. **Pleomorphic hyalinizing angiectatic tumor of soft parts** (hemosiderotic fibrohistiocytic lipomatous lesion), a slowly growing tumor, usually arises in the subcutis of the lower extremity in adults. There is a predilection for the foot and ankle. The neoplasm is characterized by a background of thin-walled ectatic blood vessels within a stroma that contains large, pleomorphic, plump spindled to round tumor cells with a low mitotic rate. Although the tumor may recur after excision, aggressively in some cases, its potential for metastatic spread appears limited (*Am J Surg Pathol.* 2004;28:1417).

B. **Intermediate (rarely metastasizing)**

1. **Angiomatoid fibrous histiocytoma (AFH)**, a slowly growing tumor usually arising in the lower dermis or subcutis of the limbs, trunk, or head and neck, occurs in children and young adults (*Arch Pathol Lab Med.* 2008;132:273). Most cases measure 4 cm or less. The cut surface is multinodular and hemorrhagic; blood-filled cystic spaces are a common feature, but nonhemorrhagic tumors are also seen. The neoplastic population consists of plump to spindled cells, with interspersed pseudoangiomatoid or aneurysmal spaces (e-**Fig. 46.51**). A minority of cases feature nodules without hemorrhage that are composed of cells with enlarged hyperchromatic nuclei. A minority of cases also feature prominent mitotic figures. The tumor cells express vimentin, desmin, CD99 (with membranous staining), and CD68. This tumor is one of several STTs that harbor an *EWSR1* translocation (*Virchows Arch.* 2010;456:219).

2. **Ossifying fibromyxoid tumor** is seen in adults as a long-standing painless extremity mass measuring 3 to 5 cm in greatest dimension. The extremities (70% of cases), head and neck, and retroperitoneum are various primary sites of the tumor (*Am J Surg Pathol.* 2008;32:996). Microscopically, lobules of uniform, round to spindled cells are arranged in cords and nests in a fibromyxoid to collagenous matrix. An incomplete fibrous pseudocapsule or shell of lamellar bone is present around the periphery. Although microscopic features do not reliably predict behavior, increased cellularity (resembling EWS/PNET) and an increased mitotic rate (up to 10 mitotic figures per 10 HPFs) are associated with a higher rate of recurrence. These tumors have a variable immunophenotype, but can express cytokeratin, S-100 protein, glial fibrillary acidic protein, and CD99.

3. **Myoepithelial neoplasms** have a number of different designations including **soft tissue myoepithelioma**, **parachordoma**, and **cutaneous mixed tumor**. These tumors comprise a heterogenous clinicopathologic group of neoplasms, all of which display varying proportions of epithelial and/or myoepithelial elements (*Ann Diagn Pathol.* 2007;11:190; *Am J Surg Pathol.* 2003;27:1183). All present as a painless swelling in the subcutis or deep soft tissues of the extremities that has often been present for several years. Most tumors present primarily in adults, but up to 20% of cases are seen in children under 10 years old (*Am J Surg Pathol.* 1997; 21:13).

There is a resemblance to pleomorphic adenoma of the salivary glands in that the epithelial and myoepithelial elements characteristically form a wide range of architectural patterns, divergent differentiation, and a low mitotic rate. Malignant degeneration into either a carcinoma or sarcoma is occasionally observed, although it is clear that morphologic features cannot be used to reliably predict prognosis since a subset of histologically benign cases also recur and metastasize. Despite the similarities between soft tissue myoepithelial tumors and pleomorphic adenoma of the salivary glands, the presence of *EWSR1* rearrangements in myoepithelial neoplasms (rather than the *PLAG1* and *HMGA2* rearrangements characteristic of pleomorphic adenoma) emphasizes that there is no pathogenic relationship between the tumor types (*Genes Chromosomes Cancer.* 2010;49:1114).

4. **Giant cell fibroblastoma** is the unique morphologic manifestation of dermatofibrosarcoma protuberans that presents in early childhood as a soft tissue mass in the subcutis of the trunk, thigh, and perineum. It is an ill-defined tumor composed of delicate to spindle cells within a fibrous to fibromyxoid to hyalinized stroma, with scattered multinucleated giant cells associated with nonvascularized spaces. Similar cells are found in giant angiofibroma, pleomorphic lipoma, neurofibroma, and collagenoma (*Diagn Pathol.* 2007;2:47; *Am J Dermatopathol.* 2004;26:141). A subset of giant cell fibroblastomas are accompanied by classic dermofibrosarcoma protuberans, which is not surprising since these tumors share the same t(17;22)(q22;q13) translocation.

5. **Perivascular epithelioid cell tumors (PEComas)** are a family of presumably related neoplasms with morphologic and immunophenotypic similarities (*Histopathology.* 2006;48:75; *Semin Diagn Pathol.* 2009;26:123; *Virchows Arch.* 2008;452:119). Angiomyolipoma, lymphangiomyomatosis, clear cell "sugar" tumor of the lung, and so-called myomelanocytic tumor of the ligamentum teres are the various specific morphologic subtypes of PEComa; generic-type PEComas are commonly found in the female reproductive tract, kidney, heart, bladder, and bone. Microscopically, PEComas are composed of variable proportions of epithelioid and spindle cells with clear to eosinophilic granular cytoplasm and round nuclei. The tumor cells can have a perivascular orientation around a thin-walled blood vessel, or a vague nesting pattern with a resemblance to a paraganglioma. Necrosis and vascular invasion are seemingly reliable features of malignancy.

The tumor cells are immunopositive for the melanocytic markers HMB-45 and melan-A, for SMA, and less often for desmin. The tumor cells are nonreactive for S-100, neuroendocrine markers, and cytokeratin. A subset of PEComas harbor *TFE3* fusion transcripts, which suggests a molecular relationship to melanotic Xp11 translocation renal carcinoma and alveolar soft part sarcoma (*Am J Surg Pathol.* 2010;34:1395; *Am J Surg Pathol.* 2009;33:609; *Arch Pathol Lab Med.* 2010;134:124).

C. Malignant

1. **Ewing sarcoma/primitive neuroectodermal tumor (EWS/PNET)** presents in the soft tissue, bone, viscera, skin, and other anatomic sites in children, adolescents, and young adults. This tumor accounts for about 20% of STS in the first two decades of life, but is also recognized throughout adulthood. Whether in bone or soft tissue, the tumor is usually in excess of 6 cm; larger tumors occur in anatomically silent locations like the paraspinal region or pelvic retroperitoneum.

A biopsy followed by posttreatment resection is the management sequence in most cases (since few of these tumors are candidates for primary resection); these biopsies offer many diagnostic challenges because of the frequently associated necrosis and compression artifact. Typically, the tumor is composed of uniform round cells with clear to finely vacuolated cytoplasm, and a central nucleus with fine to slightly coarse chromatin. Mitotic figures are present but are not numerous in most cases. Architecturally, broad sheets, lobules, nests, and strands are some of the growth patterns (e-Fig. 46.52); other features include Homer-Wright rosettes, condensed small cellular nodules within otherwise monotonous sheets of round cells, some spindling (possibly an artifact), and a pale mucoid background. Clear cytoplasm is usually an indication of abundant diastase digestible glycogen. Vimentin and CD99 immunostains are diffusely positive with

TABLE 46.7	Differential Immunohistochemical Phenotypes of Malignant Round Cell Tumors									
	VIM	**CK**	**CD45**	**DES**	**CD99**	**WT-I**	**CHR**	**TDT**	**CD43**	**MPX/CD68**
RMS	+	−	−	+	−	−	−	−	−	−
NB	±	−	−	−	−	−	+	−	−	+
HLM	+	−	+	−	+[a]	−	−	+	+	±[b]
EWS/PNET	+	±	−	−	+	−	+	−	−	−
DSRCT	+	+	−	+	±	+	±	−	−	−
BWT	+	−	−	±	−	+	−	−	−	−
NEC	−	+	−	−	−	−	+	−	−	−

[a]CD99 is expressed in lymphoblastic leukemia/lymphoma.
[b]MPX is expressed in acute myeloid leukemia (M1, M2) and CD68 in acute monocytic leukemia (M5).
RMS, rhabdomyosaroma; NB, neuroblastoma; HLM, hematolymphoid malignancy (leukemia, lymphoma, granulocytic sarcoma); EWS-PNET, Ewing sarcoma/peripheral neuroectodermal tumor; DSRCT, desmoplastic small round cell tumor; BWT, blastemal Wilms tumor; NEC, neuroendocrine carcinoma; VIM, vimentin; CK, cytokeratin; DES, desmin; CHR, chromogranin; TdT, terminal desoxynucleotidyl transferase; MPX, myeloperoxidase.

a cytoplasmic and membrane pattern, respectively (Table 46.7). Punctate cytokeratin reactivity is seen focally in 20% to 25% of cases.

Chromosomal translocations that form fusions between the *EWSR1* gene and a member of the *Ets* family of transcription factors are characteristic of EWS/PNET (Table 46.1). Demonstration of the translocation by molecular techniques is a valuable aid for diagnosis (*Virchows Arch.* 2010;456:219), although a small fraction of tumors have variant translocation or cryptic fusions that introduce diagnostic uncertainty (*Cancer Genet Cytogenet.* 2010;200:60; *Mod Pathol.* 2011;24:333). Secondary structural rearrangements, mainly deletions and trisomy, have been correlated with a poor outcome (*Genes Chromosomes Cancer.* 2008;47:207).

2. **Desmoplastic small round cell tumor (DSRCT),** a tumor that was originally reported as presenting as peritoneal masses in males in their second or third decade, is now recognized to occur in peripheral soft tissues and various organs including salivary gland, kidney, ovary, bone, and brain. This tumor, like EWS/PNET, is composed of malignant round cells with a nested pattern within a desmoplastic stroma (e-Fig. 46.53); rosette and glandular formations may be seen. Since several other malignant round cell neoplasms also can have desmoplastic stroma, including blastemal predominant Wilms tumor, EWS/PNET, and ERMS or ARMS, caution in diagnosis is warranted. The unique immunophenotype of DSRCT (Table 46.7) is helpful in this regard, as is the presence of a characteristic *EWSR1-WTI* fusion in DSRCT.

3. **Synovial sarcoma (SS)** typically presents in the periarticular soft tissues in patients between the ages of 15 and 40 years, but it is now recognized that the tumor can arise in virtually any organ or anatomic site. Consequently, it is prudent to consider the possibility that any spindle cell sarcoma may be a synovial sarcoma. Approximately 8% to 10% of all STS in the first two decades are synovial sarcoma, but the tumor is uncommon in individuals over 50 years of age.

A well-circumscribed mass with a gray-tan surface is the usual gross appearance; however, cystic and calcific foci may be seen. Tumors >5 cm tend to have a worse outcome (*J Pediatr Hematol Oncol.* 2005;27:207; *Orthopedics.* 2007;30:1020). The two classic histologic subtypes are the monophasic type (which is a spindle cell sarcoma with hemangiopericytoma-like foci) and the biphasic type [which contains epithelial-like glands (**e-Fig. 46.54**) or nests]. A third type, poorly differentiated SS, has features of a primitive round cell sarcoma. The immunophenotype, regardless of subtype, includes the expression of vimentin, cytokeratin (CK7), and/or epithelial membrane antigen and CD99. The t(X;18) is characteristic of the tumor, which can be helpful for distinguishing the tumor from fibrosarcoma, MPNST, LGFMS, and SFT/hemangiopericytoma.

4. **Clear cell sarcoma** of tendon and aponeuroses (melanoma of soft parts) typically presents in the soft tissues of the foot and ankle of children and young adults. However, the neoplasm is also recognized in the intestinal tract (often with osteoclast-like giant cells), kidney, and other sites including the head and neck (*Arch Pathol Lab Med.* 2007;131:152; *J Clin Pathol.* 2010;63:416; *Ann Diagn Pathol.* 2009;13:30). Nests to broad fascicles of plump spindled to polygonal cells with abundant eosinophilic to clear cytoplasm, with vesicular nuclei with a prominent eosinophilic nucleolus, are the histologic features (**e-Fig. 46.55**). Multinucleated cells may be found. Like cutaneous melanoma, the immunophenotype includes vimentin, HMB-45 and melan-A (MART-1) immunopositivity, but these two tumors are distinctively different at the molecular genetic level. The balanced translocations involving the *EWSR1* gene in clear cell sarcoma (Table 46.1) are not present in cutaneous melanoma (*Virchows Arch.* 2010;456:219).

5. **Alveolar soft part sarcoma,** most commonly seen in patients between the ages of 15 to 35 years, has a predilection for the orbit and base of the tongue in children, and the deep soft tissue of the extremities (especially the thigh) in adults (*Arch Pathol Lab Med.* 2007;131:488). Other than a mass with varying dimension, there is nothing specific about the gross features of the tumor. Microscopically, uniform large epithelioid or polygonal cells with abundant eosinophilic granular to clear cytoplasm are typically arranged in nests separated by delicate fibrous septa and sinusoidal vessels (**e-Fig. 46.56**). However, the tumor may have a more diffuse, nonalveolar pattern, especially in children; anaplasia, mitotic activity, necrosis, and vascular invasion are other common features (*J Clin Pathol.* 2006;59:1127). Rod-shaped or rhomboid crystalline inclusions, when present, are highlighted by a PAS stain after diastase digestion. The nonreciprocal der(17)t(X;17) translocation is the characteristic cytogenetic feature of this tumor (*Virchows Arch.* 2010;456:153).

6. **Extraskeletal myxoid chondrosarcoma,** typically arising in the deep soft tissues of the proximal extremities, usually presents between 35 and 60 years of age and has a male predilection. Uncommon other primary sites include the nasopharynx, vulva, heart, and retroperitoneum. Grossly, the tumor is multilobulated, and its myxoid gross appearance is reflected in its microscopic composition of small, uniform, round cells with minimal atypia, finely granular eosinophilic cytoplasm, and bland round to oval nuclei that are arranged in clusters, cords, and delicate networks within a prominent myxoid matrix (**e-Fig. 46.57**). Cartilaginous differentiation is not present despite the appellation.

   The tumor is associated with a limited set of translocations (Table 46.1) that produce rearrangements of the *CHN* gene (*Pathol Int.* 2005;55:453). The same rearrangements are not present in chondrosarcoma of skeletal origin or extraskeletal mesenchymal chondrosarcoma.

7. **Extrarenal malignant rhabdoid tumor** is an extremely aggressive neoplasm of the liver, axial soft tissues, and central nervous system (in the latter location it is named atypical teratoid–rhabdoid tumor) in children, typically under the age of 2 years (*Cancer.* 2007;110:2061; *Pathol Int.* 2006;56:287). This tumor can present in newborns with disseminated disease including placental involvement, and is in all respects identical to renal malignant

rhabdoid tumor. Grossly, it is a poorly circumscribed, highly infiltrative neoplasm has a soft, grayish tan, and often necrotic cut surface. Various microscopic patterns may be associated with this high-grade malignant round cell neoplasm. Few or many obvious rhabdoid cells that have an eccentric vesicular nucleus, prominent nucleolus, and the characteristic eosinophilic filamentous inclusion (which contains vimentin or cytokeratin) may be present. Oftentimes, immunostaining for vimentin and/or cytokeratin highlights the fact that many more cells have inclusions. The tumor cells also express CD99 with a patchy or focal pattern.

Somatic biallelic inactivation of the *hSNF5/INI1* gene is the underlying genetic feature which can be demonstrated by an absence of nuclear immunoreactivity for BAF47. Molecular demonstration of alterations involving this locus can be used to differentiate extrarenal malignant rhabdoid tumor from poorly differentiated carcinomas and sarcomas in adults that have a rhabdoid phenotype as an epiphenomenon. The distinction between extrarenal malignant rhabdoid tumor and epithelioid sarcoma has become blurred on the basis of recent immunophenotype and molecular genetic findings.

8. **Epithelioid sarcoma** typically presents in individuals in the second through the fourth decade. The distal or conventional type of epithelioid sarcoma is found in the fingers, hand, or wrist, or the equivalent sites in the distal lower extremity. The more aggressive proximal type involves the pelvis, perineum, and genital tract with overlapping clinical and pathologic features of extrarenal malignant rhabdoid tumor (*Cancer Res.* 2005;65:4012).

In the distal type, arcades and nodules of uniform epithelioid cells with an eosinophilic cytoplasm may show a transition into areas of spindled cells, both set in a background of abundant collagen (e-**Fig. 46.58**). The nodules can undergo central necrosis, creating an appearance that resembles a necrobiotic granuloma (with the potential misinterpretation as granuloma annulare since both lesions present in the fingers or toes) (*Adv Anat Pathol.* 2006;13:114). Recurrent epithelioid sarcoma may have features of a high-grade pleomorphic sarcoma with only a remote resemblance to the primary tumor.

In the proximal type, the tumor is composed of sheets of large cells with prominent rhabdoid morphology in the absence of a granuloma-like pattern (e-**Fig. 46.58**).

Both the distal and proximal types of tumor express EMA, vimentin, cytokeratins, and CD34 (in 40% to 50% of cases). There is general agreement that both types consistently display loss of BAF47 reactivity (80% to 90% of cases) that reflects inactivation of the *hSNF5/INI1* gene (*Am J Clin Pathol.* 2009;131:222; *Am J Surg Pathol.* 2009;33:542; *Hum Pathol.* 2009;40:349).

9. **Undifferentiated–poorly differentiated sarcoma** is a pathologic diagnosis of last resort. The morphologic scenario usually differs on the basis of age: in children, the problematic tumor is usually a primitive or high-grade round cell neoplasm, while in adults it is an equally high-grade pleomorphic neoplasm with anaplasia, bizarre mitoses, and necrosis.

In children, the diagnosis of "undifferentiated round cell sarcoma" or "sarcoma of undermined histogenesis" becomes the interpretation once the various differentiated malignant round cell neoplasms have been excluded by immunohistochemical and molecular testing (Table 46.7), and both are ever shrinking categories (*J Pediatr Hematol Oncol.* 2001;23:215; *Hum Pathol.* 2009;40:1600). In these undifferentiated tumors, loss of *hSNF5/INI1* expression in infants and young children seems to be associated with a better prognosis (*Mod Pathol.* 2009;22:142).

TABLE 46.8	Staging of Soft Tissue Sarcoma			

Definition of TNM
Primary tumor (T)

TX	Primary tumor cannot be assessed			
T0	No evidence of primary tumor			
T1	Tumor ≤5 cm in greatest dimension[a]			
T1a	Superficial tumor			
T1b	Deep tumor			
T2	Tumor >5 cm in great dimension[a]			
T2a	Superficial tumor			
T2b	Deep tumor			

Regional lymph nodes (N)

NX	Regional lymph nodes cannot be assessed			
N0	No regional lymph node metastasis			
N1	Regional lymph node metastasis			

Distant metastasis (M)

M0	No distant metastasis			
M1	Distant metastasis			

Anatomic stage/prognostic groups

Stage 1A	T1a	N0	M0	G1, GX[b]
	T1b	N0	M0	G1, GX
Stage 1B	T2a	N0	M0	G1, GX
	T2b	N0	M0	G1, GX
Stage IIA	T1a	N0	M0	G2, G3
	T1b	N0	M0	G2, G3
Stage IIB	T2a	N0	M0	G2
	T2b	N0	M0	G2
Stage III	T2a, T2b	N0	M0	G3
	Any T	N1	M0	Any G
Stage IV	Any T	Any N	M1	Any G

[a]A superficial tumor is located exclusively above the superficial fascia without invasion of the fascia; a deep tumor is located either exclusively beneath the superficial fascia, superficial to the fascia with invasion of or through the fascia, or both superficial and beneath the fascia.
[b]See Table 46.3.
From: Edge SB, Byrd DR, Compton CC, et al., eds. *AJCC Cancer Staging Manual.* 7th ed. New York, NY: Springer; 2010. Used with permission.

In adults, once sarcomatoid carcinoma and melanoma have been excluded on the basis of a thorough immunohistochemical evaluation, "undifferentiated high-grade pleomorphic sarcoma" or "pleomorphic MFH sarcoma" is often the diagnosis.

XIII. **REPORTING.** The surgical pathology report of a soft tissue tumor should include the location of the tumor, the grade of the tumor (as per the College of American Pathologists recommendations, the FNCLCC system is preferred for ease of use and responsibility; see Table 46.3), depth of the tumor (see Table 46.8), the surgical procedure, the size of the tumor, the histologic type of tumor, and the biologic potential or managerial category (clinically benign, clinically intermediate, or clinically sarcoma). The extent of tumor necrosis should be noted, as well as the status of the surgical margins and the presence of neurovascular invasion. The results of any ancillary studies, including immunohistochemistry, electron microscopy, routine cytogenetic analysis, and/or molecular testing should also be reported in the microscopic section of the surgical pathology report (*Mod Pathol.* 1998;11:1257).

SUGGESTED READINGS

Dehner LP. Soft tissue. In: Stocker T, Dehner LP, Husain AN, eds. *Stocker and Dehner Pediatric Pathology*, 3rd ed. Philadelphia: Lippincott, Williams & Wilkins; 2011.

Fletcher CDM, Unni KK, Mertens F. *Pathology and Genetics of Tumors of Soft Tissue and Bone. World Health Organization Classification of Tumors*. Lyon: IARC Press; 2002.

Kempson RL, Fletcher CDM, Evans HL, et al. *Tumors of the Soft Tissues. Atlas of Tumor Pathology, 3rd Series, Fascicle 30*. Washington, DC: Armed Forces Institute of Pathology; 2001.

Pfeifer JD. *Molecular Genetic Testing in Surgical Pathology*. Philadelphia: Lippincott, Williams & Wilkins; 2006.

Weiss SW, Goldblum JR. *Soft Tissue Tumors*, 5th ed. St. Louis: Mosby; 2008.

47 Retroperitoneum

Catalina Amador-Ortiz, Louis P. Dehner, and John D. Pfeifer

I. **NORMAL ANATOMY.** The retroperitoneal space (in some respects a virtual space) is located between the posterior parietal peritoneum and the fascia that covers the muscles of the lumbar region. It extends upward to the diaphragm, downward to the base of the sacrum and iliac crests, and laterally to the external borders of the lumbar muscles and the ascending and descending colon. The retroperitoneum contains loose connective tissue surrounding lymph nodes, the aorta and inferior vena cava with their vascular branches, the adrenal glands, the kidneys and ureters, the pancreas, and portions of the duodenum. This chapter will focus on the entities that arise from the tissues of the retroperitoneal space; disorders arising from the organs that are completely or partially retroperitoneal are covered in the respective chapters.

II. **NONNEOPLASTIC DISEASES**

A. **Inflammatory**

1. **Idiopathic fibroinflammatory lesions** constitute a morphologically similar category of tumefactive processes, and a variety of diagnostic terms such as sclerosing mesenteritis and/or panniculitis have been applied. The usual presentation is a mass in the retroperitoneum and/or root of the mesentery; sclerosing changes may extend into the inferior retroperitoneum with similar features, if not identical, to idiopathic retroperitoneal fibrosis. A biopsy reveals a variably intense mixed lymphocytic and plasmacellular infiltrate in a dense, relatively hypocellular collagenous background. Residual adipose tissue may have the features of fat necrosis with dystrophic calcification and panniculitis. In the presence of lymphadenopathy, the possibility of lymphoma should be excluded. Metastatic disease including poorly differentiated adenocarcinoma of the pancreas, carcinoid, lobular carcinoma of the breast, and acinar carcinoma of the prostate may be accompanied by disproportionate fibroinflammatory reaction to the actual volume of tumor, and thus also need to be excluded. If the biopsy has a prominently spindle cell component, inflammatory pseudotumor, inflammatory myofibroblastic tumor (IMT), sarcomatoid carcinoma, pleomorphic spindle cell sarcoma, and IgG4-related sclerosing disorder are also in the differential diagnosis (*Nat Rev Gastroenterol Hepatol.* 2010;7:401; *J Clin Pathol.* 2008;61:1093). Since the histologic findings of idiopathic fibroinflammatory lesions are nonspecific, even after the other possibilities have been excluded, the diagnostic line in the report may simply read "chronic inflammation and fibrosis."

2. **Malakoplakia** occasionally affects the retroperitoneal soft tissues. The process is a response to infection and grossly appears as a yellow plaque-like lesion. Microscopically, it is composed of abundant inflammatory cells and sheets of granular and vacuolated histiocytes that contain lamellated, PAS-positive diastase-resistant inclusions known as Michaelis–Gutmann bodies. These distinctive inclusions (**e-Fig. 47.1**)* are thought to represent the remnants of bacteria within phagosomes that have been mineralized by calcium and iron.

---

*All e-figures are available online via the Solution Site Image Bank.

3. **Retroperitoneal abscesses** are generally secondary to infectious processes of adjacent organs, most commonly of the kidneys. Less frequently, abscesses originate from distant septic foci that propagate via a hematogenous route.

4. **Other nonneoplastic conditions** including hemorrhage, bile collection, and extravasation of urine can be occasionally encountered in the retroperitoneal space. Endometriosis may also involve the retroperitoneum.

B. **Idiopathic retroperitoneal fibrosis (sclerosing retroperitoneal fibrosis, Ormond disease)** is an uncommon inflammatory process characterized by sclerosing fibrosis of the retroperitoneum that can ultimately cause constriction and obliteration of the ureters.

Grossly, there is poorly circumscribed fibrosis, usually at the level of the lower abdominal aorta and its bifurcation. Microscopically, the process is characterized by dense fibrosis with collagen entrapment, with associated alternating areas of prominent inflammation primarily consisting of plasma cells, histiocytes, eosinophils, and lymphocytes (e-**Fig. 47.2**). The plasma cells may be IgG4 positive in which case the disorder may be a member of the IgG4-related sclerosing disorders, especially in affected males (*Am J Surg Pathol.* 2009;33:1833); periaortitis in association with retroperitoneal fibrosis may be part of the same sclerosing disease spectrum (*Am J Surg Pathol.* 2008;32:197), as are sclerosing inflammatory diseases in the thyroid, mediastinum, and bile ducts. In the remaining cases, the etiology is undetermined or associated with methysergide and other drugs (and often regresses after cessation of the drug).

C. **Cystic lesions.** While most cystic lesions of the retroperitoneum represent a secondary or degenerative change within a benign or malignant neoplasm, several benign primary cystic lesions also occur.

1. **Cystic lymphangioma** or **cystic lymphatic malformation** of the retroperitoneum accounts for 5% of all retroperitoneal cystic lesions and can occur at any age. Involvement of the mesentery is an associated feature since this malformation is not well circumscribed (*J Surg Oncol.* 1996;61:234). Pathologically, multi- or unilocular cysts contain clear or milky fluid, and are lined with a single layer of flattened endothelium, which is D2-40 immunopositive (*J Pediatr Surg.* 1999;34;1164).

2. **Multicystic peritoneal inclusion cyst** occurs predominantly in women of reproductive age and, even though rarely seen in the retroperitoneum, is seen in the differential diagnosis of cystic lesions (especially of multilocular cystic lymphangioma). Prior abdominal surgery is common. Histopathologically, the lesion consists of mesothelial-lined cystic spaces usually containing watery secretions, separated by a delicate fibromuscular stroma. The lining epithelium is usually immunoreactive for calretinin. As discussed in some detail in Chapter 11 (Section IV.B), some confusion exists regarding the proper classification of multicystic peritoneal inclusion cyst, as demonstrated by the fact that the lesion is also known as multicystic mesothelioma (*Ann Diagn Pathol.* 2000;4:308).

3. **Bronchogenic cysts** can rarely occur in a subdiaphragmatic location, including the retroperitoneum, as part of the morphologic spectrum of bronchopulmonary foregut malformations. The related anomaly, extralobar sequestration with features of congenital cystic adenomatoid malformation type 2 presents a solid mass in the same site, usually in infants and young children; its suprarenal location can lead to confusion with neuroblastoma (*J Pediatr Surg.* 2007;42:1627). The cysts are lined by respiratory-type, pseudostratified, ciliated columnar epithelium that can focally contain seromucous glands and nodules of hyaline cartilage.

4. **Müllerian cysts** of the retroperitoneum are usually in excess of 10 cm in greatest dimension and are lined by cuboidal to columnar epithelium that often contains ciliated cells; there is no atypia, although stratification and epithelial

tufting can be present as in tubal epithelium. Beneath the lining of a müllerian cyst, loose fibrous tissue, dilated vessels, and incomplete smooth muscle bundles can be seen (*Hum Pathol.* 2003;34:194). Mucinous cystadenoma with ovarian type stroma (which is inhibin immunopositive) occurs rarely as an extrapancreatic cyst in the retroperitoneum.

5. **Enteric duplication cyst (EDC)** is an extremely uncommon congenital lesion and may be detected prenatally (*Pediatr Radiol.* 2000;30:671). Although usually intra-abdominal and associated with the small intestine, it has sporadically been described in the retroperitoneum. A spherical, tubular, or dumbbell-shaped cyst with a smooth lining and viscous contents is the gross appearance. Microscopically, the cyst wall has a variably differentiated enteric mucosa consisting of a simplified cuboidal or cylindrical epithelium, to a more normal appearing mucosa with a muscularis mucosa and a muscularis propria. Focal areas of squamous metaplasia and gastric-type mucosa have also been described in retroperitoneal EDCs (*JOP.* 2006;7:492). Heterotopic pancreas is another infrequent finding.

III. **NEOPLASMS.** Primary retroperitoneal tumors arise from the extravisceral tissues that comprise the retroperitoneum; the neoplasms for the most part are malignant in adults and originate from lymphoid and various soft tissue elements including fat and neural structures. The histogenesis of some of the high-grade sarcomas is not apparent, and the immunophenotype often does provide information that is specific in terms of lineage.

In children and young adults, germ cell neoplasms can present in the retroperitoneum, but the most common neoplasms of the retroperitoneum in children include the neuroblastic tumors (neuroblastoma and its variants) and high-grade lymphomas, in particular Burkitt lymphoma, large cell lymphoma, and Hodgkin lymphoma. The most commonly encountered primary retroperitoneal tumors in adults are sarcomas, followed by lymphomas and germ cell tumors (*Sarcoma.* 2001;5:5). Overall, 70% to 80% of retroperitoneal tumors are malignant (and thus the retroperitoneum is the only body site where the frequency of malignant neoplasms exceeds that of benign tumors).

The anatomy of the retroperitoneal space makes it possible for primary (as well as metastatic) tumors to attain substantial dimensions before clinical manifestations become evident. Malignant retroperitoneal tumors have a generally poor prognosis since they are often found at an advanced stage of disease, and even resectable tumors often recur.

A. **Soft tissue tumors.** Primary sarcomas arising in the retroperitoneum constitute 10% to 20% of all soft tissue sarcomas in adults: liposarcoma (40% of cases), leiomyosarcoma (30%), and pleomorphic sarcoma—malignant fibrous histiocytoma (25%) (*Expert Rev Anticancer Ther.* 2009;9:1145). As a group, retroperitoneal sarcomas are often in excess of 10 cm and weigh in excess of 400 to 500 g. Complete resection is associated with the most favorable outcome, but size and involvement of other structures often limits the extent and completeness of the resection; local recurrence is guaranteed in the latter cases. With complete resection and no local recurrences, the 5-year survival is 40% to 50%. As for soft tissue sarcomas arising in other anatomic sites, the American Joint Committed on Cancer (AJCC) staging system is utilized for staging of retroperitoneal sarcomas (see Chap. 46).

1. **Adipocytic tumors**
   a. **Benign**
      i. **Myolipoma,** one of the more common benign retroperitoneal lipomatous tumors, is more common than pure retroperitoneal lipomas. This encapsulated lesion has a lobulated fatty appearance with bands and nodules of white to gray-white tissue (*World J Surg Oncol.* 2005;3:72); the large size, usually 10 cm or greater, often raises the question of

liposarcoma. Microscopically, the tumor contains an admixture of mature adipocytes and bundles of smooth muscle (which usually predominate), but there is an absence of mitotic activity and atypia. The tumor is diffusely and strongly immunopositive for smooth muscle actin (SMA) and desmin.

ii. **Other mixed-type benign fatty tumors** in the retroperitoneum include **myelolipoma** and **angiomyolipoma (AML)** arising in the adrenal and kidney, respectively; as these tumors enlarge, both may convey the impression of a tumor based in the retroperitoneum. Examples of purely retroperitoneal AMLs have been described (*Abdom Imaging.* 2004;29:721). Microscopically, the presence of myeloid elements characterizes myelolipoma; atypical appearing lipoblasts may lead to a misinterpretation of liposarcoma in a largely fatty AML, but thick-walled vessels should be the clue to the latter diagnosis. HMB-45 and Melan-A immunopositivity in the nonadipocytic areas of AML also can be used to establish the diagnosis. Nuclear staining for TFE3 is another feature of AML. **Perivascular epithelioid cell neoplasm,** a related entity to AML, has also been reported as a primary tumor of the pelvis, mesentery, or retroperitoneum (*Am J Surg Pathol.* 2005;29: 1558).

iii. **Lipoblastoma,** a tumor of early childhood, presents in the retroperitoneum in 5% to 10% of the cases. From the retroperitoneum, the tumor may extend into the mesentery and omentum. Lipoblastoma is commonly in excess of 6 cm in diameter, and grossly has a glistening gray-white mucoid surface with faint lobulation. Microscopically, the lobules contain a mixture of mature adipocytes and immature fetal adipocytic cells with progressive differentiation toward mature adipose cells. The lobules are usually separated by connective tissue septa that contain small vessels. Some tumors have a striking resemblance to myxoid liposarcoma, but lipoblastoma contains desmin-positive cells and a *PLAG1* mutation.

b. **Malignant.** As a group, liposarcoma is the most common primary nonvisceral malignant neoplasm of the retroperitoneum and accounts for 30% to 50% of retroperitoneal sarcomas.

i. **Atypical lipomatous tumor/well-differentiated liposarcoma (ALT/WDLPS)** is the most common subtype of liposarcoma in the retroperitoneum. It is the largest neoplasm of this site and can measure in excess of 15 cm and weigh 1 kg or more. Grossly, a thin external membrane is usually the only structure serving as a "capsule" for an otherwise well-circumscribed yellowish-white lipomatous mass. The diagnostic challenge of ALT/WDLPS is the identification of atypical lipoblasts with enlarged, hyperchromatic, irregular nuclei with indented or scalloped nuclear membranes, especially in those cases with a predominant mature lipomatous appearance and few classic lipoblasts (e-**Fig. 47.3**). The paucity of lipoblasts may be accompanied by fibrosclerotic foci containing atypical stromal cells, a feature of equal diagnostic importance to the atypical lipoblasts.

ii. **Dedifferentiated liposarcoma** is identified by the presence of sharply demarcated areas of nonlipogenic sarcoma adjacent to areas of well-differentiated liposarcoma (e-**Fig. 47.4**). In the retroperitoneum, the nonlipogenic sarcomatous component has a fibrosarcomatous or undifferentiated morphology. Both ALT/WDLPS and dedifferentiated liposarcoma harbor amplification of the *MDM2* and *CDK4* genes, and immunohistochemically, both are positive for MDM2 and CDK4 expression.

iii. **Myxoid/round cell liposarcoma** is uncommon in the retroperitoneum. On the basis of immunohistochemical and molecular analysis, it has been shown that most presumed primary retroperitoneal myxoid/ round cell liposarcomas actually represent well-differentiated/ dedifferentiated liposarcomas (*Mod Pathol.* 2009;22:223).

iv. **Pleomorphic liposarcoma** in the retroperitoneum presents the differential diagnosis of pleomorphic undifferentiated sarcoma. Correct classification is often a matter of identifying convincing lipoblasts.

2. **Smooth muscle tumors**
   a. **Deep-seated leiomyoma (leiomyoma of deep soft tissue)** is an extremely uncommon benign tumor that primarily occurs in perimenopausal women; only isolated cases have been reported in males. Microscopically, the tumor resembles a uterine leiomyoma, exhibiting intersecting fascicles of bland appearing smooth muscle cells. Mitotic activity is low (<5 mitoses per 50 high-power fields [HPFs]), and the tumor is commonly positive for estrogen and progesterone receptor expression. Deep-seated leiomyoma will occasionally recur after incomplete excision, but metastasis does not occur (*Adv Anat Pathol.* 2002;9:351). Explanations for a deep smooth muscle tumor in the abdomen or retroperitoneum of a female include a so-called parasitized leiomyoma from the uterus, which has essentially separated from the outer portion of the uterus and gained its principal blood supply from an adjacent structure. **Intravenous leiomyomatosis** from the uterus also presents as benign appearing smooth muscle tumors in the pelvic soft tissues, often with extension into adjacent lymph nodes. The essential pathologic feature is the identification of circumscribed nodules of benign-appearing smooth muscle within vascular or lymphatic spaces.
   b. **Leiomyosarcoma (LMS)** accounts for 20% to 30% of all retroperitoneal sarcomas, is the most aggressive of retroperitoneum sarcomas, and in some series is the most common sarcoma of this site. Like the other retroperitoneal sarcomas, dimensions and weights often exceed 15 cm and 500 g, respectively. There is commonly a pseudoencapsule and a nodular surface with areas of hemorrhage, necrosis, and cystic degeneration. Histologically, the tumor is composed of highly atypical-appearing spindle cells with elongated, blunt-ended nuclei and eosinophilic cytoplasm (**e-Fig. 47.5**). The presence of any cytological atypia, significant mitotic activity, or coagulative necrosis in a retroperitoneal smooth muscle neoplasm warrants a diagnosis of LMS. Aggressive metastatic disease and a poor prognosis are characteristic of retroperitoneal LMSs with even very low mitotic activity (1 to 4 mitoses per 10 HPFs). It is worth mentioning that LMSs in the retroperitoneum may present in the inferior vena cava, or as a metastasis from a primary LMS of the uterus or paratesticular soft tissues.

3. **Skeletal muscle tumors**
   a. Benign skeletal muscle tumors of the retroperitoneum are extremely rare. Only isolated cases of **rhabdomyoma** have been reported, with similar pathologic characteristics as when the tumor occurs elsewhere.
   b. **Rhabdomyosarcoma (RMS)** of the embryonal or alveolar subtypes in the retroperitoneum–pelvis is a neoplasm of children between 2 and 10 years of age (**e-Fig. 47.6**). Approximately 10% to 15% of childhood RMSs arise in the soft tissues of the pelvis and/or retroperitoneum, and are usually 10 cm or greater in maximal dimension (*Pediatr Blood Cancer.* 2004;42: 618); the retroperitoneum is an unfavorable site for a childhood RMS (*J Pediatr Hematol Oncol.* 2001;23:215). Pleomorphic RMS in the retroperitoneum may represent a component of a dedifferentiated liposarcoma, a nongerminal pattern of malignancy in a germ cell tumor, or spread of a malignant mixed müllerian tumor (*Am J Surg Pathol.* 2007;31:1557).

4. **Fibroblastic tumors**
   a. **Benign fibroblastic tumors** other than desmoid fibromatosis are rare in the retroperitoneum. It may be difficult to differentiate between a presumed fibrous tumor and a nonneoplastic fibroinflammatory process (e.g., an IgG4 fibrosclerosing process).
   b. **Desmoid fibromatosis, IMT, extrapleural solitary fibrous tumor/hemangio-pericytoma, and gastrointestinal stromal tumors (GISTs)** are several examples of intermediate behavior tumors that may involve the retroperitoneum.

      Desmoid fibromatosis usually arises in the mesentery-omentum with extension into the retroperitoneum, but occasionally is limited to the retroperitoneum. Those desmoid tumors arising in the proximal lower extremity can, in the course of several local recurrences, extend through sciatic notch into the retroperitoneum as well; the presence of familial adenomatous polyposis in these patients should be addressed. Desmoid fibromatosis is not encapsulated but is well circumscribed, except in these cases, which represent a local recurrence. Its cut surface shows a firm, trabeculated pattern resembling a smooth muscle tumor. Microscopically, dense interlacing bundles of uniform spindle-shaped fibroblasts are present in a collagenous, keloid-like, or myxoid stroma with no evidence of nuclear atypia. Scattered mitotic figures may be identified and should not be a source of concern unless they are atypical (e-**Fig. 47.7**). The tumor is immunopositive for vimentin, SMA, and nuclear β-catenin staining. If the tumor is positive for CD34 and CD117 (c-kit), GIST is the favored diagnosis as either a local recurrence or a rare primary extraintestinal GIST (*J Gastrointest Surg.* 2009;13:1094).

      Primary retroperitoneal extrapleural solitary fibrous tumor/hemangio-pericytoma is uncommon, but documented (*J Am Coll Surg.* 2004;198: 322; *Hum Pathol.* 2000;31:1108). These CD34-positive (but CD117-negative) neoplasms may be quite cellular and mitotically active, in which case the most appropriate diagnosis is malignant solitary fibrous tumor. Although grouped together as related (if not identical) tumors in the current World Health Organization (WHO) scheme (see Chap. 46), the diagnosis of hemangiopericytoma is reserved for tumors that resemble the cellular areas of solitary fibrous tumor with the characteristic network of vascular profiles.

      IMT, like desmoid fibromatosis, may present in the mesentery-omentum with extension into the retroperitoneum. IMT typically presents in children and young adults. Grossly, it is a circumscribed firm, gray-white mass that measures 5to 10 cm. Microscopically, it has a varied microscopic pattern of spindle cells with accompanying plasma cells, myxoid foci resembling nodular fasciitis, and dense hyalinized collagen. In addition to immunopositivity for vimentin and SMA, 50% or more of cases are anaplastic lymphoma kinase (ALK-1) positive (*Am J Surg Pathol.* 2007;31:509). The presence of IgG4 plasma cells in IMT is seen in some cases (*Mod Pathol.* 2011;24:606).
   c. **Malignant fibroblastic tumors** are very rare in the retroperitoneum. **Adult fibrosarcoma** is currently a diagnosis of exclusion and, according to recent series, accounts for <5% of all retroperitoneal sarcomas; sarcomatous transformation of a solitary fibrous tumor should be considered in the differential diagnosis (*Am J Surg Pathol.* 2009;33:1314). Microscopically, fibrosarcoma is composed of spindle-shaped cells with large elongated nuclei and scant cytoplasm, arranged in a classic herringbone pattern. **Infantile fibrosarcoma** is known to occur in the retroperitoneum, but most commonly presents in the extremities; the identical neoplasm arising in the kidney in infancy, **cellular mesoblastic nephroma,** has the

same morphology and also harbors the t(12;15) translocation (*J Clin Oncol.* 2010;28:318–323). Other variants of fibrosarcoma, such as low-grade fibromyxoid sarcoma and myxoid-type fibrosarcoma, are rarely encountered in the retroperitoneum. In fact, most retroperitoneal tumors that present histologic features of myxofibrosarcoma may actually represent dedifferentiated liposarcomas (*Virchows Arch.* 2001;439:141).

5. Fibrohistiocytic tumors

   a. Pleomorphic undifferentiated sarcoma—malignant fibrous histiocytoma (MFH) formerly accounted for up to 30% of sarcomas of the retroperitoneum. Recent studies would seem to imply that many of these high-grade sarcomas actually represent dedifferentiated liposarcomas. Thus, a careful search for focal ALT/WDLPS, as well as immunostains for MDM2 and CDK4 expression and/or cytogenetic analysis for chromosome 12 abnormalities (as discussed in Section III.A.1.b) should be performed to confirm the diagnosis.

   b. Inflammatory MFH is most commonly found in the retroperitoneum. Microscopically, it is characterized by atypical spindle cells admixed with xanthomatous cells within an extensive acute and chronic inflammatory infiltrate composed of neutrophils, eosinophils, lymphocytes, and plasma cells (e-**Fig. 47.8**). The differential diagnosis includes LMS and liposarcoma, both of which may have similar inflammatory reactions.

6. Neural tumors

   a. Benign. Schwannoma accounts for approximately 1% to 5% of all retroperitoneal tumors, and grossly appears as a large (>10 cm) solitary, well-encapsulated, firm, round mass. Histologically, it presents with alternating cellular areas with palisading nuclei (Antoni A areas), and myxoid hypocellular areas (Antoni B areas). A characteristic feature of schwannomas of the retroperitoneum is the presence of cystic change (*Urology.* 1986;28:529), as well as thickened hyalinized vessels. **Ganglioneuroma** is a tumor with dispersed ganglion cells in a background neuromatous stroma. Ganglioneuroma can be mistaken for a schwannoma in those areas of the tumor with a paucity or absence of ganglion cells.

   b. Malignant. Malignant peripheral nerve sheath tumor (MPNST) represents 5% to 10% of all retroperitoneal sarcomas. Microscopically, the tumor features asymmetric spindle-shaped cells arranged in dense fascicles with hyperchromatic nuclei and frequent mitoses (e-**Fig. 47.9**). In the setting of neurofibromatosis type I, the tumor often has a plexiform growth pattern.

   c. Tumors of sympathetic nervous tissue

      i. Neuroblastoma may originate from the sympathetic nervous system chain of ganglia, commonly in the retroperitoneum and without involvement of the adrenal gland. In fact, the extraadrenal retroperitoneum is the site of origin of 30% to 35% of neuroblastomas in the pediatric population. **Adult neuroblastoma,** though rare, is nonetheless in the differential diagnosis of malignant round cell tumors of the retroperitoneum of adults. Nonetheless, there is a greater likelihood that a paraspinal malignant round cell neoplasm in a young adult is Ewing sarcoma/peripheral neuroectodermal tumor (EWS/PNET) or lymphoma than a neuroblastoma.

      ii. Extraadrenal retroperitoneal paraganglioma is an uncommon tumor, and arises from the chromaffin cells located in the paraaortic sympathetic chain and at the aortic bifurcation. Similar to adrenal pheochromocytomas and extraadrenal paragangliomas elsewhere, the tumor may be functional with associated characteristic signs and symptoms, but most cases are nonfunctional. Grossly, the tumor is rubbery with firm brown to tan cut surfaces, and in large specimens can exhibit a cystic component secondary to central necrosis or hemorrhage. The tumor is composed of well-defined nests of cells surrounded by sustentacular cells; the nests are usually composed of round cells with abundant granular eosinophilic or basophilic cytoplasm (e-**Fig. 47.10**). Nuclear atypia and vascular invasion may also be present. In the retroperitoneum, these tumors tend to have an aggressive course with local invasion and a high incidence of local recurrence, and a higher rate of metastasis than adrenal pheochromocytoma (20% to 42% for the former versus 2% to 10% for the latter) (*Urol Ann.* 2010;2:12).

7. **Vascular tumors.** Most vascular tumors, ranging from hemangiomas to angiosarcomas, have been reported as isolated cases in the retroperitoneum. The vascular tumor that is particularly common in the retroperitoneum is **Kaposiform hemangioendothelioma**, a tumor of childhood that is frequently complicated by the Kasabach–Merritt phenomenon. Although initially described as a distinctive vascular neoplasm of the retroperitoneum, it is now recognized to occur in skin and soft tissues of the extremities (*Am J Surg Pathol.* 1991;15:982). In the retroperitoneum, the tumor tends to be large, poorly circumscribed, and may involve adjacent structures including the colon. Microscopically, the tumor is composed of fascicles of spindle cells and narrow vascular spaces that have a lobular arrangement; microthrombi, slit-like endothelial-lined vascular channels, and hyaline globules are also present, and thus the tumor resembles Kaposi sarcoma. However, Kaposiform hemangioendothelioma lacks nuclear positivity for human herpes virus 8 (HHV-8).

8. **Miscellaneous soft tissue tumors**
   a. **Synovial sarcoma** represents ~1% of all retroperitoneal sarcomas. The true incidence may be higher since cases formerly diagnosed as fibrosarcoma may have represented examples of monophasic synovial sarcoma. A firm, gray-pink, circumscribed mass measuring 8 to 10 cm in greatest dimension is the typical gross appearance. In contrast to synovial sarcomas elsewhere, retroperitoneal synovial sarcomas tend not to metastasize remotely, but are difficult to control locally and thus have an overall poor prognosis (*Histopathology.* 2004;45:245; *J BUON.* 2008;13:211). A potential diagnostic pitfall may arise since retroperitoneal schwannomas are often AE1/AE3 cytokeratin immunopositive, but schwannomas are also glial fibrillary acidic protein immunopositive unlike synovial sarcomas (*Mod Pathol.* 2006;19:115).
   b. Virtually all **malignant round cell tumors** have been described as primary tumors of the retroperitoneum. **EWS/PNET** presents in this location in ~5% of cases, usually as a paraspinal mass. **Desmoplastic small round cell tumor** usually arises in the peritoneal cavity, but in some series up to 15% of cases originate in the retroperitoneum.

B. **Germ cell tumors**
   1. Primary **retroperitoneal teratomas** typically occur in infancy and childhood but are rare in adults. About 75% of cases occur in children younger than 5 years, and the incidence in females is twice that of males, as is also the case for sacrococcygeal teratomas in children. Grossly, these tumors have a mixed cystic solid appearance.
      a. As elsewhere, **mature teratomas** contain mature tissue, often from all three germ layers, with occasional calcification or ossification. Mature cystic teratomas should be thoroughly sampled (one section per centimeter) in order to exclude the presence of yolk sac tumor, especially in a young child. Immature somatic elements such as primitive neural tubules or sheets of neuroblasts with a fibrillary background should not be viewed with concern in an infant or young child.

b. **Immature teratomas** contain immature or primitive tissue (derived from any or all three germ cell layers) that is usually mixed with areas of mature tissue. The most common immature neural tissues form rosettes, sheets of neuroblasts, or tubules of primitive neural cells. The pathologic grading of retroperitoneal teratomas, specifically in children, on the basis of the extent of immature somatic tissues has no prognostic significance. On the other hand, the presence of yolk sac tumor or endodermal sinus tumor establishes the malignant nature of the neoplasm.

2. **Secondary germ cell neoplasms.** A teratoma in an adolescent or young male may be a posttreatment "growing teratoma," which represents residual metastatic disease from a malignant germ cell tumor of the testis. Similarly, the presence of a retroperitoneal tumor in the absence of a known primary testicular germ cell tumor should lead to careful evaluation of the testes since they may harbor a scar with or without intratubular germ cell neoplasia as evidence of spontaneous regression of a primary testicular neoplasm. In fact, a retroperitoneal germ cell tumor, in a male, whether seminoma or of another pattern, is metastatic disease from the testis until proven otherwise.

C. **Lymphomas and other lymphoproliferative disorders**

1. Both **non-Hodgkin** and **Hodgkin lymphoma** present in retroperitoneum with lymphadenopathy, as a localized mass, or as retroperitoneal fibrosis. Bulky retroperitoneal lymphadenopathy with or without intestinal or other organ involvement in the first two decades of life usually represents Burkitt lymphoma. In adults, the same presentation usually represents small lymphocytic lymphoma/chronic lymphocytic leukemia or one of the other B-cell lymphomas including follicular lymphoma. Diagnosis can be challenging due to limitations on the adequacy of the specimen, a prominent fibrous reaction, necrosis, or a nonrepresentative biopsy.

2. **Castleman disease** also occasionally presents in the retroperitoneum. The hyaline type, which is most common in the retroperitoneum as elsewhere, is usually localized to a single lymph node and tends to be asymptomatic. The plasma cell type is multifocal and usually presents with a more aggressive course and systemic manifestations. The hyaline type is characterized grossly by homogenous orange-yellowish cut surfaces, and microscopically by giant lymphoid follicles centered on a markedly hyalinized vessel surrounded by lymphocytes arranged in an onion-skin pattern (e-**Fig. 47.11**). The plasma cell type is grossly similar, but on microscopic examination contains more plasma cells with less vascular hyalinization.

D. **Tumors of müllerian type** are occasionally described in the retroperitoneum. As in the ovary, they are usually of serous, mucinous, or endometrioid type, and can be benign borderline or malignant. In the retroperitoneum, borderline and malignant tumors appear to be more common than their benign counterparts. Tumors are usually large and unilateral, and tend to present with no concomitant ovarian lesions.

E. **Metastatic tumors.** Various primary malignant neoplasms arising in retroperitoneal or posterior abdominal wall organs such as the pancreas, kidney, liver, and adrenal gland often present with or are accompanied by direct extravisceral invasion into the retroperitoneum. Retroperitoneal lymph node metastases are also seen in association with many primary tumors of other sites.

48 Bone Neoplasms and Other Nonmetabolic Disorders

Omar Hameed and Michael J. Klein

I. **NORMAL MICROSCOPIC ANATOMY.** The bones are composed of compact bone, which is derived from intramembranous ossification, and coarse cancellous bone, which is the osseous remnant of endochondral ossification. Compact bone makes up the cortices of long bones and constitutes their diaphyses and the surface portion of their metaphyses, as well as the compacta of the flat and irregular bones. Cancellous bone is present in the medullary cavity and is abundant at the ends of the long bones. In bone, form follows function (Wolff's law). In the shafts of bones, most of the forces act upon the surface. Here, the compact bone, which is 90% solid and only 10% space, bears the compression, tension, shear, and torsional forces. The medulla, shielded from forces, contains practically no bone at all. The ends of the bones are supported by the vertical plates and horizontal struts of the cancellous bone, yet cancellous bone is only 25% bone and 75% marrow by volume; here the cortex is very thin.

Bone matrix is classified as woven or lamellar depending on the predominant fiber arrangement of its collagen. In woven bone, the collagen fiber pattern is random. This type of bone is found in the fetal skeleton and in processes in which there is very rapid bone production. In lamellar bone, the bone collagen fibers are arranged in stacks of tightly packed fibers that are parallel in the same stack. In the next layer, the collagen fibers are also parallel to one another, but their direction is different from the collagen in the previous stack so that the bone appears to be layered. Both compact bone and cancellous bone consist of lamellar bone after the age of 3 years. After this age, woven bone is almost always pathologic, although the etiology is often not discernible without imaging studies (Bullough PG. *Orthopedic Pathology*. 5th ed. St. Louis: CV Mosby; 2010). In compact bone, the lamellae are arranged concentrically around central vascular canals termed Haversian canals; each vascular canal and its associated lamellae are referred to an osteon or Haversian system. In cancellous bone, the lamellae are arranged in linear, parallel plates (e-Fig. 48.1).* Adjacent osteons are separated from each other and from interstitial lamellae (see the section on circulatory diseases) and circumferential lamellae (which encircle the inner and outer cortex and are remnants of periosteal intramembranous ossification) by basophilic staining cement lines. Cement lines are sliding planes that are richer in calcium than surrounding bone matrix but the exact composition of which is unknown; they are produced by osteoblasts when bone is synthesized following osteoclast resorption (reversal cement lines) or after a period of inactivity (arrest cement lines). In the former type, the lamellae are discontinuous on either side of the cement line and in the latter the lamellae are continuous on either side (e-Fig. 48.2).

II. **SPECIMEN PROCESSING**

A. **Gross handling and selection of sections.** The approach to specimen handling is largely one of common sense. Small biopsy specimens should be submitted for sectioning in their entirety. If there is any doubt about whether they

---

*All e-figures are available online via the Solution site image bank.

contain bone, they should be fixed, briefly decalcified, and rinsed. Most bone biopsies performed with needles are sufficiently thin for adequate fixation and decalcification, whereas curettings may sometimes need to be sliced into thinner fragments. The amount of curettings to submit for sectioning depends on their volume and the uniformity of the curettings. When it is feasible, all curettings should be submitted. If the lesion curetted is a hyaline cartilage tumor, as much of the histology as possible should be reviewed to identify atypical chondrocytes as well as any subtle interface with normal surrounding bone.

Other large specimens such as total joint replacements and bone resections also need to be sliced into thinner fragments. Although this may be accomplished with large band saws or other power-type saws, motorized saws are dangerous and somewhat time-consuming to maintain properly, especially in a laboratory that receives a limited number of bone specimens. Vibrating or oscillating saws, which are usually available in autopsy suites, should be avoided if possible, because they do not section uniformly and their oscillating movement creates tension and compression artifacts that often make bone sections impossible to interpret properly. A very easy approach is to hold bone specimens steadily in a tabletop vise or clamp and to cut them with a hacksaw in which two fine-tooth blades are separated by 2- to 3-mm-thick washers. Such an apparatus is easily and cheaply made, although there are commercial instruments available for the same purpose. It must be emphasized that double-bladed instruments should be scrupulously cleaned between every specimen to avoid tissue cross-contamination between different cases.

The handling and disposition of larger resection specimens depends on the reason for the procedure. For malignant tumors in which patients have not received neoadjuvant chemotherapy (after biopsy but prior to resection), grading, staging, and adequacy of resection are the major clinical issues. Amputations from these patients should include sections from the soft tissue and vascular margins as well as those from the tumor itself. Tumor sections should be taken in such a way as to document the pertinent tumor histology, whether the tumor involves the medulla and/or cortex, and how far the tumor extends into soft tissues. The specimen should be cut in such a way as to disclose the greatest extent of tumor; review of the imaging studies can guide the selection process. Careful attention should be paid to taking sections from any areas that are grossly disparate from the appearance of the majority of the tumor. Radical resections for malignant tumors that are not amputations need the same sectioning methods, but any area of the resection constituting a margin must be sectioned and appropriately designated. This includes the bone resection margin, overlying soft tissue dissection margins, and the margins of any skin and soft tissue encompassing a prior biopsy site.

Specimens resected from patients who have received neoadjuvant chemotherapy (currently used in osteosarcoma and in Ewing sarcoma/primitive neuroectodermal tumor [EWS/PNET]) need more extensive sampling to estimate the extent of treatment-associated necrosis. This means that one or more thin slabs should be cut through the entire extent of the bone and tumor, and that the entire slab or slabs should be fixed, decalcified, mapped, and examined not only for tumor stage, but also for the extent of necrosis. The slabs should be photographed so as to produce a section map; if a specimen x-ray machine is available, specimen radiographs can be used both as section maps and as controls for adequate specimen decalcification (e-Fig. 48.3). Additional sections may be taken if there are areas not in the slab selected that appear as though they might be viable; the pathologist's task in this enterprise is to find viable tumor if any is present. It is worthwhile to remember that to extrapolate the degree of necrosis in a single slab into necrosis of the tumor as a whole makes the assumption that what is present in that particular slab is representative of the entire lesion.

B. Decalcification. The main difference between processing of bone specimens and of softer tissues is the requirement for an extra step of decalcification. Removal of calcium insures that bone collagen is no harder than the paraffin in which it is embedded, and that microtomy of bone tissues will approximate that for other types of specimens. Decalcification may be performed in a number of ways. In acid decalcification, hydrogen ions are in effect substituted for calcium ions. Electrolysis in effect accomplishes the same end, but is performed in an electrolyte solution with a weak electrical current. Ionic exchange is the slowest method but is the most gentle on tissue and results in the fewest artifacts. In practice, most histology laboratories rely on weak acid decalcification because it is the quickest and there is pressure from eager clinicians for rapid turnaround times in diagnosis. With use of acid decalcification methods, a few caveats must be kept in mind. First, the tissue must always be fixed adequately prior to decalcification to prevent artifacts that interfere with adequate staining or that can degrade the tissue after sections are prepared. This means that the tissue must be adequately thin (no more than 3- to 4-mm thick) prior to fixation, and that the tissue has remained in formalin or some other suitable fixative for an interval adequate to coagulate the proteins for routine staining. In addition, if immunohistochemistry needs to be performed, adequate fixation helps to insure that the decalcification process will less alter immune antigens. Second, when decalcification is performed with acid solutions, specimens must be rinsed in running water to ensure that the residual pH of the tissue is sufficiently neutral for hematoxylin staining. Failure to neutralize the acid not only results in understaining with hematoxylin, but also will cause stained sections to lose their hematoxylin staining in an accelerated manner. If time is insufficient for adequate specimen rinsing, the specimen should be neutralized in a dilute basic solution such as sodium bicarbonate. Third, if sections are left in dilute acid for a much longer period than necessary for calcium removal, tissue hydrolysis will remove the nucleic acids that cause nuclear hematoxylin staining and nuclei will appear acidophilic. This so-called overdecalcification artifact is generally not reversible. Overdecalcification may not interfere with many diagnostic interpretations, but it is important not to mistake this artifact for tissue necrosis, particularly in postchemotherapy specimen interpretation.

Adequate decalcification will vary by the tissue being decalcified. For example, woven bone, even though it tends to have higher calcium concentrations than lamellar bone, will often section adequately with incomplete decalcification because the former has less organization and less cutting resistance. The decision regarding whether the tissue is ready for embedding is often subjective and revolves around whether the tissue is pliable, trims easily, or can be penetrated with a needle. Complete decalcification is best judged either by testing the supernatant fluid with a colorimetric indicator or by comparing specimen radiographs prior to and after decalcification. These tests are seldom practical in a very busy general surgical pathology practice.

C. Approach to the interpretation of bone specimens. Patient complaints related to the musculoskeletal system constitute nearly one-third of physician office visits in the United States, so orthopedic problems are extremely common. While surgical pathologists are often asked to rule out bone tumors as the etiology of a clinical problem, it is useful to keep in mind that fractures alone are about 3000 to 4000 times more common than all primary bone tumors combined, and that metastatic tumors to bone are at least 20 times more common than primary bone tumors. The accurate diagnosis of bone diseases requires the correlation of patient demographics along with the clinical history and imaging studies to put the problem in its correct context prior to any histologic examination of the tissue. Symptoms and signs are fairly similar in orthopedic diseases; these consist of pain, loss of function, deformities, and (in the case of tumors) sometimes a mass or a sense of fullness. Pain is the most common symptom, and although it may vary considerably, pain severe enough to wake a patient from sleep is the type suspicious for neoplastic diseases.

D. Importance of radiologic findings. The surgical pathology of orthopedic diseases most often consists of defining the nature of bone lesions that are space occupying on imaging studies, advising the clinician if an infection may be present, and histologically documenting miscellaneous bone diseases that are not diagnosable by imaging studies alone. Because surgical pathologists usually render biopsy diagnoses with the assumption that a biopsy is representative of the pathologic process, it is natural to assume the same parameters in bone biopsies. This is a potentially dangerous assumption, because most orthopedic diseases are invisible without imaging studies. This means that to assure that a biopsy is representative of a process, the smaller the biopsy specimen, the greater the need to review the imaging studies defining that process. Because bones are deep seated, imaging studies are required to grasp the extent and behavior of bone lesions. For a surgical pathologist, correlating imaging studies with histologic findings depends on knowledge of normal bone and joint anatomy, normal anatomy as represented in radiographic images or other imaging studies, and the rudimentary alterations in imaging studies produced by pathologic processes (not only what a process does to normal bone, but also how normal bone alters the process) (*Adv Anat Pathol.* 2005;12:155). The majority of the radiographic image produced by long bones is due to beam attenuation by cortical bone in the shafts and by cancellous bone in the ends (e-**Fig. 48.4**). The attenuation produced by flat bones is primarily due to cortical bone, and that of irregular bones depends on the proportion of bone elements in any given part of the bone.

Space-occupying lesions within bone usually cause bone destruction, bone production, or some combination of the two. Destructive lesions are not seen in a single radiographic view until at least 40% of the bone in the path of the x-ray beam is destroyed. This means that almost an entire thickness of cortex must be destroyed to see the lesion if an intact and a destroyed cortex are superimposed in one view, or that at least 40% of cancellous bone must be destroyed in a bone end. It is partly for this reason that orthogonal views of bones are taken (e.g., posteroanterior and lateral views) so that destructive lesions may be isolated in routine radiographs. Radiodense lesions superimpose on the extant bone, causing more attenuation and easier visibility on a routine radiograph. In contrast, a lesion that is less dense than bone may fill the entire medullary cavity of a bone, but if it does not destroy the cortex it will be invisible regardless of the view because the dominant attenuator of the x-ray beam is the cortex, not the medullary fat or marrow. It is for these reasons that other imaging studies such as computed tomography (CT) scans and magnetic resonance imaging (MRI) are performed. These studies yield information that is complementary to that derived from routine radiographs. While they may be more sensitive in yielding information, a particular type of imaging modality should be used in concert with routine radiographs to answer a particular clinical question not answered by the radiographs.

III. DIAGNOSTIC FEATURES OF BONE LESIONS. There are very few general categories of bone disease (Table 48.1), although there are many individual diseases (McCarthy EF, Frassica FJ. *Pathology of Bone and Joint Disorders with Clinical and Radiographic Correlation.* Philadelphia: WB Saunders; 1998). Most patients can be separated into general diagnostic categories on the basis of their imaging studies. For example, traumatic diseases, which are among the commonest problems, will demonstrate fractures (with or without bone displacement) or dislocations on routine radiographs. Metabolic bone diseases (discussed in Chap. 49), which

TABLE 48.1	Bone Diseases by Category
Congenital	
Developmental/acquired	
Traumatic	
Circulatory	
Metabolic and Paget disease	
Infectious	
Iatrogenic	
Neoplastic and tumor-like	

characteristically affect the entire skeleton, usually demonstrate generalized radiolucency or osteopenia. Congenital and developmental diseases will usually affect more than one bone, are often symmetrical, and often demonstrate modeling deformities. Infections show a variety of radiographic abnormalities, depending on the type of organism present, the localization of the infection, and its chronicity. Avascular necrosis and idiopathic infarction demonstrate radiodensity in end arterial distributions; they are wedge-shaped at the convex ends of long bones and medullary in their diaphyses. Primary tumors of bone are usually localized defects that vary in their radiographic appearance in accordance with their biologic behavior. Metastatic tumors are usually localized defects that affect more than one bone or more than one focus in one bone, but they can be mistaken for primary tumors if they are solitary. Joint diseases change the quality or quantity of the space between the bone ends normally seen in radiographs; they may also produce joint erosions or joint deformities. The salient features of some miscellaneous bone diseases that pathologists sometimes encounter are presented in Table 48.2.

A. **Congenital and developmental diseases.** Very few of these disorders come to the attention of surgical pathologists, since most are diagnosed on the basis of their clinical and imaging appearances. Some of them, such as the histiocytoses and storage disorders, may be confirmed histologically, or may be seen incidentally, such as when there is a hip replacement for avascular necrosis associated with Gaucher disease. Many others, such as most of the sclerosing dysplasias exclusive of diseases with specific histologies (e.g., osteopetrosis), demonstrate bone of increased density but are not specific or separable from one another histologically without demonstrating the changes seen in the radiographs (e-Fig. 48.5).

B. **Traumatic disorders.** Fractures are numerically the most frequent bone and joint disorders. They do not usually come to the attention of surgical pathologists because most treatments are closed or do not produce tissue for diagnosis. In contrast, open fractures requiring debridement and acute fractures of the femoral neck undergoing joint replacement are sometimes received in pathology laboratories. Acute fractures usually demonstrate some degree of accompanying hemorrhage, reactive changes such as dilated sinusoids in still viable nearby marrow, and fragmented bone trabeculae. Subacute fractures will also demonstrate devitalization of the bone at the fracture site (empty osteocyte lacunae and necrosis of marrow), although histologic evidence of healing is usually not evident for 7 to 10 days. Fractures that do not heal and fractures that are thought to be pathologic are sometimes sampled to rule out the presence of tumor or infection. It is very important to know that there is a history of trauma when reviewing tissue, or there is some danger of misinterpreting microcallus or reactive changes as matrix production by a tumor. Even if the history is not available, imaging studies will reveal if a tumor is present, and it is worthwhile to remember that primary bone tumors that produce bone matrix are rarely the sites of fracture. There are histologic parameters to separate bone and cartilage

TABLE 48.2 Salient Features of Miscellaneous Nonneoplastic Bone Diseases That Pathologists May Occasionally Encounter

Tumor/Lesion	Location	Age	Radiologic findings	Pathologic findings	Differential diagnosis
Congenital/ developmental	Diffuse, sometimes localized; usually symmetrical	<10	Modeling abnormality	Disease-dependent	Very broad
Traumatic	Any part of any bone	Any	Fracture lines; dislocations	Hemorrhage; organization; woven bone and chondroid matrix	Osteosarcoma and chondrosarcoma
Circulatory					
Avascular necrosis	Convex ends of LBs	5–40	Wedge-shaped radio-density; crescent sign; collapse of articular cartilage	Necrotic marrow and bone; subarticular plate fracture	None
Idiopathic infarction	Medulla of LBs	>20	Hazy density sometimes resembling smoke	Necrotic marrow and bone; calcification and ossification of marrow fat	Enchondroma[a]
Paget disease	Any portion of any bone; almost always extending to articular ends	>50	Early: bone resorption in wedge-shaped edge Later: course trabeculation; loss of corticomedullary demarcations	Osteoclastic resorption + increased vascularity and marrow fibrosis; "mosaic" cement lines in middle to late stages	Hyperparathyroidism; myelodysplasia and myelofibrosis; metastatic carcinoma with fibrosis
Infectious					
Hematogenous	Cortex of LBs	2–15	Early: ↑ uptake on bone scan; change of marrow signal on MRI; Later: mixed sclerosis and radiolucency	Marrow fibrosis with osteonecrosis and exudate/ mixed inflammatory cell infiltrate	Round cell tumors and Langerhans cell histiocytosis
Direct	Any; open trauma or deep ulcer	Varies	Mixed sclerosis and radiolucency	Marrow fibrosis with osteonecrosis and exudate/ mixed inflammatory cell infiltrate	Round cell tumors and Langerhans cell histiocytosis

[a]Radiologic differential diagnosis.
LBs, long bones; MRI, magnetic resonance imaging.

formation by tumor from that of trauma, although it takes some experience to recognize them. Bone or osteoid production by tumor matrix is often lace-like and becomes sheetlike as more bone is produced. Bone produced as a repair phenomenon may be focally lacelike, but more often it rapidly acquires a micro-trabecular architecture and then becomes trabecular as it matures. In reactive bone there is almost always a zonation of maturity that is dependent on both the area in the lesion sampled and the time from trauma. While bone and cartilage are common findings in both osteosarcoma and fracture callus, cartilage tends to disappear as callus matures but it persists in osteosarcoma (e-Fig. 48.6). In addition, the progression from bone to cartilage and back to bone is orderly in reactive processes but is totally random in bone tumors.

C. Circulatory disturbances

1. **Bone necrosis.** Osteonecrosis occurs in areas where the bone circulation has an end arterial distribution. The most common sites are near the convex surfaces of joints where epiphyseal arterial branches supply the cancellous bone in the distribution of a cone. When this area of bone is deprived of circula-tion, avascular or aseptic necrosis of the bone results. The cancellous bone up to the calcified zone of the articular cartilage, deriving its blood supply from nutrient arteries to the epiphysis, undergoes infarction. The overlying articular cartilage, which derives oxygen and nutrients from the synovial fluid, remains viable. These changes are not immediately visible on routine radiographs because there are no changes in density of the necrotic bone. However, radionuclide bone scans do demonstrate early hypervascularity in the zone surrounding the necrotic area, and MRI demonstrates edema and loss of marrow fat because of early adipocyte necrosis. The wedge-shaped area of radiodensity characteristic of late osteonecrosis develops for a vari-ety of reasons, but deposition of calcium salts due to saponification of free fatty acid esters may be of greatest importance (although it is often difficult to recognize calcium salts in decalcified sections because they are dissolved by the decalcification process). Clinical symptoms become severe when the necrosis has extended to the articular cartilage with loss of congruency of the usual convex–concave joint surface and destruction of the subarticular plate. It is not uncommon for the articular cartilage and superficial subartic-ular plate to detach from the underlying cancellous bone (because dead bone matrix and living bone have the same inherent strength and stiffness, this probably happens because the subarticular bone no longer has the capacity for remodeling in the face of repetitive forces, and accumulated shear stress causes it to detach). When detachment occurs, the radiodense subarticular bone attached to the articular cartilage forms a crescentic shadow that may be seen radiographically (e-Fig. 48.7).

2. **Bone infarctions.** Infarcts are also presumably the result of a disruption in end arterial circulation. In the diaphysis, a bone infarct is largely confined to the medulla. This portion of the bone derives its blood supply from nutrient arteries that penetrate the cortex to supply the sinusoids of the medullary cavity and the inner cortex. The saponified marrowfat resulting from fat necrosis may appear to contain hazy or smoky radiodensities, and biopsies will reveal fat necrosis and a few scant trabeculae with empty osteocyte lacunae (e-Fig. 48.8).

   The outer cortex is supplied mainly by perforating arterioles derived from arteriae comitantes of the periosteum. The cortical portions of this circulation travel longitudinally via Haversian canals and interconnect within the cor-tex via the Volkmann canals. Because the circulation in the cortex is thereby microscopically collateralized, the cortex of long bones is somewhat more protected against infarction than is the medullary cavity. It is important to remember that within the cortex there are interstitial lamellae derived from the remnants of old Haversian systems, and inner or outer circumferential lamellae that have not fully resorbed but have no active blood supply, and because of this, physiologically there are lamellae that are devoid of osteocytes and are physiologically dead (e-Fig. 48.9); since all cortical bone is compact bone, this means that small foci of empty osteocyte lacunae within the cortex do not necessarily imply that there is avascular necrosis even though the bone is histologically dead. Ordinarily, it is necessary for both nutrient and periosteal blood supplies to be disrupted to cause a true cortical infarction. This happens most often in conjunction with trauma and with infections.

D. **Paget disease.** This disease has some histologic features in common with high-turnover metabolic bone diseases, but it is not a metabolic disease because it does not diffusely affect the entire skeleton and has no known associated metabolic defect (metabolic bone diseases are covered in Chap. 49). Paget disease is characterized by an imbalance or uncoupling of osteoclastic and osteoblastic activities, with osteoclastic bone resorption predominating early in the disease and osteoblastic activity persisting late in the disease. These histologic manifestations are correlated radiographically with characteristic radiolucency early in the disease, radiodensity in the late stages, and a mixed pattern for most of the interval between (*Skeletal Radiol.* 1995;24:173). Because the bone microarchitecture is altered, there is loss of the normal bone contour radiographically, and there is gradual loss of the normal cortical appearance and an increasingly coarse appearance to the bone trabeculations. A biopsy from an early radiolucent lesion demonstrates large bizarre osteoclasts producing large and irregular resorption pits (Howship's lacunae) on trabecular surfaces. These are often accompanied by paratrabecular fibrosis and dilated marrow sinusoids. As the resorption pits become filled in by osteoblast activity, irregularly shaped cement lines (sometimes likened to grout lines in a mosaic) mark the demarcation between the old and new bone. The bone on either side of these cement lines demonstrates either lamellar bone, in which the layers are discontinuous on either side, or lamellar bone on one side and woven bone on the other side. As the disease progresses and osteoclast activity slows, the bone becomes thicker and more interconnected than normal, but its arrangement and increased irregular cement lines make it more prone to deformities and fractures (e-Fig. 48.10).

E. **Infectious disorders.** Infections of bone arise either by direct introduction of organisms into the bone due to open trauma or overlying infections of soft tissue, or by secondary hematogenous spread. Most hematogenous osteomyelitis occurs in the first two decades of life. Its usual site in the bone is in the metaphysis adjoining the growth plate of a long bone because the microcirculation is stagnant in this area. Osteomyelitis due to open trauma can occur at any age; osteomyelitis associated with overlying infections is most often associated with peripheral vascular disease and so is seen later in life. Most infections of the bone are bacterial, but infections with fungi and lower virulence organisms may occur in immunocompromised hosts.

The vast majority of hematogenous osteomyelitis is due to coagulase-positive *Staphylococcus aureus,* but many other organisms may infect bones. Histologically, microorganisms are seldom seen in bone biopsies of patients with osteomyelitis because the sheer number of organisms required for the sensitivity of high-power or oil-immersion microscopy to detect bacteria is very high. Because of this, bacterial cultures should always be taken when infections of bone are suspected clinically—preferably prior to the institution of antibiotic therapy. A single bacterial culture is on the order of 10 million times more sensitive than histology—even when special stains for organisms are added to the regimen. Infections in bone are often accompanied by necrosis of at least some of the affected bone; the primary reason for this is that edema accompanies inflammation, and edema in the closed confines of the cortex compromises the medullary nutrient arteries and sinusoids due to resulting increased pressure. The innermost cortical circulation may be similarly compromised by increased intramedullary pressure. If the pressurized exudate finds its way into empty Haversian and Volkmann canals, it may push its way through these intracortical spaces and eventually dissect the periosteum, and its perforating arteries, from the cortex. If the cortex is deprived of its dual circulation, then it in turn becomes necrotic; this necrotic bone is called sequestrum. The combination of necrotic bone sequestrum, marrow fibrosis and/or fat necrosis, and mixed inflammatory infiltrates (usually including neutrophils and plasma cells) provides good histologic corroboration of osteomyelitis, but the demonstration of organisms is the gold standard for the diagnosis of infections (e-**Fig. 48.11**).

F. Iatrogenic disorders. Treatment-related disorders are seldom a major problem in the pathologic diagnosis of orthopedic disease, provided that an accurate clinical history is communicated to the surgical pathologist. For example, the diagnosis of osteosarcoma would be very unusual in a patient of the sixth decade without prior radiation of the site, or without some other underlying premalignant bone lesion. Administration of various therapeutic regimens may lead to secondary alterations in bones; perhaps the most notable of these is the amyloidosis of bones, tendon sheaths, and ligaments that develops from β2-microglobulin accumulation in long-term hemodialysis patients. Substances that have been given parenterally but that are not metabolized may also be deposited in bones or joints; without prior knowledge of therapeutic treatment, it may be difficult to make an accurate diagnosis (e-**Fig. 48.12**).

G. Neoplastic and tumor-like lesions. Primary tumors of bone are quite rare, accounting for only 0.2% of all malignancies, or an incidence of 1 per 100,000 individuals per year (Fletcher, CDM, Unni K, Mertens K, eds. *Tumors of Soft Tissues and Bone.* Lyon, France: IARC Press; 2002). There is a bimodal age distribution, with one peak in adolescence and a smaller one in patients older than 60 years. Among other characteristics, each bone tumor has its own age predilection, which is very useful from a differential diagnostic standpoint. Primary benign bone tumors are probably less common than primary malignant tumors if the very common nonossifying fibroma, osteochondroma, and enchondromas of the hands are excluded. In addition to benign and malignant bone neoplasms, there are a number of nonneoplastic lesions that can present in a manner similar to neoplastic conditions (Table 48.3); all of these lesions are discussed below, and their main features are presented in Tables 48.4 and 48.5. Pathologic stage is among the findings that are recommended to be reported for bone tumors (*Hum Pathol.* 2004;35:1173) and the American Joint Committee on Cancer (AJCC) Tumor, Node, Metastasis (TNM) staging scheme (Table 48.6) and/or the simpler Musculoskeletal Tumor Society scheme (Table 48.7) can be used for this purpose.

1. Cartilage-forming tumors

a. Osteochondroma is a cartilage-capped bony protrusion (e-**Fig. 48.13**) that arises from the surface of any bone that models or grows by endochondral ossification. On imaging, osteochondromas demonstrate a marrow cavity and a cortex continuous with those of the host bone. Although classified as bone neoplasms, osteochondromas may also result from displacements of the cartilaginous grown plate. This is consistent with their metaphyseal location and the fact that they cease to grow after skeletal maturation. Most osteochondromas are sporadic and solitary; however, multiple lesions are present in osteochondromatosis, which is an autosomal dominant hereditary condition. The presence of *EXT-1* mutations in the germline of these patients has been used as evidence of the classification of osteochondroma as a neoplasm (*J Clin Invest.*

TABLE 48.3	WHO Classification of Bone Tumors

Cartilage tumors

Osteochondroma
Chondroma
Enchondroma
Periosteal chondroma
Multiple chondromatosis
Chondroblastoma
Chondromyxoid fibroma
Chondrosarcoma
   Central, primary, and secondary
   Peripheral
   Dedifferentiated
   Mesenchymal
   Clear cell

Osteogenic tumors

Osteoid osteoma
Osteoblastoma
Osteosarcoma
Conventional
   Chondroblastic
   Fibroblastic
   Osteoblastic
Telangiectatic
Small cell
Low-grade central
Secondary
Parosteal
Periosteal
High-grade surface

Fibrogenic tumors

Desmoplastic fibroma
Fibrosarcoma

Fibrohistiocytic tumors

Benign fibrous histiocytoma
Malignant fibrous histiocytoma

Ewing sarcoma/primitive

Neuroectodermal tumor

Ewing sarcoma

Hematopoietic tumors

Plasma cell myeloma
Malignant lymphoma, not otherwise specified

Cell tumor

Giant cell tumor
Malignancy in giant cell tumor

Notochordal tumors

Chordoma

Vascular tumors

Hemangioma
Angiosarcoma

Smooth muscle tumors

Leiomyoma
Leiomyosarcoma

Lipogenic tumors

Lipoma
Liposarcoma

Neural tumors

Neurilemmoma

Miscellaneous tumors

Adamantinoma
Metastatic malignancy

Miscellaneous lesions

Aneurysmal bone cyst
Simple cyst
Fibrous dysplasia
Osteofibrous dysplasia
Langerhans cell histiocytosis
Erdheim–Chester disease
Chest wall hamartoma

From: Fletcher CDM, Unni K, Mertens K, eds. *World Health Organization Classification of Tumours. Pathology and Genetics. Tumours of Soft Tissues and Bone.* Lyon: France; IARC Press; 2002. Used with permission.

2001;108:511). While multiple hereditary osteochondromas are associated with an increased incidence of secondary chondrosarcoma, the malignant change also takes place in solitary osteochondromas, most of which do not harbor *EXT-1* mutations.

b. Chondromas comprise a group of lesions that are composed of variably cellular mature hyaline cartilage (e-**Fig. 48.14**). Enchondromas arise within the medullary cavity and most commonly involve the small bones of the hand and feet or long tubular bones, whereas periosteal chondromas arise on the cortical surface (about half of which involve the humerus). Most chondromas are incidental, but some, especially in long bones, can present with pathologic fractures. Radiographically,

TABLE 48.4	Commonest Location(s), Usual Age Distribution, and Salient Pathologic Features of Benign Bone Tumors and Tumor-like Lesions		
Tumor/lesion	**Location**	**Age**	**Salient pathologic findings**
Cartilaginous			
Osteochondroma	Metaphysis of LBs	10–30	Cartilage-capped bony protrusion
Chondroma	Hands/feet; medulla of LBs	Any	Variably cellular hyaline cartilage
Chondroblastoma	Epiphysis/apophysis of LBs	10–20	Chondroid-like matrix; S-100-positive cells with grooved nuclei
Chondromyxoid fibroma	Metaphysis of LBs	10–30	Hypocellular chondromyxoid lobules surrounded by more cellular spindle-cell areas
Osseous			
Osteoma	Facial bones	Adults	Mineralized compact bone
Osteoid osteoma	Cortex of LBs	10–30	"Nidus" of immature bone surrounded by sclerotic bone
Osteoblastoma	Vertebrae; cortex of LBs	10–30	Identical to osteoid osteoma but larger; often no sclerosis
Fibrous			
Fibrous dysplasia	Ribs; jaw; LBs-medullary	10–30	Irregular woven bone within fibroblastic stroma
Osteofibrous dysplasia	Tibial cortex	<20	Similar to fibrous dysplasia but with appositional osteoblasts
Desmoplastic fibroma	LBs; jaw; pelvis	20–30	Fibromatosis-like proliferation
Nonossifying fibroma	LBs	5–15	Bland spindle cells in storiform pattern + histiocytes + giant cells
Histiocytic			
Benign fibrous histiocytoma	LBs; pelvis	>20	Identical to nonossifying fibroma but variable
Langerhans cell histiocytosis	Skull; jaw; metaphysis and diaphysis of LBs	5–15	Mixed inflammatory cells and eosinophils; S-100/CD1a-positive cells with grooved/multilobated nuclei
Erdheim–Chester disease	LBs	>40	Foamy histiocytes and fibrosis
Giant cell tumor	Epiphysis/metaphysis of LBs	20–45	Evenly placed giant cells among mononuclear cells with identical nuclei; normal serum calcium/phosphate/blood urea nitrogen/creatinine
Others			
Aneurysmal bone cyst	Vertebrae; flat and LBs	10–20	Blood-filled spaces separated by fibrous septae; giant cells
Simple cyst	Metaphysis of LBs	10–20	Fluid-filled "cysts" lined by connective tissue
Hemangioma	Vertebrae; flat and LBs	20–50	Capillary and/or cavernous sized vessels

LBs, long bones.

TABLE 48.5 Commonest Location(s), Usual Age Distribution, and Salient Pathologic Features of Malignant Bone Tumors

Tumor/lesion	Location	Age	Salient pathologic findings
Cartilaginous			
Chondrosarcoma	Flat bones; metaphysis, and epiphysis of LBs		
Conventional (NOS)	Metaphysis	20–80	Variably cellular hyaline cartilage permeating bone
Dedifferentiated	Metaphysis	>30	Conventional chondrosarcoma + high-grade spindle cell sarcoma
Mesenchymal	Metaphysis	20–50	Undifferentiated small cell tumor + hyaline cartilage
Clear cell	Epiphysis	20–70	Conventional tumor with abundant large clear tumor cells
Osseous			
Osteosarcoma	Metaphysis of LBs; jaw	10–20; >40	
Conventional	Medullary		Osteoid formed directly by malignant cells
Low-grade central	Medullary		Mildly atypical fibroblastic proliferation + thick bone trabeculae
Telangiectatic	Medullary		Blood-filled spaces + fibrous septae + highly malignant osteoid
Parosteal	Cortex outside periosteum		Mildly atypical fibroblastic proliferation + thick bone trabeculae
Periosteal	Cortex inside periosteum		Abundant cartilage matrix with variable malignant osteoid
Fibrous/fibrohistiocytic			
Fibrosarcoma	Metaphysis of LBs; may extend to end of bone	20–60	Malignant spindle cells in a fascicular pattern
Malignant fibrous histiocytoma	Metaphysis of LBs; may extend to end of bone	20–80	Malignant spindle cells in storiform pattern + histiocytic cells (other patterns may be seen)
Hematolymphoid			
Myeloma	Skull; vertebrae; pelvis; LBs	>40	Variably atypical (monoclonal) plasma cells
Lymphoma	Any	Any	Lymphoid proliferations similar to nonbony lesions
Epithelial			
Adamantinoma	Cortex of tibia and/or fibula	25–35	Epithelial cells + fibroblasts + woven or lamellar bone
Metastatic carcinoma	Any	>40	Malignant epithelial cells; morphology/ IHC helps confirm origin
Others			
Ewing sarcoma	Diaphysis of LBs	5–20	Small round blue cells ± rosettes; characteristic IHC; translocation
Chordoma	Base of skull; sacrum	>30	Lobules of vacuolated cells embedded in myxoid matrix
Angiosarcoma and hemangioen- dothelioma		20–60	Anastomosing vascular channels lined by highly atypical cells OR vacuolated cells in myxoid background; characteristic IHC

LBs, long bones; NOS, not otherwise specified; IHC, immunohistochemistry.

TABLE 48.6	Tumor, Node, Metastasis (TNM) Staging Scheme for Malignant Bone Tumors (Excluding Myeloma and Lymphoma)

Histologic grade (G)

GX	Grade cannot be assessed
G1	Well differentiated—low grade
G2	Moderately differentiated—low grade
G3	Poorly differentiated—high grade
G4	Undifferentiated—high grade

Primary tumor (T)

TX	Primary tumor cannot be assessed
T0	No evidence of primary tumor
T1	Tumor ≤8 cm in greatest dimension
T2	Tumor >8 cm in greatest dimension
T3	Discontinuous tumors in the primary bone site

Regional lymph nodes (N)

NX	Regional lymph nodes cannot be assessed
N0	No regional lymph node metastasis
N1	Regional lymph node metastasis

Distant metastasis (M)

MX	Distant metastasis cannot be assessed
M0	No distant metastasis
M1	Distant metastasis
M1a	Lung
M1b	Other distant sites

American Joint Committee on Cancer (AJCC) stage groupings

Stage IA	T1	N0	M0	G1, 2 Low grade, GX
Stage IB	T2	N0	M0	G1, 2 Low grade, GX
	T3	N0	M0	G1, 2 Low grade, GX
Stage IIA	T1	N0	M0	G3, 4 High grade
Stage IIB	T2	N0	M0	G3, 4 High grade
Stage III	T3	N0	M0	G3, 4
Stage IVA	Any T	N0	M1a	Any G
Stage IVB	Any T	N1	Any M	Any G
	Any T	Any N	M1b	Any G

From: Edge SB, Byrd DR, Compton CC, et al., eds, *AJCC Cancer Staging Manual.* 7th ed. New York, NY: Springer; 2010. Used with permission.

chondromas appear as well-demarcated lucent lesions with variable amounts of stippled mineralization (e-**Fig. 48.15**).

Ollier disease is characterized by multiple widespread enchondromas associated with bone deformities that develop early in life, whereas Maffucci syndrome is characterized by multiple enchondromas with associated soft tissue angiomas. Both of these developmental disorders are associated with a significantly increased incidence of secondary chondrosarcoma, although the incidence is higher in patients with Maffucci syndrome. Enchondromas in these patients tend to be more cellular and myxoid, so the histologic appearances alone cannot always be used to diagnose malignant transformation. In such cases, clinical (e.g., rapid growth), radiologic (e.g., cortical destruction, soft tissue masses), and/or pathologic (e.g., necrosis, permeation of bone trabeculae) findings must be used in combination to arrive at the correct diagnosis.

TABLE 48.7	Musculoskeletal Tumor Society Staging Scheme for Malignant Bone Tumors (Excluding Myeloma, Lymphoma and Ewing Sarcoma)
Grade	
G1	Low grade
G2	High grade
Site	
T1	Intracompartmental (within the bone)
T2	Extracompartmental (spread beyond the bone)
Distant metastasis (M)	
M0	No regional or distant metastasis
M1	Regional or distant metastasis

Stage groupings			
Stage IA	G1	T1	M0
Stage IB	G1	T2	M0
Stage IIA	G2	T1	M0
Stage IIB	G2	T2	M0
Stage III	Any	Any	M1

Modified from Enneking WF. A system of staging musculoskeletal neoplasms. *Clin Orthop Relat Res.* 1986;204:9–24.

c. **Chondroblastoma** is a benign neoplasm, which is characteristically an epiphyseal or apophyseal tumor that often presents with arthritic pain and/or joint stiffness due to its close proximity to joints. Histologically, the tumor is composed of discrete, round mononuclear cells with ovoid, folded, or grooved nuclei (e-**Fig. 48.16**). A pink extracellular material resembling early cartilage is also present, sometimes with "chicken-wire" calcification, but the lesion very seldom produces true hyaline cartilage. Giant cells are often present; if they are abundant, and the matrix is scant, the lesion can be confused with a giant cell tumor. However, the radiologic identification of a sclerotic rim or a demarcated edge with or without calcification (e-**Fig. 48.17**), as well as the fact that almost all patients with this lesion are young and still have open growth plates, helps distinguish chondroblastoma from giant cell tumor. In addition, immunohistochemistry demonstrates that the neoplastic chondroblasts are usually S-100 positive.

d. **Chondromyxoid fibroma** presents in the metaphyses of growing individuals. It is characteristically well circumscribed, eccentric, and may demonstrate bone expansion (e-**Fig. 48.18**). Histologically, there are lobular aggregates of spindle-shaped to stellate cells arranged within a chondroid to myxoid matrix. Importantly, these lobules are surrounded by zones of hypercellularity in which mononuclear and multinucleated giant cells are evident (e-**Fig. 48.19**). The behavior is benign.

e. **Chondrosarcoma (not otherwise specified)** is one of the few primary malignant tumors that affects adults with fully mature skeletons. It is classified as primary when there is no preexisting lesion or secondary when it arises in a preexisting bone lesion such as osteochondroma or Ollier disease. Chondrosarcoma most commonly involves the flat bones of the trunk and proximal tubular bones of the extremities. Radiographically, it tends to be large and radiolucent, with radiodense stippling, curlicues, and rings due to matrix calcification or ossification. When it is a central (medullary) lesion, there is often cortical destruction and sometimes cortical thickening. When peripheral, the cartilage matrix is usually >3 cm in thickness (e-Fig. 48.20).

Histologically, chondrosarcoma is composed of mature-appearing hyaline cartilage except that the chondrocytes have varying degrees of increased cellularity, nuclear atypia, and even mitotic activity. Chondrosarcoma can show variable degrees of differentiation, ranging from minimally hypercellular tumors resembling enchondromas with scattered enlarged hyperchromatic tumor cell nuclei that are sometimes binucleate (grade I), to unequivocally malignant tumors with markedly atypical cells and easily identifiable mitotic figures (grade III). Grade II tumors have features intermediate between the two (e-Fig. 48.21). Regardless of their grade, chondrosarcomas (when sampled adequately) invariably show permeation of existing marrow spaces between bony trabeculae (e-Fig. 48.22); this is a very helpful feature for distinguishing low-grade tumors from enchondromas, especially in the small bones of the hands and feet where enchondromas may show a degree of hypercellularity and/or binucleation quite reminiscent of that seen in low-grade chondrosarcomas of larger, more proximal bones. The presence of tumor cell necrosis can also point to a diagnosis of chondrosarcoma. Nevertheless, there are cartilaginous tumors that remain difficult to accurately categorize, especially when the radiologic features of malignancy are not clearly evident. Occasionally, complementary imaging studies such as CT scans may help to identify true bone destruction in a central cartilage tumor, or MRI will demonstrate the extent of a cartilage cap in a peripheral cartilage tumor, which in turn can help to identify the true biologic nature of the lesion when a small biopsy cannot (e-Fig. 48.23). The prognosis of chondrosarcoma is mostly dependent on grade and completeness of resection (as no other modality of treatment is effective), with 5-year survival rates ranging from 90% for low-grade tumors to 53% for higher-grade tumors.

f. **Dedifferentiated chondrosarcoma.** In addition to areas of classic chondrosarcoma (usually low grade), this tumor is characterized by the presence of a distinct, second, clearly defined, high-grade, noncartilaginous sarcomatous component (e-Fig. 48.24). The later is most frequently represented by a malignant fibrous histiocytoma-like component, but osteosarcoma, fibrosarcoma, and rhabdomyosarcoma have also been reported. The tumor has a very poor prognosis.

g. **Mesenchymal chondrosarcoma** is a rare tumor also characterized by a dimorphic pattern and is composed of a highly undifferentiated small round cell component that is often arranged in a hemangiopericytomatous pattern, intermixed with a variable number of islands of hyaline cartilage (e-Fig. 48.25). Although it may occur at any age, the peak age incidence of patients with this tumor (second and third decades) is earlier than that seen in patients with other chondrosarcomas. Mesenchymal chondrosarcoma has a high incidence of local recurrence and distant metastasis, although the latter may not occur for 5 to 10 years.

h. **Clear cell chondrosarcoma** is another rare type of chondrosarcoma; this tumor shows a predilection for the ends of long bones after the growth plates have closed (e-Fig. 48.26). It is characterized histologically by the presence of abundant large round clear cells with well-defined cell borders, intermixed with areas of conventional low-grade chondrosarcoma (e-Fig. 48.27). The clear cells contain large amounts of intracellular glycogen and stain strongly for S-100 protein. The prognosis is similar to that of low-grade chondrosarcoma. Metastases occur in about 20% of patients, and may behave indolently or aggressively. Clear cell chondrosarcoma has a high predilection for metastasis to other bones.

2. Bone-forming tumors

a. Osteoma is a well-circumscribed, radiodense, benign lesion that most frequently arises in the jaws and paranasal sinuses (e-Fig. 48.28), but can also be seen in long bones. Some cases are sporadic, whereas others arise in association with familial polyposis coli (see Chap. 14). Histologically, osteomas are composed of mineralized compact bone matrix with a variable admixture of mature and immature bone but no cellular stroma (e-Fig. 48.28).

b. Osteoid osteoma. This benign, self-limited tumor usually presents with pain that often wakes patients from sleep, but is relieved by aspirin. Although it usually involves the cortices of long bones, osteoid osteoma has been reported in almost every skeletal site. Radiographically, there is a central area of radiolucency surrounded by dense reactive sclerosis (e-Fig. 48.29). The quantity of sclerosis varies by location in the bone. If the lesion is cortical, the reactive sclerosis may obscure the lesion such that it can only be seen by thin-cut CT scans. In the medullary cavity, there may be little or no sclerosis.

Histologically, the radiolucent area, termed the "nidus," is composed of vascularized fibroconnective tissue in which immature new bone is being formed. This new bone is usually arranged in microtrabecular arrays lined by plump appositional osteoblasts that lack nuclear pleomorphism (e-Fig. 48.30). Simple excision or curettage of the nidus of an osteoid osteoma is curative.

c. Osteoblastoma is virtually identical histologically to osteoid osteoma but, unlike the latter, is not limited in growth potential. When diagnosed, osteoblastomas are usually >2 cm in diameter. Radiographically, they may resemble large osteoid osteomas, they may be expansile like aneurysmal bone cysts (ABCs), or they may even appear as aggressive as malignant tumors. There is also a predilection to involve the axial skeleton, especially the vertebral pedicles and arches. Occasionally, osteoblastomas may be very cellular, and their osteoblasts may be several times the size of usual osteoblasts. Tumors having predominant areas of this histologic feature have been termed "aggressive osteoblastoma" or "epithelioid osteoblastoma" (e-Fig. 48.31). The prognosis of osteoblastomas is excellent if amenable to excision.

d. Osteosarcoma is the most common nonhematopoietic primary malignant neoplasm of bone. The peak incidence of this tumor is late childhood and adolescence; however, there is a second peak in patients older than 40 years, most cases of which develop secondarily in preexisting bone lesions (e.g., Paget disease) or following irradiation. The metaphyses of long bones (femur, tibia, and humerus) are the most common sites of involvement; isolated diaphyseal involvement is rare, and involvement of the epiphyses of long bones or small bones of the hands and feet is exceptionally rare. Other sites of involvement include the jaws, skull, and axial skeleton. Most cases of osteosarcoma present with pain (often dull and unremitting) with or without a palpable mass. Radiologically, there is almost always evidence of a destructive bony lesion, often with evidence of new bone formation. There may also be an interrupted periosteal reaction and soft tissue involvement (e-Fig. 48.32).

The histologic hallmark of osteosarcoma is the presence of osteoid or bone formation directly by tumor cells. Osteoid appears as dense, pink, amorphous material (resembling collagen or amyloid) that has a lacelike or sheetlike appearance (e-Fig. 48.33). Intermixed within, and often in direct contact with this osteoid matrix, are the neoplastic tumor cells which can be quite variable in appearance and include polyhedral cells, spindle cells with variable nuclear atypia, small blue cells (resembling EWS, see below), and large markedly atypical cells. The predominant matrix produced by the tumor can be bone or osteoid, cartilaginous, or fibrous. Historically, osteosarcomas have been subclassified on the basis of the predominant matrix production (osteoblastic, chondroblastic, or fibroblastic), but this classification has no prognostic importance. Instead, as described below, osteosarcomas are best classified on the basis of radiologic and/or pathologic features that have been shown to have distinct prognostic implications (*Am J Clin Pathol.* 2006;125:555).

i. **Central osteosarcomas** arise within the medullary cavity and include the following:

(a) **Conventional intramedullary osteosarcoma** is the prototypical osteosarcoma, for which most of the above information refers. Neoplastic tumor cells in conventional osteosarcoma are often polyhedral or spindle-shaped with unequivocally malignant features. Given that preoperative chemotherapy for these tumors is the current standard of care (and has significantly improved the 5-year survival rate of this tumor from 20% to over 80%), it is important to carefully map the tumor in the resection specimen (as discussed earlier) to determine the extent of tumor necrosis compared to the volume of viable plus nonviable tumor since a favorable long-term outcome is associated with >90% tumor necrosis. Additional chemotherapy is often offered to patients with less necrosis as a second-line attempt to further improve survival.

(b) **Low-grade central osteosarcoma** is a rare type of osteosarcoma (1% to 2%) composed of a variably cellular spindle cell/fibroblastic proliferation that lacks the degree of cytologic atypia seen in conventional osteosarcoma. In addition, bone production is usually evident as irregular, somewhat thick, anastomosing, or branching bony trabeculae. These trabeculae simulate the woven bone of fibrous dysplasia or the longitudinal seams of bone in parosteal osteosarcoma (see below), and are separated by a spindle-cell stroma. Review of the radiologic findings often reveals subtle signs of malignancy that are useful in making the diagnosis (e-**Fig. 48.34**). This tumor has a much more indolent course compared with conventional osteosarcoma; however, there is still a high recurrence rate if the tumor is inadequately excised, often with associated grade progression.

(c) **Telangiectatic osteosarcoma** is characterized by large, blood-filled spaces separated by highly cellular fibrous septae that contain markedly pleomorphic cells with a variable amount of osteoid production (e-**Fig. 48.35**). Radiologically, this tumor is radiolucent and expansile, and resembles ABC. Compared to other osteosarcomas, it is more likely to present with a pathologic fracture. Although not necessarily associated with improved survival, this aggressive osteosarcoma is very sensitive to chemotherapy.

(d) **Small cell osteosarcoma** is composed of small round blue cells and histologically resembles EWS except that there is histologic evidence for osteoid formation (although it is often scant). It is usually entirely radiolucent. It has a capricious clinical behavior, often but not always resistant to usual osteosarcoma chemotherapy. Although the usual reciprocal chromosomal translocation described in EWS (see below) has not been generally observed, this lesion has been shown to have membrane positivity for CD99, which has led some authors to theorize that it is a variant of EWS with divergent differentiation.

ii. **Surface osteosarcomas.** About 1 in 20 osteosarcomas occurs in association with the bone surface rather than in the medullary cavity. The vast majority of these are low-grade tumors showing radiodensity and osseous differentiation. They include:

(a) **Parosteal osteosarcoma** accounts for ~4% of osteosarcomas and the majority of surface osteosarcomas. It characteristically involves the posterior distal femur, is associated with the outer fibrous layer of the periosteum, and tends to wrap around the bone. Histologically, it consists of well-formed bony trabeculae, often arranged in parallel streamers separated by a hypocellular spindle stroma as seen in low-grade central osteosarcoma (**e-Fig. 48.36**). Cartilaginous differentiation is also common, often seen as a cartilage cap and sometimes causing confusion with osteochondroma. Radiographically, however, there is no continuity of the interior of parosteal osteosarcoma and the medullary cavity, the adjacent bony cortex is not continuous with the outside of parosteal osteosarcoma (**e-Fig. 48.37**), and the intertrabecular spaces do not contain fatty or hematopoietic marrow. The prognosis of parosteal osteosarcoma is similar to that of low-grade intramedullary osteosarcoma. If inaccurately diagnosed as benign, or if inadequately excised, these lesions will recur. Recurrences may be low grade, but they may also be high grade; low-grade parosteal sarcoma undergoing high-grade transformation is termed *dedifferentiated parosteal osteosarcoma* and has a prognosis similar to conventional osteosarcoma.

(b) **Periosteal osteosarcoma** arises between the cortex and overlying periosteum most commonly in the tibial or femoral diaphysis, and is characterized by abundant cartilaginous matrix and a somewhat greater degree of cytologic atypia than is seen in parosteal osteosarcoma.

(c) **High-grade surface osteosarcoma** is histologically identical to conventional intramedullary osteosarcoma, except that it arises on the bone surface. The prognosis is similar to that of conventional intramedullary osteosarcoma.

3. **Fibrous tumors and tumor-like conditions**

a. **Fibrous dysplasia.** This space-occupying lesion has been classified variously as developmental, tumorous, or tumor-like. It usually presents as a solitary lesion, although it may affect multiple bones in a single limb bud distribution, or multiple bones without limb bud distribution. The polyostotic form is one of the manifestations of the McCune–Albright syndrome, which includes pigmented skin lesions and endocrinopathies. The presence of activating G-protein mutations in both monostatic lesions and McCune-Albright syndrome suggests that fibrous dysplasia represents a true neoplasm (*J Pediatr.* 1993;123:509). Fibrous dysplasia may be asymptomatic, but deformities, secondary fractures, and even pain may be the presenting manifestation. Radiographically, the lesion is almost always intramedullary, and it tends to affect those portions of bone formed by endochondral ossification. While secondary cortical atrophy may take place because of intramedullary expansion of the lesion, fibrous dysplasia usually does not involve the cortex. Fibrous dysplasia is often expansile and results in modeling deformities of the host bone. It is well circumscribed and radiolucent, but less radiolucent than the underlying bone that it has replaced; radiologists often refer to its appearance as having a ground glass quality (e-**Fig. 48.38**).

Histologically, fibrous dysplasia consists of various combinations of any tissue present in bone, so fibrous tissue, bone, cartilage, and vascular tissues are produced in various combinations. The usual microscopic pattern, however, consists of loosely arranged, vascularized fibrous tissue in which disconnected curved microtrabeculae of bone are disposed. These trabeculae are not only woven in their collagen fiber pattern, but when a section is examined under polarized light, the fabric of their collagenous background forms a continuum with the fabric of the fibrous tissue (e-**Fig. 48.39**). Cartilage formation is not unusual, and occasionally cartilage is formed in such excess that lesions may be mistaken radiographically and histologically for cartilaginous neoplasms. Treatment is usually focused on relief of deformities or other morbid symptomatology. The prognosis is usually excellent.

b. **Osteofibrous dysplasia** is a fibro-osseous lesion and is invariably seen in the tibia, fibula, or both. Its peak incidence is in the first two decades of life. Radiographically, the lesion is radiolucent and usually based on the cortex; it may extend to the medullary cavity. The lesion may be unilocular or multilocular; while it tends to be circumscribed, it may also diffusely involve the diaphysis and cause secondary bowing deformities (e-**Fig. 48.40**). Histologically, osteofibrous dysplasia resembles fibrous dysplasia except that the microtrabeculae of bone tend to be rimmed by appositional osteoblasts even at their very earliest synthesis (e-**Fig. 48.41**). The fibrous stroma tends to be more cellular than in fibrous dysplasia, and is less contiguous with the trabeculae under polarized light. The lesional bone also tends to mature at the periphery with the surrounding normal bone. The lesional bone tends to undergo spontaneous involution with time, although sometimes it behaves more aggressively.

c. **Nonossifying fibroma (fibrous cortical defect)** is the commonest space-occupying lesion of bone, estimated to affect one in four individuals. Even though it is thought to be developmental, in rare cases, the lesion behaves as a tumor of limited biologic potential. Unless it is associated with a fracture, patients are generally without symptoms; the lesions are typically discovered incidentally during the course of evaluation for some other condition and the routine radiographs are virtually diagnostic. The lesion is a well-circumscribed radiolucent defect in the metaphyseal cortex with scalloped sclerotic borders, and it is almost always longer in the cephalocaudal than axial direction (e-**Fig. 48.42**).

Histologically, the lesion consists of spindle cells arranged in a distinctly storiform pattern. A fair number of multinucleated giant cells, histiocytic cells with foamy cytoplasm, and histiocytes containing hemosiderin pigment (e-**Fig. 48.43**) may also be present. While bone formation is not observed (hence the name), lesions that have fractures or microscopic infarctions are admixed with reactive bone. Because this lesion may be focally cellular, it is important to review the radiographs to avoid misdiagnosis. Most nonossifying fibromas are self-healing and do not require clinical intervention.

d. **Desmoplastic fibroma.** This rare tumor occurs in adolescents and young adults, with the mandible being the most commonly affected site. Radiologically, it often expands the involved bone, is entirely radiolucent, and is usually well circumscribed. Histologically, it is composed of bland fibroblastic or myofibroblastic cells in a background of collagen identical to that found in desmoid tumors and/or soft tissue fibromatosis (e-Fig. 48.44). Although it is benign, it behaves similarly to fibromatosis of soft tissue in that there is a high recurrence rate when not completely excised.

   e. **Fibrosarcoma** constitutes ~5% of all primary malignant bone tumors with a relatively uniform age distribution between the second and sixth decades. It usually involves the metaphyses of long bones resulting in pain, swelling, and a destructive radiologic lesion without radiographically detectable matrix. Histologically, fibrosarcomas are usually quite cellular with malignant spindle cells arranged in a fascicular or herringbone pattern (e-Fig. 48.45). The differential diagnosis includes other malignant spindle-cell tumors such as fibroblastic osteosarcoma, leiomyosarcoma, malignant fibrous histiocytoma, and desmoplastic fibroma.

4. **Histiocytic and fibrohistiocytic tumors**

   a. **Benign fibrous histiocytoma** is a rare bone lesion that is histologically similar to its soft tissue counterpart. There is a wide age distribution, with more than half of the cases developing in patients older than 20 years. The tumor most commonly involves either the epiphysis or the diaphysis of long bones, or the pelvis. Radiographically, the lesion is well defined and radiolucent, and may expand the bone. Similar to benign fibrous histiocytoma elsewhere, the lesion is composed of spindle-shaped fibroblasts at least focally arranged in a whorled or storiform pattern, intermixed with histiocytes and giant cells (e-Fig. 48.46). Mitoses may be evident. The main differential diagnosis is a secondary fibrohistiocytic reaction within another primary bone lesion, such as giant cell tumor or nonossifying fibroma.

   b. **Malignant fibrous histiocytoma** is also similar to its soft tissue counterpart, with most cases developing in patients older than 40 years. It can also complicate Paget disease, or occur after irradiation or infarction. Most cases involve the long bones of the extremities or the pelvis. Histologically, there is a mixed population of spindle cells, histiocytic cells, and giant cells. Pleomorphic tumor cells, abnormal mitotic figures, and the characteristic storiform pattern of growth are also evident (e-Fig. 48.47). Almost all of the histologic subtypes described in soft tissue have also been described in bone. The management and prognosis of this tumor most closely resemble osteosarcoma; the focal identification of osteoid or bone matrix is sometimes the only histologic difference between these two tumors, although most osteosarcomas arising in this age group are secondary to a prior disease or treatment.

   c. **Langerhans cell histiocytosis** comprises a group of neoplastic Langerhans cell proliferations that can be unifocal (solitary eosinophilic granuloma), multifocal (Hand–Schüller–Christian disease), or disseminated (Letterer–Siwe disease). All can produce bone lesions that tend to present early in multifocal and disseminated forms. Langerhans cell histiocytosis most frequently involves the craniofacial bones, but other bones such as the femur, pelvis, and ribs may also be involved. Radiographically, the lesions appear radiolucent and rapidly destructive, sometimes with associated exuberant periosteal new bone formation when they occur in long bones (e-Fig. 48.48).

      Histologically, there is a mixed inflammatory infiltrate including neutrophils, eosinophils, lymphocytes, and histiocytes (with or without giant cells) in which Langerhans cells are identified. Langerhans cells have eosinophilic to clear cytoplasm and contain oval, grooved, or multilobated nuclei (e-Fig. 48.49); immunohistochemically, they characteristically express S-100 and CD1a. Because there is a histologic similarity to chronic osteomyelitis, lesions thought to be Langerhans cell histiocytosis should be cultured, and the culture results should be known before formulating a final diagnosis. Langerhans cell histiocytosis has a very good prognosis except in the disseminated form, which is associated with a poor outcome (*Pediatr Blood Cancer.* 2005;45:37).

d. Erdheim–Chester disease is a rare disorder of unknown etiology characterized by the presence of skeletal and extraskeletal foamy histiocytic infiltrates with associated fibrosis (e-**Fig. 48.50**). Most patients are older than 40 years, and there is usually bilateral symmetric or patchy sclerosis of the medullary cavity of the involved bones (most frequently the long bones of the extremity). Given the frequent and progressive infiltration of vital organs (such as the kidney, heart, or lung), most patients succumb within a few years.

e. Giant cell tumor comprises around 4% to 5% of all primary bone tumors and has a peak incidence between 20 and 45 years of age; it is rarely seen in skeletally immature individuals or in patients older than 50 years. Although there is some controversy as to its exact origin, it is placed in the histiocytic category because its giant cells are modified histiocytes and at least some of its stromal cells also express histiocytic markers. Giant cell tumor typically affects the ends of long bones and extends to the articular or apophyseal portions of the bone. The pelvis or small bones of the hand or feet are more rarely affected. Given the often juxta-articular location of the tumor, joint swelling and limitation of movement are common presenting symptoms. Radiologically, the tumor is radiolucent and eccentric, may expand the bone, and is well demarcated (e-**Fig. 48.51**). There is almost never a periosteal reaction associated with the tumor.

The histologic hallmark of the tumor is the presence of sheets of round, oval, or elongated mononuclear cells with an open chromatin pattern, evenly intermixed with numerous osteoclast-like giant cells with nuclei similar to those of the mononuclear cells (e-**Fig. 48.52**). The cell borders are often indistinct, so that on low power the lesion appears as a syncytium. Mitoses are variable in number; atypical mitoses are occasionally seen and do not necessarily predict malignant behavior. The presence of the characteristic mononuclear cells and the even interposition of the giant cells are essential for the diagnosis, since giant cells can be a component of many bone lesions. Other histologic features occasionally seen in giant cell tumors include a focal storiform pattern, which, when abundant foam cells are present, can easily be confused with benign fibrous histiocytoma. There also may be areas of fibrosis, as well as secondary cystic areas resembling ABC (see below). The most important differential diagnosis is the so-called brown tumor of hyperparathyroidism (see Chap. 49); the lack of radiologic or biochemical evidence of hyperparathyroidism, as well as the absence of additional bone lesions, can be very helpful in this regard. Another important differential diagnosis is the so-called giant-cell reparative granuloma that characteristically involves the mandible and is composed of granuloma-like aggregates of giant cells in a fibrovascular stroma, but which lacks the mononuclear cells characteristic of giant cell tumor (e-**Fig. 48.53**).

Most cases of giant cell tumor behave in a benign fashion; some, however, are associated with local aggressiveness and occasionally (~2%) with distant metastasis. Most of these metastases grow slowly and are rarely lethal. There are no reliable histologic features that can predict a malignant outcome.

Malignant giant cell tumor is defined as a sarcomatous lesion arising within a giant cell tumor, or as a sarcoma that appears in the same area in which a bona fide giant cell tumor was treated (e-**Fig. 48.54**). The former instance is sometimes referred to as a primary malignant giant cell tumor; the latter as a secondary malignant giant cell tumor. The prognosis is related to the histology, size, and grade of the malignant component.

5. **Hematolymphoid tumors**
   a. **Solitary plasmacytoma and multiple myeloma.** These tumors are malignant proliferations of plasma cells that account for the majority of tumors arising primarily in bone. The presentation of myeloma is quite variable (see Chap. 44), but involvement of the skeletal system is usually manifested by bone pain and/or pathologic fractures. Radiologically, plasmacytoma and the lesions of multiple myeloma are lytic, well demarcated, and without a rim of sclerotic bone; however, multiple myeloma may also present with generalized osteoporosis without any detectable foci of discrete bone destruction. Histologically, the tumors are composed of plasma cells and their precursors at various stages of development (e-**Fig. 48.55**). The main differential diagnosis is often other hematolymphoid tumors, although myeloma cells are occasionally quite anaplastic and can resemble carcinoma or high-grade sarcoma. Accordingly, immunohistochemical reactivity for CD138 or CD38 (among other markers; see Chap. 44) can be useful to confirm the diagnosis.
   b. **Lymphoma.** Most bone lymphomas are secondary to disease elsewhere, but primary bone lymphomas also occur. In general, lymphomas presenting in bone are classified as primary provided no lymph node involvement is present both at the time of presentation and for a long interval afterward (the length of this interval varies according to different authors). Most primary lymphomas of bone represent examples of diffuse large B-cell lymphoma or other high-grade tumor, because most lower-grade lymphomas and leukemias present with diffuse marrow involvement rather than as a tumorous mass. Primary Hodgkin lymphoma of bone is exceedingly rare. Radiologically, lymphomas usually present as radiolucent lesions, sometimes disproportionately destructive when compared with the patient's clinical symptoms (e-**Fig. 48.56**). In about 20% of cases, the lesions present as radiodensities. The histologic findings recapitulate those seen in extraskeletal sites. The prognosis is dependent on the type of lymphoma and stage.

6. **Vascular tumors**
   a. **Hemangioma.** Although incidental hemangiomas are relatively common, clinically symptomatic tumors account for <1% of primary bone tumors and tend to present in late adulthood. Hemangioma is most frequently seen in the vertebrae, followed by the craniofacial skeleton and metaphyses of long bones. It appears as a radiolucent, often expansive lesion in long bones but as a vertically striate "corduroy pattern" lesion in intact vertebrae. Histologically, it is composed of capillary sized or cavernous vessels that permeate the marrow and are lined by bland endothelial cells (e-**Fig. 48.57**). As the name indicates, this tumor, as well as the closely related lymphangioma, is benign with low rates of recurrence following excision.
   b. **Angiosarcoma and hemangioendothelioma.** These two neoplasms account for <1% of bone tumors and may present at any age group, although the peak incidence is in young adulthood. They constitute a spectrum of lesions ranging from locally destructive but indolent tumors with a good response to surgery or local radiation, to poorly differentiated malignant

tumors with a high metastatic rate. Most tumors are radiolucent with poor margination; however, a sclerotic rim is occasionally identified. While angiosarcomas are often solitary, hemangioendotheliomas tend to present as multifocal lesions in the same bone or in the same limb bud distribution and may be mistaken for skeletal metastases (e-**Fig. 48.58**).

Angiosarcomas are usually characterized, at least focally, by the presence of irregularly anastomosing vascular channels that are lined by highly atypical endothelial cells, but they may largely consist of solid, patternless aggregates of polyhedral or spindle cells (e-**Fig. 48.59**). Poorly differentiated angiosarcomas may fail to express vascular markers. It should be noted that angiosarcomas are known to express cytokeratins, which is an important consideration when metastatic carcinoma is in the differential diagnosis. Most angiosarcomas are associated with a poor outcome.

Epithelioid hemangioendothelioma is composed of cords, nests, or sheets of plump cells that, in their attempt to form vessels, are often vacuolated, and some of the vacuoles may contain erythrocytes. An extracellular myxoid or hyalinized stroma is characteristic, although not always identified. Immunohistochemical reactivity with vascular markers such as CD31, CD34, and Factor VIII–related antigen can be used to confirm endothelial differentiation, and may help to exclude a diagnosis of metastatic signet-ring cell adenocarcinoma. Epithelioid hemangioendothelioma may have an indolent course.

7. Epithelial tumors

a. Adamantinoma comprises <1% of malignant bone tumors. There is a wide age distribution, with the median age of patients between 25 and 35 years. The tibia is most frequently involved, followed by the fibula, and both sites synchronously. Radiologically, an intracortical radiolucent lesion is evident, which may involve the medullary cavity (e-**Fig. 48.60**).

Histologically, classic adamantinoma is composed of epithelial cells having a basaloid, tubular, or squamoid appearance; has a predominantly spindle cell pattern; or consists of a mixture of the two patterns (e-**Fig. 48.61**); a storiform fibroblastic proliferation that contains variable amounts of woven or lamellar bone may also be present. Rarely, the tumor is predominantly composed of the latter component, with only rare scattered epithelial cells (single or in small nests, sometimes only detected by immunohistochemistry); such tumors have been termed as having an "osteofibrous dysplasia-like pattern" or as "differentiated adamantinomas," and usually present in patients younger than 20 years. Adamantinomas are invariably immunopositive for various keratins and epithelial membrane antigen, and often also for vimentin. Classic adamantinomas are indolent tumors with a high local recurrence rate and metastasis in only about 20% of patients; differentiated adamantinomas almost never metastasize.

b. Metastatic carcinoma is the most common tumor affecting the skeleton, which is the third most common site to be involved by metastatic carcinoma after the lungs and liver. Primary carcinomas of the breast, lung, prostate, kidney, and thyroid gland compose >80% of all bone metastases. Radiologically, metastatic deposits can be radiolucent or radiodense or can display a mixed pattern (e-**Fig. 48.62**). Given its high incidence, metastatic carcinoma should always be in the differential diagnosis of solitary or multiple bone lesions in patients older than 40 years.

The histology usually resembles that of the primary carcinoma, if it is known. It should be noted that a fibroblastic, osteoblastic, or vascular response to the metastatic tumor may occasionally be quite prominent and overshadow the tumor cells, which may only be focally evident (e-**Fig. 48.63**). Consequently, immunohistochemistry may reveal isolated subtle tumor cells that are not obvious in small biopsy specimens.

8. **Miscellaneous neoplasms**

a. **EWS/PNET.** In addition to its classic presentation in the diaphyses of long bones, the tumor can involve axial bones such as the pelvis and ribs, as well as soft tissues (see Chap. 46) and other organs. EWS/PNET has been described at various ages, but most patients are younger than 20 years. Although patients usually have pain and a mass, they may also present with fever and leukocytosis suggestive of an infectious process. Radiologically, a destructive, permeative lesion is usually evident, often with an overlying multilayered but discontinuous "onion-skin" periosteal reaction (e-**Fig. 48.64**). Occasionally, there is a large soft-tissue mass with no obvious bone destruction on the routine radiographs, but the intraosseous component becomes evident on a CT scan or MRI.

Histologically, EWS/PNET is the prototype for "small blue round cell tumors" as it is composed of sheets of such cells, often with glycogen-containing clear cytoplasm (e-**Fig. 48.65**). Evidence of neuroectodermal differentiation may be manifested by extracellular eosinophilic neuropil-like structures or Homer–Wright rosettes (composed of groups of tumor cells that surround a central core of eosinophilic extracellular material). Immunohistochemically, EWS/PNET shows characteristic strong cell membrane immunoreactivity for CD99, negativity for CD45, and variable reactivity for neural markers such as neuron-specific enolase, synaptophysin, CD57, neurofilament, and S-100 protein. Cytokeratins may also be positive.

A characteristic feature of this tumor is the presence of a recurrent balanced reciprocal translocation involving the *EWS* gene on chromosome 22 and a member of the *Ets* family of genes, the most common of which (85% of cases) is the *FLI1* gene on chromosome 11 (*Br J Cancer.* 1994;70:908). Immunohistochemistry, polymerase chain reaction, and fluorescent in situ hybridization have all been used to confirm the diagnosis by detecting expressed *FLI1*, the fusion transcript, or the translocation itself, respectively. The prognosis of EWS has greatly improved with multimodality treatment, and 5-year survival rates now approach 70%.

b. **Chordomas** are derived from notochordal remnants and account for ~4% of malignant bone tumors. Most tumors present after 30 years of age with a peak incidence between 50 and 60 years of age. The midline of the axial skeleton, particularly the sacrum and the base of the skull, is usually affected. Radiologically, a lucent lesion is seen with scattered calcifications; there is often a large associated soft-tissue component (e-**Fig. 48.66**). Histologically, chordomas are composed of lobules of tumor in which sheets, cords, or nests of vacuolated, eosinophilic to clear cells are embedded in a myxoid matrix (e-**Fig. 48.67**). Chordomas express cytokeratins, epithelial membrane antigen, and S-100 protein, an immunohistochemical profile that is helpful in distinguishing this tumor from chondrosarcoma (which is cytokeratin and epithelial membrane antigen negative). Chordomas are aggressive tumors that are most notable for local recurrence when incompletely excised, but also have a metastatic potential. A controversial entity, "chondroid chordoma," characterized by areas of mimicking hyaline cartilage, appears to have a better prognosis, whereas "dedifferentiated chordoma," with its high-grade sarcomatous component, is associated with a very poor outcome.

9. Cystic/cyst-like lesions

a. **Simple bone cyst** is an intraosseous space-occupying lesion consisting of an accumulation of fluid. The lesion is usually lined by a thin membrane composed of flattened cells of unknown type that may be involved in the production of the fluid, which usually appears serous. The base of the lesion is usually situated at an active growth plate, and the cyst is more or less maintained by continuous remodeling of the bone around the area of fluid pressure. The lesion is circumscribed and radiolucent, and usually involves the proximal humeral, femoral, or tibial region (e-**Fig. 48.68**). It does not expand the bone or cause deformity unless there has been a fracture with displacement before healing, and it tends to be symmetric. While fluid may not be obvious radiographically, the contents are demonstrable by MRI. Histologically, the diagnosis is one of exclusion and depends upon correlation of the imaging, operative findings, and lack of any other diagnostic tissue. Because most simple cysts are treated conservatively by injection of steroids or other sclerosing agents, it is unusual to see the lining of a simple cyst histologically unless there has been repeated fracture.

b. **Intraosseous ganglion.** This is a subarticular defect in the cancellous bone filled with mucoid fluid. The bone surrounding the defect is remodeled and sometimes sclerotic (e-**Fig. 48.69**). The defect is histologically similar to the subarticular cysts associated with overlying osteoarthritis (geodes) except that the subarticular plate and articular cartilage are radiographically intact in patients with intraosseous ganglia. The lesion is presumed to arise from a microscopic continuity of the subarticular plate with the joint space that either cannot be detected by imaging studies or that has healed; this etiology would allow pressurized synovial fluid to come in contact with the intertrabecular medullary space. There are no diagnostic features histologically as the concentrated fluid is practically acellular and resembles the contents of tenosynovial ganglia.

c. **Aneurysmal bone cyst.** This peculiar lesion derives its name from its expansile character. It is not a true cyst, but rather a collection of blood-filled spaces that are separated by fibro-osseous tissue septa containing a varying amount of multinucleated giant cells and immature bone. Most ABCs occur prior to 20 years of age. The lesion usually arises as an eccentric radiolucent lesion in metaphyses of long bones (e-**Fig. 48.70**). When it is central and symmetric it can often be distinguished from a simple cyst because it causes the bone to become wider than the growth plate. The bone destruction associated with ABC is perhaps the most rapid associated with any osseous lesion. While its internal edge tends to be well margined radiographically, ABC sometimes extends across adjacent bones, particularly if it arises in the spine. Complementary imaging studies, particularly MRI, reveal peculiar fluid–fluid levels on T2-weighted axial and sagittal views (e-**Fig. 48.71**); these levels are caused by the signal differences in erythrocytes and plasma, reflect erythrocyte sedimentation, and demonstrate that blood in intact ABC is both unclotted and stagnant or slow moving.

Histologically, the lesion has vascular spaces that progress from very small capillary spaces to very large sinusoids separated by fibrous septae and sometimes by bone (e-**Fig. 48.72**). Within the septae are fibroblasts, scattered multinucleated giant cells, and osteoblasts associated with the bone production. Rarely, the lesion is almost entirely solid, although sometimes the solid variant may demonstrate fluid levels on imaging. In about half the cases, there is some other lesion associated with the cyst and admixed with curetted fragments; this has been termed secondary

ABC. The associated lesion is usually benign, although malignant tumors have also been described in association with ABC. Gene rearrangements of the *USP6* gene on chromosome 17, and/or the *CDH11* gene of chromosome 16, have been described in ABC, raising the possibility that the lesion is truly neoplastic. The genetic abnormalities thus far seem to apply mainly to the primary variety of this lesion, and have also been found in the solid variant (*Am J Pathol.* 2004;165:1773).

10. **Other rare primary bone neoplasms.** There are other benign and malignant soft-tissue neoplasms that can primarily arise in bone, including leiomyoma, leiomyosarcoma, lipoma, liposarcoma, and schwannoma. All of these are histologically similar to their soft-tissue counterparts (see Chap. 46).

49 Metabolic Diseases of Bone

Deborah Novack

I. NORMAL ANATOMY. Because of its accessibility and composition of both cortical and trabecular (cancellous) bone, the iliac crest is the site of choice for evaluation of systemic metabolic bone diseases. Cortex forms the external layer of all bones, comprises ~80% of bone mass, and supports most of the tissue's mechanical function. Trabecular bone, the meshwork surrounded by marrow or fat, is much more metabolically active than cortex. To support both its mechanical and metabolic functions, bone is dynamically regulated, and the skeleton is replaced completely every 10 years. The process of replacement, known as remodeling or turnover, is accomplished by the coordinated action of bone-forming osteoblasts (OBs) and bone-resorbing osteoclasts (OCs), and is regulated by a variety of systemic factors including calcium, phosphorus, and parathyroid hormone (PTH). The goal of iliac crest trochar biopsy is to assess this process.

In either the cortex or the trabeculum, remodeling begins when mononuclear OC precursors (derived from hematopoietic progenitors) arrive at a bone surface, fuse, and differentiate into functional polykaryons (Fig. 49.1). Mature OCs polarize and secrete acid and proteases onto an isolated microenvironment of the bone surface, excavating a pit known as Howship's lacuna. This resorption phase ends with the OCs' apoptosis, and a reversal phase follows, characterized by activation of OBs (of mesenchymal origin) to replace the excavated bone; the activity of OCs and OBs is normally tightly coupled, and the amount of bone synthesized matches the amount resorbed. Newly secreted matrix called osteoid becomes mineralized to form mature bone. The remodeling cycle ends when new bone formation is complete, and the OBs are either incorporated into the new bone matrix as osteocytes or become quiescent surface bone lining cells. The net result of each cycle is the formation of a new osteon, a packet of bone delineated by a "cement line" in which the collagen fibers are aligned. These lamellae of bone are easily seen when decalcified hematoxylin and eosin (H&E)-stained sections are examined under polarized light (e-Fig. 49.1).*

OCs can be identified by their characteristic appearance as multinucleated cells on the bone surface, with discrete nuclei (in contrast to megakaryocytes, which have fused nuclei). The most sensitive method of identifying OCs histologically is expression of tartrate-resistant acid phosphatase (TRAP), which stains OCs bright red (e-Fig. 49.2), although this is not usually necessary for diagnosis. OBs appear as cuboidal cells on the bone surface, often in rows, with abundant cytoplasm and an eccentric nucleus (e-Fig. 49.3). However, the strength of the undecalcified biopsy is in the evaluation of the function of these cells rather than their morphology.

OBs secrete matrix proteins onto the bone surface, but several days are required for mineral deposition. Therefore, the extent of bone surface covered by osteoid (osteoid surface) is one indicator of OB activity. The thickness of the osteoid seams reflects the rate of mineral apposition, because mineralization converts osteoid to

---

*All e-figures are available online via the Solution Site Image Bank.

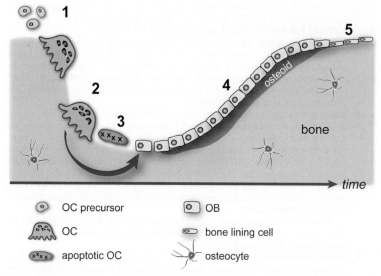

Figure 49.1 The bone remodeling cycle. **A:** OC precursors are recruited to the bone surface, where they fuse and differentiate into mature polykaryons. **B:** The OCs resorb both organic and inorganic matrix of bone. **C:** The resorption phase ends with OC apoptosis. **D:** During the reversal phase, OBs differentiate from mesenchymal precursors under the influence of factors from OCs (*curved arrow*) and secrete new bone matrix known as osteoid. **E:** At the end of the remodeling cycle, some OBs have been incorporated into the bone and become osteocytes, whereas others remain on the surface as synthetically quiescent bone-lining cells.

bone. Decalcification required for standard paraffin processing removes the distinction between newly synthesized osteoid and mature calcified bone. In contrast, undecalcified plastic sections can be stained in several ways to demonstrate osteoid. The von Kossa stain, a silver-based stain used with a basic fuchsin counterstain, shows calcified bone matrix as dark brown or black, whereas the unmineralized matrix (osteoid) appears pink-red (**e-Fig. 49.4A**). A trichrome stain, either Goldner (**e-Fig. 49.3**) or modified Masson (**e-Fig. 49.4B**), also distinguishes mineralized bone from osteoid. These latter stains allow easier interpretation of cellular morphology than the von Kossa, and also highlight peritrabecular or marrow fibrosis.

A second critical marker of OB function is tetracycline labeling. Tetracycline family antibiotics are calcium-chelating fluorochromes that bind to actively mineralizing bone surfaces, can be taken orally, and are well-tolerated. They are given in two courses, separated by 2 weeks (see below). If bone formation is active during both intervals, examination of unstained sections by fluorescence microscopy demonstrates two bright bands of labeling (a double label) (**e-Fig. 49.5**). Similarly, active bone formation during only one of the labeling periods yields a single tetracycline label (**e-Fig. 49.5**). Combination of the extent of labeled trabecular bone surface and the distance between labels provides the mineral apposition rate and bone formation rate. In a normal subject, most surfaces with osteoid, as seen on trichrome or von Kossa stains, have single or double labels.

During normal endochondral bone development, cartilage formed at the growth plate is replaced by bone in the primary spongiosa through the action of OCs. Toluidine blue stains cartilage purple, and cartilage may be found within trabeculae near the growth plate in children (**e-Fig. 49.6**). However, a finding of entrapped cartilage in an iliac crest bone biopsy in an adult, or >1 cm from the growth plate in a child, is indicative of OC dysfunction such as in osteopetrosis.

II. INDICATIONS FOR BIOPSY, TISSUE SAMPLING, AND PREPARATION

A. **Indications for biopsy.** The most common indications for metabolic bone biopsy are end-stage renal disease (ESRD) and unexplained hypercalcemia or hyperphosphatemia, osteoporosis unresponsive to therapy, or suspected osteomalacia. Patients who have multiple or unexplained fractures (particularly if they are failing to heal), unexplained bone pain, or an elevation in serum alkaline phosphatase may also be candidates.

B. **Biopsy procedure.** A critical component of evaluation of metabolic bone biopsies is in vivo fluorochrome labeling of bone via use of a regimen of tetracycline (250 mg orally four times a day [PO qid]) for 3 days, followed by a 14-day interval, then 3 more days of therapy (250 mg PO qid). Biopsy is performed on the third day after the last dose (biopsy interpretation may therefore be confounded by recent therapeutic use of antibiotic drugs in the tetracycline family; similarly, inadequate labeling can be caused by malabsorption syndromes or by taking tetracycline with meals, dairy products, iron-containing medications, antacids, or calcium supplements).

Biopsy is performed as an outpatient procedure; the most accessible site for biopsy is the anterior iliac crest. When obtained, the specimen should be placed directly into 70% ethanol.

C. **Sample preparation.** The specimen should be fixed in 70% ethanol for at least 48 hours, and this solution is suitable for shipping and long-term storage at room temperature. Following dehydration with xylene, the specimen is mounted in methyl methacrylate, and the tissue core is sectioned parallel to its long axis at 5 to 7 μm thickness using a tungsten blade. Undecalcified sections are stained with von Kossa, Goldner or modified Masson trichrome, and toluidine blue. One section is decalcified and stained with H&E. Thicker 10-μm sections are coverslipped without staining for examination under fluorescence.

D. **Quantitative versus qualitative evaluation.** The American Society for Bone and Mineral Research has described a nomenclature for a basic set of structural and kinetic features identified by nondecalcified bone biopsy (*J Bone Miner Res.* 1987;2:595), and there are two commercially available systems that allow quantitative analysis based on these standards (OsteoMeasure, OsteoMetrics, Inc. and Bioquant Osteo II, BIOQUANT Image Analysis Corporation). Reference values, based on somewhat limited populations, have been published (*Engl J Med.* 1988;319:1698; *J Bone Miner Res.* 1988;3:133; *Bone.* 2000;26:103; *J Bone Miner Res.* 2004;19:1628). Although some laboratories perform quantitative analysis on all specimens, qualitative assessments are often adequate for diagnosis of individual patients. Quantitative analysis is most useful in the setting of research studies.

III. DIAGNOSTIC FEATURES OF METABOLIC BONE DISORDERS

A. **Osteoporosis.** In the setting of osteoporosis or osteopenia, biopsy establishes the rate of bone remodeling (turnover), degree of mineralization, architectural integrity, and effects of treatment. Iliac crest bone biopsy is a poor indicator of bone mass, as bone volume/tissue volume (BV/TV) is variable within this region. However, trabecular connectivity, which describes the intactness of the trabecular meshwork, correlates with bone mass. In osteoporosis/osteopenia, trabeculae are very small and often appear as isolated islands (low connectivity), rather than as an interconnected grid (good connectivity) (e-**Fig. 49.7**). In high-turnover osteoporosis, osteoid surface is enhanced (e-**Fig. 49.8A**), with normal or increased numbers of OCs and OBs. The extent of double tetracycline-labeled trabecular bone surface is also increased, although the distance between the double labels is usually normal (e-**Fig. 49.8B**). In low-turnover osteoporosis or osteopenia, there is little osteoid, few OCs or OBs, and rare or absent trabecular double tetracycline labels (e-Fig. 49.9). Even in low-turnover states, double labeling in the cortex is usually present, and is a good positive control for adequate tetracycline dosing and specimen processing.

Many patients with osteoporosis have been treated with bisphosphonates, often for several years. Although biopsy studies have shown that normal turnover is intact in most patients (*JAMA*. 2006;296:2927), some cases of severely suppressed bone turnover have been reported and are associated with increased fractures (*J Clin Endocrinol Metab*. 2005;90:1294; *N Engl J Med*. 2006;355:2048). Bisphosphonates target the OC, decreasing resorption and enhancing apoptosis, producing changes that can readily be seen in tissue sections with OCs appearing either hyperchromatic with pyknotic nuclei (e-Fig. 49.10A) or round and unpolarized (e-Fig. 49.10B).

B. Osteomalacia. In osteomalacia, newly formed organic bone matrix fails to mineralize normally, and the result is wide osteoid seams, often greatly increased in extent along the trabecular bone surface (e-Fig. 49.11A). Some osteoid may be completely unlabeled by tetracycline (e-Fig. 49.11B), whereas other surfaces may show irregular and diffuse fluorescence (e-Fig. 49.11C); double tetracycline labels are rare. Florid osteomalacia due to nutritional rickets (vitamin D deficiency) is rare, but milder cases may be found unexpectedly and bone biopsy is the only definitive diagnostic tool. Osteomalacia is also seen in fluorosis, usually caused by excessive fluoride in drinking water (e-Fig. 49.11D and E). The degree of osteomalacia in hypophosphatasia, a rare deficiency of alkaline phosphatase activity, can be quite severe (e-Fig. 49.11F).

Tumor-induced osteomalacia (TIO, also known as oncogenic osteomalacia) is a rare form of osteomalacia that can occur in both adults and children. Iliac crest bone biopsy in TIO shows the typical features of osteomalacia described above (e-Fig. 49.12A). The bone manifestations of TIO are caused by mesenchymal tumors that secrete the phosphatonin FGF-23, leading to hypophosphatemia due to renal phosphate wasting. The tumors are typically small and slow-growing, and can be difficult to detect. If not visible by CT or MRI, sestamibi or octreotide scans may be useful, as well as targeted venous sampling for FGF-23 (*Expert Rev Endocrinol Metab*. 2009;4:435). Histologically, the majority of the tumors in cases of TIO are best characterized as **phosphaturic mesenchymal tumor (mixed connective tissue variant)** and have low cellularity, bland spindled cells, distinctive "grungy" calcified matrix, and an incomplete rim of membranous ossification and/or formation of an osteoid-like matrix at least focally (*Am J Surg Pathol*. 2004;28:1) (e-Fig. 49.12B). They may be locally infiltrative into muscle or fat (e-Fig. 49.12C), have prominent vessels reminiscent of hemangiopericytoma, myxoid change, hemorrhage, or OCs. TIO tumors typically stain for FGF23 but not S100, CD34, or smooth muscle actin. Resection of the solitary tumor mass results in complete resolution of hypophosphatemia and clinical symptoms in the majority of cases.

C. Renal osteodystrophy. Chronic kidney disease-metabolic bone disease (CKD-MBD) has been defined as a systemic disorder of bone and mineral metabolism due to CKD manifested by one or more of the following: (i) abnormalities of calcium, phosphorus, PTH, or vitamin D metabolism; (ii) abnormalities of bone turnover, mineralization, volume, linear growth, or strength; (iii) vascular or other soft tissue calcification (*Kidney Int*. 2006;69:1945). CKD-MBD is associated with increased morbidity and mortality. Three predominant patterns in bone biopsy have been described: high bone turnover with osteitis fibrosa (hyperparathyroid bone disease), low bone turnover (including low-turnover osteomalacia and adynamic bone disease), and mixed uremic osteodystrophy.

1. The most important role of biopsy is in the setting of **hypercalcemia,** in which a finding of PTH-driven high turnover indicates a need for parathyroidectomy, whereas a finding of low turnover is a contraindication for this surgery. Bone changes can occur relatively early in CKD, and low turnover correlates with increased vascular calcification.

2. In **high-turnover renal osteodystrophy,** elevated PTH levels drive bone resorption by many OCs; peritrabecular fibrosis, also known as osteitis fibrosa, may also be present (e-**Fig. 49.13A**). Bone formation is accelerated, often with formation of disorganized woven bone (seen on polarization; e-**Fig. 49.13B**) and increased tetracycline double labels (e-**Fig. 49.13C**). Trabeculae may be irregular in shape, and the cortex may be porous due to increased resorption.

3. In either form of **low-turnover osteodystrophy,** trabecular surfaces appear quiescent, with few OBs or OCs. Trabecular connectivity may also be decreased, and this parameter is more useful than the overall BV/TV (as mentioned earlier in the discussion of osteoporosis). In the osteomalacic form of renal osteodystrophy, mineralization is delayed and wide osteoid seams identified by von Kossa or trichrome staining (e-**Fig. 49.14A**) are not tetracycline labeled (e-**Fig. 49.14B**). In adynamic bone disease, both osteoid (e-**Fig. 49.14C**) and tetracycline labels (e-**Fig. 49.14D**) are minimal or absent. In the past, aluminum toxicity from dialysis was often the cause of low-turnover renal osteodystrophy, but the etiology of the adynamic changes seen more recently is not known.

4. **Mixed uremic osteodystrophy,** as the name implies, shows features of increased PTH and defective mineralization. Additionally, the appearance may vary considerably within the specimen (e-**Fig. 49.15A**), with areas of increased turnover adjacent to more quiescent regions with poor mineralization. Some areas may show abundant osteoid and robust tetracycline double labels (e-**Fig. 49.15B** and **C**) adjacent to broad single labels or unlabeled osteoid (e-**Fig. 49.15D**).

D. **Glucocorticoid-induced osteoporosis.** Because long-term glucocorticoid therapy is widely used in chronic inflammatory diseases and in organ transplantation, there is a high prevalence of glucocorticoid-induced bone disease. Early in treatment, glucocorticoids increase bone resorption, but more prolonged therapy eventuates in adynamic bone in which the number of OCs and OBs is decreased, as is tetracycline double labeling.

E. **Primary hyperparathyroidism.** Diagnosis of most cases of primary hyperparathyroidism is based on elevated serum calcium and PTH levels. However, in normocalcemic patients with variable or borderline PTH levels, bone biopsy can be useful in making the diagnosis because histologic findings represent the net effect of PTH over time. As in secondary hyperparathyroidism, such as in high-turnover renal osteodystrophy, sections typically show increased osteoid surfaces (some with woven bone), increased tetracycline labeling, and elevated numbers of OCs and OBs. Osteitis fibrosa cystica, the formation of cystic bone loss due to elevated OC activity associated with marrow fibrosis, is found only in severe cases and due to routine testing of serum calcium is rarely seen. However, peritrabecular fibrosis may be present. Another effect of PTH is to increase the porosity of the cortex, which may be difficult to distinguish from trabecular bone.

Focal well-demarcated osteolytic lesions known as **brown tumors** are also associated with hyperparathyroidism (e-Fig 49.16). Brown tumors consist of clusters of multinucleated giant cells in a fibrotic stroma, and the associated islands of bone are often woven rather than lamellar. Brown tumors can occur in any bone as a single lesion, or be multifocal. They generally resolve when PTH levels are restored to normal.

SUGGESTED READINGS

Monier-Faugere MC, Langub MC, et al. Bone biopsies: a modern approach. In: Avioli LV, Krane SM, eds. *Metabolic Bone Disease and Clinically Related Disorders*. San Diego, CA: Academic Press; 1998:237–273.

Recker RR, Barger-Lux MJ. Bone biopsy and histomorphometry in clinical practice. In: Favus M, ed. *Primer on the Metabolic Bone Diseases and Disorders of Mineral Metabolism*. Washington, DC: American Society for Bone and Mineral Research; 2006:161–169.

50 Joints and Synovium

Peter A. Humphrey

I. **NORMAL ANATOMY.** Joints are composed of the ends of contiguous bones and the associated soft tissue elements, including cartilage, ligaments, tendons, and synovium. Diarthrodial movable joints, which are the most common type, are usually covered by hyaline cartilage. Histologically, this articular cartilage is hypocellular with a glassy extracellular matrix composed mainly of collagen, proteoglycan, and water. Embedded within the matrix are chondrocytes within surrounding spaces (lacunae). There are four zones in articular cartilage—superficial, intermediate, deep, and calcified (**e-Fig. 50.1**)* and chondrocytes have a different appearance depending on their location. Those near the surface of the articular cartilage are small and flattened; in the middle zones, the chondrocytes are more rounded and arranged in columns. The deep and calcified layers of articular cartilage are separated by a thin, basophilic line known as the tidemark, which represents the mineralized front. The calcified cartilage base interdigitates with underlying subchondral bone.

Ligaments, which join two adjacent bones, are formed mainly of collagen. At the insertion site onto bone the ligamentous tissue is calcified. Tendons are connective tissue structures connecting muscle to bone. Microscopically, scant fibroblasts are found within parallel collagen bundles.

Synovium is a glistening white membrane with delicate villous projections that lines the inner surface of the joint capsule (*Am J Clin Pathol.* 2000;14:773) (**e-Fig. 50.2**). The inner lining surface is created by synovial cells, including fibroblastlike cells and histiocytes, which are arranged as a thin two- to three-cell layer of closely packed cells with elliptical nuclei and abundant cytoplasm. A fibrous or fibroadipose supporting layer lies beneath the synovial cell layer. Synovium also lines the flexor tendons of the hand and bursae (subcutaneous and subtendinous sacs).

II. **GROSS EXAMINATION AND TISSUE SAMPLING.** Joint or synovial soft tissue is received as needle core tissue, as fragments from arthroscopic or open synovectomy, as fragments from revised total joint arthroplasty, or as excisions of soft tissue tendon sheath or extra-articular masses. If fragments are received, the number, color, shape, and aggregate size of the fragments should be recorded. If meniscus tissue is submitted, fibrillations or tears should be noted. If chalky white deposits are identified, some of the tissue should be placed into absolute (100%) alcohol to preserve the crystals. Decalcification may be required for calcified cartilage, bone, or soft tissue. Fragments that appear different from normal should be selected for embedding, along with representative unremarkable-appearing fragments.

A. **Revision arthroplasties.** The presence or absence of necrosis, purulent exudate, and foreign material should be recorded. The explanted prosthesis should be described, including any identification numbers or defects.

B. **Soft tissue tumors.** For excised soft tissue tendon sheath or juxta-articular masses size, color, consistency, shape, and nodularity (single vs. multiple) should be provided. The outer surface of the specimen should then be inked, and cut sections should be characterized as to color, presence or absence of hemorrhage and necrosis, and distance of tumor to inked margin. One section per centimeter

---

*All e-figures are available online via the Solution Site Image Bank.

of tumor is a useful guide for section submission. Demonstration of tumor in relation to the closest inked margin(s) and to any recognizable normal tissue is important.

C. **Joint replacement surgeries.** Joint tissue may also be removed along with bone in orthopedic joint replacement surgeries, such as knee and total hip replacement procedures, which are most often performed for osteoarthritis. In such cases, where there is identifiable bone and attached articular cartilage, gross examination is particularly important. The overall dimensions and shape of the submitted bone and soft tissue should be recorded. Articular cartilage presence or absence, color, thickness, and abnormalities such as loss, cleft, or tuft formation, crystalline deposits, and bony and cartilaginous overgrowths (osteophytes or exostosis) should be documented. Synovium color, thickness, and consistency, and any nodules or villous projections should be described. One or several sections of synovium should be submitted for formalin fixation. Any associated gross bone defects, such as subchondral cyst formation and superficial bony necrosis, should be noted. Again, if chalky white deposits are identified, tissue should be placed into absolute (100%) alcohol to preserve the crystals. Sections of macroscopically abnormal areas should be submitted for histologic examination as follows. The bone and overlying cartilage should be fixed overnight in formalin, decalcified, and sectioned into 3- to 5-mm slices; one or two sections are usually sufficient to document cartilaginous and associated bone abnormalities. Junctions of normal and abnormal cartilage with underlying bone should be demonstrated by the sections.

D. **Synovial fluid.** Examination can be extremely useful in the diagnosis of different types of arthritis, especially infectious arthritis.

III. **DIAGNOSTIC FEATURES OF COMMON DISEASES OF JOINTS AND SYNOVIUM**

A. **Osteoarthritis** (also known as degenerative joint disease) is defined by the American College of Rheumatology as a "heterogeneous group of conditions that leads to joint symptoms and signs which are associated with defective integrity of articular cartilage, in addition to related changes in the underlying bone at the joint margins" (*Semin Arthritis Rheum.* 2005;3:1). It is the most common disease of the joints after the age of 65 years, with a prevalence of about 60% in men and 70% in women. The etiology of osteoarthritis is multifactorial, with inflammatory, metabolic, and mechanical causes. Major trauma, repetitive joint use, chronic inflammatory arthritis, and congenital malformations are major risk factors. The diagnosis is usually based on clinical and radiographic features. Pathologically, although the name osteoarthritis indicates an inflammatory condition, disruption of the articular cartilage is the fundamental finding. The joints most commonly affected are the distal and proximal interphalangeal joints of the hands, the hips and knees, and the cervical and lumbar spine.

Grossly, cartilaginous thinning, disruption, and fibrillation can be seen. In areas of complete cartilage loss, the underlying bone is exposed; this bone has a dense polished appearance like marble (known as eburnation). Microscopically, vertical clefts in the cartilage are characteristic (**e-Fig. 50.3**). There may be associated villous hyperplasia and mild chronic inflammation of the synovium (which should not be confused with rheumatoid arthritis). Papillary masses of metaplastic cartilage, bone, or adipose tissue may form in the synovial membrane; detachment of the masses results in intra-articular loose bodies (known as rice bodies). In eburnated areas, the bone may show sclerotic thickened bony trabeculae, cysts with fluid and fibromyxoid tissue, and superficial bony necrosis. It should be noted that in the vast majority of cases, the pathologic findings are confirmatory of the clinical diagnosis, so it has been suggested that routine pathologic examination in uncomplicated total hip and total knee arthroplasties may not be necessary. In only a small percentage of cases is the pathologic diagnosis different from the clinical impression; in these discrepant cases, the pathologic diagnosis in most cases is avascular necrosis, rheumatoid arthritis, pseudogout, or pigmented villonodular synovitis (*J Arthroplasty*. 2000;15:69; *Bone Joint Surg Am*. 2000;82:1531). Although rare, these cases with unexpected findings argue that microscopic examination of all cases of osteoarthritis is warranted.

B. **Rheumatoid arthritis** is a chronic multisystem disease of unknown cause. The hallmark of rheumatoid arthritis is a persistent inflammatory synovitis, typically involving the peripheral joints in a symmetric distribution. Clinically, the synovial inflammation causes swelling, tenderness, and limitation of motion. Histologically, the main attribute is joint destruction. There is hypertrophy and hyperplasia of the synovium along with a lymphoplasmacytic infiltrate, which together generate a papillary/polypoid chronic synovitis (e-Fig. 50.4). Lymphoid follicles and acute fibrinous surface exudate (e-Fig. 50.5) can also be seen. Synovial giant cells and bone and cartilage fragments may be present in the synovium. This overall histologic picture is not specific for rheumatoid arthritis, and similar changes may be seen in other arthritides such as systemic lupus erythematosus and psoriasis. Destruction of cartilage and joint fusion (ankylosis) can occur due to the formation of pannus (inflamed synovium and granulation tissue) over the surface of the articular cartilage, with invasion into cartilage and even bone and joint capsule.

Extra-articular manifestations of rheumatoid arthritis, which usually occur in patients with high titers of rheumatoid factor, include rheumatoid nodules, vasculitis, pleuropulmonary involvement (such as fibrosis and serositis), and splenomegaly with neutropenia in Felty syndrome. Rheumatoid nodules develop in ~25% of patients with rheumatoid arthritis. Although common locations include the olecranon bursa, proximal ulna, and Achilles tendon, they can also be found in the heart, lung, pleura, kidney, and meninges. Histologically, there is a central zone of fibrinoid necrosis surrounded by palisading histiocytes (e-Fig. 50.6).

C. **Synovitis associated with loose large joint arthroplasty** can be seen when there is failure of a total joint replacement, and can be related to a foreign body-type inflammatory response or infection. The foreign material can be metal, plastic/polyethylene, and/or methyl methacrylate cement. Microscopically, metallic particles are present as 1- to 3-μm particles within macrophages. Needle-shaped, polarizable fragments of polyethylene plastic are usually found in foreign body giant cells. Methyl methacrylate cement is lost upon processing, and consequently the cement causes empty spaces within foreign body-type giant cells in histologic sections after routine processing. These different types of foreign material can also elicit an exuberant fibrohistiocytic response (e-Fig. 50.7).

When neutrophils are seen, particularly when they are numerous, the possibility of infection should be considered. Frozen section of the inflamed tissue from a failed joint replacement may be requested, and the number of neutrophils per high-power field (HPF) should be reported. At least 5 HPFs on at least two sections should be examined. Observation of ≤5 neutrophils per HPF in tissue (not fibrin) is associated with high specificity (of about 95%) for the absence of infection, whereas the presence of >5 neutrophils per HPF has a sensitivity of up to 69% in identification of the presence of infection (*Mod Pathol*. 1998;11:427).

D. **In crystal-induced synovitis,** deposition of microcrystals in joints and periarticular tissues results in gout (urate crystals), pseudogout (also known as chondrocalcinosis—calcium pyrophosphate dihydrate crystals), and apatite disease (hydroxyapatite crystals) (*Am J Clin Pathol*. 2000;14:773). Gout and pseudogout are definitively diagnosed by light microscopic detection of crystals in joint fluid. Gouty tophi are formed when urate crystals are deposited in subcutaneous soft tissue, synovium, bone, or bursae, with a granulomatous response dominated by histiocytes and foreign body giant cells (e-Fig. 50.8); fixation of the tissue in alcohol is necessary to preserve the crystals. A de Galantha histochemical stain can be used to highlight the crystals. The crystals of pseudogout appear rhomboid and purple in nondecalcified H&E-stained slides (e-**Fig. 50.9**); with decalcification, the crystals are lost and what is left are rounded pools of basophilic material surrounding rhomboid areas that mark the prior site of the crystals. These crystal deposits do not typically elicit a histiocytic or foreign body giant cell reaction (*Semin Diagn Pathol.* 2011;28:37).

E. **Infectious arthritis** is diagnosed by clinical history and joint fluid examination, including Gram stain of a centrifuged cell pellet and microbiologic culture.

F. **Hemosiderotic synovitis** follows chronic intra-articular hemorrhage, which can occur in patients with hemophilia and synovial hemangioma. Microscopically, there are fine villous projections early in the disease course. Hemosiderin is present within synoviocytes and macrophages (e-**Fig. 50.10**). Osteoarthritis usually ensues.

G. **Baker cyst**, which can be found in osteoarthritis and rheumatoid arthritis, is a synovial-lined cyst in the popliteal space that is formed by herniation. In contrast, ganglia (ganglion cysts), located near a joint capsule or tendon sheath, are not synovial-lined cysts and do not communicate with the joint cavity.

H. Tissue from a **torn meniscus** from the knee may be submitted as tissue shavings or as a fibrocartilaginous loose body. Histologically, there are few changes in the avascular and collagenized tissue because reparative fibrosis and neovascularization are uncommon.

I. Each **intervertebral disc** is a type of joint (amphiarthrodial), and tissue fragments from a prolapsed disc may be submitted. Microscopically, fibrous tissue, fibrocartilage, and cartilaginous tissue can be seen. Chondrocyte necrosis and/or groups of proliferating chondrocytes may be found. The presence of neovascularization indicates herniation (*Hum Pathol.* 1988;19:406).

J. **Synovial tumors** are uncommon and can arise from synovium of the tendon sheaths, bursae, and joint spaces (*Semin Diagn Pathol.* 2011;28:37). Regardless of their articular or extra-articular location, this family of neoplasms shares translocations of chromosome 1p13 (Table 46.1), which often also involve 2q35 resulting in formation of a *COL6A3-CSF1* fusion gene (*Proc Natl Acad Sci USA.* 2006;103:690). It is uncertain whether synovial tumors are best classified as fibrohistiocytic tumors (as in the WHO classification) or as tumors differentiating toward synovial cells.

   1. **Giant cell tumor of tendon sheath, localized type** (localized tenosynovial tumor, nodular tenosynovitis) is the most common benign tumor of the tendon sheath and synovium. It appears to be a neoplasm rather than a reactive process. These giant cell tumors are usually found in adults on the fingers, and uncommonly on the ankle and knee (*Cancer.* 1986;57:875). Grossly, they are circumscribed lobulated masses a few centimeters in diameter, with mottled pink-gray cut surfaces that often show flecks of yellow or brown (representing lipid and hemosiderin, respectively). Microscopically, there is a vague nodularity at low magnification; at higher powers of magnification, rounded mononuclear cells, giant cells, foam cells, and collagen are seen in varying proportions (e-**Fig. 50.11**). Hemosiderin deposition may be present. Mitotic figures are uncommon, and when they exceed two figures per 10 HPFs, the likelihood of recurrence is greater. Immunohistochemistry and electron microscopy have demonstrated macrophage and synovial cell features in the lesional cells (and osteoclast attributes in the giant cells), but neither technique is required for the diagnosis. Similarly, although cytogenetic studies have demonstrated clonal abnormalities (especially involving 1p11–13) in the lesional cells, karyotypic analysis is not needed for diagnosis.

   Tenosynovial giant cell tumors are benign, with a recurrence rate of about 10% to 20% related to mitotic activity (as noted earlier), cellularity, and incomplete excision. Accordingly, margin status and a high mitotic rate should be reported.

2. **Giant cell tumor of tendon sheath, diffuse type** (pigmented villonodular synovitis) presents as an intra-articular or extra-articular tumor. The gene expression profile of the neoplasm resembles that of activated macrophages (*Arthritis Rheum.* 2006;54:1009), and structural rearrangements of 1p11–12 have been reported in the lesion; however, these special studies are not needed to establish the diagnosis.

   a. The **intra-articular** form typically involves the joint space of the knee of young adults, although ankle, hip, and shoulder involvement have also been reported. Involvement of the synovium can be localized with the formation of either nodular or pedunculated masses; the more common diffuse form affects virtually the entire synovium. Grossly, tissue from the diffuse form removed by open synovectomy is spongy, diffusely thickened, and brownish-yellow. Microscopically, subsynovial fibrohistiocytic cells with uniform round to oval nuclei are seen. Foam cells and iron pigment are always present, and giant cells are common and tend to be arranged in groups. Aside from the villous structures, the overall appearance is similar to nodular tenosynovitis (**e-Fig. 50.12**).

      The localized form has an excellent prognosis and a low recurrence rate when managed surgically, whereas the diffuse form has a reported recurrence rate of up to 46%. Radiation treatment has shown mixed results. Combined surgical and nonsurgical approaches may be necessary, and in some patients, total joint arthroplasty may be the only effective treatment (*J Am Acad Orthop Surg.* 2006;14:376).

   b. The **extra-articular** form is much less common; the knee, ankle, and foot are predominant sites of occurrence. Some, but not all, cases are extensions of the intra-articular form; the rare exclusively extra-articular cases likely arise from the synovium of bursa or tendon sheaths. Grossly, the tumor is a large, multinodular, and white to yellow-brown mass, without villous projections. Microscopically, there are sheets of rounded to polygonal mononuclear cells with the formation of clefts and pseudoglandular spaces. Giant cells are fewer in number compared with the giant cell tumor of tendor sheath, localized type. Xanthoma cells, spindle cells, and chronic inflammatory cells are present. Scant data exist on outcome for these patients, although recurrence rates appear high, at 40% to 50%.

3. **Malignant giant cell tumor of tendon sheath** is rare type of sarcoma and can be diagnosed when a histologically benign giant cell tumor of tendon sheath is admixed with overtly malignant areas, or when malignancy is seen in a recurrence of the benign tumor. Histologic indicators of malignancy include diffuse infiltrative growth, scant giant cells, cytologic atypia, necrosis, and a mitotic count of >10 per 10 HPFs.

4. **Synovial chondromatosis** is a benign nodular cartilaginous proliferation arising in the synovium of joints, bursae, or tendon sheaths. It is usually monoarticular in distribution, involving the knee or hip in adults. Grossly, there are multiple osteocartilaginous nodules, each measuring <1 mm to several millimeters in diameter, which may be embedded within synovium and/or mobile as loose bodies (note that loose bodies can also be seen in epiphyseal osteonecrosis, osteochondral fracture, and osteochondritis dissecans, so their presence is not diagnostic). Microscopically, the nodules of hyaline cartilage show clusters of chondrocytes that can show nuclear atypia with nuclear enlargement, hyperchromasia, and binucleation (**e-Fig. 50.13**), findings that should not be viewed as evidence of malignancy. Clonal chromosomal abnormalities have been cited as evidence for a neoplastic process, but cytogenetics is not used for diagnosis. Local recurrence after excision occurs in ~15% of

cases. Rare cases of chondrosarcoma arising in synovial chondromatosis have been reported.

5. **Synovial chondrosarcoma** is extremely rare, and can be classified as primary or secondary to synovial chondromatosis. Histologic features of malignancy include loss of the "clustering" growth pattern typical of synovial chondromatosis (e-Fig. 50.14), with replacement by a sheetlike arrangement of chondrocytes, myxoid change in the matrix, areas of necrosis, and spindling at the periphery of chondroid lobules (*Cancer.* 1991;67:155). The prognosis is poor.

6. **Synovial hemangioma** is very rare and usually found in the knee of young adults. Microscopically, most are cavernous hemangiomas; some are capillary or arteriovenous hemangiomas (e-Fig. 50.15).

7. **Synovial lipoma** is rare. Grossly, the synovium is yellow, thickened, and exhibits excrescences (lipoma arborescens). Microscopically, the synovium is infiltrated by mature adipose tissue (e-Fig. 50.16). Recurrence is rare.

8. Rare case reports of other synovial tumors include intra-articular hemangiopericytoma, intracapsular chondroma, synovial sarcoma, epithelioid sarcoma, malignant fibrous histiocytoma, and lymphoma.

Cytopathology

51 General Principles of Cytopathology

Brian Collins

I. **INTRODUCTION.** Cytopathology has developed into a discipline that examines cellular elements from throughout the body collected by a wide variety of methods and procedures. It shares with other anatomic pathology disciplines a morphologic study of cells utilizing patterns and cellular features to identify specific pathologic conditions. Cytopathology provides diagnostic information in a wide variety of clinical settings, and can thus be used to guide patient management both at the time of initial diagnosis and during the course of treatment. In broad terms, there are three main areas of cytopathology, specifically (i) gynecologic/Pap slides, (ii) nongynecologic (Non-Gyn), and (iii) fine needle aspiration (FNA).

The utility of cytopathology is underscored by the fact that virtually all ancillary laboratory techniques used in surgical pathology can also be performed on cytology specimens.

A. **Immunocytochemistry.** Special stains are commonly applied to cytologic samples, often to confirm the morphologic diagnosis, to help in determining the possible primary sites of a tumor, or to determine the presence of specific prognostic markers. In general, cell block sections are preferred for immunocytochemical staining because most laboratories have experience in processing the formalin-fixed, paraffin-embedded (FFPE) tissue sections that are generated from cell blocks.

B. **Flow cytometry.** In the presence of a lymphocyte-rich sample, the possibility of a lymphoproliferative process may need to be addressed by flow cytometry. Body fluids, particularly effusions, are amenable to this type of analysis.

C. **Molecular genetic methods.** Cytological preparations, including fluid specimens, brushings, washings, and scrapings, are suitable substrates for molecular analysis. Regardless of the method used to process samples (e.g., whether air dried, ethanol fixed, or used to produce a cell block) it is possible to extract nucleic acids that can be analyzed by a wide variety of genetic assays, including polymerase chain reaction (PCR), DNA sequence analysis, gene expression analysis, and fluorescence in situ hybridization (FISH).

II. **GYNECOLOGIC/PAP SLIDES.** The "Pap test" is the most successful cancer screening test in medicine. After the wide introduction of the Pap smear, the incidence of cervical carcinoma dropped significantly and it remains the mainstay of screening women for cervical carcinoma. Standardized terminology and categorizations for the Pap smear have been developed (*The Bethesda System for Reporting Cervical Cytology.* New York, Springer-Verlag, Inc.; 2004). The Bethesda Reporting System for Cervical Smears is covered in more detail in the cytopathology section of Chapter 34.

III. NONGYNECOLOGIC CYTOPATHOLOGY encompasses a wide variety of body sites, organs, and types of specimens. In general, any lesion that can be drained, brushed, washed, or scraped can be a "non-gyn" cytopathology specimen.

A. Specimen types

1. **Fluid.** These constitute a major category of non-gyn specimens and include pleural fluid, ascites/peritoneal fluid, pericardial fluid, and cerebrospinal fluid. Any loculated fluid can be drained and submitted for analysis (neck cyst, hepatic cyst, etc.) including synovial and vitreous fluid. Urine specimens, either voided or catheterized, are also commonly examined.

2. **Brush.** The endoscope makes it possible to introduce a brush and collect cells and tissue from a wide variety of internal locations. These include the bronchopulmonary tree (bronchial brush), alimentary tract (esophageal brush, gastric brush, and common/pancreatic/hepatic bile duct brushes), peritoneal cavity, and genitourinary tract (urethra brush, ureter brush, and renal pelvic brush).

3. **Wash.** Lesions sampled by a brush are usually accompanied by a "wash" specimen, which can be collected to sample additional cells. These specimens commonly include lung (bronchial wash, bronchoalveolar lavage), peritoneal cavity (pelvic wash), and urinary bladder (bladder wash, ureter wash, and renal pelvic wash).

4. **Scrape.** The Tzanck smear of the skin is utilized for the identification of mucocutaneous herpes virus effect.

B. Preparation and processing

1. **Submission.** Material can be submitted fresh or fixed. In general, unfixed material should be refrigerated until it can be delivered to the cytopathology lab. Even after arrival, it should be refrigerated until processed since unfixed cells in a fluid environment are in a constant state of degeneration, both in situ and after being collected. Specimens delayed in processing that have not properly handled can be uninterpretable.

2. **Fixative and stain.** Alcohol is the standard fixative. Alcohol fixation can be utilized at a variety of steps in specimen handling, including at the time of collection (slides prepared from a brush can be placed in 95% ethanol at the patient's bedside, or the brush itself can be placed directly into a liquid fixative container) or after initial processing of the specimen (after preparation of cytospin slides from a fluid sample). Regardless, once cellular material is placed on a slide, it needs to be alcohol fixed as soon as possible. A delay of more than a few seconds can cause air drying artifact, which renders the cells indistinct and the nuclei "washed out" when subsequently Pap stained. Severe air drying artifact can render a slide uninterpretable.

   a. The **Pap stain** highlights nuclear morphologic details including distinct chromatin and nuclear membrane detail. The cytoplasm tends to have a blue-green coloration with keratinization showing organophilic decoration.

   b. A modified **Wright–Giemsa,** commonly referred to as **Diff-Quik**^{TM}, is the other main cytopathology stain. It is performed on slides which are first air dried. Once completely air dried, slides are placed in a methanol fixative and then stained (total time to complete the stain can be less than a minute). The **Diff-Quik**^{TM} stain highlights lymphoid elements and a variety of extracellular elements (colloid, matrix, mucin, and so on).

   c. The Pap stain and Diff-Quik^{TM} stain are complementary and both are frequently utilized in combination on non-gyn and FNA specimens.

C. Reporting. Standardized recommendations for reporting the findings in non-gyn cytopathology specimens have recently been developed (*Arch Pathol Lab Med.* 2009;133:1743). Uniform reporting enhances patient care and thus implementation of these guidelines in routine practice is strongly recommended.

IV. **FNA.** One of the most challenging and dynamic areas of cytopathology is FNA. Virtually any organ or abnormality (either palpable or localized by imaging techniques) can be subjected to FNA. The technique essentially provides a microbiopsy of cellular material (cells and tissue) for microscopic examination and a wide variety of ancillary tests. The method permits immediate interpretive evaluation which makes possible real-time adjustments of the biopsy procedure, appropriate specimen triage, and directed ancillary testing.

A. **Principles.** The procedure is minimally invasive and accurate. At its core, FNA involves the use of a thin bore needle with a cutting end moved in a piston motion to obtain cells and tissue. The cellular elements present within the needle are then processed for diagnosis (e-**Fig. 51.1**).*

B. **Technique.** While simple, proficiency and adequacy require an understanding of the procedure and experience in its use. It is the cutting, bevelled end of the needle and capillary action of a repetitive "piston-like" motion movement which provides the cellular elements necessary for diagnosis. The appropriate application of needle movement is critical since insufficient movement will not adequately sample the tissue, and prolonged movement can lead to hemodilution and entrapment of tissue in clot. The appropriate number of tissue passes and appropriate negative pressure will vary for each individual case and clinical presentation.

Negative pressure during the procedure (typically applied by an empty 10- or 20-cc plastic syringe attached to the needle) can be useful but is not always necessary. There are many solid cellular lesions/neoplasms that can be adequately sampled without aspiration, including lymph nodes and the thyroid. Vascular organs and neoplasms benefit from a nonaspiration FNA technique since aspiration can lead to bleeding and specimen hemodilution.

Needles utilized can range from 22 to 27 gauge. Larger gauge needles tend to cause more bleeding and paradoxically tend to be less diagnostic. Needle length can vary significantly (5/8th in. up to 8 in.) and will depend on what is required to reach the lesion.

C. **Procedure.** In broad terms, the needle is directed to the area of interest by either palpation or under image guidance.

1. **Palpable.** This method involves any lesion that can be localized or identified by manual palpation. It must be stressed that FNA of every location requires an understanding of the associated local anatomy, especially for areas in the head and neck, thyroid, chest wall, and various soft tissue locations. Superficial FNA of palpable lesions is well tolerated, minimally invasive, and has a very low complication rate.

2. **Image guidance.** This method involves utilizing an imaging modality to direct the needle, most commonly, ultrasound and CT imaging. The principles of the FNA biopsy itself remain the same. In some cases, a stylet within the needle is helpful; it is used to prevent sampling of organs as the needle moves toward the lesion, and then removed once the needle tip is in the desired location. An immediate assessment of the FNA sample makes it possible for the pathologist to guide the clinician to ensure that a diagnostic sample is collected and that the appropriate ancillary studies are initiated at the time of the procedure.

D. **Materials**

1. **Palpable.** The materials required are simple and readily available. They can be conveniently organized in a small basket or box, which can be easily transported from the laboratory (e-**Fig 51.2**).

---

*All e-figures are available online via the Solution Site Image Bank.

2. **Image guidance.** The appropriate type of needle and the FNA approach are determined by the clinical setting. On-site presence of the cytopathology team with glass slides, fixative (alcohol), needle rinse tube (normal saline or RPMI), stains (Diff-Quik™), and a microscope, will help optimize the likelihood that a diagnostic sample is obtained and that appropriate ancillary studies are initiated.

E. **Clinical application**

1. **Immediate evaluation.** Immediate evaluation is the standard of care because it provides several advantages. First, it guides the procedure and thus ensures a maximum effort to obtain a diagnosis. By examining the slides during the procedure, immediate evaluation can be used to help decide if more FNAs are necessary; guide the needle position placement by determining if lesion or nonlesional material is present; and if nondiagnostic, support a decision to move to a potential second site. Second, with immediate evaluation, the trade-off between the length of the procedure and number of biopsies can be managed to balance the requirement for diagnostic tissue without unnecessarily extending the length of the procedure. By assuring a diagnostic procedure, the number of nondiagnostic samples can be minimized and repeat procedures and delays in diagnosis can be avoided. Third, the cytopathologist can identify those cases where tissue for appropriate ancillary studies needs to be collected to enhance diagnostic accuracy. These situations include identifying a lymphoproliferative process where rinse material is sent for flow cytometry analysis, abscess/granulomatous inflammation where microbiologic cultures are indicated, poorly differentiated neoplasms where a cell block can provide material for immunohistochemical evaluation, and lesions where cytogenetics/molecular diagnostics can contribute to diagnosis and treatment.

F. **Specimen processing**

1. **Direct smears** are stained by the Papanicolaou and Diff-Quik™ methods.

2. **Liquid medium.** FNA samples that are collected in a liquid medium provide a wide variety of options for further analysis. While it is helpful to perform needle washes during the FNA procedure, the best chance for a sufficient cell block involves direct (no slides prepared) dedicated FNA samples placed in the liquid medium (saline or RPMI). Cell block preparation affords a variety of options and advantages; sections of the cell block contribute to the morphologic evaluation of the lesion, and also provide cellular material for immunohistochemical analysis, interphase FISH, and for a wide range of PCR-based molecular tests.

SUGGESTED READINGS

Crothers BA, Tench WD, Schwartz MR, et al. Guidelines for the reporting of nongynecologic cytopathology specimens. *Arch Pathol Lab Med.* 1999;133:1743–1756.

Gupta PK. University of Pennsylvania aspiration cart (Penn-A-Cart): an innovative journey in fine needle aspiration service. *Acta Cytol.* 2010a;54:165–168.

Gupta PK. Progression from on-site to point-of-care fine needle aspiration service: opportunities and challenges. *Cytojournal.* 2010b;7:6.

Wright TC, Massad LS, Dunton CJ, et al. 2006 consensus guidelines for the management of women with abnormal cervical cancer screening tests. *Am J Obstet Gynecol.* 2007;197:346–355.

SECTION XIII

Ancillary Methods

Frozen Sections and Other Intraoperative Consultations

Michael E. Hull, Peter A. Humphrey, and John D. Pfeifer

I. **INTRODUCTION.** Intraoperative consultations fall into two general categories. Microscopic consultations, usually performed as frozen sections, are undertaken to establish a tissue diagnosis, determine the nature of a lesion that may require ancillary testing, establish that sufficient diagnostic tissue has been obtained, identify metastatic disease, and assess surgical margins or extent of disease. Microscopic consultation can also be performed using touch preparations, a practice that has the advantage of preserving valuable tissue. Nonmicroscopic consultations are gross examinations of a specimen that provide the surgeon with real-time information on tissue margins and the anatomic extent of disease processes. They also facilitate the triage of fresh tissue for ancillary diagnostic studies or research protocols.

II. **FROZEN SECTIONS.** High-quality frozen sections can be performed with remarkable speed if equipment is kept in optimum working condition and if the operator is well versed in the technique. In experienced hands, the entire consultation can often be performed in 10 to 15 minutes from the time of the arrival of the specimen in the frozen section room to the notification of the surgeon of the diagnosis. For larger tissue specimens, proper interpretation requires a thorough gross examination of the tissue before sectioning. Good communication with the surgeon regarding operative findings and knowledge of pertinent clinical history are also absolutely essential for optimization of the process.

A. **Indications.** Frozen sections are indicated to establish a tissue diagnosis (such as the presence of malignancy, which will guide intraoperative patient management and extent of surgery); for tissue identification (e.g., to confirm the presence of parathyroid tissue in a parathyroidectomy specimen); to determine the nature of a lesion that may require ancillary testing that requires special fixatives or media (e.g., RPMI for flow cytometry or glutaraldehyde for electron microscopy); to establish that sufficient diagnostic tissue has been obtained; to identify metastatic disease; and to assess surgical margins or extent of disease.

Frozen sections should not be used merely to satisfy a surgeon's curiosity, to compensate for inadequate preoperative evaluation, or as a mechanism to communicate information more quickly to the patient or the patient's family.

B. **The frozen section procedure.** Frozen sections are performed by freezing the tissue in a block of specialized embedding medium, followed by cutting thin (usually 5 μm) sections from the block using a cryostat (refrigerated microtome). The sections are adhered to glass slides, fixed in ethanol, and stained with hematoxylin and eosin (H&E). Small specimens may be completely utilized for frozen section slide preparation, but if possible, a portion of the tissue should be preserved for routine handling to avoid freezing artifacts that can compromise interpretation of the permanent sections (e.g., in the case of brain biopsies). For larger tissue samples, judgment must be exercised in gross sampling so that the area(s) of highest diagnostic yield is selected for frozen section. Cytological imprints from tissues can be an important adjunct in diagnosis, especially for hematolymphoid abnormalities, lymph node biopsies, and thyroid lesions.

C. **Interpretation.** The interpretation of frozen sections requires integration of the histologic morphology in the H&E-stained sections; the gross features of the specimen; information from the surgeon regarding the origin of the tissue, the indication for the consultation (including the clinical history, radiological findings, and intraoperative observations); and the ways in which the frozen section diagnosis will affect the operative strategy. In some difficult cases, it may be necessary to request additional tissue for frozen section analysis. If additional tissue cannot be obtained, deferral of a definitive diagnosis pending examination of formalin-fixed paraffin-embedded sections is acceptable. In routine clinical practice, such deferrals are employed in <5% of frozen section diagnoses.

D. **Communication of findings.** Clear communication of a concise diagnosis to the surgeon is the last step of the intraoperative consultation. Usually, there is a narrowly defined clinical problem that frozen section is to solve; this should be specifically and unambiguously addressed in the diagnosis. The diagnosis is written and signed, with the date and time, by all interpreting pathologists and made part of the final pathology report. If the written diagnosis is verbally transmitted, the pathologist should first confirm with the recipient of the information the identity of the patient (using two identifiers) and the surgeon. The operating room staff member taking the diagnosis should repeat it back to the pathologist to confirm accurate communication.

Certain phraseologies tend to be resistant to misinterpretation. For instance, "negative for malignancy" or "positive for malignancy" are generally understood well. Since some diagnosis can easily be incompletely heard or misunderstood in a busy operating room, the diagnosis should always be repeated back as a safeguard.

E. **Accuracy of frozen sections.** The accuracy of frozen sections will vary from institution to institution on the basis of the types of surgical cases evaluated and the experience of the involved pathologists. Table 52.1 highlights the fact that the accuracy of frozen section diagnosis is dependent on the anatomic site. Regular self-audits of the frozen section service are desirable so that surgeons and pathologists are aware of the performance characteristics of the modality in their own hands. Such audits of single institutions, and pooled data across hundreds of institutions, show that accurate diagnoses are made overall in >95% of cases, while discordance with the final diagnosis occurs in 1% to 2% of cases. Deferral of the diagnosis until permanent section diagnosis occurs in 1% to 4% of cases.

F. **Sources of error in frozen sections.** Errors can be divided into errors of interpretation and errors of sampling; both usually result in false-negative diagnoses. False-positive diagnoses are rarer, likely because experienced pathologists tend to appropriately defer to permanent section rather than making an incorrect diagnosis on substandard material.

Misinterpretation accounts for about 40% of errors overall (*Arch Pathol Lab Med.* 1996;120:804; *Arch Pathol Lab Med.* 1996;120:19). Interpretations of frozen sections are more prone to this error than interpretation of permanent sections due to the presence of artifacts that are not encountered in routinely fixed, paraffin-embedded sections. Some tissues are more likely to show significant artifact, especially those with high fat content, such as most pelvic lymph nodes.

TABLE 52.1 Examples of Frozen Section Evaluation

Tissue	Concordance with permanent section diagnosis	False negative	Comments on utility
Breast			Limited (see text)
Cervix	73% for evaluation of dysplasia		Poor for evaluation of dysplasia
Gallbladder	95% when used to evaluate a mural lesion		Useful in the rare instances in which it is required
Liver			Diagnostic dilemmas that generate deferrals: 1. Hamartoma vs. cholangiocarcinoma 2. Regenerative nodule vs. hepatocellular carcinoma 3. Adenoma vs. hepatocellular carcinoma
Lung	99%		Useful; deferral rate of only 3–4%
Axillary sentinel lymph nodes for metastatic breast cancer	90[a]–96%[b]	15[a]–37%[b]	Possibly useful (see text)
Lymph nodes for staging	~100%[c]	20–40%[c]	Limited and dependent upon the lymph node location (see text)
Ovary	92%	5%	Useful; errors are disproportionately represented among mucinous tumors
Pancreas	98% when used for diagnosis of primary lesion; almost 100% for margins	1%	Atypical ductal structures, especially in the setting of pancreatitis, may mimic carcinoma; deferral rate of 6–7%
Parathyroid	99% (for parathyroid vs. nonparathyroid tissue)		Useful for distinction of parathyroid versus nonparathyroid tissue; inadequate for diagnosis of parathyroid carcinoma, or for differentiating adenoma from hyperplasia
Skin, melanoma		Up to 50%	Strongly discouraged (see text)
Skin, nonmelanoma		About 2%, based on recurrence rates following Mohs' microsurgery[d]	Useful for the evaluation of margins in the resection of tumors with infiltrating borders and tumors of the face, especially eyes, ears, and nose.
Thyroid	98%	10%	Inadequate for follicular lesions, as the sampling required is not practical (see text); better for lesions with papillary architecture; deferral rate is 6%

[a]When nodes with submicrometastases (<0.2 mm) are considered "positive."
[b]When nodes with submicrometastases are considered "negative."
[c]Staging pelvic lymph nodes at prostatectomy.
[d]Data on correlation with permanent sections is sparse, as follow-up permanent sections are not performed.

Sampling errors occur in two ways. The first is sectioning error. Diagnostic tissue may be present in the frozen block, but the block may not be faced sufficiently for the lesion to be present on the actual frozen section slides; the diagnostic material may then be found in routine permanent sections of the residual frozen block, a scenario that accounts for 10% to 15% of errors. The second type of sampling error is gross sampling error. This accounts for about 45% of errors overall, and is seen when the diagnostic tissue is not in the portion of the specimen sampled by the frozen section; good gross pathology skills will minimize, but never eliminate, this problem. Furthermore, it is not feasible to completely sample larger lesions by frozen section, and so sampling errors will always exist for large lesions with heterogeneous composition.

Discrepancies between a frozen section and the final (permanent section) diagnosis should be documented in the final surgical pathology report, along with the reason for the discrepancy. If the discrepancy is of clinical significance, the pathologist should immediately alert the surgeon to the change in diagnosis.

G. **Anatomic sites deserving special mention.** The anatomic sites with the most discrepancies between frozen and permanent sections are skin, breast, lymph nodes for metastatic disease, the female genital tract, and thyroid. Frozen sections do have a role in the surgical management of disease in these sites, but since loss of diagnostic material during the performance of frozen sections is unavoidable, each case must be critically evaluated as to whether the frozen section diagnosis will add enough value to warrant this loss.

1. **Skin.** Frozen sections for margin assessment in the excisions of large nonmelanoma skin cancers such as basal cell carcinoma and squamous cell carcinoma are indicated if the lesion has vague infiltrative borders or is in a location in which wide excision is not possible, as in the case of tumors of the eyelid, nose, or ear (*Arch Pathol Lab Med.* 2005;129:1536). If the borders of a lesion are well defined, frozen sections are not as necessary.

   It is widely agreed that the intraoperative primary diagnosis of pigmented lesions is ill-advised. The determination of prognosis and subsequent management of melanoma requires an accurate assessment of Breslow thickness, and frozen artifact may cause so much specimen distortion as to make a depth of invasion assessment meaningless in both permanent and frozen sections. Freezing artifact compounded by actinic damage, frequent in patients with pigmented lesions, also conspires to obscure histology. Subtle changes, such as intraepidermal spread by single melanocytes, are very difficult to appreciate in frozen sections, making the method a poor choice for margin assessment as well. For example, the false-negative rate for lentiginous spread of melanoma by frozen section evaluation may be as high as 50%.

2. **Breast.** Once commonplace, the initial pathologic diagnosis of breast tumors is now very rarely made during surgery, since methods for detection of smaller tumors and more sophisticated treatment algorithms (as opposed to mastectomy only) now usually lead to diagnosis on the basis of needle core biopsy or aspiration cytology. Margin evaluation is sometimes requested during breast-conserving procedures, but the high fat content of breast tissue makes frozen specimens technically difficult to section and prone to freezing artifact. Evaluation of margins by imprint histology is an alternative to frozen section, but it is insensitive unless the margins are grossly involved, in which case the examination is unnecessary (*Arch Pathol Lab Med.* 2005;129:1565). As a rule, an intraoperative gross examination of a lumpectomy specimen is used to determine whether or not there will be additional excisions.

3. **Lymph nodes for metastatic disease (including axillary sentinel lymph nodes for breast carcinoma)**

   a. **Sentinel lymph nodes.** Although current diagnostic modalities have reduced the need for breast frozen sections, requests for frozen sections of breast sentinel lymph nodes have increased (e-**Fig. 52.1A** and **B**).* Unfortunately, frozen sections on sentinel nodes consume considerable tissue; if no metastases are identified, further evaluation of the node has therefore been significantly hampered (e-**Fig. 52.2**).

Numerous studies have indicated that the sensitivity of frozen section evaluation of sentinel nodes is about 60%, although the specificity is near 100% (*Mod Path.* 2005; 18:58). It has been argued that the metastases that are typically missed by frozen section are submicroscopic (<0.2 mm in greatest dimension) or are detected by cytokeratin immunohistochemistry alone, and that since the significance of these classes of metastases is not yet clear, the low sensitivity of the approach underestimates its clinical utility. A sensible middle ground seems to be to perform frozen sections when the clinical history and gross examination of the node give a high degree of suspicion for metastasis. Imprint cytology, as a routine measure, is another possible approach to intraoperative sentinel lymph node evaluation.

b. Other lymph node frozen sections. The intraoperative evaluation of lymph nodes can be performed by frozen section or by imprint cytology, and if indicated, tissue should be allocated for flow cytometric analysis, routine histology, and molecular diagnostics.

4. Thyroid. The widespread use of fine needle aspiration has altered the approach to frozen section evaluation of the thyroid. Frozen section evaluation of thyroid excision specimens is best performed in conjunction with imprint cytology, the latter of which is more sensitive for the nuclear grooves, inclusions, and chromatin-clearing characteristic of papillary carcinoma. Since the distinction between follicular adenoma and carcinoma by frozen section (e-**Fig. 52.3**) would require thorough sampling of the tumor and capsule for invasion and angioinvasion, frozen section is poorly suited to this application (*Can J Surg.* 2004;47:29).

5. Female genital tract. Of all the neoplastic processes of the female genital tract, ovarian neoplasms are probably the best suited to intraoperative frozen section diagnosis (*Arch Pathol Lab Med.* 2005;129:1544; *Int J Gynecol Cancer.* 2005;15:192). Even so, borderline mucinous neoplasms of the ovary have a significant rate of discordance between the frozen section and permanent section diagnoses, primarily due to sampling error. The diagnosis of cervical dysplasia is fraught with difficulties due to frozen section artifact and low concordance with permanent section diagnosis.

III. OTHER INTRAOPERATIVE CONSULTATIONS. Intraoperative nonmicroscopic consultations are often required even though no frozen section is needed. Indications include gross diagnosis (such as benign simple ovarian cyst or leiomyoma of uterus); gross confirmation of the presence of a lesion or mass; identification of a margin or region of interest that requires special sampling for permanent sections; specimen orientation; triage of tissue for ancillary testing modalities that require special processing or fixatives (in which case good judgment is required to ensure a balance between the need for tissue for routine histopathologic evaluation and the need for tissue for specialized testing); and collection of tissue for tumor banking or research studies.

A. Opening of a viscus organ for gross examination and fixation. Gastrointestinal specimens commonly require opening in the operating room so that the surgeon can see whether or not lesional tissue has been excised. In partial intestinal excisions for inflammatory disease, in which the risk for malignancy is increased, a careful intraoperative examination may inform the surgeon of a previously undetected tumor, which may have implications for additional surgical therapy.

---

*All e-figures are available online via the Solution Site Image Bank.

Similarly, gross examination and opening of the adnexa and/or uterus can aid in determining the extent of surgery that is required. Such gross examination often leads to frozen sections when ovarian surface papillary excrescences are identified, or when solid or complex architecture features are discovered in an ovarian cyst.

B. Tumor for banking must be chosen so that the remaining lesional tissue material will still be suitable for a complete diagnostic evaluation. The banked tissue should not include a surgical margin, or have an important relationship to an anatomic structure that would impact staging or the need for adjuvant therapy. In cases of small specimens, it may be necessary to defer banking for the sake of a thorough diagnostic evaluation.

SUGGESTED READINGS

Lechago J. Frozen section examination of liver, gallbladder, and pancreas. *Arch Pathol Lab Med.* 2005;129:1610.

Marchevsky, AM, Changsri C, Gupta I, et al. Frozen section diagnoses of small pulmonary nodules: accuracy and clinical implications. *Ann Thorac Surg.* 2004;78:1755.

Young MP, Kirby RS, O'Donoghue EP, et al. Accuracy and cost of intraoperative lymph node frozen sections at radical prostatectomy. *J Clin Pathol.* 1999;52:925.

53 Electron Microscopy

Ashima Agarwal and Frances V. White

I. **INTRODUCTION.** Transmission electron microscopy (EM) has been used by surgical pathologists over the past 50 years for the diagnosis of a wide range of diseases in various organ systems (Table 53.1). The method allows for the visualization of subcellular morphology, with appreciation of disease processes and structural abnormalities that cannot be resolved by light microscopy. EM is an essential part of the work-up of medical renal diseases, peripheral nerve diseases, muscle diseases, and primary ciliary dyskinesia. It is also useful in evaluating metabolic and inherited diseases, providing an initial differential diagnosis, or ruling in or out a specific disease process. The role of EM in the diagnosis of neoplasms has decreased since the advent of immunohistochemical and molecular techniques, but it is still an ancillary tool for the evaluation of atypical tumors or when other techniques yield indeterminate results. Although not usually needed, EM is occasionally used to demonstrate infectious agents or evidence of drug toxicity.

In recent years, EM has been combined with immunohistochemical and in situ hybridization methods, allowing antigen detection and localization at the subcellular level. These combined methods require special fixation and processing protocols. Although immunoelectron microscopy is currently used primarily in research laboratories, the method is now considered to be a promising diagnostic technique in oncologic surgical pathology, in particular, for the identification and localization of targets for gene therapy.

II. **METHODOLOGY.** Tissue for EM must be immediately fixed. A thin slice of tissue should be immersed in a cold fixative such as buffered glutaraldehyde 2% to 4%, or buffered glutaraldehyde plus paraformaldehyde, and then diced into 1-mm cubes using a sharp, clean scalpel blade. Specimens are usually postfixed in osmium tetroxide, dehydrated in ethanol, and then embedded in an epoxy resin or plastic. Semithin (1-μm-thick) sections are cut from the blocks and stained with toluidine blue or methylene blue, and light microscopic examination of the semithin sections is used to select the blocks from which thin sections are cut and placed on grids. The thin sections are usually stained with uranyl acetate and lead citrate; other stains, however, may be selected to enhance electron contrast of specific particles or structures depending on the tissue type and diagnostic question. Tissue processing typically takes a couple of days, but with microwave techniques, grids can be ready within 5 hours postfixation.

For some disease processes, if glutaraldehyde-fixed tissue is not available, EM can be performed on formalin-fixed wet tissue or paraffin-embedded tissue. Wet tissue is preferable to paraffin-embedded tissue, but previous prompt fixation in formalin is essential. Autopsy material, whether fixed in glutaraldehyde or formalin, is often unsatisfactory due to the prolonged postmortem interval prior to fixation.

A focused differential diagnosis based on integration of the clinical history and light microscopic findings is essential for the correct interpretation of ultrastructural findings. Except for the most routine specimens, the pathologist should personally review the semithin sections by light microscopy and select the blocks for further processing. In addition, the pathologist should communicate his differential diagnosis to the electron microscopist and specify the cell type and subcellular structures of interest. Obviously, sampling error is minimized and the most

TABLE 53.1	Examples of Subcellular Features Used for Classification of Disease by EM	
Subcellular feature	**Cell/tissue type**	**Diagnostic setting**
Peroxisomes	Liver	Increased number in alcoholic liver disease, chronic passive congestion, oral contraceptive use, various hepatitides
Siderosomes	Mitochondria	Sideroblastic anemia
Genetic diseases		
Cilia	Epithelial cells	Primary ciliary dyskinesia
Lysosomes	Neurons	Identification of lipoidosis and several types of mucopolysaccharidoses
	Hepatocytes	Identification of several types of mucopolysaccharidoses
Peroxisomes	Liver and kidney	Absence in Zellweger syndrome and neonatal adrenoleukodystrophy
Neoplasms		
Intercellular junctions	Epithelial cells; selected mesenchymal and nonlymphoid tumors	Distinction between lymphoma and carcinoma
Intracellular or intercellular lumina	Glandular epithelium	Identification of adenocarcinomas
Microvillous core rootlets	Glandular epithelium of alimentary tract	Identification of gastrointestinal origin of metastatic carcinomas
Cytoplasmic tonofibrils	Squamous epithelium	Identification of squamous differentiation in epithelial tumors
Premelanosomes and melanosomes	Melanocytic cells	Identification of melanomas
Neurosecretory granules	Neuroendocrine and neuroectodermal cells	Identification of neuroendocrine and neuroectodermal neoplasms
Birbeck granules	Langerhans cells	Identification of Langerhans proliferations such as Langerhans cell histiocytosis
Other		
Viruses and parasites	Solid tissues, fecal specimens, body fluids	Identification of infectious agent
Electron-dense deposits and/or other basement membrane alterations	Glomeruli	Identification and classification of glomerular diseases
	Adjacent to vascular smooth muscle	CADASIL syndrome

CADASIL, cerebral autosomal dominant arteriopathy with subcortical infarcts and leukoencephalopathy.

information is obtained when the pathologist is directly involved in scanning the tissue grids.

III. **KIDNEY.** EM, in conjunction with routine histology and immunofluorescence, is an essential part of the work-up of medical renal biopsies to diagnose glomerular disease. It is also performed on renal allograft biopsies when recurrent or de novo glomerular disease is suspected. The protocol for triaging renal biopsies is presented in detail elsewhere in this manual. Because EM makes it possible to visualize the individual components of the glomerular capillary wall, including endothelium, glomerular basement membrane, and visceral epithelial cells, it is used for identification and localization of discrete electron-dense deposits in glomeruli, either of immunoglobulins or amyloid and amyloid-like proteins. The glomerular basement membrane can also be evaluated for abnormal thickening, thinning, and/or splitting and for the presence of electron lucent, granular, or other deposits. Tubular basement membranes, arterioles, and the interstitium can also be evaluated by EM for pathogenic changes, for example, nonimmune deposits such as amyloid, light chain dense deposits, and cryoglobulins. Chapter 19 describes in detail the ultrastructural findings in specific renal diseases.

IV. **NEOPLASMS.** The role of EM in the diagnosis of neoplasms has decreased since the advent of immunohistochemical and molecular markers. EM, however, is still a useful ancillary method in selected cases and for poorly differentiated tumors for which immunohistochemical and molecular studies are inconclusive. In general, a differential diagnosis is first developed on the basis of light microscopic findings, and EM is then used to look for evidence of cellular differentiation toward the tumors in the differential diagnosis (e-Fig. 53.1).* For example, desmosomes, tonofilaments, melanosomes, and premelanosomes may be sought in the differential diagnosis of carcinoma versus melanoma. EM does not differentiate reactive, benign, neoplastic, and malignant processes.

V. **INHERITED METABOLIC DISEASES.** Initial studies in the work-up of inherited metabolic diseases often include a biopsy of affected organs (such as liver, muscle, or peripheral nerve). For select diseases, EM findings may be pathognomonic. In most cases, however, light microscopy and EM findings are useful in narrowing the differential diagnosis and providing direction for further laboratory studies. Definitive diagnosis typically requires enzyme studies of fibroblast cultures and/or molecular studies.

A. **Prenatal studies.** EM can be performed on amniotic cells and chorionic villous tissue obtained for prenatal diagnosis. Ultrastructural studies on noncultured amniotic cells can yield a rapid diagnosis or differential for certain metabolic diseases, including type 2 glycogen storage disease, lysosomal storage diseases, and peroxisomal disorders.

B. **Liver.** Inherited metabolic diseases often result in hepatocellular dysfunction, either as part of a systemic disorder or as part of disease limited to the liver. In the work-up of hepatitis and cholestatic liver disease in infancy and childhood, a portion of the liver biopsy is routinely placed in glutaraldehyde for possible ultrastructural studies. In cases where obstruction and infection have been ruled out, EM is performed to look for evidence of primary metabolic disease. Certain metabolic diseases have pathognomonic or near-pathognomonic findings, such as type 2 and 4 glycogen storage diseases, alpha-1-antitrypsin disease, and Wilson disease (e-Fig. 53.2). Abnormalities in the number and structure of mitochondria and peroxisomes are characteristic of other specific diseases, as are lysosomal inclusions. Ultrastructural findings are always interpreted in conjunction with light microscopic findings, clinical history, biochemical assays, and other laboratory studies.

C. **Lung.** The protocol for lung biopsy in the work-up of interstitial lung disease in infancy includes placing a portion of the specimen in EM fixative so that tissue is available for ultrastructural analysis if needed, based on the light microscopic findings. Diseases that have characteristic ultrastructural findings (e-Fig. 53.3)

---

*All e-figures are available online via the Solution Site Image Bank.

include pulmonary interstitial glycogenosis and surfactant processing abnormalities (surfactant protein B [SPB] deficiency and adenosine 5′-triphosphate [ATP]-binding cassette transporter A3 [ABCA3] mutations).

D. Heart. Glycogen storage disease type 2 (Pompe disease) can be diagnosed on the basis of ultrastructural findings in cardiac biopsies. Adriamycin toxicity involving the heart results in characteristic cytoplasmic changes that can be seen by light microscopy in semithin sections prepared for EM.

VI. NEUROPATHOLOGY SPECIMENS. EM is critical for the evaluation of peripheral nerve biopsies and muscle biopsies (*Can J Vet Res.* 1990;54:1) and is also useful in the evaluation of selected neuro-oncologic specimens (*J Neuropathol Exp Neurol.* 2002;61:1027). EM examination of skin and conjunctival biopsies is used in the diagnosis of neuronal ceroid lipofuscinosis, infantile neuroaxonal dystrophy, and cerebral autosomal dominant arteriopathy with subcortical infarcts and leukoencephalopathy (CADASIL) (**e-Fig. 53.4**).

VII. PRIMARY CILIARY DYSKINESIA. At present, EM is the method of choice for the diagnosis of primary ciliary dyskinesia (*Acta Otorhinolaryngol Belg.* 2000;54:309 and *Nat Rev Mol Cell Biol.* 2007;8:880) using ciliary biopsies and brushings obtained from the nasal mucosa and lower airway. The most frequent ultrastructural abnormalities are decreased numbers or absence of outer and/or inner dynein arms, some of which are associated with specific genetic abnormalities that have an autosomal recessive inheritance pattern (*Respiration.* 2007;74:252) (**e-Fig. 53.5**). Ultrastructural abnormalities in other ciliary components have also been reported, but not in a consistent manner. Difficulties in interpretation result from significant overlap of EM findings in chronic inflammatory processes and an inherent difficulty in the visualization of inner dynein arms.

VIII. MICROVILLUS INCLUSION DISEASE. Microvillus inclusion disease presents as intractable secretory diarrhea in the neonate. Characteristic light microscopic findings include villous atrophy and loss of the brush border, but EM is required for diagnosis. Pathognomonic ultrastructural findings include absent or decreased numbers of stubby microvilli on the apical cytoplasmic membrane of enterocytes, along with cytoplasmic membrane–bound inclusions with microvillus projections. Morphologic variants have been reported.

SUGGESTED READINGS

D'Agati VD, Jennette JC, Silva FG. *Non-neoplastic Kidney Disease. Atlas of Nontumor Pathology* (*First series, Fascicle 4*). Washington, DC: American Registry of Pathology Press; 2005.

Iancu TC. The ultrastructural spectrum of lysosomal storage diseases. *Ultrastruct Pathol.* 1992;16:231–244.

Sherman PM, Mitchell DJ, Cutz E. Neonatal enteropathies: defining the causes of protracted diarrhea of infancy. *J Pediatr Gastroenterol Nutr.* 2004;38:16–26.

54 Histology and Histochemical Stains

Kevin Selle

I. **RECEIPT, ACCESSIONING, AND GROSS DISSECTION.** Most, if not all, biopsies and large tissue specimens are routed to the pathology laboratory. Under normal circumstances, the specimens are received in 10% neutral buffered formalin (formalin begins the fixation process and prevents autolysis and decomposition). The specimen is first logged into the surgical pathology computer system and given a unique identifying number, referred to as an accession number or case number. Once accessioned, the specimen is taken to the gross dissection room; depending on the practice setting, residents, fellows, pathologist assistants, and/or trained technicians are responsible for gross processing of the specimen under the supervision of an attending pathologist. Gross processing entails describing the specimen by its size, shape, color, and overall general appearance, followed by placing samples of the tissue in processing cassettes (for biopsies, the entire tissue specimen is placed in a cassette; for larger specimens, regions of tissue are sampled according to established protocols). Each cassette is labeled with the accession number as well as a part designator and number; this numbering scheme is designed to allow the location of a particular section of tissue within the context of the whole specimen.

II. **PROCESSING.** The loaded cassettes are stored in 10% neutral buffered formalin until automated tissue processing. The normal processing cycle is ~8 hours long and in general is designed to remove the water from the specimen and replace it with paraffin. Automated, closed-system tissue processors utilize agitation, vacuum, and increased temperature to optimize the process. In general terms, the process is as follows. First, the tissue is subjected to 10% neutral buffered formalin to ensure complete fixation. Complete fixation aids in the dehydration steps and prevents tissue shrinkage and other artifacts caused by excessive or rapid dehydration; chemically, formalin fixation produces methylene cross-links between nucleic acids and/or proteins. Once the tissue is well fixed, it is subjected to several changes of graduated alcohols in a gradient starting at 70% and ending at 100%, a process that removes water from the tissue at a slow controlled rate designed to prevent excessive shrinkage and disruption of the architecture and cellular components. After complete dehydration of the tissue has been accomplished, a clearing agent is used to remove the alcohol and allow tissue infiltration by paraffin; this clearing agent must therefore be miscible in both alcohol and paraffin. Xylene is most often used for this purpose, although commercial xylene substitutes are available. In the next step of processing, heated paraffin infiltrates into the tissue. Paraffin is a solid at room temperature but has a relatively low melting point, and so is a good choice as an infiltration and embedding media. While pure paraffin wax was used in the past, current commercially available paraffins are formulated with various plastic polymers to allow better infiltration and a more rigid crystalline structure, both of which aid subsequent microtomy.

III. **EMBEDDING.** Properly fixed and processed tissue sections are embedded in molds to prepare them for microtomy. The tissue is removed from the cassette and oriented in the base of a mold that is of a size to allow paraffin to surround the tissue section. During embedding, the tissue is oriented with the understanding that the surface placed down in the mold will become the face of the tissue block, and will thus be the surface cut into first by the microtome blade. Attention must be given to tissues requiring specific orientation such as tubular structures requiring complete cross sections (e.g., ureteral margins). Orientation is critical to proper tissue representation on the finished slide and leads to proper pathologic diagnosis, and so the importance of proper embedding cannot be overstated. After proper orientation, the mold and tissue are touched to a cold plate to begin to solidify the paraffin so that the tissue is held in place as the mold is filled with paraffin. The empty cassette is placed on top of the mold so that it becomes the back of the tissue block, conveniently retaining the identification of that tissue sample. Finally, the mold is allowed to cool so that the paraffin block containing the oriented tissue can be easily removed.

IV. **MICROTOMY.** Proper microtomy requires a well-trained and highly skilled micro-tomist, usually a trained histotechnician or histotechnologist. The microtome instrument is designed to hold the paraffin tissue block firmly in place as it is cyclically presented to a stationary microtome blade. Each turn of the microtome handle (each cycle) advances the tissue block a set distance, so microtomes must be kept clean and in good working order. Most tissues are sectioned at 4 to 5 μm thick; however, some tissues are cut thinner at 3 μm (e.g., kidney biopsies and lymph node biopsies), and others thicker at 5 to 6 μm (e.g., bone and brain).

In practice, the paraffin block is first "faced in" to reach a level within the tissue where there is a representative tissue section plane; the block is then cooled on wet ice to further harden the paraffin and aid microtomy. If proper care is taken, individual sections come off of the microtome blade connected to each other, a string of tissue sections called a "ribbon." The tissue ribbon is then floated on a warm water bath at a temperature 6°C to 8°C below the melting point of the paraffin to make the paraffin very pliable. This aids in mounting the sections on a glass microscope slide labeled with the corresponding accession number and part identifier for that particular block (in addition, the convection currents formed in the water bath help gently stretch the tissue sections, removing any wrinkles).

V. **HEMATOXYLIN AND EOSIN (H&E) STAINING.** Slides that have been sectioned are stained to reveal their histologic detail. The primary stain used for pathologic diagnosis is the H&E stain. Hematoxylin is derived from the log wood tree, and has long been in use in the pathology laboratory. By itself it is not a dye, but once it is oxidized to hematein and combined with a metallic mordant, it acquires a strong affinity for nuclear chromatin. Eosin is a dye that at a pH of approximately 4.6 to 5.0 is a strong anion and thus has an affinity for positively charged, cationic, tissue protein groups. At the proper pH, eosin combines at different rates to tissue proteins and thus produces a graduation of distinct shades from light pink to pinkish red.

There are several methods for performing the H&E staining that can be used to achieve slight variations in the end stain to match the preference of the pathologist. The two general variations of H&E staining in common use are progressive and regressive methods. Progressive methods involve staining slides for a designated period of time, and then stopping the reaction as soon as optimal staining has occurred; every tissue stains slightly differently with hematoxylin on the basis of its type, fixation, and prior decalcification, and therefore the length of time in hematoxylin is critical using the progressive method. Regressive methods overstain the tissue sections with hematoxylin, and then differentiate the hematoxylin using acid alcohol; by overstaining and then differentiating the hematoxylin by the regressive method, a darker, crisper stain can be achieved with the assurance that all hematoxylin-positive elements are represented.

The routine regressive staining protocol for the H&E stain is briefly as follows. The tissue sections are dried completely in an oven since water left on or under the tissue sections can allow the sections to fall off of the slide during the staining process. The slides are then deparaffinized by soaking in xylene, the xylene is removed by alcohol, and the slides are rehydrated by 95% alcohol and then water before staining with hematoxylin. Excess hematoxylin is then removed with a water rinse, the slides are differentiated using acid alcohol, rinsed, and the hematoxylin is "blued" by immersion in a weak ammonia water solution. The slides are rinsed again, placed in 80% alcohol, and stained with eosin. Excess eosin is removed by alcohol rinses, and the slide is prepared for mounting with a coverslip and resinous media by removal of the alcohol using xylene rinses.

VI. OTHER FREQUENTLY USED HISTOCHEMICAL STAINS. Tissue stains range from very simple to complex in methodology, and can be used to demonstrate most major tissue elements relevant to pathologic diagnosis. They are based on the chemistry of various dyes and metals, and most were developed prior to the advent of immunohistochemistry. In general, a histochemical stain consists of the main chemical reaction that demonstrates the specific tissue element of interest, followed by chemical reactions that provide staining of the background uninvolved tissue elements, often including nuclear detail. Histochemical stains are usually grouped by the tissue element they stain.

A. Carbohydrates. In humans, carbohydrates exist as various sugars and polymers linked to proteins. Simple sugars cannot be detected by standard histochemical procedures because they are water soluble and thus removed during processing; however, polymers such as glycogen can be detected. Naturally occurring polysaccharides can be classified into four groups on the basis of their histochemical staining differences: neutral polysaccharides (Group I), acid mucopolysaccharides (Group II), glycoproteins (Group III), and glycolipids (Group IV). Amyloid must also be included because, even though it is not a carbohydrate, its histochemical staining properties are similar to those of polysaccharides. The histochemical stains most often used to detect carbohydrates and differentiate various types of carbohydrates are Alcian blue, colloidal iron, mucicarmine, the periodic acid-Schiff (PAS) reaction, Congo red, and Thioflavin T.

   1. Mucicarmine. The mucicarmine method is used to detect tissue mucins and utilizes the tissue dye carmine. When carmine is reacted with aluminum, it forms a compound that has a net positive charge and is attracted to the negative acid groups of epithelial mucins. Metanil Yellow and Weigert's hematoxylin are used as counterstains and produce yellow staining of the background tissue elements and blue-black nuclear staining (e-**Fig. 54.1**).*

   2. Alcian blue, a phthalocyanine basic dye, forms salt bridges with the acid groups in mucopolysaccharides. Staining tissue sections in an Alcian blue solution at pH 1.0 produces staining of only sulfated mucopolysaccharides, while staining at pH 2.5 produces staining of all mucopolysaccharides. These two methods make it possible to differentiate sulfated from carboxylated mucopolysaccharides; further differentiation between mucosubstances of connective tissue origin and that of epithelial origin can be achieved by the addition of hyaluronidase digestion (e-**Fig. 54.2**).

   3. Colloidal iron. The colloidal iron stain is based on the chemical principle that at low pH colloidal ferric ions can be absorbed by both carboxylated and sulfated mucopolysaccharides, as well as other glycoproteins. The absorbed ferric ions are detected by use of the Prussian blue reaction (see below).

   4. Congo red. Congo red reacts with cellulose and amyloid. The dye is a linear molecule that attaches to amyloid in a sheet-like fashion resulting in so-called apple green birefringence when subjected to polarized light. This "apple green" birefringence is considered specific for amyloid in Congo red–stained tissue sections (e-**Fig. 54.3**).

   5. Thioflavin T. Thioflavin T is a fluorescent tissue dye that has an affinity for amyloid. Thioflavin T fluoresces yellow to yellow-green when the tissue

---

*All e-figures are available online via the Solution Site Image Bank.

section is viewed by fluorescent microscopy, but the dye is not as specific for amyloid as Congo red.

6. **PAS.** The PAS reaction is invaluable in histochemistry because of its versatility. In this reaction, the glycol groups of polysaccharides, mucosubstances, and basement membranes are subjected to oxidation by a solution of periodic acid. The oxidation of the glycols results in the formation of dialdehydes. The dialdehydes are then reacted with Schiff's reagent, a colorless solution created by reducing basic fuchsin in the presence of sulfurous acid. When reacted with the previously oxidized tissue, Schiff's reagent is bound to the dialdehyde groups and gains a red color (e-**Fig. 54.4**).

   The differentiation of glycogen from other mucosubstances can be achieved using the PAS stain as follows: Two identical tissue sections are cut. The first section is treated (or digested) with either amylase or diastase to remove any glycogen in the tissue, and then both sections are stained following the PAS procedure. If the substance in question is glycogen, it will be present in the undigested section but not in the digested one (e-**Fig. 54.5**).

B. **Connective tissues.** Connective tissue is made up of three elements in varying amounts, namely cells, a variety of protein fibers, and so-called ground substance. The commonly used connective tissue stains are used to demonstrate cells and various protein fibers, and include the reticulin stain, trichrome stain, Jones' methenamine stain, phosphotungstic acid hematoxylin (PTAH) stain, Verhoeff Van Gieson (VVG) stain, and Oil red O stain. Each of these stains has many different modifications on the basis of the preferences of the lab and pathologists involved. Since ground substance is principally composed of mucopolysaccharides, it can be demonstrated by the carbohydrate stains mentioned previously.

   1. **Reticulin.** The reticulin stain is similar to the PAS stain in that glycols are first reduced to dialdehydes by the use of an acid. The tissue is next sensitized to accept metallic silver ions with an ammoniacal silver solution, and the silver ions that are attached on and around the dialdehyde groups are then reduced to metallic silver. Finally, the tissue sections are toned from brown to black by replacing the metallic silver with metallic gold; sodium thiosulfate is used to remove any remaining unreacted silver in the tissue to prevent darkening of the slide over time. The end result is that reticulin fibers are stained black against a clear background (e-**Fig. 54.6**).

   2. **Jones' methenamine silver (JMS).** The JMS stain uses methenamine to form a complex with silver, which is then reacted with dialdehyde groups formed by the reduction of glycol units in the basement membrane in a process similar to that of the reticulin stain (e-**Fig. 54.7**).

   3. **Trichrome.** There are a number of variations of the trichrome stain; in general, they all use three dyes with affinities for different connective tissue elements. The first step in the trichrome stain involves mordanting the tissue with a heavy metal fixative such as Bouin's Fixative. The tissue is then dyed with a nuclear stain, most often an iron hematoxylin. Next, an acidic dye such as acid fuchsin or Biebrich scarlet is used to stain the cytoplasm of cells, collagen, and muscle; either phosphotungstic acid or phosphomolybdic acid is then used to remove the acid dye from the collagen (since the cytoplasm of cells is less permeable than collagen, with proper timing the dye can be removed from collagen without complete removal from other tissue elements). Finally, collagen is stained using aniline blue. As the name suggests, the method produces tissue sections that are stained in three colors: black cell nuclei; red cell cytoplasm and muscle; and blue collagen and mucus (e-**Fig. 54.8**).

   4. **VVG.** The VVG is another compound stain. The tissue section is first overstained with an iron hematoxylin solution, and then the hematoxylin is differentiated by removal with ferric chloride; since elastic fibers have the greatest affinity for iron hematoxylin, they are the last to decolorize, and so it is

possible to halt the differentiation at the point when the elastic fibers are the only tissue elements still stained. The tissue section is then treated with van Gieson's solution, which contains the dye acid fuchsin; in a very strong acid solution the dye selectively stains only collagen. Picric acid, used to maintain the proper pH during staining, stains the rest of the tissue elements yellow. The VVG stain demonstrates red-stained collagen, black elastic fibers, and a yellow background (e-Fig. 54.9).

5. **PTAH.** The PTAH stain requires mordanting of the tissue section in Zenker's fixative before staining. Because phosphotungstic acid is present in the staining solution in excess over hematoxylin, all of the hematoxylin is bound into a tungsten–hematein lake, which selectively binds to cell nuclei, fibrin, and cross-striations in muscle fibers. The excess unreacted phosphotungstic acid stains the remaining tissue elements red to red-brown.

6. **Pentachrome.** The pentachrome stain is a compound stain that essentially combines the elastic fiber staining of a modified VVG stain with a modified trichrome stain. Alcian blue is first used to stain mucosubstances, and then iron hematoxylin is used to stain elastic fibers. Following the differentiation of the iron hematoxylin, a combined crocein scarlet and acid fuchsin solution is used to stain muscle, cellular cytoplasm, amorphous ground substance, and collagen red. Phosphotungstic acid in solution is then used to decolorize the collagen and amorphous ground substance, which is then subsequently stained yellow using a saturated alcoholic safran solution.

7. **Oil red O.** This stain is used to demonstrate fat in tissue sections, or lipid droplets in cell cytoplasm. The dye Oil red O is highly soluble in lipids, and when used in solution with isopropanol is actually more soluble in fat than in alcohol.

   This stain requires the use of frozen section tissues because the alcohol and xylene steps in standard paraffin processing remove virtually all lipids from the tissue. The staining itself is fairly straightforward: frozen tissue sections are cut, fixed with formaldehyde, and then stained in the Oil red O solution. The sections are next rinsed free from any excess stain and then counterstained using hematoxylin. The stain results in blue cell nuclei and bright red staining of fat droplets.

C. **Microorganisms.** There are many different stains that can be performed to demonstrate microorganisms, specifically bacteria and fungi, in tissue sections. The most commonly used stains are the acid-fast bacteria (AFB), the Fite modification of the AFB, Gram, Grocott methenamine silver (GMS), Warthin–Starry, and PAS.

1. **Gram stain.** The tissue Gram stain is not much different from the standard Gram stain performed in the microbiology lab. In the tissue Gram stain, however, after the use of crystal violet to demonstrate gram-positive bacteria by a blue color, basic fuchsin (a red dye) is used to demonstrate gram-negative organisms as well as cell nuclei. Differentiation of gram-positive and gram-negative bacteria is still a critical step; overdifferentiation is a common staining error. The final step in the Brown–Hopps Gram stain involves treating the tissue with a picric acid solution that renders the background yellow. In addition to identification of bacteria, the stains can be used to demonstrate some cases of actinomyces, *Nocardia* infections, coccidioidomycosis, blastomycosis, cryptococcosis, aspergillosis, rhinosporidiosis, and amebiasis (e-Fig. 54.10).

2. **AFB.** The tissue AFB stain is simply a modification of the standard Ziehl–Neelsen and Kinyoun stains that are based on the fact that carbol-fuchsin, a solution created by reacting basic fuchsin with phenol in alcohol, is soluble in lipids. Tissue sections are first treated with the carbol-fuchsin solution and then differentiated using acid alcohol; bacteria that have waxy,

lipid-containing cell walls resist decolorization with acid alcohol and are said to be "acid fast." A methylene blue counterstain is used to highlight other tissue elements and provide a background to highlight the red microorganisms (e-**Fig. 54.11**). A slight modification of this procedure can be used to specifically stain for *Nocardia* species in tissue sections. Another modification of this stain, known as the Fite AFB stain, is used when *Mycobacterium leprae* is suspected (e-**Fig. 54.12**).

3. **GMS.** This stain utilizes most of the same chemical reactions and principles as the JMS stain. In the GMS stain, however, a stronger oxidizer, chromic acid, is used instead of the weaker periodic acid. Since the cellular walls of fungi are very thick and contain much more carbohydrate than basement membranes and reticulin fibers of the surrounding tissue, the stronger oxidizer allows for creation of dialdehyde groups from the carbohydrates of the fungi cell walls with overoxidation and subsequent destruction in basement membranes and other carbohydrate structures in the tissue section. The GMS stain utilizes a light green counterstain, resulting in fungus cell walls that are various shades of black to taupe in a light green background (e-**Fig. 54.13**).

4. **Warthin–Starry.** The Warthin–Starry method is used primarily for the demonstration of spirochetes, but other bacteria are also stained. The procedure is based on the principle that bacteria in general and spirochetes in particular have the ability to bind silver ions.

 The staining procedure therefore involves impregnation of the spirochetes in the tissue with silver ions, with subsequent reduction of these ions to metallic silver using a developer containing hydroquinone. The stain demonstrates black spirochetes against a yellow to pale brown background. The spiral morphology of this form of bacteria can be fully appreciated by the use of this method (e-**Figs. 54.14** and **54.15**).

5. **PAS.** This stain is often used for the demonstration of fungi in tissue, but is most helpful when a counterstain of light green is applied. The method used in stains for microorganisms is no different than when used for carbohydrates.

D. **Nervous system.** Most of the stains used on tissues from the nervous system are for demonstration of either nerve fibers or myelin sheath. Two commonly used stains for central nervous system tissues are the Bielschowsky and the Luxol fast blue.

1. **Bielschowsky.** The Bielschowsky and all of its modifications are silver stains that follow the principles and general steps of the reticulin stain. In the Bielschowsky technique, the tissue sections are impregnated with a 20% silver nitrate solution and then treated with an ammoniacal silver solution to which formaldehyde has been added. Nerve endings, neurofibrils, neurofibrillary tangles, and neuritic plaques are all stained black.

2. **Luxol fast blue.** Luxol fast blue, a phthalocyanine dye that is soluble in alcohol, is attracted to bases found in the lipoproteins of the myelin sheath. For this stain, tissue sections are treated with Luxol fast blue over an extended period of time (usually overnight) and then differentiated with a lithium carbonate solution. Since Luxol fast blue has a strong affinity for the lipoproteins of the myelin sheath, it remains bound to these lipoproteins even after removal from other tissue elements. The myelin sheath is stained blue against a colorless background.

E. **Pigments and minerals.** Pigments are substances deposited in the interstitium of tissues, or as inclusions or granules in the cytoplasm of cells. Pigments can be derived from minerals such as iron and calcium, or can be endogenous such as melanin. The following staining techniques are used for the demonstration of the most commonly encountered pigments.

1. **Iron.** The Prussian blue reaction is the most common staining technique for the demonstration of iron in tissue sections. Prussian blue stains only weakly

bound iron. Strongly bound iron, such as iron in hemoglobin, will not stain. The principle of this stain is simple: when treated with potassium ferrocyanide in an acidic solution, ferrous ions in tissue react to form an insoluble blue pigment. A nuclear fast red counterstain is usually applied to demonstrate the background tissue morphology (e-**Fig. 54.16**).

2. **Urates.** A modified GMS stain can be used to demonstrate uric acid crystals. No oxidation of the tissue sections is performed; instead, the sections are reacted in the methenamine solution for an extended period at an elevated temperature. Silver ions deposit on the uric acid crystals which in turn reduce the silver ions to metallic silver, so no toning is necessary. A light green counterstain is usually applied, and the resulting stained section demonstrates black uric acid crystals in a green background.

This stain requires the use of alcohol-fixed tissues because uric acid is soluble in water.

3. **Calcium (von Kossa method).** The von Kossa method to stain for calcium is very simple. Tissue sections are incubated in a 5% silver nitrate solution under a very strong light source. The silver ions deposit on the calcium and are reduced to metallic silver by the strong light, in much the same process as occurs in photographic film. The stained section is rinsed free of any unreacted silver ions by a sodium thiosulfate wash, and then counterstained with nuclear fast red to highlight the background tissue morphology (e-**Fig. 54.17**).

4. **Copper (Rhodanine method).** Copper can be demonstrated in tissues using several methods, but the most sensitive method employs rhodanine. Tissue sections are subjected to a saturated solution of 5-(*p*-dimethylaminobenzylidene) rhodanine in aqueous solution. The rhodanine reacts with proteins that have bound copper rather than directly with the copper itself. The excess stain is rinsed from the sections, and the sections are counterstained with Mayer's hematoxylin, an aqueous hematoxylin that will not overstain the rhodanine reaction. This tissue stain demonstrates bound copper as a granular red pigment with pale blue cell nuclei (e-**Fig. 54.18**).

5. **Argyrophil staining.** Argyrophil substances within a cell bind silver ions. They are "silver loving" but do not reduce silver to its visible metallic form. There are several different techniques for the demonstration of argyrophil substances, all of which are chemically similar to the Warthin–Starry technique. A solution of silver nitrate is used to impregnate the argyrophilic substances in the tissue, and a reducing solution containing hydroquinone is then used to reduce the bound silver ions to metallic silver. Nuclear fast red is often used as a counterstain. By this approach, argyrophilic substances are stained black.

6. **Argentaffin staining (Fontana–Masson method).** Argentaffin substances not only bind silver ions like argyrophilic substances, but also reduce bound ionic silver to metallic silver without the use of a developer or other reducing agent. This property of argentaffin substances, which include melanin, underlies the Fontana–Masson stain. An ammoniacal silver solution is used to treat tissue sections, and the argentaffin substances within the tissue not only bind the silver ions in the solution, but also reduce them to metallic silver. Gold chloride is used as in the reticulin stain to tone the metallic silver from brown to black. Nuclear fast red is the counterstain of choice for this stain (e-**Fig. 54.19**).

7. **Bile pigments.** Bile pigment stains are used on liver sections to distinguish bile pigments from lipofuchsin. Fouchet's reaction demonstrates biliverdin, bilirubin, and most other bile pigments. The tissue sections are treated with an aqueous solution of trichloroacetic acid and ferric chloride, which renders an emerald green precipitate, and von Gieson's solution is used as a counterstain

(as in the VVG procedure). Stained tissue sections show bile pigments as emerald green, collagen as red, and other tissue elements as yellow.

F. **Enzymes.** Most enzyme stains require the use of frozen section tissues because formalin fixation and paraffin processing tends to inactivate cellular enzymes. The vast majority of enzyme stains are used in the evaluation of diseases that affect skeletal muscle.

The only enzyme stain performed on routinely processed tissue is the Leder stain, which demonstrates the presence of chloroacetate esterase in cells of myeloid lineage (chloroacetate esterase is an enzyme that can survive the

TABLE 54.1 | Common Histochemical Stains

Stain	Tissue element demonstrated	Result
Alcian blue pH 2.5	All acidic mucopolysaccharides	Blue
Alcian blue pH 1.0	Only sulfated acid mucopolysaccharides	Blue
Colloidal iron	Both carboxylated and sulfated mucopoly-saccharides and all glycoproteins	Blue
Mucicarmine	Epithelial mucins; *Cryptococcus* capsule	Red
PAS	Neutral mucopolysaccharides, glycogen basement membranes, and fungi	Rose-red
Congo red	Amyloid	Apple-green
Thioflavin T	Amyloid	Yellow
Reticulin	Reticulin fibers	Black
Trichrome	Nuclei, collagen, muscle	Black, blue, red
JMS	Basement membranes	Black
PTAH	Fibrin, muscle striations	Deep purple
Pentachrome	Nuclei, collagen, muscle, elastic fibers Fibrin, muscle, mucin	Black, yellow, red Black, red, blue
Oil red O	Fat	Red
VVG	Elastic fibers	Black
AFB	Acid fast bacilli	Red
Fite AFB	*Mycobacterium leprae*	Red
Gram	Differentiating gram-positive from gram-negative bacilli	Gram-positive bacteria: blue Gram-negative bacilli: red
GMS	Fungi	Taupe to black
Warthin–Starry	Spirochetes	Black
Steiner	Bacteria, particularly *Helicobacter pylori*	Black
Dieterle	Spirochetes and *Legionella*	Black
Giemsa	Bacteria, primarily *H. pylori*	Blue
Bielschowsky	Nerve endings, neuron fibrils, tangles and plaques	Black
Luxol fast blue	Myelin	Blue
Iron (Prussian blue)	Iron	Blue
Copper (Rhodanine)	Copper	Red to red-orange
Calcium (von Kossa)	Calcium	Black
Calcium(Alizarin red S)	Calcium	Red
Uric acid (Gomori's)	Urate crystals	Black
(Fontana–Masson)	Argentaffin granules Melanin	Black
Bile pigments (Hall's bile)	Bile pigments	Emerald green
Churukian–Schenk	Argyrophil granules	Black
Leder	Cells of myeloid lineage	Red

rigors of formalin fixation and paraffin processing but not acid decalcification; therefore, application of the stain to bone marrow specimens requires the use of nonacid decalcification). In the Leder method, tissue is treated with a solution of naphthol-chloroacetate and pararosaniline, and reaction with the cellular chloroacetate esterase forms a red precipitate. Hematoxylin is used as the counterstain to demonstrate nuclear detail (e-Fig. 54.20).

G. Staining. Table 54.1 presents tissue stains listed by their most common name, the tissue element that they demonstrate, and the resulting coloration or specific result.

SUGGESTED READINGS

Bancroft JD, Gamble M, eds. *Theory and Practice of Histological Techniques.* 5th ed. Edinburgh, UK: Churchill Livingston; 2002.

Carson FL. *Histotechnology: A Self-Instructional Text.* 2nd ed. Chicago: ASCP Press; 1997.

Sheehan DC, Hrapchak BB, eds. *Theory and Practice of Histotechnology.* 2nd ed. Columbus, OH: Battelle Press; 1980.

55 Immunohistochemistry

Peter A. Humphrey

I. **INTRODUCTION.** Immunohistochemistry is one of the most powerful and widely used ancillary methods in surgical pathology. The technique makes it possible to simultaneously visualize cell type and differentiation markers in standard tissue sections by light microscopy, and has revolutionized diagnostic surgical pathology.

Antigens in tissue sections were first detected using antibodies via immunofluorescence performed on frozen sections (*Proc Soc Exp Biol Med.* 1941;47:200). Although immunofluorescence is still used in the evaluation of medical kidney biopsies (see Chap. 19), currently the most common approach for diagnostic detection of antigens uses formalin-fixed paraffin-embedded (FFPE) tissue sections and immunoperoxidase methodology. This enzymatic labeling technique has evolved from simple direct peroxidase conjugation of the primary antibody, to the use of multistep peroxidase–antiperoxidase (PAP), avidin–biotin (and related) conjugate methods, which, along with amplification techniques such as tyramide and polymer-based labeling, allow for much greater sensitivity in antigen detection.

The laboratory utilization of immunohistochemistry (also known as immunohistology and immunostaining) requires appropriate test selection, specimen acquisition and management, methodology, validation, reporting, and interpretation. This chapter provides a concise overview of these elements. Guidelines pertaining to these elements were published in 2011 by the Clinical and Laboratory Standards Institute (CLSI) (www.clsi.org) in a comprehensive document entitled "Quality Assurance for Design Control and Implementation of Immunohistochemistry Assays; Approved Guideline–Second Edition."

II. **TEST SELECTION (PREANALYTICAL PHASE).** Immunohistochemical stains are usually ordered after examination of hematoxylin and eosin (H&E)-stained sections. Common indications for immunohistochemistry are the diagnosis and characterization of neoplasms, but there are other indications as well, such as detection of infectious organisms and evaluation of prognostic and/or predictive factors.

The use of specific immunostains is driven by the clinical and morphological context of each individual case. Panels of antibodies are often used, and these panels should be devised on the basis of the anticipated value added to the clinical, radiographic, and pathological differential diagnosis. Panels of antibodies should thus be directed toward a specific question. Various approaches have been used to help construct appropriate immunostain panels, including algorithmic approaches and tabular approaches. Web sites with information on the specificity and sensitivity of various immunostains, and on construction of immunostain panels based on differential diagnosis of specific neoplasms, also exist (see below).

III. **SPECIMEN TYPE AND TISSUE MANAGEMENT.** Immunostains can also be performed on cytological specimens, although they are usually performed on standard histological tissue sections. Whereas the use of FFPE tissue sections offers obvious logistical advantages, some antigens require the use of fresh tissue or tissue preserved with ethanol-based fixatives. The discussion here focuses on tissues fixed in 10% neutral buffered formalin, because this is the tissue type most commonly available for analysis in routine clinical practice.

Immediate fixation in neutral pH formalin for 12 to 48 hours at room temperature is desirable. However, it must be noted that formalin induces cross-links that may mask some epitopes, resulting in loss of immunoreactivity. Acid decalcification of bone samples can also cause loss of immunoreactivity. "Unmasking" of some epitopes from FFPE tissue (and tissue treated with acid decalcification) can be accomplished by antigen retrieval techniques. Enzyme digestion was used for this purpose in the past, but now simple heat treatment (heat-induced antigen retrieval) is the most commonly used approach to optimize antigen detection. Unstained tissue sections cut onto charged slides or poly-L-lysine-coated slides (or gelatin- or albumin-coated slides) are typically used for immunohistochemistry, but it is possible to perform immunostains on sections that have already been stained with H&E (*Am J Clin Pathol.* 2005;124:708); because success with such restaining protocols is variable, unstained tissue sections remain the best resource for immunostains. Immunostaining should be performed on freshly cut sections from the paraffin block, because unstained sections exposed to air may lose antigen immunoreactivity over the course of days to weeks.

IV. METHODOLOGY

A. The primary antibody is an immunoglobulin molecule that binds to the target antigen in the tissue sections. The primary antibody may be either a monoclonal antibody derived via the hybridoma technique, or a polyclonal antibody from an antiserum. In general, polyclonal antibodies tend to be more sensitive but less specific than monoclonal antibodies. Unlike monoclonal antibodies, polyclonal antibodies are not uniform reagents of unlimited supply; different batches of antisera may result in polyclonal antibody heterogeneity.

Each antibody, whether polyclonal or monoclonal in origin, needs to be tested for sensitivity and specificity in target antigen detection, and the reaction conditions for its use need to be optimized. Titration experiments must be performed to achieve a working dilution of the primary antibody that yields the greatest contrast between specific staining and nonspecific staining. If prediluted reagents and kits are used, it is recommended that the manufacturer protocol be followed because validation was performed with those reaction conditions.

B. Background staining results from nonspecific antibody binding and from endogenous enzymes that nonspecifically interact with the chromogenic substrate. Nonspecific antibody binding is more likely to occur with polyclonal antibodies. Endogenous enzymes that cause background staining are found in normal cells including erythrocytes, neutrophils, eosinophils, hepatocytes, plasma cells, and neoplastic cells; their activity can often be blocked (e.g., endogenous peroxidase can be blocked by incubation with hydrogen peroxide).

C. Detection systems

1. Direct conjugate-labeled antibody method. In this method, the label—such as peroxidase or fluorescein—is directly chemically linked to the primary antibody. Disadvantages of this approach include a requirement for a large amount of primary antibody for labeling and a lack of signal amplification.

2. Indirect or sandwich method. The primary antibody is unlabeled, and a secondary antibody, reactive against the primary antibody, carries the label.

3. Unlabeled antibody method. Also known as the PAP method. This procedure uses an unlabeled primary antibody, an unlabeled bridge antibody, and a complex of an antiperoxidase antibody and the peroxidase molecule itself. The bridge antibody, directed against both the primary antibody and the antiperoxidase antibody, links the primary antibody–tissue antigen reaction to the signal generated by the peroxidase. This approach has largely been replaced by the more sensitive approaches below.

4. Avidin–biotin or streptavidin–biotin conjugate method. A biotinylated secondary antibody is used to recognize the primary antibody; avidin or streptavidin complexed with biotinylated peroxidase is then bound to the secondary antibody (both avidin and streptavidin have extremely high affinity for biotin). These reactions deliver several peroxidase molecules to the primary antibody binding site and so boost sensitivity. Streptavidin has several advantages over avidin, including decreased background staining.

5. **Tyramine amplification (catalyzed signal amplification [CSA]) methods.** With these methods, there is increased sensitivity due to greater accumulation of biotin at the antigen–primary antibody reaction site as a result of the catalytic activity of peroxidase on biotinylated tyramine.

6. **Polymer-based labels.** This approach uses dextran chain polymers to localize numerous enzyme molecules to the antigen site by linking multiple antibody and enzyme molecules together along the polymer chain (Fig. 55.1). This method avoids problems due to endogenous biotin.

7. **Alkaline phosphatase** can be used instead of peroxidase when the target antigen is in tissues rich in myeloid cells that contain high levels of endogenous peroxidases, such as bone marrow.

8. **Chromogens** are the color-producing reactants in the detection system. Methods using peroxidase, diaminobenzidine (DAB, produces a brown color), and 3-amino-9-ethyl carbazole (AEC, produces a red color) are commonly used.

9. **Counterstaining** is most often accomplished using the nuclear stain hematoxylin. Care must be taken not to overstain the tissue sections, especially when the target antigen is located in the nucleus.

10. **Antibody cocktails** can be used to detect two or more antigens at the same time. Single-color (*Am J Surg Pathol.* 2005;29:579) or two-color (*Am J Clin Pathol.* 2005;123:231) approaches can be used.

11. **Automation.** Automated immunostaining devices are in routine use in many laboratories and can improve standardization, throughput, and reproducibility of immunohistochemical procedures.

12. **Quantitative immunohistochemistry.** In the past, immunohistochemical reactions have been manually scored in a semiquantitative manner by pathologists, via analysis of the staining intensity and estimates of the percentage of cells stained in the area of interest. Such scoring has been particularly important for a few markers, for example, detection of HER2/*neu* immunoreactivity in breast carcinoma to determine the eligibility of breast cancer patients for trastuzumab (Herceptin) therapy (*J Clin Oncol.* 2007;25:118). Because image analysis improves the consistency of quantitative immunohistochemical scoring, it is likely that digital microscopy (see Chap. 63) with image analysis will be increasingly used in this context in the future.

V. **VALIDATION.** Positive and negative controls should be included in every sample run and reviewed along with the test immunohistochemical reaction. A positive tissue or cell control known to express the antigen under investigation should be used, and should be subjected to the same reaction conditions in the same analytical run as the test tissues or cells. Some laboratories place a positive control tissue section on the same slide as the test tissue section; for some immunostains, there may be an internal positive control in the test tissue. A negative control can be generated using a tissue known to lack the antigen of interest or by replacing the primary antibody with an irrelevant nonimmune antibody or antiserum; a search should also be made in the test tissues for negative internal controls.

VI. **REPORTING.** Immunohistochemical stain reports should include specific content elements (Table 55.1).

VII. **INTERPRETATION.** Interpretation of immunostains, including their significance, should be integrated with the interpretation of the clinical, radiographic, gross, and histopathologic findings of the case, as well as the results of any additional

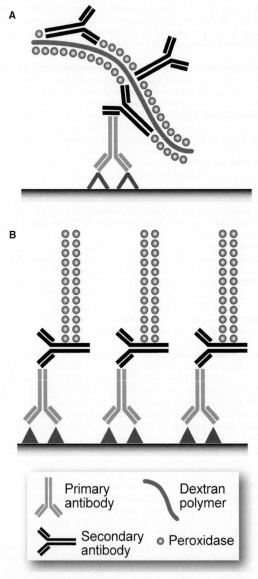

Figure 55.1 Immunohistochemical detection using the polymer method. This technique allows linkage of numerous molecules of enzyme (either peroxidase or alkaline phosphatase) to one (**B**) or more (**A**) molecules of secondary antibody. Delivery of a large number of enzyme molecules to the antigen–primary antibody reaction site yields high sensitivity. (Modified from Taylor CR, Cote RJ, eds. *Immunomicroscopy. A Diagnostic Tool for the Surgical Pathologist*, 3rd ed. Philadelphia: Elsevier, 2006.)

TABLE 55.1	Guidelines for Incorporation of Results of Immunohistochemical Stains in Surgical Pathology Reports

1. All immunostain results should be reported, whether positive, negative, or noncontributory
2. A differential diagnosis justifying immunostain selection should be given
3. The report should also include the following:
   - The nature of the specimen tested: frozen section, paraffin section, cytoprep, etc.
   - The paraffin block number used to obtain sections for immunostaining
   - The antibodies used, including where appropriate, the clone number
   - The result of staining for each antibody, including cellular localization when relevant
4. An interpretation of the findings in the context of the diagnosis, with reference to the associated surgical pathology report if immunohistochemical results are reported separately
5. Exact protocols, antigen retrieval methods, and reaction conditions need not be part of the report but must be available in laboratory manuals and records.

Modified from Taylor CR, Cote RJ, eds. *Immunomicroscopy. A Diagnostic Tool for the Surgical Pathologist,* 3rd ed. Philadelphia, PA: Elsevier; 2006:41, Table 1.8.

ancillary tests (such as molecular genetic tests). After evaluation of positive and negative controls, the test tissue sections should be assessed for presence of the area(s) of interest, localization of immunohistochemical signal, intensity of signal, and number of immunoreactive cells or foci. In some cases, especially for limited and small tissue samples, the area of interest may not be present in the additional sections used for immunohistochemistry. Specific attention should be directed toward background staining, and artifacts such as localization of signal along tissue edges (edge artifact) or in areas of necrosis. Appropriate location of the signal—for example, cytoplasm versus nucleus—should be noted.

Immunostain results can profoundly influence a diagnosis or can be noncontributory; so, the role of immunostains in arriving at the final diagnosis should be specified in the report. For example, a comment in the report should indicate that immunostains were used to establish, confirm, or support a diagnosis, or that they were noncontributory. For predictive markers such as HER2/*neu*, guidelines for reporting should be followed (*J Clin Oncol.* 2007;25:118).

VIII. **SOURCES OF DATA ON ANTIBODIES AND ANTIGENS, INCLUDING CONSTRUCTION OF MARKER PANELS.** The chapters in this book provide information on the most useful immunostains for the evaluation of diseases of each organ system and/or tissue type. Other sources for detailed information on useful marker panels include books (common panels for immunohistochemical studies can be found in Tables 7.3 to 7.41 in Lester SC, ed. *Manual of Surgical Pathology,* 3rd ed. Philadelphia: Elsevier; 2010:73–106) as well as internet sites (one helpful commercial site is PATHIQ Immunoquery at www.immunoquery.com).

SUGGESTED READINGS

Dabbs DJ, ed. *Diagnostic Immunohistochemistry.* Philadelphia: Elsevier; 2010:1–41.
Taylor CR, Cote RJ, eds. *Immunomicroscopy. A Diagnostic Tool for the Surgical Pathologist.* 3rd ed. Philadelphia: Elsevier; 2006.

56 Immunofluorescence

Anne C. Lind, Joseph P. Gaut, and Rosa M. Dávila

I. **INTRODUCTION.** Immunofluorescence studies are used to support fixed tissue diagnoses and to provide additional diagnostic and prognostic information as it relates to autoimmune diseases, vesiculobullous diseases, transplantation, and glomerular disease. Immunofluorescence requires fresh tissue submitted in a preservative nonfixative transport medium such as Michel's medium, or fresh frozen tissue; currently, immunofluorescence is not routinely performed on formalin-fixed paraffin-embedded (FFPE) tissue. For fresh tissue, the transport medium should be held at room temperature; temperature extremes should be avoided. A specialized microscope and a room where the majority of ambient light can be extinguished are required for either direct or indirect immunofluorescence examination.

II. **DIRECT IMMUNOFLUORESCENCE**
   A. **Skin/mucosa.** Cutaneous/mucosal biopsies for immunofluorescence are stained with fluorescein-labeled antibodies to immunoglobulin (IgG, IgA, IgM), complement (C′3), and collagen IV. The patterns of staining that correlate with specific diseases are discussed in more detail with the corresponding diagnoses in the chapter on inflammatory disorders of the skin (Chap. 38). Patterns of staining include basement membrane (e-**Fig. 56.1**)* and intercellular (e-**Fig. 56.2**) positivity.
      1. **Bullous pemphigoid.** A biopsy of perilesional tissue to include the edge of a blister is optimal. Some studies have reported a high false-negative rate for tissue from the lower extremity; if possible, tissue for direct immunofluorescence should be obtained from above the knee. Direct immunofluorescence is positive in approximately 85% to 90% of cases of bullous pemphigoid.
      2. **Pemphigus vulgaris.** A biopsy of perilesional tissue, without including the edge of a blister, is optimal. Direct immunofluorescence is positive in approximately 90% to 95% of cases of pemphigus vulgaris.
      3. **Dermatitis herpetiformis.** A biopsy of perilesional tissue, avoiding excoriated areas, is optimal. Direct immunofluorescence is positive in ~80% of cases of dermatitis herpetiformis.
      4. **Vasculitis.** A biopsy of lesional tissue is required. Sources vary on recommendations regarding age of lesion; however, the majority favors a lesion that has been present for <48 hours.
      5. **Lupus.** A biopsy of an established lesion that has been present for at least 8 weeks, preferably 12, is required to detect immunofluorescence positivity in discoid lupus. In the past, prognostic information regarding disease activity was associated with immunofluorescence positivity in sun-protected, nonlesional skin in systemic lupus.
   B. **Kidney.** It is the current standard of practice to obtain a minimum of two tissue cores to distribute for light microscopy, immunofluorescence, and electron microscopic analysis (*Kidney Int.* 1999;55:713; *Mod Pathol.* 2004;17:1555). Renal biopsies are usually performed under ultrasound guidance, and the tissue cores are evaluated in the ultrasound suite with a dissecting microscope. Since it is important to avoid air drying of the tissue, the biopsy is placed in a petri

---

*All e-figures are available online via the Solution Site Image Bank.

dish with a balanced salt solution while it is examined with the dissecting micro-scope. Because glomerular diseases are a common indication for renal biopsy, the tissue is distributed in such a way that approximately two or more glomeruli are examined by electron microscopy, two or more by immunofluorescence, and 10 or more by light microscopy. The tissue assigned to electron microscopy is placed in glutaraldehyde; tissue for immunofluorescence is frozen, and tissue for light microscopy is placed in formalin. When a biopsy needs to be trans-ported to the laboratory from a remote site, it should be placed in a container with transport medium such as Michel's medium. Although it has been shown that immunofluorescence can be performed on FFPE tissue for the evaluation of renal biopsies (*Kidney Int.* 2006;70:2148), FFPE tissue is not routinely used for immunofluorescence evaluation.

Light microscopic evaluation of the renal biopsy is performed using hema-toxylin and eosin, periodic acid–Schiff (PAS), trichrome, and methenamine silver–stained sections. The PAS and silver stains facilitate examination of the basement membranes, and the trichrome stain highlights areas of interstitial fibrosis. Evaluation with fluorescein isothiocyanate (FITC)–conjugated antibod-ies against IgG, IgM, IgA, C'3, C1q, fibrinogen, albumin, κ, and λ are performed by direct immunofluorescence. Transplant kidney biopsies are also stained for C4d using an indirect immunofluorescence technique. C4d is used to assess for humoral rejection, usually seen as immunopositivity of the peritubular capillar-ies. Addition of a 3% Evans Blue counterstain (Health Scientific, Saint Louis, MO) is helpful to decrease the FITC background and to enhance visualization of the tissue (*Am J Transplant.* 2009;9:812) (e-**Fig. 56.3**).

C. Lung. In the event of suspected humoral rejection after pulmonary transplan-tation, biopsy of pulmonary parenchymal tissue acquired via transbronchial biopsy can be submitted in Michel's medium for evaluation of complement (C4d) by direct immunofluorescence. It is worth noting that evaluation for the presence of C4d can also be accomplished using an immunoperoxidase method on formalin-fixed tissue.

III. INDIRECT IMMUNOFLUORESCENCE. Blood (5 to 10 mL) drawn into a tube without anticoagulant is required for all indirect immunofluorescence studies. The serum is removed and is applied to an epithelial substrate. The substrate varies with the clinical diagnosis, and the clinical diagnosis should guide the decision to pursue the appropriate indirect immunofluorescence study. For indirect immunofluorescence, serial dilutions (1:10 to 1:1280) of serum are inoculated onto the tissue substrate together with fluorescein-labeled anti-IgG.

A. Pemphigus vulgaris. The primary utility for indirect immunofluorescence is for the diagnosis of pemphigus vulgaris and to follow response to therapy. Serial dilutions are performed and the end point of positivity of intercellular IgG is reported (e-**Fig. 56.2**). Commercially prepared slides using guinea pig or mon-key esophagus are used. As in other serologic tests, it is possible to get a pro-zone effect in patients with pemphigus vulgaris, so additional dilutions may be required to avoid a false-negative result.

B. Paraneoplastic pemphigus. The substrate for evaluation of paraneoplastic pem-phigus is murine/rat bladder epithelium. Because this test is not commonly ordered, it is usually only performed at reference laboratories.

C. Bullous and/or cicatricial pemphigoid. Circulating antibodies that produce a linear basement membrane zone positivity (e-**Fig. 56.1**) are detected in fewer than half of the patients with documented pemphigoid, making ancil-lary testing by indirect immunofluorescence minimally useful for this disease process.

D. Dermatitis herpetiformis. Circulating antibodies are not detectable in the serum of patients with dermatitis herpetiformis; therefore, indirect immunofluorescence is not indicated.

E. Reference laboratories. Reference laboratories are a useful resource for indirect immunofluorescence testing for rare diseases. Evaluation of epidermolysis bullosa is performed by Beutner Laboratories (Buffalo, NY). Testing for paraneoplastic pemphigus is performed by Mayo Clinical Laboratories (Rochester, MN). Some research laboratories also perform specialized testing for rare vesiculobullous dermatoses; however, testing in this setting may not be approved for clinical use.

57 Flow Cytometry

Friederike Kreisel

I. **BASIC PRINCIPLE.** Flow cytometry simultaneously measures and analyzes multiple physical and/or chemical characteristics of single particles, usually cells, as they flow in a fluid stream through a beam of light. With this technique, any suspended microparticle, ranging in size from 0.2 to 150 μm, can be analyzed. Peripheral blood or bone marrow aspirate specimens already represent a suspension of single cells but they must be prevented from clotting by using collection tubes containing disodium ethylenediaminetetraacetic acid (EDTA), sodium citrate, or heparin. Enrichment of leukocytes can be achieved by lysis of accompanying red blood cells with ammonium chloride buffer or use of density-gradient separation. Many protocols also exist for producing cell suspensions from solid tissue suspensions.

II. **FLOW CYTOMETER.** The flow cytometer is composed of three main systems (**Fig. 57.1**).

A. **The flow system.** The sample is injected into a stream of sheath fluid within the flow chamber. Through the principle of hydrodynamic focusing, the particles are forced into the center of the stream and transported through a laser beam for analysis, one particle or cell at a time. A higher flow rate is generally used for the immunophenotyping of cells. A lower flow rate is important in applications where greater resolution is needed, such as DNA analysis.

B. **The optical system.** Lasers illuminate the particles in the sample stream and optical mirrors and filters route the different wavelengths of the generated light scatter and fluorescent signals to the appropriate photodetectors.

1. **Light scatter.** Light scattering occurs when a particle or cell deflects laser light. Forward-scattered (FSC) light is in line with the laser light beam and represents a measurement of the cell surface size. Side-scattered (SSC) light is collected perpendicular to the laser light beam and analyzes the granularity or internal complexity of a cell. Leukocytes can be separated into different subpopulations using FSC and SSC. For example, lymphocytes will show both a low forward scatter and a low side scatter due to the small size and lack of cytoplasmic granulation. In contrast, neutrophils are larger in size and show granular cytoplasm as well as a complex nucleus, and therefore will show both a high forward and a side scatter (**e-Fig. 57.1**).*

2. **Fluorescence.** Another way to identify particular subpopulations is to conjugate fluorescent dyes to monoclonal antibodies directed toward antigens on a particular cell subset. The staining procedure can be carried out in a direct or indirect staining process. The direct staining procedure involves a single staining incubation, followed by several washes to remove nonspecifically bound antibodies. The indirect staining procedure involves the incubation of cells with a nonfluorescent monoclonal antibody directed toward the specific antigen. After washing to remove nonspecifically bound antibody, there is a second incubation with a fluorescent antibody directed against the monoclonal antibody. Although more time-consuming, the indirect staining procedure is less expensive.

Argon ion lasers are the most common lasers used in flow cytometry because the 488-nm light emitted can be absorbed by more than one

---

*All e-figures are available online via the Solution Site Image Bank.

Electronic System

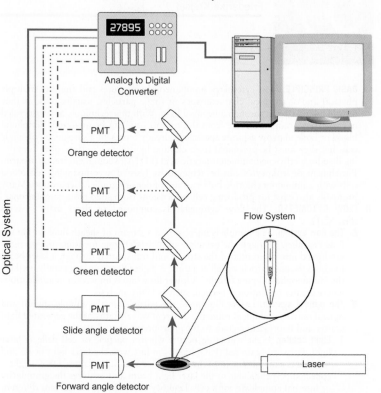

Figure 57.1 The flow cytometer is composed of a flow system, optical system, and electronic system. The flow system transports cells in a stream to the laser beam for analysis. The optical system consists of lasers to illuminate the cells in the sample stream and optical filters to direct the resulting light signals to the appropriate detectors. The electronic system converts light signals into electronic signals that are processed by the computer.

fluorochrome. Examples of fluorochromes that are conjugated to antibodies are fluorescein isothiocyanate (FITC) and phycoerythrin (PE). FITC absorbs light in the range of 460 to 510 nm and then fluoresces in the range of 510 to 560 nm, with a peak at ~525 nm, giving a green fluorescent color. PE absorbs light in the range of 480 to 565 nm and fluoresces at ~570 nm, giving a red fluorescent color. Although both fluorochromes absorb light at ~488 nm, the resulting different peak emission wavelengths can be detected by different detectors, which make it possible to use more than one fluorochrome in one sample to simultaneously collect information on the expression of several markers in a specific cell. Combined with the FSC and SSC data, the staining pattern of each subpopulation will aid in delineating which cells are present in a sample and in what percentage they are present (e-**Fig. 57.2**).

C. **The electronic system.** Photodetectors convert the generated FSC, SSC, and fluorescent light signals into electrical impulses.

1. **Photodetectors.** Generally, two types of photodetectors are used in flow cytometry: photomultiplier tubes (PMTs) and photodiodes. PMTs amplify the electrical current generated from the light signals, and are mostly used to detect weaker signals generated by SSC and fluorescence. Photodiodes are less sensitive to light signals and are used to detect stronger FSC signals. Amplification of a signal detected by a photodetector can be achieved by means of log amplification or linear amplification. Log amplifiers are usually used to separate negative from dim positive signals, and are commonly used for signals from cells stained with fluorochrome-labeled antibodies because these cells often exhibit a great range of fluorescence intensities. Linear amplifiers are generally used to analyze forward and side scatter signals.

2. **Conversion into a digital value.** The intensity of the electronic impulses derived from the photodetectors is assigned a digital value by means of an analog to digital converter (ADC). The role of the ADC is to analyze a continuous distribution of signals falling into a channel of a certain light intensity range and to organize these signals into a data plot.

   An electronic threshold is used to limit the number of events to the population of interest. For example, the threshold can be set on FSC to eliminate events that represent debris smaller than the threshold channel number. After the acquired data are saved, the cell populations can be displayed by several different types of data plots. A single parameter such as FSC or FITC (FL1) can be displayed as a single-parameter histogram, on which the horizontal axis represents the signal intensity (expressed as the parameter's signal value in channel numbers) and the vertical axis represents the number of events per channel (e-**Fig. 57.3**). Two parameters such as FITC (FL1) and PE (FL2) can be displayed simultaneously in a dot plot in which one parameter is displayed on the *x*-axis and the other on the *y*-axis (e-**Fig. 57.4**).

   Finally, a subset of data can be defined through a gate. On the basis of FSC and SSC, an electronic gate can be set on a selected population of interest and analysis restricted to only that subset.

III. **USES**

   A. **Cell markers.** Flow cytometry has become a valuable ancillary method for classifying acute leukemias and lymphomas. Monoclonal antibody technology has provided flow cytometry with a large variety of antibodies specific to nuclear, cytoplasmic, and surface antigens characteristic of particular cell subsets. These are organized as clusters of differentiation (CD) antigens, which help differentiate cells into the different subpopulations of the hematopoietic and lymphoid system. Selected CD markers that are used in the diagnosis of acute leukemias and lymphomas are discussed in Chapters 42 and 43. Flow cytometric scattergrams of an example of precursor B-lymphoblastic leukemia are shown in e-**Figure 57.5**. Typical flow cytometric findings of chronic lymphocytic leukemia (CLL) are shown in e-**Figures 57.6** and **57.7**.

   B. **DNA content.** Besides analyzing surface or cytoplasmic properties of a cell, flow cytometry can also be used to analyze the DNA content of a cell. Several types of fluorescent stains are available that target different DNA bases within the double helix, most of which require the use of laser with significant ultraviolet output to be specific. For example, HOECHST 33342 or 4′,6-diamidino-2-phenylindole (DAPI) are specific for the adenine/thymine base pairs, whereas mithramycin and chromomycin A3 preferentially target guanine/cytosine base pairs. Propidium iodide is not very specific because it stains all double-stranded nucleic acids, but it can be included as a DNA stain in conventional cytometers with low-power argon lasers because it absorbs light at 488 nm.

   DNA staining is generally performed to assess the amount of DNA in the nucleus of a cell or to analyze cell division. Because most normal cells contain the same amount of DNA (diploid or euploid), measurement of DNA content

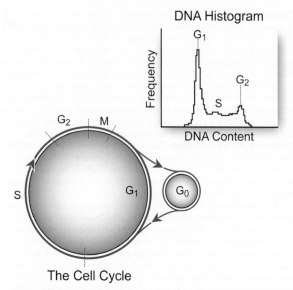

Figure 57.2 Histogram of the DNA distribution in a cycling population of cells that illustrate the distribution of nuclear DNA content present at a particular moment in the population of cells.

of a cell will differentiate normal cells from aneuploid malignant cells. The histograms from malignant tumors will show abnormal peaks corresponding to more (hyperdiploid) or less (hypodiploid) DNA than normal cells.

C. **Cell cycle analysis.** The cell cycle is composed of four phases. Cells in G1 are recovering from division or are preparing for division; cells in S phase are in the process of synthesizing new DNA. Cells in G2 phase have finished DNA synthesis and therefore have double the normal amount of DNA (tetraploid). M phase encompasses division into two similar daughter cells. (Note that cells in G0 phase are not cycling at all). The cell cycle can be plotted as a histogram with the number of cells per channel on the y-axis and the fluorescence intensity of cells stained for DNA content on the x-axis (Fig. 57.2).

SUGGESTED READINGS

Keren DF, McCoy JP, Carey JL, eds. *Flow Cytometry in Clinical Diagnosis.* 3rd ed. Chicago: ASCP Press; 2001:31–65.

Givan AL. *Flow Cytometry, First Principles.* New York: Wiley-Liss; 1992:75–102.

Ormerod MG, ed. *Flow Cytometry.* 3rd ed. Oxford: Oxford University Press; 2005:23–33.

58

Cytogenetics
Shashikant Kulkarni, Hussam Al-Kateb, and Catherine Cottrell

I. **INTRODUCTION.** The three significant milestones in the history of clinical cytogenetics are the preparation of chromosome spreads from peripheral blood cultures (*Exp Cell Res.* 1960;20:613), the development of hypotonic methods to obtain enhanced chromosome spreads (*Cancer Res.* 1960;20:462), and the discovery that fluorescent quinacrine compounds could be used to demonstrate a unique banding pattern for each human chromosome pair (*Hereditas.* 1971;67:89). The remarkable advancement of the field of human cytogenetics is emphasized by the fact that it has been only 50 years since the correct number of human chromosomes was established. The various banding methods in current use not only permit identification of each chromosome, but also make it possible to detect specific alterations associated with hereditary syndromes and neoplasms.

II. **TRADITIONAL CYTOGENETIC ANALYSIS.** While cytogenetic analysis is commonly used in the evaluation of congenital disorders (specifically, to diagnose syndromes associated with abnormalities of chromosomal number or structure, to establish the chromosomal sex in cases of sexual ambiguity, and to screen for karyotypic abnormalities in patients with multiple birth defects) and for prenatal diagnosis, the technique's primary application in surgical pathology is in the evaluation of neoplastic disorders. The utility of the technique in surgical pathology rests on the fact that specific cytogenetic abnormalities have been recognized that are closely, and sometimes uniquely, associated with morphologically and clinically distinct subsets of lymphoma and leukemia, or with soft tissue neoplasms. Cancer cytogenetic studies have greatly aided targeted therapy, prognosis, and risk-based stratification of intensity of therapy.

A. **Advantages.** The power of conventional cytogenetics lies in its ability to provide simultaneous analysis of the entire genome without any foreknowledge of the chromosomal regions involved in the disease process. In most cases, the type and location of an identified chromosomal abnormality is either directly diagnostic or can be used to direct additional testing. Contrary to some predictions, the advent of technologies such as array comparative genomic hybridization (aCGH) has not diminished the importance of traditional cytogenetics; in fact, these novel molecular techniques achieve some of their greatest utility when they are utilized in conjunction with traditional clinical cytogenetics.

B. **Limitations.** The clinical utility of traditional cytogenetic analysis is restricted by two general features of the method. From a technical standpoint, analysis can only be performed on viable tissue specimens that contain proliferating cells (discussed in more detail below). From a sensitivity standpoint, analysis has resolution of only about 3 to 4 Mb at an 850-band level, and only about 7 to 8 Mb at a 400-band level. Traditional cytogenetic analysis is therefore only suited for detection of numerical abnormalities and gross structural rearrangements. The method does not have the sensitivity to detect mutations such as small deletions and amplifications, single base pair substitutions, and so on.

C. **Basic laboratory procedures.** Chromosomes that can be individually distinguished by light microscopy can only be obtained during cell division, and so the fundamental requirement for traditional cytogenetic analysis is a tissue specimen that contains actively proliferating cells, or cells that can be induced to proliferate in vitro. The basic method for production of metaphase chromosomes for cytogenetic analysis is shown in Figure 58.1.

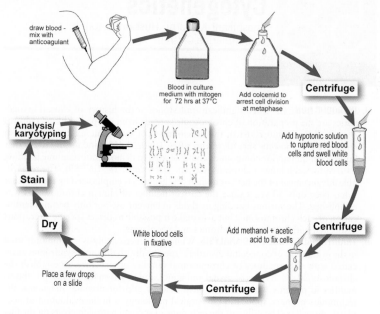

Figure 58.1 Overall scheme for the production of metaphase chromosomes for traditional cytogenetic analysis.

1. **Culture initiation.** Different specimen types have different sample and handling requirements (Table 58.1). Inappropriate handling, as well as delay between specimen collection and culture initiation, can markedly decrease the likelihood that the sample will grow in vitro, so communication and coordination with the cytogenetics laboratory are essential.

   In vitro culture relies on a sterile microenvironment, and so specimens should be collected under sterile conditions. In practice, sterility is most difficult to achieve when sampling solid tissues; in this setting, clean instruments and a clean cutting surface, together with transport of the specimen in medium supplemented with broad-spectrum antibiotics, can be used to minimize contamination.

TABLE 58.1	Specimen Requirements
Tissue type	**Sample collection**
Peripheral blood	Preservative-free sodium heparin; transport refrigerated or at room temperature
Bone marrow aspirate	Preservative-free sodium heparin; the first several milliliters of the aspirate usually contains the greatest proportion of cells and so is the optimal sample for cytogenetic analysis; transport at room temperature
Solid tissue	Collect and transport in sterile culture medium containing broad-spectrum antibiotics; carefully select maximally viable tumor for analysis; transport on ice to minimize autolysis and microbial overgrowth

Bone marrow and solid tissue neoplasms consist of cell types that proliferate spontaneously in culture, although often at a low rate. Lymph nodes are composed of cells that have a low intrinsic proliferative rate but that can be induced to divide much more rapidly by the addition of mitogens. Phytohemagglutinin (PHA) stimulates proliferation of T-lymphocytes. Lipopolysaccharide (LPS), protein A, 12-O-tetradecanoly-phorbol-13-acetate (TPA), Epstein–Barr virus, synthetic oligonucleotides, and pokeweed mitogen induce proliferation of B-lymphocytes, and are also required for successful culture of some leukemias and lymphomas of B-cell origin.

2. **Culture maintenance.** The length of in vitro culture depends on cell type. Since bone marrow cultures contain spontaneously proliferating cells, they can be harvested after only a 24- to 48-hour culture interval, if not directly after specimen collection. Peripheral blood cultures usually require a 72-hour culture interval. The growth rate of solid tissue specimens is difficult to predict; some solid tumors require culture periods of 2 weeks or longer.

3. **Cell harvest.** Colcemid, a synthetic analogue of colchicine (an alkaloid from the bulb of the Mediterranean plant *Colchicum*), prevents separation of sister chromatids and is used to block the proliferating cells in metaphase, thus allowing an accumulation of cells at metaphase stage. A hypotonic solution is then used to swell the cells so that, after fixation, the chromosomes are adequately spread for microscopic analysis.

   Since cells in culture do not proceed through the cell cycle in synchrony, chemical synchronization of cell division is often required to obtain an acceptable mitotic index. A common chemical approach involves addition of excess thymidine, which stalls cells at the S-phase of the cell cycle by decreasing the amount of dCTP available for DNA synthesis. When the excess thymidine is removed (or the effect of excess thymidine is eliminated by the addition of deoxycytidine), normal DNA replication resumes, and the collective release of the cells from S-phase produces a transiently high mitotic index. Alternatively, 5-fluorodeoxyuridine (which inhibits the enzyme thymidylate synthetase) can be used to stall cells at the G1/S boundary; in this method, addition of thymidine releases the block.

4. **Banding.** The different techniques that can be used to stain metaphase chromosomes can be divided into two general categories: methods that produce specific alternating white and dark regions (bands) along the length of each chromosome and methods that stain only a defined region of specific chromosomes (Table 58.2). In general, the dark bands are gene-poor AT-rich regions, whereas the light bands are composed of gene-rich GC-rich regions. The quality of staining depends on several technical factors, including sufficient separation of the chromosomes in the metaphase spread to allow clear visualization. Although there are no internationally accepted standards for banding resolution, ideograms are used as reference points (e-**Fig. 58.1**).* Many countries, including the United States, Canada, UK, France, Japan, and Australia have established standards that specify the minimum requirements for the number and quality of cells that must be processed for chromosome analysis depending on sample type, although many cases require even more detailed analysis.

5. **Microscopic analysis.** The method used to stain the chromosomes dictates whether bright-field microscopy or fluorescence microscopy is used to visualize the chromosomes. Conventional photography has traditionally been used to produce high-resolution prints of the stained chromosomes, but

---

*All e-figures are available online via the Solution Site Image Bank.

TABLE 58.2	Major Chromosome Staining and Banding Techniques
Method	**Staining pattern**
Techniques that produce specific alternating bands along each chromosome	
Giemsa banding (G-banding)	Dark bands are AT rich; light bands are CG rich
Quinacrine banding (Q-banding)	Bright regions are AT rich
Reverse banding (R-banding)	AT-rich regions stain lightly (have dull fluorescence), CG-rich regions staining darkly (have bright fluorescence)
4,6-Diamidino-2-phenylindole (DAPI) staining	DAPI binds AT-rich regions; produces a pattern similar to Q-banding
Techniques that stain selective chromosome regions	
Constitutive heterochromatin banding (C-banding)	Stains heterochromatin (α-satellite DNA) around the centromeres; can also be used to demonstrate some inherited polymorphisms
Telomere banding (T-banding)	Technical variation of R-banding used to stain telomeres
Silver staining for nucleolar organizer regions (NOR staining)	Stains the NORs (which contain rRNA genes) on the satellite stalks of acrocentric chromosomes
Fluorescence in situ hybridization (FISH)	Staining pattern is dependent on the probe

electronic imaging systems have now replaced conventional photographic processes.

6. The final step in cytogenetic analysis is the production of a *karyotype*, which consists of the chromosomal complement of the cell displayed in a standard sequence on the basis of size, centromere location, and banding pattern (e-**Fig.** 58.2).

D. **Assay failure.** Many of the common causes of failure to obtain a cytogenetic result (Table 58.3) can be avoided by careful selection of viable tissue with prompt specimen transport to the cytogenetics laboratory in the appropriate medium. Nonetheless, several causes of assay failure are inherent to in vitro culture and cannot be eliminated by even the most meticulous laboratory technique.

TABLE 58.3	Common Reasons for Failure of Traditional Cytogenetic Analysis

Culture failure

No viable cells present in the sample (necrotic tumor sample or improper specimen handling)
Inappropriate sample (peripheral blood without blasts is submitted instead of bone marrow)
Overgrowth by nonneoplastic cells
Overgrowth by a nonrepresentative clone of tumor cells
Microbial overgrowth
Post culture failure
Technical errors involving cell harvest, slide preparation, or staining
Misdiagnosis (an abnormality is overlooked, or an abnormality is incorrectly interpreted)

Cytogenetic analysis of solid tumors highlights a number of these intrinsic technical limitations. First, since benign solid tumors contain few mitotic cells, cultures are susceptible to overgrowth by nonneoplastic cells. Second, even high-grade malignant solid tumors often grow poorly in vitro, especially if grown without the appropriate culture medium and growth factor supplementation. Third, the number of neoplastic cells in a solid tumor sample can be difficult to determine on the basis of gross examination, and the material submitted to the cytogenetics laboratory may consist primarily of stromal cells and inflammatory cells. Fourth, the viability of the neoplastic cells is often uncertain; even tumor samples that are not grossly necrotic may contain predominantly nonviable tumor cells. Fifth, in vitro culture selects for subclones within the neoplastic population that have a growth advantage, and so the karyotype may not be representative of the entire neoplasm. Sixth, contamination is often unavoidable for samples collected in the frozen section area or gross room, or from specimens arising from anatomic sites normally colonized by bacteria, such as the oral cavity, gastrointestinal tract, and skin.

The overall failure rate of conventional cytogenetic analysis is difficult to quantify for many tissue types, neoplasms, and diseases, and so it is difficult to provide objective statements regarding the utility of analysis in routine surgical pathology. In studies that specifically address this issue for hematolymphoid neoplasms, cytogenetic analysis has a success rate for detecting characteristic chromosomal aberrations that varies from 33% to 100% depending on the specific diagnosis, but is about 70% overall (*Am J Clin Pathol.* 2004;121:826). For solid tumors, the success rate of analysis is less certain; reports describing cytogenetic abnormalities of many solid tumors often do not provide data on failed analyses or negative cases. Objective measures (including sensitivity, specificity, predictive value of a positive or negative result, etc.) of traditional cytogenetic analysis as an ancillary testing methodology in routine clinical practice are therefore often unknown.

III. **METAPHASE FLUORESCENCE IN SITU HYBRIDIZATION (FISH).** Virtually, all metaphase chromosome in situ hybridization analysis is performed using probes that are directly or indirectly labeled with fluorophores. Guidelines for the use of metaphase FISH in clinical laboratory testing have been developed by the American College of Medical Genetics (http://www.acmg.net/StaticContent/SGs/Section_E_2010.pdf), and standardized nomenclature for reporting results has been developed (discussed in more detail below).

Metaphase FISH is essentially a modified Southern blot in which the target DNA consists of chromosomes rather than membrane-bound DNA. Technically, the method has four steps: the probe and metaphase target are denatured by a high temperature and formamide, the probe is hybridized to the chromosomal target, unbound probe is removed by posthybridization washes, and finally, the bound probe is detected by fluorescence microscopy. A fluorochrome-based counterstain is virtually always used to help detect the chromosomes during microscopic examination; the use of 4,6-diamidino-2-phenylindole (DAPI) as a counterstain makes it possible to localize the position of the bound probe to specific chromosomal bands.

A. **Probes.** A variety of fluorophores can be incorporated into metaphase FISH probes either directly or indirectly. The choice of labels is largely governed by practical issues, such as the excitation and emission filters on the microscope that will be used to view the chromosome spreads.

A few probe kits have been cleared by the United States Food and Drug Administration (FDA) for in vitro diagnostic testing, although many probes for metaphase FISH are classified as analyte-specific reagents (ASRs) and so are exempt from FDA approval. Standards and guidelines for clinical use of ASRs have been established by the American College of Medical Genetics, as have recommendations for interpretation of a metaphase FISH result (see http://www.acmg.net/StaticContent/SGs/Section_E_2010.pdf).

1. **Repetitive sequence probes.** The most widely used repetitive sequence probes bind to α-satellite sequences of centromeres; these probes produce strong signals since α-satellite sequences are present in hundreds of thousands of copies. Chromosome-specific centromere-specific probes have been developed for most human chromosomes on the basis of differences in α-satellite sequences, and are particularly useful for demonstrating aneuploidy. These FISH probes can be used on both metaphase and interphase preparations, and simultaneous analysis of more than one locus is possible when a cocktail of differentially labeled probes is used in the same hybridization. Other repetitive sequence probes include probes that recognize β-satellite sequences (located on the short arms of acrocentric chromosomes), and probes that recognize the telomeric repeat sequence TTAGGG.

2. **Unique sequence probes.** Probes of this type are used to detect sequences that are present only once on a given chromosome homologue. They are usually derived from genomic clones, but can also be produced from cDNA or by *polymerase chain reaction* (PCR). Different cloning vectors are used to produce unique sequence probes of different length, including plasmids for probes 1 to 10 kb long, bacteriophage λ for probes up to 25 kb long, bacterial artificial chromosomes (BACs) for probes up to about 300 kb long, and yeast artificial chromosomes (YACs) for probes from 100 kb to 2 Mb long. The availability of mapped BAC libraries, originally developed as part of the Human Genome Project, has greatly simplified the production of probes for any locus under study (http://genome.ucsc.edu/cgi-bin/hgGateway and http://bacpac.chori.org/).

   Unique sequence probes (also known as locus-specific identifier [LSI] probes) are used primarily to detect changes in the copy number of a specific locus, to confirm the presence of rearrangements involving a specific locus, or to detect so-called cryptic rearrangements that cannot be identified by examination of chromosomes stained by routine banding methods (e-**Fig. 58.3**). The advantages and disadvantages of metaphase FISH analysis using unique sequence probes directly parallel those of interphase FISH (as discussed in Chap. 59).

3. **Whole chromosome probes (WCPs).** WCPs, also known as chromosome painting probes or chromosome libraries, consist of thousands of overlapping probes that recognize unique and moderately repetitive sequences along the entire length of individual chromosomes. They are isolated through flow sorting of specific chromosomes, microdissection of specific chromosomes accompanied by PCR amplification, or via production of somatic cell hybrids. WCPs are used to identify rearrangements that are not evident by routine banding methods, to confirm the interpretation of aberrations identified by routine banding methods, or to establish the chromosomal origin of rearrangements that are difficult to evaluate by other approaches. These probes are designed for use with metaphase chromosome preparations because hybridization to the decondensed chromatin in interphase nuclei gives a splotchy, undefined hybridization pattern. WCPs for each human chromosome are commercially available.

IV. **MULTIPLEX METAPHASE FISH.** Multiplex FISH (also known as multicolor FISH) and spectral karyotyping (SKY) are related techniques in which metaphase chromosome spreads are hybridized with a combination of probes labeled with different fluorophores. Since N different fluorophores can produce $(2^N - 1)$ different color combinations, five different fluorophores yield sufficient different color combinations to uniquely label WCPs so that all 24 different human chromosomes can be identified in one hybridization (1-22 autosomes, X and Y chromosomes).

For both multiplex FISH and SKY, a cocktail consisting of labeled probes for each of the 24 chromosomes is hybridized to metaphase chromosome spreads, and the fluorescent emissions are measured by computerized imaging systems. Specialized software is used to determine the combination of fluorophores present along the length of each chromosome, which makes it possible to assemble a karyotype.

A. **Advantages.** Multiplex FISH and SKY are used to detect aneuploidy, detect interchromosomal rearrangements, and identify marker chromosomes (extra-chromsomal material of unknown origin). In many cases, multiplex-FISH or SKY make it possible to establish the chromosomal origin of rearrangements that cannot be defined on the basis of routine cytogenetic analysis. A web-based database has been developed to facilitate identification of chromosomal aberrations detected by multiplex FISH (http://www.ncbi.nlm.nih.gov/sky/), a database that contains links to other websites that can be used to integrate the cytogenetic map with physical and sequence maps.

B. **Disadvantages.** The lower limit of the size of individual DNA chromosomal fragments that can be visualized by either technique is in the range of 1 to 2 Mb, although neither technique provides direct information on the involved chromosomal bands. Similarly, multiplex FISH and SKY will only reveal intrachromosomal deletions and duplications that are large enough to result in a change in size of the affected chromosome; neither technique is designed to detect intrachromosomal rearrangements such as inversions, and neither is informative in regions with repetitive DNA.

C. **Modifications of multiplex FISH and SKY.** Mixtures of so-called partial chromosome paints, each of which hybridizes to only a band or subband of an individual chromosome, can be used to produce a pseudocolor-banded karyotype at a resolution of about 550 bands (*Cytogenet Cell Genet.* 84:156, 1999). The use of partial chromosome paints makes it possible to employ multiplex FISH and SKY methodology to identify translocation breakpoints and to detect interchromosomal rearrangements.

V. **COMPARATIVE GENOMIC HYBRIDIZATION (CGH).** While CGH often has a higher sensitivity than conventional cytogenetic analysis, of even greater significance is the fact that CGH can be performed using DNA extracted from fixed as well as fresh tumor samples. The technique therefore makes it possible to perform a genome-wide scan for structural alterations even on those cases for which conventional cytogenetic analysis is not feasible or is unsuccessful. CGH essentially opens the entire formalin-fixed tissue archive to at least limited cytogenetic analysis.

For a typical CGH test, genomic DNA from a tumor sample is labeled with a red fluorophore, and genomic DNA from a paired normal tissue sample is labeled with a green fluorophore. The green and red probes are mixed and used in a single hybridization.

A. **Metaphase CGH.** This technique is basically a variation of metaphase FISH used to survey the entire genome for chromosomal deletions and amplifications (*Science.* 1992;258:818; *Trends Genet.* 1997;13:405). The labeled probe mixture is used in a hybridization to metaphase chromosomes prepared from normal cells, and the ratio of the green to red fluorescent signals is measured along the length of each chromosome. Areas where the ratio deviates significantly from the expected one-to-one relationship indicate a change in DNA copy number in the tumor; areas where the red to green ratio is significantly > 1 are areas of chromosomal gain (usually amplifications), and areas where the red to green ratio is significantly < 1 are areas of chromosomal loss (deletions). The smallest chromosomal alterations that can be reproducibly detected are about 3 Mb long.

B. **Array CGH (aCGH).** This approach utilizes a microarray consisting of an ordered arrangement of DNA molecules (features) linked to a solid matrix support. The labeled probe mixture is hybridized to the microarray, and the ratio of the green

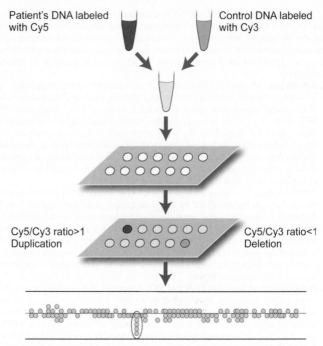

Figure 58.2 Array CGH methodology. **Top:** Method. A patient's DNA is labeled with a red dye and a control genomic DNA preparation is labeled with green dye. The DNA preparations are mixed and cohybridized to an array of BACs or oligonucleotides on a glass slide. The DNA bound to each spot (known as a feature) of the array is quantified using a laser scanner. In the patient's DNA, normal regions will be indicated by a yellow balanced color; regions of duplication will be identified as red, and regions of deletion will be identified as green. **Bottom:** Data presentation. The data from each feature of the array (represented by *circles*) are plotted in relation to the features' positions along the chromosome and a balanced copy number (*horizontal line*). In this illustration, a cluster of adjacent features that falls significantly below a balanced copy number result (*oval*) indicates the presence of a deletion. The resolution of array CGH is in theory limited only by the number of features in the array; commercially available arrays currently provide a resolution of <10 kb. (Adapted from Beaudet et al. *Annu Rev Med.* 2008;59:113.)

to red fluorescent signals is measured for each feature (Fig. 58.2). Because each DNA feature has been mapped to a specific region of the genome, the ratio of the green to red fluorescent signal for each feature provides information on the gain or loss of the corresponding chromosomal region. The resolution of aCGH is in theory limited only by the number of features in the array; commercially available arrays currently provide a resolution of <10 kb. Genomic microarrays (aCGH and related microarray-based methods) are currently clinically applied to detect genomic copy number changes as well as copy neutral changes (uniparental disomy [UPD]/loss of heterozygosity [LOH]).

VI. **MICROARRAY ANALYSIS.** Since the advent of the use of genomic microarrays in the clinical laboratory, the technology has rapidly become the standard of care to evaluate patients for genomic imbalance, especially in diagnostic testing for patients with congenital anomalies, developmental delay, and intellectual disabilities. However, adaptation of genomic microarrays in cancer diagnostics, especially in solid tumors, is not currently widespread.

A. Advantages. Microarray testing offers several advantages over traditional cytogenetic techniques. With a markedly increased resolution over conventional chromosome analysis, genomic imbalances less than 50 to 100 kb are routinely detectable using array-based copy number methodology. Additionally, there is no requirement for cell viability since DNA serves as the starting material. Testing can therefore be performed on a variety of specimen types including peripheral blood lymphocytes, bone marrow, lymph nodes, formalin fixed paraffin embedded tumor tissue, amniocytes, products of conception, and buccal cells, among others.

Although BAC arrays utilizing cloned DNA targets of ~160 kb served as the first generation of aCGH diagnostics in the clinical laboratory, oligonucleotide arrays (utilizing probes that are 25 to 75 bp long) are easier to design and manufacture, and provide markedly increased probe coverage across the genome. Consequently, oligonucleotide arrays have replaced BAC arrays in clinical laboratories, where their use employs two general strategies, namely CGH and single nucleotide polymorphism (SNP) analysis. Although the aim of both techniques is the detection of genomic gain or loss, the method for doing so differs between each assay.

As discussed above, aCGH detects copy number imbalances through the comparison of a normal control sample against a patient sample. In contrast, SNPs are evaluated by comparing signal intensities from the assay substrate (derived from the DNA of the patient sample) to that of an in silico reference model in order to determine relative gains and losses. The ability to probe for SNPs is advantageous for several reasons. First, the approach makes it possible to perform simultaneous copy number quantification and SNP detection. Second, the use of SNP arrays allows for detection of regions with a copy neutral LOH, which may be used to identify genetic alterations in tumor samples,

TABLE 58.4	Comparison Between SNP and Oligo Arrays	
Array attributes	Single nucleotide polymorphism arrays	Oligonucleotide arrays
Number of markers	1,000,000 Markers	<200,000 Markers
DNA input requirement	200–500 ng	1–5 μg
Probe types	SNP and oligo probes	Oligo probes
Limits of resolution	<10–20 kb	As low as 10–20 kb
Threshold for detection of mosaicism	May be as low as 5%	20–30%
Ability to detect copy neutral LOH	Yes	No
Ability to detect uniparental disomy	Yes	No
Ability to detect consanguinity	Yes	No
Method of assessment of copy number imbalance	Probe signal intensities (derived from the patient sample) compared to an in silico reference model	Patient sample directly hybridized against control DNA to detect relative gains and losses
Detection of balanced chromosomal rearrangements	No	No

heterodisomy, the parental chromosome of origin for a de novo deletion or duplication, and more generally, consanguinity and UPD. Ultimately, SNP detection helps maximize the potential for detecting disease-associated abnormalities and also offers mechanistic evidence for the molecular basis of the disease. A comparison of SNP and oligoarrays is shown in Table 58.4.

The technique of allelic discrimination by SNP analysis differs between commercially available platforms, but nonetheless involves hybridization of fragmented single-stranded DNA (derived from the patient sample) to arrays that contain unique nucleotide probe sequences (two million or more). One widespread commercial approach is based on allele-specific hybridization to probes representing the possible alleles; signal intensities that correspond to the level of binding (Fig. 58.3) are measured by scanning technology. The other

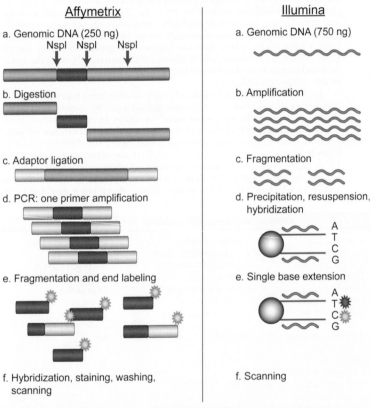

Figure 58.3 SNP array procedures. In the Affymetrix platform (Affymetrix; Santa Clara, CA), genomic DNA is digested with the NspI restriction enzyme and the resulted DNA fragments are ligated to adaptors and subsequently amplified; the amplification products are fragmented, end-labeled, and hybridized to the array. In the Illumina platform (Illumina, Inc., San Diego, CA), the entire genome is amplified and then hybridized to a bead array; allelic discrimination is achieved by a single base extension reaction. In both platforms, the probe intensity is measured and compared with an in silico reference to evaluate DNA copy number. (Adapted from Schoumans and Ruivenkamp. *Methods Mol Biol.* 2010;628:53.)

widespread commercial approach utilizes a single base extension technique with differentially labeled nucleotide terminators to distinguish the SNP alleles; the signal intensity generated from this reaction is used to make a base call at that SNP (Fig. 58.3).

    B. **Limitations.** As with any technology, microarray-based copy number analysis has limitations. While copy number changes are often readily discernable, balanced chromosomal rearrangements cannot be detected with this technology, including balanced translocations, inversions, and insertions. Additionally, regions containing segmental duplications, those with a complex genomic structure, and those containing other repetitive sequences will have limited detection. Low-level mosaicism may not be detectable, and LOH is demonstrable only using SNP-based platforms.

VII. **HUMAN CHROMOSOME NOMENCLATURE.** Technical advancements, together with an even more complete understanding of human chromosomal structure, necessitate periodic revision of nomenclature guidelines. The document in current use is the *International System for Human Cytogenetic Nomenclature* from 2009, abbreviated ISCN 2009, which includes ideograms for all of the chromosomes that serve as useful reference points because of their universal acceptance and availability.

    A. **Chromosome region and band designations.** The centromere divides each chromosome into a short or p arm and a long or q arm. Each chromosome arm ends in a terminus, designated pter and qter for the short and long arms, respectively. A list of the more frequent symbols and abbreviations used to describe human karyotypes is shown in Table 58.5.

TABLE 58.5	Common Symbols and Abbreviations Used in Karyotype Designations
Abbreviation or Symbol	**Description**
add	Additional material of unknown origin
square brackets []	Number of cells in each clone
cen	Centromere
single colon (:)	Break
double colon (: :)	Break and reunion
comma (,)	Separates chromosome number, sex chromosomes and abnormalities
del	Deletion
der	Derivative chromosome
dmin	Double minute(s)
dup	Duplication
i	Isochromosome
idem	Identical abnormalities as in prior clone
inv	Inversion
ins	Insertion
mar	Marker chromosome
minus sign (−)	Loss
multiplication sign (×)	Multiple copies, also designates copy number with ISH
plus sign (+)	Gain
question mark (?)	Uncertainty of chromosome identification or abnormality
r	Ring chromosome
rcp	Reciprocal
slash (/)	Separates cell lines or clones
semicolon (;)	Separates chromosomes and breakpoints in rearrangements involving more than one chromosome
t	Translocation

Chromosome arms are divided into regions on the basis of landmarks, defined as consistent and distinct morphologic areas that aid in the identification of that chromosome. The regions adjacent to the centromere of the short arm and long arm are designated as p1 and q1, respectively, the next distal as p2 and q2, and so on. Chromosome regions are divided into bands, and the bands are divided into subbands, both of which are numbered sequentially. The terminal band on the long arm of chromosome 11 is therefore written as 11q25, indicating chromosome 11, long arm, region 2, band 5, and is referred to as "eleven q two-five."

B. Description of karyotypes. ISCN nomenclature provides rules for karyotype designations. The first item of the designation is the total number of chromosomes followed by abnormalities in the autosomal chromosomes in numerical order. For each chromosome described, numerical changes are listed before structural aberrations. Table 58.6 provides examples of the karyotypic designation of numerical and structural abnormalities detected by traditional cytogenetic analysis. The rules for designating the karyotype of constitutional abnormalities are also used for designating the abnormalities associated with neoplasms, although the biology of tumors requires additional definitions and guidelines.

C. Description of FISH results. ISCN 2009 also includes rules for designating cytogenetic findings derived from various in situ hybridization techniques

TABLE 58.6 Examples of Human Chromosome Nomenclature

Designation	Description
Description of karyotypes	
Constitutional sex chromosome aneuploidies	
45,X	Turner syndrome
47,XXY	Klinefelter syndrome
Autosomal chromosome aneuploidies	
47,XY,+21	Male with trisomy 21 (Down syndrome)
48,XY,+21c,+21[20]	Male with trisomy 21, with gain of an additional chromosome 21 in his tumor cells. The number in brackets designates the number of cells that were analyzed and contain the additional chromosome 21.
Abnormalities in neoplasms	
47,XX,+10,t(11;22)(q24;q12)[5/20]	Female whose tumor cells have two cytogenetic abnormalities: an additional chromosome 10, and a reciprocal translocation between the long arm (q) of chromosome 11 at region 2, band 4, and the long arm (q) of chromosome 22 at region 1, band 2. The first number in brackets designates the number of cells with the observed abnormalities and the last number designates the total number of cells that were analyzed.
Description of metaphase FISH results	
47,XY,+mar.ish der(3)(wcp3+)	In this tumor, traditional cytogenetic analysis shows a marker chromosome; metaphase FISH using a whole chromosome paint for chromosome 3 shows that the marker is derived from chromosome 3

(a summary of the more common symbols and abbreviations is shown in Table 58.5). For metaphase chromosome in situ hybridization, the results of conventional cytogenetic analysis (if performed) are listed first, followed by the results of in situ hybridization analysis. Ideally, loci are designated according to the HUGO Gene Nomenclature Committee (http://www.genenames.org/); when HUGO designations are unavailable, probe names are used.

SUGGESTED READINGS

Beaudet AL, Belmont JW. Array-based DNA diagnostics: let the revolution begin. *Annu Rev Med.* 2008;59:113–129.

Gersen SL, Keagle MB, eds. *The Principles of Clinical Cytogenetics.* 2nd ed. Totowa: Humana Press; 2005.

Kallioniemi OP, Kallioniemi A, Sudar D, et al. Comparative genomic hybridization: a rapid new method for detecting and mapping DNA amplification in tumors. *Semin Cancer Biol.* 1993;4:41–46.

LaFramboise T. Single nucleotide polymorphism arrays: a decade of biological, computational and technological advances. *Nucleic Acids Res.* 2009;37:4181–193.

Miller DT, Adam MP, Aradhya S, et al. Consensus statement: chromosomal microarray is a first-tier clinical diagnostic test for individuals with developmental disabilities or congenital anomalies. *Am J Hum Genet.* 2010;86:749–764.

Rooney DE, ed. *Human Cytogenetics: Constitutional Analysis: A Practical Approach.* 3rd ed. Oxford: Oxford University Press; 2001.

Schoumans J, Ruivenkamp C. Laboratory methods for the detection of chromosomal abnormalities. *Methods Mol Biol.* 2010;628:53–73.

Shaffer LG Slovak ML, Campbell LJ, eds. *ISCN 2009: An International System for Human Cytogenetic Nomenclature.* Basel: S Karger; 2009.

59 Fluorescence in Situ Hybridization

TuDong Nguyen, Arie Perry, and Anjum Hassan

Fluorescence in situ hybridization (FISH) utilizes tagged probes that bind to chromosome-specific DNA sequences of interest, thereby allowing for the identification of both structural and numeric aberrations characteristic of certain hematopoietic and nonhematopoietic malignancies. While FISH can be performed on dividing (metaphase) cells, it has several major advantages over conventional cytogenetics in that it can be applied in many clinical settings (Table 59.1), can be performed on nondividing (interphase) cells, can be performed on air-dried or formalin fixed specimens, can facilitate detection of molecular abnormalities in neoplasms with low proliferation rates such as multiple myeloma, and can facilitate detection of numeric abnormalities. In surgical pathology, the technique is used primarily to detect somatic cancer-associated alterations with known diagnostic, prognostic, or therapeutic implications.

FISH provides insight into intranuclear target DNA localization and copy number. Therefore, using locus-specific probes (with the exception of XY sex chromosome determinations in males), two signals per nucleus are expected and so four common alterations are readily detectable: aneusomy (gain or loss of a chromosome), gene deletion, gene amplification, and translocation (e-**Figs. 59.1** through **59.4**).* Sex chromosome determinations can be useful in patients with sex mismatched bone marrow or organ transplants (e-**Fig. 59.5**), in order to monitor engraftment success or failure.

I. ADVANTAGES AND LIMITATIONS OF FISH

A. **Specimens, retained morphology, and combined FISH/immunohistochemistry.** FISH is applicable to a variety of specimen types, including fresh or frozen tissue, cytologic preparations, and formalin-fixed paraffin-embedded (FFPE) tissue (Table 59.2). The latter provides a particularly rich source of archival material.

In clinical diagnostic testing, morphologic preservation is one of the principal advantages of FISH, particularly for studies on heterogeneous tissue samples in that it eliminates the need for microdissection (e-**Fig. 59.6**). An extension of this morphologic advantage comes from the possibility of combining FISH with immunohistochemistry, wherein separate assessments can be rendered in immunopositive and immunonegative cellular populations.

B. **FISH versus other cytogenetic and molecular techniques.** When compared with metaphase cytogenetics (see Chap. 58), interphase FISH has several clear advantages. One advantage is the lack of a requirement for mitotically active cells via cell culture, which removes potential artifacts due to in vitro growth selection biases such as overgrowth of nonneoplastic stromal elements. On the other hand, FISH is not a genomic screening tool; it provides a targeted approach for alterations that have been initially identified by more global molecular techniques, such as classic cytogenetics, loss of heterozygosity (LOH) screening, comparative genomic hybridization (CGH), array CGH (aCGH), array single nucleotide polymorphism (SNP) analysis, and gene expression profiling.

In terms of resolution, FISH is more sensitive than conventional karyotypic analysis and CGH (both of which are limited to alterations of several Mb in size)

---

*All e-figures are available online via the Solution Site Image Bank.

TABLE 59.1	Examples of Diagnostic Tests by FISH

Prenatal testing
  Trisomy 13, 18, 21
  XY aneusomies

Microdeletion syndromes
  Cri-du-Chat (5p)
  Prader-Wili/Angelman (15q)
  Di George syndrome (22q)

Transplant pathology
  XY FISH on sex mismatched organ transplant
  Disease relapse using known genetic alterations in primary tumor

Oncology (diagnostic, prognostic, and/or predictive markers)
  Chromosomal aneusomies
  Gene/locus deletions
  Gene amplifications
  Translocations

but less sensitive than PCR-based assays for detecting small alterations (which can be designed to detect even single base pair mutations). Since FISH probes are typically at least 20 kb long, and most average 100 to 200 Kb long, alterations need to be fairly large for reliable detection by FISH, and consequently FISH cannot detect small intragenic mutations, deletions, or insertions.

Minimal residual disease or early recurrences are better detected by PCR of blood or fresh tissue specimens rather than FISH. Minimal residual disease detection usually involves detection of as few as one abnormal per million normal cells, a level of sensitivity that cannot be attained by FISH techniques to date. In contrast, FISH is very sensitive for identifying gene deletions or amplifications from samples of mixed cellularity, such as neoplasms with clonal heterogeneity or contaminating nonneoplastic elements (*J Neuropathol Exp Neurol.* 1997;56:999); in this setting, FISH can typically detect gains, translocations, or amplifications in as few as 5% and deletions in 15% to 30% of the cells within a sample.

C. **Tissue microarray–FISH.** This technology takes advantage of multi-specimen paraffin blocks (tissue microarrays, or TMAs) constructed from hundreds of 0.6 to 2.0 mm neoplastic, nonneoplastic, and control tissue cores of interest. TMA–FISH markedly increases efficiency by reducing data acquisition time, as well as probe, reagent, and storage space requirements. TMA studies have shown excellent morphologic, antigenic, and genomic concordance compared

TABLE 59.2	Examples of Specimen Types Applicable to FISH

Fresh/Frozen tissue

Cytology specimens
  Body Fluids (e.g., urine)
  Intraoperative smears
  Cell culture preparations

Formalin fixed paraffin embedded tissue
  Thin sections (4–6 μm)
  Disaggregated nuclei
  Archived unstained sections
  Previously stained sections (e.g., negative immunohistochemistry controls)

to the traditional whole slide approaches (*Adv Anat Pathol.* 2001;8:14), and although complications due to tumor heterogeneity can be problematic, adequate sampling can be optimized by incorporating multiple cores from each specimen. TMA–FISH is an excellent method for new probe validation, proficiency testing, interlaboratory comparisons, and quality assurance/quality control (*J Histochem Cytochem.* 2004;52:501).

D. **Disadvantages and pitfalls of FISH.** Although recent technical advances have greatly enhanced the clinical applicability of FISH, a number of limitations remain. Signal fading is one of the main disadvantages. Clinical labs typically circumvent this pitfall by capturing digital images as a permanent record of each case; a permanent record is not otherwise possible unless chromogenic detection (CISH) is used. Unfortunately, multicolor CISH is not as simple as multicolor FISH; currently available chromogens lack the spectral versatility, sensitivity, and spatial resolution attainable with fluorochromes. Some commercial CISH applications bypass this problem by providing the test and reference probes separately, so that in place of one dual-color FISH assay, two single-color CISH experiments are performed. Recently developed photostable quantum dots offer a potential alternative for permanent fluorescent signals (*J Histochem Cytochem.* 2003;51:981). Other limitations include a variety of artifacts, particularly common in paraffin sections, that make correct interpretation of FISH results dependent on significant experience.

1. **Truncation artifact.** This artifact is due to the underestimation of copy number because of an incomplete DNA complement within transected nuclei, and it is therefore important to assess controls cut at the same thickness.

2. **Aneuploidy and polyploidy.** Artifacts due to aneuploidy and polyploidy can result in confusing signal counts and are a particularly common finding in malignant and even some benign neoplasms. Although the simplest approach is to interpret absolute losses (<2 copies) and gains (>2 copies), "relative" losses and gains can also be delineated on the basis of a reference ploidy, obtained either by flow cytometry or the assessment of multiple chromosomes by FISH. For example, cells with four chromosomes, nine centromeres, and two copies of the *p16* gene region on 9p21 would be interpreted as having polysomy 9 and a hemizygous p16 deletion (e-**Fig. 59.7A**); a similar tumor with no p16 signals would be interpreted as polysomy 9 with homozygous p16 deletion (e-**Fig. 59.7B**).

3. **Autofluorescence.** This is a particularly common problem in FFPE tissue sections. Although autofluorescent tissue fragments are usually larger and more irregular than true signals, some fragments may have just the right size to mimic true nuclear signals. The use of multiple filters is helpful, since autofluorescence will often appear at several wavelengths of light, whereas true signals only fluoresce at one wavelength.

4. **Partial hybridization failure.** This issue is most problematic when combining a highly robust probe (e.g., centromere) with a comparatively weak probe (e.g., small locus specific probe). This artifact can be minimized by counting only in regions where the majority of cells have discernible signals. Signals from both probes should be seen in normal cells (e.g., endothelial cells) within the region for the counts to be considered reliable.

E. **Additional technical considerations.** Many different FISH protocols are available; they vary depending on individual preferences and specimen type. Simple protocols are generally better, requiring less "hands on" time, fewer opportunities for error, and fewer troubleshooting requirements. Automated instruments are now available to minimize hands on time, though they are expensive. In general, the basic steps of the protocols are similar to those of immunohistochemistry and include deparaffinization, pretreatment/target retrieval, probe and target

DNA denaturation, hybridization (a few hours to overnight), posthybridization washes, detection, and microscopic interpretation/imaging. FISH is therefore typically a 2-day assay, although same day assays are possible if the probes are particularly robust (e.g., centromere probes).

Similar to immunohistochemistry, microwave or heat-induced target retrieval often enhances hybridization more effectively than chemical forms of pretreatment (*Anal Cell Pathol.* 1994;6:319). Nonetheless, optimal pretreatment and digestion varies from specimen to specimen and depends on a number of variables, including method of fixation and processing. Some hybridization buffers are also significantly more efficient and may lower probe concentration requirements considerably, which can be particularly beneficial with expensive commercial probes. Lastly, a variety of amplification steps are available for enhancing weak signals, although such steps are rarely necessary with robust commercial probes. One exciting advancement made possible by high-level signal amplification techniques is the potential use of smaller probes, down to the level of 1 kb or less (*Biotechniques.* 1999;27:608).

II. FISH PROBES AND PROBE DEVELOPMENT

A. **Centromere enumerating probes (CEPs)** were among the first types of probes developed and remain ideal for detecting whole chromosome gains and losses, such as monosomy, trisomy, and other polysomies. CEPs target highly repetitive 171 bp sequences of α-satellite DNA, and so are associated with excellent hybridization efficiencies and typically produce large, bright signals. Unfortunately, sequence similarities in some pericentromeric regions result in cross-hybridization artifacts with the potential for overestimating signal counts. Another artifact is caused by the interesting phenomenon observed in nonneoplastic brain specimens in which certain chromosomes in interphase nuclei are packaged such that paired centromeres are in close proximity, a process known as somatic pairing (*Hum Genet.* 1989;83:231; *Cytogenet Cell Genet.* 1991;56:214); because of the close proximity, FISH yields an unexpected fraction of cells harboring a single large signal rather than two smaller ones, potentially leading to overinterpretation of monosomy. Despite these technical limitations, CEPs remain extremely useful for detecting aneusomies and are still among the best FISH probes available. The presence of repetitive DNA sequences in subtelomeric regions has led to the development of commercially available probes for each chromosomal arm as well.

B. **A whole chromosome paint (WCP)** probe consists of a cocktail of DNA fragments that targets all the nonrepetitive DNA sequences of an entire chromosome. Because a WCP covers such a large region, it produces a diffuse signal in interphase nuclei (although some of the smaller acrocentric chromosomes yield sufficiently discrete signals for enumeration, even in interphase nuclei). For this reason, WCPs are not often used in interphase FISH, but instead are primarily utilized in advanced cytogenetic applications (see Chap. 58).

C. Currently, the most versatile FISH probes are **locus-specific identifier probes** (also known as LSI, or gene-specific, probes). These probes target distinct chromosomal regions of interest and utilize single copy rather than repetitive DNA sequences. In order to yield signals of sufficient size in interphase FFPE nuclei, the probe typically needs to be at least 20 kb long; the largest LSI probes are >1 Mb long, although most fall into the 100 to 300 kb range. The assortment of LSI probes available commercially has expanded greatly over the last few years. Additionally, cloning vectors, such as cosmids, bacterial artificial chromosomes (BACs), P1 artificial chromosomes (PACs), and yeast artificial chromosomes (YACs) are excellent sources for developing analyte specific (i.e., homemade) FISH probes. In the past, development of LSIs required a rather lengthy and tedious process of screening vector libraries, but the BAC libraries generated as part of the human genome project have made it possible to rapidly identify vectors that contain sequences of interest, gene names, or physical maps of individual chromosomes (http://www.genome.ucsc.edu). Similarly, mapped BAC clones spread throughout the human genome at 1-Mb intervals have also become available (http://mp.invitrogen.com). However, regardless of how a probe is obtained, it is important to verify its identity, either by screening for the DNA sequence of interest by PCR or by performing metaphase FISH to determine that the probe localizes to the appropriate cytogenetic band (e-**Fig. 59.8**).

III. **CLINICAL APPLICATIONS.** FISH testing is clinically useful when a cytogenetic alteration (deletion, gain, amplification, and translocation) is sensitive and specific for a single tumor type, either as a diagnostic biomarker (as in many hematopoietic malignancies) or as a prognostic biomarker helping to predict which tumors will be aggressive or indolent (*HER-2/neu* amplification testing in breast cancer). Some translocation and deletions detected by FISH are also helpful in predicting response to a specific therapy; examples include detection of t(11;18) in a subset of mucosa-associated lymphoid tissue (MALT) lymphomas (which tend to be resistant to conventional therapy), detection of *FIP1L1-PDGFRA* fusion formed as a cryptic deletion at 4q12 in chronic eosinophilic leukemia which is sensitive to imatinib therapy, and detection of del(13q) and/or t(4;14) in a subset of cases of multiple myeloma (which tend to have a worse prognosis). The most common clinical applications of FISH testing currently include *HER-2/neu* amplification testing for breast cancer, UroVysion testing in urine cytology specimens, 1p/19q deletion testing in gliomas, and testing for signature translocations associated with specific hematologic, soft tissue, and/or pediatric malignancies. Clinically relevant examples for each alteration type detectable by FISH are summarized in Table 59.3.

A. **Aneusomies and deletions.** Aneusomies represent gains and losses of whole chromosomes. Deletions are losses of distinct chromosomal regions, varying in size from loss of a specific gene or portion of a gene to an entire chromosomal arm. Aneusomies and deletions are amongst the most common alterations detected in neoplasms by FISH (Table 59.3), although it is sometimes difficult to distinguish specific tumor-associated polysomies and monosomies from nonspecific gains and losses that are secondary changes due to the genomic instability that is characteristic of many malignancies. The use of reference probes helps to distinguish such chromosomal gains or high-level polysomies from true gene amplification (e-**Fig. 59.3**).

One of the most common FISH applications is testing for deletions of 1p and 19q in diffuse gliomas. The presence of 1p and 19q codeletion (typically, loss of the entire arm of each) has diagnostic, prognostic, and predictive value in that this genetic signature (e-**Fig. 59.2A** and **B**) is associated predominantly with pure oligodendrogliomas with enhanced therapeutic responsiveness and overall survival time (*J Neuropathol Exp Neurol.* 2003;62:111). There is no current consensus for the optimal way to enumerate signals for chromosomal losses and gains, though in clinical cases a common approach is to use two individuals who count signals in 100 cells each; when the counts are concordant, they are simply added for a total enumeration of 200 cells, but when there is a discrepancy or the counts are borderline for an alteration, then either the same individuals count additional cells or a third enumerator is utilized. Despite the clinical utility of 1p and 19q testing, the precise gene targets on these chromosomes remain unclear.

In other tumor types, a specific tumor suppressor is known to be targeted by various chromosomal deletions (Table 59.3). Notable examples include the *INI1/hSNF5* gene on 22q11.2 in malignant rhabdoid tumors and atypical teratoid/rhabdoid tumors, the *NF2* gene at 22q12 in meningiomas, the *RB1* gene at 13q14, the *TP53* gene at 17p13.1 in multiple myeloma, and the *NF1* gene at 17q11.2 in malignant peripheral nerve sheath tumors.

TABLE 59.3	Cancer-Associated Alterations Commonly Detected by FISH		
Type	**Tumor type (references)**	**Alterations/probes**	**Association**
Aneusomies/deletions	Oligodendroglioma	1p− with 19q−	Diagnostic, prognostic, predictive
	Urothelial Carcinoma	+3, 7, or 17; 9p−	Diagnostic
	Lung Carcinoma	+7p, 8q, 5p, or 6	Diagnostic
	CLL	13q−, 11q−, 17q−	Diagnostic, prognostic
	GBM	+7, −10	Diagnostic
	Prostatic carcinoma	8p−, 8q+	Prognostic
	Medulloblastoma	17p−, 17q+; (i17q)	Diagnostic
	Leukemias/MDS	+8, +12; −5, −7	Diagnostic, prognostic
	MRT, AT/RT	*INI1/hSNF5* (22q−)	Diagnostic
	Meningioma	*NF2* (22q−)	Diagnostic
	Multiple myeloma	*RB1* (13q−), *TP53* (17p−)	Prognostic
	MPNST	*NF1* (17q−)	Diagnostic
Amplifications	Breast carcinoma	*HER-2/neu*	Prognostic, predictive
	Neuroblastoma	*N-myc*	Diagnostic, prognostic
	GBM	*EGFR*	Diagnostic
	Medulloblastoma	*MYCN, c-myc*	Diagnostic, prognostic
	Gastric carcinoma	*HER-2/neu*	Prognostic, predictive
Translocations	EWS/PNET	*EWS-FLI1*, EWS-BA	Diagnostic
	Synovial sarcoma	*SYT-SSX*, SYT-BA	Diagnostic
	Alveolar RMS	*PAX3-FKHR*, FKHR-BA	Diagnostic
	DSRCT	*EWS-WT1*, EWS-BA	Diagnostic
	M/RC liposarcoma	CHOP-BA	Diagnostic
	Clear cell sarcoma	*EWS-ATF1*, EWS-BA	Diagnostic
	IMT	*ALK-TPM3, ALK-TPM4, ALK-CARS*, ALK-BA	Diagnostic, prognostic
	Burkitt lymphoma	*MYC-IGH*, MYC-BA	Diagnostic
	MALT lymphoma	*API2-MALT1, IGH-MALT1*, MALT1-BA	Diagnostic
	Follicular lymphoma	*IGH-BCL2*	Diagnostic
	ALCL	ALK-BA	Diagnostic, prognostic, predictive
	Mantle cell lymphoma	*IGH-CCND1*	Diagnostic
	Multiple myeloma	*IGH-CCND1, IGH-FGFR3*, IGH-BA	Prognostic
	CML	*BCR-ABL*	Diagnostic, MRD, predictive
	AML	*AML1-ETO*, CBFB-BA, *PML-RARA*, RARA-BA, MLL-BA, *BCR-ABL*	Diagnostic, prognostic, predictive
	ALL	*TEL-AML1, BCR-ABL*, MLL-BA	Diagnostic, prognostic, predictive
	BCL, unclassifiable with features intermediate between DLBCL and Burkitt lymphoma	*IGH-BCL2; MYC-IGH*, MYC-BA	Diagnostic; prognostic
	Myeloid and lymphoid neoplasms with eosinophilia	*PDGFRA, PGDFRB, FGFR1; FIP1L1-PDGFRA*	Diagnostic; prognostic; predictive

CLL, chronic lymphocytic leukemia; GBM, glioblastoma; MDS, myelodysplastic syndrome; MRT, malignant rhabdoid tumor; AT/RT, atypical teratoid/rhabdoid tumor; MPNST, malignant peripheral nerve sheath tumor; EWS, Ewing Sarcoma; PNET, primitive neuroectodermal tumor; RMS, rhabdomyosarcoma; DSRCT, desmoplastic small round cell tumor; M/RC, myxoid/round cell; IMT, inflammatory myofibroblastic tumor; ALCL, anaplastic large cell lymphoma; CML, chronic myelogenous leukemia; AML, acute myelogenous leukemia; ALL, acute lymphoblastic leukemia; BCL, B cell lymphoma; DLBCL, diffuse large B cell lymphoma; BA, break apart probe set; MRD, minimal residual disease assessment.

In terms of tumor-specific chromosomal gains and losses, Vysis (http://www. vysis.com) markets a number of multicolor probe cocktails for clinical and translational studies, each with different recommendations for minimum number of nuclei counted and cutoffs for alterations. For example, the UroVysion (e-**Fig. 59.9**) and LAVysion probe sets have been shown to increase diagnostic sensitivities in body fluid cytology specimens for urothelial carcinoma (*J Urol.* 2003;169:2101) and lung carcinoma (*Am J Clin Pathol.* 2005;123:516), respectively. Similarly, the CLL and ProVysion FISH assays have been shown to identify prognostically relevant subsets of chronic lymphocytic leukemia (*Cancer Gen Cytogenet.* 2005;158:88) and prostatic adenocarcinoma (*Genes Chrom Cancer.* 2002;34:363) patients, respectively. Likewise, the detection of specific aneusomies and deletions by FISH has been clinically useful in identifying diagnostically challenging cases of glioblastoma (particularly the small cell variant), medulloblastoma (especially the anaplastic/large cell variant), and prognostically relevant subsets of leukemia/myelodysplastic syndrome.

B. **Gene amplifications.** High level gene amplifications typically occur in one of two patterns. If the amplified gene is present on small extra-chromosomal segments known as double minutes , FISH will show numerous individual signals (e-**Fig. 59.3A and C**). If the gene amplification consists of contiguously arranged gene copies within a single chromosomal region manifested as a homogenously stained region on chromosomal banding, FISH will show regions of hybridization so close together that they coalesce into abnormally large linear or globular signals (e-**Fig. 59.3B**); rough estimates are made regarding how many signals are contained within the coalescent signals on the basis of their overall size. In both settings, CEP probes are often used as references for chromosome number in order to distinguish polysomies (i.e., gains of the entire chromosome; e-**Fig. 59.3D**) from true gene amplification.

Of the current clinical applications of FISH in surgical pathology, the assessment of *HER-2/neu* amplification status in breast cancer is one of the most common applications (*Cancer.* 2003;98:2547). Although there is agreement that *HER-2/neu* assessment provides clinically useful information, the optimal diagnostic approach is still much debated. Recently, the American Society of Clinical Oncology and College of American Pathologist recommended guidelines for testing of *HER-2/neu* amplification in breast cancer (*Arch Pathol Lab Med.* 2007;131:18). *HER-2/neu* gene amplification is present in 20% to 35% of breast carcinomas (e-**Figs. 59.3C and 59.10**) and provides both prognostic and predictive information with the following associations for positive tumors: reduced patient survival, especially in lymph node positive cases; increased responsiveness to Adriamycin-based therapeutic regimens; increased responsiveness to Herceptin (trastuzumab), which specifically targets the overexpressed surface protein; and decreased responsiveness to radiation therapy, cyclophosphamide, methotrexate, 5-FU, hormonal therapy, and Taxol. Additionally, due to the significant risk of cardiotoxicity with combined Adriamycin and Herceptin therapy, testing is justified to identify patients with a low probability of response. New methods using chromogenic in situ hybridization methods for *HER-2/neu* gene status assessment in breast cancer are also being explored (*Am J Clin Pathol.* 2009;131:490). Since trastuzumab-based therapies have also been shown to be beneficial in *HER-2/neu*, positive patients with advanced gastric cancers, guidelines for testing for *HER-2/neu* amplification are also being developed for gastric carcinomas (*Virchows Arch.* 2010;457:299; *Adv Anat Pathol.* 2011;18:53).

In pediatric pathology, testing of neuroblastomas for *MYCN* amplification has similarly become standard of care, with positive cases typically showing an aggressive biology (*J Pathol* 2002;198:83). A similar pattern is encountered in a subset of the CNS counterpart medulloblastoma; *MYCN* and *CMYC* amplifications are particularly common in the highly aggressive anaplastic/large cell variant.

EGFR amplification, often in combination with monosomy 10 or chromosome 10q deletion, helps to distinguish the clinically aggressive and therapeutically refractory small cell variant of glioblastoma from the more biologically favorable and chemotherapeutically responsive look-alike anaplastic oligodendroglioma.

C. Translocations. The list of known tumor-associated chromosomal translocations is already extensive and continues to grow. Translocation analysis by FISH is particularly useful as an ancillary diagnostic aid in primitive-appearing hematopoietic and soft tissue malignancies (Table 59.3). Chromosomal translocation analyses are unique among FISH assays in that interpretation relies on the spatial relationships of the signals rather than their number. For optimal probe design, detailed knowledge of the breakpoints is needed, though reliable probes are commercially available for most of the common translocations.

  1. Fusion FISH. Also known as FISH-F, this strategy employs two locus specific probes with different fluors (color tags), targeting two different partners in a translocation (e.g., *BCR* on 22q and *ABL* on 9q). Separated or "split" signals (e.g., two green, two red signals; e-**Fig. 59.4A**) are therefore present in translocation-negative cells, but "fusion" yellow or red–green signals are present in translocation-positive cells due to the juxtaposition of the target loci by the translocation (e.g., one fusion, one green, one red signal; e-**Fig. 59.4B**). FISH-F results must be scored carefully to avoid overinterpreting small cellular populations where green and red signals overlap purely by chance. On the basis of signal proximities in normal controls, typical conservative cutoffs for positive test results require the presence of fused signals in >30% cells for FISH-F (*Mod Pathol.* 2006;19:1).

  2. Break apart FISH. Also known as FISH-BA, this strategy utilizes two probes localizing just proximal and distal to one of the two breakpoints of interest. The two probes are therefore in close proximity to one another in normal cells, resulting in fusion signals (e.g., two fusion signals; e-**Fig. 59.4C**). Cells harboring the translocation will contain at least one pair of split signals (e.g., one fusion, one green, one red signal; e-**Fig. 59.4D**). The advantages of FISH-BA are that split signals don't occur purely by chance, the test yields a positive result even when the translocation can involve multiple partner genes (e.g., *C-MYC* at chromosome 8q24 can fuse with multiple partner genes in Burkitt lymphomas including *IGH* at 14q32, or less commonly the light chain loci on 2q11 or 22q11), and commercial break apart probes yield large easily interpretable signals (e-**Fig. 59.11** through e-**Fig. 59.14**). Disadvantages of FISH-BA include that it provides no information regarding the identity of the fusion partner. On the basis of signal proximities in normal controls, typical conservative cutoffs for positive test results require the presence of split signals in >15% of cells for FISH-BA (*Mod Pathol.* 2006;19:1).

  3. Other approaches. A strategy that has been used to increase the sensitivity of FISH-F is to include one particularly large FISH probe that spans a breakpoint region. In the presence of a translocation, the large DNA probe is split, leading to an extra signal (hence the name FISH-ES) smaller than the remaining nonsplit, nonfused signals (e.g., one fusion, one normal green, one normal red, and one ES red signal). Since it is unlikely that individual cells will contain both a fusion signal and an extra signal, smaller populations of tumor cells can be confidently identified in heterogeneous specimens (e.g., minimal residual disease in CML).

  An even more reliable method to increase the sensitivity of FISH-F is to use two large probes that span both breakpoint regions. By this approach, a tumor harboring the target translocation will harbor two fusion or "double fusion" signals marking the two derivative chromosomes (hence the name D-FISH). However, if a positive tumor additionally has superimposed changes such as polyploidy, the deletion of one of the derivative chromosomes, an unbalanced translocation, and so on, the FISH pattern becomes considerably more complex and difficult to interpret with certainty.

To improve the accuracy of analyzing the cell of interest, FISH can be analyzed in FFPE tissue sections with simultaneous antibody immunofluorescence. This approach is used in plasma cell myelomas where simultaneous CD138 immunofluorescence is used in conjunction with FISH evaluations of *IGH* translocations, to assess the cytogenetic abnormalities in the malignant plasma cells (*J Mol Diagn.* 2006;8:459).

IV. **DEVELOPMENT OF A FISH TEST FOR CLINICAL USE.** The clinical utility of FISH, together with the ease of assay development, makes the methodology an ideal basis for development of new molecular genetic tests. The basic format for developing a new FISH test is outlined in Table 59.4.

The first critical step is the identification of distinct molecular cytogenetic alterations known to be associated with a particular tumor type or genetic syndrome; these data typically come from genomic screening studies. Next, DNA probe availability must be addressed; acquisition is simple if a probe is commercially available; if not, analytic specific (i.e., homemade) probes can be developed as described above. For deletions, regional chromosomal gains, or gene amplifications, the CEP from the same chromosome is often utilized as the reference probe; alternatively, a marker on the opposite chromosomal arm as the locus under study can serve as a copy number reference. Depending on the frequencies of various translocations, breakpoint inconsistencies, and variant translocations, FISH-F, FISH-BA, FISH-ES, D-FISH, or a combination strategy can be designed.

TABLE 59.4	Development of New FISH Tests

Identify a cytogenetic biomarker
Chromosomal gain/loss
Gene/locus deletion
Gene amplification
Translocation

Obtain test and reference DNA probes
Commercial
Analyte specific (e.g., BAC clones)

Assess potential clinical relevance
Diagnostic aid
Prognostic aid
Predicts response or lack of response to patient therapy

Determine appropriate specimen cohort to test and clinical endpoints needed
Archival paraffin-embedded tissue versus fresh/frozen versus cytology
Retrospective versus prospective
Morphologically overlapping tumor entities to assess specificity
Times to disease progression, metastasis, and/or patient death
Patient age or other demographically relevant prognosticators
Extent of resection/surgical margin status
Types of adjuvant therapy administered
Biostatistics needed to answer study questions?
Statistical power analysis: number of specimens needed for statistical significance

Once the appropriate DNA probes are obtained, diagnostic accuracy is evaluated using tumor types with overlapping morphologic features. If prognostic value is the issue, there must be sufficient clinical follow-up to accurately determine statistical associations to patient outcomes, such as time to tumor recurrence, presence/absence of metastases, and patient death. If responsiveness to a specific form of therapy is being tested, patients must be treated uniformly, and data on times to recurrence, parameters of response versus progression, and/or survival times must be collected; confounding variables that often affect prognosis should also be considered (e.g., patient age, demographics, extent of surgery, forms of adjuvant therapy, etc.). Depending on the clinical setting, biostatistical support may be required to determine the sample numbers required to provide sufficient statistical power.

V. FISH NOMENCLATURE. Technical advancements, together with an ever more complete understanding of human chromosomal structure, necessitate periodic revision of nomenclature guidelines. The document in current use is the *International System for Human Cytogenetic Nomenclature* from 2009, abbreviated ISCN 2009, which includes rules for designating cytogenetic findings derived from various in situ hybridization techniques, including interphase FISH. A summary of the more common symbols and abbreviations is shown in Table 59.5.

If interphase in situ hybridization is performed, results are presented in the following order: the abbreviation nuc ish is listed first, followed by the chromosome band to which the probe maps, followed by the locus designation, a multiplication sign, and the number of signals present (Table 59.6). If both conventional cytogenetic analysis and metaphase in situ hybridization are performed, the results of the conventional cytogenetic analysis is listed first, followed by a period, followed by the abbreviation ish, followed by the in situ hybridization results presented in the same order described above. If conventional cytogenetic analysis is performed in conjunction with interphase in situ hybridization, the results are described on separate lines of nomenclature. Ideally, loci are designated according to Genome Data Base (GDB) nomenclature (http://gdbwww.gdb.org). When GDB designations are unavailable, probe names are used. If two or more probes for the same or different loci are used, they are separated by commas.

By these guidelines, simultaneous analysis by FISH-F utilizing probes on different chromosomes expected to produce separate signals in normal cells, but

TABLE 59.5	Examples of Symbols and Abbreviations Used in Interphase FISH Nomenclature
Abbreviation or Symbol	**Description**
Plus sign (+)	Present on a specific chromosome
Minus sign (−)	Absent on a specific chromosome
++	Duplication on a specific chromosome
X	Precedes numbers of signals seen
Semicolon (;)	Separates probes on different derivative chromosomes
Period (.)	Separates cytogenetic results from ish results
amp	Amplified signal
con	Connected or adjacent signals
ish	When used by itself, refers to hybridization to chromosomes
nuc ish	Nuclear or interphase in situ hybridization
pcp	Partial chromosome paint
sep	Separated signals (which are usually adjacent in normal cells)
subtel	Subtelomeric
wcp	Whole chromosome paint

TABLE 59.6	Examples of Nomenclature Used for Neoplasms Evaluated by Interphase FISH[a]
Designation	**Description**
nuc ish 11p13(WT1x2),22q12(EWSx2), (WT1 con EWSx1)	Interphase FISH of a tumor cell using single-fusion probes. A probe for WT1 at 11p13 shows two signals, as does a probe for EWS at 22q12. However, one WT1 and one EWS signal are juxtaposed (or connected) suggesting they lie on the same chromosome, consistent with a t(11;22)(p13;q12) translocation
nuc ish 22q12(EWSR1x2)(5′EWSR1sep 3′EWSR1x1)	Interphase FISH of a tumor cell using a break-apart probe set for the EWS locus at 22q12. Two sets of EWS signals are present, but on one copy of chromosome 22, the probes are separated (most likely as a result of a rearrangement of the EWS locus)
nuc ish 22q12(5′EWS,3′EWS con 5′EWS,3′EWS)x2[169/200]	Interphase FISH using the same break-apart probe set as in the above example. However, in this tumor, the two probes remain juxtaposed on both copies of chromosome 22 (which provides no evidence of a rearrangement of the EWS locus). The indicated results are present in 169 of 200 nuclei evaluated
nuc ish 8q24(MYCx2)(5′MYC sep 3′MYCx1)[119/200]	Interphase FISH using a break-apart probe set. In this tumor, a split of red and green signals was detected. This is consistent with a c-myc-containing chromosomal rearrangement in 119 of 200 nuclei evaluated
nuc ish 8q24(5′MYC,3′MYC con 5′MYC,3′MYC)x2[174/200]	Interphase FISH was performed utilizing a commercial c-myc (8q24) break-apart probe set. In this particular case, a split of red and green signals was not detected in 174 of 200 nuclei evaluated

[a]The assistance of Diane Robirds, CLSp(CG) in the preparation of this table is gratefully acknowledged.

juxtaposed signals in cells harboring the target rearrangement, employs the abbreviation con (for connected) to indicate juxtaposed signals; this finding suggests that the target loci are present on the same chromosome (Table 59.6). Similarly, analysis by FISH-BA utilizing probes that are juxtaposed in normal cells, but that become separated in cells that harbor the target chromosomal rearrangement, employs the abbreviation sep to indicate separated signals; this finding suggests that a rearrangement of the target region is present.

60 Direct and Indirect Methods for DNA Sequence Analysis

TuDong Nguyen, Barbara Zehnbauer, and John D. Pfeifer

I. **INTRODUCTION.** Clinical molecular diagnostic methods have been integrated into many laboratory disciplines, and guidelines and recommendations from both professional societies and regulatory agencies have been developed to assist in the development and performance of clinical molecular pathology testing (Table 60.1). Most molecular tests performed in surgical pathology focus on somatic or acquired DNA variations in the cells of the disease process that provide information that aids in diagnosis, identifies prognostic indicators, stratifies patients into effective treatment options, helps monitor treatment response, and/or identifies patients at increased risk of disease. Because polymerase chain reaction (PCR)-based approaches are quick, reliable, and sensitive, PCR has become a central technology for much of clinical molecular genetic testing.

II. **SPECIMEN REQUIREMENTS, HANDLING, AND PROCESSING.** Clinical PCR-based molecular testing in the setting of surgical pathology requires the same attention to detail regarding efficient specimen collection, identification, preparation, and routing as any other pathology test.

A. **Specimens.** Specimen requirements are dictated by the disease process, including the type of tissue, amount of tissue, type of sample (fresh or frozen tissue, formalin-fixed paraffin-embedded tissue [FFPE], cytology specimen, and so on), and the extent of the disease in the sample. The amount of tissue required for PCR-based testing is relatively small, which contributes to the clinical utility of the technique.

Regardless of specimen type, two general features of the tissue sample influence molecular assays. First, there must be a sufficient quantity of the specific target cell (and therefore target DNA or RNA) in the sample. Second, the size or integrity of the nucleic acid molecules after isolation from the tissue can dramatically affect the sensitivity of the detection of specific alterations, thus nucleic acid degradation (whether due to fixation, or enzymatic, heat, pH, or mechanical forces) can reduce the sensitivity of testing.

1. **Tissue type.** Fresh peripheral blood, bone marrow, solid tissue biopsies, cytology specimens, enriched cell populations (e.g., from flow cytometry), and FFPE tissue sections are all sources of nucleic acids for molecular analysis. Specimens should be collected and transported to the molecular pathology laboratory using aseptic techniques, if possible. Transport on ice reduces cell lysis, minimizes nuclease activity, and reduces nucleic acid degradation.

2. **Tissue quality**

a. Fresh tissue and cell suspensions are the optimal templates for PCR. The preferred method of preservation of fresh tissue prior to isolation of nucleic acids is ultra-low-temperature frozen storage at $-70°C$, which permits indefinite preservation with virtually no effect on the quality of the extracted nucleic acids. Low-temperature frozen storage around $-20°C$ can adequately preserve DNA and RNA for several months.

Cell suspensions (including hematologic specimens such as peripheral blood and bone marrow) should be collected in the presence of an

TABLE 60.1	Selected Resources for Clinical Molecular Pathology Laboratory Operational Guidelines	

Entity	Site	Tool(s)
Clinical Laboratory Improvement Amendments '88	http://www.cms.hhs.gov/clia/ Centers for Medicare and Medicaid Services	Clinical Laboratory Accreditation requirements and compliance lists 57 Federal Register 7137–7186 (1992)
College of American Pathologists (CAP)	http://www.cap.org	Laboratory Accreditation (LAP) Molecular Pathology Laboratory Inspection Checklist Proficiency surveys • Molecular oncology (MO) • Medical genetics (MGL) • Pharmacogenetics (PGX) • Monitoring engraftment (ME) • Molecular microbiology (HIV, HCV, ID) • Microsatellite instability (MSI) • Sarcoma translocation (SARC) • Nucleic acid testing (viral; NAT)
Clinical and Laboratory Standards Institute (CLSI; *formerly National Committee for Clinical Laboratory Standards, NCCLS*)	http://www.nccls.org	Molecular Methods Guidelines • Genetic diseases • IGH & TCR gene rearrangements • Nucleic acid amplification • Nucleic acid sequencing • Collection and handling of specimens • Proficiency testing
American College of Medical Genetics (ACMG)	http://www.acmg.net	Standards and Guidelines for Clinical Genetics Laboratories Policy Statements for Molecular testing of genetic diseases
US Food and Drug Administration (FDA)	http://www.fda.gov	Medical Devices 21CFR809.30 In Vitro Diagnostic Products for Human Use • Analyte-specific reagents (ASRs)
Association for Molecular Pathology (AMP)	http://www.amp.org	Molecular Pathology professional organization (incl. genetics, hematopathology, infectious disease, solid tumors) CHAMP listserve for AMP members Test directories • Solid tumors • Hematopathology • Infectious disease

anticoagulant, preferably ethylenediaminetetraacetic acid (EDTA) or acid citrate dextrose (ACD); heparin should be avoided because heparin carryover after nucleic acid isolation may inhibit subsequent PCR steps. Freezing of hematologic specimens presents distinct obstacles to the preparation of good quality nucleic acid and should generally be avoided.

b. Nucleic acids extracted from fixed tissue can also be used in PCR, although the type of fixative and length of fixation both have a profound effect on their recovery. Non-cross-linking fixatives such as ethanol provide the most consistent preservation of amplifiable DNA, with more variability from tissues fixed with formalin, Zamboni's and Clark's fixatives, paraformaldehyde, and formalin–alcohol–acetic acid. Tissues processed in Carnoy's, Zenker's, Bouin's and B-5 fixatives are poor substrates for PCR testing since little amplifiable DNA can be recovered from them.

The effects of formalin fixation on PCR-based testing have been evaluated in some detail, not surprising given that most surgical specimens are fixed in formalin. Formaldehyde reacts with nucleic acids and proteins to form a mixture of end products that are covalently linked by methylene bridges. Thus, the quality of DNA isolated from formalin-fixed tissue is critically dependent on the length of fixation, with a deterioration of PCR signal with increasing fixation time. In general, tissue fixed in neutral buffered formalin for <8 hours contains DNA and RNA from which PCR products >600 bp in length can be reliably amplified, but fixation extended for greater than 8 to 12 hours decreases the length of PCR products that can consistently be amplified.

3. Tissue quantity. Minimum sample requirements are determined by the assay methodology and extent of target cell involvement in the tissue. A typical PCR-based assay requires only 20 to 200 ng of DNA (about 10^3 to 10^4 cells), although multiplexed PCR may require a bit more DNA in order to equally represent all targets. The sensitivity of PCR for detection of a few target molecules in a large background of unaltered DNA molecules (1 in 10^5) is one of the principle strengths of the methodology.

III. ANALYTIC/TECHNICAL VERSUS DIAGNOSTIC AND OPERATIONAL ASPECTS OF TESTING. The familiar probabilistic model used to define the likelihood that a particular patient is correctly classified on the basis of a test result (Table 60.2) can be applied to molecular genetic tests as with any other laboratory test. However, it is important to recognize that the quantitative performance of a lab test can be evaluated at four different levels (Table 60.3), and that test performance at one of the four levels does not necessarily predict performance at the other levels. Differences between these four levels of analysis are often overlooked even though they account for many of the confusing or seemingly conflicting results regarding the utility of molecular genetic testing in surgical pathology.

IV. BASIC PCR METHODOLOGY

A. Amplification. Selective amplification of the target sequence is achieved through the use of oligonucleotide primers that hybridize to the 5′ and 3′ ends of the DNA target sequence (Fig. 60.1). In addition to the two primers and input (template) DNA, the reaction mixture also includes the four deoxynucleotide triphosphates (dATP, dCTP, dGTP, dTTP) and a heat-stable (thermostable) DNA polymerase. The first step of the PCR itself involves heating the mixture to a high temperature to denature the target DNA; in the second step, the reaction is cooled to allow the primers to anneal to their complementary sequence in the target DNA; in the third step, the reaction is heated to the temperature at which the heat-stable DNA polymerase has optimal activity. As a result of this three step denaturation, annealing, and polymerization cycle, the two primers will initiate synthesis of new DNA molecules from opposite strands of the input DNA heteroduplex. With each repetition of the three-step cycle, the newly synthesized DNA strands

TABLE 60.2	Nomenclature When Bayes' Theorem for One Variate Is Applied in Laboratory Testing	
	Number of subjects with positive test result	**Number of subjects with negative test result**
Number of subjects with disease	TP	FN
Number of subjects without disease	FP	TN

TP, True positives *or* number of diseased patients correctly classified by the test; FP, false positives *or* number of patients without the disease misclassified by the test; FN, false negatives *or* number of diseased patients misclassified by the test; TN, true negatives *or* number of patients without the disease correctly classified by the test.

Diagnostic sensitivity $= \dfrac{TP}{TP + FN}$

Diagnostic specificity $= \dfrac{TN}{FP + TN}$

Predictive value of positive test $= \dfrac{TN}{TP + FP}$

Predictive value of negative test $= \dfrac{TN}{TN + FN}$

Efficiency of the test or number fraction of patients correctly classified $= \dfrac{TP + TN}{TP + FP + FN + TN}$

Youden index $= [(\text{sensitivity} + \text{specificity}) - 1]$

will also act as templates for further DNA synthesis, and so DNA duplexes in which both strands have the fixed length of the target sequence (so-called amplicons) accumulate exponentially.

PCR makes it possible to selectively amplify a specific DNA target sequence within a background of heterogeneous DNA sequences, such as total genomic DNA or cDNA derived from unfractionated cellular RNA. However, each of the components in a PCR, including the input DNA, the oligonucleotide primers, the thermostable polymerase, the buffer, and the cycle parameters, has an effect on the sensitivity, specificity, and fidelity of the reaction.

B. Factors that affect PCR testing on an analytic/technical level
   1. Advantages of PCR
      a. **PCR is simple, quick, and inexpensive.** A single PCR cycle of melting, annealing, and extension is usually completed within several minutes, and consequently an entire PCR amplification of 25 to 35 cycles can be performed in only a few hours. Because of the high level of amplification achieved by PCR, the product DNA can be visualized after simple gel electrophoresis, avoiding the hazards and expense of radiolabeling methods.

TABLE 60.3	Four Levels at Which a Laboratory Test Can Be Evaluated
Level	**Measures**
Analytic/technical	Technical sensitivity, technical specificity, precision, accuracy, proficiency
Diagnostic	Diagnostic sensitivity, diagnostic specificity, Youden index
Operational	Predictive value of a positive result, predictive value of a negative result, efficiency
Medical decision making	Cost–benefit analysis, stratification to optimal treatment regimen, stratification to gene-targeted treatment regimen

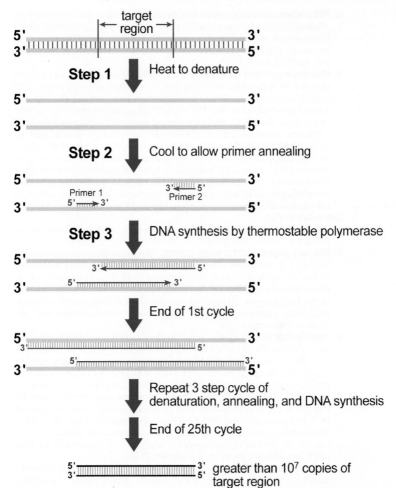

Figure 60.1 Schematic diagram of PCR. Each cycle consists of three steps: The reaction mix is heated to denature the double-stranded DNA template, the reaction mix is cooled to permit annealing of oligonucleotide primers to sequences that flank the target region, and then the reaction mix is warmed to permit the heat-stable polymerase to synthesize new DNA strands. Each newly synthesized DNA strand then acts as a template in subsequent three-step cycles of denaturation, annealing, and DNA synthesis, producing exponential amplification of the target region.

b. **PCR has high sensitivity and specificity.** When optimized, PCR can detect one abnormal cell in a background of 10^5 normal cells, and can even be used to analyze single copy genes from individual cells (*Methods Enzymol.* 2002;356:295, 334). PCR can also be used to detect a broad range of genetic abnormalities ranging from gross structural alterations such as translocations to single base-pair changes.

c. **PCR products are easily labeled for detection.** For primer-mediated labeling, a labeled chemical group (usually a fluorophore) is attached to the 5′ end of either or both oligonucleotide primers. Alternatively, the PCR product can be directly labeled by including one or more labeled nucleotide precursors into the PCR mix.

d. **Phenotype–genotype correlations are possible.** When performed on tissue sections, PCR provides only an indirect correlation of morphology with underlying genetic abnormalities. Microdissection, in which the region of interest is carved out of the FFPE tissue block, scraped from tissue sections or cytology slides, or collected more precisely with a micromanipulator apparatus, provides some enrichment for morphologic–genetic correlations. More precise phenotypic–genotypic analysis is achieved by collecting individual cells by laser capture microdissection, by flow cytometry, or even by immunomagnetic methods. In situ PCR performed on histologic tissue sections themselves is perhaps the ultimate method for providing morphologic localization of genotypic expression; however, the technique is so technically demanding that it has limited use in clinical laboratories.

2. **Limitations of PCR**

a. **PCR only analyzes the target region.** Testing only provides information on the target segment amplified by the specific primer set employed.

b. **PCR only amplifies intact target regions.** Mutations that damage a primer binding site (including insertions, deletions, and even point mutations) preclude amplification of the target region by PCR and can easily lead to errors in test interpretation. Similarly, mutations that alter the structure of the target region in ways not accounted for during primer set design (e.g., large insertions, deletions, inversions, or translocations) may preclude amplification.

c. **Amplification bias.** PCR bias refers to the fact that some DNA templates are preferentially amplified versus other templates within the same reaction. PCR bias can be caused by differences in template length, random variations in template number (especially with very low target abundance, producing an artifact known as allele dropout), and random variations in PCR efficiency with each cycle. Amplification bias can even result from differences in the target sequence itself as small as a single base substitution. PCR bias can cause over tenfold differences in amplification efficiency in some settings, a difference that can influence quantitative PCR (Q-PCR) test results and loss of heterozygosity analysis. PCR bias can be a particularly troublesome problem in multiplex PCR.

d. **Technical factors.** There are several technical factors that can lower the sensitivity and specificity of PCR in routine clinical practice below that obtained in optimized research settings. Nonspecific inhibitors of PCR are sometimes present in patient samples, including heparin and uncharacterized components of CSF, urine, and sputum. With the extreme sensitivity of PCR, strict attention to the physical organization and methodologies of the laboratory are required to avoid cross-contamination of specimens.

However, the most important technical limitations are introduced when fixed rather than fresh tissue specimens are used for testing due to the degradation of DNA and mRNA that occurs prior to and during fixation, as noted earlier. Test sensitivity and specificity are compromised by degradation since it makes it necessary to amplify shorter target sequences or employ a nested PCR approach, both of which increase the risk of amplification of nonspecific sequences and cross-contamination (*Am J Surg Pathol.* 2002;26:965).

C. **Factors that affect testing on a diagnostic level.** The intrinsic biologic variability of disease has the greatest impact on the diagnostic sensitivity and specificity of molecular testing. Since only a subset of patients with a specific disease may harbor a characteristic mutation, more than one genetic variant may characterize a specific disease, the same mutation may be characteristic of more than one disease, a mutation characteristic of disease may be present in healthy individuals (reduced penetrance), and so on, even a molecular genetic method with perfect analytic performance will have a lower sensitivity and specificity when used for diagnostic testing of patient samples.

Another diagnostic limitation of the use of PCR in routine clinical testing is a result of the fact that the technique is so sensitive that it amplifies target DNA and RNA sequences from cellular debris as well as viable cells (*Cancer.* 1997;80:1393). Consequently, in the absence of histologic confirmation of the presence of live tumor cells, the significance of PCR-based detection of tumor-derived nucleic acids in lymph nodes or even peripheral blood is uncertain.

D. **Factors that affect testing on an operational level.** Purely operational factors can introduce uncertainty into the interpretation of results when testing is performed prospectively in routine clinical practice. If the probability that a case is subjected to additional analysis depends on the initial test result itself, clinical variables, or both, selection bias (also called verification bias, posttest referral bias, and work-up bias) is introduced into the test. Discrepant analysis (also known as discordant analysis) can also introduce uncertainty in the interpretation of test results. Finally, even mundane factors such as differences in disease prevalence can have a marked effect on the predictive value of positive and negative test results.

E. **Implications for clinical testing.** Taken together, the analytic/technical features of molecular genetic assays, biologic variability, variation in assay design, and differences in distribution of disease in the patient populations have many implications for testing applied in routine clinical practice.

   1. **Characteristics of tests with clinical utility.** The criteria used to evaluate the clinical utility of other hospital laboratory tests should also be applied when considering the role of the molecular pathology laboratory in patient care (Table 60.4).

TABLE 60.4	Characteristics of Molecular Tests with Clinical Utility
Criterion	**Utility**
The disorder must be a significant health problem.	Disease prevalence and adverse effect on affected individuals are measurable and serious.
Treatment alternatives are available to alter disease course.	The genotype does affect the patient's clinical outcome.
A reliable molecular test is available to distinguish true positive and false positive results.	Focus on molecular changes known to be associated with disease pathology.
Pretest and posttest counseling resources are available.	Interpretation of molecular findings with the data from the clinical presentation and other pathology tests.
The test is cost-effective and/or cost-beneficial.	More costly or invasive disease monitoring methods are unnecessary. Specific treatment options and/or prognostic outcomes are indicated by the molecular results.
Referring clinicians accept the test as worthwhile to aid their decision making.	Diagnosis, treatment, and/or clinical outcome are enhanced by the addition of the molecular pathology results to other medical tests.

a. The relative merit of the molecular testing should focus on the ability of the test findings to improve patient care. For clinical utility, the molecular diagnostic test must provide an improvement in the standard of patient care by providing new or refined information with the potential for clinical stratification of disease subtypes, prognostic categories, treatment regimens, gene-targeted therapies, survival statistics, or disease progression. The test results should complement the findings of established tests, such as cytogenetics, immunohistochemistry, and cell surface marker analysis. In the context of surgical pathology, the test results must be correlated with the histopathologic features of the case.

b. Routine clinical use of molecular tests must consider practical aspects of clinical prevalence (the disease should represent a significant health problem or diagnostic dilemma), test run frequency, clinically relevant turn-around-time, sensitivity, and specificity. Testing for diseases which are common in many populations (e.g., cancer, microbial infections, and genetic predispositions) and have well-defined molecular markers will be performed in many laboratories. Molecular genetic testing for rare disorders will be routinely available only at selected laboratories with specific clinical programs or areas of institutional focus and expertise.

c. Testing must include steps to validate the result, and will include positive and negative assay controls, definition of the details and limits of interpretation of test results, and provisions for proficiency testing of the analytic method, competency of the technologists, and interpretive expertise of the laboratory director.

d. Results must be reported in a context that explains the molecular assay data and integrates the findings with other pathology results to avoid seemingly contradictory reports in comparison with other laboratory tests that possess different levels of resolution or detection.

e. Biosafety, legal, ethical, and privacy issues must consistently be observed.

2. **Discordant cases.** Cases will arise in which there is a lack of concordance between the diagnosis suggested by the molecular test results and the morphologic diagnosis. The debate over the best approach to resolve the ambiguity presented by these cases reflects the fundament impact of molecular genetics on the classification of disease as well as the status of morphology as the historical standard of diagnosis by which new methods are measured. Rather than arbitrarily assuming that genetic testing or morphology is superior in all cases, the most reasonable way to handle discordant cases is to acknowledge the presence of the discrepancy, and then reappraise the clinical data, pathological findings, and therapeutic implications of all the test results.

For those cases in which the diagnosis suggested by morphology and genetic testing are different, prospective clinical trials are required to assess whether stage, prognosis, and response to treatment are more accurately predicted by the molecular test results than by the morphologic findings on which most staging and treatment protocols are based. Epidemiologically, there is a distinction between diagnostic testing and prognostic testing, with different study designs required to assess the performance of tests in these different settings (*J Clin Epidemiol.* 2002;55:1178; *Ann Intern Med.* 2003;139:950).

V. VARIATIONS OF PCR

A. **Nested PCR.** In this technique, two consecutive PCRs are performed on the same DNA sample; an initial amplification of a longer target sequence followed by a second amplification of a shorter sequence contained within the first amplicon. The second PCR may involve two internal primers (fully nested) or one internal primer and one of the original primers (seminested). Nested PCR provides a marked increase in sensitivity compared with traditional PCR, and is desirable when the target sequence is present at an extremely low copy number, such as when the mutation is present in only a small subset of the cell population under study, when the nucleic acids have been degraded as a result of tissue fixation, or, for reverse transcriptase-PCR (RT-PCR) as discussed below, when the target mRNA is expressed at an extremely low level. Since the increased sensitivity carries an increased risk of cross-contamination, reproducible nested PCR results require strict attention to laboratory technique, rigorous use of controls, and confirmation of product identity.

B. RT-PCR. RT-PCR makes it possible to amplify RNA extracted from a tissue sample; a complementary DNA (cDNA) strand is synthesized from the RNA template using the enzyme RT, and the cDNA is then amplified by conventional PCR. Fresh (or fresh frozen) tissue is the preferred source of RNA for RT-PCR. RNA from fixed tissue is an acceptable substrate for testing (e-**Fig. 60.1**),* even though it always suffers some degree of degradation depending on the prefixation interval, the type of fixative, the length of fixation, and the method used to isolate the RNA.

1. **Advantages of RT-PCR.** RT-PCR permits direct amplification of multiexon sequences by eliminating the intervening introns, and thus greatly simplifies mutation scanning methods. Similarly, RT-PCR makes it much simpler to demonstrate the presence of translocations that create fusion genes by making it possible to directly detect the fusion transcripts encoded by the translocations (e-**Fig. 60.2**). RT-PCR can also be used to detect changes in mRNA structure that result from alternative splicing, to demonstrate aberrant splicing due to mutations, and to evaluate the level of gene expression through the quantitative methods discussed below.

2. **Limitations of RT-PCR.** RNA is a more technically demanding substrate with less stability than DNA. Tissue samples must be processed rapidly (ideally, within 20 minutes) to avoid mRNA degradation, especially since many mutations render transcripts more susceptible to cellular mechanisms that clear abnormal transcripts from the cell and result in unstable mRNA. A nested PCR approach is often necessary when the target RNA is present at very low levels, but RT-PCR carries an increased risk of contamination and amplification of nonspecific sequences because the transfer of the first PCR product to a separate tube for the nested PCR entails transmission of a highly amplified DNA preparation.

C. Q-PCR. An ideal PCR would generate a perfect twofold increase in the number of copies of the amplicon in each cycle of the reaction. In reality, inhibitors of the reaction, accumulation of pyrophosphate molecules, decreasing polymerase activity, and reagent consumption all contribute to a plateau phase in the later stages of the reaction during which the amplicon is no longer accumulating at an exponential rate (*Clin Chem Lab Med.* 2000;38:833). Reliable quantitation of PCR therefore involves more than simple measurement of the amount of product DNA present at the end of 30 to 40 cycles of the reaction. Real-time PCR, also referred to as Q-PCR, employs real-time measurements of DNA accumulation (usually via fluorescence-based approaches) during the early exponential phases of PCR progress to provide precise estimates of the initial concentration of the target sequence(s).

A wide variety of different chemistries for Q-PCR are in routine use, including the so-called *Taq*Man (also known as 5′ exonuclease or hydrolysis real-time PCR), molecular beacon (which can be designed to distinguish targets differing by only a single nucleotide), scorpion (also known as self-probing amplicons),

---

*All e-figures are available online via the Solution Site Image Bank.

hybridization probe, and intercalating dye methods. Regardless of the chemistry, changes in fluorescence that result from target amplification are measured by a detector for each cycle of the reaction, and used by a computer to construct an amplification plot of fluorescence versus the cycle number to quantify the concentration of the input target DNA sequence.

1. **Advantages of Q-PCR.** The method can be applied to fresh as well as FFPE tissue, and phenotype–genotype correlations are possible through analysis of specific cell populations collected via microdissection, laser capture microdissection, and so on. Q-RT-PCR is also a robust analytic approach (e-**Fig. 60.3**).

2. **Disadvantages of Q-PCR.** Even for optimized assays, testing can be complicated by amplification bias, which in the context of Q-PCR has two major sources; PCR drift due to random fluctuations in amplification efficiency in the early cycles of the reaction when the templates are present at very low concentration, and PCR selection due to mechanisms that systematically favor amplification of some particular target(s). For Q-RT-PCR, the reverse transcription reaction can introduce additional variables into the analysis.

3. **Use of Q-PCR in nonquantitative settings.** Since the probes used in Q-PCR (and Q-RT-PCR) have specificity for the target amplicon, the amplification plot confirms not only the presence of the DNA product, but also its identity. Intercalating dyes can also provide confirmation of both the presence and the identity of the DNA product when coupled with subsequent melting curve analysis. Because Q-PCR eliminates the need for gel electrophoresis to demonstrate successful amplification while simultaneously confirming product identity, Q-PCR is often used as a "one-step" alternative to conventional PCR or RT-PCR even when quantitation is not required.

D. **Multiplex PCR.** Multiplex PCR is the simultaneous amplification of multiple target sequences in a single reaction through the simultaneous use of multiple primer pairs. The technique saves time and money, is ideal for conserving templates that are in short supply, and has been successfully applied to many amplification approaches including nested PCR and Q-PCR. However, even in optimized reactions, multiplex PCR may be complicated by amplification bias due to PCR drift and PCR selection. Rigorous optimization of primer design and careful titration of the relative primer concentration among separate primer pairs are essential for robust, reproducible multiplex PCR.

E. **Methylation-specific PCR.** Methylation of CpG sites in human DNA has been associated with transcriptional inactivation of imprinted genes, is important for X chromosome inactivation, and is an important mechanism for developmentally regulated and tissue-specific gene regulation. An altered pattern of methylation is also characteristic of many human diseases (e-**Figs. 60.4** and **60.5**). Changes in the CpG methylation pattern in some malignancies have been associated with differences in response to specific chemotherapeutic agents and overall survival.

Recently developed methylation-specific PCR techniques exploit the sequence differences produced when methylated CpG (meCpG) and unmethylated CpG are treated with sodium bisulfite (*Proc Natl Acad Sci USA.* 1996;93:9821). This chemical modification will not alter methyl cytosine but will depurinate cytosine to produce a transversion, which results in replacement by thymidine in subsequent DNA synthesis during PCR. Since the two strands of genomic DNA are no longer complimentary after sodium bisulfite treatment, PCR with specifically designed primers for meC and T substituted sequences makes it possible to infer the methylation status of the original untreated DNA. Methylation-specific PCR can be applied to DNA extracted from fresh tissue, FFPE tissue, and even archival cytology specimens.

F. Telomerase repeat amplification protocol (TRAP). The hexanucleotide TTAGGG repeat sequence of human telomeres is essential for the maintenance of chromosome stability and integrity, and abnormalities of telomere length have been associated with a number of developmental abnormalities and malignancies. The PCR-based TRAP assay is a simple, sensitive, and reproducible method for measurement of telomerase activity as an adjunct in early diagnosis, for prognostic testing, or as a means to identify drugs that inhibit telomerase function.

The technique has limitations; the protein extract used for testing can only be prepared from fresh cells or tissue samples, false-negative and false-positive reactions are commonly encountered, and heterogeneity within a tumor can lead to significant variability in the test result. Although early studies suggested that altered telomerase activity is a characteristic finding in a variety of neoplasms, a growing body of evidence suggests that telomerase activity demonstrated by the TRAP assay is neither a consistent feature of malignancy nor specific for a malignant phenotype (*Hum Pathol.* 2004;5:393). Attempts to correlate a malignant phenotype with telomerase activity measured by other techniques (such as RT-PCR-based measurement of the level of expression of mRNA encoding the hTERT catalytic subunit of telomerase, or immunohistochemical analysis of hTERT) have likewise produced mixed results.

VI. DNA SEQUENCE ANALYSIS

A. Direct DNA sequence analysis

1. The **dye terminator cycle sequencing method** for direct DNA sequencing is currently used for virtually all routine DNA sequence analyses. This technique (e-**Fig. 60.6**) utilizes synthetic oligonucleotide primers complimentary to a known sequence of the template strand to be analyzed, and is greatly simplified by the use of fluorescently labeled, chain-terminating dideoxynucleotide triphosphates. As initially described, enzymatic extension of the primer was performed only once per sequencing reaction, but the utility of the method is greatly increased by the modification known as cycle sequencing (or linear amplification sequencing). Cycle sequencing is similar to conventional PCR in that it employs a thermostable DNA polymerase and a temperature cycling format for DNA denaturation, annealing, and enzymatic DNA synthesis, but only one primer (the sequencing primer) is added to the reaction mixture.

2. **Next-generation sequencing (NGS).** Recent developments in the technology of so-called next-generation DNA sequencing (also known as deep sequencing) using several different platforms can generate millions of short sequence reads per run, making it possible to sequence gene panels, all expressed genes (known as the exome), or even the entire human genome at an extremely low cost (*Brief Bioinform.* 2010;2:484; *Protein Cell.* 2010;1:520). The many genetic variations that can be detected by NGS include single-nucleotide polymorphisms (SNPs), indels (small insertions and deletions), structural variants (SVs), and copy number variations (CNVs). Massive sequencing of cDNA libraries, also known as RNA-Seq, is an application of NGS technologies focused on the transcribed portions of the human genome (known as the transcriptome), which provides a comprehensive readout of gene expression that exceeds the sensitivity of microarray-based methods. And through the use of sodium bisulfite treatment of DNA, NGS technologies also offer the potential to study genome-wide DNA methylation patterns (epigenomic analysis).

Complete whole genome sequences have already been published from several human cancers, including acute myeloid leukemia, breast cancer, melanoma, lung cancer, and glioblastoma. Recent demonstration of whole genome sequencing of a proband with Charcot–Marie tooth syndrome demonstrates that NGS also has significant diagnostic potential in clinical settings besides cancer biology, such as the diagnosis of inherited diseases.

As with all other molecular diagnostic tests, significant attention must be paid to NGS results to ensure data quality, including the incorporation of controls that allow the identification of sample contaminations, library chimeras, sample mix-ups, tumor-normal switches, and variable run quality.

B. **Indirect DNA sequence analysis.** Indirect identification of normal and mutant alleles at a specific locus, which correlate with the presence of disease can be of clinical utility and substitute for direct determination of specific nucleotide sequences. Virtually all of the indirect methods are based on PCR and can be applied to a broad range of clinical specimens. Examples of indirect methods include the following.

1. **Allelic discrimination by size.** Alleles that vary by small insertions or deletions can be distinguished on the basis of the size of the PCR product after gel electrophoresis, perhaps the most straightforward method for indirect DNA sequence analysis (e-**Figs. 60.4, 60.7**, and **60.8**).

2. **Allelic discrimination based on susceptibility to a restriction enzyme.** Using the technique known as restriction fragment length polymorphism (RFLP) analysis, mutations that either create or destroy a restriction endonuclease site can easily be distinguished by a two-step process that involves DNA digestion with the restriction endonuclease followed by gel electrophoresis to size fractionate the digested DNA. Virtually all RFLP analysis is performed on PCR product DNA (e-**Figs. 60.7, 60.9**, and **60.10**).

3. **Allele-specific PCR.** Allele-specific PCR (also known as the amplification refractory mutation system [ARMS]) employs oligonucleotide primers designed to discriminate between normal and mutant target DNA sequences that may differ by a single base (*J Mol Diagn.* 2007;9:272). Simultaneous analysis of multiple loci via a multiplex PCR format is possible if the amplicons from different loci are of different sizes. PCR conditions must be optimized with sufficient stringency so that amplification only occurs when complete DNA sequence complementarity exists between primer and target molecules.

4. **Single-strand conformational polymorphism (SSCP) analysis.** SSCP is one of the most simple and widely used techniques used as a mutation scanning system. Single-stranded DNA molecules fold into complex three-dimensional structures, stabilized primarily by intrastrand base-pairing hydrogen bond formation, that alter the mobility of the molecule during nondenaturing gel electrophoresis. SSCP has limited resolution of DNA fragment sizes (100 to 400 bp long is optimal), and while a base sequence may be indicated by the altered mobility, SSCP does not provide information about either the location of the base change within the DNA fragment or the chemical identity of the base change. In practice, the DNA fragments evaluated by SSCP are generated by PCR.

5. **Melting curve analysis.** Every DNA duplex has a characteristic melting temperature (dependent on sequence and duplex length) and though small, the differences in melting temperature between the duplexes can be reliably detected by high-resolution melting analysis. Differences in the melting transition of PCR products can therefore be used to infer sequence variations such as SNPs, small deletions, and small insertions. The most straightforward methods melt unlabeled PCR products in the presence of DNA-binding dyes such as SYBR Green that differentiate double-stranded from single-stranded DNA during melting by changes in fluorescence intensity (*Nature Protocols.* 2007;2:59).

C. **Clonality assays.** Demonstration that the cells in a lesion share a common genetic alteration can be used to support classification as a neoplasm rather than as a polyclonal reactive process, although it is important to emphasize that clonal neoplasms are not necessarily malignant.

1. **Assays based on immunoglobulin and T-cell receptor genes.** Most PCR clonality assays performed clinically are used to assess lymphoid infiltrates on the basis of evaluation of immunoglobulin gene or T-cell receptor gene rearrangements. PCR primer design is an important component of these assays; since generation of immunoglobulin and T-cell receptors involves deletions, template-independent nucleotide additions, and single base-pair changes, consensus primers are designed to bind to conserved sequence regions, and multiple sets of primers are used in order to insure that a broad range of rearrangements can be detected. Demonstration of a monoclonal or oligoclonal population of cells within an infiltrate is very often, but not always, indicative of malignancy since oligoclonal or monoclonal gene rearrangements may characterize reactive lymphoid proliferations.

2. **Clonality assays based on specific gene mutations.** This class of assays focuses on detection of specific mutations in individual genes, including single base-pair changes and larger-scale structural changes (such as deletions or insertions of viral genomes). This type of analysis can be useful when attempting to show that two neoplasms represent independent synchronous tumors rather than one tumor with metastases.

D. **Microsatellite instability (MSI) assays.** Defects in the DNA mismatch repair system produce a characteristic pattern of mutations known as MSI. Direct analysis of the genes responsible for mismatch repair is not desirable in routine clinical practice because it requires complete DNA sequencing of (at least) four causative genes; there are no specific mutation "hot spots," and the genes may be inactive as a result of epigenetic silencing rather than mutation. PCR-based analysis offers a more efficient, though indirect, method to identify defects in the DNA mismatch repair system via detection of the short increases or decreases in the length of the short tandem repeat (STR, or microsatellite) sequences that are the characteristic feature of MSI. Mutations in the genes which normally monitor the fidelity of DNA replication of these repeated sequences is defective and allows for the generation of the variable lengths of repeats in the tumor cells.

Laboratory testing regimens for MSI have only been formally addressed in the context of colorectal cancer (*Cancer Res.* 1998;58:5248). For all other tumor types, MSI testing is not yet standardized in terms of the number and identity of microsatellite loci that must be analyzed, or in terms of the number of loci that need to show length alterations to be considered indicative of MSI.

DNA derived from either fresh or FFPE tissue can be analyzed in the MSI assay. Comparison of the size of the PCR products from the target STR loci in the neoplasm versus normal tissue is used to detect changes in the length of the microsatellite sequences indicative of MSI. In most cases, the profile of PCR-amplified sequences permits straightforward classification as indicative of MSI or not; however, there are no uniform criteria for interpretation of marginal test results, although standards have been proposed (*Mutat Res.* 2001;461:249). Sources of variation in MSI analysis include the presence of contaminating non-neoplastic tissue (which can limit test reliability because demonstration of MSI in even the most sensitive testing regimens requires that neoplastic cells comprise at least 10% of the total population), the identity of the microsatellite markers used in the analysis (the susceptibility of a given microsatellite to instability is highly dependent on both the number of repeats and the length of the repeat units), and the potential for biased amplification of some alleles.

E. **Infectious disease testing.** PCR-based molecular genetic approaches frequently have higher sensitivity than standard special stains, and can often provide information not typically available from special stains such as species-specific identification and drug sensitivity. Molecular methods are also a useful way to detect organisms that cannot be cultured (e.g., human papilloma virus [HPV]) or that are notorious for their slow growth in culture (e.g., *Mycobacterium tuberculosis*).

1. **Bacteria**
   a. **Mycobacteria.** In most assays, PCR targets the highly conserved gene that encodes the 65 kDa heat shock protein, but other target loci include the genes encoding 16S rRNA or the repetitive insertion element IS6110. PCR testing has been successfully applied to FFPE tissue from a wide variety of sites, including the respiratory tract, GI tract, GU tract, skin, bone, liver, and lymph nodes, and also to cytology specimens. Alternative isothermal amplification approaches originally developed for use in the clinical microbiology laboratory have also been adapted for use with processed tissue specimens (*Expert Rev Mol Diagn.* 2004;4:251).
   b. **Helicobacter pylori.** Although the genome of *H. pylori* is remarkable for the polymorphism between different clinical isolates, PCR-based methods have nonetheless been developed that permit successful detection of virtually all reported forms of *H. pylori* by PCR from either fresh or FFPE tissue, including the nonculturable coccoid form. The most common target loci in PCR assays include the 16S rRNA gene, urease gene, or arbitrary regions chosen empirically based on their utility. Recently developed real-time Q-PCR methods that target the 23S rRNA gene permit simultaneous detection of *H. pylori* and antibiotic-resistant testing.
   c. **Other bacterial pathogens.** PCR has been used to detect *Bacillus anthracis* organisms in patient specimens associated with bioterrorism or accidental environmental release from bioweapons facilities (*J Clin Microbiol.* 2002;40:4360).

2. **Fungi.** Most PCR assays target sequences within the fungal rRNA genes. PCR can be performed using universal primers that bind to highly conserved sequences in the region, followed by direct or indirect DNA sequence analysis of the PCR product to identify the specific fungal pathogen. Alternatively, sequence differences in the 18S rRNA gene can be used to design primers that are specific for individual fungal pathogens. Sequence polymorphisms of the mitochondrial large subunit rRNA gene have also been used as a target in PCR tests to identify fungal pathogens in tissue specimens, and Q-PCR methods have also been developed for detection of fungal pathogens in tissue specimens.

3. **Viruses**
   a. **HPV.** Most PCR protocols for HPV testing make use of consensus primers targeted to the viral L1 gene that are potentially capable of detecting all HPV types that affect the anogenital region. Following amplification using consensus primers, the HPV type can be determined by either DNA sequence analysis or membrane hybridization with type-specific probes. However, both approaches are labor intensive and difficult to automate, which makes them poorly suited for screening a large volume of patient specimens. For this reason, HPV testing of cytology specimens is usually performed using liquid-based methodologies (as is discussed in more detail in the cytopathology section of Chap. 34).
   b. **Hepatitis C virus (HCV).** RT-PCR methods used to detect HCV in liver biopsy specimens focus on the 5′ noncoding region of the virus that is highly conserved between the (at least) six genotypes and more than 90 subtypes of HCV that have been described worldwide. Maximal RT-PCR test sensitivity can only be achieved via a nested RT-PCR approach, or when the PCR products are evaluated by Southern blot hybridization.
   c. **Epstein–Barr virus (EBV).** A Q-PCR methodology has been described that targets five highly conserved segments of the EBV genome (*J Mol Diagn.*

2004;6:378). The method can be applied to FFPE tissue, but maximum test sensitivity is only obtained when analysis involves all five marker loci.

d. **Respiratory viruses.** Although PCR assays have been developed for many individual viruses, a multiplex RT-PCR assay for seven common respiratory viruses (specifically, adenovirus, influenza types A and B, respiratory syncytial virus, and parainfluenza types 1 to 3) is one of the most efficient molecular approaches thus far described (*J Mol Diagn.* 2004;6:125). The multiplex assay not only has a specificity of 100% for each viral pathogen, but also has sensitivity for each virus that is superior to either direct immunofluorescent antibody staining alone or antibody staining combined with viral culture.

A nested RT-PCR assay has been described for detection of the coronavirus responsible for severe acute respiratory syndrome (SARS) (*Am J Clin Pathol.* 2004;121:574). The method can be applied to FFPE tissue from both open-lung biopsies and necropsy specimens, a feature of the assay that is important given the virulence of the pathogen. The rapidity and simplicity of the approach make it ideally suited for diagnosis given the epidemiology of SARS outbreaks.

4. **Protozoans**

a. **Toxoplasmosis.** Several different PCR-based assays (for use with either fresh or FFPE tissue) have been developed for detection of *Toxoplasma gondii*, the etiologic agent of toxoplasmosis. The assays have clinical utility because serologic diagnosis of active infection is unreliable since IgM levels do not correlate with recent infection, and since reactivation of disease is not always accompanied by changes in antibody levels.

b. **Leishmaniasis.** A number of different loci serve as targets in PCR-based tests for leishmaniasis, including repetitive nuclear DNA sequences, genes encoding rRNA, and kinetoplast DNA. In fact, PCR utilizing primers that amplify a 120-bp fragment of kinetoplast DNA has a higher sensitivity than all other diagnostic methods that have been evaluated, including serologic testing, microbiologic culture, routine histopathologic evaluation, and immunohistochemical staining.

c. **Intestinal parasites.** A nested PCR that targets the gene encoding the small subunit rRNA gene of microsporidia has been described that can be used with fresh tissue for species-specific detection of four different pathogenic microsporidia; since different pathogenic microsporidia can have different sensitivities to antimicrobial agents, testing provides an opportunity to establish the diagnosis as well as direct therapy. PCR targeted to genes encoding 18S rRNA or oocyst wall proteins can be used to document infection with *Cryptosporidium*.

F. **Identity determination.** Although the advantages of DNA-based identification analysis have been most widely publicized in forensics and parentage studies, this testing also has a role in the routine practice of surgical pathology including resolution of specimen identity issues (*Am J Clin Pathol.* 2011;135:132), differentiation of synchronous and metachronous tumors from metastases, evaluation of tumors in transplant recipients, evaluation of bone marrow engraftment, diagnosis of hydatidiform moles (e-**Fig. 60.11**), and demonstration of natural chimerism.

PCR-based approaches for DNA typing have greatly expanded the range of testing because they require such small amounts of DNA and can be performed on fresh, fixed, or even partially degraded specimens. Virtually all DNA typing is currently performed on the basis of a core set of STR loci chosen by the Federal Bureau of Investigation of the United States for use in a national database of convicted felons known as the Combined DNA Index System (CODIS).

Commercial kits for either monoplex or multiplex PCR amplification of CODIS loci have greatly simplified STR typing and made the method accessible to most molecular genetic laboratories.

SUGGESTED READINGS

Leonard DGB. *Molecular Pathology in Clinical Practice*. New York: Springer; 2006.

Pfeifer JD. *Molecular Genetic Testing in Surgical Pathology*. Philadelphia: Lippincott Williams & Wilkins; 2006.

Rudin N, Inman K, eds. *An Introduction to Forensic DNA Analysis*. 2nd ed. Boca Raton: CRC Press; 2002.

Strachan T, Read AP. *Human Molecular Genetics*. 4th ed. London: Garland Science; 2010.

61 Microarrays

Mark Watson

I. **INTRODUCTION.** Nucleic acid microarrays are an ordered arrangement of DNA molecules (*probes* or *features*) on a solid surface. A sample of DNA or RNA derived from cells or tissue (*target*) is then hybridized to the array to quantify the level of nucleic acid corresponding to each probe. Microarrays can be utilized for a number of different experimental and clinical applications (Fig. 61.1).

A. **Array comparative genomic hybridization (aCGH).** This microarray-based assay is used to compare genome copy numbers between biospecimens. Often, a patient tumor DNA sample is directly compared with a corresponding nonmalignant or germline DNA sample from the same individual to assess quantitative changes in a tumor genome. This approach is routinely used in clinical molecular diagnostics and provides a higher-resolution complement to more traditional cytogenetic and fluorescent in situ hybridization (FISH) assays.

B. **Genotyping.** Microarray technology can be used to assay single nucleotide polymorphism (SNP) genotypes or copy number variation (CNV) across 1 to 2 million genomic loci in a single DNA sample. This approach is useful for identifying correlations between phenotype and genotype in familial linkage or genome-wide association (population-based) studies and can be used clinically to identify CNV polymorphisms associated with inherited or constitutional traits.

C. **Sequencing.** Sequencing by hybridization utilizes microarray technology to determine the complete nucleotide sequence of a DNA target, usually 100 to 300 kilobases in length. Unlike conventional sequencing chemistry using capillary gel electrophoresis, the target sequence need not be a contiguous stretch of DNA, but may consist of a set of regions of diagnostic relevance distributed throughout the genome.

D. **Genome tiling.** Very high density microarray designs contain nucleotide probes with 10 to 35 nucleotides spaced across the entire genome. These high-resolution probe arrays allow for identification of methylation and DNA–protein binding patterns at the single nucleotide level.

E. **Gene expression.** By hybridizing cellular RNA to microarrays with probes directed to mRNA or microRNA (miRNA) targets, it is possible to perform qualitative (i.e., detection of alternative splicing) and quantitative gene expression analysis simultaneously on 30,000 to 50,000 genes from a single-RNA specimen. Measurement of transcript abundance (i.e., gene expression profiling) has been the most common use of microarray technology in investigative and diagnostic pathology to date.

II. **MICROARRAY TECHNOLOGY.** Nucleic acids microarrays are fabricated using several different technologies and probe types, depending upon the intended application (Fig. 61.1).

A. **Bacterial artificial chromosome (BAC) arrays.** BAC-cloned DNA is deposited onto a solid surface (usually a glass microscope slide) by a robotic, mechanical spotting device. Each BAC clone represents a large stretch of genomic DNA from a specific chromosomal region, usually several hundred kilobases in length. BAC arrays have been particularly useful in assessing genome-wide DNA copy number changes in tumor specimens, and when employed in a CGH have enhanced the resolution of traditional cytogenetic studies. Validated BAC arrays

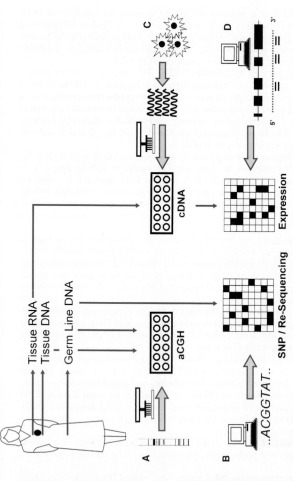

Figure 61.1 Microarray applications and technology. Microarray technology can be used for many different applications, depending upon the nucleic acid composition of the array (probes) and the test material (target) that is hybridized to it. **A:** For aCGH assays, fragments of genomic DNA (i.e., BACs) are spotted as probes onto the microarray surface using robotics. Genomic DNA from the patient's tissue and germ line are then cohybridized to the array to identify regions of chromosomal gain or loss. **B:** Alternatively, genomic DNA sequence can be used to computationally design oligonucleotide probes that detect specific alterations in DNA samples (either germ line or tissue) for either SNP genotyping or DNA resequencing studies. **C:** cDNA clones generated from cellular RNA also can be spotted as probes onto the microarray and patient tissue RNA subsequently hybridized to quantify relative mRNA transcript abundance for gene expression profiling experiments. **D:** Similarly, oligonucleotides can be designed based upon known gene exon structure and spotted on the array surface to perform quantitative or qualitative assessment of mRNA or miRNA expression.

are used in a number of clinical laboratories, although compared with newer, oligonucleotide-based platforms, they suffer from poor resolution and require a sufficient laboratory infrastructure to grow and maintain BAC libraries which are used to generate the DNA probes. BAC arrays have been largely supplanted by oligonucleotide arrays for these reasons.

B. **cDNA microarrays.** Some of the earliest microarray designs utilized cDNA probes. Messenger RNA (mRNA) from a defined tissue or cell source is converted into a double stranded cDNA clone library. Plasmid DNA from each clone is then spotted onto the microarray surface. Genome sequence information is not necessarily required for microarray design, a particular advantage for studying the few remaining experimental organisms where genome sequence information is not available. However, because cDNA probes correspond to relatively long stretches of transcribed mRNA, cross-hybridization and lack of specificity can often limit the accuracy of cDNA microarray results. Like BAC arrays, the effort and infrastructure necessary to grow, grow, purify, monitor quality control, and track individual cDNA clones are considerable and not easily standardized. This last constraint has and will continue to limit the use of cDNA microarrays as clinical diagnostic tools.

C. **Oligonucleotide microarrays.** The availability of the completely sequenced and annotated human genome, coupled with improved synthesis chemistries, has shifted the fabrication of nucleic acid microarrays toward the use of synthetic oligonucleotide probes, usually 60 to 75 nucleotides in length. Probe sequences may be customized for specific genes, gene transcripts, or gene transcript segments using defined nucleic acid sequences. Sophisticated bioinformatics programs can select optimized oligonucleotide sequences for any gene or transcript of interest while minimizing cross reactivity with other sequences, and at the same time standardizing hybridization properties such as melting temperature and G/C sequence content. This level of customization has provided a new level of standardization and flexibility to the design of sequence content on nucleic acid microarrays that is aptly suited for clinical diagnostic assays.

D. **In situ synthesized microarrays.** Another strategy for microarray design involves simultaneously synthesizing specific oligonucleotide probes in situ using combinatorial photochemistry. Affymetrix GeneChip® microarrays use a series of micron-scale "masks" to direct light to specific locations on the microarray surface. Photoreactive nucleotides (A,C,G,T) are sequentially passed over the array surface in the presence of each mask. Depending upon the mask pattern, a specific nucleotide is added to the growing chain of oligonucleotides at a specific position. In this combinatorial method, the use of 25 different masks sets (A, C, G, T) in 100 sequential nucleotide addition steps can result in 4^{25} (1×10^{15}) different sequences that are simultaneously created on the array surface.

Alternate methods use a "maskless" approach for in situ probe synthesis in which a sheet composed of micron-scale electronic mirror is programmed to direct light to specific areas of the microarray during sequential steps of photochemical oligonucleotide synthesis. The method is similar to GeneChip® fabrication, but does not rely on the creation of fixed lithographic masks and therefore allows for flexible design on a single array basis.

E. **Bead arrays.** An alternate approach to traditional microarray design involves the use of a beaded microarray. In this approach, micron-sized beads, each containing a unique oligonucleotide gene sequence in tandem with a unique nucleotide address sequence, are allowed to randomly assemble onto a solid surface. By repeated interrogation of each bead address sequence, the identity of each bead at each position is deduced. The "decoded" array can then be used for its intended hybridization assay.

III. **MICROARRAY ASSAYS.** Microarray assays are complex (**e-Fig. 61.1**)*, both because of the amount of data generated and the exacting specimen requirements that are necessary to produce high quality data.

A. **Study design.** To date, most microarray-based studies have been designed as biomarker discovery experiments, with the aim of defining a panel of multiple biomarkers that can then be transitioned into a more conventional clinical assay. Microarray experiments generally fall into several classes.

1. **Class discovery.** In such studies, experimental specimens are classified based solely upon their microarray data values, and the results of the classification are reviewed to identify new, previously unappreciated clinical or pathologic classifications. Perhaps the most elegant illustration of this approach has been the reclassification of breast adenocarcinoma based upon microarray-generated gene expression profiles (*Clin Cancer Res.* 2005;11:5678). Similar studies have effectively identified other molecular subtypes of tumors as well (*J Clin Oncol.* 2006;24:5079; *N Engl J Med.* 2003;348:1777).

2. **Class distinction.** This type of study is designed to identify novel predictive biomarkers, patterns of gene expression, CNVs, or sequence alterations that demonstrate a correlation to an already known parameter such as clinical outcome or treatment response (*J Clin Oncol.* 2009;27:1160).

3. **Single sample classification.** Ultimately, to achieve clinical utility, it is necessary to create a robust molecular signature that can be prospectively applied to individual patient specimens to accurately predict clinical phenotype. Typically, a specific subset of probes on a microarray (sometimes a customized array designed for a specific diagnostic purpose) is examined and a weighted discriminate index is calculated. The resulting index provides a probability measure that a given specimen falls into a specific, predefined diagnostic category. Studies which independently validate a previously identified signature are relatively rare to date, but are obviously a critical step in transitioning any assay into routine clinical use (*Clin Cancer Res.* 2010;16:5222).

B. **Statistical considerations.** In principle, microarray data analysis is no different than evaluating whether a single biomarker demonstrates a statistically significant difference between defined sample classes using traditional statistics. By definition, a traditional significance threshold of $p = 0.05$ allows for a 5% false-positive (false discovery) rate. Therefore, when analyzing 50,000 to 2,000,000 independent biomarker values obtained by a microarray assay, as many as 100,000 values will appear to be "significant" by chance alone. To contend with this problem of multiple testing, several methods have been applied to calculate a true significance threshold when analyzing thousands of variables in relatively few numbers of samples (*Genome Biol.* 2003;4:210). Although these approaches minimize false-positive results for a given sample set, they can in no way substitute for data validation using multiple, independent sets of samples across different technology platforms and laboratories.

C. **Specimen requirements.** Because of the inherent complexity of microarray-based assays, specimen quality assurance is essential.

1. **Specimen collection.** Careful consideration must be given to specimen collection for microarray studies. While DNA and DNA methylation patterns are relatively stable and probably less sensitive to environmental conditions, the same is not true for mRNA and miRNA when targeted in microarray-based gene expression profile assays. Global changes in gene expression can occur in tissue biospecimens as a result of tissue warm ischemia time (*J Clin Oncol.* 2006;24:3763), creating artificial differences in gene expression patterns seen between specimens based on collection procedures rather than important

---

*All e-figures are available online via the Solution Site Image Bank.

clinical differences. For peripheral blood and bone marrow specimens, the method in which a specimen is collected and processed can also influence gene expression signatures (*Physiol Genomics* 2004;19:247). Finally, most tissue specimens are inherently heterogeneous collections of many cell types. Variable cellular composition between tissue specimens may lead to differences in genomic and transcriptional profiles generated from microarray assays. For example, two prostate tumor samples, one of which contains 5% neoplastic cellularity and a second which contains 70% neoplastic cellularity, may demonstrate two different gene expression signatures based simply on the content of neoplastic epithelial cells present in the tissue. Similarly, measurement of a tumor-associated change in DNA copy number will vary considerably depending upon the content of neoplastic epithelial cells. For this reason, many investigators use techniques such as laser microdissection to isolate more homogeneous cell populations for both gene expression and DNA copy number microarray analysis (see Chap. 62).

    2. Specimen processing. Generally, diagnostic surgical pathology tissue specimens are subjected to formalin fixation and paraffin embedding, a process that results in chemical cross-linking and degradation of nucleic acids. DNA extracted from formalin-fixed, paraffin-embedded (FFPE) tissue may be suitable for some microarray-based DNA analyses (*Methods Mol Biol.* 2011;724:127). However, most investigators have found that RNA derived from FFPE tissue is unsuitable for traditional gene expression microarray-based assays, although novel molecular amplification procedures and microarray platforms suggest that this may no longer be true (*J Mol Diagn.* 2011;13:48; *BMC Cancer.* 2011;11:253). Nonetheless, freshly procured, snap frozen biospecimens remain the "gold standard" for microarray analysis, particularly for RNA-based gene expression assays. Since many clinical centers do not have access to resources needed for the processing and storage of frozen samples, a number of solutions have been proposed to circumvent the limited availability of fresh-frozen biospecimens for microarray analysis (*J Mol Diagn.* 2006;8:31). Such advances enable routine prospective analysis of clinical specimens for RNA- or DNA-based microarray assays.

  D. Target preparation. To prepare samples for microarray assays, RNA or DNA derived from a tissue or cell specimen is converted into a synthetic target in the presence of labeled deoxynucleotides. In order to analyze clinical specimens containing small amounts of cellular material, such as diagnostic core or needle aspiration biopsies, most protocols for microarray target synthesis employ some method of molecular amplification including PCR, isothermal DNA polymerization, or in vitro transcription (*Br J Cancer.* 2004;90:1111).

IV. DATA ANALYSIS. Data analysis is by far the most complicated aspect of any microarray study (*Nat Rev Genet.* 2001;2:418; *BMC Bioinform.* 2005;6:115). The principal steps in microarray data analysis involve the following:

  A. Image analysis. Current microarray technology allows for laser scanning of several square centimeters of microarray surface at the resolution of micron-sized image elements. The result is a primary image data file that can be hundreds of megabytes in size. While a number of software solutions and data repositories have been developed to hold and distribute experimental microarray data, regulatory issues related to storage and transfer of data in a clinical setting have yet to be fully addressed.

    The first step in microarray analysis involves the conversion of these raw, pixilated images into numerical values that relate to hybridization signal intensity at each feature (probe). For two color arrays, the fluorescence intensity must be sequentially captured and analyzed for each emission spectrum. In other microarray platforms such as the Affymetrix GeneChip, multiple probes are used to assay for a single transcript or genomic locus and the signal from the multiple different probes must be integrated to create a single, averaged intensity value. Due to the widespread use of the Affymetrix platform, several different algorithms have been developed to translate raw hybridization data into gene expression values. Using standardized data sets, the sensitivity and specificity of each of these algorithms to detect known changes in copy number between samples have been evaluated at length.

B. Normalization. Once image data have been converted into numerical values for each probe or probe set represented on the array, the composite set of data is usually normalized to a reference point to allow for comparison between sets of array data (e-**Fig. 61.2**). For example, inter-array normalization algorithms compensate for global differences in the signal intensity between arrays. Inter-gene normalization algorithms are useful for identifying common patterns of gene expression between study samples, even when absolute gene expression values are considerably different. Other types of data transformation techniques, such as log transformation of two-color signal ratios, may also be appropriate depending upon the nature of the primary microarray data set.

C. Visualization and data reduction. After normalization, data must be visualized and statistically analyzed to address a specific research question (e-**Fig. 61.2**). There are a number of relatively standard methods in which voluminous and multidimensional microarray data may be visualized.

1. **Hierarchical clustering.** Samples are organized based upon their similarity in gene marker values, and genes are organized based upon their similarity across samples. Several different measures of similarity can be used and several different algorithms can be applied to perform the clustering, and no particular algorithm can be considered to be the gold standard. In fact, while hierarchical clustering is a useful tool to provide a manageable view of immense data sets, it does not necessarily impart any underlying "truth" to microarray data.

2. **Heat maps.** A colorimetric representation of numerical data, usually presented in combination with hierarchical clustering. This visualization scheme provides a convenient method to identify patterns or blocks of similarity between gene markers and/or samples.

3. ***k*-means clustering** and **principal components analysis (PCA).** These data reduction methods are particularly useful for reducing the level of microarray data complexity. A large number of variables (i.e., microarray probe values) are placed into a finite number of "bins" based upon their similarity of values across a much smaller number of observations (i.e., target samples). The number of bins created (the "k" in k-means) can be adjusted to create a much smaller set of similar, collective values which can then be used as the basis for further analysis.

   In PCA, samples are plotted in "gene marker space" where the distance between samples in this space is related to their similarity based upon gene marker values. However, for a 47,000-element microarray, gene marker space is represented in 47,000 different dimensions. Therefore, the goal of principal component analysis is to reduce 47,000 dimensions into two to three principal components. Then, relatedness between samples can be plotted.

D. Annotation. A final significant challenge in data analysis is to determine how patterns of gene expression can be related to biologically meaningful results. As annotation and understanding of the human genome continue to improve, investigators have been able to classify a large number of human genes into ontologies based on function, cellular location, and structural determinants. Several software programs are available that can map lists of biomarkers to these ontologies, which often results in a clearer view of altered biologic processes associated with differential gene expression. For single cellular and simple multicellular organisms, this approach has led to sophisticated models for cell signaling and transcriptional regulatory networks, whereas for humans this type of analysis is still evolving.

E. **Validation.** Like any other diagnostic test, the results of a microarray assay must be validated through independent testing. Validation of microarray assays is particularly problematic for many reasons. First, microarray assays are relatively expensive ($200 to $800 per sample), which creates financial constraints on the number of samples that can be analyzed. Second, given the stringent specimen requirements needed to perform most microarray assays, availability of suitable specimens is often limiting. Finally, as discussed above, the large number of variables associated with a microarray data set requires that a relatively large number of observations (e.g., samples) must be analyzed to create any degree of statistical confidence. To perform data validation for microarray results in the face of these limitations, investigators have devised a number of approaches (*Expert Rev Mol Diagn.* 2003;3:587).

1. **Cross validation.** One of the most popular approaches for data validation is sequential sampling or "leave-one-out" cross validation analysis in a single sample set. In an analysis of N study samples, $N - 1$ samples are used for the initial statistical analysis to identify groups of signature genes. The ability of these genes to correctly classify the Nth sample is then calculated and the gene list modified, discarding biomarkers that perform poorly and solidifying those with the best performance. This process is repeated, removing all N samples, one at a time, until a list of genes with the best class prediction score is created. The advantage of this method is that no additional data or experimentation is needed for validation. However, because the cross-validation is still applied to a single set of samples (i.e., the "test" and "validation" sets are one in the same), the ability to generalize conclusions to independent or larger sample sets may still be limited.

2. **Sample set splitting.** If an initial microarray sample set is large enough, it is also possible to divide the experiment into independent sets of test data and validation data. In this scheme, patterns of "significant" gene expression are identified using the first set of samples, and patterns are validated in a second set of arrays. Although this approach utilizes two truly independent data sets, it necessarily limits the number of independent samples available for the discovery phase and validation phase. The desire to split a limited number of samples into test and validation sets raises the question of sample size requirement for performing microarray analyses with sufficient statistical power (*Physiol Genomics.* 2003;16:24). While multiple methods have been proposed to calculate required sample sizes, the number of samples required will ultimately depend upon the expected biologic effect. For example, relatively few study samples may be necessary to identify fundamental genomic differences between acute myelogenous leukemia (AML) and acute lymphocytic leukemia (ALL), as these tumor cell types are biologically very distinct. On the other hand, a considerably larger study set may be required to identify reliable differences in molecular signatures associated with clinical outcome within ALL patients if the intrinsic biologic basis for patient outcome is more subtle (*BMC Med Genomics.* 2011;4:31).

3. **Meta-analyses.** Microarray data results can be validated using multiple, independent study data sets. As an increasing number of microarray studies are published and corresponding data sets are made publicly available in microarray data repositories, it has become increasingly possible to validate patterns of gene expression identified in one experiment using other microarray experiments in the published literature (*PLoS Med.* 2008;5:e184). In fact, meta-analyses of microarray data are becoming more frequent, and while some studies have shown that significant patterns of gene expression can be

validated in experiments conducted by independent investigators (*N Engl J Med.* 2006;355:560), other such analyses have demonstrated clear differences between studies (*J Natl Cancer Inst.* 2005;97:927).

V. CLINICAL APPLICATIONS. Microarray technology was initially utilized primarily for basic science studies that involved whole genome analyses to identify novel biomarkers or elucidate biologic signaling pathways. However, as this technology has evolved, nucleic acid microarrays are now being utilized as a clinical diagnostic platform.

A. Gene expression profiling as an ancillary diagnostic tool for the pathologist. Perhaps one of the most useful applications of gene expression microarray technology has been its use in the diagnosis of histologically ambiguous tumor specimens. Gene expression profiles can molecularly define the cell lineage of metastases of unknown origin (particularly adenocarcinoma) with 80% to 90% accuracy based upon thorough retrospective analysis of clinical data (*Expert Rev Mol Diagn.* 2010;10:17). Gene expression data can also be used to discriminate histologic "look-alikes" with distinct cell origins, such as small round blue cell tumors (*Nat Med.* 2001;7:673). Of greater interest are results demonstrating that molecular profiling can subclassify histologically indistinguishable tumors into biologically relevant subtypes. The first study to define this principle was conducted in diffuse large B-cell lymphoma, where gene expression patterns clearly segregate tumors with aggressive and indolent molecular profiles that also have significance for patient survival (*N Engl J Med.* 2003;348:1777). Gene expression profiles of invasive ductal breast carcinoma can also clearly define "basal-cell" and "luminal cell" tumor types (among others) that have unique biologic characteristics and therapeutic response profiles (*Clin Cancer Res.* 2005;11:5678). An even more intriguing application of microarray-based molecular profiling involves complete tumor reclassification based not on anatomic site or histopathologic features, but by patterns or modules of gene expression (*Cancer Res.* 2008;68:369). Given that the phenotypic behavior of tumor cells and their response to molecular therapies may be more dependent upon molecular profiles than organ site of origin, this approach has the potential to significantly modify the role of pathology and the practice of clinical oncology.

B. Predicting disease behavior. Gene expression profiles of primary tumor samples have been used to develop predictive signatures of local and distant metastasis, for both specific and more global tumor types (*Cancer Genomics Proteomics.* 2007;4:211). Further clinical validation of such signatures could, for example, define a new diagnostic category of "lymph node potential positive" tumors which might play an equal if not more important role than traditional histopathology for staging cancer patients and therapeutic decision making.

C. Predicting survival. Several large clinical studies have identified gene expression signatures that predict patient survival in breast cancer, lung cancer, leukemia, lymphoma, and many other tumor types. While results from these studies are usually individually validated using statistical methodology or through independent training and test patient populations, an increasingly worrisome finding is that clinically predictive gene expression signatures are not reproducible across multiple studies of the same tumor type (*PLoS Med.* 2008;5:e34). Proposed explanations for these discordant findings include the use of differing and nonstandardized microarray platforms, the examination of patient cohorts that are not matched for clinical and treatment parameters, and the relatively complex phenotype of survival which is dependent upon many variables in addition to tumor molecular signatures.

D. Predicting therapeutic response. In the context of neoadjuvant chemotherapy trials, gene expression microarray analyses of pretreatment tumor biopsy specimens have been used to develop predictive signatures of treatment response

(*Clin Cancer Res. 2005*;11:5678). To date, these studies have been small and retrospective. However, the ability to use tumor gene expression data to prospectively manage patient treatment will be an important step toward the concept of personalized medicine.

E. **Nontumor pathology.** Microarray technology has been applied to biomarker discovery in other fields of pathology and clinical medicine such as neuropathology (Alzheimer disease, Parkinson disease, epilepsy, schizophrenia), immunopathology (systemic lupus, multiple sclerosis), organ transplantation, reproductive endocrinology, trauma and sepsis, and cardiovascular disease. However, in multiorgan disease processes, the appropriate target cell population for study is often not obvious, or often difficult to obtain from a large number of patients. Therefore, many microarray studies focusing on noncancer disease processes have been limited to very small sample sizes. Known and unknown variability within these disease processes and between patient participants makes it difficult to establish definitive associations between patterns of gene expression and disease phenotype.

F. **Genotyping.** DNA sequence alterations, either single nucleotide polymorphisms (SNPs) present in germline DNA or somatic point mutations which occur in tumor cells, are important diagnostic markers for disease predisposition, diagnosis, and treatment. Microarray technology is a high-throughput method for genotyping individuals at as many as one million loci across the genome, and is beginning to have enormous implications in clinical genetics. For example, familial linkage studies designed to identify inherited disease genes associated with tumor syndromes have greatly benefited from this technology. Microarray-based genotyping has also been used in genetic association studies to define loci associated with disease predisposition and clinical phenotype. Although most applications of genotyping microarrays have been used to discover a single disease locus of interest, it is likely that complex multigenic diseases will require genotyping at multiple loci in order to accurately classify a genetic phenotype.

G. **Genome copy number.** Another major application of microarray technology involves assessment of genome copy number (*Nature. 2008*;452:553). Tumor cells experience a wide variety of chromosomal gains and losses, and while these events have been traditionally measured using cytogenetic techniques, microarrays are becoming an increasingly useful method to correlate gene copy number changes with clinical and pathologic features of tumors. Microarray-based gene copy number assessment has been used to define critical regions, and even single genes, whose gain or loss has previously been measured only on the scale of chromosome arm losses or gains, which has led to the rapid identification of new oncogenes and tumor suppressor genes. Microarray analysis of gene copy number has also identified genomic alterations that are characteristic of particular tumor types and which can be associated with clinical outcome.

Microarray analysis of gene copy number has also demonstrated that the germline genome of normal populations contains a large number of copy number polymorphisms as well (*Nat Genet. 2007*;39:S16). This normal variability in locus copy number has known significance for disease predisposition and pharmacogenomics, making the use of copy number–based microarray analysis a useful tool for patient management.

H. **Methylation.** Methylation of CpG dinucleotides occurs frequently in tumor genomes and is associated with transcriptional silencing of key tumor suppressor genes. Microarray measurement of methylation patterns has many potential applications; for example, it has allowed for whole-genome methylation profiling to distinguish subtypes of leukemia, and has made it possible to identify patterns of methylation associated with treatment response.

I. **DNA resequencing.** A final, but perhaps most promising, application of microarrays involves their use in gene resequencing. Oligonucleotide microarrays can be constructed to interrogate individual bases of DNA sequence, thus providing a method for sequencing clinical samples by hybridization. Microarrays have been designed to sequence the genomes of the SARS and HIV virus for the purposes of strain classification and predicting response to antiviral agents, respectively. In another application, investigators have developed a "MitoChip," a microarray designed to sequence the entire mitochondrial genome since specific mitochondrial mutations occur frequently in human cancer cells and therefore have become intriguing candidates for tumor biomarkers. As a final example, a microarray designed to resequence the entire p53 tumor suppressor gene has been used to predict clinical outcome and therapeutic response in patients, based on the spectrum of somatic p53 sequence alterations in their primary tumors; the sensitivity of this approach is >90% and, with the exception of detecting nucleotide insertions and deletions, is comparable to that of traditional dideoxy sequencing (*Breast Cancer Res Treat.* 2011;128).

Now that the cancer genome is being characterized in detail using whole genome sequencing technologies (see Chap. 60), there is compelling evidence that specific gene sequence alterations in tumors will predict vulnerability and resistance to specific therapies such as the epidermal growth factor receptor inhibitor, gefitinib (*J Clin Oncol.* 2007;25:587). As more and more clinically relevant somatic sequence alterations are identified in viruses, tumor cells, and other pathologic specimens, the ability to perform rapid resequencing of multiple genetic loci on a single clinical specimen will be an important requirement for the clinical pathology laboratory. In this respect, as compared with traditional sequencing methodologies, microarrays and the sequencing by hybridization approach could become routine clinical molecular diagnostic tools that supplement many traditional histopathologic and immunohistochemical approaches currently used to evaluate pathology specimens. Alternatively, as the cost of next-generation sequencing technology continues to fall, assays that employ quantitative RNA-sequencing or targeted genome sequencing could eventually obviate the use of any microarray technology in the clinical laboratory altogether.

VI. USE OF MICROARRAYS IN THE CLINICAL LABORATORY. While nucleic acid microarrays have been used for numerous research studies with potential clinical significance, the routine use of this technology platform in the clinical laboratory still requires several significant advancements.

A. Array content. Since the microarray format is well suited to measure multiple markers from a single sample, it is ideal for the clinical laboratory that performs prospective analysis on single clinical specimens. For discovery experiments, thousands of individual genetic markers can be simultaneously assayed, but in doing so, each marker is optimized for neither sensitivity nor specificity. In clinical testing, this may be problematic for measuring low levels or subtle alterations of gene expression, or for detecting genomic alterations that may be present in only a subset of cell populations. By designing disease-specific marker sets, optimizing hybridization conditions for each marker and placing redundant probes for each marker on the same array, it may be possible to increase the sensitivity and precision of microarray assays for clinical use, although this has only recently become a microarray design consideration. A microarray used for discovery purposes may assay 10,000 genes using a single set of probes; a similarly sized array could assay 100 genes using 100 different probe measurements. Thus, the ability to create large number of redundant probe sets and control sequences could provide a level of precision not currently available from most research-based microarrays.

B. Automation and standardization. Another potential advantage of microarray technology is that it can be highly automated and regulated, attributes that are critical for any clinical laboratory test. Newer sample preparation methods utilize single tube, "hands-off" chemistries that facilitate routine use in the clinical laboratory. Self-contained microarray cassettes, such as those manufactured by Affymetrix and other vendors, also provide an acceptable format for regulated clinical tests. Finally, as diagnostic biomarkers become more established, microarray platforms will need to evolve into clinical diagnostic tools which meet all regulatory requirements of standard clinical tests, including additional standardization and inter-laboratory assay validation, which are both now receiving appropriate attention (*Nat Biotechnol.* 2010;28:827).

C. **Assay complexity.** Microarrays are indisputably high complexity assays, and although streamlined protocols, automation, and standardized array manufacturing can mitigate some inherent technical complexity, microarray assays still remain in the domain of specialized clinical laboratories. Like most hybridization-based assays, the time required to perform microarray analysis even in its most automated format may still be three to four days. Assay turnaround time could be problematic when assay results are needed to guide immediate therapy. Finally, because microarray assays are based on signal detection by hybridization, there is an inherent limit to sensitivity as compared with amplification-based PCR detection assays.

D. **Sample requirements.** Another technical limitation of microarray assays is their requirement for high sample quality. Although exact specimen requirements depend upon the analyte measured (i.e., mRNA, genomic DNA, methylated DNA), the use of formalin-fixed tissue or other specimens that have been collected under routine hospital conditions currently limits the use of microarray technology in a number of clinical settings. Methods are available for amplifying and labeling nanogram quantities of nucleic acids samples (both DNA and RNA), so the ability to utilize small numbers of cells obtained from minimally invasive procedures such as fine needle aspiration, swabs, or lavages allows microarray-based assays to be used for diagnostics in an increasing number of different clinical scenarios. Refinements in the use of routine pathology tissue specimens that have been fixed and embedded in paraffin will allow full integration of this technology with routine histopathologic assessment.

E. **Clinical relevance.** The biggest challenge for implementing microarray technology in the clinical laboratory, however, is not array technology itself but rather the clinical validity of the array biomarker content. To date, the majority of microarray platforms have been designed as whole genome discovery tools. Studies have used a relatively small number of observations (patients) and a large number of variables (genes), an approach which has consistently led to high false-positive rates that are unacceptable for clinical assay validation. A considerable amount of microarray data generated and reported in the literature (particularly gene expression data) has not been reproducible in independent samples sets (*PLoS Med.* 2008;5:e184). Therefore, while microarray technology itself still holds promise for use in a clinical laboratory, there is a need for many larger, prospective correlative studies to support the use of microarray-based biomarker panels in routine diagnostic pathology.

62

Biospecimen Banking
Mark Watson

I. **SIGNIFICANCE TO PATHOLOGY AND TRANSLATIONAL RESEARCH.** National initiatives such as The Cancer Genome Atlas (http://cancergenome.nih.gov) and the 1,000 Genomes Project (http://www.1000genomes.org/) have greatly enhanced the resources available to better understand the molecular and genetic basis of human disease. Technologies such as gene expression profiling, methylation scanning, comparative genome hybridization, and high-throughput resequencing have also made it possible to harness genomic information to identify disease-specific molecular alterations that occur in human tissues. However, to ultimately understand the significance of basic biological findings toward the improved diagnosis and treatment of human disease, primary human biospecimens (i.e., tissue and body fluids) must be available for clinico-genomic correlative studies. Six important principles embody the rationale for biospecimen banks.

A. **Availability of large biospecimen cohorts.** The number of specimens available must be relatively large to generate statistically significant findings. For example, because of the large number of variables (e.g., gene expression values) generated from DNA microarray experiments compared to the much smaller number of observations (patients), traditional statistical approaches generate a large number of false positive results, that is, genes whose expression appears to classify subpopulations of patients but only does so by mere chance. Validating findings from such whole genome approaches requires large numbers of patient specimens.

B. **Accurately diagnosed biospecimens.** Several anecdotal examples have illustrated how gene expression profiling can correctly classify specimens that were histologically misidentified by routine clinical pathology (*Am J Pathol.* 2001;159:1231). However, initial diagnostic mislabeling can seriously impede supervised learning approaches to identify new biomarkers. In addition to issues of diagnostic accuracy, knowledge of the precise cellular makeup of specimens (particularly for heterogeneous tissues) is important to properly interpret both gene expression profile and DNA sequencing data. Techniques such as laser capture microdissection (LCM) can be used to isolate homogeneous cell populations (*Acta Histochem.* 2007;109:171), but requires considerable technical expertise. An added level of complexity in longitudinal studies is that multiple specimens collected from the same patient need to be accurately coded and tracked to ensure that the intended specimen (e.g., initial presentation vs. relapse) is used for downstream analyses.

C. **Availability of specimens with high molecular integrity.** Although genomic DNA is relatively stable and unaffected by variables in clinical specimen processing and storage, the same is not true for cellular RNA and protein. Cellular RNA and protein may be degraded in cells ex vivo, if clinical specimens are not rapidly and properly processed and stored (*Am J Clin Pathol.* 2002;118:733). More insidiously, the mRNA and protein complement of cells may rapidly change as a function of processing time and methodology (*J Clin Oncol.* 2006;10;24: 3763).

D. **Maximal utilization of diverse biospecimens.** Because of the number and diversity of potential biomarkers that can be evaluated from banked biospecimens, repositories should contain a wide variety of specimens in a format that can be distributed as widely as possible. For example, preoperative serum from cancer patients may be useful for identifying tumor-associated serum markers for early detection, while nucleated cell fractions from bone marrow, peripheral blood, or cavity washings from the same patient may be used to evaluate markers for tumor metastasis detection (Figure 62-1). Collected specimens may be rare or small in size, so strategies to efficiently consolidate specimen resources (such as tissue microarrays [TMAs]) or to molecularly amplify limiting amounts of genomic material from needle biopsies, tissue touch preps, or washings are critical to providing a useful specimen resource.

E. Biospecimen annotation. Given the cost and effort associated with next generation sequence analyses of clinical specimens (or proteomic or metabolomic analysis), molecular data associated with human biospecimens is arguably more valuable than the specimen itself. A data system that can accurately track individual samples within large clinical specimen sets and that allows for accurate integration and correlation of sequence, expression, biomarker, and clinical data is obviously crucial. A large and viable specimen resource is only useful if it is linked to complete and accurate clinical data that can be used to substantiate or refute clinical hypotheses. At the same time, increasing concerns for medical record privacy and, in particular, genetic data privacy require proper measures to protect patient confidentiality.

F. Biospecimen custodianship. There have been increasing concerns regarding ownership of tissue specimens (*Clin Chem.* 2010;56:1675) and the intellectual property that is generated from their use. There is also a continuing need to appropriately honor the intent and privacy of patient donors. This requires the establishment of an unbiased agent who can judiciously administrate and regulate the collection and distribution of specimens.

The biospecimen bank is such an integral part of medical research, and is becoming such an integral part of clinical medicine, that several national and international agencies, such as the National Cancer Institute (NCI), have created dedicated offices and guidelines for bank operation (http://biospecimens. cancer.gov). The principles of biospecimen banking obviously relate to the general practice of pathology and, therefore, it is almost exclusively the pathologist and the pathology department that have sufficient expertise to govern these activities. The development and maintenance of a biospecimen resource involves many policies and processes which are outlined in Figure 62-2, summarized in this chapter, and described in more detail elsewhere (*Br J Cancer.* 2004;90:1115; *Methods Mol Biol.* 2010;576:1).

II. BIOSPECIMEN COLLECTION. The types of biospecimens collected and the methods used to process and store them depends greatly on their projected use, although for many specimens the intended use is unknown. Since the cost associated with biospecimen procurement and storage is not insignificant ($20 to $150 per specimen), careful consideration should be given to the scope and focus of the bank's operation (*Clin Transl Sci.* 2009;2:172).

A. Defining the scope of operation. The type and number of participants from whom biospecimens are collected depends upon the stated mission and available resources of the biospecimen bank. In some cases, small banks may collect only defined specimens from participants enrolled in specific clinical trials. In other cases, the bank may be disease-based and seek to generically collect all available tissue specimens for a given disease type. When resources or institutional barriers do not permit the creation of a large centralized facility, several small banks may elect to create a federated system where each bank operates independently, but is linked by a common informatics network (*Adv Exp Med Biol.* 2006;587:65). A biospecimen bank need not be a "bank" at all, but may simply serve to collect, process, deidentify, and immediately distribute biospecimens; the Cooperative Human Tissue Network frequently operates as such a

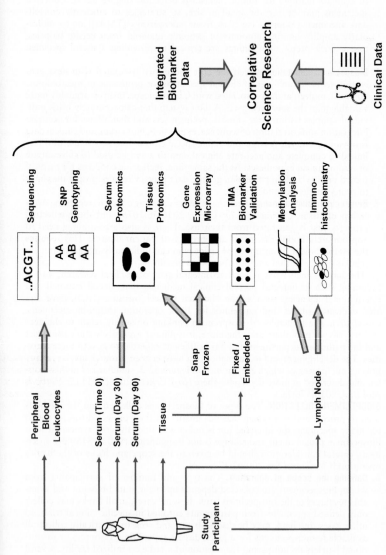

Figure 62.1 From a single participant, a biospecimen resource may collect multiple specimen types and corresponding data to enable a wide variety of translational research projects. A corresponding informatics system is often required to track and maintain these data.

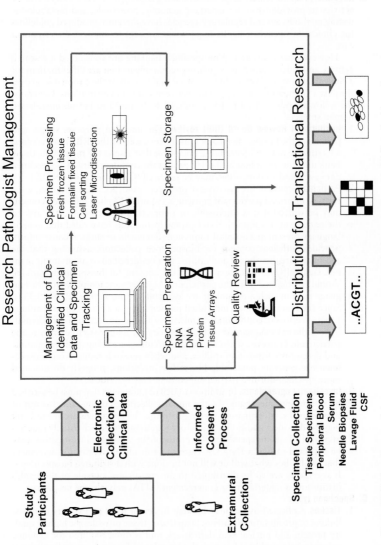

Research Pathologist Management

Management of De-Identified Clinical Data and Specimen Tracking

Specimen Processing
Fresh frozen tissue
Formalin fixed tissue
Cell sorting
Laser Microdissection

Specimen Storage

Specimen Preparation
RNA
DNA
Protein
Tissue Arrays

Quality Review

Distribution for Translational Research

..ACGT..

Electronic Collection of Clinical Data

Informed Consent Process

Specimen Collection
Tissue Specimens
Peripheral Blood
Serum
Needle Biopsies
Lavage Fluid
CSF

Study Participants

Extramural Collection

Figure 62.2 Flow diagram of the many processes and resources required to operate a typical full service biospecimen resource

tissue broker (*Cancer Epidemiol Biomarkers Prev.* 2009;18:1676). A biospecimen bank may also simply exist as a more formal representation of diagnostic paraffin block specimens already available in the pathology department.

B. Regulatory requirements. Biospecimen banking is going to be a necessary ancillary activity to provide tissue for emerging genomic, proteomic, and metabolomic testing methods. Several regulatory agencies have therefore produced guidelines for clinical biospecimen banks (e.g., www.cap.org) to support direct patient care.

However, many aspects of biospecimen banking are considered a research activity and must conform to regulatory requirements that are different than for a clinical laboratory. Policies have evolved significantly at the national level over the past 5 years, and also vary greatly between states and institutions. Generally, the following points need to be considered with regard to biospecimen-based human subjects' research.

1. Institutional Review Board (IRB) review. The intended purpose, scope, and policies of the biospecimen bank must be reviewed by the IRB. In some cases, a Certificate of Confidentiality, a document that asserts the right of the tissue bank director (or honest broker) to protect the confidentiality of biospecimen data even under court order, may be required (*Genet Test.* 2004:8:209).

2. Participant consent. In most cases of prospective biospecimen collection, some form of informed participant consent is required. Explicit informed consent may be waived if it is impossible or impractical to obtain and the risk to the participant is minimal. Rarely, some institutions have ruled that generic language present in a hospital admissions document or surgical consent form provides sufficient consent for biospecimen collection, assuming that the specimens are distributed and utilized in a de-identified or anonymous manner. Generally, however, explicit written consent for biospecimen banking should be obtained from the participant. Many generic templates for the language used in such a document are available (*J Clin Pathol.* 2006;59:335). Since the main risk to an individual participating in a biospecimen banking program is loss of confidentiality, measures used to protect such confidentiality and the risks associated with this loss are the main risks to convey to the participant. However, when human biospecimens are being used for genomic and disease-predisposition studies, and when research results from biospecimen use generate patentable biomarker inventions, properly documented more specific informed participant consent may be critical.

3. Investigator agreements. In addition to IRB requirements that must be satisfied by the biospecimen bank for the initial collection, coding, and storage of biospecimens, investigators seeking to utilize biospecimens from the bank may need to meet additional regulatory requirements, which usually requires approval of an independent IRB protocol. In addition, investigators may be expected to sign a Data Use Agreement or other investigator agreement that establishes what will or will not be done with distributed biospecimens. If specimens are to be distributed to an investigator outside of the bank's institution, a material transfer agreement (MTA) may also be necessary.

C. Specimen types

1. Tissues. Collected tissues may be snap-frozen or fixed in a variety of cross-linking or precipitating fixatives. Snap frozen tissue provides the highest quality protein and nucleic acid derivatives, and is often required for genomic or proteomic studies. However, the logistics of frozen tissue collection are difficult and proper storage is relatively expensive. Formalin-fixed, paraffin embedded (FFPE) tissue blocks are easy to obtain, easy to store, and very familiar to any pathology service. The quality of molecular derivatives from such tissues is vastly inferior, although several recent technical advances allow FFPE tissue to be used for the generation of DNA sequence and RNA expression data (*PLoS One.* 2011;11;6:e17163; *J Mol Diagn.* 2011;13: 325). Fixation of tissue in precipitating fixatives such as ethanol, acetone, and others (*Mod Pathol.* 2001;14:116; *Diagn Mol Pathol.* 2011;20:52), followed by embedding in low temperature polymers (*J Mod Diagn.* 1999;1:17), provides tissue with excellent histologic detail and molecular material that is superior to that of traditional FFPE tissue (**e-Fig. 62.1**).* However, RNA and protein quality still do not match that of material derived from frozen tissue.

2. **Blood components.** Serum and plasma (often collected at multiple time points throughout a patient's clinical course) are often banked. They are the preferred biospecimen for proteomic analysis, but when properly aliquoted from multiple patients from multiple time points, can occupy a large amount of storage space. Peripheral blood leukocytes are the ideal source for germline DNA, and can be stored or processed without the need for additional cell separation protocols such as mononuclear cell isolation. Bone marrow may also be banked, particularly for analysis involving hematologic malignancies, other bone marrow dyscrasias, or occult tumor cell detection.

3. **Other body fluids.** Urine, sputum, cavity lavages, and effusions serve as useful analytes. However, large fluid volume specimens (such as urine) may be difficult and expensive to process and store for long periods of time, particularly for a future unknown use. Furthermore, analysis of such biospecimens may require only a small amount of material per assay, which then necessitates that collections be excessively aliquoted to prevent multiple freeze/thaw cycles of the same specimen. As an alternative, the cellular component of these fluids may be isolated by centrifugation and stored as cell pellets.

D. **Collection methods.** Depending on the biospecimen type and its intended application, there are a number of important considerations involved in collecting specimens for a biospecimen bank.

1. **Specimen acquisition.** For most general tissue bank activities, tissue specimens are collected in the course of routine treatment, such as a surgical resection of a solid tumor, a therapeutic needle aspiration to remove joint or body cavity fluid, or a diagnostic bone marrow biopsy. In these cases, it is important that biospecimen collection for research purposes do not compromise the diagnostic utility of the specimen. In many cases, such as the resection of a small breast tumor or malignant prostate gland, it is important that biospecimen procurement occur under the direct guidance of a pathologist who can supervise and assure that diagnostic integrity (e.g., an intact tumor margin) is not compromised. In cases where the diagnostic tissue specimen is limiting, properly supervised ex vivo sampling by core needle biopsy instrument or skin punch may be used to acquire sufficient material for research without compromising the diagnostic specimen. Other protocols may allow for redundant tissue sampling at the time of a diagnostic procedure; for example, for a patient with a suspicious liver mass, standard of care may dictate that two specimens from a CT-guided needle biopsy be submitted for diagnostic evaluation, while two additional needle cores may be taken for the research tissue bank. In certain cases, the research bank may receive tissue samples that harbor clinically relevant diagnostic findings that are not present in the routinely processed tissue samples; for this reason, every pathology department will need to develop policies regarding clinical versus research specimen collection, which may include holding all research specimens in escrow until a final clinical diagnosis is rendered. Finally, an IRB-approved study protocol may require the collection of biospecimens above and beyond what is needed for routine standard of care; for example, a tissue biopsy or peripheral

---

*All e-figures are available online via the Solution Site Image Bank.

blood specimen collected before and at multiple time points after a course of therapy.

2. **Biospecimen preservation.** For molecular and genomic analyses, proper tissue preservation is critical. A specimen's molecular profile (i.e., gene expression, protein phosphorylation) can rapidly change from the time it is first collected until the time when it is ultimately preserved by freezing or fixation (*J Clin Oncol.* 2006;10;24:3763) due to so-called "warm ischemia time". Although few evidence-based guidelines exist, warm ischemia time should be limited and at least documented so as not to introduce additional preanalytical variability. Although snap-frozen tissue is the preferred substrate for many studies, several commercial and "home-brew" tissue preservatives are available that provide acceptable biospecimen preservation (*BMC Genomics.* 2004;5:88). Delays in blood processing can affect proteomic biomarker profiles (*Expert Rev Proteomics.* 2006;3:409); unlike tissue, whole blood cannot be immediately snap frozen, but must be centrifuged to remove the specific plasma or serum component which then, in turn, must be aliquoted and rapidly frozen. As with tissue, a number of commercial products are available to preserve blood cell components at ambient temperature without freezing, although these products are relatively expensive and require specialized downstream isolation procedures (*Cytometry A.* 2004;59:191; *Physiol Genomics.* 2004;19:247).

3. **Remote site collection.** For multi-institutional research protocols, it may be necessary to collect biospecimens from remote sites, often from health centers or medical offices which have little experience in dealing with intricate biospecimen requirements such as snap-frozen tissue. Proper and efficient collection of biospecimens from such sites may require preassembled specimen procurement kits (e-**Fig. 62.2**) and personnel training to ensure the uniform collection of biospecimens.

4. **Specimen quantity.** New molecular amplification strategies such as PCR, whole genome amplification, and transcript amplification allow investigators to use nanogram quantities of DNA and RNA for analysis. Instrumentation for proteomic analysis has also become considerably more advanced and, although it is not possible to amplify protein analytes from biospecimens, tissue requirements have been minimized even for these technologies. Therefore, even limited size biospecimens such as needle aspirates, tissue touch preps, and core biopsies are valuable and frequently amenable to molecular analyses. Obviously, however, such specimens must be judiciously distributed to maximize their research potential. Conversely, the collection of large tissue specimens is not necessarily desirable; for example, large resected carcinoma specimens are often not properly preserved when fixed or frozen in their entirety. For such cases, tissue specimens should be divided into samples no >1 cm^3 for fixation and/or freezing.

5. **Associated data collection.** Clinical and pathologic data corresponding to the patient and specimen (for clinical applications), and the participant and specimen (for research applications), are as important as the specimen itself. Without these associated data, the utility of the specimens for clinical or correlative studies is lost. The scope of the data that are collected and stored with the biospecimen will depend upon the mission of the biospecimen bank. It is usually impractical to gather detailed clinical information represented as written notes in a clinical chart or report; instead, it may be more efficient to rely on electronic sources of data. Although data are usually represented in text format, surgical pathology reports provide an accurate and detailed source of pathology information for tissue specimens that are collected and diagnosed as part of routine clinical care. In some centers, an electronic medical record may provide access to basic patient demographics and clinical

diagnostic data. For cancer patients and their specimens, the hospital tumor registry is often a reasonably detailed and standardized source for cancer-related clinical and pathology data. Except for specific studies, it is generally advisable to collect a limited but standardized data set corresponding to each collected case, rather than an exhaustive (and inevitably incomplete) data set for every specimen.

E. **Biospecimen data management.** As depicted in Figure 62.1, biospecimen banks may house a complex array of specimens and associated data. It is critical that specimens be accurately tracked and annotated if they are to be useful (*Cancer Inform.* 2008;6:127). While smaller banks may rely on written log books and electronic spreadsheets to track specimen information, these methods become rapidly constraining as the bank becomes larger and more diversified. Basic data types that may be required in a biospecimen bank information system include the following:

1. **Receipt, study association, and consent tracking.** An accurate record must be maintained of when and from where biospecimens were received, and whether they are intended for clinical or research use. For the latter, the intended protocol must also be recorded, as well as the consent under which the specimens were collected, since the consent likely regulates how the specimens may be used.

2. **Inventory and storage.** It is important to accurately maintain the availability and storage location of every specimen so that it can be rapidly retrieved on demand.

3. **Quality assurance.** Quality assurance measures such as tissue histology review, warm ischemia time, details of specimen processing, and nucleic acid quality should be maintained for each specimen.

4. **Clinical annotation.** As discussed above, a minimal set of clinical and pathology annotation data should be associated with each specimen.

5. **Distribution and utilization.** The efficacy of a biospecimen bank is judged almost entirely upon its distribution of biospecimens for clinical testing or productive translational research. Therefore, detailed data concerning specimen distribution is essential in justifying the activity and operation of the bank.

   Several commercial software packages are available to assist in the management of biospecimen banks. More frequently, individual centers develop their own data systems, often creating rather arbitrary and custom data schemes and data definitions. While such applications may serve the immediate needs of the bank, they present a significant obstacle to collaboration among different biospecimen resource centers. To address this challenge, the NCI's Cancer Biomedical Informatics Grid (caBIG) program has fostered a group of pathologists, biologists, and informatics specialists working to develop data standards and tools for pathology and biospecimen resources (https://cabig.nci.nih.gov/workspaces/TBPT). Among these tools is the caTissue software application, a freely available web-based tool for managing biospecimen inventory (https://cabig.nci.nih.gov/tools/catissuesuite).

III. **BIOSPECIMEN PROCESSING.** The same principles of specimen processing used in the clinical laboratory apply to biospecimens banked for clinical and/or research purposes. However, since specimens collected for research purposes may be used for experimental studies that are not a part of traditional diagnostic histopathology, special specimen processing needs must be considered.

A. **Frozen tissue.** Although the histologic quality of frozen tissue is inferior to that of FFPE tissue, most molecular studies require high grade DNA, RNA, and protein that can only be obtained from frozen specimens. Tissue may be frozen in liquid nitrogen, an isopentane cryobath (such as is available in most pathology frozen section rooms), or a make-shift dry ice ethanol bath. Tissue specimens should be no >1 cm^3 to ensure rapid and consistent freezing throughout the specimen. If the specimen is to be used for histologic sectioning for quality review or laser microdissection (LM), it may first be embedded in freezing media such as optimal cutting temperature (OCT) compound. Since OCT material does not interfere with nucleic acid isolation, but may have an effect on proteomic studies, it may be advisable to freeze both embedded and nonembedded tissue for the widest range of downstream uses. Once frozen, tissue may be stored in cassettes in −80° ultralow freezers or liquid nitrogen (LN$_2$) vapor inventory systems. While the latter is more expensive and difficult to maintain, specimens stored in LN$_2$ are immune to the power failures and mechanical breakdowns that can occur with electric freezers. Any frozen storage system should be equipped with a temperature recording device to document appropriate storage conditions and a remote alarm system that can contact the laboratory supervisor in the event of machine failure or power loss.

B. Fixed tissue. FFPE tissue specimens are not as well suited for molecular and genomic analyses as frozen tissue. However, the quality of fixed tissue specimens can be improved using several quality control measures.

1. **Control and documentation of fixation and processing times.** By minimizing the time for which tissues are fixed, over-fixation (which leads to excessive antigen crosslinking and molecular degradation) can be avoided. Documentation of processing times for each specimen can remove this preanalytical variable from tissue specimens collected over different time periods or from different locations.

2. **Use of "molecularly friendly" fixatives.** Several commercially available and "home brew" precipitating fixatives preserve tissue and tissue histology while minimizing the damaging effects to protein antigens and nucleic acids, caused by cross-linking fixatives such as formalin (*Mod Pathol.* 2001;14:116; *Diagn Mol Pathol.* 2011;20:52).

3. **Vacuum storage.** Although there are no convincing data to suggest an added benefit, many biospecimen repositories recommend that paraffin tissue blocks and, more importantly, cut unstained sections, be vacuumed, sealed, and stored at 4°. The premise of this storage approach is that antigenicity and nucleic acids are protected from further degradation by both removal of oxygen and reduced temperature.

C. Blood components. For isolation and storage of serum and plasma, whole blood must be immediately spun and the appropriate liquid component removed from cellular material, aliquoted, and frozen. Processing must be performed rapidly before cell lysis and protein degradation occurs. Consortia of proteomics investigators have published recommendations on blood processing for proteomic studies (*Expert Rev Proteomics.* 2006;3:409) and while some of these guidelines are evidence based, robust guidelines have not been firmly established. Many institutions freeze whole blood at the site of collection as a convenient way to store blood for future genomic DNA isolation; however, freezing blood in glass Vacutainer tubes presents a safety hazard, requires considerably more freezer space to store, and inevitably causes cell lysis which results in DNA that is frequently lower in yield, degraded, and contaminated with heme products that can effect downstream assays. Although more labor intensive, immediate spinning of whole blood followed by selective removal, washing, aliquoting, and freezing of the buffy coat creates a high-quality specimen that is easy to store and results in higher DNA yield and quality. In some cases, it may be desirable to isolate the peripheral blood mononuclear cell (PBMC) fraction and preserve these cells; this approach has the advantage of removing peripheral blood granulocytes and preserving the monocyte fraction which can be manipulated for future uses such as flow cytometry and cell immortalization. However, viable preservation of PBMC is expensive, requires additional expertise, and is seldom necessary for simple DNA isolation. When PBMC isolation is not a consideration, whole blood may be stored at 4° for as long as 72 hours with little loss in PBMC viability (*Ann Epidemiol.* 2000;10:538).

D. **Laser microdissection.** For some types of genomic analysis, it may be desirable to have material derived from homogeneous cell populations. Laser microdissection (LM) is a method that makes it possible to use a laser to either "capture" or cut the desired cells away from surrounding tissue under direct microscopic visualization (e-**Fig. 62.3**). The isolated cells may then be used for DNA, RNA, or protein isolation for molecular analysis (*Acta Histochem.* 2007;109:171; *Methods Mol Biol.* 2005;293:187). Although LM instrumentation is expensive, and the technique is time-consuming and requires expertise, it has become routine in many biospecimen banks.

E. **Tissue microarrays.** TMAs provide another format to maximize utilization of limiting tissue specimens (*Methods Mod Med.* 103:89, 2005). TMAs are constructed by sampling one to three 0.8 mm (up to as large as 3 mm) tissue cores from a donor paraffin tissue block, and assembling them into an array of as many as 300 cores in a recipient block (e-**Fig. 62.4**). The resulting recipient block can then be sectioned as a traditional tissue block, making it possible to perform simultaneous immunohistochemistry or fluorescence in situ hybridization on each of the 300 cores on a single slide. TMAs allow researchers to easily validate patterns of biomarker expression in a large sample series using relatively inexpensive technology. Few special reagents are required and basic TMA instrumentation is relatively inexpensive, but expert review and informatics tracking of the 300 cores per slides is required. A recognized disadvantage of the TMA format is that it is prone to sampling error as only a small sample from each tissue block is incorporated into the array.

F. **Nucleic acid.** Genomic technologies have shifted requirements from fixed tissue sections to derivative nucleic acids, and so many biospecimen banks now produce DNA and RNA for research investigators. Nucleic acid can be effectively derived from frozen and fixed tissue using several standard protocols, although the quality from the later is often inferior, as discussed above. In some cases, it may be desirable to isolate nucleic acid directly from collected specimens, such as DNA from peripheral blood. Nucleic acids (RNA and DNA) are more stable once isolated and can be more conveniently stored as compared to the parent tissue or fluid. However, the initial cost and effort to generate DNA and/or RNA from every banked specimen as it is received is great, and so prospective preparation of nucleic acids should only be considered when material will be of immediate use.

IV. **QUALITY ASSURANCE.** A biospecimen resource should only provide material that is subject to rigorous quality control. In fact, one of the main reasons for a pathologist-supervised biospecimen resource is that it is pathologists who best understand the approach to and importance of clinical specimen quality control.

A. **Specimen identification.** Just as in any clinical laboratory, proper specimen labeling and identification are critical, because a biospecimen bank may store biospecimens for prolonged periods of time; maintenance of proper specimen identification is important. As biospecimen banks become subject to regulatory review as with any clinical laboratory (as noted above), they will need to implement standard clinical laboratory practices to prevent sample mislabeling including use of preprinted barcode labels, double data entry, and routine data auditing.

B. **Representative tissue sampling.** In most cases, biospecimens that are submitted for clinical diagnosis and those that are submitted to a bank are not identical. They may be collected at slightly different times or locations, or may involve sampling bias. For example, in a heterogeneous prostate tumor, a tissue biopsy banked for research may contain no neoplastic cells although the routinely processed tissue for diagnosis shows adenocarcinoma; distribution of the banked specimen under the assumption that it truly reflects the diagnostic material may result in a compromised research study. Consequently, it is important that individual biospecimens received by the bank undergo individual diagnostic review, either prospectively or prior to distribution. Such a review of tissue or cellular samples may involve confirmation of a histopathologic diagnosis as well as notation of general cellular features such as histologic preservation, tissue cellularity, and necrosis. A special circumstance arises when a novel finding or diagnosis is observed in a banked research specimen that was not reported from the material for diagnosis; resolution of such a problematic circumstance will depend upon the policies of both the IRB and pathology service, and should be documented as part of the bank's standard operating procedures.

C. **Tissue preservation and molecular integrity.** When the bank will be responsible for generating and distributing nucleic acids (DNA and RNA), it is important that molecular integrity is verified. As discussed above, the quality of nucleic acid is directly related to the manner in which the biospecimen was collected and preserved. Fixation and delays in specimen processing (warm ischemia time) can compromise nucleic acid quality as can repeated freeze/thaw cycles (**e-Fig. 62.5**). Inherent necrosis and tissue cellularity in the specimen can also affect the quality of nucleic acids. Documentation of molecular specimen quality can be accomplished by readily available (albeit often expensive) instrumentation designed for quality review of small amounts of nucleic acid, including fiberoptic spectrophotometers and capillary microelectrophoresis systems. Metrics have been developed which relate quantitative results from these instruments to expected performance in downstream applications and assays (*BMC Mol Biol.* 2007;22:8).

V. **BIOSPECIMEN UTILIZATION.** The success of any biospecimen bank is measured by the utilization of collected biospecimens. Distribution of biospecimens for patient care or funded research projects is also an important revenue source to support the larger biospecimen banking effort. Although there is often a 3 to 5 year lag phase before a new biospecimen bank is routinely utilized, while the bank is developing and maturing its collection, a fundamental principle of biospecimen banking is that the collection should be biased in favor of those biospecimens that will be used for funded research projects. Measures which can help promote the productive utilization of a biospecimen resource include the following.

A. **Advertisement of available resources.** This is best accomplished through a web-based catalog of available sources.

B. **Streamlined administrative processes.** Often, clinics and researchers are unfamiliar with procedures for requesting specimens, obtaining appropriate IRB approval, and creating necessary MTAs. Having a standardized and facilitated process for dealing with regulatory steps necessary for biospecimen banking and subsequent distribution will greatly enhance utilization of a biospecimen resource.

C. **High quality annotated specimens.** Clinical testing and translational research can only be accelerated when the biospecimens distributed are properly quality controlled and "assay ready." Minimal but sufficient clinical and/or pathology data should be supplied with each specimen in order to easily enable the correlative analysis.

D. **Facilitated and judicious distribution.** The process of case selection, specimen retrieval and processing, specimen annotation, and distribution can be time-consuming and expensive. As a biospecimen bank matures, increasing requests may overtax the bank's available resources and can result in significant delays in providing specimens. Competing interests for limited biospecimens may also become problematic as bank utilization increases. Therefore, a biospecimen bank should establish a utilization review committee so that the finite effort and physical resources of the bank can be fairly allocated to the clinical and research committees. These committees should be an unbiased representation of pathologists and scientists, with allocation decisions based on clinical necessity, scientific merit of proposed projects, investigator track record with previous requests, funding status, and likelihood that distributed biospecimens will meaningfully contribute to patient care or grant or scientific publication development.

VI. **SUPPORT.** The biospecimen bank must find its own means of financial support. Frequent sources of support include the following:

A. **Clinical activities.** Biospecimen banking to support direct patient care (i.e., for diagnosis and to direct therapy) should be compensated in a way consistent with its value. Possible mechanisms include the following:

1. **Hospitals.** The costs can be borne by hospitals, since clinical biobanking is part of the general hospital infrastructure required to support best patient care.

2. **Specific billing codes.** Clinical tissue banking can be compensated via establishment of specific billing codes that reflect the technical components (specimen handling, quality assurance, informatics, and storage) and professional components (selection of appropriate tissue, microscopic review of banked specimens) of biospecimen banking. Such codes currently do not exist.

B. **Research activities**

1. **Institutional support.** Academic institutions or departments often support the initial development and operation of a biospecimen bank, which is not surprising considering the central importance of the bank in the mission of translational research. In return, the institution expects a return on its investment in terms of the number of biospecimen-based projects, publications, and research grants that can be enabled through such a resource.

2. **Extramural funding.** Unlike traditional, hypothesis-based research grants, there are a few extramural (noninstitutional) funding mechanisms to specifically support biospecimen banks. A bank or tissue procurement shared resource facility may, however, be a key funded component of larger initiatives such as NIH program project grants, center grants, or disease-focused programs (e.g., Specialized Programs of Research Excellence, or SPOREs).

3. **Investigator fees.** A viable specimen resource will need to develop investigator fees for the services it provides, including biospecimen collection, storage, and processing. These fees should be calculated realistically and take into account all operations and resources that are required from the initial collection of a biospecimen to its final distribution to an investigator. Such fees should be structured to also allow for bank growth and further development. At the same time, fees should not be so burdensome as to deter the conduct of sound research, particularly for pilot translational studies where investigator funding may be limited, or where a unique opportunity exists to collect biospecimens (perhaps in the context of a clinical trial), store them, and utilize them at a later date once additional research funding is obtained. Obviously, the greater a bank's participation in funded research, the easier it will be to maintain long-term support for the operation, and the more likely it will be that the bank will significantly contribute to translational research.

SUGGESTED READINGS

Handbook of Human Tissue Source: A National Resource of Human Tissue Samples. Elisa Eiseman and Susanne B. Haga. RAND Corporation. ISBN: 0-8330-2766-2. http://www.rand.org/pubs/monograph_reports/MR954/.

NCI Office of Biorepositories and Biospecimen Research. http://biospecimens.cancer.gov.

NCI Specimen Resource Locator. http://pluto3.nci.nih.gov/tissue/expediter.cfm.

International Society for Biological and Environmental Repositories. http://www.isber.org/.

63 Imaging Technologies in Surgical Pathology: Virtual Microscopy and Telepathology

Jochen K. Lennerz, Michael Isaacs, Erika Crouch, and John D. Pfeifer

I. **CONVENTIONAL LIGHT MICROSCOPY** remains the core tool in diagnostic surgical pathology. The future of surgical pathology will, however, include electronic modes of image presentation to support diagnoses rendered by viewing the cells or tissue on a computer screen rather than with an optical microscope, since digitized images of glass slides increase the clinically useful information that can be obtained from a pathologic specimen, and permit modes of analysis including electronic consultations, morphometry, and slide storage that go beyond the capabilities of current microscopy-based diagnostic pathology.

II. **VIRTUAL MICROSCOPY** is the technique whereby entire glass slides or selected areas of slides are scanned and converted to digital data files (also known as virtual slides), which can then be viewed on a computer screen. The characteristics of the displayed image, in terms of resolution and range of magnification, are primarily determined by the optical features of the scanning system and are overall comparable with those of glass slide microscopy. However, in contrast to conventional light microscopy where the magnification, focus, and condenser setting can be adjusted at any time, for digital scanning, the "scanning depth" must be determined prior to image acquisition. The scanning depth includes the region of interest, the scanning power, and the number of horizontal levels to be obtained in the plane of the tissue section (scanning power includes the physical magnification [e.g., $20\times$] and resolution [e.g., 2048×4800 pixels], while the number of horizontal levels [so-called z-stacking] is dependent on the section thickness and the need to be able to focus up and down through the tissue and cells in the final virtual image). Depth of focus is a requirement for interpretation of specimens that rely on a three-dimensional assessment of cellular morphology, for example, cytology specimens (*Cancer Cytopathol.* 2007;111:203).

Average scanning time for a single horizontal level of a slide (non-z-stacked) is about 5 minutes and generates a data file that is enormous (ranging from about 200 MB to 1.5 GB). Unfortunately, no uniform (open-source) virtual slide file format is currently available, although interfaces are available that can convert image files between the different virtual slide formats.

Each virtual file consists of multiple parts, called file segments, which include an identification tag, a scanned barcode linked to the laboratory information system (LIS), a low-power overview, and the images at the selected power. While image acquisition methods vary (linear, meander, array), currently all available systems produce tiled images, that is, small images that are retrieved and stitched together to form the final image on the computer screen at the selected power. Most interfaces allow electronic zooming (i.e., additional magnification) beyond the original scanned power.

Resolution and functionality of virtual slides have achieved levels that are comparable with conventional light microscopes. Scanning time, on the other hand, is still time-consuming, since scanning time is mainly dependent on computational speed and optical physics, the latter of which is determined by the magnification of the scanning objective. The actual image acquisition step occurs via a charge-coupled device (CCD), which consists of several hundred thousand individual picture elements (pixels) that transform the optical image into a virtual image; whole slide images are therefore acquired via a single optical lens that moves over the slide. Some scanners shorten scanning time by using a meander rather than a linear scanning pattern to acquire images, but both the meander and the linear methods have inherent physical limitations that become most apparent when acquiring multiple images within each plane of section (i.e., when z-stacking). An emerging technology, so-called lens array microscopy that uses arrays of detectors (miniaturized lenses) to simultaneously capture information from larger areas of the tissue section, may be able to markedly shorten scanning times but still meet the high standards of diagnostic pathology (*Hum Pathol*. 2004;35:1303).

A. **Setting up virtual microscopy** in the surgical pathology laboratory requires an electronic and organizational infrastructure as well as a slide scanning instrument. The infrastructure requires an efficient interaction between information technology (IT) and LIS personnel, and dedicated and trained technical personnel (an image technologist) are required to load and maintain the scanning instrument, perform initial screening (and rescanning if necessary), monitor scan quality, and distribute the virtual files in a manner that can be conveniently viewed by the pathologist (*J. Pathol Inform*. 2011;2:39). A file server with the necessary storage capability (upgradeable tera- to petabyte range or beyond), databases for the virtual files (linked and updated to the LIS), and the necessary maintenance and updates must be managed by a knowledgeable IT person (*Human Pathol*. 2003;34:968). For optimal use in routine patient care, high-quality LCD monitors of sufficient size (at least 53 cm diagonal) for peripheral vision are required (*Hum Pathol*. 2006;37:1543), with extended desktop computer functionality to be able to simultaneously view the LIS, the gross description and gross images of the specimen, and the virtual slide viewer.

B. **Diagnostic and clinical applications** of virtual microscopy include diagnostic consultations, archiving, primary diagnosis, and quality assurance (QA).

1. The use of virtual microscopy for **diagnostic consultation** (so-called e-consultation) is one of the most useful applications of virtual slide microscopy. In addition to convenience (no packing or mailing of slides is required), there are several advantages to e-consultations. Electronic distribution is virtually instantaneous and allows consulting pathologists to review the scanned slides at any time and location. Online, real-time conferencing and simultaneous viewing by two or more pathologists is easily achieved. In addition, there are no risks of losing the primary data (i.e., tissue blocks or glass slides).

2. **Scanning of selected cases for archiving.** Virtual slide creation of selected slides sent in consultation (the medicolegal climate in the United States dictates return of all diagnostic materials to the referring institution) makes it possible for the consulting institution to have a permanent record of the diagnostic slides. Such an archive enhances patient care by providing an immediately available permanent record of the slides to guide frozen section diagnosis, or final diagnosis at the time of definitive excision. In addition, the virtual slides are available for subsequent clinicopathologic conferences (*Hum Pathol*. 2010;41:751).

3. **Primary diagnosis** based on review of virtual slides has been shown to have the same accuracy as primary diagnosis based on routine light microscopy (*Arch Path Lab Med*. 2011;135:372), although the use of virtual slides for primary diagnosis requires an extensive validation procedure. While the use of virtual slides has clear applications for improved pathology services to underserved areas (*Natl Med J India*. 2002;15:363; *Ethiop Med J*. 2005;43:51), there is

little evidence that digitizing all slides in routine practice results in cost or time savings (*J Path Inform.* 2011;2:39; *Anal Cell Pathol.* 2011;34:1).

4. **QA programs** may be enhanced by review of virtual slides from cases with diagnostic discrepancies. Files can be flagged for subsequent review, and trends in diagnostic errors easily identified (*Dis Mark.* 2007;23:459).

C. **Education.** Virtual microscopy is already an indispensable tool for medical education in pathology, including medical student teaching, teaching of pathology residents and fellows, and continuing medical education for practicing pathologists. Many national pathology conferences and slide seminars now post virtual slides on websites before the meeting, and some organizations are building a collection of teaching cases (e.g., see the United States and Canadian Academy of Pathology [USCAP] Virtual Slide Box at www.uscap.org). Other examples of educational activities based on virtual slides include teaching of histology to medical students (*Anat Rec.* 2006;289B:128), a tutorial on Gleason grading of prostatic adenocarcinoma (*Hum Pathol.* 2005;36:381), didactic presentations using a combination of text and virtual microscopy (*Ann Diagn Pathol.* 2003;7:67), and online virtual atlases (e.g., of breast pathology at www.webmicroscope.net).

Education and experience with interpretation of virtual slides is critical for pathology residents and fellows; at the very least, it prepares trainees for the American Board of Pathology virtual microscopy practice examination (www.abpath.org/VMInstr.htm).

D. **Research applications** for virtual microscopy in surgical pathology include quantitative image analysis, and imaging of tissue microarrays used to study patterns of gene and protein expression. Virtual images can also provide documentation of specimens or tissue microarrays retained in tissue banks (*Eur J Cancer.* 2006;42:3110), or for patients enrolled in clinical trials. As for diagnostic pathology, virtual slides make it possible to easily share specimens among investigators at different sites, anytime. Virtual slides also allow for the electronic publication of whole slides rather than selected fields of slides, which facilitate the transfer of new information to practicing pathologists.

Image analysis can be performed on any of the virtual slide file formats produced by the current generation of slide scanners, and widely accepted freeware and a variety of subprograms are available to support clinical applications. The most versatile solution for image processing and analysis is the NIH freeware named ImageJ (*Biophot Int.* 2004;11:36, available at http://rsb.info.nih.gov/ij/). The versatility of this program derives from its open architecture that allows users to implement small and typically customized subprograms (called "plug-ins"). Over the years, many plug-ins (mostly research-derived) have been developed; for example, 'Image J for microscopy' (www.macbiophotonics.ca/imagej) includes numerous tools such as intensity and time analysis, particle analysis, colocalization analysis, intensity processing, color processing, stack-slice manipulation, z-functions, t-functions, deconvolution, and annotation.

III. **TELEPATHOLOGY** is the practice whereby pathologists render diagnoses from a distance by viewing electronically transmitted images rather than by examination of the glass slides themselves by light microscopy. Electronic Images can be transmitted by ordinary telephone lines, high-speed digital lines, or satellites, but increasingly the images are transmitted via the Internet. With some overlap, three systems are currently available: dynamic, static, and virtual.

A. **Dynamic telepathology systems.** In these systems, pathologists view images in real time by electronic control of a distant robotic microscope that has motorized optics and a motorized stage. Dynamic-robotic telepathology has been primarily used to provide intraoperative frozen section diagnoses to hospitals without on-site pathologists (*Hum Pathol.* 2007;38:1330). Typically, in less than a minute, a digital overview of the slide is created; virtual controls enable the pathologist to remotely control the movement of the slide on the microscope. Reported diagnostic accuracy is comparable to that of conventional light microscopy.

A variation of the dynamic method is the submission of a live ("streaming") image from the remotely located microscope either with or without robotic control; in the latter paradigm, manipulation of the slide and magnification are simply controlled via instructions to the person using the microscope.

One important disadvantage of either of the dynamic telepathology method is the extra time needed to review the virtual slides compared with standard slides. In one study (*J Neuropathol Exp Neurol.* 2007;66:750), the lack of an on-site presence affected every stage of the intraoperative consultation including the gathering of patient information, gross specimen examination and handling, frozen section and smear preparation, communication between various parties involved, and documentation of the consultation process. Thus, implementation of telepathology requires substantial planning, communication, and training of both pathologists and support personnel.

B. **Static telepathology systems** use images that have been selected, stored, and forwarded to the pathologist. Static systems are mainly used to obtain second opinions on difficult cases. Overall, the diagnostic accuracy approaches conventional glass slide optical microscopy. Problems leading to discordance include field selection and poor image quality (*Hum Pathol.* 2003;34:1228). For large or complex specimens, the handicaps of preselected images are more pronounced.

C. **Virtual slide telepathology.** The use of virtual microscopy in telepathology has been shown to have clinical utility, even in time-sensitive settings such as intraoperative frozen section diagnosis (*Hum Pathol.* 2009;40:1070). However, the scanning time to produce a whole slide image, the required infrastructure, and the large file sizes may limit the usefulness of virtual slide telepathology in many practice settings.

IV. **EMERGING IMAGING-RELATED TECHNOLOGIES** include spectral imaging (*Cytometry* A. 2006;69:735), nonconventional optical techniques, computer-aided detection (e.g., visual field tracking, pattern recognition, image segmentation), and the application of artificial intelligence to image analysis. However, these techniques remain largely experimental and have yet to be tested in routine surgical pathology.

V. **OBSTACLES.** Significant issues must be addressed to allow the routine implementation of virtual microscopy and telepathology in diagnostic surgical pathology. First, there are unresolved licensure and reimbursement issues concerning diagnostic surgical pathology practice from a distance. Second, there is debate as to whether virtual microscopy instrumentation is subject to governmental approval, and whether users must be certified prior to rendering diagnoses using these technologies. Third, validation and incorporation of digital pathology images into the electronic medical record are haphazard and not standardized (*J. Biomed Opt.* 2007;12:051801). Despite these uncertainties, there is little question that recent advances in imaging technologies provide unique opportunities to improve patient care.

SUGGESTED READINGS

European Virtual Microscopy network at http://www.webmicroscope.net
Pathology informatics at http://www.pathologyinfromatics.org

Index